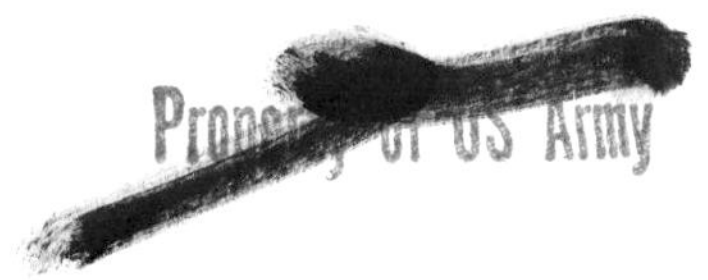

Hepatobiliary and Pancreatic Malignancies

With Contributions by

K. R. Aigner
H. G. Beger
J. M. Bigot
J. W. Braasch
C. E. Broelsch
M. Büchler
J. W. ten Cate
R. A. F. M. Chamuleau
T. K. Choi
J. A. Diaz
J. C. Emond
L. Engelholm
A. E. M. Floor
I. G. Garcia
J. S. González
D. González González
G. Gozzetti
H. Grimm
D. Henne-Bruns
M. N. van der Heyde
H. J. Houthoff
T. J. Howard
K. Huibregtse
S. Iwatsuki
J. James
P. L. M. Jansen

S. N. Joffe
G. Klose
C. Koedooder
B. Kremer
J. S. Laméris
B. Launois
D. J. van Leeuwen
A. Lensing
M. Levi
N. J. Lygidakis
D. Mathieu
A. Mazziotti
N. Moerman
R. Montz
E. Moreno González
H. W. Müller-Gärtner
P. Neuhaus
M. H. Pascual
E. Passaro, Jr.
J. W. A. J. Reeders
G. Rosenbusch
R. L. Rossi
D. A. Rouch
E. A. van Royen
A. C. Santiuste
R. G. Sanz

J. Scheele
W. Schmiegel
K. H. Schuur
C. Segebarth
P. R. Selas
W. U. Shipley
N. J. Smits
N. Soehendra
T. E. Starzl
L. te Strake
R. S. Swanson
J. E. Tepper
J. R. Thistlethwaite, Jr.
T. L. Tio
J. de Toeuf
G. N. J. Tytgat
C. H. N. Veenhof
A. L. Warshaw
J. Weber
C. Willett
J. Wong
M. Zalcman
W. W. A. Zuurmond

Hepatobiliary and Pancreatic Malignancies

Diagnosis, Medical and Surgical Management

Edited by N. J. Lygidakis and G. N. J. Tytgat

with the cooperation of M. N. van der Heyde, B. Kremer,
E. Moreno González, K. Huibregtse and J. W. A. J. Reeders

Foreword by D. B. Skinner

730 Illustrations

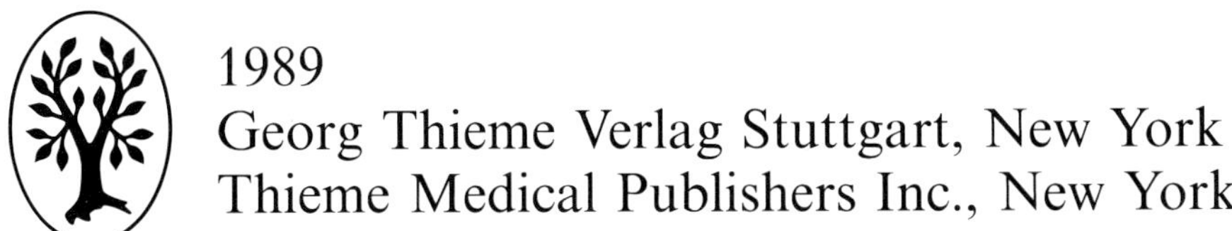

1989
Georg Thieme Verlag Stuttgart, New York
Thieme Medical Publishers Inc., New York

Library of Congress Cataloging-in-Publication Data

Hepatobiliary and pancreatic malignancies : diagnosis, medical, and surgical management / edited by N. J. Lygidakis and G. N. J. Tytgat, in cooperation with M. N. van der Heyde ... [et al.] ; with contributions by K. R. Aigner ... [et al.].
    p. cm.
    Includes bibliographies an index.
    1. Liver–Cancer. 2. Biliary tract–Cancer. 3. Pancreas–Cancer.
I. Lygidakis, N.J. II. Tytgat, G.N.J. III. Aigner, K. (Karl), 1947–   .
    [DNLM; 1. Biliary Tract Neoplasms.
    2. Liver Neoplasms.
3. Pancreatic Neoplasms. WI 735 H528]
RC280.L5H445   1989
616.99′436–dc20
DNLM/DLC
for Library of Congress   89–5186
                                        CIP

© 1989 Georg Thieme Verlag, Rüdigerstraße 14, D-7000 Stuttgart 30, Germany
Thieme Medical Publishers, Inc., 381 Park Avenue South, New York, N.Y. 10016
Typesetting by Tutte Druckerei GmbH, Salzweg-Passau (Monophoto Lasercomp)
Printed in West Germany by Grammlich, Pliezhausen
Cover drawing by Renate Stockinger

ISBN 3-13-724701-3 (GTV, Stuttgart)
ISBN 0-86577-327-0 (TMP, New York)
                    2 3 4 5 6

Illustrations in Chapters 6.4, 7.1–7.4, 7.7, 8.1 and 8.2
by A. A. van Horssen
Anne Franklaan 23
1403 HP Bussum
The Netherlands

Foreword

Malignancies of the liver, bile ducts, gall bladder, and pancreas are among the most dismal of neoplasms. Early diagnosis, at a time when curative treatment can be employed, is rare. In fact, until recently, tissue diagnosis of more advanced cases has been difficult. Any biliary or pancreatic surgeon with experience is occasionally frustrated by the inability to obtain a tissue diagnosis even when a mass in the pancreas, or a biliary stricture, is exposed. Similarly, the surgical techniques required for attempted cure or palliation are difficult, and the results discouraging. Even within the last decade, several centers have advocated that only palliation should be the goal of treatment in patients with these tumors.

As we approach a new decade and a new millennium, much is changing rapidly in this challenging field. This outstanding book brings together new technologies for diagnosis and treatment in an admirable way. The Academic Medical Center of Amsterdam, with its vast experience and outstanding leadership in gastroenterology, digestive tract surgery, and diagnostic imaging, is recognized worldwide as a center for the management of hepatobiliary and pancreatic neoplasms. The staff of this great institution, led by the editors, Professors Lygidakis and Tytgat, and their colleagues including the Chairman of Surgery, Professor M.N. van der Heyde, contributed a substantial portion of this book based solidly upon personal experiences. The editors have wisely supplemented authorship by calling upon other internationally recognized contributors for particular chapters. As I read through the proofs of this elegant book, I was struck by the authority with which each chapter is presented, and the consistent style throughout the book, a tribute to the editors of a multiauthored text.

The initial chapters present the fundamental anatomy, histology, and pathology of the organs in a way that lends a new perspective on function for the clinician. The most important recent advances in this field are in diagnostic methods, and the extensive section edited by Professor Reeders covers the entire spectrum of methods available up to the present moment. This includes ultrasonography, endoultrasonography, CT and MRI scans, ERCP, percutaneous transhepatic cholangiography and drainage, angiography, radionuclide investigations including monoclonal antibody techniques, radioscintigraphy, and biochemical tumor markers. Each of these chapters is extensively illustrated, well-referenced, succinct, and informative.

The remaining two-thirds of the volume describe in detail the full repertoire of treatment approaches, with particular emphasis on surgical management. The surgical chapters are well illustrated with both examples and clear diagrams describing the surgical techniques. These are completely up to date, including recent technical advances made by the authors.

In spite of the surgical advances, complication rates and an inability to offer curative surgery remain high for patients with these diseases. Accordingly, a detailed knowledge of the potential complications and their management, and techniques for palliation in incurable cases, is essential for the clinician treating such patients. Fortunately, full discussions of the complications and palliative approaches are provided, as well as an appropriate emphasis on attempts at curative therapy.

This volume presents an amazing amount of well-documented material in a succinct fashion, and in a well-organized and readable style. To my knowledge, there is no other book like it in any language which brings this rapidly evolving field so much up to date. I predict that this book will be adopted as essential for students of hepatobiliary pancreatic disease at any age, and will become recognized as a watermark volume in the evolution of this difficult subspecialty.

New York, July 1989 *David B. Skinner, M.D.*

Preface

During the last ten to fifteen years, major changes have occurred in the field of hepatobiliary and pancreatic malignant diseases. These changes involve our understanding of basic pathophysiology, the incidence of disease, approaches to diagnosis through new diagnostic developments, approaches to medical and surgical treatment, and possibilities and expectations regarding the results of management.

These developments encouraged and more than justified the idea of producing a book in which we could include the new methods of diagnostic and therapeutic approach in an interdisciplinary way, combining the efforts of the Departments of Gastroenterology and Surgery in Amsterdam. The need for such a book is greater now than before. The paucity of similar joint experience today suggests a real demand for a ready reference work. Furthermore, there is still some controversy concerning the indications and results of surgical versus medical management for a number of malignancies in the liver, pancreas and biliary tree. We have attempted to make a comprehensive presentation by including most, if not all, of these controversies.

We have attempted to offer the reader, whether a surgeon or a gastroenterologist, the possibility of evaluating the facts objectively.

All of the chapters have been written by experts in their fields, reflecting their personal attitudes towards the diagnosis and management of specific pathological entities. New material for biliary and pancreatic endoscopy, new surgical modalities in dealing with biliary and pancreatic cancer, and new concepts regarding the pathological staging of these diseases, are presented in this book. We believe that the present work will be a valuable contribution for a broad spectrum of readers involved in the subject, and we hope that surgeons, endoscopists, radiologists, and pathologists will each find areas of interest in it.

Writing a book is an experience. Now, having passed through the tunnel, we cannot move on without mentioning a few of the many people who have assisted us in fulfilling this project. First of all, we would like to thank our patients, both the patients we remember and those whom we have forgotten, for entrusting their lives to us and thus offering part of the experience which is presented in this book. Secondly, we would like to thank our parents for inspiring in us our love for and dedication to medicine, and for guiding us on the path of what we call duty and obligation. Last but not least, we wish to express our thanks and sincere appreciation to our wives Despina and Christiane, for sharing with courage, optimism, faith and determination the ups and downs of our professional life, and for giving us the support needed to continue our activities.

We wish to express our appreciation to Margaret Hadler, of Georg Thieme Verlag, for her patience, advice and understanding, and to Dr. Michael Robertson for his outstanding job of supervision and editorial production. Warmest thanks are due to Lammegien Kok-Noorman (Dept. of Surgery, Academic Medical Center) for her continuous editorial support. Finally, our grateful thanks are due to all our co-editors and co-authors for their contributions and continuous support. We feel very honored to have their trust and understanding.

Amsterdam, June 1989   N. J. Lygidakis
G. N. J. Tytgat

Contributors

Dr. med. *K. R. Aigner*
Dept. of Surgery
Kreiskrankenhaus Trostberg
Siegerthöhe 1
8223 Trostberg
Federal Republic of Germany

Prof. Dr. *H. G. Beger*
Dept. of General Surgery
University of Ulm
Steinhoevelstr. 9
7900 Ulm
Federal Republic of Germany

Dr. *J. M. Bigot*
Service de Radiologie
Hôpital Tenon
Paris
France

Dr. *J. W. Braasch*
Dept. of General Surgery
Lahey Clinic Medical Center
41 Mall Road
Burlington, MA 01805
USA

Prof. Dr. *Ch. E. Broelsch*
Dept. of Surgery
University of Chicago
Box 259
5841 South Maryland Avenue
Chicago, IL 60637
USA

Dr. med. *M. Büchler*
Dept. of General Surgery
University of Ulm
Steinhoevelstr. 9
7900 Ulm
Federal Republic of Germany

Dr. *J. W. ten Cate*
Dept. of Hematology
Academic Medical Center
University of Amsterdam
Meibergdreef 9
1105 AZ Amsterdam
The Netherlands

Dr. *R. A. F. M. Chamuleau*
Dept. of Gastroenterology – Hepatology
Academic Medical Center
University of Amsterdam
Meibergdreef 9
1105 AZ Amsterdam
The Netherlands

Dr. *T. K. Choi*
Dept. of Surgery
University of Hong Kong
Queen Mary Hospital
Hong Kong

J. A. Diaz
Hospital de la Seguridad Social 'Doce de Octubre'
Carretera de Andalucia, km 5,500
28041 Madrid
Spain

Dr. *J. C. Emond*
Dept. of Surgery
University of Chicago
Box 259
5841 South Maryland Avenue
Chicago, IL 60637
USA

Dr. *L. Engelholm*
Unité de Résonance Magnétique
Cliniques Universitaires de Bruxelles
Hôpital Erasme
Route de Lennik 808
1070 Brussels
Belgium

Dr. *A. E. M. Floor*
Dept. of Anesthesiology
Academic Medical Center
University of Amsterdam
Meibergdreef 9
1105 AZ Amsterdam
The Netherlands

I. G. Garcia
Hospital de la Seguridad Social 'Doce de Octubre'
Carretera de Andalucia, km 5,500
28041 Madrid
Spain

J. S. González
Hospital de la Seguridad Social 'Doce de Octubre'
Carretera de Andalucia, km 5,500
28041 Madrid
Spain

Prof. Dr. *D. González González*
Dept. of Radiotherapy
Academic Medical Center
University of Amsterdam
Meibergdreef 9
1105 AZ Amsterdam
The Netherlands

Prof. Dr. *G. Gozzetti*
Clinica Chirurgica 2
University of Bologna
Policlinico S. Orsola
Via Massarenti 9
40138 Bologna
Italy

Dr. med. *H. Grimm*
Endoscopy Unit
Dept. of Surgery
University Hospital, Eppendorf
Martinistr. 52
2000 Hamburg 20
Federal Republic of Germany

Dr. med. *D. Henne-Bruns*
Dept. of Surgery
University Hospital, Eppendorf
Martinistr. 52
2000 Hamburg 20
Federal Republic of Germany

Prof. Dr. *M. N. van der Heyde*
Dept. of Surgery
Academic Medical Center
University of Amsterdam
Meibergdreef 9
1105 AZ Amsterdam
The Netherlands

Prof. Dr. *H. J. Houthoff*
Dept. of Pathology
Academic Medical Center
University of Amsterdam
Meibergdreef 15
1105 AZ Amsterdam
The Netherlands

Dr. *T. J. Howard*
Dept. of Surgery
UCLA School of Medicine
Centre for the Health Sciences
Los Angeles, CA 90024
USA

Dr. *K. Huibregtse*
Dept. of Gastroenterology – Hepatology
Academic Medical Center
University of Amsterdam
Meibergdreef 9
1105 AZ Amsterdam
The Netherlands

Prof. Dr. *S. Iwatsuki*
School of Medicine
University of Pittsburgh
3601 Fifth Avenue
Pittsburg, PA 15213
USA

Prof. Dr. *J. James*
Laboratory of Histology and Cell Biology
Academic Medical Center
University of Amsterdam
Meibergdreef 15
1105 AZ Amsterdam
The Netherlands

Dr. *P. L. M. Jansen*
Dept. of Gastroenterology – Hepatology
Academic Medical Center
University of Amsterdam
Meibergdreef 9
1105 AZ Amsterdam
The Netherlands

Prof. Dr. *S. N. Joffe*
Dept. of Surgery
University of Cincinnati Medical Center
231 Bethesda Avenue
Cincinnati, OH 45267
USA

Prof. Dr. *G. Klose*
Zentralkrankenhaus links der Weser
Senator-Wessling-Str. 1
2800 Bremen 61
Federal Republic of Germany

Dr. *C. Koedooder*
Dept. of Radiology
Academic Medical Center
University of Amsterdam
Meibergdreef 9
1105 AZ Amsterdam
The Netherlands

Prof. Dr. *B. Kremer*
Dept. of Surgery
University Hospital, Eppendorf
Martinistr. 52
2000 Hamburg 20
Federal Republic of Germany

Dr. *J.S. Laméris*
Dept. of Radiology
Academic Hospital Rotterdam Dijkzigt
Dr. Molewaterplein 40
3015 GD Rotterdam
The Netherlands

Prof. Dr. *B. Launois*
Centre de Chirurgie Digestive et Unité
de Transplantation
Centre Hospitalier et Universitaire de Rennes
Bloc Hôpital de Pontchaillou
Rue Henri Le Guilloux
35033 Rennes
France

Dr. *D.J. van Leeuwen*
Dept. of Gastroenterology – Hepatology
Academic Medical Center
University of Amsterdam
Meibergdreef 9
1105 AZ Amsterdam
The Netherlands

Dr. *A. Lensing*
Dept. of Hematology
Academic Medical Center
University of Amsterdam
Meibergdreef 9
1105 AZ Amsterdam
The Netherlands

Dr. *M. Levi*
Dept. of Hematology
Academic Medical Center
University of Amsterdam
Meibergdreef 9
1105 AZ Amsterdam
The Netherlands

Dr. *N.J. Lygidakis*
Professeur agrégé
Dept. of Surgery
Academic Medical Center
University of Amsterdam
Meibergdreef 9
1105 AZ Amsterdam
The Netherlands

Dr. *D. Mathieu*
Service de Radiologie
Hôpital Henri Mondor
Créteil
France

Dr. *A. Mazziotti*
Clinica Chirurgica 2
University of Bologna
Policlinico S. Orsola
Via Massarenti 9
40138 Bologna
Italy

Dr. *N. Moerman*
Dept. of Anesthesiology
Academic Medical Center
University of Amsterdam
Meibergdreef 9
1105 AZ Amsterdam
The Netherlands

Prof. Dr. *R. Montz*
Dept. of Nuclear Medicine
University Hospital, Eppendorf
Martinistr. 52
2000 Hamburg 20
Federal Republic of Germany

Prof. Dr. *E. Moreno González*
University of Madrid
General Diaz-Porlier 39
Madrid 28001
Spain

Dr. Med. *H.-W. Müller-Gärtner*
Dept. of Nuclear Medicine
University Hospital, Eppendorf
Martinistr. 52
2000 Hamburg 20
Federal Republic of Germany

Prof. Dr. *P. Neuhaus*
Chirurgische Klinik
Klinikum Braunschweig
Salzdahlumerstr. 90
3200 Braunschweig
Federal Republic of Germany

M.H. Pascual
Hospital de la Seguridad Social 'Doce de Octubre'
Carretera de Andalucia, km 5,500
28041 Madrid
Spain

Prof. Dr. *E. Passaro, Jr.*
Dept. of Surgery
UCLA School of Medicine
Centre for the Health Sciences
Los Angeles, CA 90024
USA

Dr. *J. W. A. J. Reeders*
Dept. of Radiology
Academic Medical Center
University of Amsterdam
Meibergdreef 9
1105 AZ Amsterdam
The Netherlands

Prof. Dr. *G. Rosenbusch*
Dept. of Diagnostic Radiology
University Hospital Sint Radboud
Geert Grooteplein Zuid 18
6500 HB Nijmegen
The Netherlands

Dr. *R. L. Rossi*
Dept. of General Surgery
Lahey Clinic Medical Center
41 Mall Road
Burlington, MA 01805
USA

Dr. *D. A. Rouch*
Dept. of Transplantation
Methodist Hospital of Indiana
1801 N. Senate Blvd.
Suite 635
Indianapolis, JN 46202
USA

Dr. *E. A. van Royen*
Dept. of Nuclear Medicine
Academic Medical Center
University of Amsterdam
Meibergdreef 9
1105 AZ Amsterdam
The Netherlands

A. C. Santiuste
Hospital de la Seguridad Social 'Doce de Octubre'
Carretera de Andalucia, km 5,500
28041 Madrid
Spain

R. G. Sanz
Hospital de la Seguridad Social 'Doce de Octubre'
Carretera de Andalucia, km 5,500
28041 Madrid
Spain

Prof. Dr. *J. Scheele*
Dept. of Surgery
University-Clinic of Erlangen-Nuremberg
Maximiliansplatz 1
8520 Erlangen
Federal Republic of Germany

Dr. med. *W. Schmiegel*
I. Medizinische Klinik
University Hospital, Eppendorf
Martinistr. 52
2000 Hamburg 20
Federal Republic of Germany

Dr. *K. H. Schuur*
Dept. of Radiology
St Elisabeth Hospital
Hilvarenbeekseweg 60
5022 GC Tilburg
The Netherlands

Dr. *C. Segebarth*
Unité de Résonance Magnétique
Cliniques Universitaires de Bruxelles
Hôpital Erasme
Route de Lennik 808
1070 Brussels
Belgium

P. R. Selas
Hospital de la Seguridad Social 'Doce de Octubre'
Carretera de Andalucia, km 5,500
28041 Madrid
Spain

Dr. *W. U. Shipley*
Dept. of Radiology
Harvard Medical School
Massachusetts General Hospital
15 Parkman Street
Boston, MA 02114
USA

Dr. *N. J. Smits*
Dept. of Radiology
Academic Medical Center
University of Amsterdam
Meibergdreef 9
1105 AZ Amsterdam
The Netherlands

Prof. Dr. *N. Soehendra*
Endoscopy Unit
Dept. of Surgery
University Hospital, Eppendorf
Martinistr. 52
2000 Hamburg 20
Federal Republic of Germany

Prof. Dr. *T. E. Starzl*
School of Medicine
University of Pittsburgh
3601 Fifth Avenue
Pittsburgh, PA 15213
USA

Dr. *L. te Strake*
Dept. of Radiology
Academic Medical Center
University of Amsterdam
Meibergdreef 9
1105 AZ Amsterdam
The Netherlands

Prof. Dr. *R. S. Swanson*
Dept. of Surgery
University of Massachusetts Medical School
55 Lake Ave.,
North Worchester, MA 01655
USA

Dr. *J. E. Tepper*
Dept. of Radiology
Harvard Medical School
Massachusetts General Hospital
15 Parkman Street
Boston, MA 02114
USA

Dr. *J. R. Thistlethwaite, Jr.*
Dept. of Surgery
University of Chicago
Box 259
5841 South Maryland Avenue
Chicago, IL 60637
USA

Dr. *T. L. Tio*
Dept. of Gastroenterology – Hepatology
Academic Medical Center
University of Amsterdam
Meibergdreef 9
1105 AZ Amsterdam
The Netherlands

Dr. *J. de Toeuf*
Unité de Résonance Magnétique
Cliniques Universitaires de Bruxelles
Hôpital Erasme
Route de Lennik 808
1070 Brussels
Belgium

Prof. Dr. *G. N. J. Tytgat*
Dept. of Gastroenterology – Hepatology
Academic Medical Center
University of Amsterdam
Meibergdreef 9
1105 AZ Amsterdam
The Netherlands

Dr. *C. H. N. Veenhof*
Division of Medical Oncology
Dept. of Internal Medicine
Academic Medical Center
University of Amsterdam
Meibergdreef 9
1105 AZ Amsterdam
The Netherlands

Prof. Dr. *A. L. Warshaw*
Dept. of Surgery
Harvard Medical School
Massachusetts General Hospital
15 Parkman Street
Boston, MA 02114
USA

Dr. med. *J. Weber*
Dept. of Diagnostic Radiology
Rissen Hospital
Suurheid 20
2000 Hamburg 56
Federal Republic of Germany

Dr. *C. Willett*
Dept. of Radiology
Harvard Medical School
Massachusetts General Hospital
15 Parkman Street
Boston, MA 02114
USA

Prof. Dr. *J. Wong*
Dept. of Surgery
University of Hong Kong
Queen Mary Hospital
Hong Kong

Dr. *M. Zalcman*
Unité de Résonance Magnétique
Cliniques Universitaires de Bruxelles
Hôpital Erasme
Route de Lennik 808
1070 Brussels
Belgium

Dr. *W. W. A. Zuurmond*
Dept. of Anesthesiology
Academic Medical Center
University of Amsterdam
Meibergdreef 9
1105 AZ Amsterdam
The Netherlands

Table of Contents

8 Surgical Management of Malignancies of the Biliary Tree 341

9 Clinical Applications of the SLT Contact Nd:YAG Laser in Hepatobiliary and Pancreatic Malignancy 383

10 Postoperative and Palliative Management 391

1 Functional Histology of the Liver and Biliary Tree

J. James

Introduction

The liver is the largest gland in the human body, weighing about 1500 g in the adult. It functions both as an exocrine gland, secreting bile which passes through a converging system of bile ducts into the duodenum, and as an endocrine gland, producing a bewildering variety of substances which are released into the blood stream. Of essential importance for these blood-related functions is the fairly complex vascular system of the liver, with a major contribution of venous blood from the portal vein and a minor one from the hepatic artery flowing together through a system of sinusoidal vessels to central veins (Fig. 1.1), which ultimately form the hepatic vein. Parenchymal cells communicate with the blood stream, secreting in it hormones, protein components of the plasma,

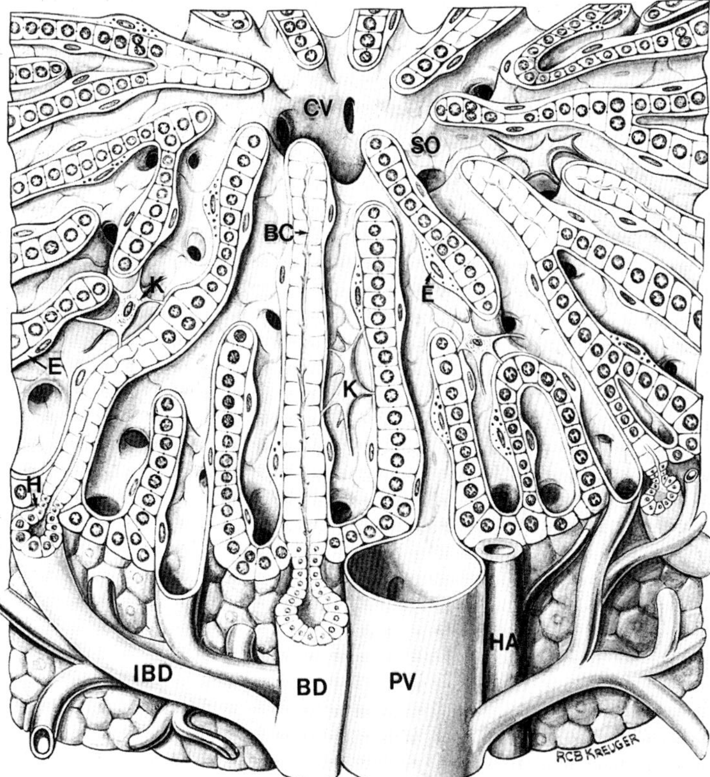

Fig. 1.**1** **Schematic view of a hepatic lobule with a portal strand in front. PV**, portal vein; **HA**, hepatic artery; **BD**, bile ductule joined in the portal strand by a smaller interlobular bile ductule (**IBD**), joined by a ductule of Hering (**H**). **BC**, bile canaliculi; **E**, endothelial cells; **K**, Kupffer's cells; **SO**, sinusoidal opening into the central vein (**CV**).
Some qualitative and quantitative relations have been modified for purposes of legibility, e.g. regarding the size of the hepatocytes which are too small in relation to the littoral cells, and the Kupffer's cells which are drawn too large and in too low a frequency compared to endothelial cells

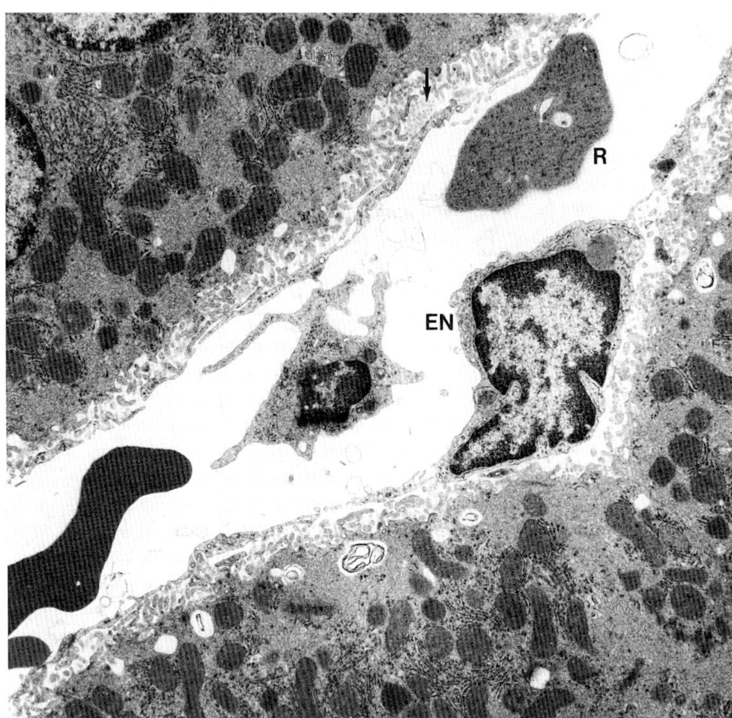

Fig. 1.**2** **Electron microscopic image from a section through a liver sinusoid**, containing an erythrocyte and a reticulocyte (R), showing an endothelial cell (EN) forming the fenestrated lining of the vascular wall. The arrow points to a bundle of thin collagenous fibrils in the subendothelial space of Disse

clotting factors, vitamins, etc. The sinusoidal wall permits uptake and absorption, metabolization, conjugation, etc., of the most widely different compounds, conveyed to the liver via the portal vein and partly returned to the circulation in modified form. Some products of degradation and/or conjugation are secreted into the bile and transported to the gut, where they may have a useful function in digestion, or may simply be carried away for elimination. With some of the exchanges of hepatocytes with the blood stream, non-parenchymal cells in or around the sinusoidal wall play a major or minor part.

An important fact in these functional relations is the circumstance that the blood plasma passes the hepatocytes in a secondary pathway beneath the fenestrated endothelium, the subendothelial space of Disse, in which the hepatocytes protrude with numerous microvilli, thus enlarging their exchange surface (Fig. 1.**2**). The other cells in and around the hepatic sinusoid wall (Kupffer cells, fat-storing cells and pit-cells), which partly also participate in this exchange, will not be dealt with in this chapter (for recent reviews, see Horn et al. 1986, Jones and Spring-Mills 1983, and Kirn et al. 1986). When considering the relation between the cell plates in the parenchyma as radiating from the central vein towards the sinusoidal capillaries, as formed in the periphery of the lobule with a 75% contribution from portal blood and a mere 25% influx from arterial origin, it is striking that the one-cell-thick "muralium" formed by hepatocytes in mammals is

exposed at two sides to circulating blood plasma in the Disse spaces (Elias and Bengelsdorf 1952, Elias and Sherrick 1969). This is a typical situation for mammals, as is the circumstance that the endothelium carries fenestrae without a diaphragm, thus enabling a totally free exchange of plasma and small particles to and from the subendothelial space (Horn et al. 1986, Wisse et al. 1985).

The exocrine secretion products of hepatocytes pass the cell membrane of adjacent hepatocytes to be collected in the 1 µm thick canaliculi formed by neighboring hepatocytes in the one-cell-thick muralium. In lower vertebrates such as amphibia and fishes, the muralium is two cells thick, leaving more space for bile canaliculi in between (Elias and Bengelsdorf 1952). In the primitive hagfish, *Myxine glutinosa*, liver tissue even forms a true tubular gland (Mugnaini and Harboe 1967). Under these circumstances, however, the contact surface between hepatocytes and blood stream is of a much lower order than with the situation in mammals; this might be related to a less important function of the liver as an endocrine organ and intermediary station in metabolism in these animals. During embryonic development in man, when the entodermal cell mass of the liver anlage is broken up into plates and trabeculae by invading mesenchyme, a two-cell-thick primitive muralium is formed at first, in which no canaliculi are found at all (Fig. 1.**3**); these are formed only in a later stage in the definitive muralium, when their lumen comes to communicate with the duct system.

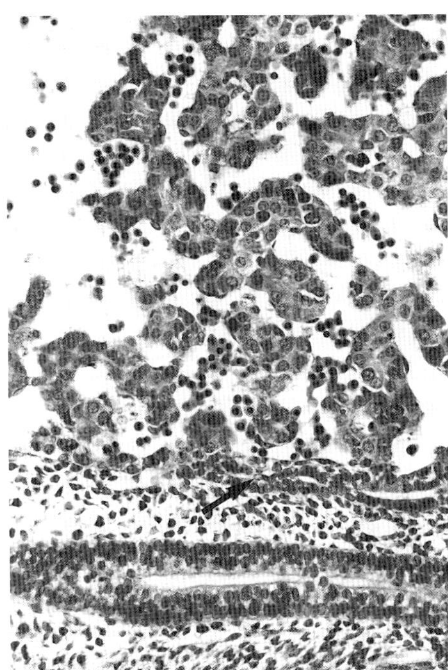

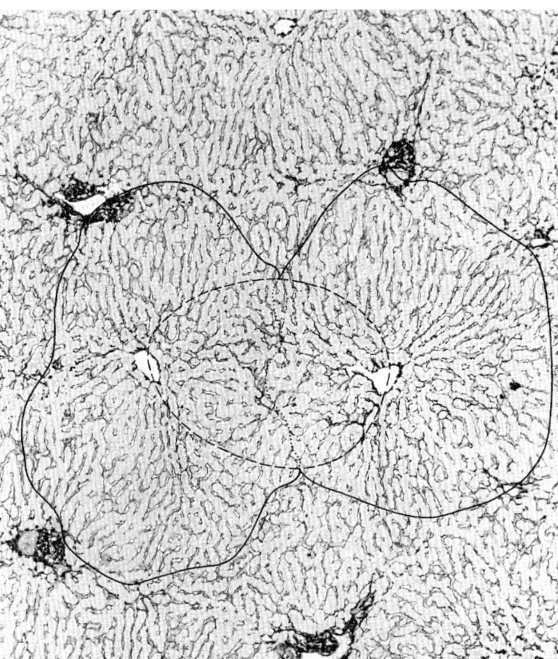

Fig. 1.**3**   **Photomicrograph from the liver region of a 13 mm human embryo** (sagittal section). Hematoxylin-phloxine, 460 ×. At left: choledic duct with, at the right, a developing intrahepatic duct (arrow), both provided with a lumen. The primitive hepatic cords, separated by open spaces with blood vessels (and with nucleated erythrocytes) and mesenchyme strands, show no signs of specific widening of intercellular clefts to form canaliculi.
Preparation kindly provided by Dr. W. Lamers, Department of Anatomy and Embryology, University of Amsterdam

Fig. 1.**4**   **The collagenous skeleton of human liver**, shown in a section stained with Sirius red according to James et al. (1986). Contours of two adjoining lobuli (uninterrupted lines) and an acinus (dotted lines)

The adult situation in man and most other mammals entails the exocrine secretion product having to pass for a distance up to a millimeter through a chickenwire-like system of narrow intercellular clefts before emptying into interlobular ductules (Fig. 1.**1**); there is no intralobular duct system as in a salivary gland, for example. These circumstances might predispose the liver to disturbances of the bile flow. The amount of connective tissue in the adult liver is generally scant and is, apart from the capsule, mainly limited to the portal strands which can be considered as branching from the hilar region into the organ, carrying branches of the portal vein, the hepatic artery and the hepatic duct. The terminal branches of the portal vein, forming the sinusoidal capillaries together with the influx from the arterial system, converge between the parenchymal cell plates towards the central vein, also called terminal hepatic venule (vein). This first root of the hepatic vein is so called because of its central position in the prismatic unit of liver tissue that constitutes the so-called classic liver lobule (Fig. 1.**1**). In many mammals, and certainly in man, this lobule is not delineated easily, as the

amount of interlobular connective tissue – apart from the portal strands – is scanty, and cell cords may pass from one lobule to a neighboring one (Fig. 1.**4**). Although the lobule is widely used as a functional unit of liver structure, a smaller unit, the acinus, without clear structural boundaries, is often propagated as more practical. An acinus such as proposed by Rappaport (1958) contains segments of two adjacent lobules, the center being formed by the course of terminal branches of the portal vein and artery and the first interlobular branches of the bile duct system, although these elements cannot always be found (Fig. 1.**4**). In the acinar concept, zones I, II and III represent areas of parenchyma with an increasing distance to this center and thus a decreasing call on the nutrient, oxygen and hormone content of the blood in the sinusoids. Both of these conceptual models represent different interpretations of the hepatic structure and function; they are not per se conflicting alternatives. In dealing with bile formation, the lobular unit concept is the most easy to use.

The comparative scarcity of collagenous liver connective tissue in the normal human liver as compared, for example, with the situation in the pig (where the lobules can be clearly discerned due to development of connective tissue partitions between the lobules) is remarkable for an organ of its size and weight. Apart from the portal strands branching in all directions from the hilar stroma which consists of dense connective tissue, the organ is enclosed in a thin but firm capsule of dense connective tissue, Glisson's capsule, which is continuous with the hilar stroma. Within the lobular parenchyma, the only support is given by the fine meshwork of thin collagenous ("reticular") fibers lining the cell plates (Fig. 1.**4**), which can be observed as bundles of fine fibrils in the Disse spaces under the electron microscope (Fig. 1.**2**, arrow).

The liver parenchyma forms a stable population of cells which have a very slow turnover; the average lifespan of a hepatocyte in the adult human is 10–18 months or more. It is typical for such a so-called renewing population of cells that mitoses take place in fully differentiated cells; liver parenchyma is, however, capable of spectacular regeneration when an adequate stimulus such as removal of a considerable part of the liver is applied. In rats this process has been studied extensively: two thirds of the liver can be removed and within ten days all lost tissue is replaced by correlated waves of mitotic and synthetic activity in parenchymal, littoral and ductular cells. The parenchyma shows a range of typical changes under these circumstances (James et al. 1986a) which may also be found on a lesser scale in the human following all kinds of more extensive injury. The causes of this regenerative activity, and the factors regulating its coming to a standstill when a certain "critical mass" of the liver has been attained, remain obscure.

Microscopic Aspects of Bile Formation and Secretion in Hepatocytes

It is a surprising fact that after so many years of intensive study, our knowledge about the cellular pathway of bile formation in the hepatocyte and the organelles involved in this process must still be described as scanty (Erlinger 1987, Jones et al. 1980). There is an extensive body of knowledge about the chemistry and (patho-)physiology of bile secretion on the one hand, and on the other, detailed insight into structural and functional aspects of the hepatocyte. In the recent edition of the handbook by Arias et al. (1988) on the liver, more than 400 pages are devoted to the hepatocyte. An explanation for this curious state of affairs might be that bile contains no components that are themselves electron-dense, or can be shown indirectly by contrast-enhancing measures.

All hepatocytes seem to be able to secrete bile, and no clear indications are known of differences in the behavior of hepatocytes with regard to bile secretion in periportal (zone I) or centrolobular (zone III) regions, for example. Bile acids are found in a somewhat greater concentration in zone I, compared to zone III. As is the case with so many zonal differences in the liver parenchyma (van Noorden 1984), it may be questioned whether such a difference, as well as data obtained from radioactively marked bile components (Jones et al. 1980), represents anything more than a reflection of the functional state of the hepatocytes depending on locally available substrates, blood flow, stimulating factors, etc.

There are some indications that bile formation takes place in the cytoplasm somewhere away from the 1 μm wide "pericanalicular cytoplasm" (Jones et al. 1979) immediately surrounding the bile canaliculus. This area is usually comparatively poor in organelles, apart from lysosomes, which are generally found concentrated in this region of the hepatocyte cytoplasm. In the transport of the bile towards this zone, a role seems to be played by microtubuli and microfilaments (Erlinger 1987, Jones and Spring-Mills 1983, Schaffner and Popper 1985). Reduction of these cytoskeletal components by the action of certain drugs (colchicine, vinblastine, cytochalasin B) greatly reduces bile secretion. With regard to organelles which seem to play a role in bile secretion, the Golgi complex as well as vesicular complexes related to it, and the smooth endoplasmic reticulum have been mentioned, all with sound arguments. An obscure role is played by the lysosomes in and around the pericanalicular cytoplasm (Fig. 1.**10**). It has been suggested that these organelles might degrade or otherwise metabolize certain substances to be secreted in the bile (Sewell et al. 1986). Likewise unclear is the role of vesicles of unknown origin which occur in the pericanalicular region and increase in frequency during taurocholate-induced choleresis (Jones et al. 1980, Renston et al. 1980). Although these vesicles seem to play a role in the transport of proteins towards the bile canaliculus, the events are *not* comparable with an exocytotic extrusion mechanism, as occurs in the exocrine (or endocrine) pancreas. The bile, with many lipophilic components and very low protein and other macromolecule content apparently can be brought to the extracellular space (i.e. the bile canaliculus) by a complex process of active transport mechanisms withouth microscopically detectable changes in the canalicular membrane. The high content of ATPase and other enzymes (Fig. 1.**7**) in this region of the hepatocyte membrane produces arguments in favor of this.

The Intralobular Gal Transport System

As mentioned in the first section, the human liver parenchyma is characteristically arranged in a tunneled continuum of perforated and anastomizing cell plates forming a *muralium simplex* (Elias

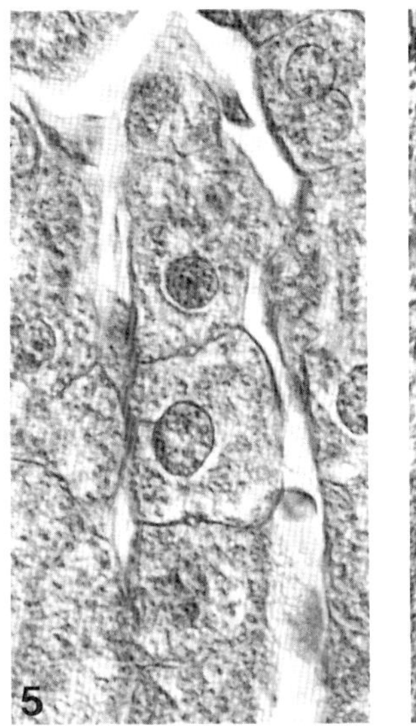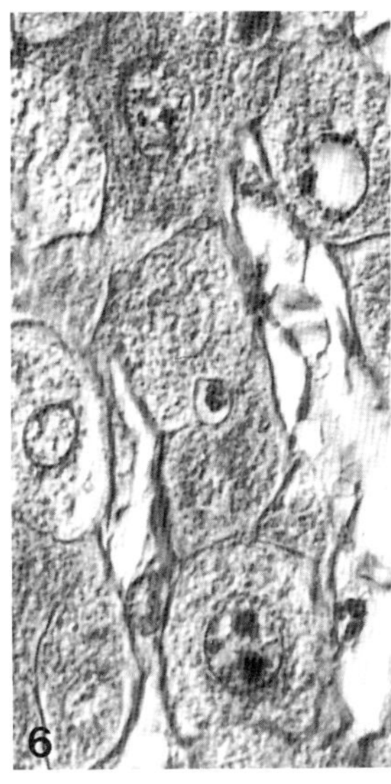

Fig. 1.**5** **Section of the muralium in normal human liver parenchyma**, with a canaliculus in between. Shoobridge stain with contrast enhancement by differential interference contrast; 880 ×

Fig. 1.**6** **A case of cholestasis due to a tumor in the bifurcation of the hepatic duct.** The greatly distended canaliculus contains a plug of condensed bile. 880 ×

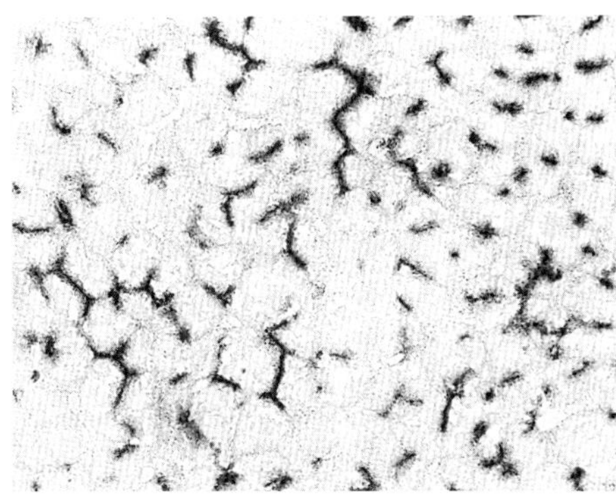

Fig. 1.**7** **Location of alkaline phosphatase activity** (indoxyltetrazolium method performed on a cryostat section) shows the pattern of bile canaliculi in rat liver parenchymal cell plates; 120 ×

and Bengelsdorf 1952, Elias and Sherrick 1969). The lacunae between the cell plates are occupied centrally by the thin-walled sinusoids, separated from the cell plates by the perisinusoidal spaces of Disse. Through the openings in the cell plates, sinusoids communicate so that they form a three-dimensional meshwork, loosely fitting within the labyrinth formed by the cell plates (Fig. 1.**1**). The geometric shapes and volume of parenchymal cells depend on their position in the muralium, apart from their ploidy degree (James et al. 1979, Jones and Spring-Mills 1983).

The bile canaliculi which are closed at one end (near the central vein, Fig. 1.**1**) form an integral part of the muralium: as a rule a single canaliculus is observed between each adjacent pair of cells (Fig. 1.**5**). In a plate of liver cells one cell thick, the bile canaliculi form a network having a more or less hexagonal mesh with a hepatocyte in each mesh. As a consequence of the branching and anastomizing of the cells in the muralium, a kind of chickenwire-like meshwork is formed of these closed expansions of the intracellular space.

The wall of the canaliculi can thus be considered as a local specialization of the plasma membrane of two (sometimes three, at the site of anastomoses of the muralium) adjoining hepatocytes. In the canalicular membrane, different enzymes are localized, such as adenosine triphosphatase and alkaline phosphatase; a reaction for one of those enzymes can be useful for selective staining of the bile canalicular system (Fig. 1.**7**). The canalicular membrane seems to be different from that in the sinusoidal or contiguous domain of the hepatocyte cell membrane, in a physical respect as well, as it is possible to isolate the canalicular membrane parts from a liver homogenate by differential centrifugation (Storch et al. 1983). When fresh liver tissue is compressed under a coverslip or when it is teased, portions of the network remain intact, while the parenchyma and sinusoids are destroyed.

Under the electron microscope, the 0.5–1.5 µm wide canaliculi are characterized by rather long microvilli, which protrude into the lumen (Fig. 1.**8** and 1.**9**). In a sense, this seems to form a certain reserve in the hepatocyte plasma membrane domains forming the canalicular wall, enabling a fair degree of dilation. Propagation of the fluid secretion product through the canalicular network towards the periphery of the lobule is brought about by contractile actin filaments in the pericanalicular region of hepatocytes, which generate a kind of peristaltic movement. This contractile apparatus also provides a tone to the canalicular system, which shows, under normal circumstances, a certain degree of widening with intense bile secretion into the canaliculus, collapsing with decreased activity (Erlinger 1987). Apart from these variable changes, bile canaliculi in the vicinity of the central vein generally have a smaller diameter than those in the portal region, where a greater amount of fluid has to be conveyed (Wisse et al. 1985). Administration of drugs (e. g. cytochalasin B), or disease processes of hepatocytes interfering with the integrity of the circumcanalicular microfilamentous apparatus, quickly lead to canalicular distention with a flattening-out of the microvilli and a failure to contract. This aspect may be similar to

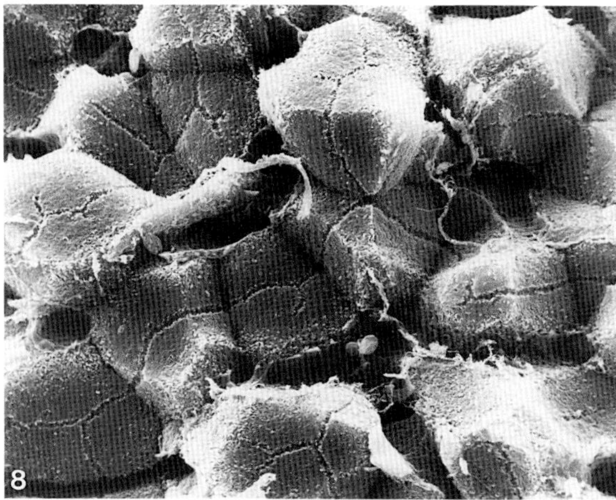

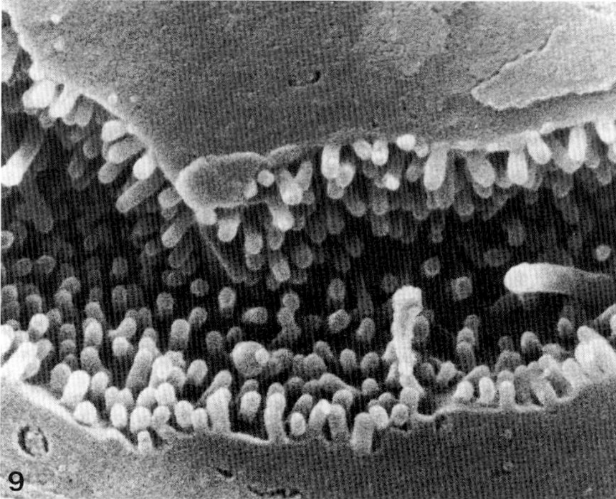

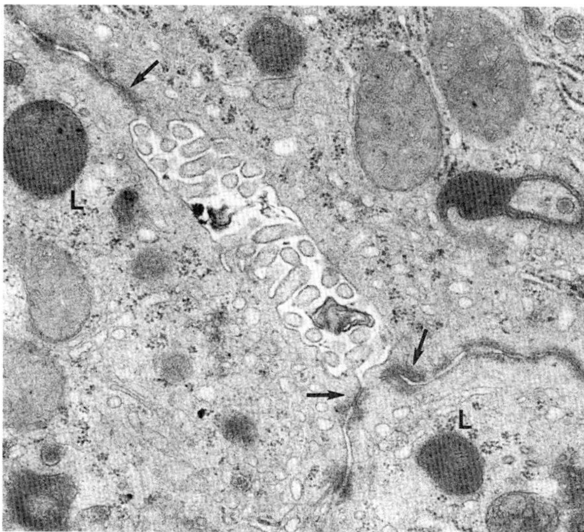

Fig. 1.**10 Electron micrograph of a slightly tangential section through a rat canaliculus** in a virtually collapsed condition, lined by three adjacent hepatocytes; 20,000 × . Note the junctional complexes sealing off the intercellular space, which can be localized by the electron-dense attachment plaques surrounding the tight junctions (arrows). L: lysosomes, which are always very numerous in the pericanalicular region

Fig. 1.**8 Scanning electron micrograph of a fracture face of rat liver;** 2300 × . Hepatocyte cords are seen, showing on their upper faces bile canaliculi, which had been enclosed between these cells and a layer of cells upon them, which have been removed in preparation of this specimen. Courtesy of Prof. E. Wisse, Brussels

Fig. 1.**9 Scanning electron micrograph at higher magnification of a face cut through a bile canaliculus of rat liver** showing the dense microvillous projections of its wall; 22,000 × . Courtesy of Prof. E. Wisse, Brussels

impairment of bile flow due to extrahepatic obstruction (Fig. 1.**6**).

The fact that increased pressure can apparently be built up in bile canaliculi with stretching of its wall (Layden et al. 1975) is due to the circumstance that, along the margins of cells enclosing a canaliculus, tight junctions occur which seal the commissures of the canaliculus and prevent its contents from escaping into the intercellular clefts on either side. Surrounding these bands of tight junctions, desmosomes with electron-dense attachment plaques are found (Fig. 1.**10**), which have a function in intercellular adhesion. In different places gap junctions occur which form a functional link (ion passage) between adjoining hepatocytes.

Tight junctions consisting of a close apposition of the outer leaflets of plasma membranes of opposing cells occur in many places elsewhere (e. g. between endothelial cells or the enterocytes in the intestinal tract). They form an effective permeability barrier at the places where the membranes are united (via specific proteins in the plasma membranes), but as they do not everywhere form a continuous sheet, small tortuous canals between sealed areas may enable a slight leakage towards the intercellular space, and from there towards the perisinusoidal space and blood stream (Erlinger 1987). These conditions are in accordance with recent data from clinical chemistry, which have shown that minimal leakage of bile constituents towards the blood stream occurs under perfectly normal circumstances.

Under conditions of increased bile pressure as provoked by bile duct ligation in experimental animals (Aronson et al. 1987), or with patients suffering from impairment of bile flow, the lumina of the bile canaliculi become greatly dilated, and often contain a bile plug (Fig. 1.**6**). Under the electron microscope, a flattening out of the microvilli can be observed under these conditions, whereas the junctional complexes seem to be pushed aside somewhat. The resistance against an opening-up of the intercellular clefts is not so much generated by the tight junctions as by the deeper lying desmosome-like structures, which often show reactive enlargement of their attachment plaques with cholestasis. As the surfaces of the tight junction between hepatocyte areas ultimately become greatly reduced and their continuity interrupted, large-scale leakage of bile occurs towards the extracellular space, and pronounced jaundice develops. Up to a point, these changes are reversible when the bile flow is restored (Metz and Bressler 1979).

Extralobular Transport of Bile Towards the Hilar Region

When bile has flown in the widening canalicular system to reach the periphery of the lobule, it is taken over by short connecting terminal bile ductules, also called cholangioles, or ductules of Hering. At first, one or two fusiform ductular cells may share a canalicular lumen with a hepatocyte. Subsequently, the ductule, now with a wall of its own lined by small cells with ovoid nuclei, conveys the bile to the interlobular space (Fig. 1.11). These ductules with a diameter of 15–20 µm empty into a larger ductule in a portal tract or in an interlobular branch of such a portal ductule (Fig. 1.12).

Organelles are sparse in cells lining the terminal ductule, apart from a certain development of the Golgi complex. Ubiquitous presence of pinocytotic vesicles suggests some metabolic activity, however, probably mainly fluid resorption. In accordance with this is the fact that these ductules have a rich vascular supply in the form of the periductular plexus, which originates from branches of the terminal hepatic arterioles (before they empty into the sinusoids). The origin of the cells of the terminal ductule is a matter of debate, as they may be considered either as deriving from cells of the larger interlobular ducts or, rather, as parenchyme-related cells. As both parenchyma and

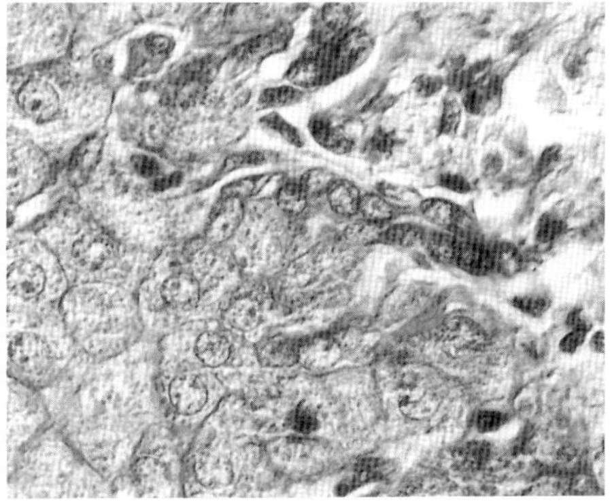

Fig. 1.**11** **Cholangiole or Hering ductule in a section of human liver** uniting the canalicular system between the liver parenchymal cells and the interlobular ductule system; 1000 ×

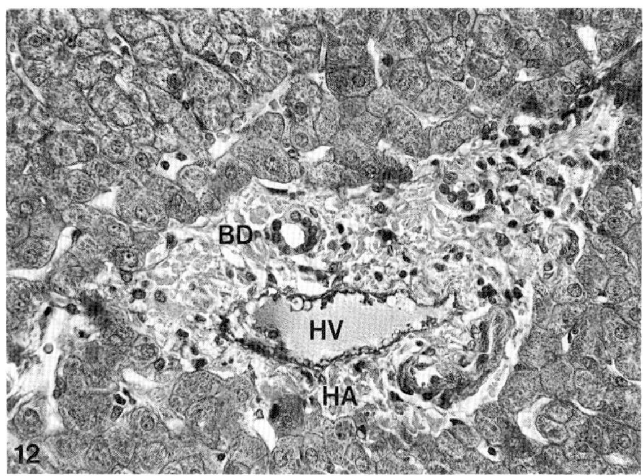

Fig. 1.**12** **Portal area in a normal liver**, showing a branch of the hepatic artery (**HA**), vein (**HV**) and bile duct (**BD**) amidst a moderate amount of connective tissue. Shoobridge stain, 680 ×

the entire ductules system are derived from the same entodermal cell mass (Fig. 1.3), such a relationship seems rather obvious, and the discussion is of limited value. Moreover, under circumstances of ductular proliferation as in cholestasis, it sometimes becomes difficult to distinguish between sections of hepatic cords enclosing widened canaliculi and the ductular complex.

The interlobular bile ductules (Aronson et al. 1987), with a diameter of 15–30 µm on their way to a portal tract (Fig. 1.1), usually follow an isolated course, i.e. are independent of interlobular blood vessels. Apart from a higher epithelium, they have a similar structure to the terminal ductules. In the portal tract, the interlobular ductules empty into the 30–40 µm thick portal ductules (Fig. 1.12) which may also receive terminal ductules directly. The cells of the bile ducts in the portal strands have a highly cuboidal to columnar epithelium. On the luminar surface, short microvilli occur, and in the apical cytoplasm, pinocytotic vesicles are found along with well-developed Golgi complex. The epithelium is surrounded by a homogeneous basal lamina with a thickness of about 50 nm, which – unlike the situation in the terminal ductules – is continuous and surrounded by a basement membrane (reticular membrane) of finely fibrillar collagen. Apart from some reabsorption of water and electrolyte exchange, no substantial changes in the bile seem to occur during the transport through the bile ducts, with increasing diameter towards the hilus. Near the hilus, the largest branches of the biliary tree may contain areas of mucous-secreting epithelium. Around these hilar ducts, smooth muscles in the wall may occur: they form the morphological basis for the narrowing of the ducts in this location, often seen in cholangiograms. The portal bile ducts remain, from the terminal portal strands

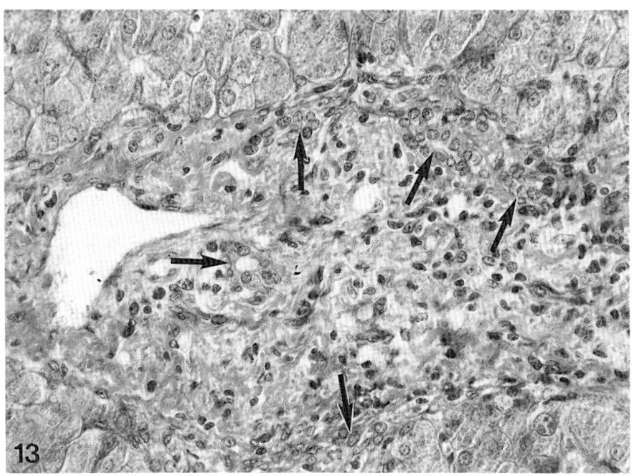

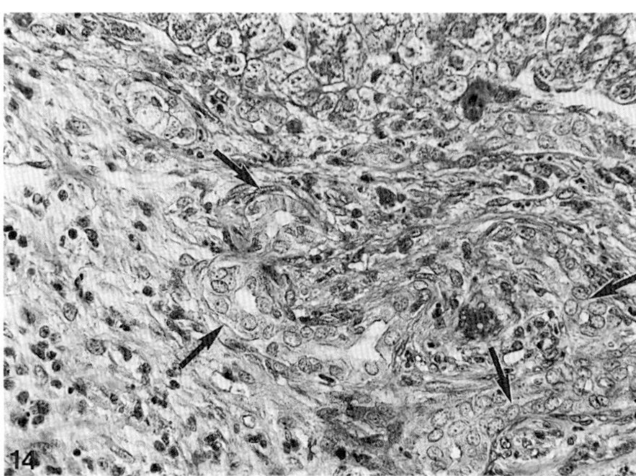

Fig. 1.**13 Portal area in a case of cholestasis due to extrahepatic obstruction** (tumor in hepatic duct bifurcation), showing proliferation of ductules (arrows) and periductal fibrosis radiating into the surrounding parenchyma

Fig. 1.**14 Enlarged and fibrotic portal area** in an infant with congenital biliary atresia (cholangiopathy), two months after birth at operation. Note the greatly expanded ductular complex (arrows) amidst a mass of fibrotic connective tissue

to the hilus, together with branches of portal vein and hepatic artery (Fig. 1.**12**). The portal connective tissue also carries the lymphatic vessels (often inconspicuous because they are collapsed) which have their origin in blind-ending lymph capillaries in the portal areas.

Portal strands in general are by far the largest accumulation of collagenous connective tissue in the liver, the collagen in the parenchyma being limited to a meshwork of bundles of fine fibrils around the hepatocyte plates (Fig. 1.**2** and 1.**4**). Under conditions of impairment of bile flow due to extrahepatic or intrahepatic causes, however, a ductular proliferation occurs which is accompanied by a progressive expansion of the connective tissue mass of the portal areas invading the parenchyma, showing typical metabolic changes (van Noorden et al. 1987). In rats submitted to ligation of the common bile duct, the volume density of collagen in the liver increases ten-fold in 4 weeks (Aronson et al. 1987). In human pathology, a similar fibrosis around expanded ductular complexes is observed, for example in patients suffering from total occlusion of the choledic duct by a tumor (Fig. 1.**13**). In extrahepatic biliary atresia consisting of destruction by unknown causes (viral infection?) of the lower part of the biliary tree during late intrauterine life, similar ductular proliferation with portal connective tissue activations and progressive fibrosis takes place (de Freitas et al. 1986, Gautier and Eliot 1981). Fig. 1.**14** gives an example of this condition two months after birth in a biopsy taken while a hepatoporto-enterostomy was performed (material kindly provided by Dr. M. Gautier of the Kremlin-Bicêtre Hospital in Paris). If the enterostomy fails to restore the communication, or no operation can be performed, the total ductular and ductal com-

plex will gradually disappear, the liver remaining as a kind of endocrine gland with minimal life expectancy for the infant. It is interesting to note that with long-standing experimental cholestasis (by ligation of the common bile duct) a tendency for the biliary tree to atrophy and disappear can also be observed (Aronson et al. 1987).

Extrahepatic Biliary Pathways

Extrahepatic bile ducts are lined with tall columnar cells. The structure of the wall has a distant relationship to that of the gut, mucosa-submucosa-muscularis and adventitia being recognizable. Mucosa and submucosa are not separated, however, by a muscularis mucosae, and the muscularis externa consists of irregularly dispersed smooth muscle fiber bundles. In the submucosa, tubular glands with mucous secretion are occasionally found; these glands are more frequently found in animals lacking a gallbladder, such as the rat. In man, these glands are found especially in the hepatic duct and its intrahepatic segments (Terada et al. 1987). Goblet cells do not occur in the epithelium, but small intramural glands not reaching the submucosa occasionally occur.

The hepatic duct (only 3 cm long in man) joins the cystic duct from the gallbladder to form the common bile duct (ductus choledochus), with a length of 6–8 cm in man, emptying into the duodenum. The anatomical situation with regard to this ending of the biliary tree in the gut and its important relation to the major pancreatic duct in the duodenal papilla is subject to considerable variation (Brown and Echenberg 1964, Healey and Schroy 1953). This will be considered in some detail

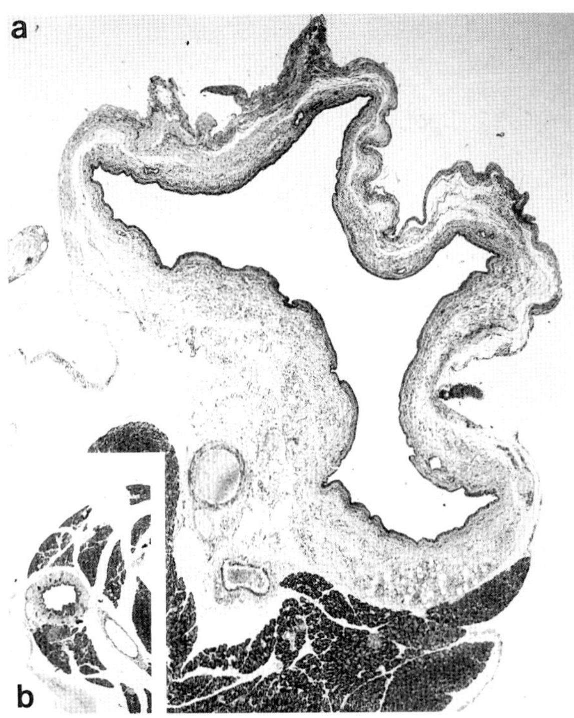

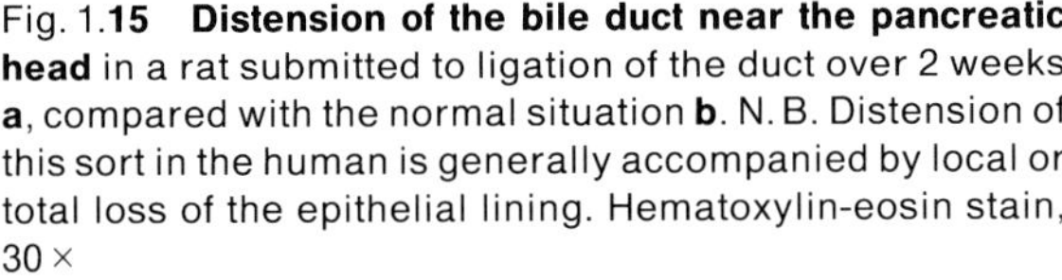

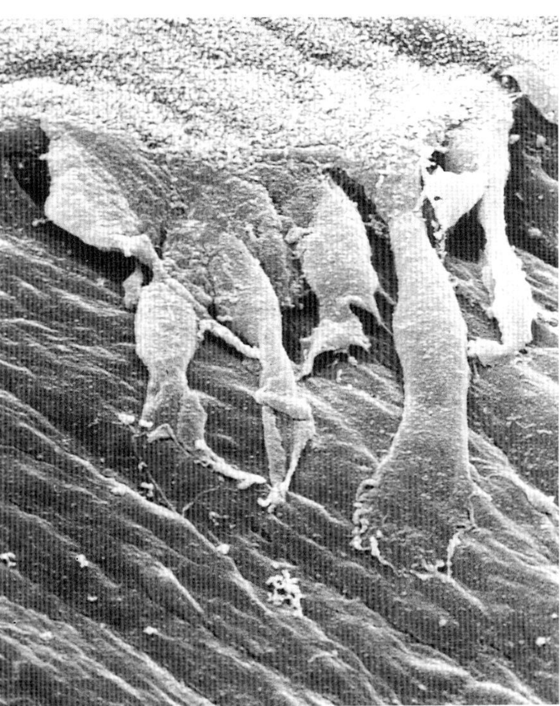

Fig. 1.**15   Distension of the bile duct near the pancreatic head** in a rat submitted to ligation of the duct over 2 weeks **a**, compared with the normal situation **b**. N. B. Distension of this sort in the human is generally accompanied by local or total loss of the epithelial lining. Hematoxylin-eosin stain, 30 ×

Fig. 1.**16   Scanning electron micrograph (4400 ×) showing movement of epithelial cells of the common bile duct** in the rabbit into the defect, 6 h after a local lesion had been made

in the following chapter. The relation of the pancreatic head to the common bile duct is of course of utmost importance for the surgical pathology of the biliary tree, and will be dealt with extensively in later chapters. In various smaller animals, such as the rat (but also in patients who have been submitted to cholecystectomy), no gallbladder exists. It is a question of nomenclature whether the only duct leading from the liver to the gut should be called common bile duct; choledic duct then seems a better name.

All these extrahepatic bile ducts have in common that they show an astonishing degree of plasticity. Behind obstructions they may extend more than 15-fold in diameter without bursting (Fig. 1.**15a**, **b**). In most cases of long-standing obstruction of the common bile duct, the epithelium disappears, so that the extended duct becomes a connective tissue sack without epithelial covering. This occurs in most cases of tumors obstructing the choledic duct (James et al., unpublished observations).

On the other hand, local damage to the extrahepatic bile duct epithelium can be repaired with astonishing rapidity, as long as the connective tissue underground is not necrotic or inflamed and the bile flow is unimpaired. It has been shown by

Van Hattum et al. (1979) in rabbit common bile duct that flattening of the epithelium in the borders after a lesion has been formed begins within hours, with transformation of the columnar epithelial cells into flattened ameboid moving cells which move into the defect (Fig. 1.**16**); a defect of 1–1.5 mm shows complete healing in 16–24 h. The reaction of these extrahepatic bile ducts to various injuries may be related to different anatomical and physiological circumstances, such as the presence or absence of a gallbladder, topographical relations between cystic and common duct bile flow and pressure, as well as the occurrence of smooth muscle tissue in the duct wall, which is absent in the rabbit, for example, but present as scattered groups of cells in dog and man (Wallraff 1969). General conclusions about the pathophysiology of the bile duct system as a whole on the basis of experimental work on animals alone must therefore be regarded with caution.

The gallbladder is a receptaculum for the bile which flows continuously from the hepatic duct (0.5–1.0 l per day). The capacity of the human gallbladder is on the average 30–60 ml. Its wall is covered by a simple columnar epithelium similar to that found in the other extrahepatic biliary pathways. It is substantially thicker, however, and shows a mucosa which is thrown into numerous

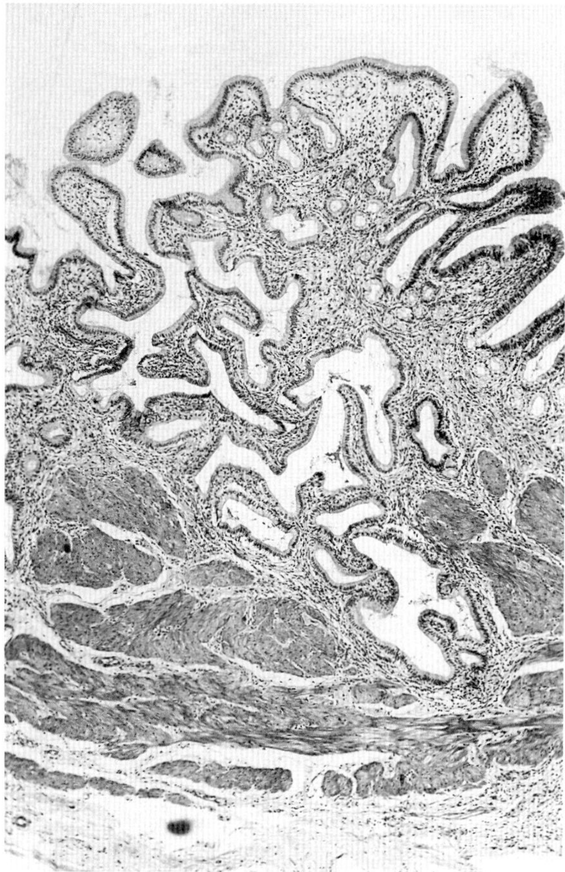

Fig. 1.**17**   **Light micrograph of a section through the wall of a human gallbladder.** Note the irregular muscular coat. At mid-right, a Rokitanski-Aschoff crypt reaching between the muscle bundles. Note the loose texture of the subserosal layer under the muscle coat. Hematoxylin-phloxine stain, 48 ×

folds of varying height which enclose bays or clefts (Fig. 1.**17**) which become reduced to low ridges at some distance apart in a distended gallbladder. The lamina propria of the mucosa contains a vascular plexus; the submucosa deep within it (a muscularis mucosa is absent) has a denser structure, with many elastic fibers. The muscularis consists of an irregular texture of loosely-connected strands of smooth muscle tissue; most of these strands follow oblique directions with regard to the longitudinal axis of the pear-shaped gallbladder. The muscular coat is rather poorly developed in man, as compared with many other mammals (cat, dog, cattle; see Wallraff 1969). The neck of the gallbladder is characteristically free of muscle fibers. In this region, tubulo-alveolar mucous-producing cells are found, which are absent in the gallbladder fundus or the extrahepatic bile ducts. The serosa lining most of the surface of the gallbladder (with the exception of the contact area with the liver) is

separated from the muscular coat by a subserosal layer from which (and from the submucosa as well) connective tissue strands radiate into the muscularis, separating the smooth muscle bundles into compartments.

Apart from its rich vascular plexus, the gallbladder has an extensive network of lymphatic vessels, among which two main plexuses can be discerned, one in the lamina propria and the other more towards the outer surface. The latter plexus has anastomoses with lymph vessels in the portal strands in the liver, which explain the pathway for hepatogenous cholecystitis. The lymph plexuses are drained into vessels accompanying the cystic and common bile duct, joining lymph nodes in the duodenal region. Nerves in the gallbladder are branches of the vagus nerve and the splanchnic sympathetic.

Apart from the clefts between the irregular folds of the mucosal wall, typical Rokitansky-Aschoff sinuses or -crypts are found which are continuations of the surface epithelium in the wall, often reaching through defects in the muscularis into the subserosal region (Fig. 1.**17**). These crypts may be confused with Luschka ducts, which are covered with mucosa of the bile duct type. The latter ducts are mainly localized in the alveolar tissue separating the hepatic surface of the liver and the gallbladder wall, but may extend into the connective tissue around the muscularis. They do *not* communicate with the lumen of the gallbladder, but have connections with intrahepatic bile ducts (hence the term aberrant bile ducts), a consequence of the developmental history of the bile ductular system. When the Luschka ducts are extensively developed, they may form an indication for drainage of the gallbladder bed following cholecystectomy.

As stated above, the gallbladder serves as a site for the storage and concentration of bile, as it is continuously secreted by the liver. The physiological aspects of its emptying under the influence of cholecystokinine, the relaxation of the sphincter of Oddi as a part of duodenal peristalsis etc. is beyond the scope of this chapter. From a histological point of view, the concentrating function of the gallbladder may give rise to typical changes in the epithelium, however, which can be explained on the basis of known cell-physiological phenomena. In gallbladders known to be active in fluid transport, a distension of the intercellular clefts is often observed. During concentration of bile, water is resorbed by the lining cells of the gallbladder. Via an active transport of Na^+ ions into the intercellular clefts, the concentration of solute is increased in this communicating network of spaces which are sealed off from the lumen by tight junctions around the apical sides of the columnar

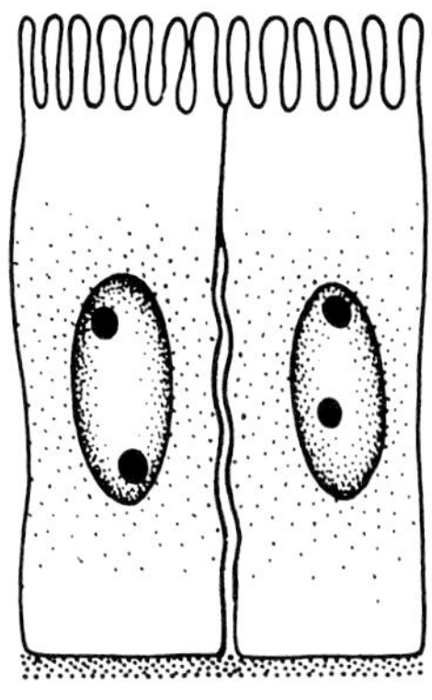

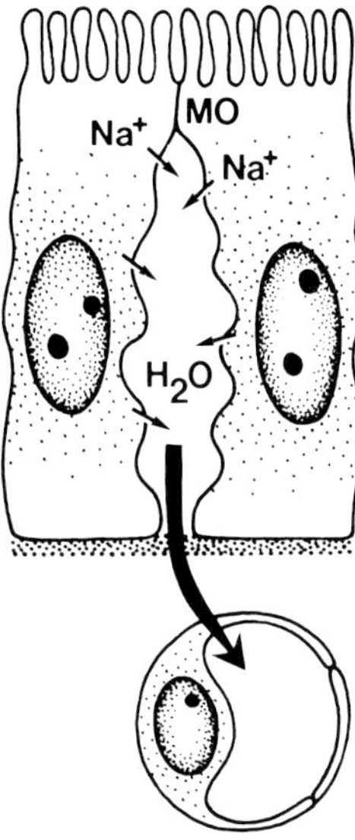

Fig. 1.**18   Schematic view of the visible effects of intensi-
fied fluid transport** across the gallbladder epithelial cells

cells. Following the osmotic gradient, water will be pulled out of the cells via the lateral cell membranes into the intercellular clefts, which can become distended when this takes place on a large scale (Fig. 1.**18**). Due to increased hydrostatic pressure, water will flow from the intercellular space through the basal lamina of the epithelium (which is freely permeable to water) towards the interstitium, where it is taken up by blood capillaries and carried away. A damaged mucosa loses its concentration power for evident reasons.

Surgical removal of the gallbladder often leads to a marked dilation of the biliary passages, which may be accompanied by a more folded pattern of the common bile duct wall. This permits a consider-able degree of distention-contraction, which can be considered as an extension of the physiological plasticity of the extrahepatic ducts (Fig. 1.**15**). Signs of the existence of compensatory mechanisms of bile concentration under these circumstances have not been reported, however.

References

Arias IM, Jakoby WB, Popper H, Schachter D, Shafritz DA, eds. Hepatocyte: organization; hepatocyte: metabolism. In: Arias IM, Jakoby WB, Popper H, Schachter D, Shafritz DA. The Liver: biology and pathobiology. 2nd ed. New York: Raven, 1988.

Aronson DC, De Haan J, James KS, Bosch KS, Ketal AG, Houtkooper JM, Heijmans HSA. Quantitative aspects of the parenchyma-stroma relationship in experimentally induced cholestasis. Liver 1988; 8: 116–126.

Brown JO, Echenberg RJ. Mucosal reduplications associated with the ampullary portion of the major duodenal papilla in humans. Anat Rec 1964; 150: 293–302.

Elias H, Bengelsdorf H. The structure of the liver of vertebrates. Acta Anat 1952; 14: 297–337.

Elias H, Sherrick JC, eds. Morphology of the liver. New York: Academic Press, 1969.

Erlinger S. Physiology of bile secretion and enterohepatic circulation. In: Johnson LR, ed. Physiology of the gastrointestinal tract. New York: Raven, 1987: 1557–1572.

de Freitas LAR, Chevallier M, Louis D, Grimaud J-A. Human extrahepatic biliary atresia: portal connective tissue activation related to ductular proliferation. Liver 1986; 6: 253–261.

Gautier M, Eliot N. Extrahepatic biliary atresia. Arch Pathol Lab Med 1981; 105: 397–403.

Healey JE Jr, Schroy PC. Anatomy of the biliary ducts within the human liver: analysis of the prevailing pattern of branchings and the major variations of the biliary ducts. AMA Arch Surg 1953; 66: 599–617.

Horn T, Henriksen, JH, Christoffersen P. The sinusoidal lining cells in "normal" human liver: a scanning electron microscopic investigation. Liver 1986; 6: 98–110.

James J, Tas J, Bosch KS, De Meere AJP, Schuyt HC. Growth patterns of rat hepatocytes during postnatal development. Eur J Cell Biol 1979; 19: 222–226.

James J, Frederiks WM, van Noorden CJF, Tas J. Detection of metabolic changes in hepatocytes by quantitative cytochemistry. Histochemistry 1986a; 84: 308–316.

James J, Bosch KS, Zuyderhoudt FMJ, Houtkooper JM, van Gool J. Histophotometric estimation of volume density of collagen as an indication of fibrosis in rat liver. Histochemistry 1986b; 85: 129–133.

Jones AL, Schmucker DL, Mooney JS, Ockner RK, Adler RD. Alterations in hepatic pericanalicular cytoplasm during enhanced bile secretory activity. Lab Invest 1979; 40: 512–517.

Jones AL, Schmucker DL, Renston RH, Murakami T. The architecture of bile secretion: a morphological perspective of physiology. Dig Dis Sci 1980; 25: 609–629.

Jones AL, Spring-Mills E. The liver and gallbladder. In: Weiss L, ed. Histology: cell and tissue biology. 5th ed. New York: MacMillan, Elsevier, 1983: 707–748.

Kirn A, Knook DL, Wisse E, eds. Cells of the hepatic sinusoid. Rijswijk: Kupffer Cell Foundation, 1986.

Layden TJ, Schwarz J, Boyer JL. Scanning electron microscopy of the rat liver: studies of the effect of taurolithocholate and other models of cholestasis. Gastroenterology 1986; 69: 724–738.

Metz J, Bressler D. Reformation of gap and tight junctions in regenerating liver after cholestasis. Cell Tissue Res 1979; 199: 257–270.

Mugnaini E, Harboe SV. The liver of myxine glutinosa: a true tubular gland. Z Zellforsch 1967; 78: 341–369.

Rappaport AM. The structural and functional unit in the human liver (liver acinus). Anat Rec 1958; 130: 673–686.

Renston RH, Maloney DG, Jones AL, Hradek GT, Wong KY, Goldfine ID. Bile secretory apparatus: evidence for a vesicular transport mechanism for proteins in the rat, using horseradish peroxidase and (^{125}I) insulin. Gastroenterology 1980; 78: 1373–1388.

Schaffner F, Popper H. Classification and mechanism of cholestasis. In: Wright R, Millward-Sadler GH, Alberti KGMM, Karran S, eds. Liver and biliary disease. 2nd ed. London: Saunders, 1985: 359–388.

Sewell RB, Dillon C, Grinpukel S, Yeomans NC, Smallwood RA. Pericanalicular location of hepatocyte lysosomes and effects of fasting: a morphometric analysis. Hepatology 1986; 6: 305–311.

Storch J, Schachter D, Inoue M, Wolkoff AW. Lipid fluidity of hepatocyte plasma membrane subfractions and their differential regulation by calcium. Biochim Biophys Acta 1983; 727: 209–212.

Terada T, Nakanuma Y, Ohta G. Glandular elements around the intrahepatic bile ducts in man; their morphology and distribution in normal livers. Liver 1987; 7: 1–8.

Van Hattum AH, James J, Klopper PJ, Muller JH. A model for the study of epithelial migration in wound healing. Virchows Arch [Cell pathol] 1979; 30: 221–230.

Van Noorden CJF. Histochemistry and cytochemistry of glucose-6-phosphate dehydrogenase. Prog Histochem Cytochem 1984; 15/4: 1–85.

Van Noorden CJF, Frederiks WM, Aronson DC, Marx F, Bosch

K, Jonges GN, Vogels IMC, James J. Changes in the acinar distribution of some enzymes involved in carbohydrate metabolism in rat liver parenchyma after experimentally induced cholestasis. Virchows Arch [Cell Pathol] 1987; 52: 501–511.

Wallraff J, ed. In: Handbuch der mikroskopischen Anatomie des Menschen. Verdauungsapparat – Atmungsapparat; vol 4. Berlin: Springer, 1969: 330–332.

Wisse E, De Zanger RB, Charels K, van der Smissen P, McCuskey RS. The liver sieve: considerations concerning the structure and function of endothelial fenestrae, the sinusoidal wall and the space of Disse. Hepatology 1985; 5: 683–692.

2 Functional Histology of the Exocrine Pancreas

J. James

Introduction: Phylogenetic and Ontogenetic Aspects

In man, the pancreas, with a weight of 75–100 g, is the second largest gland associated with the alimentary tract after the liver, which has a more than tenfold greater mass. It is an elongated, faintly pinkish organ lying in a retroperitoneal position across the upper abdominal wall at the level of the second and third lumbar vertebrae. At right, the enlarged head is curved against the middle portion of the duodenum, forming a flattened hook (Fig. 2.1). The ending of the bent part, the uncinate process, passes behind the superior mesenteric vessels to end behind the neck of the organ.

The pancreas is a mixed exocrine-endocrine gland, the exocrine secretory units forming the greatest volume (84%), the total of endocrine cells only 1–2%. The remainder is occupied by ducts, blood vessels and connective tissue. The latter do not form a true capsule, as is the case with Glisson's capsule in the liver. The overall paucity of connective tissue components in the organ, and consequently its weak consistence, is at the origin of the name pancreas (Greek pan = all, and kreas = flesh). The topographical relations between pancreas head, pancreatic duct and common bile duct are of the utmost importance with all surgical diseases in this region.

The endocrine portion of the pancreas, consisting of groups of cells with various specializations, is mainly concerned with the endocrine regulation of carbohydrate metabolism, and will be treated only in passing in this chapter. With their diffuse localization and their exclusive involvement in hormonal regulation, the islets of Langerhans do not play a role in hepatobiliary and pancreatic surgery. Tumors of the specific cell types from the endocrine pancreas are extremely rare. In man, the small part of the pancreatic volume occupied by

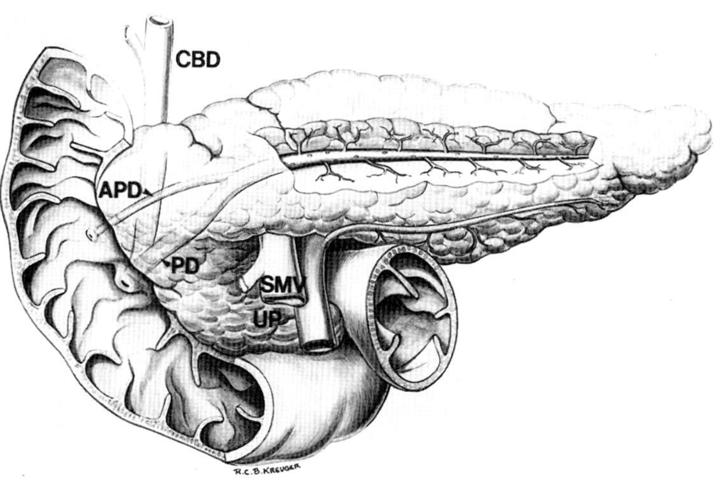

Fig. 2.**1 Three-dimensional drawing of topographical relations** between the pancreas with its main duct (PD) and accessory duct (APD), the common bile duct (CBD) and the superior mesenteric vessels (SMV). UP: uncinate process

endocrine cells is divided over roughly one million islets, with a diameter of a few tenths of a millimeter, which are dispersed throughout the organ; they are somewhat more numerous in the tail than the in body and head. Some notions with regard to the relation between the exocrine and endocrine pancreas will be dealt with at the end of this chapter.

In man, as in all mammals, pancreas and liver are two separate glands, although they usually share a common terminal pathway before entering the duodenum. This situation is not found in all vertebrates. In many primitive vertebrates the pancreatic tissue is dispersed throughout the liver; in the lamprey, the exocrine pancreas has already emerged from the liver, however (Bendayan et al. 1985). In many non-mammalian vertebrates, the pancreas consists of a group of glandular concentrations dispersed throughout the mesenterium; the anomalous occurrence of ectopic pancreatic tissue in human pathology can be considered as a

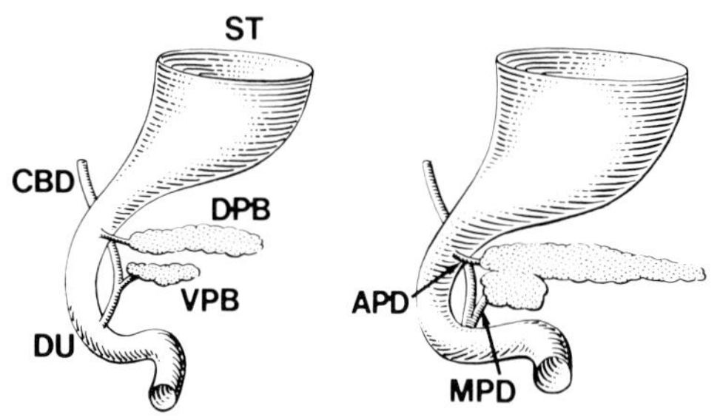

Fig. 2.2 **Schematic view of the fusion between the dorsal and ventral pancreatic buds** (DPB and VPB, respectively) before **a** and after **b** the fusion process. ST: stomach; DU: duodenum; CBD: common bile duct; MPD: major pancreatic duct; APD: accessory pancreatic duct

distant reminiscence of this. It is interesting to note that in animals with a dispersed exocrine pancreas, such as bony fishes, the endocrine pancreas may form a totally separate organ.

Embryonic development of the pancreas, which is of some importance in order to understand the topographical situation of the ducts and the genesis of developmental abnormalities, starts after the first organogenesis of the liver has taken place. At the beginning of the fifth week of intra-uterine life, two outgrowths appear in the foregut: 1) a ventral pancreatic bud arising near the entry of the bile duct into the duodenum and 2) a dorsal bud consisting of a cell mass which quickly becomes more voluminous than the ventral bud. (Strictly speaking, the names dorsal and ventral are not quite adequate; they are situated, rather, to the right and left of the gut axis.) With the intense migratory and rotatory activity in and around this part of the gut which follows this stage, both buds approach each other after some time, so that the ventral pancreatic bud comes into a position inferior and posterior to the dorsal bud (Fig. 2.**2a**). Both buds then fuse, the ventral bud forming the inferior part of the future head with the uncinate process, while the remainder of the gland with the tail differentiates from the dorsal bud. Curiously enough, although the largest part of the pancreas is derived from the dorsal bud, the main pancreatic duct, which opens together with the common bile duct in the duodenum, is formed from the duct of the ventral bud (Fig. 2.**2b**). The original duct of the dorsal pancreas mostly (but not always) persists as the much slimmer minor accessory pancreatic duct, to end higher up in the gut in the so-called minor papilla, 1–3 cm from the major papilla (of Vater) in which the common bile duct and the major pan-

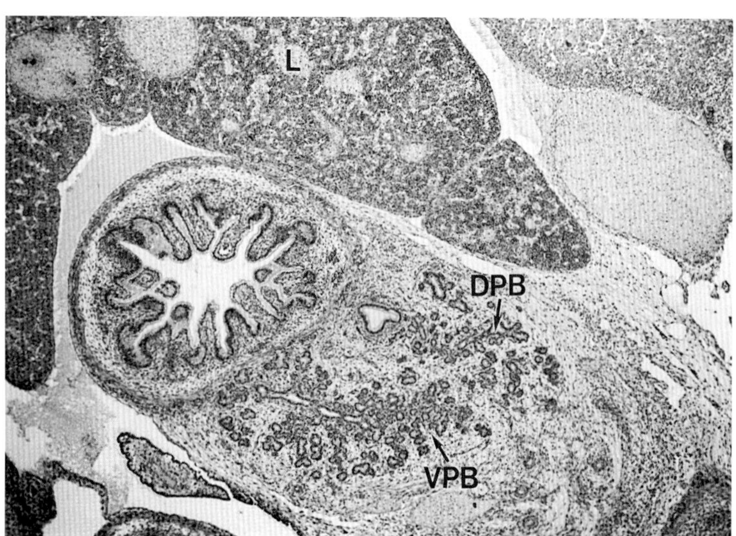

Fig. 2.3 **Photomicrograph of a transverse section of a human embryo** (36 mm, ± 8 weeks) in which dorsal and ventral buds (**DPB** and **VPB**, respectively) can be seen with their respective ducts. **L**, liver. Hematoxylineosin stain, 42×. The dorsal duct, destined to play a secondary role later on, seems the larger of the two in this section. The situation roughly corresponds with an intermediate stage between those of Figures **2a** and **b**. Material kindly provided by Prof. J. A. Los, Dept. of Anatomy and Embryology, University of Amsterdam

creatic duct empty into the duodenum (Fig. 2.**1**). In early development, before the actual fusion of the two buds, the duct of the larger dorsal pancreatic bud has a greater diameter than that of the future main duct (Fig. 2.**3**). These anatomical relations are subject to great variations, and even a persistence of both pancreatic buds as separate entities with two ducts is far from rare.

A fairly common anomaly of this development process is the annular pancreas, which consists of a ring of pancreatic tissue, which may lead to duodenal obstruction in early life or adulthood (Ravitch 1979). Just like the frequent occurrence of "ectopic" or "aberrant" pancreatic tissue within the wall of stomach, duodenum or jejunum, this is to be considered a sequel of the hectic migratory activity of material of the pancreatic buds and changes in the gut topography around the sixth week of intra-uterine life.

The Pancreatic Acinus

In the classical histological descriptions of the pancreas in textbooks (Bloom and Fawcett 1986, Jamieson 1983), the exocrine pancreas is depicted as a compound acinar gland organized in a great number of small lobules bound together by loose connective tissue, also carrying a rich meshwork of blood vessels. The functional unit of the exocrine pancreas is the acinus, which, in contrast to the liver acinus, is a sharply delineated structure composed of some 40–60 pyramidal cells around a shallow lumen (Fig. 2.**4**). Between the cells, short secretory canaliculi open into the lumen, which is somewhat wider with active secretion and is virtually collapsed during rest. The acinus is drained by a short intercalated duct lined with cuboidal cells (Fig. 2.**4**, arrow), which empties into a short, inconspicuous intralobular duct, which in its turn empties into an interlobular duct (see below). Cells of the intercalated ducts often seem to extend for some distance into the acinus, forming so-called centroacinar cells which are surrounded by acinar cells.

This situation, described as such in all textbooks, is essentially incorrect with regard to the topographical relation of acini and intercalated ducts. By serial sectioning, retrograde injection and study with the scanning electron microscope, it has emerged that the basic architecture of the pancreas does *not* correspond with a grape cluster, but with a branching complex of tubules which may end blindly as acini, but may also anastomose with other tubuli, the thicker parts of the tubule complexes corresponding with acini (Fig. 2.**5**). This situation has been shown to exist in rats and dogs, and also in man (Akao et al. 1986, Bockman et al. 1983). An acinus may thus empty into two different intercalated ducts, and secretion material could have to pass another acinus before reaching an intercalated duct emptying into a larger interlobular duct. Functionally, this might be of importance, in view of the addition of alkaline fluid to the secretory products of the acini by cells of the ducts (see below). These relations might be of importance also for the understanding of pathological changes in pancreatic tissue (Bockman et al. 1983).

While keeping these new insights in mind, pancreatic secretion can still be treated starting from the acinus as the basic unit of exocrine secretory activity. The more or less pyramid-shaped cells rest on a clear basal lamina (Fig. 2.**7**). It has been proposed that aberrations in turnover of basal lamina material might be of importance for neo-

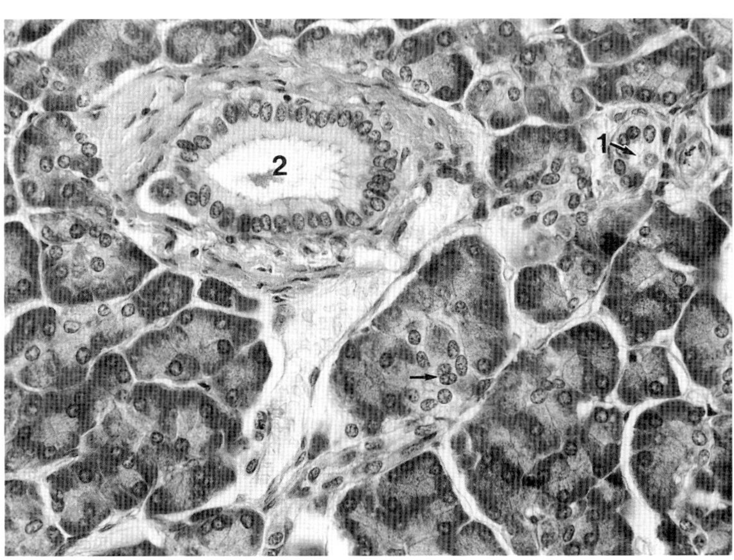

Fig. 2.**4 Section of a human pancreas.** Hematoxylin-phloxine stain, 800 × . Note the typical ergastoplasm in the basal region of the cells forming an acinus. At the lower border, an intercalated duct, which can be seen to continue within an acinus forming centroacinar cells (arrow). Note the ovoid shape of the ductular cells on longitudinal section. 1: transverse section of an intralobular/intercalated duct of this sort. 2: interlobular duct with columnar epithelium and a thick sheath of fibrous connective tissue surrounding it, which is absent from the two smaller ducts

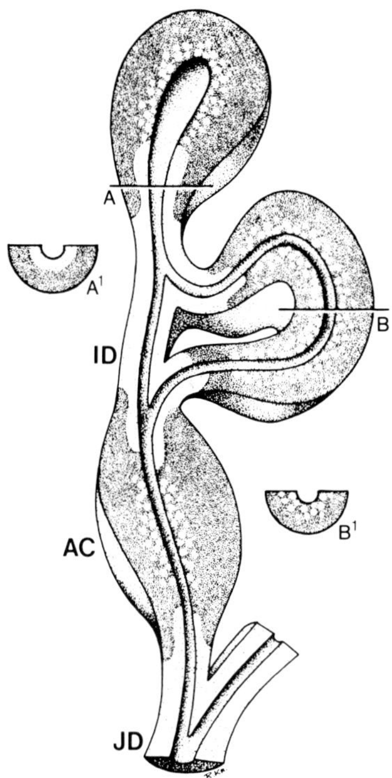

Fig. 2.**5 Semi-diagrammatic view of topographical connections** between acinus, centroacinar cells and intercalated ducts in the human pancreas according to recent views. A¹ and B¹ give a transverse section through the region A and B with and without centroacinar cells, respectively. ID, intercalated duct; AC, acinus

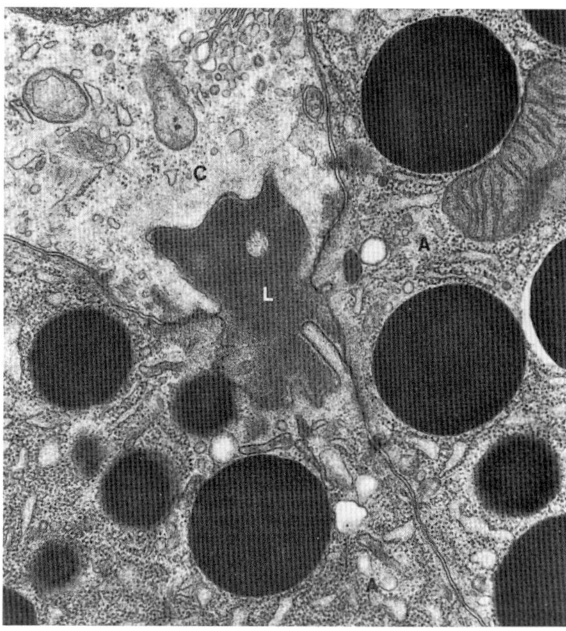

Fig. 2.**6 Electron micrograph of a section from a rat pancreas** (30,000 ×) showing a light centroacinar cell in the upper left quadrant and darker acinar cells with electron-dense ripe secretion granules lower and right. L: lumen in which, based on its electron density, extrusion of zymogen granules has taken place recently.
Reproduced from Junqueira LC, Carneiro J, Long JA; Basic histology, 5th ed., Los Altos, USA, 1986

plastic transformation (Ingber et al. 1985). The centroacinar cells, which can easily be detected in light-microscopical preparations as pale cells amidst the closed row of dark acinar cells (Fig. 2.**4**), are comparable to the cells forming intercalated ducts from which they are derived. Under the electron microscope (Fig. 2.**6**), they have an electron-translucent cytoplasm, a small Golgi complex, a few scattered cisternae of endoplasmic reticulum, and large, abundant mitochondria. It has been shown that centro-acinar cells contain the enzyme carbonic anhydrase (Spicer et al. 1982). For other reasons, these cells are also considered – together with other segments of the duct system – as producers of bicarbonate-rich fluid which mixes with the secretions from the acinar cells (Schulz 1987). The secretion of this alkaline fluid is independent from the acinar secretion (Kuijpers and De Pont 1987), and is stimulated by a specific hormone formed in so-called S-cells in the mucosa of the upper small intestine in inactive form (prosecretin). The release of active secretin from prosecretin is caused by chyme entering the intestine, especially when it is rich in hydrochloric acid from secretory activity in the stomach. Secretin has no influence on enzyme secretion by the acinus, which is stimulated by cholecystokinin (see below).

Secretory Activity of Acinar Cells

Knowledge of the secretory pathway of enzymatic proteins in pancreatic acini is very detailed, as the exocrine pancreas has served for many years as the model for a protein secreting gland in a great many cytological, cytochemical and biochemical studies. The secretion products have also been studied in detail, and it has been found that most of the enzyme products are secreted in inactive form by the acinar cells. A failure of this mechanism possibly gives a clue to the pathogenesis of acute pancreatitis. Only a few basic facts with regard to the secretory process as a whole will be dealt with here, for a better understanding of the events taking place in the pancreas under pathological conditions.

The large pyramidal acinar cells with their typical basal ergastoplasma (Fig. 2.**4**) form a closed layer around the lumen, whereas certain specializations are found between contiguous cells at the luminar side. These junctional complexes are composed (as in bile canaliculi) at the luminar side of tight junctions restricting the passage of (pro-) enzymes to the intercellular space. Although such belt-like tight junction seals are never completely impermeable to small molecules, secretory proteins

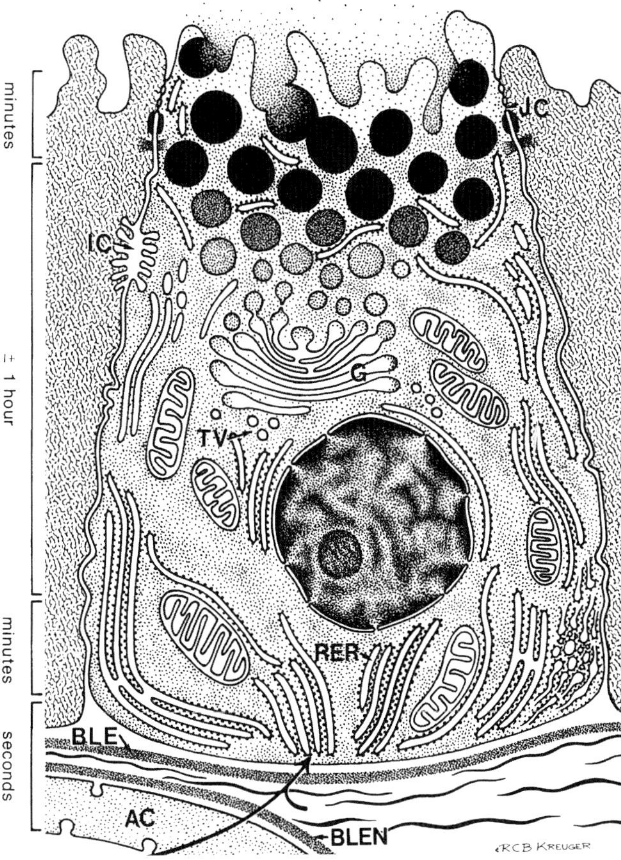

Fig. 2.**7** **Panoramic scheme of an exocrine pancreas cell**, shortly after it has become stimulated to secrete by cholecytokinin. JC: junctional complex; IC: intercellular secretory canal; G, Golgi complex; TV: transport vesicles; RER: rough endoplasmatic reticulum; BLE: basal lamina of epithelium; BLEN: basal lamina of endothelium; AC: pathway of amino acids as they are taken up by the secretory cell. At left, a rough indication of periods of time spent by incorporated radioactive amino acids in the different compartments indicated

which have a molecular weight of 20,000–90,000 are unlikely to cross this barrier (Fig. 2.7). Beneath the tight junctions, the junctional complexes consist of adherent structures (both zonulae adhaerentes and maculae adhaerentes), associated with fine filamentous structures of the cell skeleton. These structures are known to have a function in the firm adhesion of cells to each other. Intercellular secretory capillaries (Fig. 2.7) communicating with the acinar lumen may protrude over a short distance within the intercellular space, but as they are surrounded by bands of tight junctions, they do not interfere with the impermeability of the intercellular space to secretory products. Where centroacinar cells occur overlying acinar cells, the secretion products of the former also reach the lumen of the acinus via a system of intercellular clefts between the zymogen cells and the centroacinar cells.

The secretory process of pancreatic enzyme proteins as a whole is too well-known to need repetition here (for an excellent recent review, see Gorelick and Jamieson 1987). By use of radioactive amino acids and autoradiography, the different phases of secretion in rough endoplasmatic reticulum, transport vesicles, Golgi complex and se-

cretory granules are known also in their time course (Fig. 2.7).

When the prospective secretory granules leave the Golgi complex by a pinching-off process, they move – by an unknown mechanism – towards the cellular apex, during which process they undergo a certain ripening through fluid loss (Fig. 2.7). In a manner which is likewise not yet elucidated, the zymogen granules seem to recognize the plasma membrane to fuse with it, subsequently evacuating their contents (Fig. 2.**6**). As two, three or more zymogen granules may sometimes fuse in the apical cell compartment (Fig. 2.7), a fairly massive discharge of secretion products may occur when the appropriate neurohormonal stimulus reaches the cell.

The hormonal stimulus for this discharge is the polypeptide hormone cholecystokinin (which also activates contraction of the gallbladder). When acting alone, it does not significantly change the volume of outflow from the pancreatic ducts, so that coordinated action of secretin (stimulating alkaline fluid secretion) is a prerequisite for optimal flow of pancreatic juice. The acinar cells may also be stimulated directly by terminations of the vagus nerve, forming synaptic endings at the basal sides of certain zymogenic cells. Through the existence of gap junctions with lowered electrical resistance between acinar cells, propagation of the stimulus to neighboring cells is made possible.

Curiously enough, starvation or stimulation does not seem to cause drastic changes in the volume densities of zymogen granules, Golgi complex or rough endoplasmatic reticulum, although some reduction in granular processing and an enhancement of protein processing after stimulation is evident (Bendayan at al. 1985). On the whole, this indicates basically a steady state of the secretion process rather than extreme differences in synthesis rates under different circumstances. Also, a supposed role of the lysosomal apparatus in removing surplus secretory material (crinophagy), e. g. in fasting, may have been overestimated in the recent past.

A very fundamental question in the entire secretory process in the acinar cells is whether the approximately 19 different enzyme proteins (Gorelick and Jamieson 1987) are processed and discharged synchronously, or whether non-parallel secretion of enzymes may occur. The evidence is somewhat conflicting, but it seems that under certain specific conditions of stimulation, early secretion of trypsinogen and chymotrypsinogen may be found, amylase and lipase being secreted after a certain lag period (Keim et al. 1986). The difference seems to be in the efficacy of the movement of the synthesized proteins into zymogen granules and out of the cell.

The enzymes formed by the acinar cells make the digestion of all macromolecules normally occurring in food, i. e. proteins, carbohydrates, fats and nucleic acids, possible. All protein-degrading enzymes are secreted into the acinar lumen in an inactive form: trypsinogen, chymotrypsinogen, pro-carboxypolypeptidase. The enzyme enterokinase, as formed in the intestinal mucosa when chyme comes into contact with it, is able to convert trypsinogen into active trypsin, by far the most important proteolytic enzyme. Trypsinogen can also be activated autocatalytically, however, by previously formed trypsin, thus initiating a chain reaction, particularly since trypsin also converts chymotrypsinogen and pro-carboxypolypeptidase into the active enzymes. Apart from the secretion of enzymes in inactive form, another safety system exists to avoid the powerful proteolytic enzymes of the pancreatic juice becoming active before they have been secreted in the intestine. The acinar cells secrete, together with these enzymes, a substance called trypsin inhibitor, which surrounds the zymogen granules intracellularly. Although this substance only inhibits trypsin activity, it has a far-reaching effect, as trypsin also plays a dominant role in the activation of other proteolytic enzymes.

Failure of all these safety devices may result in autodigestion, such as occurs in acute pancreatitis. The conditions leading to this are not elucidated in all respects, however, nor is the precise role of the enzymes secreted in active form, such as lipase.

The Duct System

The acinar formations, which may or may not have centroacinar cells protruding into the acinus from the duct system at one or two endings (Fig. 2.**5**) continue into intercalated ducts, the cells of which have characteristics similar to those of the centroacinar cells. The intercalated ducts, which also have a function in the secretion of fluid and electrolytes, are lined with a pale-staining cuboidal epithelium with nuclei which are ovoid in longitudinal sections and round in transverse sections (Fig. 2.**4**). There is virtually no connective tissue around these ductules, which unite into short interconnecting ducts having a similar structure, and which empty into interlobular ducts with prismatic epithelium which have a thick connective tissue sheth (Fig. 2.**4**). It should be noted in passing that the difference between intralobular and interlobular ducts is not as distinct here as it is in the salivary glands, where intralobular ducts are much longer, and moreover show typical features of ion-transporting cells ("striated ducts"). This is related to their function in making saliva hypotonic by ion exchange during passage through the duct system. These devices are absent in the pancreas, which produces an alkaline, but essentially isotonic, secretion product.

The interlobular ducts fuse again into short ducts leading to side branches of the main pancreatic duct, which follows a longitudinal course centrally in the gland. These larger ducts are lined with a high cuboidal or cylindrical epithelium with occasional goblet cells, small mucous glands and a fairly thick layer of dense connective tissue with some elastin. The main duct begins in the tail and increases in size after having received numerous branches of connecting ducts; it ends as the pancreatic duct (formerly called the duct of Wirsung), fusing with the choledic duct in the manner indicated above (Fig. 2.**1**). The smaller minor or accessory duct lies cranial to the pancreatic duct, and has an identical histological aspect. The pancreatic duct at its common ending with the common bile duct becomes ensheated with thick strands of smooth muscle when they traverse the duodenal wall; the mass of this complex of smooth muscle coursing in different directions around these two ducts and uniting them (sphincter ampullae, formerly called sphincter of Oddi) causes a local thickening of the duodenal mucosa, the hepatopan-

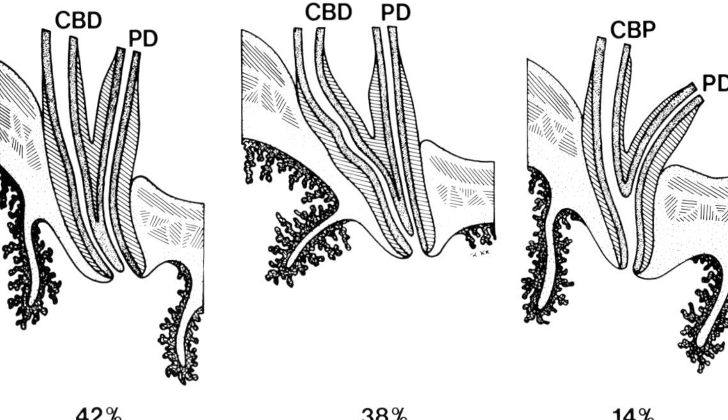

Fig. 2.**8** **Schematic transections of the major duodenal pupilla** in man, showing the frequencies of the most common interconnections between common bile duct (CBD) and pancreatic duct (PD) before they empty into the duodenum

creatic ampulla (ampulla of Vater). The relations between the openings of the two ducts within the ampulla and the structure and position of the components of the sphincter complex is subject to considerable individual variation (Boyden 1957). In view of the importance of these anatomical relations for the occurrence of regurgitation of bile into the pancreatic duct as a possible cause of pancreatitis, these variations have been studied in detail (Sterling 1954). Figure 2.**8** shows the three most common situations, redrawn after Sterling's data. In some 3% of cases the common channel even traverses more than half of the papilla (not drawn).

anlage could generate either a predominantly exocrine or a predominantly endocrine product (Pictet and Rutter 1972). All these, and many other techniques (among them the immunohistochemical localization of hormonal products) have shown that foregut entoderm, i. e. primary pancreatic bud tissue, can originate both exocrine and endocrine pancreatic tissue. In the adult situation, a common origin of this sort also appears from the occurrence of so-called intermediate cells (Mehmed 1979) which show characteristics of acinar cells, but also contain secretory granules characteristic for endocrine pancreas cells. A specific functional significance for these cells, if any, has remained obscure.

The Islets of Langerhans

As stated in the introduction above, a treatment of the structure and function of the islets of Langerhans would be beyond the scope of this chapter, which deals with the functional histology of the exocrine pancreas as a basis for the understanding of surgical disease processes. Nevertheless, a few remarks have to be made about the histological relation between exocrine and endocrine parts.

The compact cell masses, permeated by a network of capillaries which form the islets of Langerhans in the adult, arise as buddings from the developing branching duct complex (Fig. 2.**9**); the endocrine cells appear beforehand in small clumps, or as single cells amongst the primary tubular branchings which subsequently become isolated from the prospective exocrine pancreatic tissue. Alternative origins for the endocrine cells have been postulated, especially an origin from neural crest cells (Pearse and Polak 1971). This has been contradicted by different authors, however (Dieterlen-Lièvre and Beaupain 1976). It has been shown that by varying the composition of the tissue culture medium, an organ culture of pancreatic

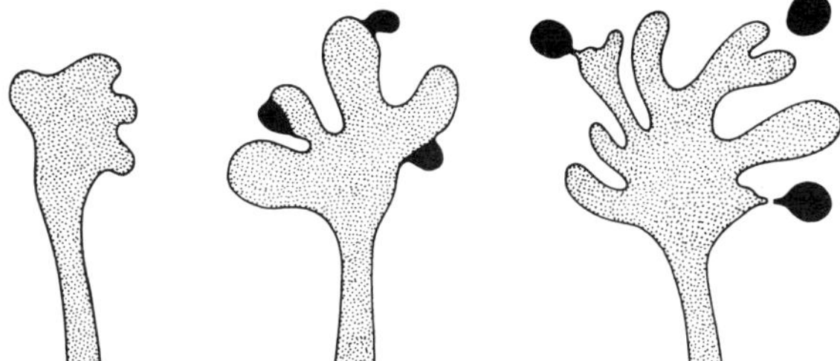

Fig. 2.**9** **Different stages in the growth of a part of the pancreatic anlage,** showing budding and segregation of islet tissue

Although the independence of the endocrine cell masses, with their dense capillary plexuses, is often symbolized by a thin sheath of connective tissue rich in collagen III (formerly called reticulin) surrounding the islets, this is not a constant phenomenon, endocrine and exocrine parts sometimes barely being separated. On the other hand, the fact that any suggested independence is illusory is shown, for example, by the fact that the vascular plexus in the islets is a derivative of the pancreatic blood vascular system as a whole, although it has been shown recently that special arterial branchings often lead to either islet or exocrine tissue (Yaginuma et al. 1986). The connection via the vascular tree cannot be entirely without functional significance, as it has been shown that the islet hormones glucagon, somatostatin, gastrin and pancreatic polypeptide have an influence on pancreatic exocrine secretion. Specific insulin receptors have been shown to exist on acinar cells of the exocrine pancreas (Gorelick and Jamieson 1987). The actual significance of these functional links has so far remained obscure, however.

References

Akao S, Bockman DE, Lechene de la Porte P, Sarles H. Three-dimensional pattern of ductuloacinar associations in normal and pathological human pancreas. Gastroenterology 1986; 90: 661–668.

Bendayan, M, Bruneau A, Morisset J. Morphometrical and immunocytochemical studies on rat pancreatic acinar cells under control and experimental conditions. Biol Cell 1985; 54: 227–234.

Bloom, W, Fawcett DW, eds. A textbook of histology. 11th ed. Philadelphia: Saunders 1986.

Bockman DE, Boydston WR, Parsa I. Architecture of human pancreas: implications for early changes in pancreatic disease. Gastroenterology 1983; 85: 55–61.

Boyden EA. The anatomy of the choledochoduodenal junction in man. Surg Gynecol Obstet 1957; 104: 641–653.

Dieterlen-Lièvre F, Beaupain D. Immunocytological study of endocrine pancreas ontogeny in the chick embryo: normal development and pancreatic potentialities in the early splanchnopleure. In: Grillo TAJ, Leibson L, Epple A, eds. The evolution of pancreatic islets. Oxford: Pergamon, 1976: 37–50.

Gorelick FS, Jamieson JD. Structure-function relationship of the pancreas. In: Johnson LR, ed. Physiology of the gastrointestinal tract. New York: Raven, 1987: 1089–1109.

Ingber DE, Madri JA, Jamieson JD. Neoplastic disorganization of pancreatic epithelial cell-cell relations: role of basement membrane. Am J Pathol 1985; 121: 248–260.

Jamieson JD. The exocrine pancreas and salivary glands. In: Weiss, L, ed. Histology: cell and tissue biology. New York: MacMillan, 1983: 749–774.

Keim V, Rohr C, Stöcken HC. Asynchronous secretion of newly synthesized pancreatic proteins in the rat. Digestion 1986; 33: 211–218.

Kuijpers GAJ, De Pont JJHHM. Role of proton and bicarbonate transport in pancreatic cell function. In: Berne BM, Hoffmann JF, eds. Annual Review of Physiology. Palo Alto: Annual Reviews, 1987: 87–105.

McLean JM. Embryology of the pancreas. In: Howat HT, Sarles H, eds. The exocrine pancreas. London: Saunders, 1979: 3–15.

Melmed RN. Intermediate cells of the pancreas: an appraisal. Gasteroenterology 1979; 76: 196–201.

Pearse AGE, Polak JM. Neural crest origin of the endocrine polypeptide (APUD) cells of the gastrointestinal tract and pancreas. 1971; Gut 12: 783–788.

Pictet R, Rutter WJ. Development of the embryonic endocrine pancreas. In: Johnson LR, ed. Handbook of physiology. Baltimore: Waverly, 1972: 25–66.

Ravitch MM. The pancreas in infants and children. Surg Clin North Am 1975; 55: 377–385.

Richardson KEY, Spooner BS. Mammalian pancreas development: regeneration and differentiation in vitro. Dev Biol 1977; 58: 402–420.

Schulz I. Electrolyte and fluid secretion in the exocrine pancreas. In: Johnson LR, ed. Physiology of the gastrointestinal tract. New York: Raven, 1987: 1147–1150.

Spicer, SS, Sens MA, Tashiam RE. Immunocytochemical demonstration of carbonic anhydrase in human epithelial cells. J Histochem Cytochem 1982; 30: 864–873.

Sterling JA. The common channel for bile and pancreatic ducts. Surg Gynecol Obstet 1954; 98: 420–424.

Yaginuma N, Takalasi T, Saito K, Kyoguko M. The microvasculature of the human pancreas and its relation to Langerhans islets and lobules. Pathol Res Pract 1986; 181: 77–84.

3 Surgical Pathology of Hepatobiliary and Pancreatic Tumors

H. J. Houthoff

New developments in the diagnosis and therapy of hepatobiliary and pancreatic malignant tumors during recent years have confronted the surgical pathologist with an increasing number of cytological preparations, biopsies and surgical resection specimens from these areas. Concomitantly, the questions to be answered in the pathology report have become more precise and have greater impact on postoperative management and on the prognosis for the patient. As the possibilities for curative surgery, or palliative treatment with relatively long survival times, are increasing, the need for adequate pathological diagnosis of surgical resection specimens (including nomenclature, staging and grading of the tumor and the radicality of resection) becomes of paramount importance for the prognosis, management and feedback between pre- and intraoperative diagnostic findings.

Relevant recent monographs and review articles on the pathology of hepatobiliary and pancreatic tumors have been listed under the general references at the end of this chapter to provide an overview of the extensive literature in this field. The aim of the present chapter is mainly to provide the essential pathologic basis for the characterization of the various tumor types, to present the experience of the Amsterdam group in relation to a selection of data from the literature, and to give practical information for tissue handling and diagnosis in surgical pathology.

General features

Parameters for Characterization of Malignant Tumors

The complete characterization of a malignant tumor consists of:

(1) Nomenclature. Site of origin, cell or tissue type of origin, and growth pattern together constitute the nomenclature of a tumor.
(2) Grading. The differentiation of the tumor cells – from highly differentiated to poorly differentiated or undifferentiated – provides the grade of a tumor, ranging from I to IV for decreasing differentiation characteristics.
(3) Staging. Clinical TNM classification (Unité Internationale pour la Lutte contre le Cancer [UICC]) (Hermanek and Sobin 1987) and histopathologic or pTNM classification provide the basis for grouping of the parameters to tumor stages.
(4) Additional parameters. These may include vasoinvasive growth, perineural growth and other characteristics of the tumor not covered by the foregoing items.

As an example, the tumor in Figure 3.1 originates from the epithelium of an extrahepatic bile duct stricture, grows as an adenocarcinoma, is highly to moderately differentiated (grade II, not shown), and has a maximal diameter of less than 1 cm but grows through the surrounding muscle coat into the adjacent fatty tissue. It has metastatic tumor islets in an adjacent regional lymph node, and extensive perineural growth, while vasoinvasive growth or distant metastases could not be detected. The appropriate "shorthand" description in the pathological diagnosis of this tumor is: adenocarcinoma of the extrahepatic bile duct epithelium, grade II, stage IVa without vasoinvasion (for the stage grouping, see next paragraph).

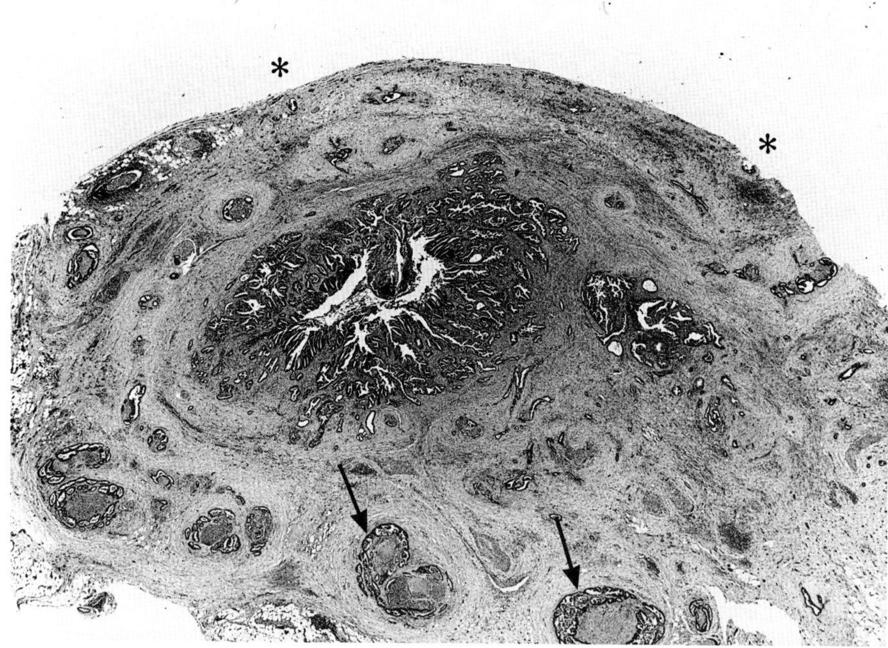

Fig. 3.**1   Adenocarcinoma originating from the middle part of the extra-hepatic bile ducts.** In **a**, the tumor is infiltrating through the muscular coat, reaching the sero-sal lining (∗).

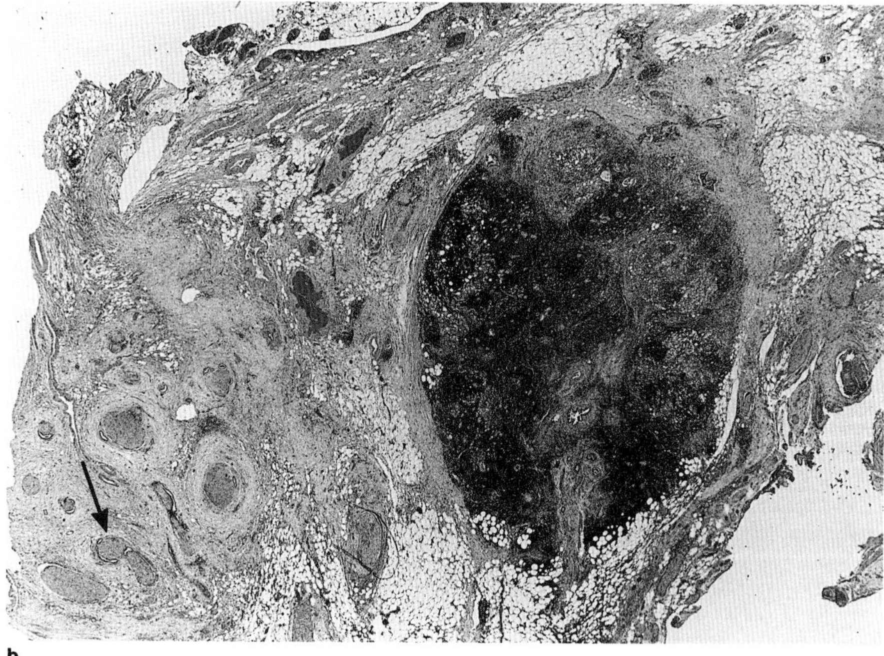

In **b**, a lymph node metastasis is shown. In both pictures, perineural invasion (→) and infiltration into the adjacent fatty tissue is obvious. Hematoxylin and eosin staining H & E, × 20

pTNM Classification and Tumor Staging

The pTNM classification (UICC) (Hermanek and Sobin 1987) is based on the histopathologic evaluation of the diameter of the tumor (pT), the presence or absence of metastatic tumor in the regional lymph nodes (pN) and the presence or absence of distant metastases of the tumor (pM). Although a properly oriented biopsy can provide information on the minimal extent of pT, a surgical resection specimen is needed for a full evaluation of pT and pN. The maximal tumor diameter can be difficult to ascertain, as many of the bile duct and pancreatic tumors are surrounded by fibrosis and chronic inflammatory changes, in which the tumor infiltrates with ill-defined tumor boundaries. It may take several sections to ascertain whether areas of fibrosis or inflammation constitute either the peri-

Table 3.1   Histopathologic classification and grading of malignant tumors

pT: Primary tumor

pTX	No histologic examination of primary tumor possible
pT0	No histologic indication of a primary tumor
pTis	Carcinoma in situ
pT1–4	Progressive diameter and spreading of primary tumor

*Stage grouping of TNM classification**

Stage 0	pTis	N0	M0
Stage 1	pT1	N0	M0
Stage 2	pT2,3	N0	M0
Stage 3	any pT	N1	M0
Stage 4	any pT	any N	M1

G: Histopathologic grading

GX	Grading of tumor differentiation not possible
G1	Well-differentiated tumor
G2	Moderately-differentiated tumor
G3	Poorly-differentiated tumor
G4	Undifferentiated tumor

* A general example; variations according to anatomical primary sites occur

pheral parts of infiltrative tumor growth or the surrounding tissue. The number of regional lymph nodes with metastatic tumor can best be expressed as the ratio between the nodes with tumor and the total number of nodes examined. The general rules for classification and grading – as proposed by the UICC committee (Hermanek and Sobin 1987) – are presented in Table 3.1; the specific rules are presented with each of the anatomic sites of tumor origin below.

Handling of Surgical Resection Specimens

For a careful examination of the margins of surgical resection specimens, to document the radicality of resection, the cleavage and resection planes should be properly marked before fixation, preferably by the surgeon who performed the operation. The distortion resulting from fixation of resection specimens of the biliary tract and pancreas is usually considerable, severely interfering with recognition of the original margins of special interest by either the surgeon or the pathologist. Therefore, a standard procedure for specimen labeling has been devised by the Amsterdam group, the essentials of which are shown in Figure 3.2. The surgeon marks the relevant planes with colored beads; the pathologist stains these planes with Indian ink after fixation to facilitate recognition of the planes in the microscopic sections. A schematic drawing of the relevant organs, as shown in Figure 3.3, is used to mark the areas of special interest, and to document the places where sections for microscopy are taken. The direction of cutting depends on the site of tumor

origin and the type of resection specimen, but sections through the center of the tumor mass showing the whole tumor in its largest diameter, and sections from the tumor mass to nearby cleavage or resection planes, should always be present for microscopic evaluation.

Cytology and Biopsies for Pre- and Intraoperative Diagnosis

When the presence of a tumor has been demonstrated by imaging techniques and other diagnostic procedures, a sample of tumor cells or tissue is most helpful in demonstrating its origin and differentiation. Such a sample can be obtained by percutaneous needle aspiration, during endoscopic retrograde cholangiopancreaticography (ERCP), or during laparotomy. A percutaneous needle biopsy or aspiration cytology, under the guidance of an imaging technique, can be obtained from tumors in the liver, bile ducts or pancreas (Schwerk et al. 1983, Hall-Craggs and Lees 1986, Soreide 1988). The complication rate is low, but includes seeding metastasis along the needle track (Rashleigh-Belcher et al. 1986) as a theoretical risk, which might be a disadvantage if radical surgery is still an option.

During ERCP, fluid from the bile and pancreatic ducts can be sampled for diagnostic cytology, brush cytology from the ampullary region and distal parts of the bile and pancreatic ducts can be obtained, and a biopsy can be taken from the ampullary region and the adjoining parts of the pancreatic head and common bile duct (Aabakken et al. 1986; Houthoff et al. 1988b; see also chapter 4.6 below). The complication rate is low, and remains essentially similar to that of ERCP alone. Although it is reported that exfoliative cytology has not fulfilled expectations for distinguishing between the various pathological entities (Gmelin and Weiss 1981, Classen and Phillip 1988), the Amsterdam group achieved superior cytological results by introducing a new cytology brush with an atraumatic flexible tip. In a series of 50 patients, bile cytology was negative in 20 cases, correlating with either a tumor-positive cytology from the pancreatic duct or inflammatory conditions such as stones, cholangitis or pancreatitis. Only two cases were inconclusive due to poor quality or lack of cells. In the 33 tumor-positive cases in either bile or pancreatic juice (Fig. 3.4), cytological grading could easily be performed and correlated to the results in surgical resection specimens. Therefore, brush cytology during ERCP might be reintroduced as a reliable method for differential diagnosis and tumor grading in pancreatic and bile duct strictures. In ampullary tumors and papillary stenosis, a biopsy during ERCP remains the first alternative.

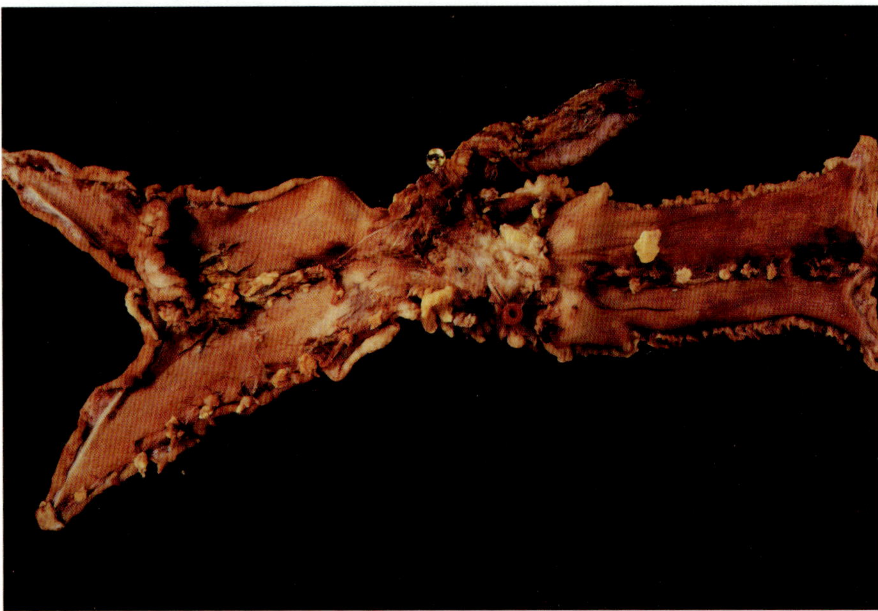

Fig. 3.2 **Partial pancreatectomy, Whipple procedure**

a An overview with the stomach (left), pancreatic head (center) and duodenum (right)

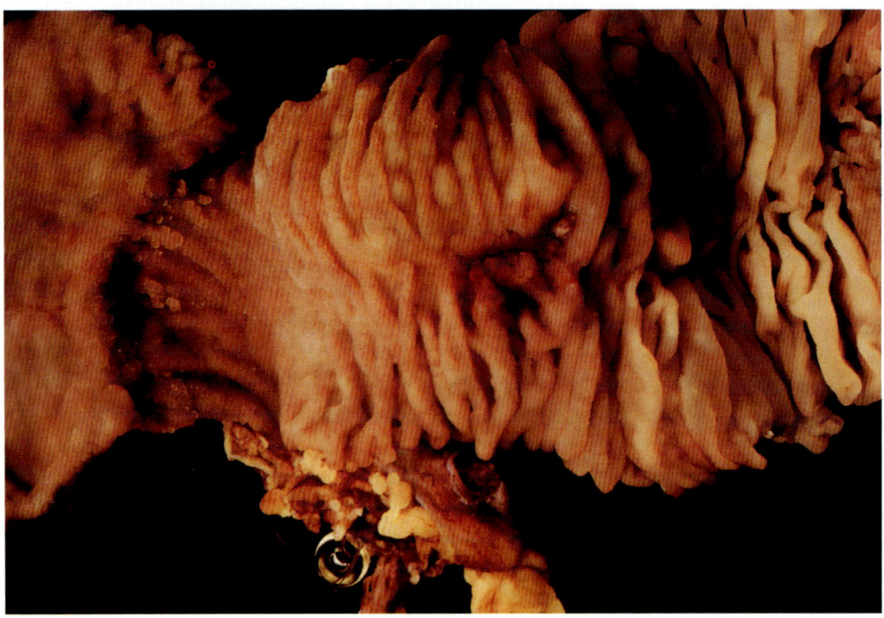

b The papilla of Vater in the duodenal mucosa

During laparotomy for exploration and surgical resection, samples of bile or pancreatic juice can be obtained at or below the site of a duct stricture for rapid cytological diagnosis during surgery (Verbeek et al. 1988). In a series of 76 patients, the results of cytological peroperative diagnosis proved to be comparable with, or even superior to, the well-established frozen section technique of tumor biopsy. Furthermore, for the intraoperative assessment of tumor growth in resection planes, simultaneous screening of frozen sections and cytological biopsy smears enhances the reliability interval of a rapid diagnosis.

Malignant Liver Tumors

Nomenclature

Liver tumors originate from the hepatocytes, from the bile ducts in the portal tracts, from the endothelial lining and Kupffer cells of the sinusoids and blood vessels, and, rarely, from the portal connec-

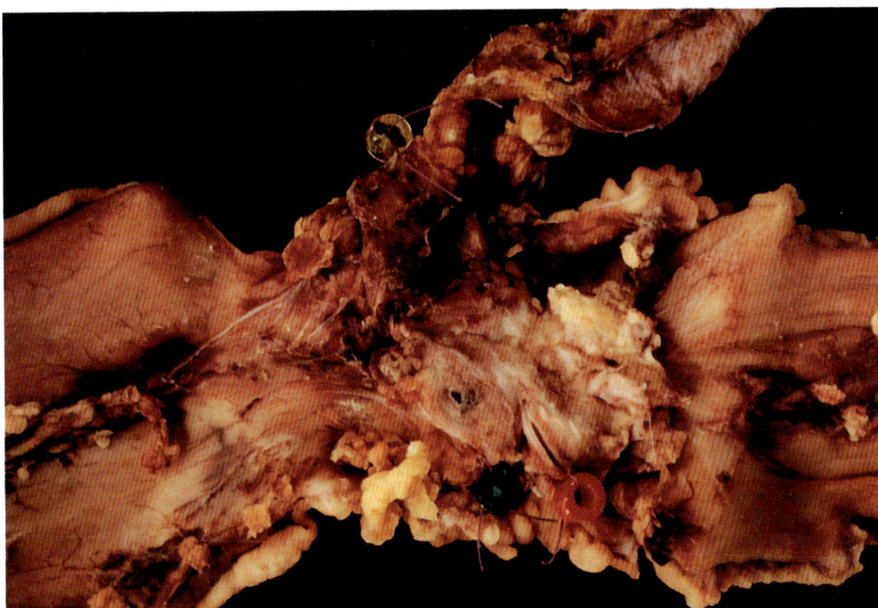

c The pancreatic head with the resection and cleavage planes. Colored beads are used as markers for the vessels and bile duct

c

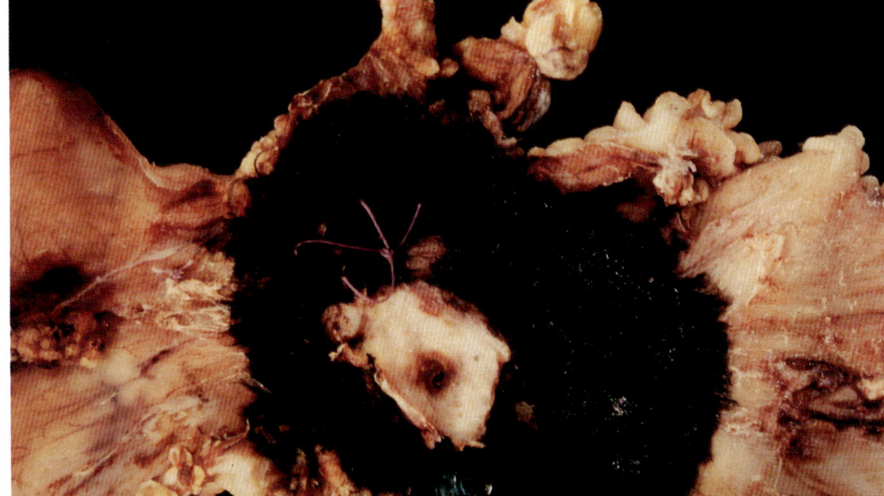

d The cleavage planes are selectively marked with Indian ink, otherwise this is comparable to **c**

d

tive tissue and nerves. A classification of primary tumors of the liver is given in Table 3.2 (Gibson and Sobin, 1978). In this section only primary liver cell (hepatocellular) carcinoma and bile duct carcinoma (cholangiocarcinoma) of intrahepatic origin will be discussed. Both tumor types are sometimes referred to as hepatoma, a non-descriptive term which should be avoided.

According to macroscopic or microscopic growth characteristics, various classifications of hepatocellular carcinomas exist (Anthony and James 1987, Weinbren 1988a, b). Of these, only the fibrolamellar type in young adults, the pedunculated type in old age and the small encapsulated type from South-East Asia deserve special attention, as these have a better prognosis than hepatocellular carcinoma in general (Caballero et al. 1985, Nakashima et al. 1983, Anthony and James 1987).

Macroscopy

In Europe and North and South America, more than 80 percent of the primary liver cell carcinomas arise in cirrhotic livers due to alcohol consumption

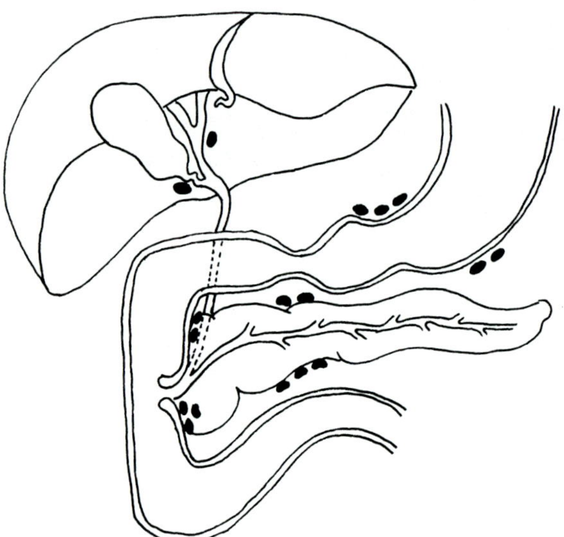

Fig. 3.3 **Diagram of the upper abdominal organs**, used for documentation of surgical specimens

or chronic hepatitis B virus infection (Anthony 1987). As both the cirrhosis and its usual etiology are relative contra-indications for surgical resection of these tumors, only a minority of the primary liver cell carcinomas will reach the pathologist in the form of surgical trisegmentectomy, hemihepatectomy or hepatectomy. Biliary obstruction with cholestasis only occurs if the tumors originate from,

or compress, the main hepatic ducts, and it is therefore mostly seen with cholangiocarcinomas. Hepatocellular carcinomas may destroy up to 80 percent of pre-existent liver tissue before cholestasis becomes obvious. Vasoinvasive growth into the large branches of the portal vein and hepatic vein is present in 65 and 23 percent of liver cell carcinomas, respectively (Nakashima et al. 1983). Intrahepatic hematogenous seeding of hepatocellular carcinoma is regularly present. Macroscopic growth patterns of hepatocellular carcinoma are only relevant for the surgical resectability of the tumor (Fig. 3.**5**). A single or expanding type, a multinodular type, a spreading type and a diffuse type can be distinguished (Nakashima et al. 1983). In the expanding and multinodular types, the tumor nodules are clearly demarcated from the surrounding liver tissue, while in the spreading type, the tumor infiltrates into the surrounding liver without clear demarcation.

Cholangiocarcinomas have no relation to liver cirrhosis. Two thirds of these carcinomas occur as solitary sclerotic tumors along the intrahepatic biliary tree, while one third arises near the portal or hilar region of the liver from the right or left hepatic ducts or their bifurcation (Fig. 3.**5**). Portal bile duct carcinomas usually remain small as they result in early duct stenosis with cholestasis and secondary biliary cirrhosis; they are referred to as Klatskin tumors (Klatskin 1965).

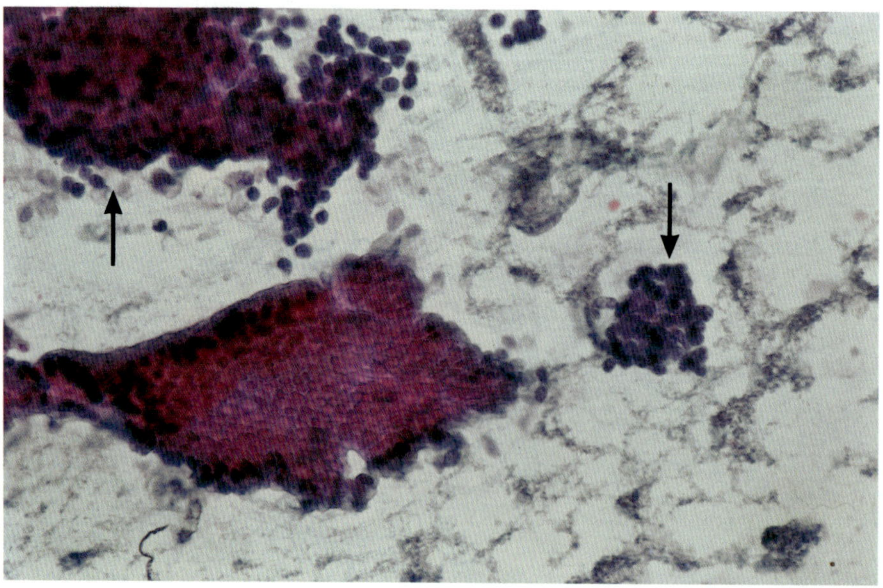

Fig. 3.4 **Bile cytology.** Giemsa (**c**, **d**) and Papanicolaou staining (**a**, **b**) × 125
a Groups of well-differentiated tumor cells (→) and a sheet of normal bile duct epthelial cells

Table 3.2 Classification of primary liver tumors (Gibson and Sobin 1978)

	benign	malignant
epithelial tumors	liver cell adenoma bile duct adenoma bile duct cystadenoma	hepatocellular carcinoma bile duct carcinoma bile duct cystadenocarcinoma hepatoblastoma carcinoid tumor
non-epithelial tumors	hemangioma hemangio-endothelioma	hemangiosarcoma epithelioid hemangio-endothelioma undifferentiated sarcoma rhabdomyosarcoma

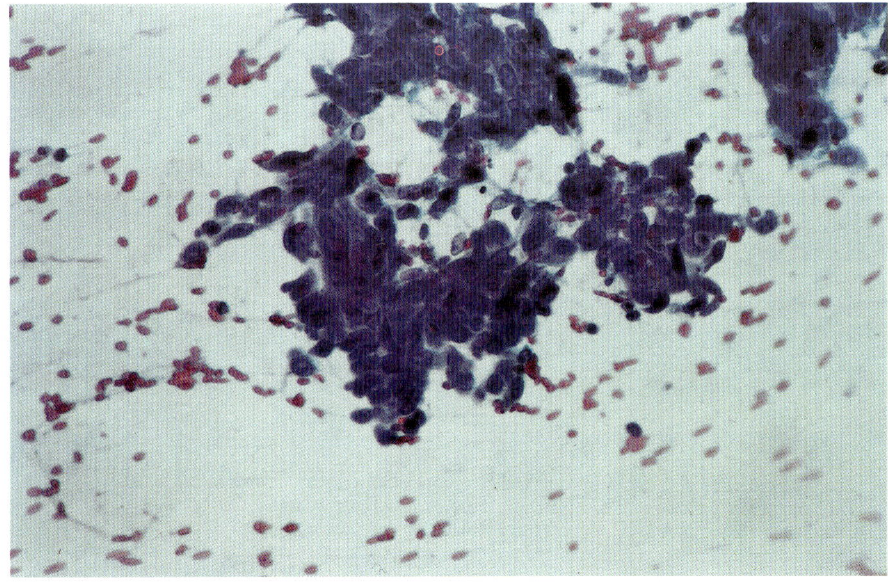

Fig. 3.4
b Poorly-differentiated
bile duct carcinoma

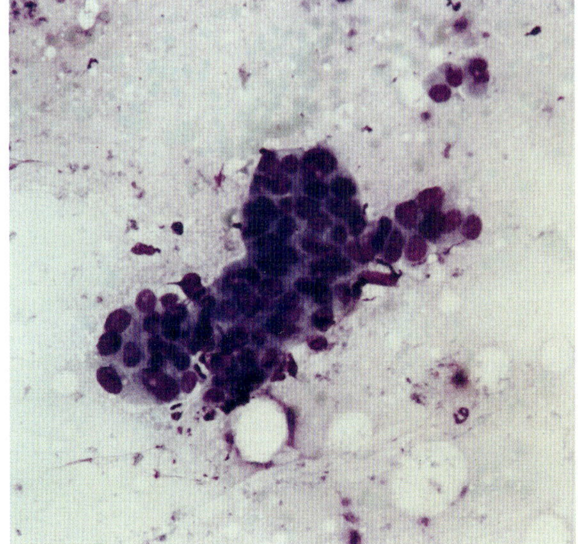

c Bile duct carcinoma with papillary formations and
moderate differentiation

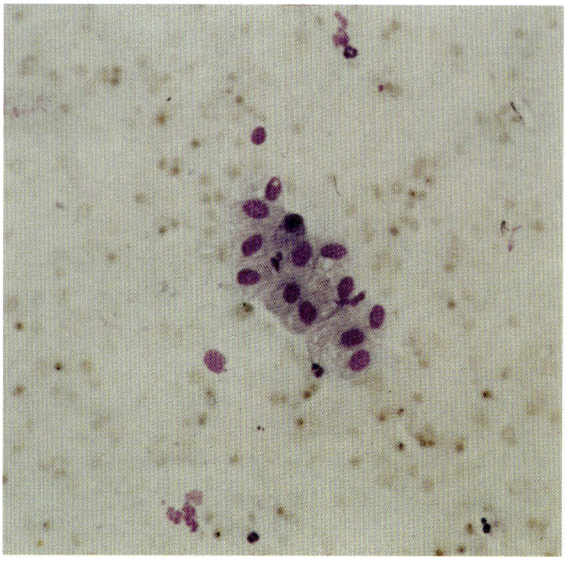

d Bile duct epithelial cells with inflammatory changes

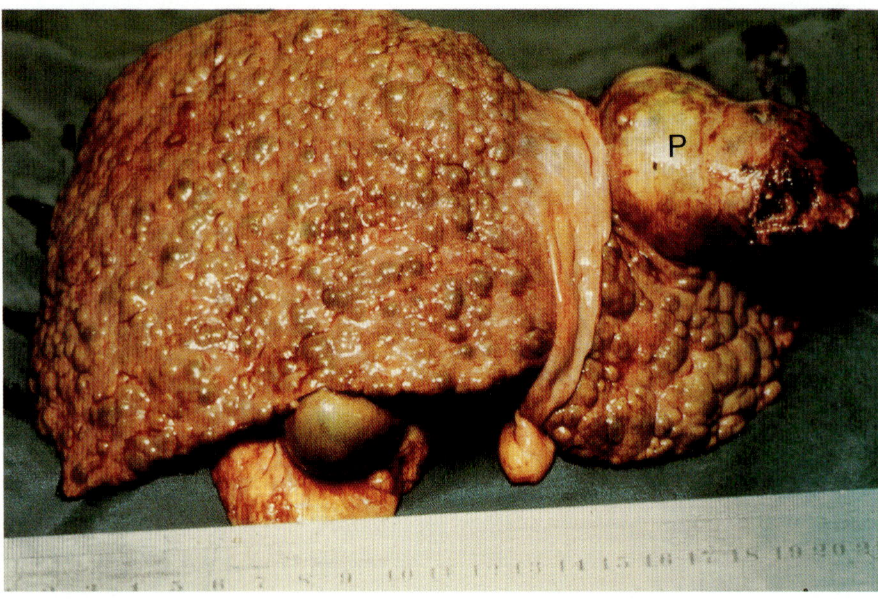

Fig. 3.**5** **Liver tumors, macroscopy**
a Pedunculated hepatocellular carcinoma (P) in a macronodular liver cirrhosis

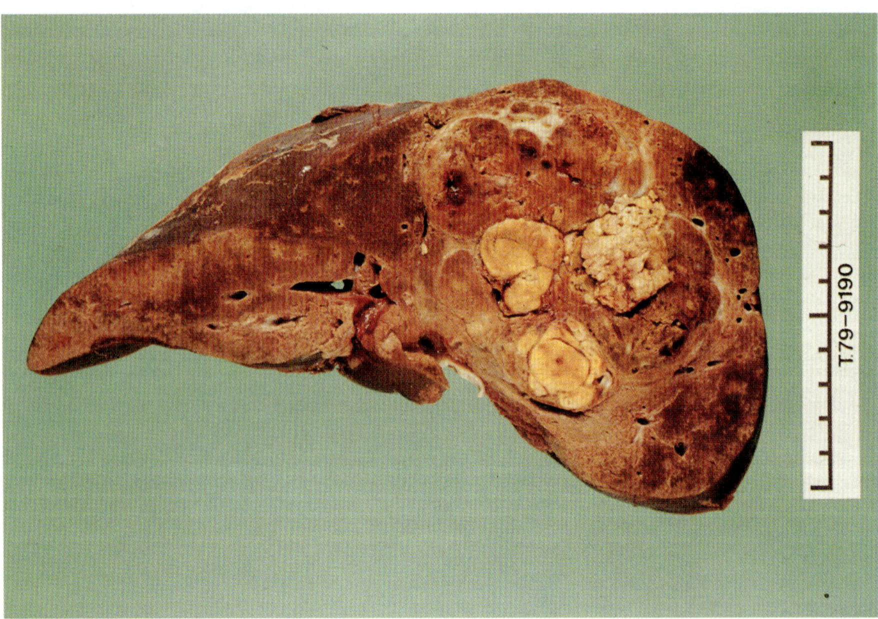

b Hepatocellular carcinoma of multinodular type in the right lobe

Microscopy

The growth pattern of liver cell carcinomas is either trabecular, pseudoglandular or solid (Fig. 3.**6**). The tumor cells resemble hepatocytes, are of clear cell type, or are pleomorphic. The presence of intracellular or canalicular bile pigment, globular hyalin bodies or Mallory's hyalin may facilitate the diagnosis (Anthony 1987). A variable amount of fibrous tissue may be present in between the strands of tumor, but a sclerosing or desmoplastic tumor stroma, as in cholangiocarcinoma, does not occur.

Thin-walled blood vessels, characteristically lacking Kupffer cells or fat-storing cells, run between the tumor strands. The fibrolamellar type of liver cell carcinoma is usually a highly differentiated tumor with cords of polygonal tumor cells with an eosinophilic cytoplasm, separated by thin strands of mature connective tissue.

The growth pattern of intrahepatic cholangiocarcinomas resembles that of extrahepatic bile duct carcinomas.

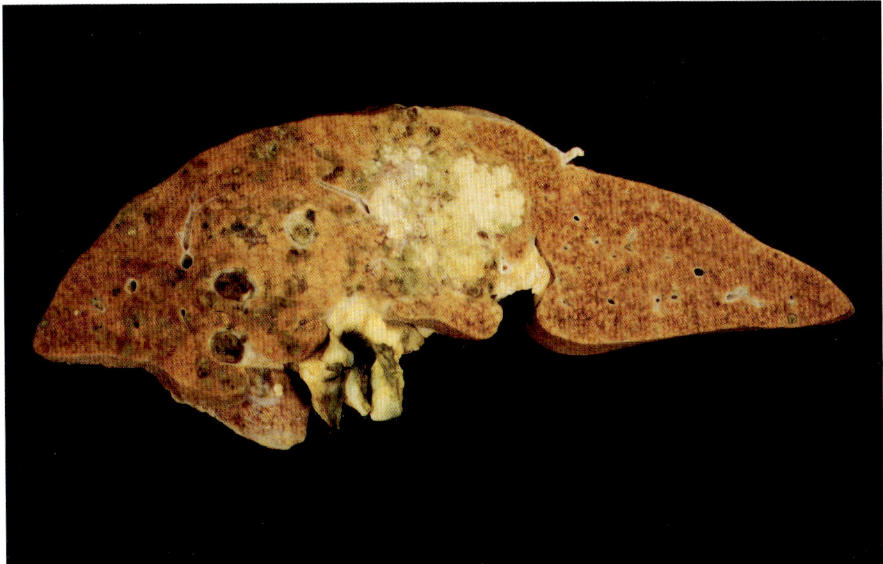

c A spreading type of
hepatocellular carci-
noma with tumor in-
filtration throughout
the right lobe

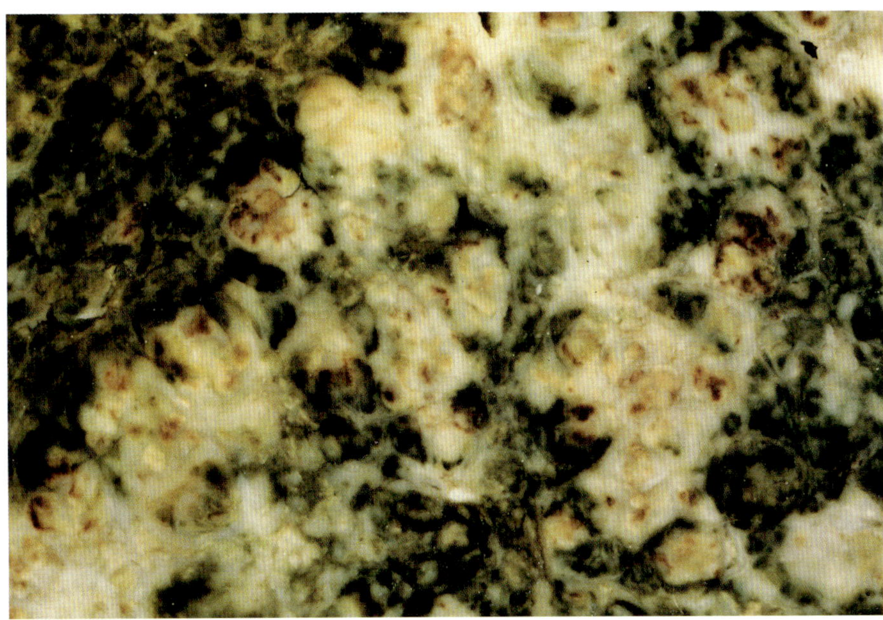

d Cholangiocarcinoma
with sclerotic portal
tracts in a cholestatic
liver

Staging and Grading

The histopathologic classification and staging of hepatocellular carcinomas and of intrahepatic cholangiocarcinomas are summarized in Table 3.3; for extrahepatic bile duct tumors see Table 3.6.

Grading of hepatocellular and intrahepatic bile duct carcinomas is reported to be of minor value for the prognosis of the patient (Anthony 1973, Anthony and James 1987).

Pathologic Findings and Prognosis

The prognosis in patients with a primary liver cell or intrahepatic bile duct carcinoma is still reported to be rather poor (Anthony and James 1987, Weinbren 1988a, b). Both tumor types are mainly found at a late stage, when the liver cell tumors tend to have intrahepatic vascular spreading or distant lymph node metastasis, and when intrahepatic cholangiocarcinomas have widespread metastasis.

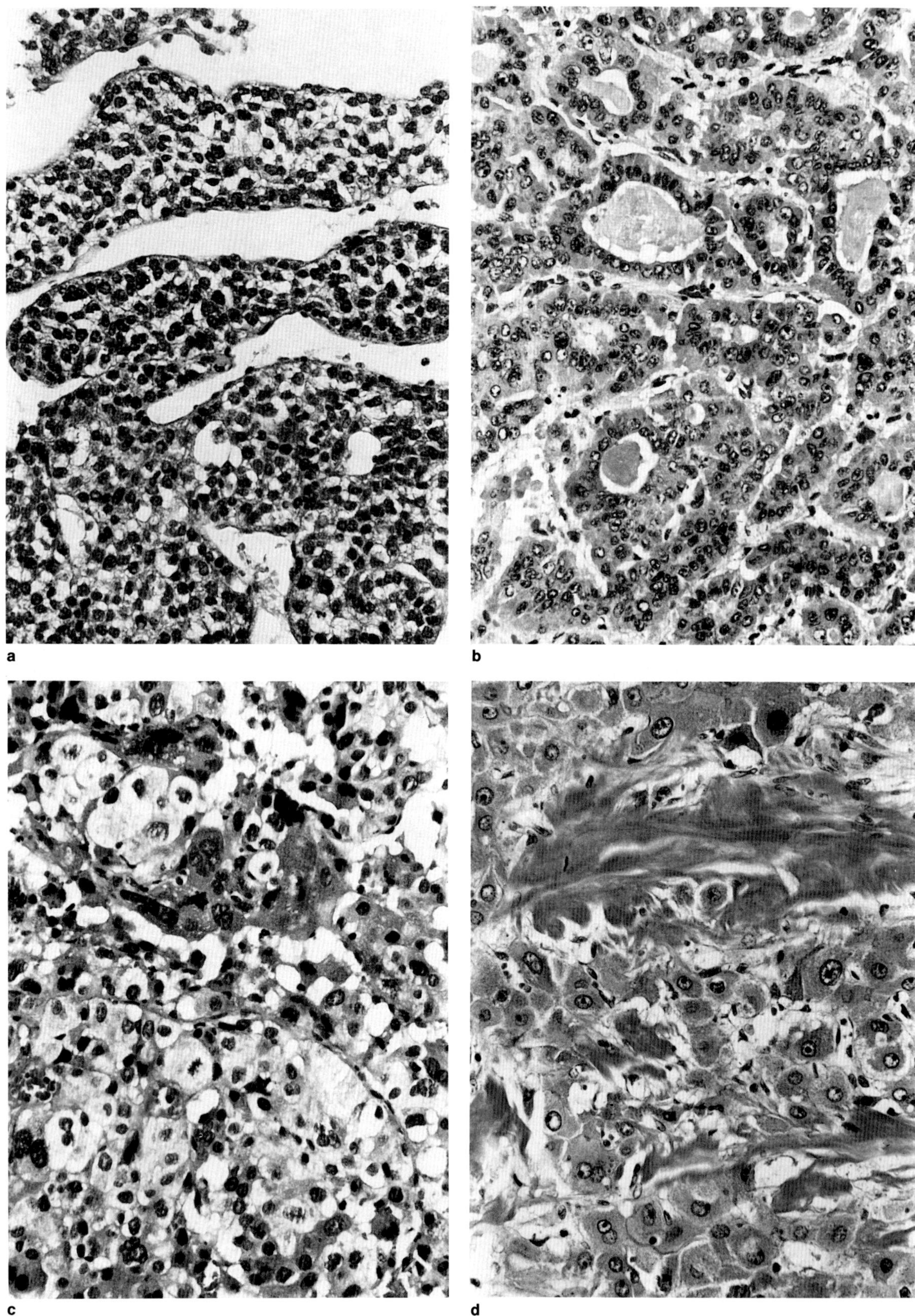

Fig. 3.6 **Liver tumors, microscopy.** Hepatocellular carcinoma of **a** the trabecular, **b** the pseudoglandular, **c** the fibrolamellar, and **d** the solid pleomorphic types. H & E, × 230

Table 3.3   TNM Classification and staging of hepatocellular and intrahepatic bile duct carcinoma

pT Classification

pTX	Histologic examination of primary tumor not possible
pT0	Primary tumor not found
pT1	Solitary tumor, ≤ 2 cm diameter, no vasoinvasion
pT2	Solitary tumor, ≤ 2 cm diameter, with vasoinvasion *or* multiple tumors in one lobe, ≤ 2 cm diameter, no vasoinvasion *or* solitary tumor, > 2 cm diameter, no vasoinvasion
pT3	Solitary tumor, > 2 cm diameter, with vasoinvasion *or* multiple tumors in one lobe, ≤ 2 cm diameter, with vasoinvasion *or* multiple tumors in one lobe, > 2 cm diameter, with or without vasoinvasion
pT4	Multiple tumors in more than one lobe *or* vasoinvasion in larger branches of portal or hepatic veins

Stage grouping of hepatocellular and intrahepatic bile duct carcinoma

Stage I	pT1	N0	M0
Stage II	pT2	N0	M0
Stage III	pT1, 2	N1	M0
	or pT3	N0, 1	M0
Stage IVa	pT4	any N	M0
Stage IVb	any pT	any N	M1

Grading of the tumors is of minor value, but the tumor stage and its site of origin are important for the evaluation of surgical resectability and prognosis (Okuda et al. 1984).

Malignant Tumors of the Biliary Tract and Gallbladder

Nomenclature

Tumors of the bile duct system originate from the epithelial lining of the ducts, from the subepithelial mucous glands, or, very rarely, from the adjoining non-epithelial tissues such as blood vessels, nerves, smooth muscle and connective tissue (Weinbren 1988a). Benign tumors of the bile duct epithelium occur very rarely and include cystadenoma, adenomatous polyp and adenomyoma. Cystadenocarcinomas of the bile duct epithelium are also reported as rare tumors, mainly occurring in the portal and intrahepatic parts of the bile duct system (Short et al. 1975).

The vast majority of primary bile duct tumors are adenocarcinomas with cellular characteristics resembling those of bile duct epithelial cells, if the tumors are highly to moderately differentiated (Fig. 3.7). According to the site of origin along the biliary tract, three preferential locations occur (Table 3.4) having implications for the surgical resection strategy.

Macroscopy

Bile duct carcinomas mainly present as a sclerosing mass along the biliary tract, with a stricture of the duct lumen (Fig. 3.8). Carcinomas of the main hepatic ducts and the bifurcation in the portal area generally grow infiltratively into the liver along the main portal tracts, clearly demarcated from the surrounding liver parenchyma. These are the areas where, in surgical resection specimens, special attention should be paid in order to document radicality. In the pancreatic area, the differentiation between carcinomas of the bile duct and the pancreatic duct is usually impossible in macroscopic serial sections of the pancreatic head: both have a tendency to form a sclerosing mass, and both are usually accompanied by chronic pancreatitis to a variable extent in the adjoining pancreatic areas. With terminal bile duct carcinomas, the surgical cleavage margins at the posterior side of resection specimens should get special attention in order to document radicality, even in small, macroscopically stage I or II tumors.

Microscopy

Although by cellular characteristics the bile duct carcinomas vary from highly- to poorly-differentiated tumors, they almost invariably retain the possibility of forming acini and secreting intraluminal mucin, at least in some areas (Fig. 3.9). The tumors nearly always induce a dense desmoplastic or sclerosing tumor stroma with a variable lympho-monocytic inflammatory infiltrate, in which the tumor acini are embedded. Remarkable perineural growth is also present in most of the tumors (Fig. 3.9). Other characteristics vary with the differentiation of the tumor, such as vasoinvasive growth (Table 3.4, 3.5; Weinbren 1988a). In a majority of the surgical resection specimens for tumors in the upper and middle parts of the bile duct system, invasive tumor growth can be found in the surgical resection or in the cleavage margins.

Staging and Grading

The histopathologic classification and staging of bile duct carcinomas is similar for those originating in the upper, middle and lower parts of the duct system and are summarized in Table 3.6. The classification of gallbladder carcinomas has been slightly modified to fit into the same table. Irrespective of tumor stage, radical surgical resection is difficult to achieve and only occurs rarely (Hout-

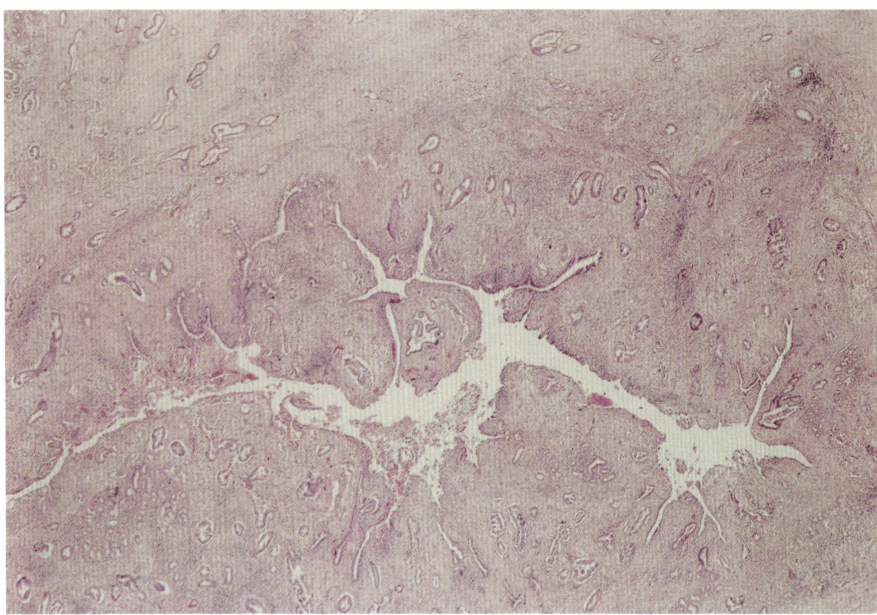

Fig. 3.**7 Well-differentiated adenocarcinoma.** H & E, × 50
a It originates from the epithelium in the lower third of the biliary tree

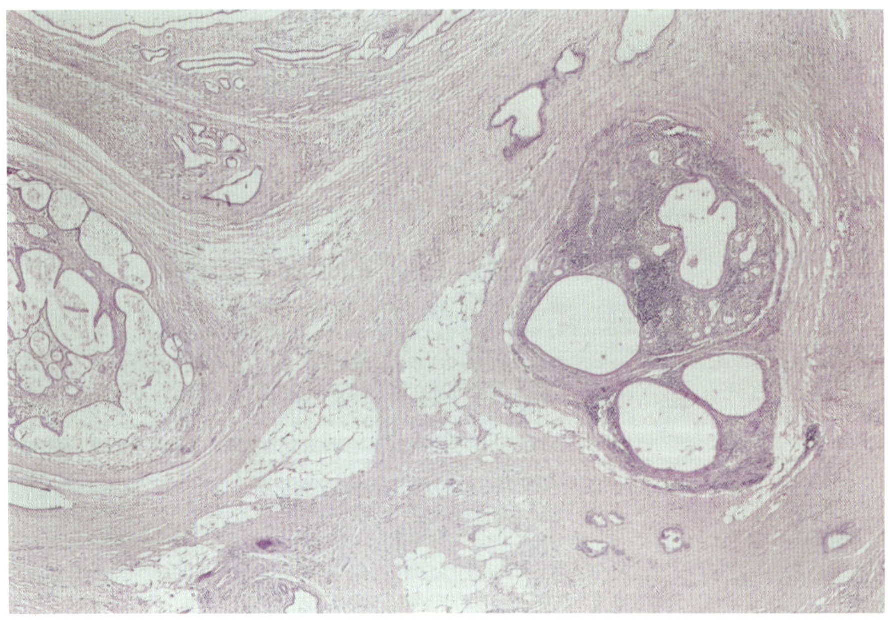

b Lymph node metastasis, perineural invasion and infiltrative growth in the pancreatic fatty tissue can be seen

Table 3.4 Adenocarcinoma of the biliary tract. Staging; results

			Stage	
Site of orgin	I	II	III	IVa
Upper third	0	8	6	25
Middle third	0	2	1	2
Lower third	1	3	4	19

hoff et al. 1988a) for tumors in the upper and middle parts.

Grading of bile duct carcinomas has proved in our series to constitute a good prognosticator for patient survival (Table 3.7). Although in the absence of radical resection the surgical treatment can not be called curative, the survival of patients with non-radical resection of a grade I or II bile duct carcinoma is remarkable. In general, the presence

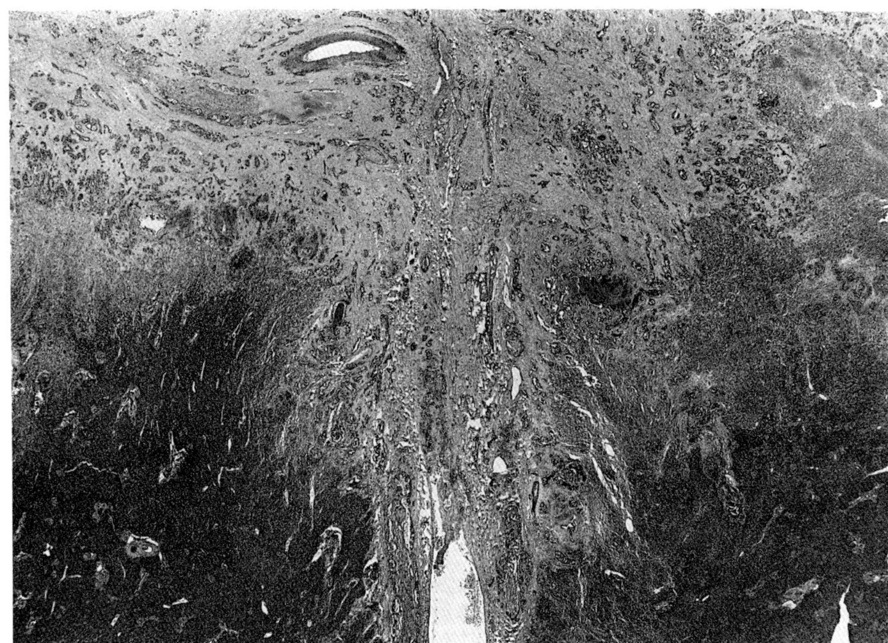

Fig. 3.**8 Adenocarcinoma of the bile duct.** H & E, × 12
a A sclerotic mass at the site of the hepatic bifurcation, with infiltrative growth into the liver

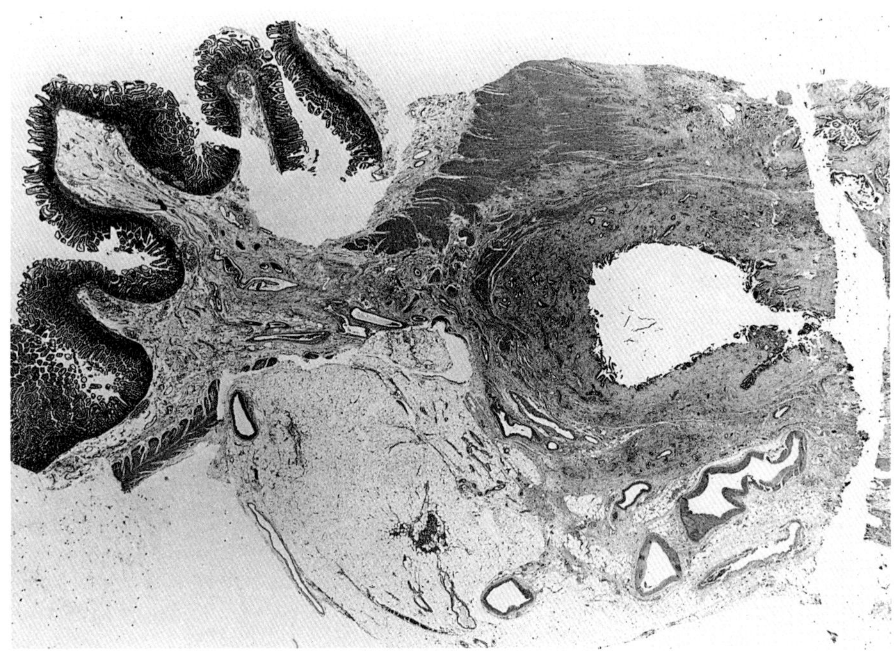

b An adenocarcinoma of the lower third underneath the duodenal wall, with infiltration into the surrounding structures

of local vasoinvasion correlated with poor differentiation, while both of these parameters were the findings most frequently present in patients who died within several months of the operation.

Pathologic Findings and Prognosis

Radical surgical resection favors a good prognosis, but in many cases cannot be achieved in carcinomas of the upper or middle parts of the bile duct system.

According to the grading, patients with a grade I or II carcinoma of the lower bile duct in the pancreatic area have an excellent prognosis, provided that a radical resection can be performed and distant metastases are absent. Patients with a grade I or II carcinoma of the middle and upper parts of the bile duct system have a good prognosis, even if a surgical resection is non-radical, provided that local vasoinvasion and distant metastases are absent.

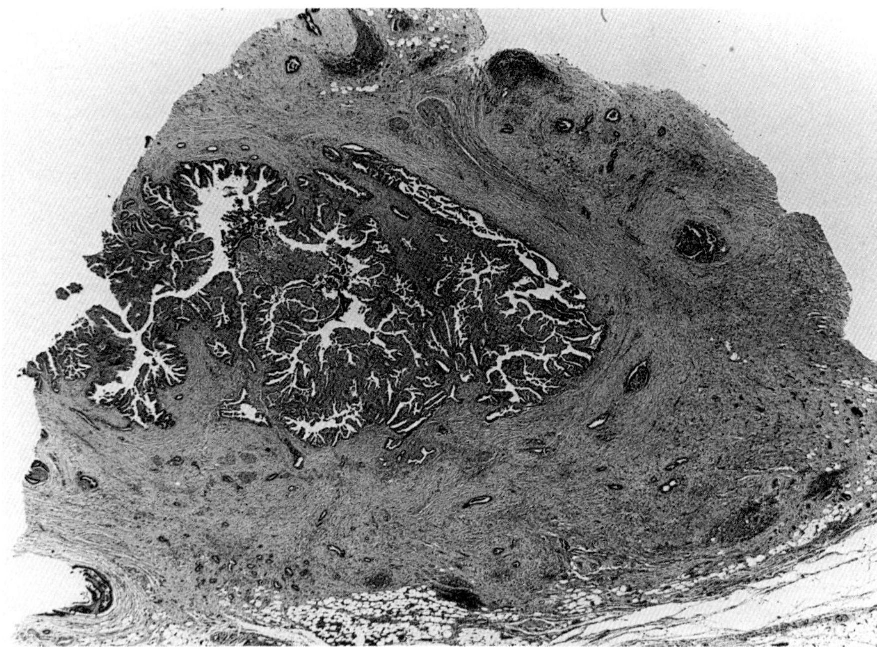

c A papillary adenocarcinoma of the middle part, surrounded by sclerotic tumor stroma

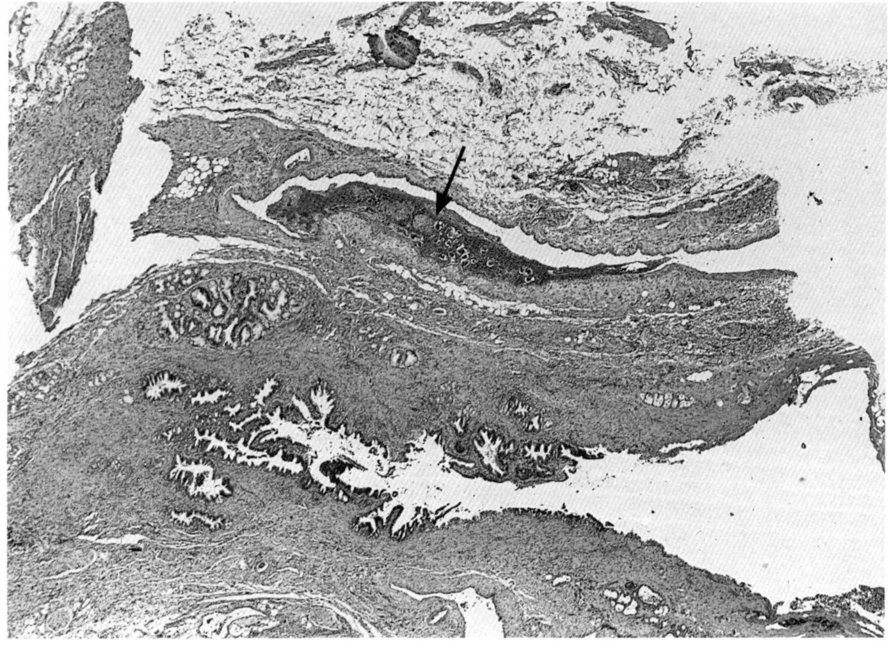

d The same tumor as in **c**, here in longitudinal transection with mural thrombosis (→) in a vein by vasoinvasive growth

According to the staging, stage I to III carcinomas in the pancreatic area have an excellent prognosis, especially when the tumors are highly differentiated.Carcinomas in the middle and upper parts of the bile duct system are mainly in stage IV a when operated; although patients with stage I and II tumors do appear to have a good prognosis, these tumors occur rarely, and staging for carcinomas in these areas at the moment still appears to be less important than grading.

Malignant Tumors of the Pancreas

Nomenclature

Pancreatic tumors originate from the pancreatic duct system, from the exocrine acini, from the endocrine islets, or, rarely, from components of the connective tissue, vessels or nerves. In addition, tumors in the pancreatic head can also originate from the common bile duct, from the ampulla, from the mucosal epithelium of the duodenum, from the

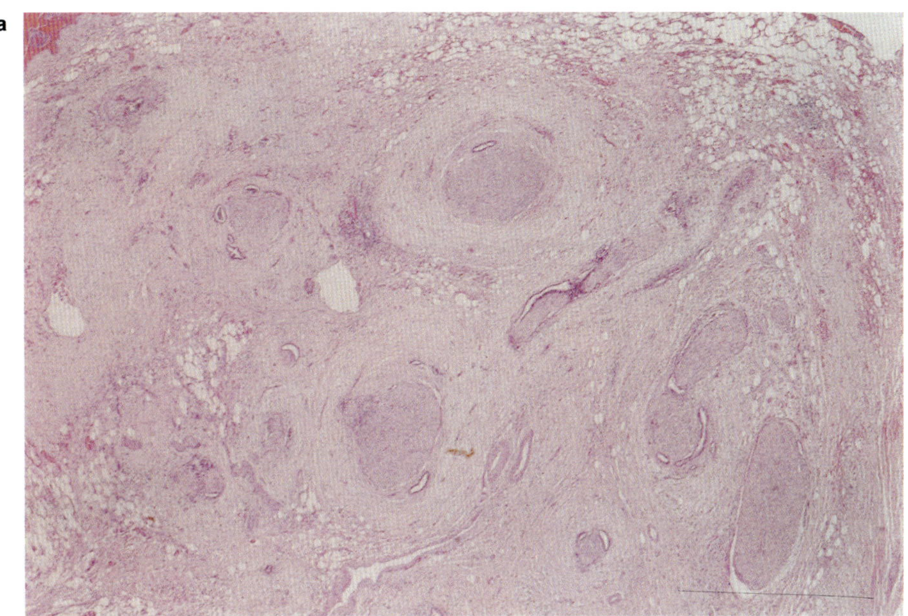

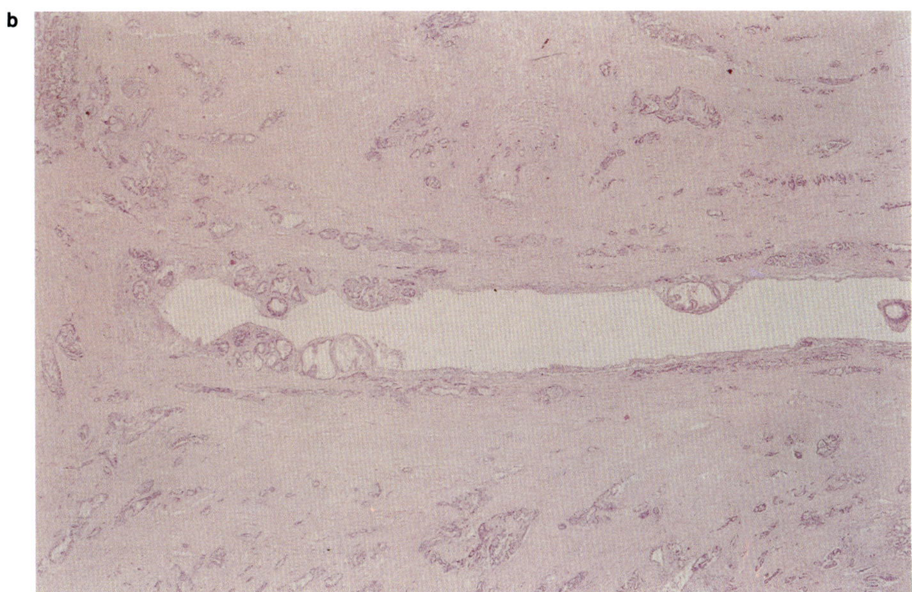

Fig. 3.**9 a** **Perineural growth** and **b vasoinvasive growth** of bile duct adenocarcinoma. H & E, × 50

Table 3.**5** **Adenocarcinoma of the biliary tract.** Comparison of parameters

Grade	Total no.	Scirrhous growth	Inflammation	Perineural invasion	Vaso-invasion	I	II	III	IVa
1	18	7	2	6	2	0	6	5	7
2	25	11	4	12	4	1	7	5	12
3	27	15	3	17	17	0	0	1	26
4	1	1	1	1	1	0	0	0	1

Table 3.6   TNM Classification and staging of carcinomas of the extrahepatic bile ducts and gallbladder

pT classification

pTX	Histologic examination of primary tumor not possible
pT0	Primary tumor not found
pTis	Carcinoma in situ
pT1	Tumor infiltration restricted to submucosa or muscular coat
pT1a	Restricted to submucosa
pT1b	Restricted to muscular coat
pT2	Tumor infiltration into perimuscular connective tissue, not reaching the serosa or liver
pT3	Tumor infiltration into adjacent organs: ≤ 2 cm into liver
pT4	Tumor infiltration into adjacent organs: liver, stomach, duodenum, pancreas, colon, omentum

Stage grouping

Stage 0	pTis	N0	M0
Stage I	pT1	N0	M0
Stage II	pT2	N0	M0
Stage III	pT1,2	N1	M0
Stage IVa	pT3	any N	M0
Stage IVb	pT4	any N	M0
	or any pT	any N	M1

endocrine cell populations in the duodenal mucosa, and occasionally from the adjoining lymphoid tissue or muscular coats. The main tumor types deriving from these tissues are summarized in Table 3.**8**. In this section, only carcinomas of the pancreas will be discussed.

The site of origin of pancreatic head carcinomas should be unequivocally determined in surgical resection specimens, as the stage grouping and prognosis are reported to be different for ampullary, duodenal, common bile duct and pancreatic duct tumors, respectively (Cubilla and Fitzgerald 1987). As their growth pattern and differentiation may be similar and resemble, for example, a diffusely infiltrating adenocarcinoma with or without differentiation characteristics, the site of origin should be deduced from the location of the tumor bulk in relation to adjoining structures and from the epithelial dysplasia nearly always present in the epithelial lining in the direct neighborhood of the site of origin. Thus, the tumor bulk may be *above* (ampullary and duodenal tumors) or *below* (common bile duct and pancreatic duct tumors) the muscularis propria of the duodenum (Fig. 3.**10**). And, although all the anatomic structures may be encompassed within a diffusely infiltrating tumor,

Table 3.7   Adenocarcinoma of the biliary tract. Upper and middle third: comparison of parameters with survival

Grade	Total no.	Stage				Radicality of resection		Survival					
		I	II	III	IVa	+	−	deceased* no.	month	(r)**	alive no.	month	(r)**
1	12	0	6	3	3	1	11	6	16	(1−42)	6	20	(7−43)
2	17	0	4	3	10	7	10	5	4	(1−9)	12	17	(3−43)
3	15	0	0	1	14	2	13	12	5	(1−14)	3	18	(2−31)
4	0	0	0	0	0	0	0	0			0		

 * hot corrected for cause of death
** range

Table 3.8   Classification of primary tumors of the pancreas

origin	*benign*	*malignant*
ductal epithelium (pancreatic duct, ampulla)	tubular adenoma	carcinoma:
	villous adenoma (papilloma)	adenocarcinoma, giant cell, adenosquamous, mucinous, undifferentiated, unclassified
	cystadenoma	cystadenocarcinoma
acinar cells	adenoma	carcinoma
islet cells	adenoma	carcinoma
non-epithelial tissue	fibroma	fibrosarcoma
	leiomyoma	leiomyosarcoma
	histiocytoma	malignant fibrous histiocytoma
	hemangioma	malignant hemangiopericytoma
	lymphangioma	malignant lymphoma

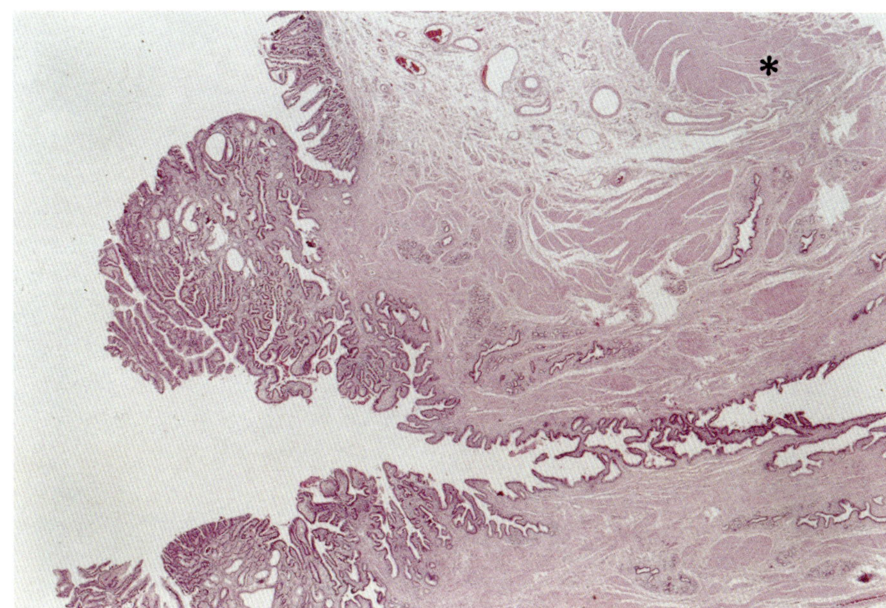

Fig. 3.**10**   In **a**, **b** and **c**, the tumors arise above the muscularis propria (∗) of the duodenum. In **d** it originates from ductal epithelium below the muscularis propria (seen at the left). H & E, × 7

a   Duodenal adenoma of the papilla of Vater

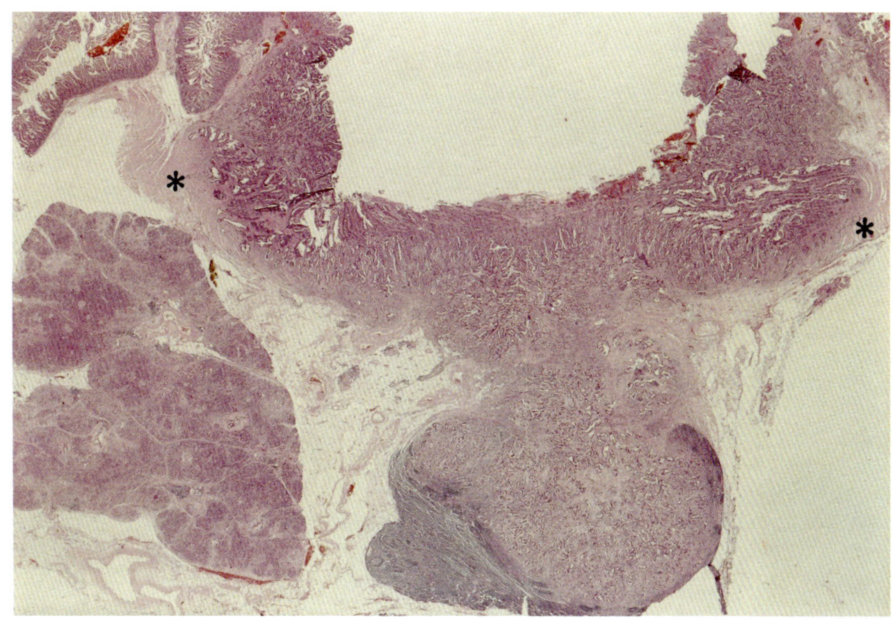

b   Ampullary adenocarcinoma with infiltrative growth above and under the muscularis propria and a lymph node metastasis

so that it appears to be impossible to determine its site of origin, it is only in the pancreatic duct or in the common bile duct etc. that epithelial dysplasia is present with increasing severity towards the site of origin of the pancreatic duct or common bile duct carcinoma, respectively (Fig. 3.**11**). Furthermore, a dilated pancreatic duct system and the presence of focal areas with papillary formations, carcinoma in situ or severe dysplasia in the pancreatic duct can provide additional information about a site of origin in the pancreatic duct (Sommers et al. 1954, Cubilla and Fitzgerald 1976, Tryka and Brooks 1979). To study these features in a surgical resection specimen, it is essential to obtain large sections for microscopy, containing the largest diameter of the tumor, cut obliquely to the duodenal surface and containing large parts of the duct system, as shown in Figure 3.**10**.

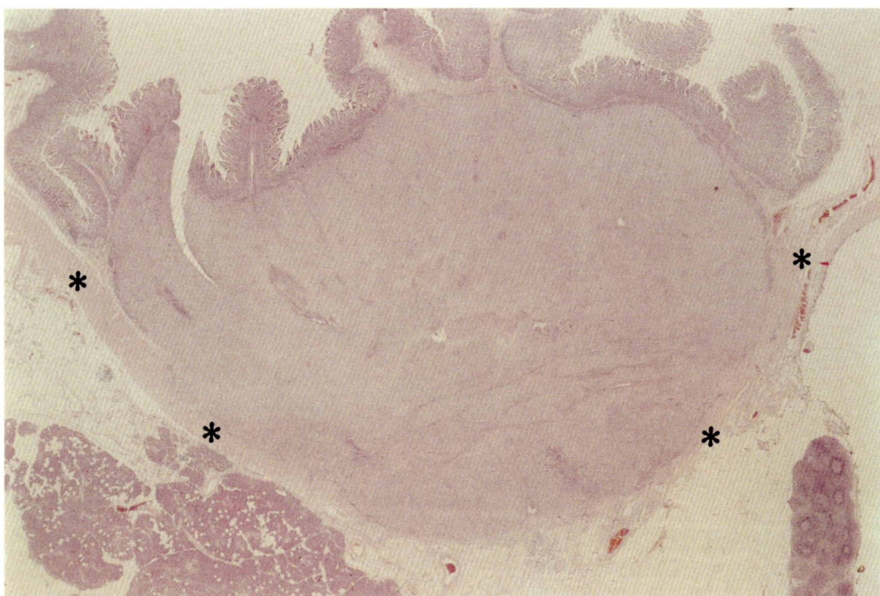

c Poorly differentiated ampullary carcinoma, restricted to the ampullary and periampullary region

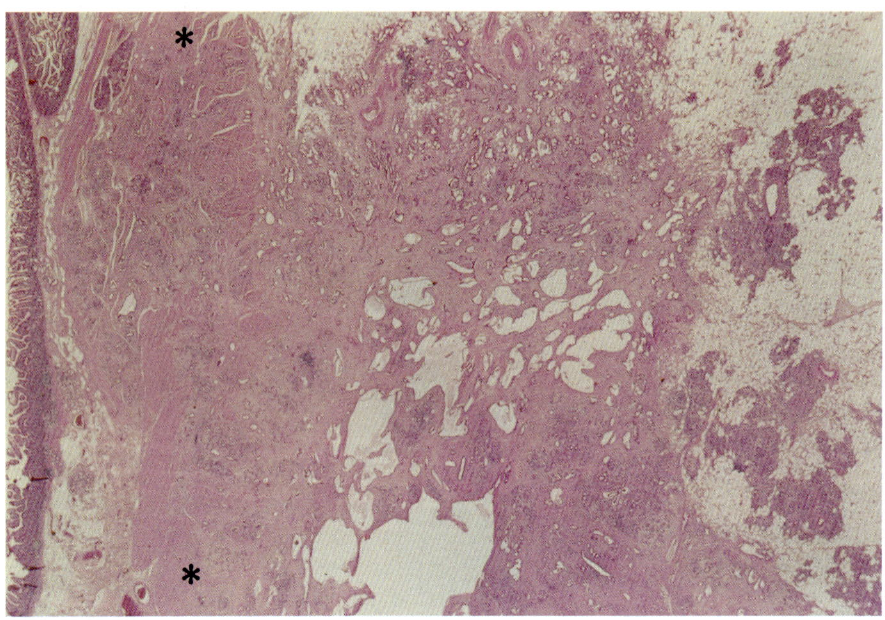

d Adenocarcinoma of the terminal part of the pancreatic duct

Macroscopy

A diagram of the pancreas and adjoining structures is given in Figure 3.3. About two thirds of pancreatic duct carcinomas occur in the pancreatic head (Cubilla and Fitzgerald 1987). The percentage is even higher in resection specimens, due to the tendency of carcinomas in the body and tail to remain symptomless till stage IV, by which time they are inoperable. In macroscopic interpretation of surgical resection specimens, care should be taken that each of the anatomical structures and groups of lymph nodes are identified and properly marked before fixation, when differences in consistency and color are still optimal and tissue distortion is minimal, as outlined in the first section of this chapter (see Fig. 3.2). In particular, the cleavage margins with the caval and portal veins should be marked, as the absence of infiltrative and vasoinvasive growth in clinical staging should be confirmed by histopathological analysis.

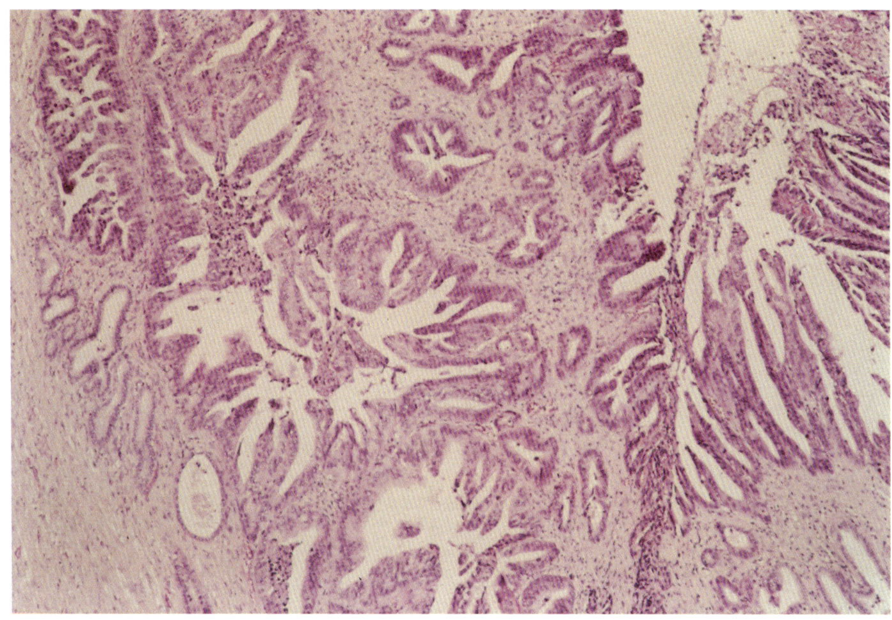

a

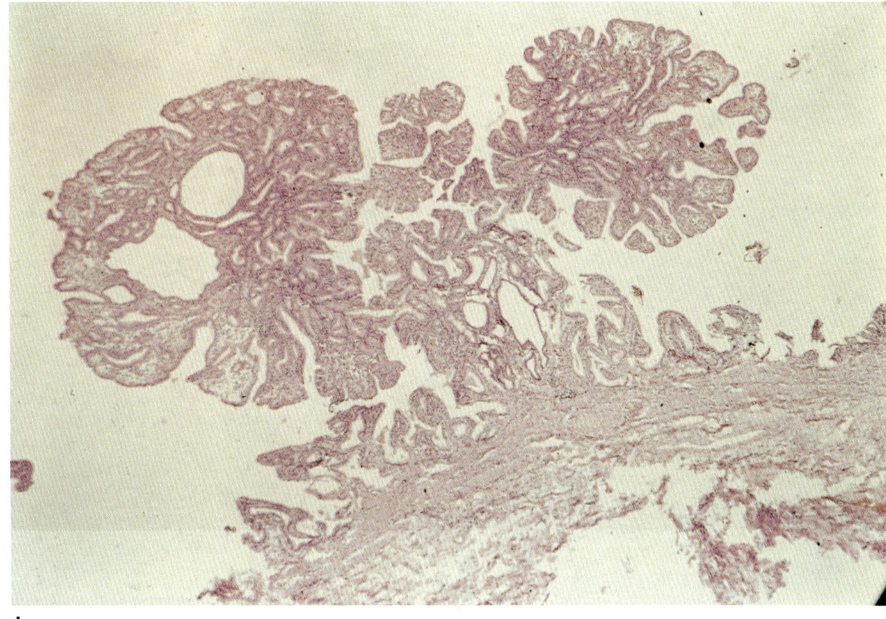

Fig. 3.**11 Epithelial dysplasia** in bile and pancreatic duct epithelium. H & E (**a**, **b**, **c**) and PAS staining (**d**), × 15
a, **c** Severe dysplasia, and **b** adenoma with light dysplasia of the bile duct epithelium in the presence of infiltrative adenocarcinoma

b

Following fixation, and taking into consideration the surgical information and markings of the specimen, the specimen can best be cut obliquely to the duodenal surface in a number of thin parallel sections, revealing the bile and pancreatic duct system with the ampullary region and the main tumor mass. Apart from surgical resection and cleavage margins, sampling for histology should include at least one of the thin parallel sections, all lymph nodes, and all areas specially marked or described by the surgeon. The surgical resection margins through the stomach and duodenum can usually be described by macroscopical inspection alone. The regional lymph nodes include the superior and inferior pancreatic nodes, the anterior and posterior pancreaticoduodenal nodes, the pyloric and proximal mesenteric nodes, the nodes along the common bile duct, and the nodes at the pancreatic tail and spleen.

Endocrine tumors of the pancreas are usually well circumscribed yellow to brown masses (Fig. 3.**12**), but may be very small and barely

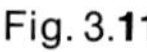
Fig. 3.**11**

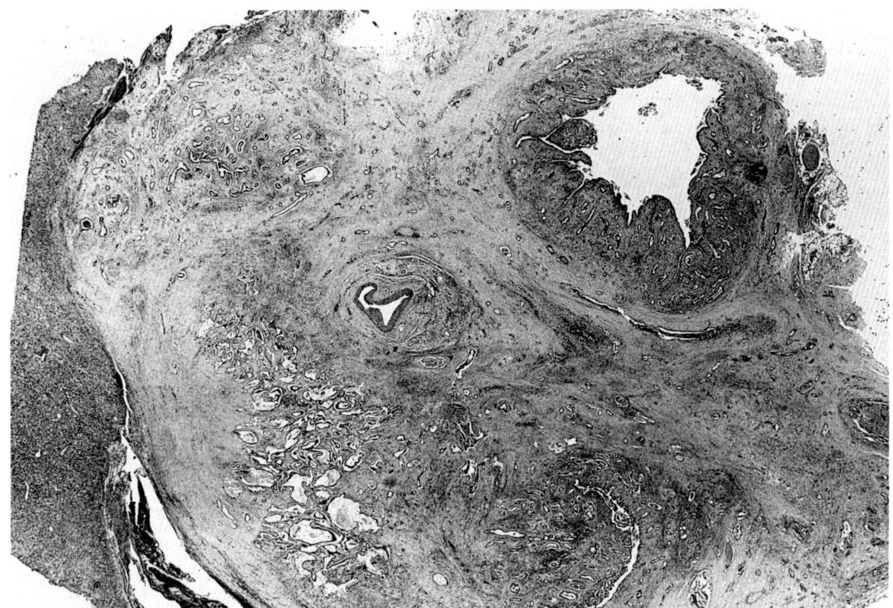

c

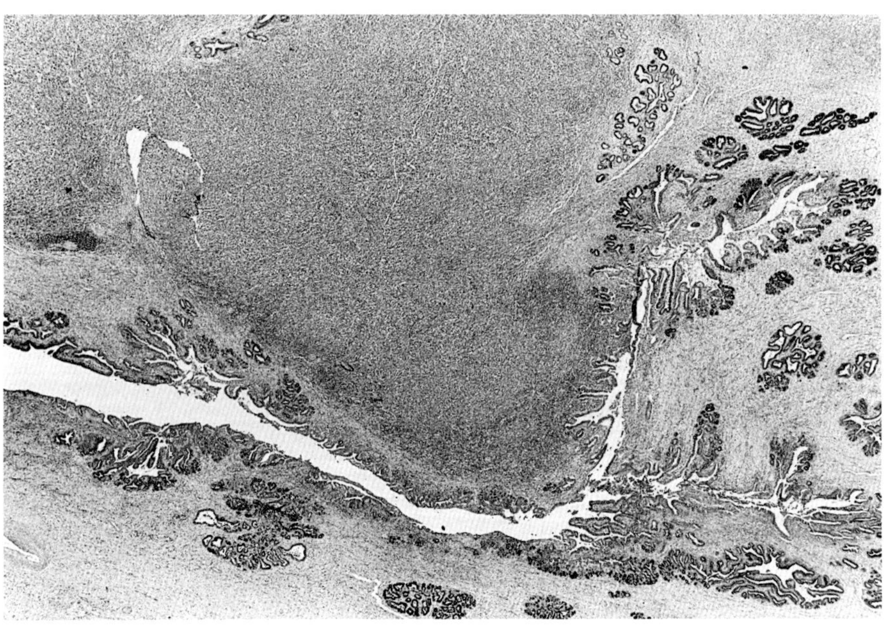

d

d Dysplasia of the pancreatic duct in pancreatic duct adenocarcinoma

detectable by the naked eye (Goudswaard et al. 1986). The surrounding exocrine pancreas usually has a normal appearance. By contrast, carcinomas of the pancreatic and bile duct system, of the ampullary region and of the acinar cells are usually diffusely infiltrating and surrounded by a variable amount of pancreatitis (Fig. 3.**13**). Reliable measurement of the largest diameter of the tumor can therefore only be made in histological sections. The color and consistency of the tumors are usually comparable to those of the surrounding pancreati-

tis, and small carcinomas may be missed altogether if mass samples are not taken for histology from many areas of the tumor and pancreatitis.

Microscopy

The growth pattern of pancreatic duct carcinomas can be classified as adenocarcinoma, giant cell carcinoma, adenosquamous carcinoma, mucinous ("colloid") carcinoma, mucinous cystadenocarcinoma or undifferentiated solid carcinoma. Of these,

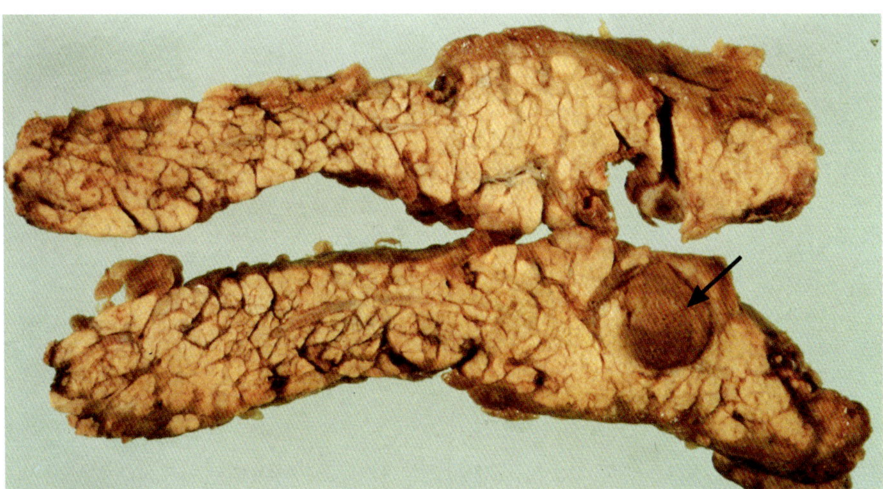

Fig. 3.**12 Macroscopy of an endocrine tumor** (→) surrounded by exocrine pancreatic tissue of normal appearance

only mucinous cystadenocarcinoma, and to a lesser extent colloid carcinoma are of clinical relevance, as they are reported to have a better prognosis in one- and five-year survival rates (Cubilla and Fitzgerald, 1987).

In our experience with a series of 71 pancreatic resection specimens following surgery for pancreatic head carcinoma (Lygidakis et al. 1986, 1988), a majority of the tumors originating from the pancreatic duct, distal common bile duct and ampulla had extensive perineural, local vasoinvasive and soft-tissue invasive growth (Table 3.**9**, Fig. 3.**14**). This was related neither to the tumor diameter nor to its site of origin, but coincided with a poor to moderate differentiation of the tumor cells. The area with pancreatitis surrounding the tumor appeared also to be related to the differentiation of the tumor cells and their potential for infiltrative growth. In fact, in many cases, scattered strands of invasively growing tumor cells could be demonstrated throughout the pancreatitis area. Therefore, the largest diameter of the tumor–pancreatitis area appears to constitute as good a measure for staging as the histologically measured diameter of the tumor alone, and correlates better with pre- and intraoperative measurements. Finally, and most importantly, the radicality of resection – estimated by the histological absence of invasive tumor growth in the surgical cleavage and resection margins – proved to correlate significantly with the tumor grading and to be independent from the tumor diameter.

Staging and Grading

The histopathologic classification and staging of ampullary carcinomas are summarized in Table 3.**10**, those of pancreatic carcinomas in Table 3.**11**. For common bile duct carcinomas in the region of the pancreas, classification and staging are summarized in the previous section of this chapter and in Table 3.**6**.

It should be noted that the criteria for tumor classification for each of these sites of origin are not the same. For instance, the tumor diameter is taken into consideration for pancreatic duct carcinomas, but not for ampullary or common bile duct tumors. The presence of perineural or local vasoinvasive growth is not taken into consideration in any of the classifications. When a common bile duct carcinoma of the terminal part of the common bile duct grows infiltratively, it almost invariably grows into the adjoining pancreatic tissue; even small bile duct carcinomas should therefore be staged as IV a under these circumstances, although they may be highly differentiated, without lymph node metastases and without vasoinvasive growth. Finally, the tumor diameter and the other parameters of the tumor stage appear not to be related, as shown in Table 3.**12**; cf. Table 3.**13**.

Grading of carcinomas from the various sites of origin in the pancreas has proved in our series to give a better insight into the possibilities of radical tumor resection and curative treatment of patients. It is the single most important prognosticator for

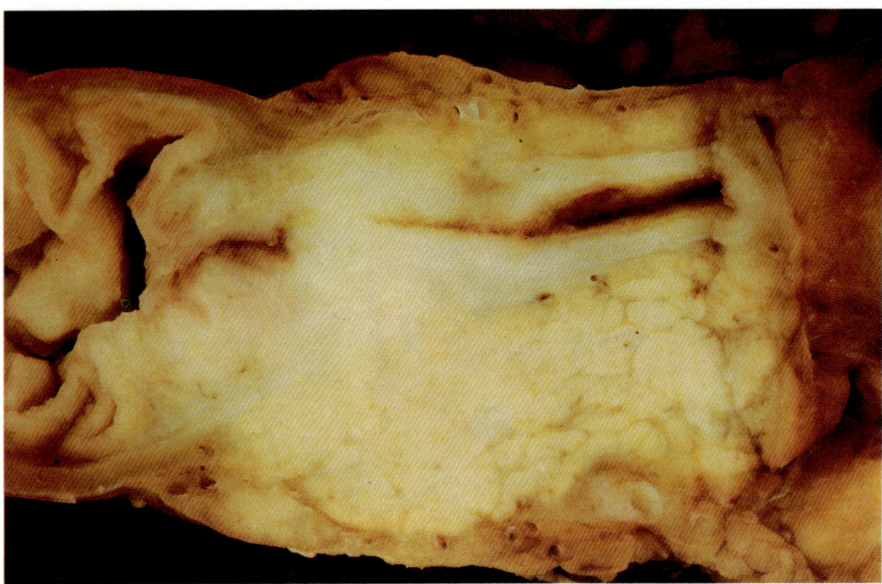

Fig. 3.**13 Macroscopy of the duodenum** (left side) and pancreatic head (to the right)

a Fibrosis and slight pancreatitis surround a pancreatic duct carcinoma

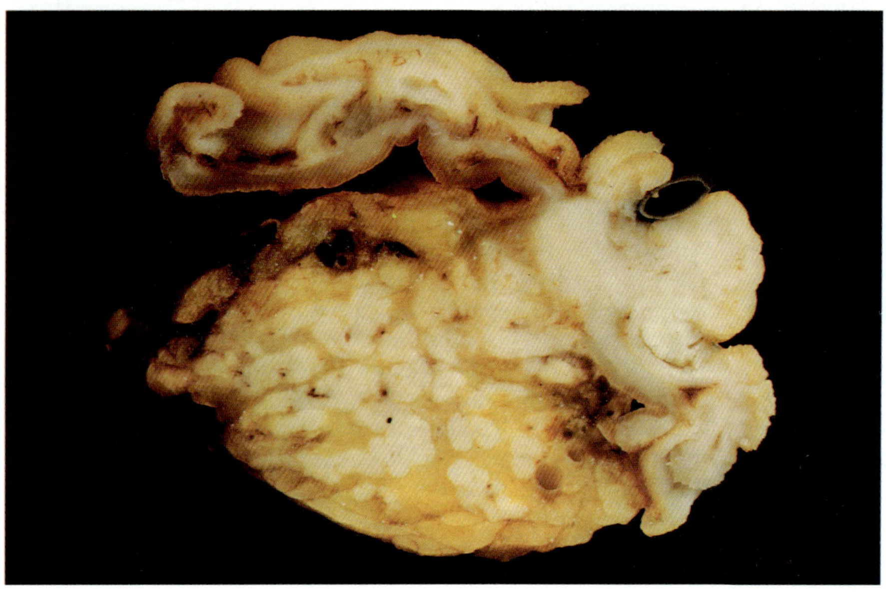

b Extensive pancreatitis is present, with an ampullary carcinoma

Table 3.**9   Histopathologic parameters in 71 surgical resection specimens with pancreatic head carcinoma**

Classification	To-tal	Grading 1	2	3/4	Tumor diameter in cm mean (range)	Invasive growth in: soft tissue	blood vessel	peri-neural	Regional lymph node metas-tasis	Surgical margins; invasive growth in: cleavage margins	blood vessels	pancre-atic ducts
Bile duct carcinoma	20	6	6	8	1.7 (0.8–2.5)	16	9	14	6	4	0	0
Pancreatic duct carcinoma	22	4	8	10	2.8 (1.2–4.5)	19	17	16	9	7	5	1
Ampulla: carcinoma	25	8	9	8	2.4 (1.0–6.5)	13	11	12	13	4	0	0
acinar cell tumor	1	0	1	0	0.5	0	0	0	1	0	0	0
carcinoid tumor	3	3	0	0	1.8 (1.5–2.0)	2	2	0	2	1	1	0
Total	71	21	24	26		50	39	42	31	16	6	1

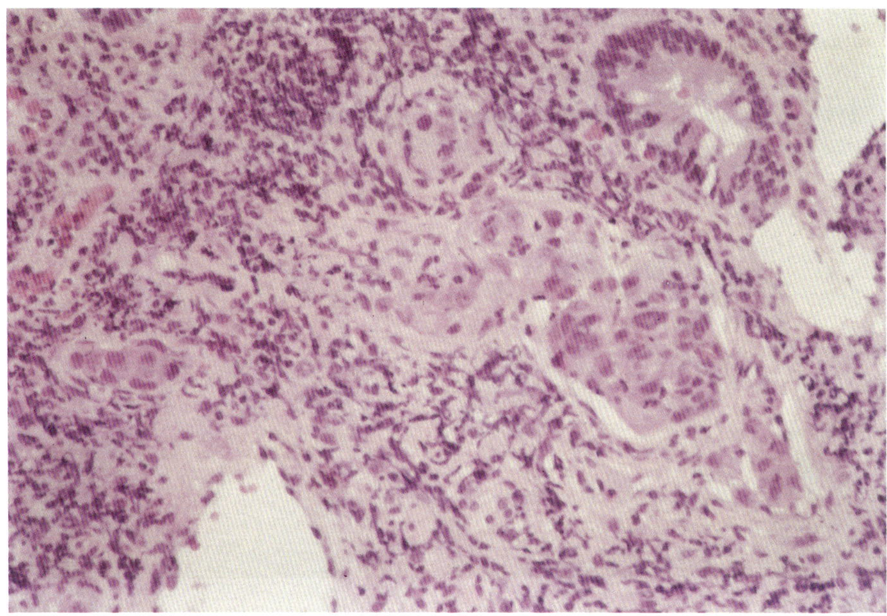

a

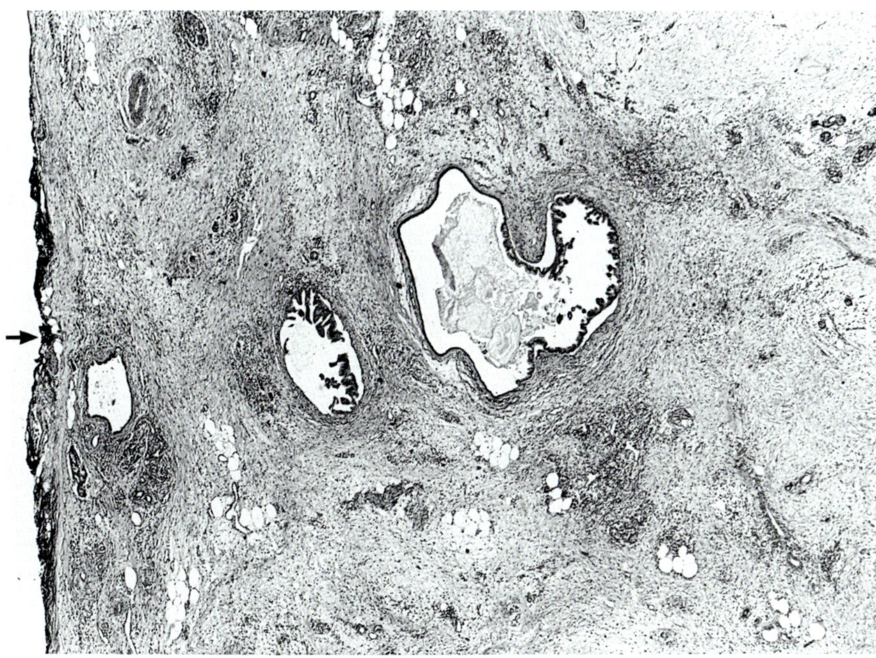

Fig. 3.**14 Infiltrative growth of pancreatic duct carcinoma**, **a** in the duodenal mucosa and **b** reaching the surgical cleavage planes ($\rightarrow$) marked with Indian ink. H & E, × 150 (**a**), × 50 (**b**)

b

long survival of patients (Lygidakis et al. 1988). In histopathology and exfoliative cytology, the grading has been based on cytological criteria such as the nucleus:cytoplasm ratio, nuclear hyperchromasia and polymorphy, and lack of cytoplasmic differentiation characteristics. In paraffin sections from surgical resection specimens, tumors were graded according to the areas with the poorest differentiation. A high differentiation (grade I) correlated in paraffin sections with a lack of vasoinvasive growth, with absent or inconspicuous perineural growth, with a less infiltrative growth pattern, with lack of desmoplastic tumor stroma and inflammation, and with near or complete absence of surrounding chronic pancreatitis. These highly differentiated carcinomas can become quite large, up to 4 cm or more in diameter, without growth into the surgical cleavage planes and consequently with a good prognosis for radical resection and curative treatment.

Table 3.10   TNM Classification and staging of ampullary carcinoma

pT Classification

pTX	Histologic examination of primary tumor not possible
pT0	Primary tumor not found
pTis	Carcinoma in situ
pT1	Tumor limited to the ampulla
pT2	Tumor infiltrating into the duodenal wall
pT3	Tumor infiltrating ≤ 2 cm into the pancreas
pT4	Tumor infiltrating > 2 cm into the pancreas or other adjoining organs

Stage grouping of ampullary carcinoma

Stage 0	pTis	N0	M0
Stage I	pT1	N0	M0
Stage II	pT2, 3	N0	M0
Stage III	pT1, 2, 3	N1	M0
Stage IV	pT4	any N	M0
	or any pT	any N	M1

Table 3.11   TNM Classification and staging of pancreatic carcinomas

pT Classification

pTX	Histologic examination of primary tumor not possible
pT0	Primary tumor not found
pT1	Tumor limited to the pancreas
pT1a	Largest diameter of the tumor ≤ 2 cm
pT1b	Largest diameter of the tumor > 2 cm
pT2	Tumor growth directly into duodenum, bile duct and/or peripancreatic tissues
pT3	Tumor growth directly into stomach, spleen, colon and/or large blood vessels

Stage grouping of pancreatic carcinomas

Stage I	pT1, 2	N0	M0
Stage II	pT3	N0	M0
Stage III	any pT	N1	M0
Stage IV	any pT	any N	M1

Table 3.12   Comparison of tumor diameter and tumor stage according to histopathological findings in 71 pancreatic resection specimens, demonstrating the lack of direct relation between these two parameters (Mantel Haenzel test, no relation)

Tumor stage:	Total no.	Diameter > 2 cm (n = 39)			Diameter < 2 cm (n = 32)		
		II	III	IVa	II	III	IVa
Bile duct carcinoma	20	3	6	3	1	4	3
Pancreatic duct carcinoma	22	1	6	4	2	6	3
Ampulla: carcinoma	25	3	8	3	3	5	3
Acinar cell tumor	1	0	0	1	0	0	0
Carcinoid tumor	3	0	1	0	0	0	2
Total	71	7	21	11	6	15	11

Table 3.13   Decision table for factors affecting prognosis

Grade	Vasoinvasion	Radicality	Prognosis

Pathologic Findings and Prognosis

Type of tumor: in cases of carcinoid tumor, mucinous cystadenocarcinoma, and to a lesser extent colloid carcinoma, the patient has a good prognosis for radical resection and long-term survival.

Grading: patients with grade I and II carcinoma have an excellent prognosis, irrespective of the site of origin and the tumor stage, provided that a radical resection can be performed and distant metastases are absent.

Staging: stage I to III carcinomas have an excellent prognosis irrespective of the site of origin, but relative to the grading, as high-grade carcinomas in stage III tend to have a worse prognosis. In stage IV carcinomas without distant metastases, ampullary and terminal bile duct tumors have a better prognosis for patient survival than pancreatic duct carcinomas (Lygidakis et al. 1988).

References

Aabakken L, Karesen R, Serck-Hanssen A, Osnes M. Transpapillary biopsies and brush cytology from the common bile duct. Endoscopy 1986; 18: 49–51.

Anthony PP. Primary carcinoma of the liver: a study of 282 cases in Uganda Africans. J Pathol 1973; 110: 37–48.

Anthony PP, James K. Pedunculated carcinoma: is it an entity? Histopathology 1987; 11: 403–414.

Anthony PP. Tumours and tumour-like lesions of the liver and biliary tract. In: Mac Sween RNM, et al., eds. Pathology of the liver. 2nd ed. Edinburgh: Churchill Livingstone, 1987: 574–645.

Brooks JR. Cancer of the pancreas. In: Brooks JR, ed. Surgery of the pancreas. Philadelphia: Saunders, 1983: 263–298.

Caballero T, Ameiros J, Lopez-Caballero J, Gomez-Morales M, Nogales F. Fibrolamellar hepatocellular carcinoma: an immunohistological and ultrastructural study. Histopathology 1985; 9: 445–456.

Classen M, Phillip J. Endoscopic retrograde choledochopancreatography. In: Blumgart LH, ed. Surgery of the liver and biliary tract; vol 1. Edinburgh: Churchill Livingstone, 1988: 257–276.

Cubilla AL, Fitzgerald PJ. Morphological lesions associated with human primary invasive non-endocrine pancreas cancer. Cancer Res 1976; 36: 2690–2696.

Cubilla AL, Fitzgerald PJ. Tumors of the exocrine pancreas. Washington: AFIP, 1984.

Cubilla AL, Fitzgerald PJ. Pathology of cancer of the exocrine pancreas. In: Howard JM, et al., eds. Surgical diseases of the pancreas. Philadelphia: Lea and Febiger, 1987: 627–640.

Fontham E, Correa P, Cohn I Jr. Epidemiology of cancer of the pancreas. In: Howard JM, et al., eds. Surgical diseases of the pancreas. Philadelphia: Lea and Febiger, 1987: 613–626.

Gibson JB, Sobin LH. Histological typing of tumours of the liver, biliary tract and pancreas. International histological classification of tumours, No 20. Geneva: WHO, 1978.

Gmelin E, Weiss HD. Tumours in the region of the papilla of Vater. Eur J Radiol 1981; 1: 301–306.

Goudswaard WB, Houthoff HJ, Koudstaal J, Zwierstra RP. Nesidioblastosis and endocrine hyperplasia of the pancreas: a secondary phenomenon. Hum Pathol 1986; 17: 46–53.

Hall-Craggs MA, Lees WR. Fine-needle aspiration biopsy: pancreatic and biliary tumors. AJR 1986; 147: 399–403.

Hermanek P, Sobin LH, eds. TNM Classification of Malignant Tumours. 4th ed. Geneva: UICC, 1987.

Houthoff HJ, Lygidakis NJ, Schipper MEI, van der Heyde MN. Surgical resection of carcinomas of the biliary tree: a comparison of staging, grading, surgical radicality and patient follow-up. 2nd World Congr Hepato-Pancreato Biliary Surgery. Neth J Surg 1988, Abstract FP 053.

Houthoff HJ, Huibregtse K, Lygidakis N, Ramsoukh T. Brush cytology of bile and pancreatic duct strictures. A new and reliable method for tumor diagnosis and grading. 2nd World Congr Hepato-Pancreato Biliary Surgery. Neth J Surg 1988, Abstract FP 244.

Klatskin G. Adenocarcinoma of the hepatic duct at its bifurcation within the porta hepatis. Am J Med 1965; 38: 241–256.

Leese T, Neoptolemos JP, West KP, Talbot IC, Carr-Locke DL. Tumours and pseudotumours of the region of the ampulla of Vater: an endoscopic, clinical and pathological study. Gut 1986; 27: 1186–1192.

Legg MA. Pathology of the pancreas. In: Brooks JR, ed. Surgery of the pancreas. Philadelphia: Saunders, 1983: 41–77.

Lygidakis NJ, Brummelkamp WH, Tytgat GH, et al. Periampullary and pancreatic head carcinoma: facts and factors influencing mortality, survival, and quality of postoperative life. Am J Gastroenterol 1986; 81: 968–974.

Lygidakis NJ, van der Heyde MN, Houthoff HJ, et al. Resectional surgical procedures for carcinoma of the head of the pancreas. Surg Gynecol Obstet 1988; 168: 157–165.

Nagai H, Kuroda A, Morioka Y. Lymphatic and local spread of T1 and T2 pancreatic cancer. Ann Surg 1986; 204: 65–71.

Nakashima T, Okuda K, Kijoro M et al. Pathology of hepatocellular carcinoma in Japan: 232 consecutive cases autopsied in ten years. Cancer 1983; 51: 863–877.

Okuda K, Obata H, Nakajima Y, Ohtsuki T, Okazaki N, Ohnishi K. Prognosis of primary hepatocellular carcinoma. Hepatology 1984; 4: 3S–6S.

Rashleigh-Belcher HJC, Russell RCG, Lees WR. Cutaneous seeding of pancreatic carcinoma by fine-needle aspiration biopsy. Br J Radiol 1986, 59: 183–185.

Schwerk WB, Durr H-K, Schmitz-Moormann P. Ultrasound guided fine-needle biopsies in pancreatic and hepatic neoplasms. Gastrointest Radiol 1983; 8: 219–225.

Short WF, Nedwick A, Levy HA, Howard JM. Biliary cystadenoma. Arch Surg 1975; 102: 78–80.

Sommers SC, Murphy SA, Warren S. Pancreatic duct hyperplasia and cancer. Gastroenterology 1954; 27: 629–635.

Soreide O. Percutaneous aspiration cytology for biliary obstruction and liver masses. In: Blumgart LH, ed. Surgery of the liver and biliary tract; vol 1. Edinburgh: Churchill Livingstone, 1988: 327–336.

Tryka AF, Brooks JR. Histopathology in the evaluation of total pancreatectomy for ductal carcinoma. Ann Surg 1979; 190: 373–382.

Verbeek PCM, Van der Heyde MN, Lygidakis NJ, et al. Clinical significance of peroperative bile cytology on patients with Klatskin tumors. 2nd World Congr Hepato-Pancreato Biliary Surgery. Neth J Surg 1988; Abstract FP 042.

Weinbren K. Tumours of the bile duct-pathological aspects. In: Blumgart LH, ed. Surgery of the liver and biliary tract; vol 2. Edinburgh: Churchill Livingstone, 1988 a: 793–806.

Weinbren K. Tumours of the liver-pathological aspects. In: Blumgart LH, ed. Surgery of the liver and biliary tract; vol 2. Edinburgh: Churchill Livingstone, 1988 b: 1093–1114.

4 Diagnostics in Hepatobiliary and Pancreatic Malignancies

Edited by J. W. A. J. Reeders

4.1 Imaging in Hepatobiliary and Pancreatic Malignancies: an Introduction

D. J. van Leeuwen, J. W. A. J. Reeders

General Introduction

Explorative laparotomy for suspected diseases of the liver, biliary tree or pancreas followed by immediate closure of the abdomen or a palliative bypass procedure has become a rare procedure since advanced imaging techniques have become widely available in the developed world. Table 4.1.1 summarizes the most important available imaging techniques; in the following chapters, each of them will be covered in detail. The variety of techniques illustrates the fact that no single imaging technique is obviously the best or sufficient. Techniques are often complementary to each other.

Human, medical and economic reasons urge the clinician to apply techniques critically. The role of the radiologist and others (the "imagers") is a major one, increasing in importance due to the fact that their role is no longer limited to imaging, since interventional options have developed. It should be realized that recommendations with respect to the best approach to a certain problem are closely related to local expertise, facilities and enthusiasm. These aspects are reflected in the literature. A preference for one approach to a particular problem seems not infrequently to be related to a lack of expertise with another technique.

Table 4.1.1 Major imaging techniques for assessment of hepatobiliary and pancreatic malignancies

Ultrasonography (US)	*Computed Tomography (CT)*
– External	(+/−) Oral or intravenous
– Peroperative	enhancement
– Endoscopic	(+/−) Arteriography
– Doppler	(+/−) Cholangiography
Cholangiography	(+/−) Lipidiol
Pancreaticography	
– Percutaneous (PTC)	*Angiography*
– Endoscopic (ERCP)	– (Selective) arteriography
– Intravenous	(+ venous phase!)
cholangiography	– Venography
	(+/− pressure)
	Scintigraphy
	– Technetium
	– HIDA
	– Labeled erythrocytes
	MRI
	(Magnetic Resonance
	Imaging)

(X-chest, abdominal film, X-barium meal/enteroclysis)

The Approach to Obstructive Jaundice in Potential Malignancies

The present approach to malignant obstructive jaundice can be used to illustrate the present state of the art and the rapid developments which have taken place in relation to this important clinical problem. There is no doubt that ultrasonography (US), "the modern stethoscope of the abdomen", should be the investigation of choice in patients presenting with jaundice. Although the quality of

US examination is strongly dependent on the investigator's expertise, improvements in technical equipment may bring improved results to such an extent that even less experienced investigators can obtain reliable results (Soiva et al. 1986).

In the 1970s, the diagnosis of obstructive jaundice as shown by US was still used to determine whether one should abstain from further treatment or refer the patient to the surgeon for confirmation of irresectability by means of an explorative laparotomy and bypass. In the 1980s, the role of US is to provide the hepatobiliary and pancreatic team (gastroenterologist, hepatologist, surgeon and radiologist) with the information they need to discuss who will proceed with further diagnostic and therapeutic steps. With regard to the question of whether malignancy might be the cause, and whether this should influence the further work-up of the patient, two major questions have to be addressed which may provide clues to diagnosis.

1. What is the likely diagnosis? Table 4.1.**2** summarizes the major points which may provide clues to the diagnosis.

Table 4.1.2   Major questions in obstructive jaundice

- known biliary stones?
- previous (complicated) biliary tract surgery?
- known malignancy elsewhere?
- inflammatory bowel disease?
- traveller?
  (chronic liver disease?)
  (alcohol abuse?)
  (drugs?)

Gallstones are a major cause of obstructive jaundice. The sensitivity and specificity of US exceeds 95 % for concrements in the gallbladder. However, stones in the common bile duct are only shown with a 22–55 % specificity and sensitivity (Einstein et al. 1984, Cronan 1986, Carr-Locke 1986). In addition to dilation of the biliary tree (if the obstruction is present for some time), US may suggest other diagnoses, such as focal liver, or pancreatic lesion and diffuse enlargements of the pancreas, or pancreatic duct dilation. At any level, obstructing tumors may be shown.

2. What are the characteristics of the patient and what consequences should follow for diagnosis and treatment?

Patients who belong to the older age group (> 75 years), who are severely ill, or suffer from widespread metastatic carcinoma, should preferably have straightforward endoscopic drainage of the biliary tract rather than further diagnostic investigations. This is due to the fact that any operation carries considerable risk per se with regard to morbidity and mortality, and surgical options may be very limited. The estimated mortality of a cholecystectomy is 0.5 %, but this increases to 4.5 % if additional common bile duct exploration is performed. This was shown in a prospective study in 1072 patients who underwent these procedures in centers with an interest in hepato-biliary disease (DenBesten and Berci 1986). Even more striking were the findings that retained stones were found in 4.5 % of the patients and the fact that in 18.5 % of the patients, a bile duct exploration did not reveal any stones. In this study the mortality and morbidity were not corrected for age, but cardiovascular problems are responsible for an estimated mortality risk exceeding 10 % in older patients. Increase in age is accompanied with the likelihood that further diagnoses are possible, as in patients with common bile duct stones and a benign or malignant biliary tract obstruction. When benign disease is associated with considerable morbidity and mortality, this is even more the case for malignant disease. The treatment of choice in our hospital is diagnostic and therapeutic endoscopic retrograde cholangiopancreatography (ERCP), which may provide cure (stone extraction) or palliation (stent).

In younger patients (biological age < 75 years), patients with good general condition and unremarkable previous medical history, in whom US suggests a limited process in the liver, liver hilum or around the distal common bile duct without evidence of metastasis elsewhere, a balance should be made with respect to the pros and cons of (immediate) biliary tract drainage. Percutaneous transhepatic cholangiography (PTC) and endoscopic retrograde cholangiopancreaticography (ERCP) are excellent techniques to assess obstructive jaundice. However, they may be life-saving modalities (stone extraction, biliary stenting) as well as life-threatening procedures when the investigator has not prepared the patient in a proper way (prophylactic antibiotic therapy if required), when he or she is not trained in therapeutic techniques (stone extraction, biliary stenting), or unexpected findings exclude the possibility of immediate biliary tract drainage. The major risk is introducing bacterial contamination of the biliary tract followed by cholangitis or a septicemia or sepsis. PTC has been increasingly abandoned due to its high complication rate. However, PTC will retain a place in the coming years 1) if endoscopic drainage is impossible and immediate drainage is required, or surgical drains are contra-indicated; 2) to introduce a guide wire which will help to insert an endoscopic stent (rendezvous procedure); and 3) as a way of applying local radiotherapy.

The need for any type of biliary drainage is related to the available surgical options. These are

Table 4.1.3 Surgical options

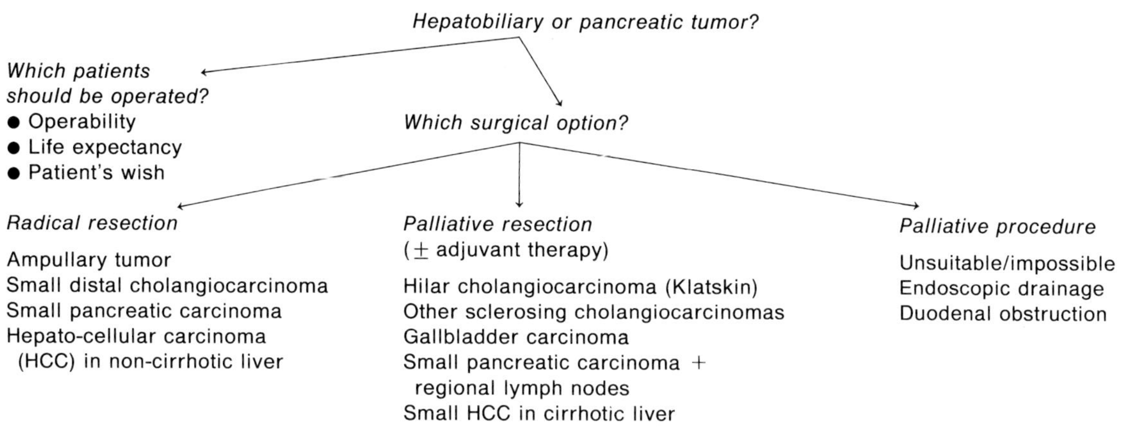

extensively discussed elsewhere in this book, and are summarized in Table 4.1.3. Surgical options include an attempt to perform a radical curative resection, an intended maximum palliative resection with the aim of improving the result by adjuvant radio- and chemotherapy, or a simple palliative procedure. The radiologist has an important task with regard to advising further useful imaging techniques and – very important! – the consecutive order in which they should preferably be carried out.

An example of a diagnostic work-up schedule for presumed malignant jaundice in an operable patient to assess resectability is given in Table 4.1.4.

The insertion of an endoprosthesis is a very serious hindrance to US and CT scan imaging. The endoprosthesis often causes major artefacts on the CT scan, and both US and CT scan will be much less likely to be able to provide the exact obstruction level after drainage. Intrahepatic gas after endoscopic drainage will hinder discrimination of intrahepatic lesions. If a CT scan is performed after a US observation of a possible distal common bile duct obstruction, optimal imaging and assessment of tumor invasion of the duodenum will be obtained if oral contrast is available in the proximal part of the small bowel. This again provides guidance on how imaging should be performed. This is one reason why, if the need is felt for both techniques, we postpone biliary tract drainage by means of an endoprosthesis until these investigations have been performed. Major resectional therapy can be offered to patients now that subtotal pancreatectomy can be performed with a mortality of less then 10%. However, US is still of major importance here: focal liver lesions must be punctured to exclude liver secondaries, which at present are a contra-indication for major resections. If palliative surgery is considered for hilar tumors

(Klatskin tumor or other hilar processes), there is a further role for US (preoperatively and intraoperatively) in predicting whether partial liver resection is feasible. Flow patterns (Doppler technique) may become increasingly relevant.

Table 4.1.4 Diagnostic work-up (1-week program) for assessing patients with presumed malignant distal common bile duct obstruction

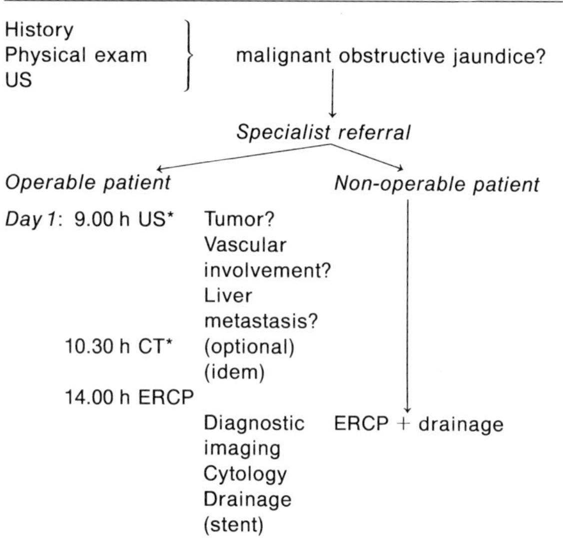

Day 2: Optional (2 days later, to avoid IV, contrast overload)
   11.00 h Endo-ultrasonography
   15.00 h Selective arteriography

Day 3: Discuss findings with hepatobiliary team and pancreatic team (gastroenterologist, hepatologist, surgeon and radiologist)

* Should precede ERCP to avoid negative interference with imaging of the endoprosthesis

Further General Considerations

A few general points with regard to the imaging of the hepatobiliary and pancreatic system should be mentioned. Various techniques (US, CT, ERCP, PTC) are very suitable in attempting to obtain cytological or histological specimens by means of brush or biopsy. It should be stressed, however, that it may be extremely difficult to obtain representative material. Even the surgeon can be faced with tremendous problems when trying to confirm malignant disease. Preoperative findings, such as the typical double duct lesion in the older age group (highly indicative of pancreas head carcinoma) should be a major guide to the surgical approach.

The importance of *quantification* of the findings should be stressed. Techniques currently available as will be outlined in the following chapters, enable investigators to obtain data with a high level of accuracy. Exact measurement allows for precise communication between various specialists. It provides the possibility of comparing patients in study groups and measuring the therapeutic response. Tumor extent may be the prognostic indicator in prospective studies. Further improvements in imaging techniques may increasingly enable US to distinguish between various components of the tumor process, such as carcinoma per se and surrounding inflammatory changes. For the investigator it may be very important and satisfying to correlate his or her own preoperative findings to those in the resected specimen.

The Future of Imaging

It is anticipated that nearly all of the currently available techniques will show further improvements in the future. These improvements include all kinds of sophisticated instruments, such as the tiny baby-endoscope used together with the large endoscope to explore the biliary tree. The resolving power of various techniques will increasingly improve, and monoclonal antibodies will be applied both for detection and classification of malignant disease as well as for specific local therapy. As mentioned in the introduction, the variety of techniques available puts a heavy responsibility on doctors' shoulders to use them selectively.

The aim should be to define the simplest but most appropriate method of diagnostic work-up for the individual patient. This requires limited use of sophisticated techniques (offered in a highly competitive market with the suggestion that they are indispensable) until the place for "improvements" has been clearly defined in prospective studies. Improvements cannot be defined by the extreme levels of accuracy resulting from optimal but expensive resolving power. For the patient's benefit, the merits of the various techniques, which will be discussed in detail below, should be assessed by the individual doctor and his local team. Reports by advocates of new techniques should be accompanied by reports indicating which techniques have become obsolete.

It is hoped that the following chapters will be read fruitfully against the background just mentioned.

References

Carr-Locke DL. In: Bateson MC, ed. Gallstone disease and its management. Lancaster: Publisher 1986: chapter 4.

Cronan JJ. U.S. Diagnosis of choledocholithiasis: a reappraisal. Radiology 1986; 161: 133–144.

DenBesten L, Berci G. The current status of biliary tract surgery: an international study of 1072 consecutive patients. World J Surg 1986; 10: 116–122.

Einstein DM, Lapin SA, Ralls PW, Halls JM. The intensity of sonography in the detection of choledocholithiasis. AJR 1984; 142: 725–728.

Soiva M, Haveri M, Taavitsainen M, Suramo I. The value of routine sonography in clinically suspected acute cholecystitis. Scand J Gastroenterol 1986; 21: 70–74.

4.2 Ultrasonography in Hepatobiliary and Pancreatic Malignancies

G. Rosenbusch, N.J. Smits, J.W.A.J. Reeders

General

Ultrasound (US) has an important place in radio-diagnostic procedures in diseases of the liver, biliary tract and pancreas. Accuracy of US has increased with technical development, i.e. higher resolution, and real-time scanning, and with growing experience among sonographers. Good anatomical knowledge is necessary for performing and interpreting the examinations.

Accuracy of US is quite good in comparison with that of other imaging procedures. As US is also cheaper than other procedures, generally available and non-invasive, it is regarded as the primary imaging method in malignancies of the liver, biliary tract and pancreas (Friedman 1987).

The tasks of US in hepatobiliary and pancreatic malignancies are:

- diagnosis/exclusion of malignancies
- localization (especially before operations)
- characterization of lesions
- diagnosis/exclusion of metastatic spread
- recognition of complications as ascites, thrombosis, abscesses
- control during therapy with cystostatics or radiation

In hepatobiliary and pancreatic malignancies the following kinds of US examination are performed:
- transcutaneous or percutaneous: imaging; Doppler; interventional (puncture under US guidance);
- via endoscope (= echo-endoscopy, endo-ultra-sonography);
- intraoperative: imaging; interventional (US guided biopsy).

For percutaneous examination, real-time scanners with 3.5 or 5 MHz transducers should be used. Sector scanners are usually better for the examination of the upper abdomen than linear arrays.

For Doppler examination of the abdominal viscera, duplex scanning is necessary, which is a combination of pulsed Doppler and image. Doppler studies are helpful in differentiating lesions and demonstrating changes in blood flow. It is possible to exclude venous thrombosis or arterial stenosis or occlusion, to study the direction of the blood flow, to identify hemodynamic disturbances, to document physiologic change from quantitative shifts in vascular impedance, to characterize tissues by their specific perfusion, and to measure absolute bloodflow (Taylor 1987a).

US is increasingly used in interventional procedures, e.g. US guided biopsy, and especially to get material for cytologic examination or for therapy in drainage procedures (Hillman et al. 1979, La Berge et al. 1984, McGahan 1987, Rowley and Cooperberg 1987). Compared with computed tomography (CT), US-guided biopsy is relatively inexpensive, as US apparatus is mobile and the biopsy can be performed anywhere in the hospital. With modern real-time scanners, the needle tip can be observed directly. Accuracy of the biopsy has therefore increased. Before starting, the procedure must be explained to the patient, and he must give his consent to it. Coagulation studies should be obtained. The patient should fast for 4–6 hours beforehand, especially if the stomach has to be transgressed. Premedication is usually not necessary, but diazepam can be indicated in some patients. When the puncture site is selected, the skin of the patient is prepared and anesthetized. The biopsy system is attached to the transducer, which is covered with a sterile glove. A 22 or 23 gauge needle is passed through the guide attachment and skin into the lesion. The needle tip can be observed sonographically. When the needle is in the correct position, suction is applied with a syringe (10–20 ml) under negative pressure. The needle is sometimes moved up and down slightly in different directions. The negative pressure is released and the needle removed. The material in the puncture needle is sent to the pathologist. Complications are rare when using fine-gauge needles. The mortality rate is reported to be 0.008% (Rowley and Cooperberg 1987).

Endoultrasonography is a very promising diagnostic modality, which is useful in staging esophageal tumors as well as in diagnosing pathology of the distal biliary tree and of the pancreas (see Chapter 4.3).

For intraoperative US, specially designed transducers, usually 5 or 7 MHz, are used. The transducer has to be sterilized or covered with a sterile glove. It is possible to examine the liver, biliary tree and pancreas intraoperatively. Small tumors are detected more easily with this method than percutaneously. Intraoperative US can also be used for guided biopsy (Machi et al. 1987).

Liver

Sonographic screening for metastatic disease of the liver in extrahepatic primary tumors is frequently done preoperatively or in the follow-up (Bernar-

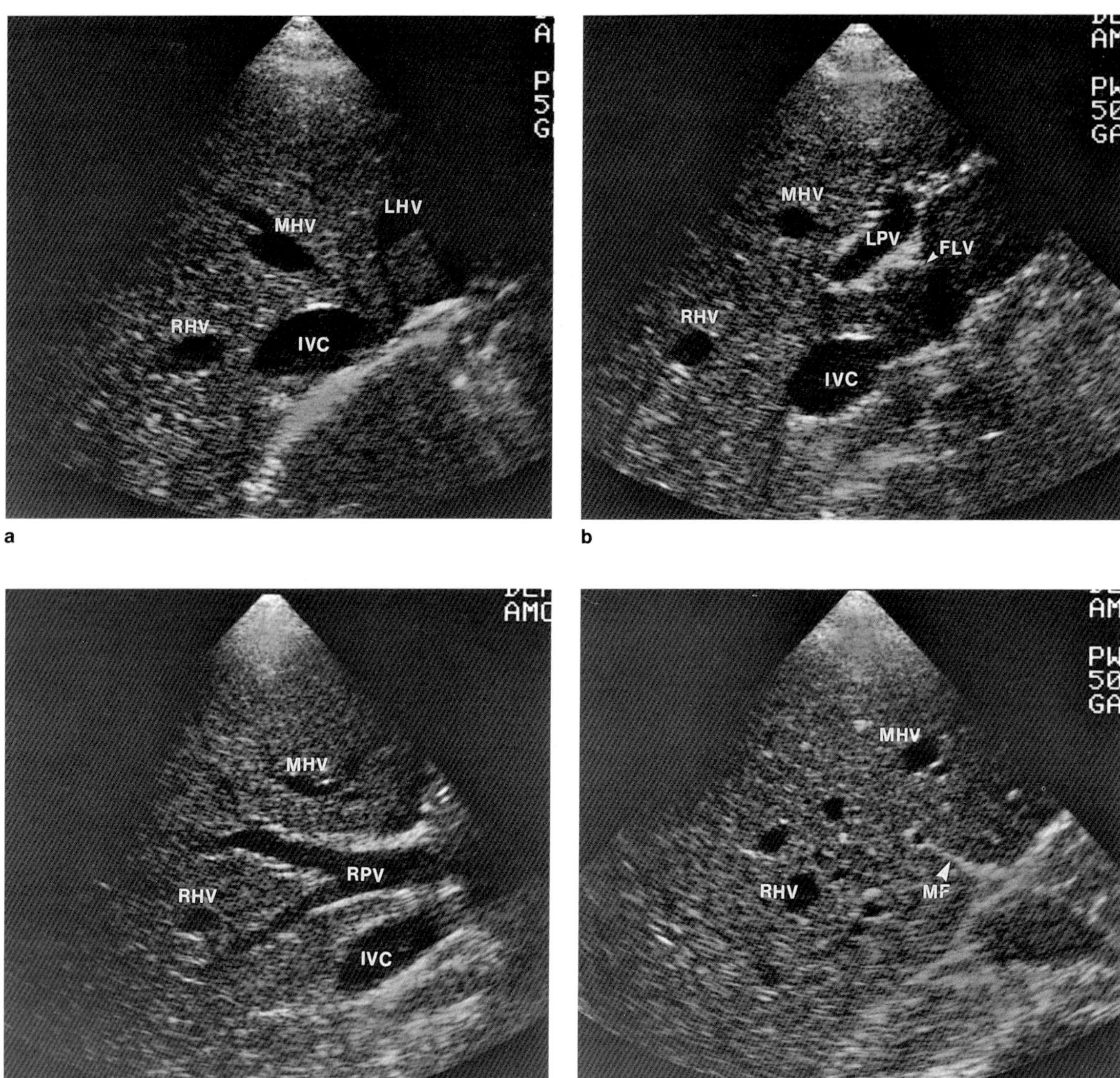

Fig. 4.2.1   Axial sonograms through the liver at four levels from cranial to caudal showing the segmental anatomy

a   At the level of the hepatic veins converging to the inferior vena cava. The hepatic veins are the boundaries of hepatic segments. RHV = right hepatic vein, MHV = middle hepatic vein, LHV = left hepatic vein, IVC = inferior vena cava

b   At the level of proximal part of left portal vein (LPV), which separates the medial segment from the lateral segment of the left lobe. The fissura for the ligamentum venosum (FLV) separates the lobus caudatum from the lateral segment of left lobe. The middle hepatic vein (MHV) and right hepatic vein (RHV) are also visible, separating respectively the medial segment of the left lobe from the anterior segment of the right lobe, and the anterior segment of the right lobe from the posterior segment of the right lobe

c   At the level of the bifurcation of the right portal vein (RPV). The middle hepatic vein (MHV) and right hepatic vein (RHV) are the boundaries of the liver segments (see above). IVC = inferior vena cava

d   At the most caudal level, the major fissure (MF) represents the boundary between the right and left lobes

dino and Green 1979, Gunvén et al. 1983, Scheible et al. 1977), as the liver is a frequent site of metastases. Primary malignant tumors of the liver are rare in Western countries.

Technical Aspects. The liver should be examined with the patient in a supine and right anterior oblique position during inspiration. Longitudinal and transverse subcostal scans as well as intercostal scans are made. The reliability of the examination decreases with obesity, high-standing liver and scars. In steatosis, the dorsal part of the liver is difficult to examine due to poor sound penetration. With real-time US "blind spots" can be reduced (the lateral part of the left lobe and the cranioventral part of the right lobe).

Anatomical Considerations in Localising Lesions. Sonography currently plays an important role in the preoperative determination of the resectability of hepatic neoplasms because of its ability to demonstrate hepatic vascular (and thus segmental) anatomy, as well as hepatic neoplasms, in a noninvasive manner (Mukai et al. 1987a, 1987b, Sexton and Zeeman 1983, Valleix et al. 1987). The boundaries of the hepatic segments are defined by the hepatic veins. Transaxial scans must be performed by lines drawn from the inferior vena cava through each hepatic vein. At lower levels of the liver, structures such as the ligamentum venosum, ligamentum teres, major fissure and gallbladder have to be defined in order to estimate the segmental boundaries (Fig. 4.2.1).

Primary Malignancies

Primary malignant hepatic tumors are almost always epithelial in origin. Of these, hepatocellular carcinoma (HCC) represents approximately 80 %. The remainder are either cholangiocarcinoma or of mixed pattern.

Hepatocellular carcinoma (HCC) is one of the most common malignancies, particularly in Southeast Asia and in Subsaharan Africa. The prognosis is very poor, with a mean survival of only a few months. Even in advanced HCCs, some patients still have normal alphafetoprotein (AFP) levels. Real-time US is more sensitive than AFP assay in the early detection of HCC, and high-risk subjects should undergo US screening at regular intervals (Sheu et al. 1985).

Ultrasonographic Findings. According to the gross pathological extent and the vascular pattern, three main types can be distinguished (Kamin et al. 1979):

– nodular type: discrete solitary or multiple lesions.
– diffuse type: hepatomegaly with diffuse distortion of the normal internal architecture. Multiple areas of increased echogenicity can be recognized throughout the distorted parenchyma of the liver, but no distinct masses can be identified.

– mixed pattern: this consists of a combination of the nodular and diffuse types. It consists of a large, densely echogenic mass associated with diffuse hepatic parenchymal disease involving the remaining liver.

Correlation between the sonographic pattern and the histomorphology (Sheu et al. 1984, 1985a, Tanaka et al. 1983). Concerning the nodular type, two main growth patterns exist sonographically. The first pattern occurs in most small HCCs, where the tumor is initially hypoechoic. Histologic examination reveals a pure cell mass without necrosis (Tanaka et al. 1983). When growing, the tumor becomes progressively more echogenic and non-homogeneous, due to non-liquefied tumor necrosis (Wooten et al. 1978), interstitial fibrosis and hemorrhage. Most of these tumors become hyperechoic when they reach a large size (Fig. 4.2.2). The second, less common, pattern is homogeneous and diffusely hyperechoic, probably due to "inherent" fatty change or dilated sinusoids; this pattern is present from the beginning, and does not change when the tumor grows. Nevertheless, it can usually be identified by a thin peripheral hypoechoic halo, which corresponds to the pseudocapsule (bull's eye appearance). Although there is some correlation between the sonographic pattern and the histomorphology, the nature of a tumor cannot be determined from the echographic features alone. US-guided needle biopsy is therefore required for conclusive diagnosis (Spamer et al. 1986, Wernecke et al. 1984, Wernecke and Peters 1985).

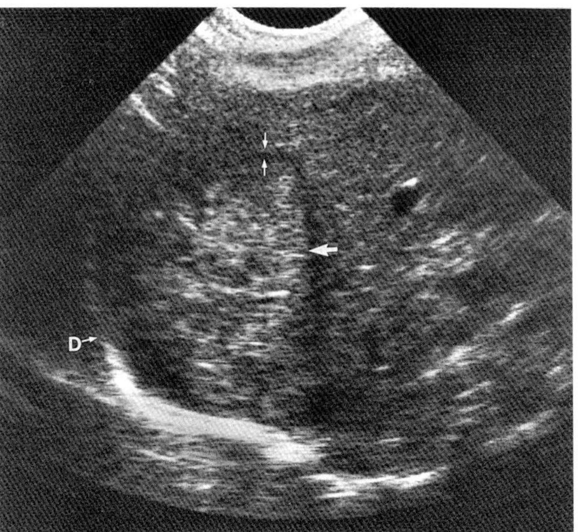

Fig. 4.2.2 Large hepatocellular carcinoma, nodular type. Sagittal sonogram (arrow) shows a large non-homogeneous hyperechoic mass 8 cm in diameter in the cranial part of the right lobe beneath the diaphragm (D). The thin peripheral hypoechoic halo (small arrows) corresponds to the pseudocapsula

Secondary signs found in HCC are hepatomegaly, ascites and lymphadenopathy. For pre-operative assessment, prognosis and possibly differential diagnosis, it is important to assess tumor extension to intrahepatic inferior vena cava, hepatic veins and portal vein branches. Sonography is very useful in depicting veins which are obscure or non-opaque in angiography. Angiography, on the other hand, may demonstrate arteriovenous shunting not noticed in sonography (Subramauyam et al. 1984).

Pulsed Doppler US is helpful in differentiating hepatocellular carcinoma from other lesions (Taylor et al. 1987). If a Doppler shift of 5 KHz or above is present, HCC is highly likely. Correlation with angiographic findings suggests that these high-velocity signals are associated with large pressure gradients due to arteriovenous shunting. In contrast, hemangioma shows either no detectable signal or a very low shift. Some metastases do not give a Doppler shift, while others give a shift of no more than 4 KHz (Taylor et al. 1987a, b). The Doppler examination has to be performed around the periphery of the lesions, i. e. on the growing edges of tumors.

Sensitivity of US in Comparison with Other Methods. Takashima et al. (1982) compared the sensitivity of various imaging methods in small HCCs. Sensitivity was 39% with RN, 50% with US, 56% with CT and 94% with angiography, including infusion hepatic angiography (IHA). IHA was essential for diagnosis of lesions of less than 2 cm. Lesions larger than 3 cm could be detected by all of these methods. In contrast, Sheu et al. (1984) found a sensitivity with US of 93.9%, with CT 84.3%, angiography 75.7% and RN 12.1%. They concluded that US was the most sensitive method for lesions of less than 2 cm. In patients with histologically proved cirrhosis and clinical suspicion of neoplastic degeneration, US prospectively diagnosed HCC in 90% (Cottone et al. 1983).

Recently, new imaging methods have been developed, such as intraoperative ultrasound (Machi et al. 1987) and computed tomography after lipiodol (iodized oil) infusion. For accurate detection of metastatic nodules of HCC, Hayashi et al. (1987) found the following results:

	Sensitivity	Specificity
Infusion hepatic angiography (IHA)	61%	100%
Computed tomography after lipiodol infusion (CT)	67%	100%
Intraoperative ultrasound (US)	94%	92%

Intraoperative US demonstrated nodules in avascular and hypovascular HCCs which both IHA and CT failed to demonstrate. The number of detected nodules with US was less than with CT, so that the resolution of intraoperative US might not be as high as that of CT. In severe liver cirrhosis, intraoperative US cannot always differentiate between small malignant nodules and regenerating nodules. In these cases, intraoperative US-guided needle biopsy is necessary (Hayashi et al. 1987).

Assessment of resectability in US compared with CT. Hepatic distribution plays a major role in determining the resectability of HCC (La Berge et al. 1984). Although both CT and US can detect HCC (96%), CT shows more extensive hepatic parenchymal involvement in 27–38% (La Berge et al. 1984, Teefey et al. 1986). In contrast, vascular invasion was seen more frequently with ultrasound (37%) than with CT (La Berge et al. 1984).

Differential Diagnosis. Metastatic disease, lymphoma, cirrhosis, hemangioma and steatosis must be mentioned in the differential diagnosis (Figs. 4.2.3, 4.2.4). As the US pattern of HCC is not specific, US-guided needle biopsy is required for definite diagnosis (Mayes and Bernardino 1981, Wernecke and Peters 1985).

Lymphoma. The liver is involved in Hodgkin's and non-Hodgkin's diseases, depending on the stage. In autopsy studies of lymphoma patients, the liver is involved in more than 50%, in Hodgkin's disease somewhat higher than in non-Hodgkin's disease. However, lesions can be detected sonographically

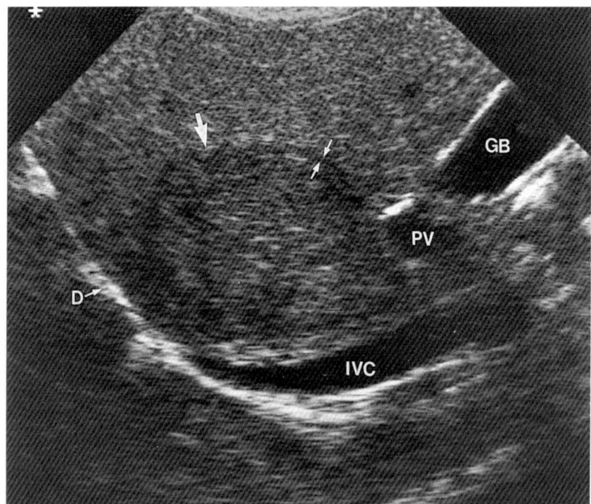

Fig. 4.2.**3 Hemangioma of the liver.** Sagittal sonogram reveals a sharply demarcated, slightly hypoechoic homogeneous lesion (large arrow) ventral of the inferior vena cava (IVC). By way of exception, this benign tumor shows a halo-like appearance along a part of its margin (small arrows). PV = portal vein, GB = gallbladder, D = diaphragm

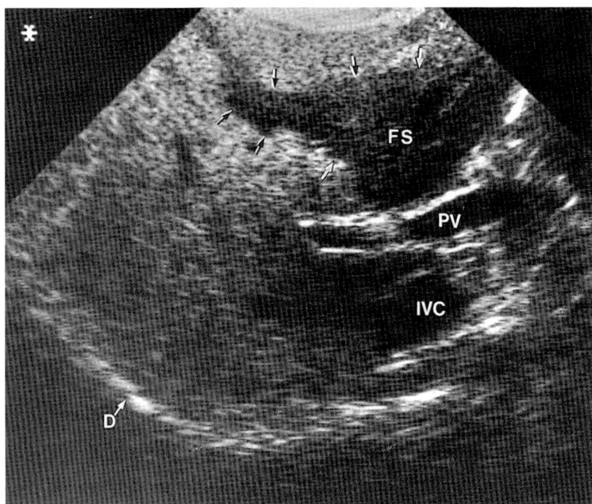

Fig. 4.2.**4** **Focal steatosis of the liver.** Transverse sonogram. The area of focal sparing (FS) within the quadrate lobe gives the impression of a tumor. Distinct from a real tumor, however, the demarcation between the hyperechoic steatotic liver tissue of the right lobe is sharp and more or less rectilinear (arrow). PV = portal vein, IVC = inferior vena cava, D = diaphragm

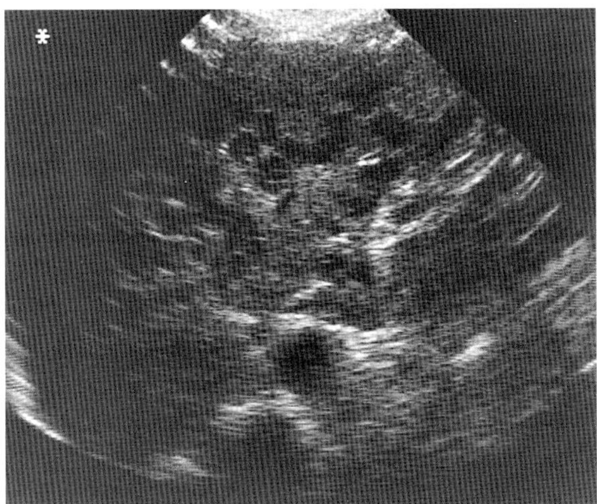

Fig. 4.2.**5** **Non-Hodgkin lymphoma of the liver.** Transverse sonogram shows numerous small round hypoechoic solid lesions throughout the whole liver

in only 5%. The sonographic findings are, in declining order of frequency (Ginaldi et al. 1980):

- hypoechoic lesions, 44%: often multiple and localized in both lobes. The lesions are 1–15 cm, round or oval, and well-defined (Fig. 4.2.**5**).
- diffuse alteration of hepatic architecture, 35%. The alteration consists of increased echogenicity, diffuse irregular alteration, or a mixture of both. Hepatomegaly occurs in this type of involvement.

- echogenic lesions, 13%. The lesions are well defined and round or oval.
- Target lesions or "bull's eye" lesions, 9%. The lesions are echogenic, surrounded by a hypoechoic ring.

It is assumed that gross pathology must be present when sonography is positive. Negative sonography does not imply a disease-free liver.

In differential diagnosis, metastases, hepatocellular carcinoma, steatosis, cirrhosis and other focal diseases must be mentioned. Correlation of sonography with clinical history and laboratory data is necessary. Definite diagnosis depends on histology.

Leukemia. Involvement of the liver in leukemia is very rare. Microscopic infiltration does not change the sonographic pattern, while focal infiltration can lead to hypoechoic nodules, often with a hyperechoic center.

Metastatic Disease

The percentage of patients with liver metastases increases from first presentation until the late stages essentially as follows: breast carcinoma from 1% to 33%, bronchus carcinoma from 15% to 45%, colorectal carcinoma from 17% to 62% and melanoma from 34% to 75% (Cosgrove 1981).

Variation in the Sonographic Appearance of Metastasis in the Liver. Corresponding to their reflectivity, these variations can be classified as follows (Koischwitz 1980, Green et al. 1977, Scheible et al. 1977).

- echo-free: rare, especially in cystic tumors of the ovary or pancreas, but also due to extensive necrosis, especially in leiomyosarcoma and in metastases of colon carcinoma and carcinoid melanoma (5%) (Fig. 4.2.**6**).
- hypoechoic: occurs in many carcinomas (31%) (Fig. 4.2.**7**).
- hyperechoic: frequent, often carcinomas of the gastrointestinal tract (43%) (Fig. 4.2.**8**).
- hyperechoic with hypoechoic area around: "bull's eye-lesion".
- hypoechoic with hyperechoic area around: "target lesion" (5%).
- hyperechoic with dorsal acoustic shadow: occurs in calcifications of necrotic metastases, especially in colorectal carcinoma (2%).
- combination of hyperechoic and hypoechoic lesions (3%).
- diffuse alteration of architecture: this occurs in diffuse tumor infiltration, especially in anaplastic carcinomas (11%).

Metastases of 1–2 cm can already be detected, and metastases larger than 2 cm are detected with high

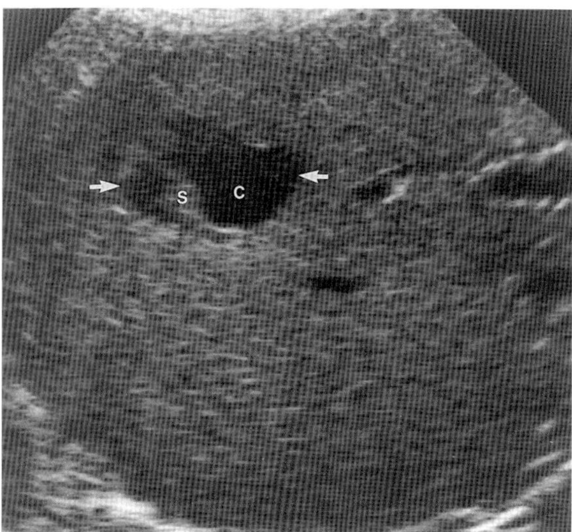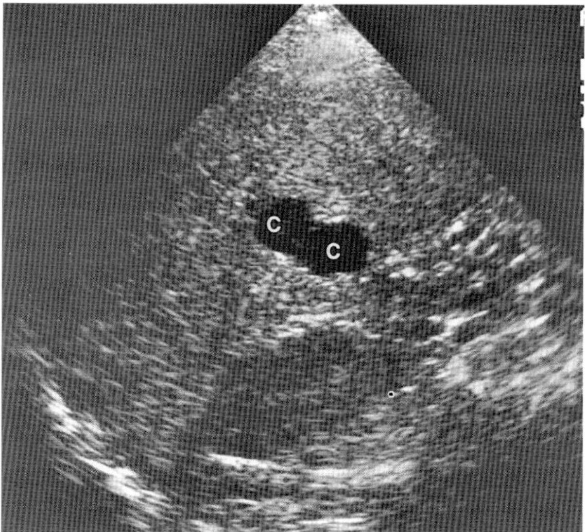

Fig. 4.2.**6 a Necrotic liver metastasis of carcinoid.** Transverse sonogram shows an almost completely echo-free cystic (C) lesion (arrows) with only a small solid portion (S)
b Liver cysts. Transverse sonogram shows two small cysts (C) close together. Note the resemblance to **a**. There is no solid portion, however

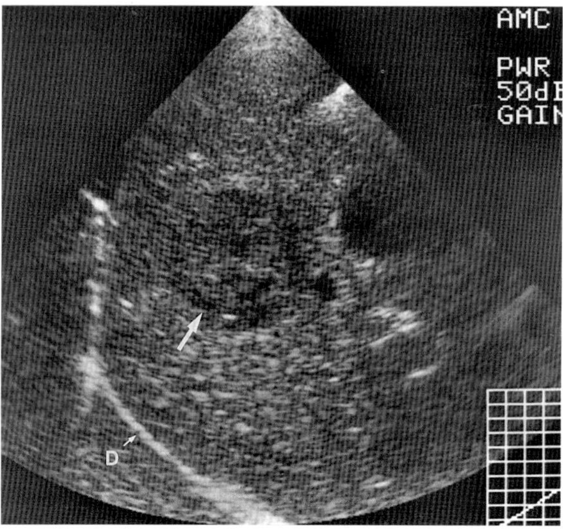

Fig. 4.2.**7 Liver metastasis of carcinoma of the pancreas.** Oblique sonogram shows a hypoechoic, sharply demarcated mass (arrow) in the right liver lobe. D = diaphragm

tissue, collagen, mucin content, necrosis and hematoma. The cell type is probably not as important as a certain pattern of the primary tumor (Hessel et al. 1982). To some authors, ultrasonography therefore lacks specificity in defining the organs of the primary tumor. For example, echogenic lesions are reported in about 50% of cases with carcinoma of the gastrointestinal and urogenital tract, but metastases of carcinomas of the gastrointestinal tract can also be hypoechoic (Fig. 4.2.**9**).

A thin hypoechoic rim is frequently seen surrounding liver metastases; it is known as the halo sign. The halo is almost always extratumoral and caused by peritumoral liver cell compression (Marchal et al. 1985). The observation of a halo of this sort suggests an expansive mass lesion. A hypoechoic halo is seldom seen around benign lesions. Differential diagnosis: hepatocellular carcinoma, lymphoma, cysts, haemangioma, steatosis.

accuracy (Becker-Gaab et al. 1987, Gunvén et al. 1985, Suramo et al. 1984). The lesions are difficult to find when located in sonographically inaccessible areas, e.g. behind the portal vein or in anterior and lateral regions. Fine-needle puncture for cytological examination under ultrasound guidance is necessary in difficult cases.
Correlation of Sonographic Pattern and Histomorphology. Most important for the sonographic appearance of metastases are vascularity, fibrous

Extrahepatic Bile Ducts

In 75–80% of patients with jaundice, it is possible to differentiate between the obstructive and non-obstructive types by laboratory tests. Patients with malignant disease of the extrahepatic bile duct usually present with jaundice (Ferrucci et al. 1983, Sample et al. 1978). Ultrasonography has changed imaging in jaundice patients dramatically, and is highly accurate in differentiating obstructive from non-obstructive jaundice (Kamin et al. 1979, Muel-

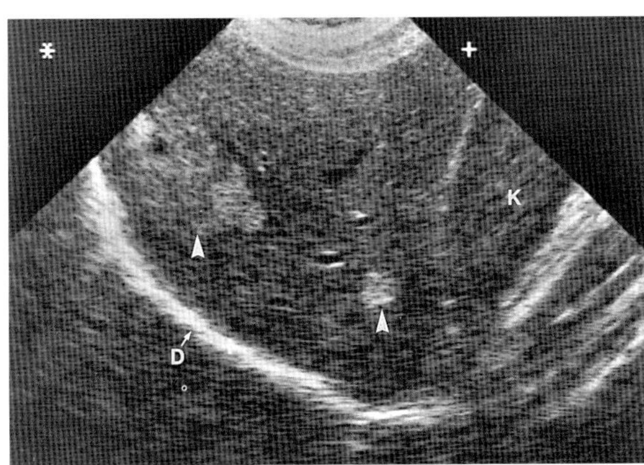 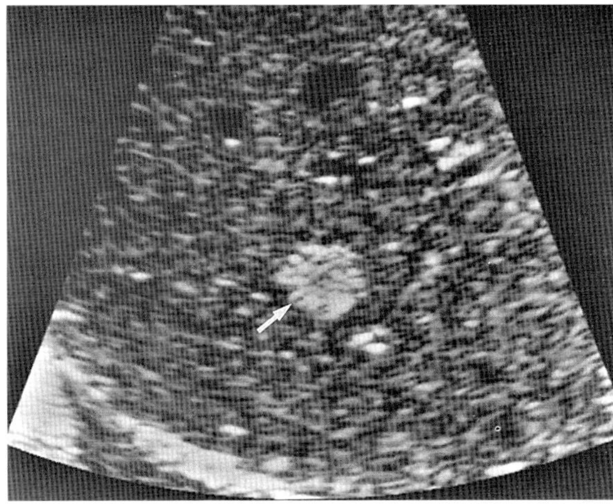

Fig. 4.2.**8a   Liver metastases of carcinoid.** Sagittal sonogram shows hyperechoic lesions (arrow heads) in the right lobe. Distinct from most malignant tumors, no clear halo is visible around the lesions in this case. D = diaphragm, K = kidney
b   Small hemangioma of the liver. The sonogram (detail) demonstrates a small, sharply demarcated, homogeneous, very hyperechoic lesion (arrow) within the right lobe. The lesion is distinct from most hyperechoic metastases in that it is more hyperechoic, and no hypoechoic halo is visible around it

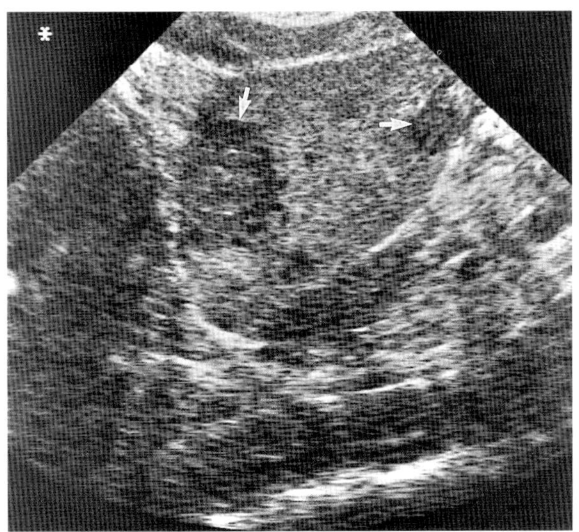

Fig. 4.2.**9   Hypoechoic liver metastases of colon carcinoma.** Sagittal sonogram reveals two hypoechoic lesions (arrows) in the left lobe. These usually hyperechoic metastases of colon carcinoma are now probably hypoechoic due to steatosis of the surrounding liver tissue

ler 1984, Mueller and Simeone 1984, Zeman 1981). In jaundiced patients, US is usually performed as the first imaging procedure to look for dilation of the bile ducts, to localize the site and cause of the obstruction. However, often more expensive and invasive diagnostic procedures have to be performed to get further information when dilated bile ducts are demonstrated (Gibbons et al. 1983,

Gibson et al. 1986, Quinn et al. 1982, Triller and Goël 1979).

Technical Aspects. The common duct lies just to the right of the hepatic artery and anterior to the portal vein. The diameter of the common bile duct should be measured at this point. A diameter of up to 5–6 mm is regarded as normal. More distally, the common bile duct can be wider, especially after cholecystectomy and in older patients, when the elasticity of tissue is decreasing. Normal intrahepatic bile ducts are only occasionally visible. The common duct is best seen when scanning the right subcostal area longitudinally with the transducer angled medially. When bile duct obstruction is suspected in normal sized ducts, or when wide bile ducts are present without clinical signs of obstruction, the functional provocative test with a fatty meal can be helpful: 30–45 min after the fatty meal in functional obstruction, the diameter of the bile duct gets smaller, while in obstruction either no change or an increase in the diameter is observed.

Primary Malignancies

Primary malignancies of the extrahepatic bile ducts are mainly carcinomas (cholangiocarcinoma) (Marchal et al. 1984). Carcinoma of the distal common bile duct occurs in 40%, and at the confluence of the cystic duct and the common hepatic duct in 24%, carcinoma of the proximal common duct occurs in 19%, of the hepatic duct and the bifurcation in 10%, and of the cystic duct in

7% (Moertel 1983). Macroscopically, two main types can be differentiated, a diffuse infiltrating type and a polypoid type.

Ultrasonographic Findings. The most important sign of malignant tumor of the extrahepatic bile ducts is dilation of the bile ducts proximal to the obstruction. Usually the more distal ducts dilate first, and the more proximal, intrahepatic ducts later.

When the tumor is localized at the junction of the two hepatic ducts (Klatskin tumor), only the intrahepatic ducts are dilated (Meyer and Weinstein 1983). The junction may not be visible when tumor infiltration extends more proximally, or when polypoid tumor masses exert compression. In this case a tumor mass may be seen around the obstruction (Fig. 4.2.**10**).

When the carcinoma is situated just distally of the confluence of the cystic ducts, the gallbladder and the cystic duct are dilated too. The dilated common bile duct usually ends abruptly in a polypoid tumor. Sometimes an echogenic intraluminal mass without shadowing can be seen. The infiltrative tumor type leads to a stricture-like lesion, which can sometimes only be differentiated by patient history from a postsurgical lesion.

Carcinoma of the distal common bile duct leads to dilation of the bile ducts, gallbladder, and pancreatic duct when the tumor is situated near the papilla of Vater. Usually there is no mass-like lesion, as in carcinoma of the pancreatic head. Due to bowel gas, the distal common duct is not seen as often sonographically as the proximal part. Water in the stomach and duodenum improves visualization of the distal common bile duct.

Early diagnosis of carcinoma of the extrahepatic bile ducts is infrequent, as jaundice is the main symptom that leads to more thorough diagnostics. Sensitivity of US can distinguish dilated bile ducts from non-dilated ones in more than 90%. However, the site and course of the obstruction are less frequently delineated (Honickman et al. 1983). Taylor et al. (1979) studied 275 jaundiced patients, 11 of them with a carcinoma of the common bile duct. In all of these patients the dilation of the bile duct could be seen, but not the tumor itself. However, in a more recent prospective study the level of obstruction (hilar or non-hilar) was correctly indicated with US in 95% and the cause in 88%, versus 90% and 63% with CT. Predicting resectability of the tumor was reported to be 71% for US and 42% for CT (Gibson et al. 1986). More invasive techniques such as ERCP or PTC have to be applied to get more details about the morphology. When a mass is identified sonographically at the site of the obstruction, percutaneous needle biopsy under US guidance can determine the histology of the underlying disease.

Differential Diagnosis. In a small percentage, obstruction of the biliary ducts occurs without dilation, probably when diagnosed early or when encasement prevents dilation. The functional provocative test with a fatty meal contributes to the diagnosis of obstruction in discrete dilation.

Hilar lymph nodes secondary to malignancy elsewhere, lymphoma in the porta hepatis, and gallbladder carcinoma growing towards the porta hepatis can obstruct bile ducts. Postoperative strictures are differentiated by patient history.

Choledocholithiasis, ampullary stenosis, pancreatitis, sclerosing cholangitis, and pancreatic malignancy are the main diseases which may show a picture similar to that of carcinoma of the distal common bile duct. Echogenic foci in bile ducts are also seen when surgical clips, intraductal air or stones (often with shadowing) are present.

Other Primary Malignancies. These are very rare. Villous adenomas grow up from the duodenum, or arise in the distal common bile duct. An echogenic mass without acoustic shadowing can be observed sonographically with proximal dilation. Carcinoids arise near the papilla of Vater. Patients present with jaundice, and US shows dilation of the bile ducts up to the papilla.

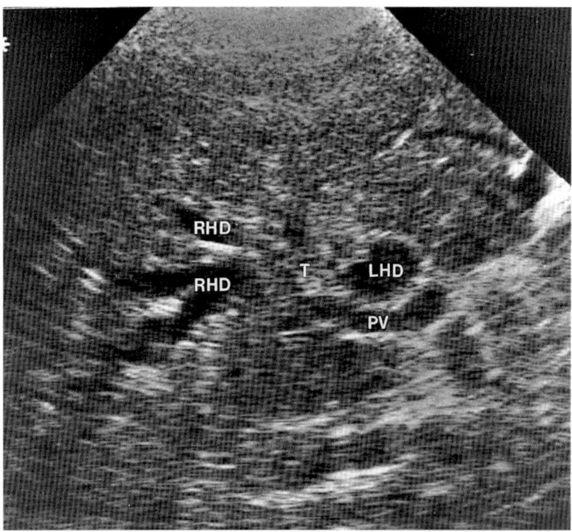

Fig. 4.2.**10 Cholangiocarcinoma (Klatskin tumor) of the liver hilum.** Transverse sonogram through the liver reveals an ill-defined isoechoic tumor (T) in the hilum of the liver at the bifurcation of the hepatic duct. The left hepatic duct (LHD) and the branches of the right hepatic duct (RHD) are dilated. PV = portal vein

Secondary Malignancies

Secondary malignancies of the extrahepatic biliary tree are mostly lymph node metastases of tumors, especially from the gastrointestinal tract, the lung, the breast and melanoma. They can arise in the ducts or can infiltrate them. When growing in the lumen, they can present as an echogenic intraluminal mass without acoustic shadowing. In lymphoma, lymph nodes in the porta hepatis or peripancreatically can cause obstruction of the biliary tree. The lymph nodes are usually sonographically echo-poor. Definite diagnosis is possible by patient history and histology (Gibson et al. 1986).

Gallbladder

Malignant tumors of the gallbladder are uncommon and usually primary.
Technical aspects. Longitudinal and transverse scans of the gallbladder region in supine position, transverse scans in left decubitus position, and longitudinal scans in sitting or standing position, are carried out.

Primary Malignancies

Primary malignancies of the gallbladder comprise only 1–3 % of all malignancies. Adenocarcinoma is the most frequent cause, while other primary malignancies such as sarcomas and carcinoids are much more seldom.
Carcinoma. Before US and CT were available, preoperative diagnosis of carcinoma of the gallbladder was rare, since no opacification was achieved with oral cholecystography due to chronic cholecystitis or obstruction of the cystic duct (Hayashi et al. 1987). These two newer diagnostic modalities have improved preoperative diagnosis of gallbladder carcinoma, and are sometimes complementary (Koenigsberg et al. 1979). As tumors are often asymptomatic, patients consult the physician at a late stage. The tumor therefore often is unresectable (Yeh 1979). The five-year patient survival rate is very poor (1–5 %).

The ultrasonic features depend on the localization of the carcinoma and are divided by Yeh (1979) into 4 types:

- Mass filling the gallbladder. The gallbladder is full of tumor, normal in size or enlarged. In the gallbladder there can be weak echos, strong echos due to stones, and echo-free areas due to necrosis or tumor-free lumen. Differentiation from the surrounding liver can be difficult. This is the most frequent finding (Fig. 4.2.11).
- Thickened gallbladder wall due to infiltrating carcinoma. The wall is often thickened irregularly and asymmetrically. This is the second most frequent finding.

- Fungating mass on the gallbladder wall. The mass is usually echogenic and without acoustic shadowing. The mass does not move with gravity. This type of carcinoma is more often found in early-diagnosed carcinoma (Koenigsberg et al. 1979).
- Combination of fungating mass on the thickened gallbladder wall, caused by infiltration of the carcinoma.

Associated US features of carcinoma of the gallbladder (Hayashi et al. 1987, Olken et al. 1987, Yeh 1979) are:

- stones in the gallbladder (in 65–95 % of cases)
- chronic cholecystitis
- cholecystitis or empyema of gallbladder (occurs when the cystic duct becomes obstructed by tumor infiltration or by a polypoid mass)
- liver abscesses
- liver involvement by carcinoma:
  - direct invasion of the liver: indistinct margin of the gallbladder at the liver side. The carcinoma invades the adjacent part of the liver (Fig. 4.2.11)
  - metastases: hematogeneous
- dilated biliary duct: by lymph node metastases in the porta hepatis or by extension of the carcinoma in the porta hepatis, especially when the carcinoma is localized in the neck of the gallbladder
- retroperitoneal or peripancreatic (celiac) lymph node metastases. Lymph node metastases are

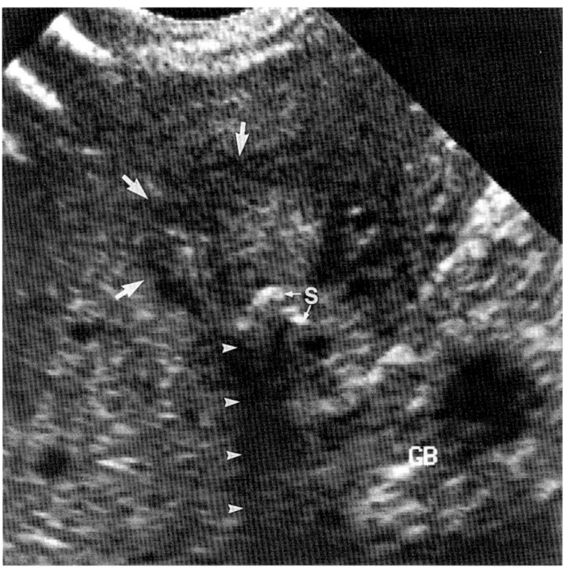

Fig. 4.2.**11 Carcinoma of the gallbladder.** Large non-homogeneous mass filling the gallbladder (arrows). The demarcation between tumor and liver is unsharp due to direct invasion of the liver. Within the tumor, stones (S) are visible. Behind them there is an acoustic shadow (large arrows)

usually sonolucent. They can cause distal obstruction of the common bile duct with proximal dilation of the bile ducts.

The sensitivity of US is reported to be 44–75% in prospective studies (Hayashi et al. 1987), and 92% retrospectively (Soiva et al. 1987).

Differential Diagnosis. The following lesions may simulate carcinoma of the gallbladder: other gallbladder malignancies which are very rare, benign tumors such as adenoma, papilloma, lipoma, cholesterol polyps, mucosal hyperplasia, inflammatory polyp, complicated cholecystitis, xanthogranulomatous cholecystitis, blood clot, sludge and even carcinoma of the pancreas (Soiva et al. 1987). Obliteration of the gallbladder lumen with stones is usually regarded as typical for chronic cholecystitis, but carcinoma can be hidden. In up to 24% of all gallbladder carcinomas, these findings are present. Solid and fungating masses in the gallbladder should be regarded as potentially malignant changes (Hayashi et al. 1987, Koenigsberg et al. 1979, Soiva et al. 1987).

Secondary Malignancies

Involvement of the gallbladder by secondary malignancies occurs mainly by blood-borne metastases and by direct extension of a carcinoma of an adjacent organ such as the colon, stomach or pancreas. Blood-borne metastases can appear as small or large filling defects, caused by subepithelial tumor growth. In two-thirds of gallbladder metastases, melanoma is the primary tumor. On the other hand, gallbladder metastases are found in 15% of patients with melanoma. These cannot usually be differentiated sonographically from primary malignancies of the gallbladder. Gallstones are present less frequently, however. In other cases of metastatic disease of the gallbladder, a primary malignancy elsewhere sometimes is found, especially in the alimentary tract (Friedman 1987, Philipps et al. 1982).

With direct extension of the tumor, localized thickening of the gallbladder wall is observed. Fistula formation in carcinoma of the transverse colon is possible.

In intra-abdominal spread of carcinoma, i.e. of carcinoma of the ovaries, stomach, or colon, the serosa of the gallbladder can be involved, leading to greater or lesser thickening of the gallbladder wall. Lymphatic spread to the gallbladder is very rare (Philipps et al. 1982).

Pancreas

In the majority of patients, the whole pancreas can be visualized sonographically. In obese patients, CT is better for imaging of the pancreas, while in thin patients, US is superior to CT. Nowadays US is regarded as the primary imaging method in pancreatic diseases, while other modalities such as CT, or endoscopic retrograde cholangiopancreatography (ERCP) are performed secondarily (Hederström and Forsberg 1987, Taylor and Taylor 1984).

Technical Aspects. To localize the pancreas, anatomic landmarks such as the superior mensenteric artery, the splenic vein, the superior mensenteric vein and the portal vein have to be identified. It is also necessary to delineate the common bile duct and the posterior wall of the stomach (Weinstein and Weinstein 1981). Transverse-oblique, longitudinal and axial scans must be carried out. Axial scans are necessary in the head of the pancreas, along the superior mesenteric vein and the portal vein. The examination is performed in supine position and after drinking water (acoustic window) in right and left oblique decubitus and in standing (sitting) position. Anteroposteriorly, the head of the pancreas measures up to 2.6 cm, and the body up to 2.2 cm. Usually the echo pattern is equal to, or greater than, that of the liver parenchyma. The normal pancreatic duct can be identified in up to 84% of cases as an echogenic line or as a very thin tubular stucture.

Primary Malignancies

Almost all primary malignancies of the pancreas are adenocarcinomas (95%), only occasionally squamous cell carcinomas, cystadenocarcinomas and islet cell carcinomas (Friedman 1987).

Adenocarcinoma. 60–70% of the carcinomas are localized in the head of the pancreas. In about 30%, the body or tail is involved. Diffuse involvement of the pancreas is rare.

Ultrasonographic Features. The carcinomas are usually less echogenic than normal pancreatic tissue. Coarse echos may be present, sometimes sonolucent lesions due to tumor necrosis or pseudocysts. In only 3% are the carcinomas echogenic. The lesions are small or large, focal, and seldom diffuse, with corresponding enlargement. The size alone is a poor diagnostic criterium. The contour of the pancreas is distorted or sometimes lobulated in bigger lesions. Usually there is no acoustic shadowing (Figs. 4.2.**12**, 4.2.**13**).

When the carcinoma is localized in the head, obstruction of the common bile duct and the pancreatic duct with dilation may occur (Figs. 4.2.**14**, 4.2.**15**). On longitudinal scans, the enlarged pancreatic head is usually better demonstrated than on transverse scans. A dilated pancreatic duct must not be mistaken for the splenic vein. Carcinomas in the tail are more difficult to detect.

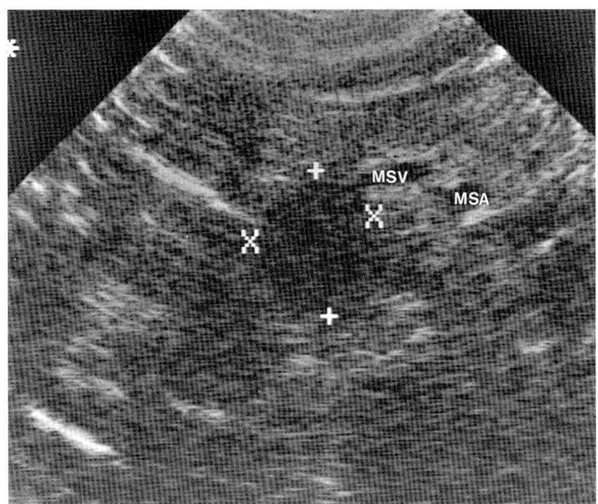

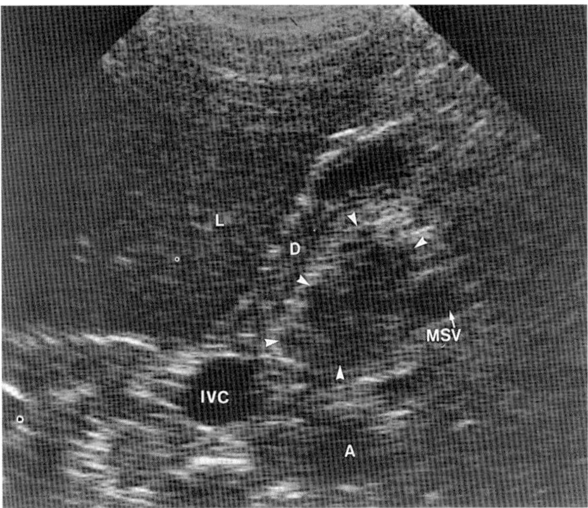

Fig. 4.2.**12** **Adenocarcinoma of the head of the pancreas;** influence of water. Transverse sonograms
a Hypoechoic lesion (between crosses) with a diameter of 3.5 cm. Due to bowel gas, there is bad demarcation with respect ot neighboring organs

b After drinking water, clear demarcation of the tumor (arrow heads) is obtained
A = aorta, IVC = inferior vena cava, MSV = mesenteric superior vein, MSA = mesenteric superior artery, D = duodenum, L = liver

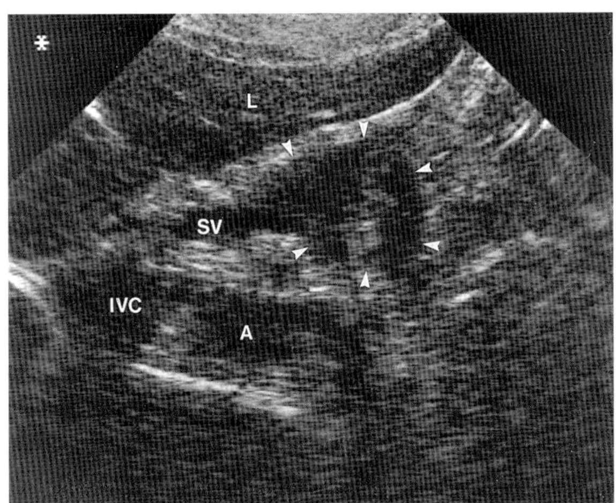

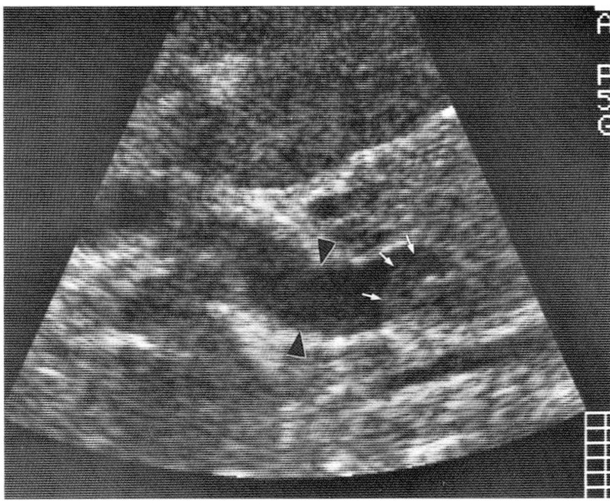

Fig. 4.2.**13** **Adenocarcinoma of the body of the pancreas.** Transverse sonogram demonstrates a hypoechoic solid tumor (arrow heads) that occludes the splenic vein (SV). A = aorta, IVC = inferior vena cava, L = left lobe of liver

Fig. 4.2.**14** **Small adenocarcinoma of the head of the pancreas.** Oblique sonogram shows a small lesion (arrows) protruding in the distal part of a dilated common bile duct (dark arrow heads)

The water-filled stomach serves as an acoustic window, especially for examining body and tail, in left decubitus or in sitting (standing) position (Taylor and Taylor 1984, White and Wittenberg 1984) (Fig. 4.2.**16**).

Secondary features of pancreatic carcinomas are distal pancreatitis with enlargement of the pancreas, displacement or obstruction of the splenic or superior mesenteric vein with collateral veins, and lymph node and liver metastases. Dilation of the common bile duct leads to dilation of the intrahepatic bile ducts and of the gallbladder.

The inferior vena cava can be compressed by a large carcinoma in the head of the pancreas.

In a prospective study the sensitivity of US for pancreatic carcinoma is reported to be 94 % and the specificity 96 %, but about 10 % of patients had to be excluded because of non-visualized or poorly visualized pancreas (Taylor and Taylor 1984). With ultrasonically guided fine-needle biopsy of pancreatic malignancy positive reports are obtained in 90 %, while false negative results are obtained in 10 % (Taavitsaien et al. 1987).

Differential Diagnosis. Chronic pancreatitis or focal

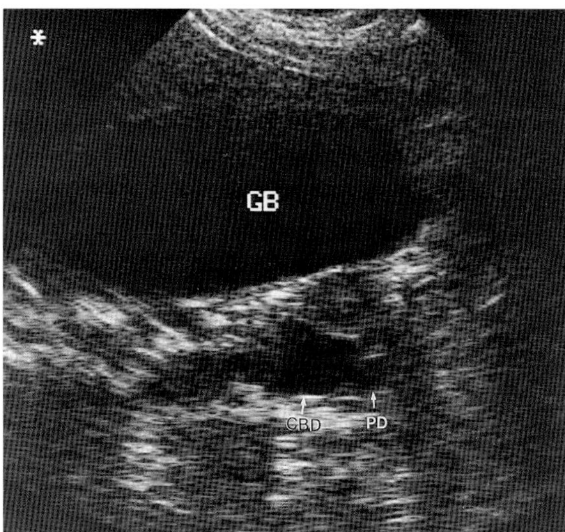

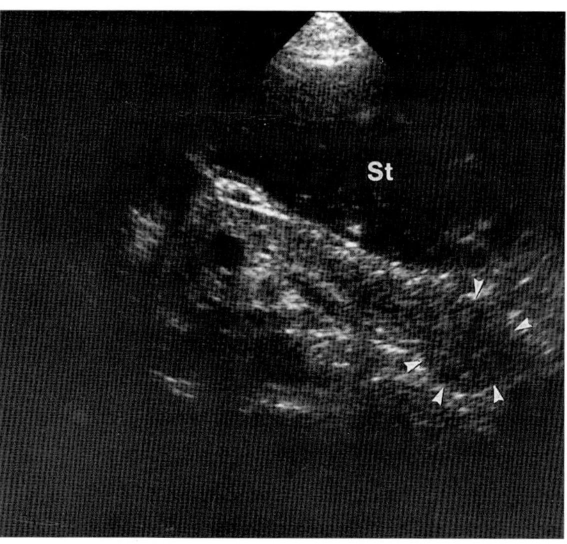

Fig. 4.2.**15 Carcinoma of the papilla of Vater.** Oblique sonogram of a patient in right anterior oblique position with an enlarged gallbladder (GB) as the window shows the distal parts of the dilated common bile duct (CBD) and the dilated pancreatic duct (PD) close together. The tumor itself, very small, cannot be visualized

Fig. 4.2.**16 Small adenocarcinoma of the tail of the pancreas.** Transverse sonogram. The small slightly hypoechoic lesion (arrow heads) in the extreme lateral part of the tail of the pancreas is difficult to visualize even with a fluid-filled stomach (St) as window

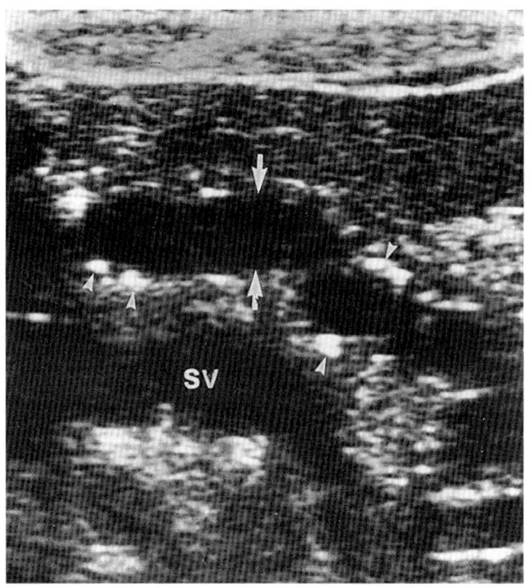

Fig. 4.2.**17 Chronic calcifying pancreatitis.** Transverse sonogram demonstrates numerous small, very hyperechoic spots (arrow heads) representing small calcifications. The pancreatic duct in the body of the pancreas is heavily dilated (arrows). SV = splenic vein

acute pancreatitis can be difficult to differentiate from carcinoma. Calcifications with acoustic shadowing are typical for chronic pancreatitis (Fig. 4.2.**17**). Lymphomatous or metastatic involvement and peripancreatic lymph nodes must be considered too. In peripancreatic lymphadenopathy, there is usually smooth lobulation and no

dilation of the pancreatic or common bile ducts. Non-pancreatic periampullary carcinoma is difficult to differentiate from pancreatic carcinoma. Endoscopy is then necessary.

Cystadenocarcinoma. This is very rare and usually localized in the pancreatic body and tail.

Ultrasonographic Features. In the body or tail, unilocular or multilocular cysts are found. The size of the cysts is 2.5 cm to 33 cm in diameter (mean: 13 cm). The septa are often difficult to see, because they are very thin. When the gain is increased, the cysts can fill in with low-level echos. Around the cysts echogenic areas can be found, sometimes focal areas with acoustic shadowing due to calcifications. Sometimes excrescences project into the cyst (Friedman 1987, Friedman et al. 1983) (Fig. 4.2.**18**).

Differential Diagnosis. Microcystic adenomas, pseudocysts, and localized ascites in the bursa omentalis can mimic cystadenocarcinomas. Biopsy of the cyst wall is necessary to prevent drainage of a resectable cystadenocarcinoma (Friedman et al. 1983).

Islet Cell Carcinoma. About 10% of islet cell tumors are malignant. In 25%, the malignant tumors are non-functioning. Non-functioning islet cell tumors are larger than functioning ones, as they present with pain, jaundice and palpable mass. Functioning tumors can be very small and multiple, as in gastrinoma (Zollinger-Ellison syndrome), and are difficult to detect.

Ultrasonographic Features. The tumors are round

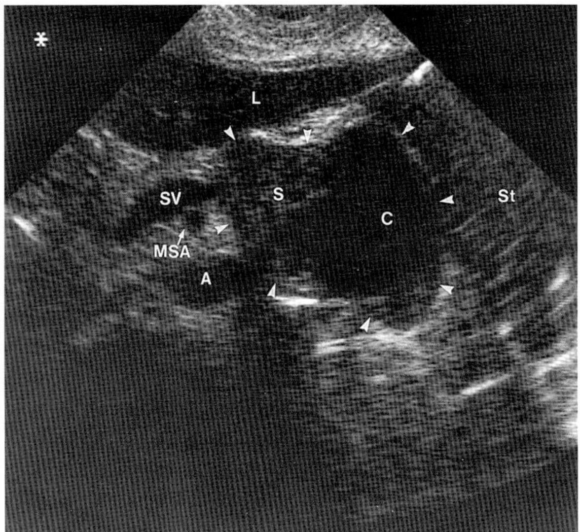

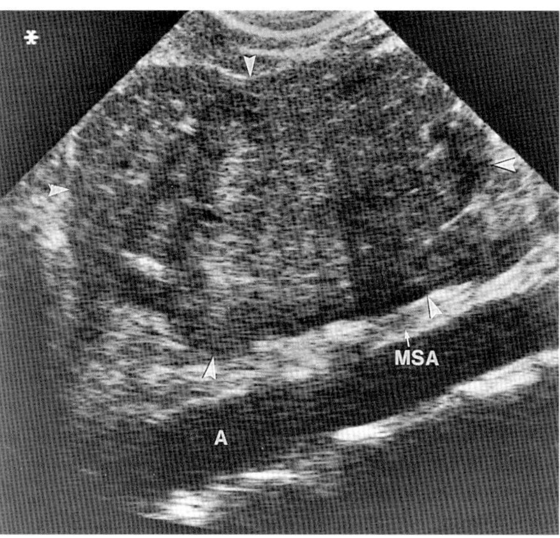

Fig. 4.2.**18** **Cystadenocarcinoma of the body and tail of the pancreas.** Transverse sonogram shows a partly solid (S), partly cystic (C) lesion (arrow heads), measuring 8 cm in diameter altogether with extension to the aorta (A). The splenic vein (SV) is occluded. L = left lobe of the liver, MSA = mesenteric superior artery, St = stomach

Fig. 4.2.**19** **Insulinoma of the pancreas.** Sagittal sonogram at the level of the aorta (A) shows a 14 cm solid mass (arrow heads) in the upper abdomen that extends to the mesenteric superior artery (MSA)

or oval, well circumscribed, and usually less echogenic than the surrounding pancreatic tissue. Acoustic shadowing caused by calcification is rarely observed (Fig. 4.2.**19**). Tumors of 7 mm or more in the head or body can be detected by ultrasonography, if there is no overlying bowel gas. Tumors in the tail are harder to find. The tumors are more easily detected on transverse scans than on longitudinal ones (Friedman 1987, Günther et al. 1983). Diagnosis of malignancy of islet cell tumors is often only possible by diagnosis of metastases in the liver or in lymph nodes. Intraoperative ultrasonography can be helpful in the diagnosis of very small islet cell tumors.

Differential Diagnosis. Adenocarcinoma, peripancreatic lymph nodes, lymphomatous involvement, and metastases have to be included in the differential diagnosis.

Secondary Malignancies

Metastases of extrapancreatic malignancies in the pancreas are rare. They can occur with carcinoma of the bronchus, the breast, or the kidney. Direct extension into the pancreas occurs in carcinoma of the stomach, colon, kidney, and duodenum. Involvement of the pancreas in non-Hodgkin lymphoma is rare, in Hodgkin's disease it is extremely rare. Peripancreatic lymphadenopathy is observed in non-Hodgkin disease. Leukemia involves the pancreas more diffusely, but usually peripancreatic lymph nodes are enlarged too (Friedman 1987).

Most of the metastases in the pancreas are echopoor. They often cannot be distinguished from primary carcinoma of the pancreas. Known primary tumor helps in the diagnosis.

References

Becker-Gaab Ch, zur Nieden J, Sauer U, Zrenner M. Sonographische Diagnostik von Lebertumoren. Digitale Bilddiagn 1987; 7: 35–42.

Bernardino ME, Green B. Ultrasonographic evaluation of chemotherapeutic response in hepatic metastases. Radiology 1979; 133: 437–441.

Cosqrove D-O. Liver. Clin Diagn Ultrasound 1981; 6: 1–20.

Cottone M, Pia Marceno M, Maringhini A et al. Ultrasound in the diagnosis of hepatocellular carcinoma associated with cirrhosis. Radiology 1983; 147: 517–519.

Ferrucci JT, Adson MA, Mueller PR, Stanley RJ, Stewart ET. Advances in the radiology of jaundice: a symposium and review. AJR 1983; 141: 1–20.

Friedman AC, ed. Radiology of the liver, biliary tract, pancreas and spleen. Baltimore: Williams and Wilkins, 1987.

Friedman AC, Lichtenstein JE, Dachman AH. Cystic neoplasms of the pancreas. Radiology 1983; 149: 45–50.

Gibbons CP, Griffiths GJ, Cormack A. Role of percutaneous cholangiography and grey-scale ultrasound in the investigation and treatment of bile duct obstructions. Br J Surg 1983; 70: 494–496.

Gibson RN, Yeung E, Thompson JN et al. Bile duct obstruction: radiologic evaluation of level, cause and tumor resectability. Radiology 1986; 160: 43–47.

Ginaldi S, Bernardino ME, Jing BS, Green B. Ultrasonographic pattern of hepatic lymphoma. Radiology 1980; 136: 427–431.

Green B, Bree RL, Goldstein HM, Stanley C. Gray scale ultrasound evaluation of hepatic neoplasms: patterns and correlations. Radiology 1977; 124: 203–208.

Günther RW, Klose KJ, Rückert K et al. Islet-cell tumours: detection of small lesions with computed tomography and ultrasound. Radiology 1983; 148: 485–488.

Gunvén P, Makunchi M, Takayasu K, Morikaura N, Yamasaki S, Hasegawa H. Preoperative imaging of liver metastases. Ann Surg 1985; 202: 573–579.

Hayashi N, Yamamoto K, Tamaki N et al. Metastatic nodules of hepatocellular carcinoma: detection with angiography, CT and US. Radiology 1987; 165: 61–63.

Hederström E, Forsberg L. Ultrasonography in carcinoma of the gallbladder. Acta Radiol Diagn 1987; 28: 715–718.

Hessel SJ, Siegelman SS, McNeil BJ et al. A prospective evaluation of computed tomography and ultrasound of the pancreas. Radiology 1982; 143: 129–133.

Hillman BJ, Smith J, Gammelgaard J, Holm HH. Ultrasonographic pathologic correlation of malignant hepatic masses. Gastrointest Radiol 1979; 4: 361–365.

Holm HH, Torp-Pedersen S, Juul N, Larsen T. Instrumentation for sonographic interventional procedures. Clin Diagn Ultrasound 1987; 21: 9–40.

Honickman SP, Mueller PR, Wittenberg J et al. Ultrasound in obstructive jaundice: prospective evaluation of site and cause. Radiology 1983; 147: 511–515.

Kamin PD, Bernardino ME, Green B. Ultrasound manifestations of hepatocellular carcinoma. Radiology 1979; 131: 459–461.

Koenigsberg M, Wiener SN, Walzer A. Accuracy of sonography in the differential diagnosis of obstructive jaundice: a comparison with cholangiography. Radiology 1979; 133: 157–165.

Koga A, Yamanchi S, Izumi Y, Hamanaka N. Ultrasonographic detection of early and curable carcinomas of the gallbladder. Br J Surg 1985; 72: 728–730.

Koischwitz D. Sonomorphologie primärer und sekundärer Leberneoplasmen. Röfo 1980; 133: 372–378.

La Berge JM, Laing FC, Federle MP, Jeffrey RB, Lim RC. Hepatocellular carcinoma: assessment of resectability by computed tomography and ultrasound. Radiology 1984; 152: 485–490.

Limpert JD, Vogelzang RL, Neiman HL. Interventional sonography of the pancreas. Clin Diagn Ultrasound 1987; 21: 103–114.

McGahan JP. Advantages of sonographic guidance. Clin Diagn Ultrasound 1987; 20: 249–267.

Machi J, Isomoto H, Yamashita Y, Kurohiji T, Shirouzu K, Kagegawa T. Intraoperative ultrasonography in screening for liver metastases from colorectal cancer: comparative accuracy with traditional procedures. Surgery 1987; 101: 678–684.

Marchal G, Gelin J, van Steenbergen W et al. Sonographic diagnosis of intraluminal bile duct neoplasm: a report of 3 cases. Gastrointest Radiol 1984; 9: 329–333.

Marchal GJ, Pylyser K, Tshibwabwa-Tumba EA et al. Anechoic halo in solid liver tumors: sonographic, microangiographic and histologic correlation. Radiology 1985; 156: 479–483.

Mayes GB, Bernardino ME. The role of ultrasound in the evaluation of hepatic neoplasms. Semin Ultrasound 1981; 3: 212–218.

Meyer DG, Weinstein BJ. Klatskin tumors of the bile ducts: sonographic appearance. Radiology 1983; 148: 803–804.

Moertel CG. Extrahepatic bile ducts: ampulla of Vater. In: Holland JF, Frei E, eds. Cancer medicine. Philadelphia: Lea and Febiger, 1983: 1551–1559.

Mueller PR. Jaundice. Clin Diagn Ultrasound 1984; 14: 25–26.

Mueller PR, Simeone JF. New concepts in biliary ultrasound. Semin Ultrasound 1984; 5: 333–348.

Mukai JK, Stack CM, Turner DA et al. Imaging of surgically relevant hepatic vascular and segmental anatomy, part 1: normal anatomy. AJR 1987a; 149: 287–292.

Mukai JK, Stack CM, Turner DA et al. Imaging of surgically relevant hepatic vascular and segmental anatomy, part 2: extent and resectability of hepatic neoplasms. AJR 1987b; 149: 293–297.

Olken SM, Bledsoe R, Newmark H. The ultrasonic diagnosis of primary carcinoma of the gallbladder. Radiology 1978; 129: 481–482.

Philipps G, Pochaczevsky R, Goodman J, Kumari S. Ultrasound patterns of metastatic tumors in the gallbladder. J Clin Ultrasound 1982; 10: 379–383.

Prando A, Goldstein HM, Bernardino ME, Green B. Ultrasonic pseudolesions of the liver. Radiology 1979; 130: 403–407.

Quinn MF, Rall PW, Boswell WD, Lapin SA, Mortis UL, Halls JM. Predicting the cause of common bile duct obstruction with sonographic data analysis of binary variables. Invest Radiol 1982; 17: 316–323.

Rowley VA, Cooperberg PL. Ultrasound guided biopsy. Clin Diagn Ultrasound 1987; 21: 59–76.

Sample WF, Sarti DA, Goldstein LI, Weiner M, Kadell BM. Gray-scale ultrasonography of the jaundiced patient. Radiology 1978; 128: 719–725.

Scheible W, Gosink BB, Leopold GR. Gray-scale echographic patterns of hepatic metastatic disease. AJR 1977; 129: 983–987.

Schmidt H, Lutz H, Heyder N, Düring A. Sonographie von malignen Hämangioendotheliomen der Leber. Ultraschall 1985; 6: 160–163.

Sexton CC, Zeman RK. Correlation of computed tomography, sonography and gross anatomy of the liver. AJR 1983; 141: 711–718.

Sheu JC, Sung JL, Chen DS et al. Ultrasonography of small hepatic tumors using high-resolution linear-array real-time instruments. Radiology 1984; 150: 797–802.

Sheu JC, Sung JL, Chen DS et al. Early detection of hepatocellular carcinoma by real-time ultrasonography. Cancer 1985a; 56: 660–666.

Sheu JC, Chen DS, Sung JL. Hepatocellular carcinoma: US evolution in the early stage. Radiology 1985b; 155: 463–467.

Snow JH, Goldstein HM, Wallace S. Comparison of scintigraphy, sonography and computed tomography in the evaluation of hepatic neoplasms. AJR 1979; 132: 915–918.

Soiva M, Aro K, Pamilo M, Paivansalo M, Suramo I, Taavitsainen M. Ultrasonography in carcinoma of the gallbladder. Acta Radiol Diagn 1987; 28: 711–714.

Spamer C, Brabss HJ, Koch HK, Gerok W. Benign circumscribed lesions of the liver diagnosed by ultrasonically guided fine-needle biopsy. J Clin Ultrasound 1986; 14: 83–88.

Subramauyam BR, Balthazar EJ, Hilton S, Lefleur RS, Hovii JC, Raghavendra BN. Hepatocellular carcinoma with venous invasion. Radiology 1984; 150: 793–796.

Suramo I, Paivansalo M, Pamilo M. Unidentified liver metastases at ultrasonography or computed tomography. Acta Radiol Diagn 1984; 25: 385–389.

Taavitsainen M, Koivuniemi A, Bondestam S, Kivisaavi L, Tierala E. Ultrasonically guided fine-needle aspiration biopsy in focal pancreatic lesions. Acta Radiol Diagn 1987; 28: 541–543.

Takashima T, Matsui O, Suzuki M, Ida M. Diagnosis and screening of small hepatocellular carcinoma. Radiology 1982; 145: 635–638.

Tanaka S, Kitamura T, Imaoka S, Sasaki Y, Taniguchi H, Ishiguro S. Hepatocellular carcinoma: sonographic and histologic correlation. AJR 1983; 140: 701–707.

Taylor KJW. Going to the depths with duplex Doppler ultrasound. Diagn Imaging Int 1987a; 3: 28–42.

Taylor KJW, Taylor CR. Pancreas. Clin Diagn Ultrasound 1984; 14: 299–326.

Taylor KJW, Ramos J, Morse SS, Fortune KL, Hammers L, Taylor CR. Focal liver masses: differential diagnosis with pulsed Doppler US. Radiology 1987b; 164: 643–647.

Taylor KW, Rosenfield AT, Spiro HM. Diagnostic accuracy of gray scale ultrasonography for the jaundiced patient: a report of 275 cases. Arch Intern Med 1979; 139: 60–63.

Teefey SA, Stephens DH, James EM, Charboneau JW, Sheedy II PF. Computed tomography and ultrasonography of hepatoma. Clin Radiol 1986; 37: 339–345.

Triller J, Goël Y. Sonographisch-radiologische Diagnostik bei obstruktivem Ikterus. Radiologe 1979; 19: 367–375.

Valleix D, Sautereau D, Pouget X et al . Ultrasonographic anatomy of the liver. Surg Radiol Anat 1987; 9: 123–134.

Weinstein DP, Weinstein BJ. Pancreas. Clin Diagn Ultrasound 1981; 6: 35–51.

Wernecke K, Peters PE. Sonographische und computertomographische Diagnostik von Lebermetastasen. Radiologe 1985; 25: 141–151.

Wernecke K, Heckemann R, Rehwald V. Ultraschallgeführte Feinnadelbiopsie herdförmiger Lebererkrankungen. Teil 1: maligne Lebertumoren. Ultraschall 1984; 5: 298–302.

White M, Wittenberg J. Pancreatic neoplasia. Semin Ultrasound 1984; 5: 401–413.

Wooten WB, Green B, Goldstein HM. Ultrasonography of necrotic hepatic metastases. Radiology 1978; 128: 447–450.

Yeh HC. Ultrasonography and computed tomography of carcinoma of the gallbladder. Radiology 1979; 133: 167–173.

Zeman RK, Dorfman GS, Burrell MI, Stein S, Berg GR, Gold JA. Disparate dilatation of the intrahepatic and extrahepatic bile ducts in surgical jaundice. Radiology 1981; 138: 129–136.

4.3   Endoscopic Ultrasonography in the Preoperative Staging of Biliopancreatic Carcinoma

T. L. Tio, G. N. J. Tytgat

Introduction

Endoscopic ultrasonography (EUS) combines endoscopy and ultrasonography – a logical and exciting combination of two high technologies in one instrument – to avoid limiting factors in conventional ultrasonography such as adipose tissue, bone, pulmonary and intestinal gas. Through the direct approach to target lesions with a high frequency real-time ultrasonic beam via the intestinal lumen, a hitherto unknown resolution can be obtained. Moreover, the real-time dynamic properties of this technique allow accurate assessment of both ductular and parenchymal abnormalities of the biliopancreatic system and particularly of vascular involvement (Di Magno et al. 1980, Strohm et al. 1980, Yamanaka et al. 1982, Lux et al. 1982, Di Magno et al. 1982, Heyder et al. 1983, Tio and Tytgat 1984, Classen and Kawai 1984, Tio et al. 1986, Tytgat and Tio 1986, Tio and Tytgat 1986, Takemoto et al. 1986). The purpose of this chapter is to document the usefulness of EUS in the preoperative assessment and staging of biliopancreatic malignant diseases and to describe the future prospects for this new diagnostic procedure.

Instrument

EUS is performed with a lateral viewing endoscope in which a small echo probe is attached to the tip (Fig. 4.3.1). Since 1983 we have been using an Olympus prototype (EU-M1) echo-endoscope and the commercially available model (EU-M2). The length of the rigid tip is 42 mm (EU-M2). The outer diameter of the echo probe is 13 mm. The frequency of the real-time mechanical sector scanner is 7.5 or 10 MHz with a penetration depth of approximately 10 or 5 cm and an axial resolution of 0.2 or 0.1 mm. The sector of images is 180 or 360 degrees. The echo probe is routinely covered with a water-filled balloon to improve ultrasonic images by making optimal contact with the mucosa, while air accumulation between the echo probe and mucosa is avoided.

Technique

After anesthetizing the throat and intravenous sedation, the echo-endoscope is inserted like any other endoscope, with the patient in left lateral position. The echo endoscope is blindly introduced into the stomach, because side viewing optics do not allow endoscopic vision in the esophagus. After endoscopic visualization of the pylorus, the echo probe is gently advanced into the duodenal bulb and then slowly into the second part of the duodenum in a manner similar to that used for insertion of the duodenoscope to perform endoscopic retrograde cholangiopancreatography (ERCP). However, the maneuvering procedure into the duodenum is usually technically more difficult than ERCP due to the rigidity of the transducer.

Pancreas

Because of the topographic anatomical relationship between the pancreas and stomach the gastric configuration plays an important role in the visualization of the pancreas (Fig. 4.3.2). An elongated stomach allows good visualization of the entire pancreas by filling the gastric lumen or the balloon with water. In the case of a small horizontal stomach, or after surgical resection, adequate examination of the pancreas is difficult or even impossible (Billroth I or II). The head of the pancreas should usually be examined from the second part of the duodenum. The body and tail of the pancreas can be examined from the middle and proximal part of the stomach using the splenic vein as a landmark (Fig. 4.3.3).

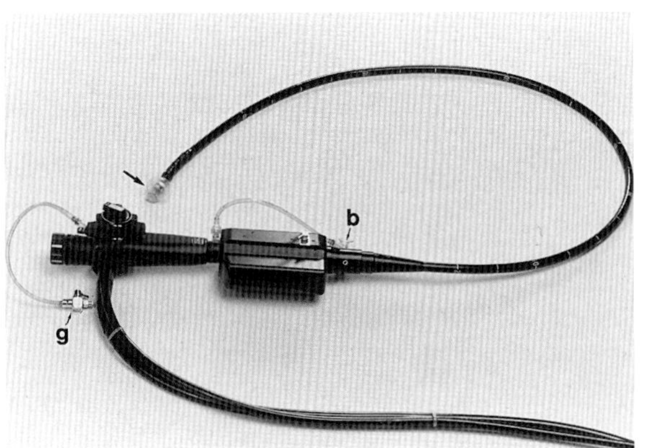

Fig. 4.3.1   **Echoendoscope** consisting of a side-viewing gastroscope (Olympus JF-B3) with a small echo probe (arrow) at its tip. Two channels are available for filling the balloon (b) and the gastric lumen (g) with water

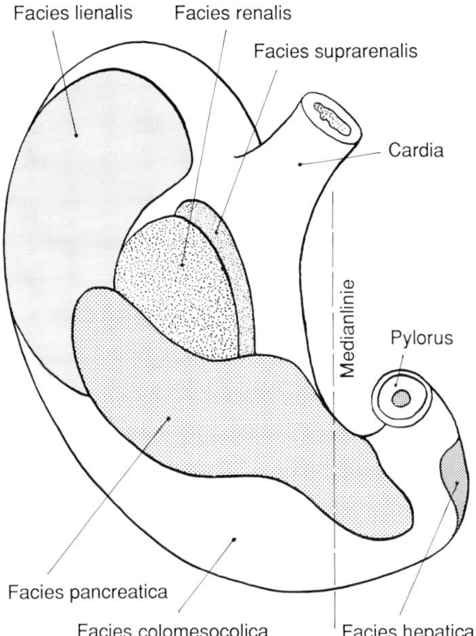

Fig. 4.3.**2 Anatomic scheme** (posterior view) shows the relationship between the stomach and the surrounding organs. Note the localization of the pancreas at the posterior wall of the antrum and corpus of the stomach

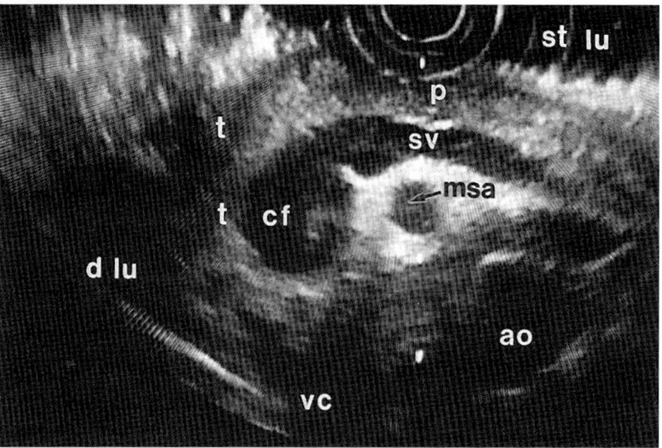

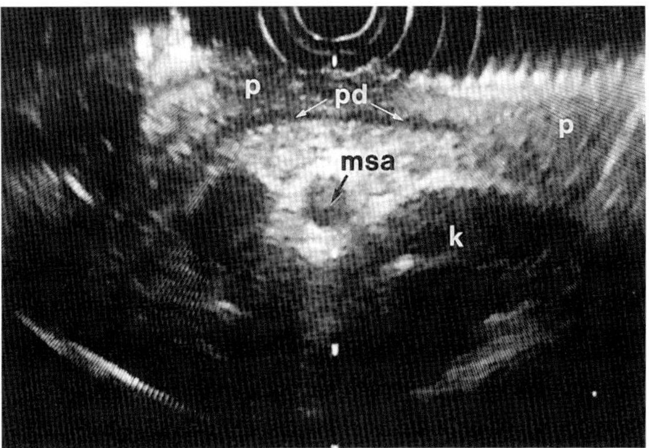

Fig. 4.3.**3a EUS picture shows the body and tail of the pancreas** visualized by filling the stomach lumen with water (st-lu) using the splenic vein (sv) as landmark; ao = aorta; cf = splenoportal confluence; dlu = duodenal lumen with water; msa = mesenteric superior artery; vc = vena cava; t = tumor
b EUS picture shows the pancreas (p) and pancreatic duct (pd) visualized from the distal part of the stomach; msa = mesenteric superior artery

Papillary Region

The papillary region must be examined from the second part of the duodenum by placing the echo probe directly adjacent to the papillary region under endoscopic control. During maneuvering into the duodenum, the rotating ultrasonic unit should not be switched, in order to avoid damage to the ultrasonic probe. The anatomical structure of the papilla of Vater can be clearly recognized because of the ability to visualize the duodenal wall layers and both the common bile duct and pancreatic duct. For accurate assessment of peripapillary tumor, cross-, longitudinal and oblique sections should be carried out. By slow withdrawal of the echo endoscope using the dilated common bile duct or the pancreatic duct for reference, the extent of tumor growth can clearly be visualized (Fig. 4.3.**4**).

Biliary System

Lesions in the distal common bile duct must be examined from the second part of the duodenum. The common bile duct can be readily identified because of its topographic relationship to the duodenum as a ductular structure immediately adjacent to the duodenal wall. Usually the portal vein is found parallel to the common bile duct. The cystic duct and gallbladder can be visualized by placing the echo probe in the duodenal bulb or in

the antrum of the stomach. The gallbladder may not always be visualized because of the limited penetration depth of ultrasound. The bifurcation of the common hepatic ducts can be visualized using the portal vein as an orientation landmark; this usually requires maneuvering of the echo probe along the lesser curvature of the duodenum and stomach.

Endosonographic Findings (Results)

Pancreas

As a rule, pancreatic carcinoma is visualized as a hypoechoic, sharply or bizarrely demarcated parenchymal structure, which appears more hypoechoic than the surrounding pancreatic tissue. The boundaries of the carcinoma may show a clear or bizarre delineation. Obstruction of the pancre-

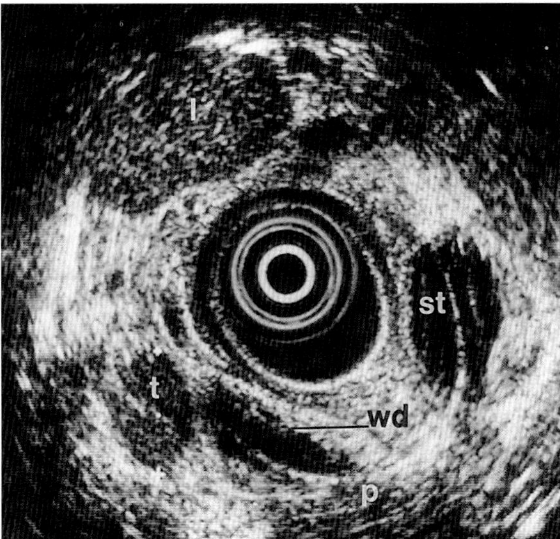

a

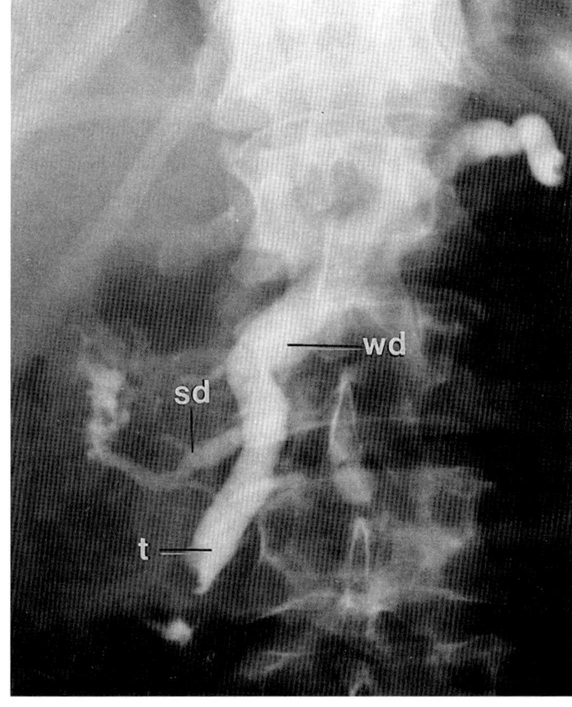

b

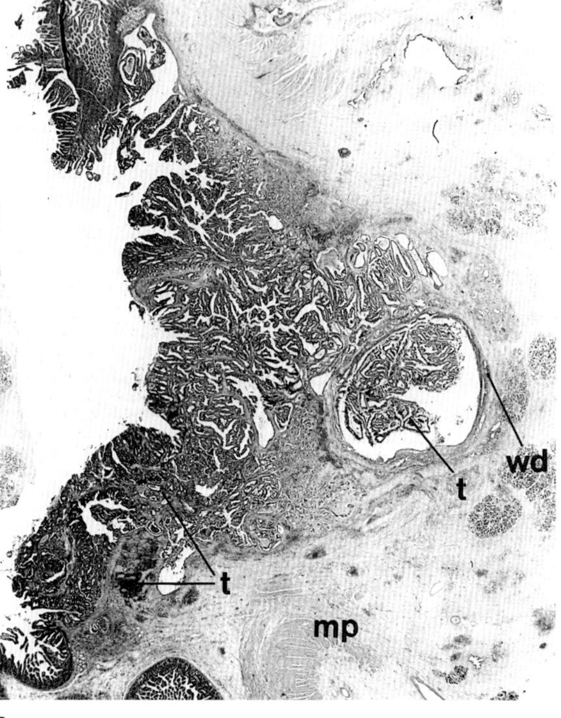

c

Fig. 4.3.**4a** **EUS picture shows a hypoechoic tumor** (t) directly adjacent to a dilated Wirsung's duct (wd); st = water-filled stomach
b **ERCP picture shows a small periampullary filling defect** (t) with prestenotic dilation of Wirsung's duct (wd) and santorini's duct (sd)
c **Corresponding histology of the resection specimen** revealing a periampullary carcinoma (t) infiltrating Wirsung's duct (wd); mp = muscularis propria of the adjacent duodenum

atic duct or of both the pancreatic and the common bile ducts are often present, corresponding to the double duct lesion often seen on ERCP (Fig. 4.3.**5**). Supplementary findings, such as prestenotic dilation of the pancreatic duct, or the common bile duct, or both, may help to assess the extent of the tumor and to characterize the malignant nature of the lesion. Exceptionally, insulinoma can be visualized as a sharply delineated hypoechoic lesion, with a central hypoechoic pattern. Carcinoid tumor in the periampullary is visualized as a hypoechoic pattern with sharp demarcation adjacent to the pancreatic duct (Tio and Tytgat 1986). Endosonographic visualization of suspicious adjacent lymph nodes and blood vessels is essential in achieving accurate staging of the malignancy. Moreover, various sections such as cross-, longitudinal and oblique section can be achieved by maneuvering the transducer endoscopically. The real-time dynamic properties of EUS are of the utmost importance, and appear to be superior to computed tomography (CT). The latter is a static imaging technique, and can only achieve cross-section images. Although ERCP is accurate in detecting and staging ductular abnormality in both the pancreatic duct or bile ducts, the extent of the tumor cannot be assessed. We divided our patients prospectively into three groups in order to assess the accuracy of EUS in comparison with other imaging modalities.

Group I consisted of lesions which appeared to be resectable, endosonographically, with the

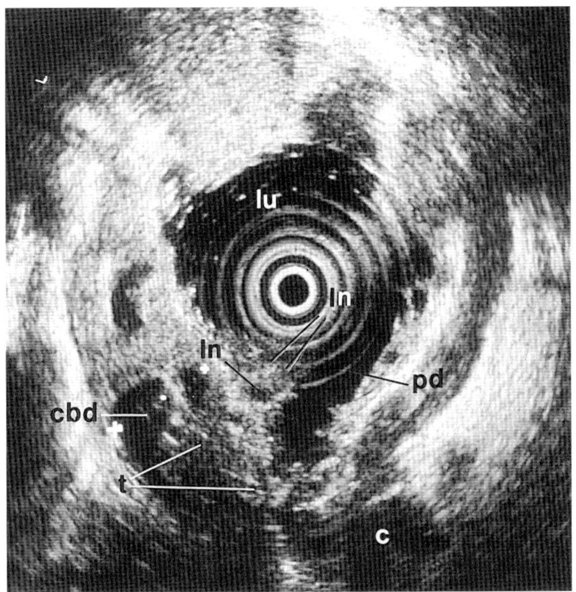
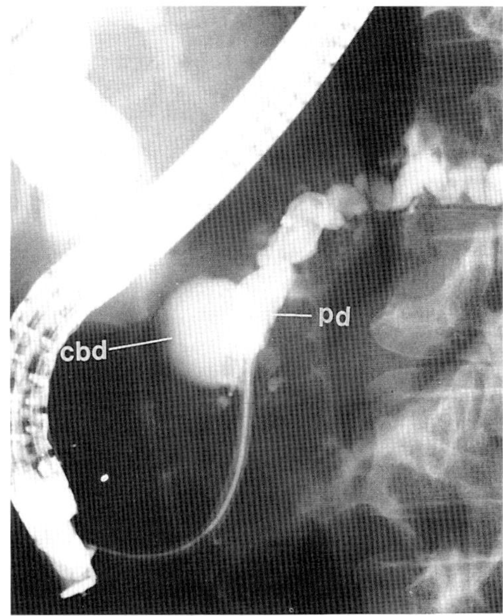

Fig. 4.3.**5a**   **EUS picture shows a hypoechoic bizarrely demarcated tumor** (t) penetrating the common bile duct (cbd) and pancreatic duct (pd) with adjacent small lymph nodes (ln); c = splenoportal confluence
b   **Corresponding ERCP shows a dilated pancreatic duct** (pd) and common bile duct (cbd), compatible with "double duct lesion"

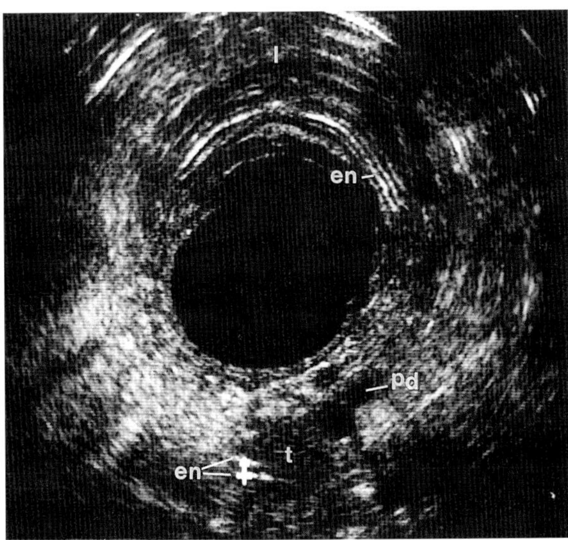

Fig. 4.3.**6a**   **EUS picture shows a hypoechoic sharply demarcated tumor** (t) approximately 1 cm in size between the pancreatic duct (pd) and biliary endoprosthesis (en)

intention of cure; this was diagnosed if a small hypoechoic lesion with a diameter of approximately 2 cm, with clearly demarcated boundaries and without evidence of penetration into the surrounding tissue and without abnormal lymph node structures was visualized endosonographically (Fig. 4.3.**6**). This definition appears to be similar with Group I according to the recent TNM system (Hermanek et al. 1987).

Group II consisted of lesions in which surgery would in all probability be palliative in nature. This was diagnosed when a clearly demarcated hypoechoic tumor mass was present with a diameter of more than 2 cm and without penetration into the adjacent major blood vessels, but with evidence of lymph node involvement (Hermanek et al. 1987) (Fig. 4.3.**7**).

Group III consisted of lesions which appeared endosonographically to be unresectable. This was diagnosed when deep penetration of carcinoma into the surrounding tissues or the major blood vessels (mesenteric artery, celiac trunc, aorta, caval vein, portal vein or splenoportal confluence) was present. Particular attention was paid to the visualization of the retroperitoneal area, which appeared to be essential because of the anatomical site of the major blood vessels (Fig. 4.3.**7**). EUS appears to be superior to CT because of its real-time dynamic properties, which allow clear visualization of vascular involvement and various sections of the main lesion (Figs. 4.3.**8**, 4.3.**9**).

Occasionally an extensive anechoic cavity can be found immediately adjacent to the main lesion, which usually suggests the presence of a necrotic mass within the malignancy. This was also usually considered to be predictive of non-resectability because of extensive spread of tumor growth. After insertion of biliary endoprosthesis, a cystic lesion can occasionally be recognized. Ultrasonically guided cytological puncture may be helpful in differentiating a carcinoma with a necrotic cavity

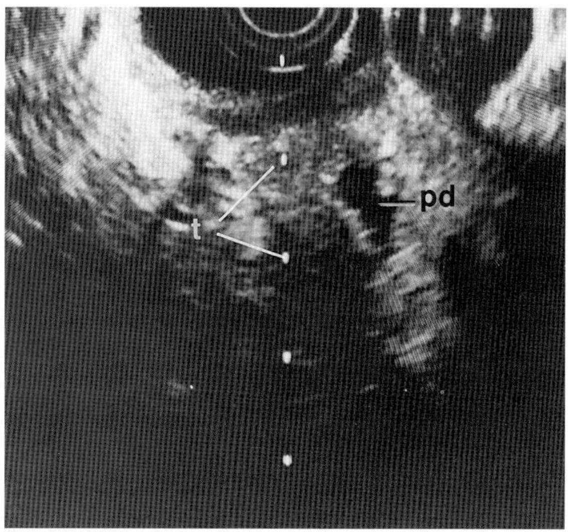
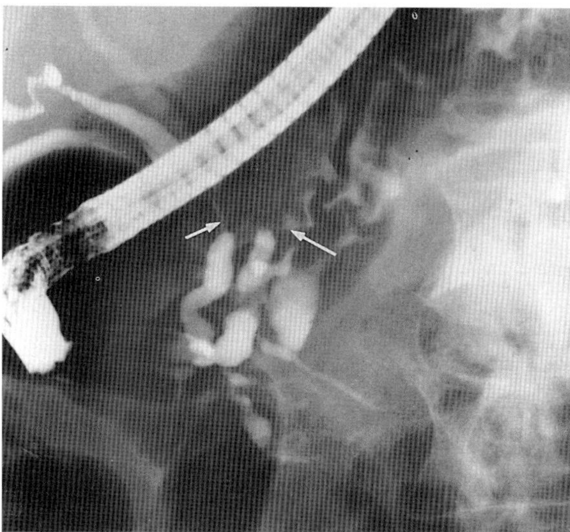

Fig. 4.3.**7 a   EUS picture shows a hypoechoic tumor** (t) 2 cm in size with dilated pancreatic duct (pd)
b   Corresponding ERCP shows an obstruction (arrows) of the pancreatic duct and common bile duct compatible with "double duct lesion"

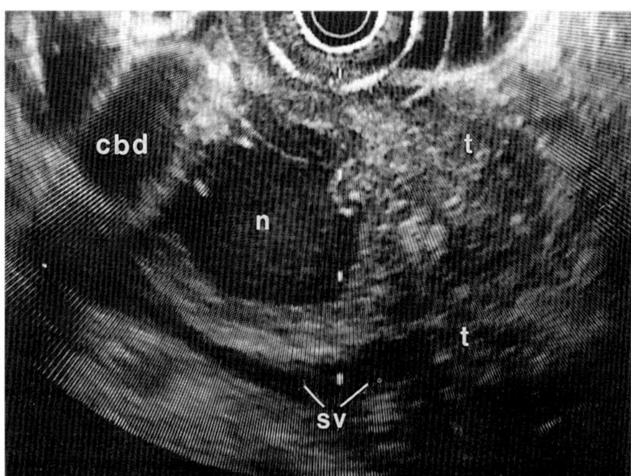
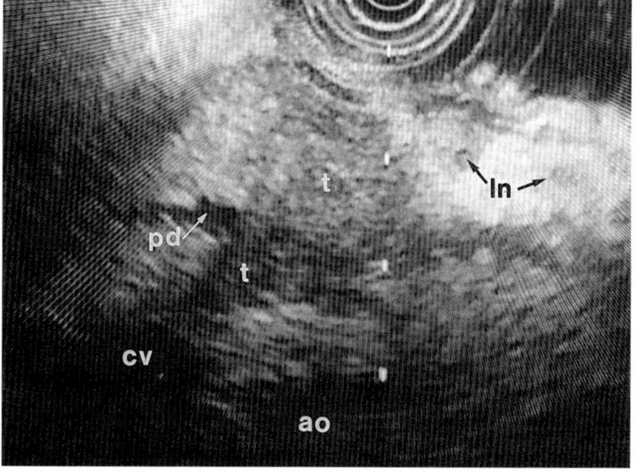

Fig. 4.3.**8 a   EUS picture shows an extensive hypoechoic non-homogeneous tumor mass** (t) adjacent to a necrotic cavity (n) penetrating into the splenic vein (sv) with dilated common bile duct (cbd)
b   EUS picture shows an extensive hypoechoic mass (t) deeply penetrating into the retroperitoneal space with adjacent lymph nodes (ln) which proved to be non-resectable at surgery. Note the hyperechoic pattern of the surrounding pancreas due to chronic pancreatitis; ao = aorta; cv = caval vein; pd = pancreatic duct

from a benign pseudocyst. Also, liver metastases, usually visualized by transcutaneous ultrasound, are considered to be a contra-indication for surgery.

Table 4.3.1 summarizes the results of EUS and surgery in predicting pancreatic carcinoma for cure, palliative resection or non-resectability. It is readily obvious from these figures that the diagnostic accuracy of EUS in pancreatic malignancy is high. EUS allows clear visualization of tumor penetration into the adjacent duodenal wall, because of its capability of visualizing the gastrointestinal wall and the pancreatic tumor. Moreover, lymph nodes can be distinguished from the primary tumor on the basis of echo pattern and configuration. In contrast, CT may recognize a pancreatic tumor as an enlargement of the pancreas. EUS therefore appears to be more accurate than CT in assessing the extent of tumor growth (Fig. 4.3.**10**). However, EUS may not always allow sonographic differentiation between fibrotic changes and infiltrating carcinomatous tissue.

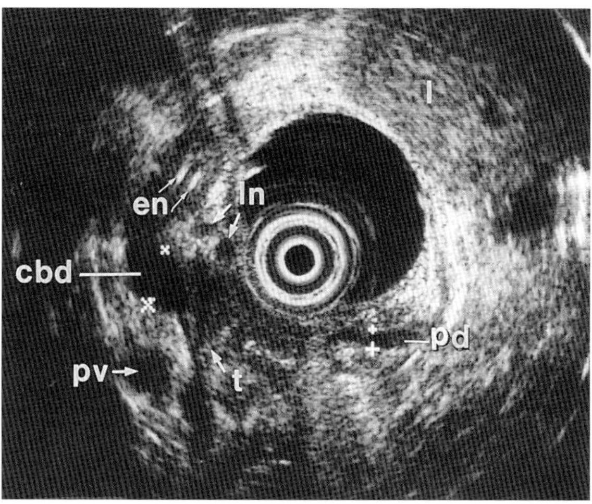

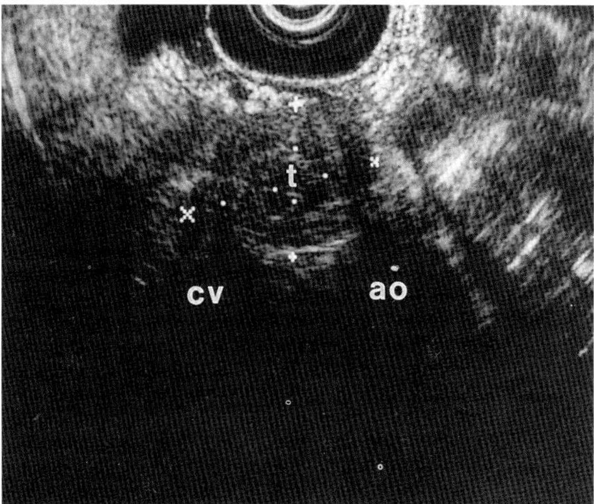

Fig. 4.3.**9a** **EUS picture shows a hypoechoic tumor mass** (t) penetrating into the dilated common bile duct (cbd) and adjacent pancreatic duct with lymph nodes (ln); en = biliary endoprosthesis; pv = portal vein
b **Another cross-section** shows the tumor mass (t) penetrating to the caval vein (cv) and aorta (ao). It proved to be non-resectable

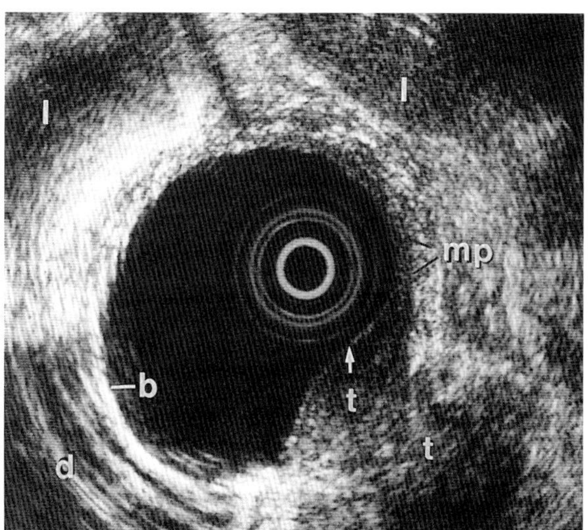

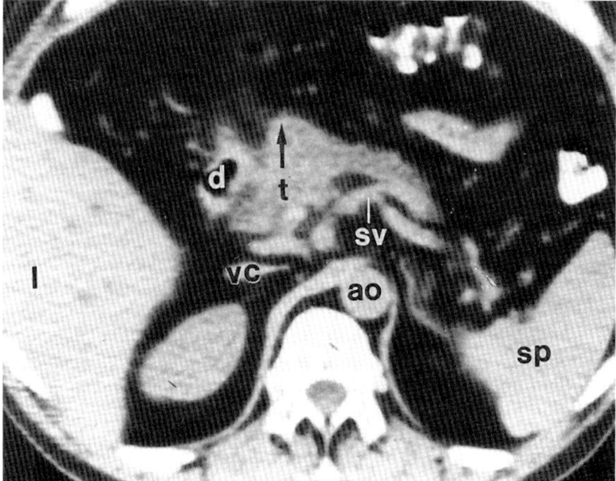

Fig. 4.3.**10a** **EUS picture shows a hypoechoic tumor mass** (t) penetrating into the adjacent duodenal wall (arrow); mp = muscularis propria; l = the right lobe of the liver
b **Corresponding CT** shows an enlargement of the pancreatic head (t) with adjacent duodenum filled with contrast (d); ao = aorta; l = liver; sp = spleen; sv = splenic vein; vc = vena cava

Table 4.3.**1** **Results of EUS in assessing resectability of pancreatic carcinoma**

	EUS No. of correct diagnoses	Surgery/ Histology
Curative	2	3
Palliative	10	11
Non-respectability	5	7
Total:	17	21

Peripapillary Carcinoma

Peripapillary lesions are visualized as hypoechoic intramural lesions, directly adjacent to the water-filled balloon or water-filled duodenal lumen. Penetration of a periampullary carcinoma into the adjacent common bile duct or pancreatic duct, or even into the adjacent pancreatic parenchyma, can readily be seen with EUS. Periampullary carcinoma can be differentiated from pancreatic cancer because of the ability of EUS to define the origin of the lesion. Periampullary tumor originates from the

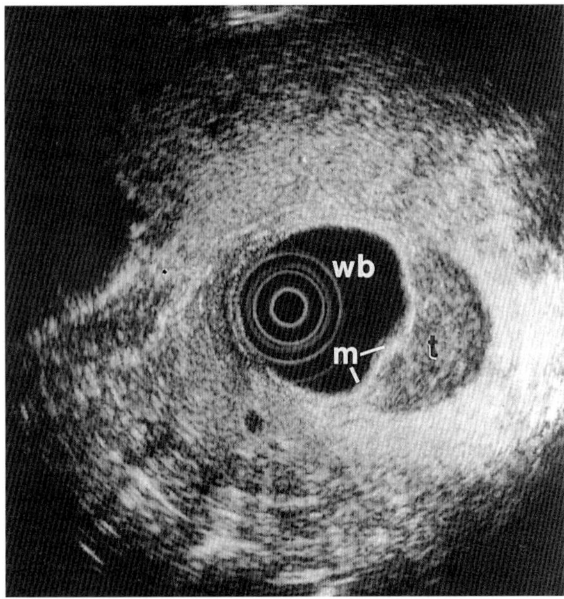

a

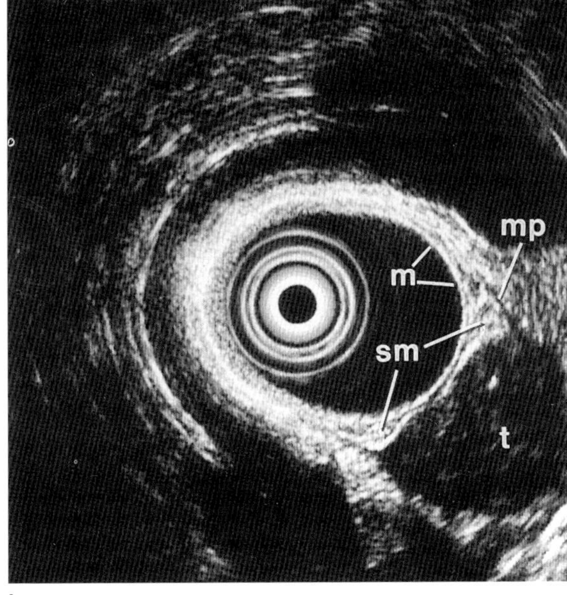

b

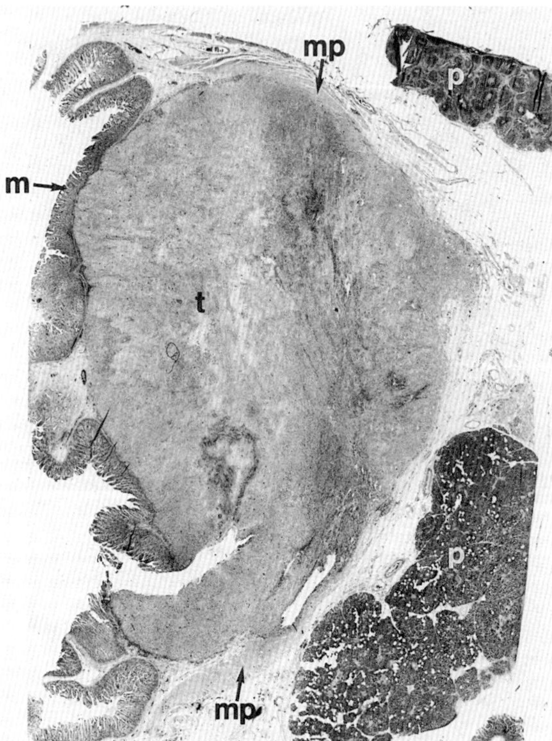

c

Fig. 4.3.**11a   Preoperative EUS picture** (EUS in vivo) shows a hypoechoic, sharply demarcated intramural lesion (t) adjacent to the papillary region

b   Corresponding EUS picture of resection specimen (EUS in vitro) shows a hypoechoic lesion (t) penetrating through the muscularis propria (mp) but without penetration into the adjacent pancreas

c   Corresponding histology of the resection specimen shows an ampullary carcinoma (t) without infiltration into the adjacent pancreas (p). Note the obvious correspondence of EUS and histology regarding the extent of tumor growth; mp = muscularis propria

papillary region, usually protruding into the duodenal lumen or penetrating into the adjacent common bile duct or pancreatic duct. In contrast, transcutaneous (conventional) ultrasonography and computed tomography (CT) may only demonstrate indirect signs of peripapillary lesions, such as dilation of the common bile duct or pancreatic duct without visualization of the primary lesion (Honickman et al. 1983, Gross et al. 1983, Marchal et al. 1984). The extent of tumor growth with or without adjacent lymph node involvement can therefore be accurately assessed only with EUS (Heyder et al. 1983, Tio and Tytgat 1986). Moreover, correlation between EUS in vivo (preoperative EUS) and EUS in vitro (EUS of resection specimen) can be achieved, showing obvious correspondence with the histology of the resection specimen (Fig. 4.3.**11**). In order to assess the accuracy of EUS in the preoperative staging of peripapillary carcinoma we subdivided our patients into three groups.

Group I patients came under the heading 'resectability with the intention of cure.' This was diagnosed when EUS visualized a hypoechoic intramural lesion without deep penetration through the organ boundaries into the adjacent structures, and without evidence of lymph node involvement (Fig. 4.3.**11**).

Group II patients came under the heading 'palliative, resectable lesions.' This was diagnosed when EUS visualized a transmural hypoechoic tumor with direct penetration into the adjacent common bile duct or pancreatic duct and pancreas, together with lymph node involvement.

Group III patients came under the heading 'non-resectable lesions.' This was diagnosed when

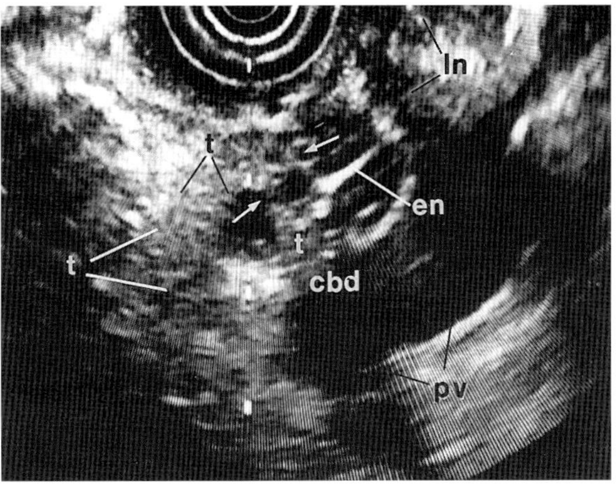

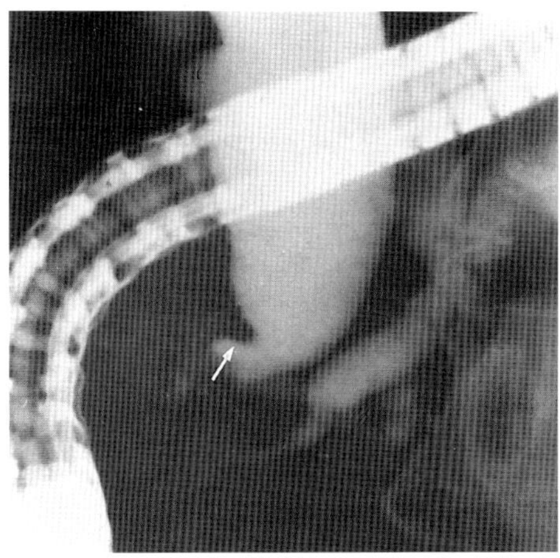

a

b

Fig. 4.3.**12a** **EUS picture shows a dilated common bile duct** (cbd) due to hypoechoic periampullary tumor mass (t) penetrating into the splenoportal confluence (pv) with multiple lymph nodes (In). Note the tumor penetration into the common bile duct (arrows) and endoprothesis (en)

b **ERCP reveals narrowing of peripapillary common bile duct** (arrow) with extensive prestenotic dilation

c **At surgery**, lymph nodes (In) along the common bile duct were removed and proven to be metastatic

c

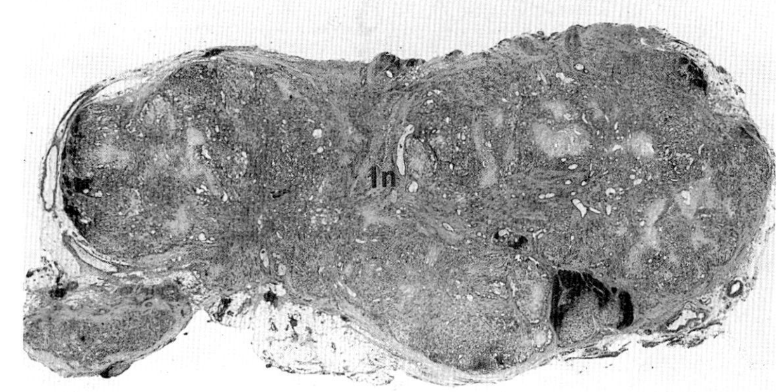

EUS visualized penetration of the tumor mass into the surrounding tissues, e.g. major blood vessels (mesenteric artery, portal vein or splenoportal confluence) or organs, e.g. pancreas or liver (Fig. 4.3.**12**).

Table 4.3.**2** summarizes the results of EUS in assessing the resectability of peripapillary carcinoma with surgery/histology.

Common bile duct tumors

A bile duct carcinoma is sonographically visualized as a polypoid tumor originating from the biliary wall and protruding into or obstructing the lumen of the bile duct. The origin of the tumor can often be clearly identified by placing the echo probe appropriately against the lesion. In the case of an extensive cholangiocarcinoma penetrating into the adjacent pancreatic parenchyma, differentiation between bile duct carcinoma and pancreatic cancer can be difficult or even impossible, particularly when the pancreatic duct is also infiltrated. Such abnormality is similar to the double duct lesion seen on ERCP. Moreover, a common bile duct car-

Table 4.3.**2** **Results of EUS in assessing resectability of peripapillary carcinoma with surgery/histology**

	EUS No. of correct diagnoses	Surgery/ Histology
Curative	7	9
Palliative	2	3
Non-resectability	2	2
Total:	11	14

cinoma adjacent to the peripapillary region can be extremely difficult to distinguish from a periampullary carcinoma. After insertion of a biliary endoprosthesis, the site of the lesion can readily be identified using the hyperechoic echo pattern of the endoprosthesis as a guide (Tytgat and Tio 1986, Tio and Tytgat 1986). A hypoechoic echo pattern adjacent to the hypoechoic structure of the endoprosthesis is characteristic of a malignant lesion. Moreover, direct tumor penetration into the adjacent lymph node can clearly be identified, usually

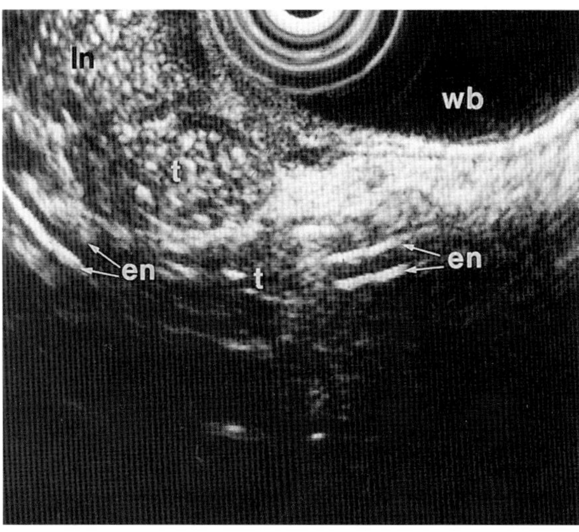

a

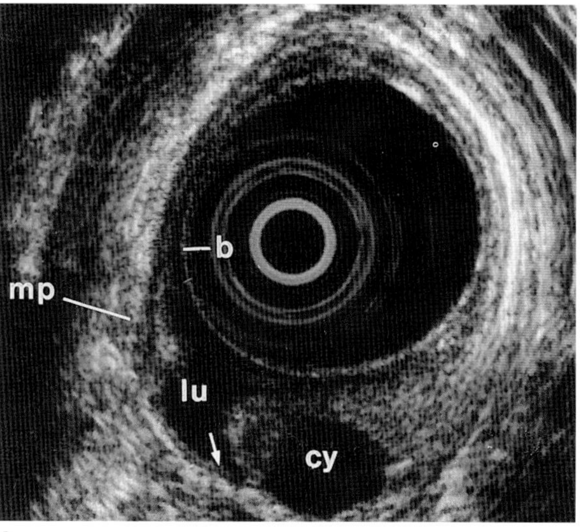

a

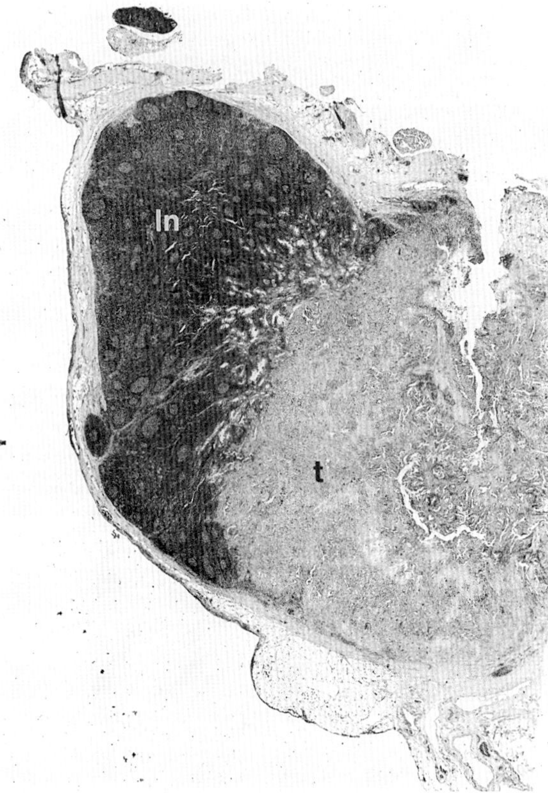

b

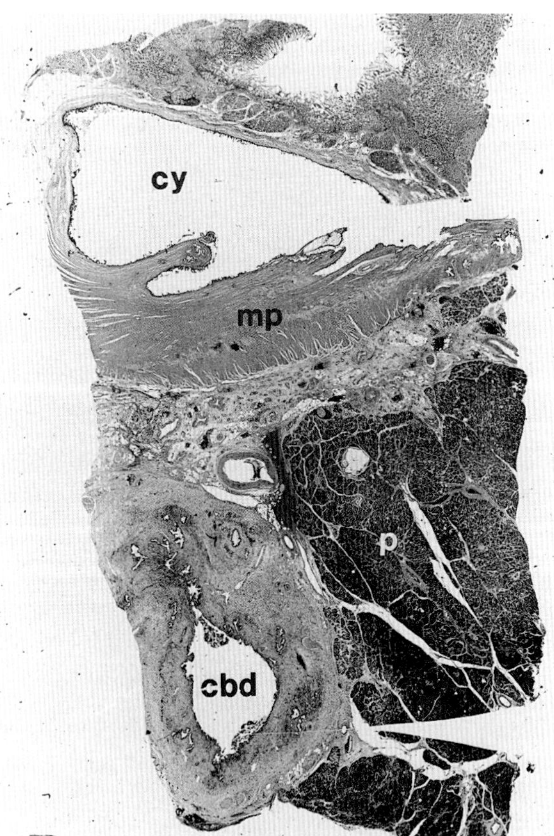

b

Fig. 4.3.**13a** **EUS picture shows an intraduodenal hypoechoic tumor** (t) adjacent to a biliary endoprosthesis (en) with an adjacent hypoechoic oval lymph node suspected to have direct tumor infiltration (arrows)
b The corresponding histology of the lymph node (ln) shows tumor infiltration (t)

Fig. 4.3.**14a** **EUS picture of a resection specimen** shows an anechoic cystic lesion (cy) bulging into the duodenal lumen (lu, arrow) immediately above the muscularis propria (mp)
b The corresponding histology shows the cystic lesion (cy) directly above the muscularis propria (mp) adjacent to the pancreas (p) and dilated common bile duct (cbd)

showing an echo pattern similar to the primary malignant lesion (Fig. 4.3.**13**). In contrast, an inserted stent often disturbs CT images. In addition, the real-time properties allow more detailed information on tumor penetration around or into major blood vessels, which is of the utmost importance in assessing resectability. After insertion of a biliary endoprosthesis, cholangitis due to periductal abscess can occur, which can be visualized as an anechoic lesion directly adjacent to the tumor (Figs. 4.3.**14**, 4.3.**15**). The most important blood vessels are the portal vein, the hepatic artery or the celiac trunk and the mesenteric artery. Criteria for assessing resectability are similar to those used to assess papillary carcinoma.

Table 4.3.**3** summarizes the results of EUS in assessing the resectability of common bile duct carcinoma in comparison with histology and surgery.

Table 4.3.**3** **Results of EUS in assessing resectability of common bile duct carcinoma with surgery/histology**

	EUS No. of correct diagnoses	Surgery/ Histology
Curative	4	6
Palliative	8	11
Non-resectability	2	2
Total:	14	19

Bifurcation (Klatskin) Tumor

Cholangiocarcinoma obstructing the bifurcation (Klatskin tumor) is visualized as a hypoechoic tumorous structure, often with polycyclic contours with round, sharply demarcated boundaries, protruding into or compressing the adjacent bile ducts and causing prestenotic dilation of the biliary tree of the left or right systems, or both. Lymph nodes can be identified directly adjacent to the tumor in the hilum, or along the common bile duct, or adjacent to the cystic duct. A tumor with sharply demarcated boundaries, without evidence of penetration into the liver parenchyma and without lymph node involvement, is considered to be resectable with the intention of cure. Tumor penetration into the adjacent liver parenchyma or extension into both sides of the biliary tree and (usually) associated with lymph node involvement, strongly suggests a non-radical (palliative) procedure (Fig. 4.3.**16**). A tumor mass deeply penetrating into both liver lobes, or penetrating into the adjacent blood vessels, is in principle predictive of non-resectability. Such extensive tumors were excluded from surgery and only treated with the insertion of a biliary endoprosthesis. Differentiation between a primary bile duct cancer and other tumor types (lymph node metastasis, non-Hodgkin lymphoma, hepatocellular carcinoma) may sometimes be difficult because of the similar echo pattern and anatomical site. In the case of proximal bile duct lesion, differentiation between benign and malignant lesions is quite difficult in ERCP, CT or conventional ultrasonography. EUS may become helpful in ruling out the presence of malignancy by clear visualization of concrement in the cystic duct (e. g. Merrizzi syndrome) or fibrosis changes after surgery (e. g. metal clips). In the near future, EUS-guided aspiration cytology may ascertain the final diagnosis.

EUS appears to be an accurate diagnostic modality during the follow-up of patients after liver resection, because of its ability to visualize both ductular and parenchymal abnormalities together with the adjacent lymph nodes. Conventional ultrasonography and computed tomography are often

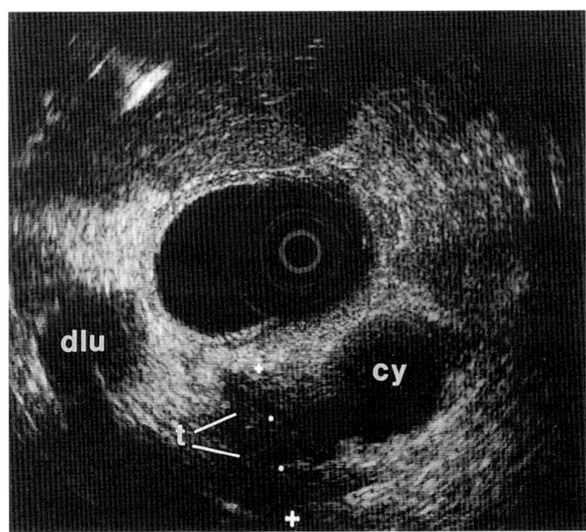

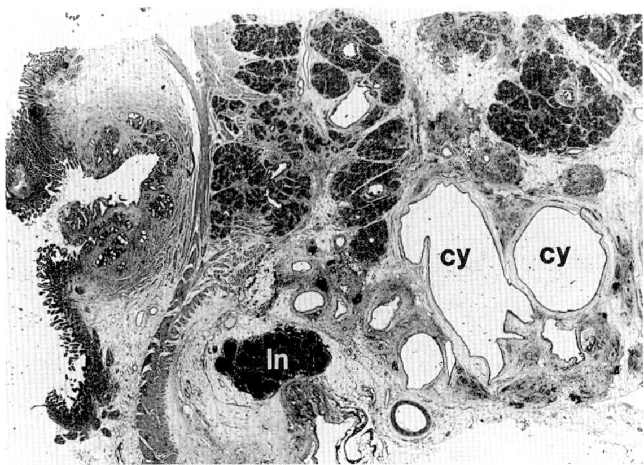

Fig. 4.3.**15 a** **EUS picture shows a hypoechoic tumor** (t) adjacent to an anechoic cystic lesion (cy) adjacent to the duodenum (dlu) and pancreas
b Corresponding histology shows the cystic lesion (cy) between the duodenal wall and the pancreas; ln = lymph nodes

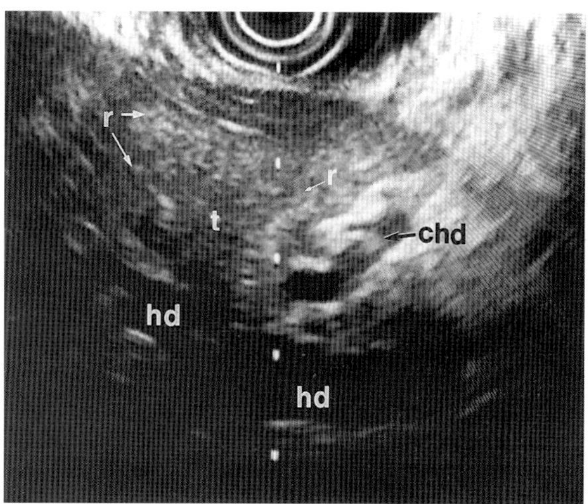

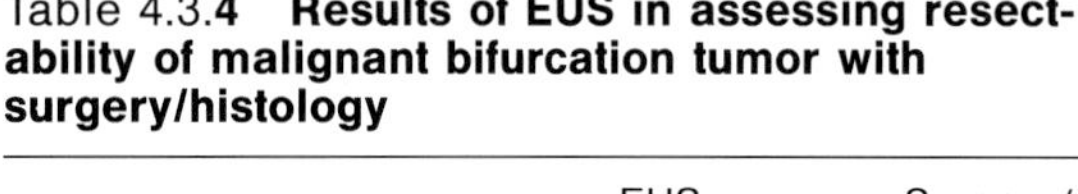

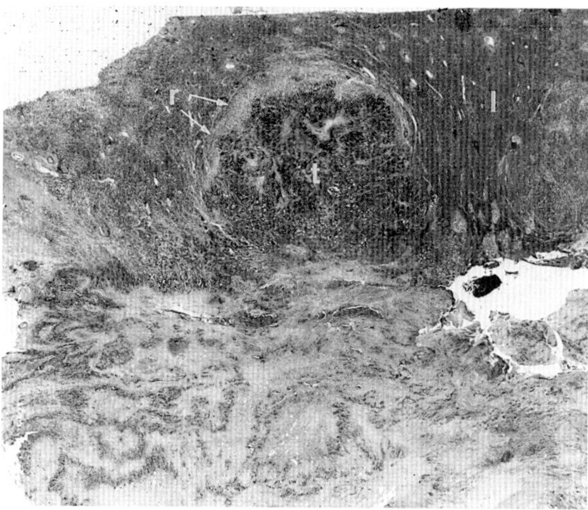

Fig. 4.3.**16a EUS picture shows a round hypoechoic tumor** (t) with a more hyperechoic rim (r) with visualization of the dilation of the hepatic duct (hd)

b Corresponding histology of the resection specimen shows a round tumor (t) with a rim (r) infiltrating into the adjacent liver parenchyma. The correspondence to the EUS image is obvious

Table 4.3.**4   Results of EUS in assessing resectability of malignant bifurcation tumor with surgery/histology**

	EUS No. of correct diagnoses	Surgery/ Histology
Curative	2	3
Palliative	12	12
Total	14	15

inadequate due to postsurgical artefacts. Also, ERCP often is impossible after biliary surgery.

Table 4.3.**4** summarizes the results of EUS in assessing curative and palliative resectability of bifurcation malignant disease in comparison with histology.

Gallbladder Tumors

Carcinoma of the gallbladder is seen as a polypoid hypoechoic structure originating from the gallbladder wall and protruding into the lumen or into the surrounding tissues. Gallbladder carcinoma without deep penetration into surrounding tissues and without evidence of distant lymph node involvement is indicative of a potential for curative resection. A carcinoma with direct penetration into the adjacent common bile duct or hepatic duct, and usually associated with lymph node involvement, strongly suggests the palliative nature of the resection. Carcinoma with deep penetration into the adjacent tissues (e.g. gallbladder bed or adjacent duodenum), or major vascular involvement, pre-

dicts non-resectability (Fig. 4.3.**17**). A carcinoma of the gallbladder with continuous spread into the proximal biliary system can occasionally be difficult to distinguish from a Klatskin tumor because of the similar echo pattern and similar intrahepatic ductular dilation. On ERCP, carcinoma penetrating into the adjacent distal bile duct and the pancreatic head may simulate pancreatic or common bile duct carcinoma, or even the presence of groove pancreatitis (Tio and Tytgat 1986, Becker 1980). EUS may be helpful in distinguishing these conditions. Occasionally, sludge in the gallbladder may simulate the presence of gallbladder malignancy because of the presence of a hypoechoic structure immediately adjacent to the wall of the gallbladder. However, a pseudotumorous lesion of this sort disappears when the position of the patient is changed.

Discussion and Future Prospects

The transduodenal and transgastric approach provides excellent sonographic visualization of the pancreas, extrahepatic bile duct and adjacent structures, because of the anatomic topographical relationship between the biliopancreatic system and the gastroduodenal tract. The direct approach to the lesion with a high-frequency ultrasonic beam allows clear imaging of both parenchymal and ductular abnormalities, together with adjacent lymph node abnormalities. The real-time dynamic properties based upon the ultrasonic character of the instrument and the ability to maneuver the transducer endoscopically to achieve various sections (dynamic quality) allows detailed visualiza-

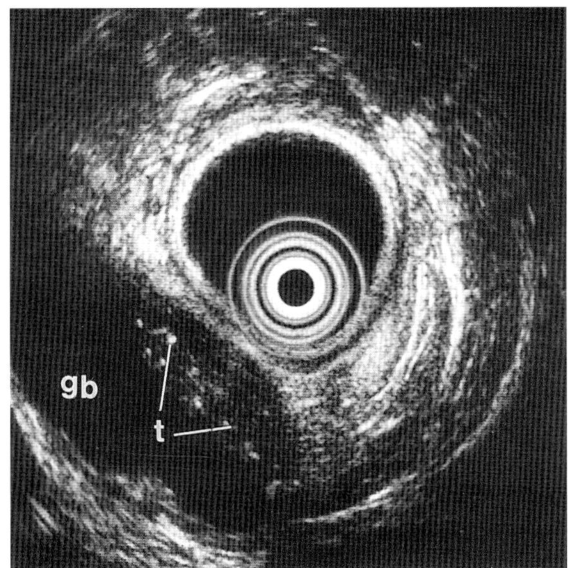

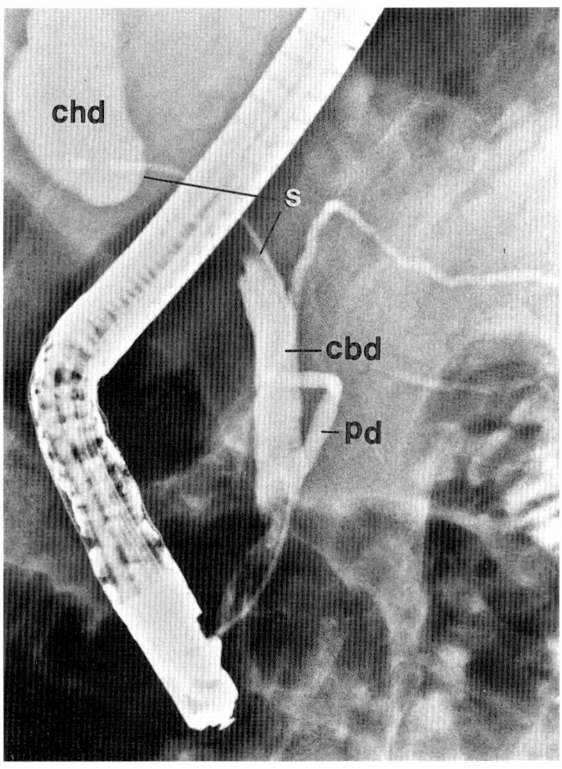

Fig. 4.3.**17 a**   **EUS picture shows a gallbladder** (gb) with polypoid tumor mass (t) penetrating into the adjacent structures
b **Corresponding ERCP** shows an obstruction in the proximal common bile duct (cbd) with proximal dilation of the common hepatic duct (chd) without visualization of the gallbladder, and a normal pancreatic duct (pd)
s = biliary stent

tion of vascular encasement, which is considered to be essential in assessing the resectability of biliopancreatic cancer. Moreover, the presence of a biliary endoprosthesis in situ and the follow-up of patients after biliopancreatic surgery do not disturb EUS images. EUS therefore has the intrinsic potential of becoming the image modality of choice for initial staging and also after endoscopic or surgical treatment. By contrast, ERCP and CT are technically inadequate in such cases. In the evaluation of peripapillary tumor (ampullary or papillary carcinoma), EUS appears to be the most accurate diagnostic procedure due to its ability to visualize the duodenal wall, the pancreatic parenchyma and both the pancreatic duct and common bile duct (Tio and Tytgat 1984, 1986). Therefore, the site, extent and indirect signs such as dilation of the common bile duct or pancreatic duct can be visualized. The shortcomings of EUS include the limited penetration depth of the ultrasound, the rigidity of the transducer and the impossibility at present of EUS-guided cytological puncture. Moreover, maneuvering the instrument into the duodenum may occasionally be difficult or impossible, particularly in case of duodenal deformity. Differentiation between benign and malignant lesions is often difficult or even impossible when only the echo pattern of the lesion is taken into consideration, despite the very clear and detailed character of the images. Definite diagnosis requires cytology or histology. The future possibility of using the biopsy channel for cytological puncture or even biopsy will further enhance the diagnostic value of this fascinating procedure. Moreover, the combination of ultrasound and Doppler or ultrasound with videoendoscope may become the trend in the near future, becoming essential to the education of medical doctors and students. In the hand of an endoscopist with extensive experience, particularly with a side-viewing instrument, this technique is safe. However, the operator must also have a lot of experience in ultrasound in order to achieve reliable images and to interpret the lesion accurately. In clinical use, EUS appears to be a most exciting diagnostic modality due to the excellent images, topographic anatomical information, and detailed information regarding the extent and spread of malignant lesion with its nodal and vascular involvement. The procedure can be performed immediately after conventional ultrasonography and before or even after ERCP, which allows the operator to draw accurate conclusions in staging biliopancreatic tumors. EUS will become an important diagnostic procedure because not only can the efficiency of diagnostic procedure be enhanced, but also the cost-benefit ratio may be made more favorable. Regarding the poor prognosis of pancreatic carcinoma, EUS will become the choice of imaging technique in selecting appropriate patients, who should benefit from surgical resection, and in differentiating papillary or distal common bile duct carcinoma from pancreatic cancer. Currently there is a prospective study of preoperative EUS in progress using the recent TNM classification to further define its role in the evaluation of biliopancreatic carcinoma.

References

Becker V. Sonderformen der chronischen Pankreatitis. Dtsch Ärzteblatt 1980; 46: 2711–2716.

Classen M, Kawai K. Frontiers of GI-endoscopy. Scand J Gastroenterol 1984; 102 (suppl).

Di Magno EP, Reagan PT, Clain JE. Ultrasonic endoscope. Lancet 1980; i: 629.

Di Magno EP, Reagan PT, Clain JE, et al. Human endoscopic ultrasonography. Gastroenterology 1982; 83: 824–829.

Gross BH, Harter LP, Core RM, Calkes PW, Filly RA, Shapirao HA, Goldberg HI. Ultrasonic evaluation of common bile duct stones: prospective comparison with endoscopic retrograde cholangiopancreaticography. Radiology 1983; 146: 471–474.

Heyder N, Lutz H, Lux G. Ultraschall-Diagnostik via Gastroscop. Ultraschall Med 1983; 4: 85–91.

Honickman SP, Mueller PR, Wittenberg J, Simeone JC, Ferruci JT, Cronan JJ, van Sonnenberg E. Ultrasound in obstructive jaundice: prospective evaluation of the site and cause. Radiology 1983; 147: 511–515.

Lux G, Heyder N, Lutz H, et al. Endoscopic ultrasonography: technique, orientation and diagnostic possibilities. Endoscopy 1982; 14: 220.

Marchal G, Gelin J, van Steenbergen W et al. Sonographic diagnosis of intraluminal bile duct neoplasm: a report of three cases. Gastrointest Radiol 1984; 9: 329–333.

Strohm WD, Phillib J, Hagenmüller F, Classen M. Ultrasonic tomography by means of an ultrasonic fiberendoscope. Endoscopy 1980; 12: 241.

Takemoto T, Aibe T, Fuji T, Okita K. Endoscopic ultrasonography. Clin Gastroenterol 1986; 15: 2.

Tio TL, Tytgat GNJ. Endoscopic ultrasonography in the assessment of intramural and transmural infiltration of tumours in the esophagus, stomach and papilla of Vater and in the detection of extraoesophageal lesions. Endoscopy 1984; 4: 220–225.

Tio TL, Tytgat GNJ, eds. Atlas of transintestinal ultrasonography. Aalsmeer, The Netherlands: Mur-Kostverloren, 1986.

Tio TL, Den Hartog Jager FCA, Tytgat GNJ. Endoscopic ultrasonography of non-Hodgkin lymphoma of the stomach. Gastroenterology 1986; 91: 401–408.

Tytgat GNJ, Tio TL. Endoscopic ultrasonography. Scand J Gastroenterol 1986; 21 (suppl 123).

UICC, Hermanek P, Sobin LH, eds. TNM classification of malignant tumours. Berlin: Springer, 1987; 53–65.

Yamanaka T, Sakai H, Yoshida Y, et al. Clinical evaluation of an ultrasonic linear scanning system (prototype). Gastroenterol Endosc 1982; 24: 598.

4.4   Computed Tomography in Hepatobiliary and Pancreatic Malignancies

L. te Strake, J.W.A.J. Reeders

Introduction

During the last decade, computed tomography (CT) has become a well-established imaging modality for the diagnosis of liver and pancreatic disease. The advantages of CT are the display of full cross-sectional anatomy with excellent spatial resolution. The administration of intravenous contrast agents enhances contrast between normal and diseased tissue. CT allows accurate distinction to be made between vascular and biliary structures, and has become a primary modality for the evaluation of metastatic spread of hepatobiliary and pancreatic malignancies. At this stage the place of magnetic resonance imaging (MRI) has yet to be determined and will depend on the results of recent improvements such as fast imaging techniques and the use of paramagnetic contrast agents. The role of CT in the diagnosis and staging of hepatobiliary and pancreatic malignant tumors is discussed in this chapter.

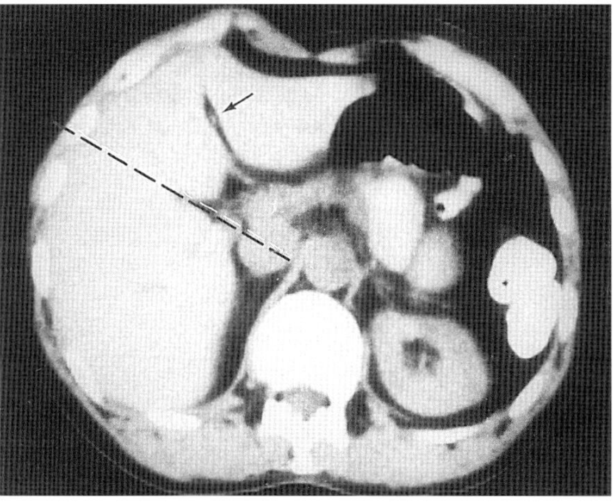

Fig. 4.4.1 **Normal liver.** The dotted line through the gallbladder fossa and the inferior vena cava represents the surgical cleavage plane between the left and right liver lobes. Note the fissure for the ligamentum teres containing low density fat (arrow)

Liver

Normal Anatomy

The normal right liver lobe is located in the right upper abdomen. The configuration of the left lobe is variable. The left liver lobe may be small or large, extending cranial and anterior to the spleen as far as the left lateral abdominal wall. Surgically the liver is divided into a left and right lobe by an imaginary plane through the gallbladder fossa and the inferior vena cava (Fig. 4.4.1). The fissure for the ligamentum teres divides the left liver lobe into a medial and lateral segment. The right lobe consists of an anterior and posterior segment. The fissure for the ligamentum venosum and the inferior vena cava are the anterior and posterior borders of the caudate lobe. Multiple venous branches drain the caudate lobe directly into the inferior vena cava. The remainder of the liver drains via the right, middle and left liver vein into the inferior vena cava. The main right and left lobar portal venous branches are well visualized as hypodense tubular structures compared to normal liver tissue. In case of diffuse fatty infiltration of the liver, blood vessels stand out as high-density structures compared to the low-density liver parenchyma.

Normal intrahepatic ducts, which run parallel to the portal venous branches, are not shown on CT. The gallbladder lies in the gallbladder fossa, extending from the liver hilum caudally along the posterior aspect of the right liver lobe. Occasionally the gallbladder may have an intrahepatic position, or may be absent in the case of agenesis. Intrahepatic branches of the hepatic artery and portal vein are well visualized during the arterial and venous phase following intravenous injection of contrast material. On these images the normal hepatic duct and common bile duct are also well shown as low-density structures within the liver hilum and hepatoduodenal ligament.

Technical Considerations

Precise determination of the number and extent of liver malignancies is particularly important for the management of those patients who are candidates for surgery. Detection of focal liver disease depends on the differences in attenuation between normal and tumor tissue. CT has been reported to be slightly more accurate than ultrasound and scintigraphy in the detection of liver metastases and as the best single test for the detection of hepatic neoplasms (Alderson et al. 1983, Zeman et al. 1985). However, the results in a single study will largely depend on the type of tumor, its vascularity and the examination technique (Fig. 4.4.2). Overall, regardless of the technique, CT appears not to be accurate enough to determine the resectability of liver tumors preoperatively (Lundstedt et al. 1987).

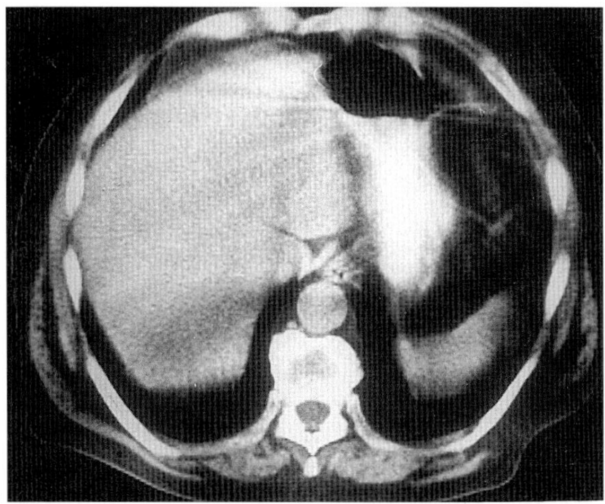

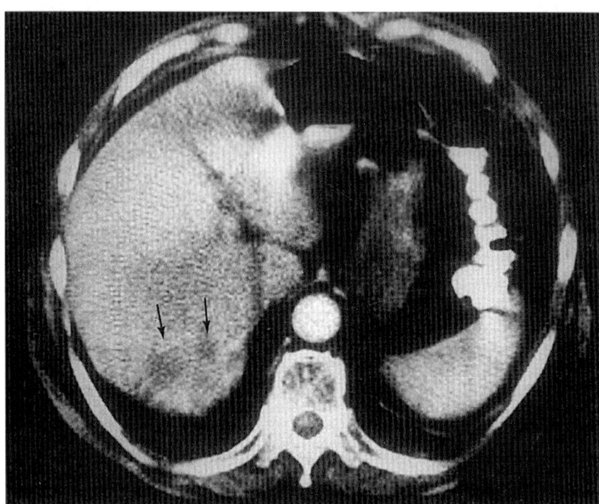

Fig. 4.4.2   Liver metastases of pancreatic carcinoma
a   Metastases, isodense on precontrast scan
b   During contrast infusion, several hypodense metastases become visible (arrows)

Dynamic incremental scanning within 4 min after intravenous injection of a high dose iodine load (50 g) increases the sensitivity of CT for the detection of focal liver disease compared to the precontrast scans (Folen et al. 1983). Using this technique of rapid sequential scanning during and immediately after contrast injection, the attenuation differences are increased between normal, rapidly enhancing liver tissue and usually hypovascular liver metastasis. However, the value of precontrast scans should not be underestimated. In a number of cases the presence of focal liver disease on precontrast scans will be sufficient to terminate the examination. Moreover, metastases from hypervascular tumors may be visible on precontrast scans only and become isodense on postcontrast, resulting in false-negative CT findings (Bressler et al. 1987).

Delayed hepatic CT scanning, 4–6 h after intravenous injection of a slightly higher dose (60 g)

of iodine than for dynamic incremental scanning, has been described as a technique which improves the detection of liver metastases compared to dynamic incremental contrast-enhanced CT, and which is helpful in questionable hepatic involvement (Bernardino et al. 1986). The contrast between tumor and normal liver is improved by delayed selective secretion into the biliary system of 1–2 % of the injected iodine by normal liver tissue. A similar effect is created by intravenous injection of an ethiodized oil emulsion (EOE-13). EOE-13 accummulates in normal liver tissue and increases the contrast between normal liver and non-enhancing metastases. The results of EOE-13 CT appear comparable to delayed hepatic scanning (Miller et al. 1987).

A more invasive and expensive procedure is CT arteriography (CTA). CT is performed immediately after selective infusion of 10–12 ml of 30 % iodinated contrast material into the hepatic artery during each scan. CTA enhances primary and secondary liver tumors, and appears to be more sensitive than dynamic incremental CT following intravenous bolus injection (Freeny and Marks 1983). CTA is more expensive and requires hospitalization, and should therefore be reserved preoperatively for patients who are candidates for liver resection.

Arterial portography CT (AP-CT) is less useful, because of a high false-positive rate (predictive value of a positive test: 63 %) (Miller et al. 1987). With AP-CT, contrast is injected into the superior mesenteric artery and reaches the liver via the portal vein.

In summary, a number of different techniques for contrast enhancement have recently been described and compared. EOE-13 is a relatively new contrast agent, which is not yet commercially available. For practical reasons at present, a precontrast scan, followed by a bolus injection and dynamic incremental scanning, depending on the findings in precontrast CT, should be considered the technique of choice rather than a single bolus injection and/or drip infusion with a non-dynamic CT examination (Zeman et al. 1985). In selected cases, delayed CT scanning 4–6 h after the initial study is a further option, as a routine procedure to improve the detection of focal liver disease.

Liver Tumors

Hepatocellular carcinoma

The appearance of hepatocellular carcinoma has been described as multicentric (50 %), solitary (40 %) or diffuse (Teefey et al. 1986). On precontrast scans, the tumor can be hypodense or isodense compared to normal liver tissue (Kunstlinger et al.

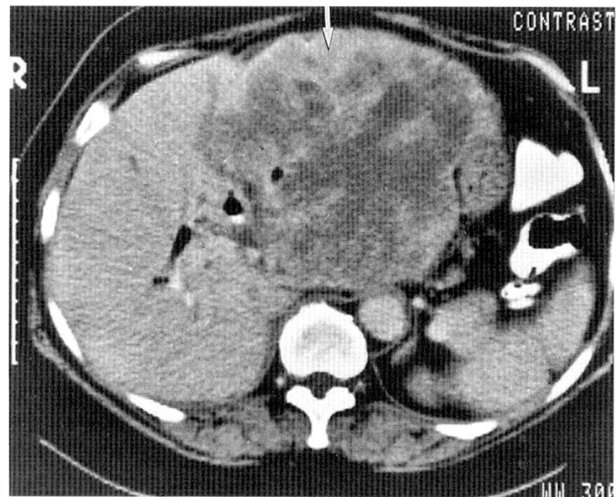

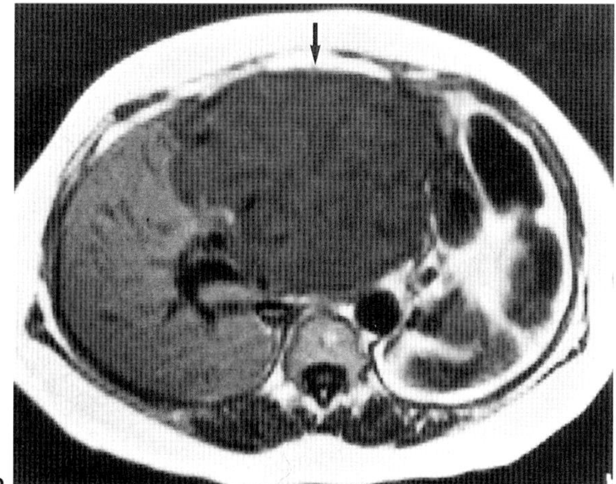

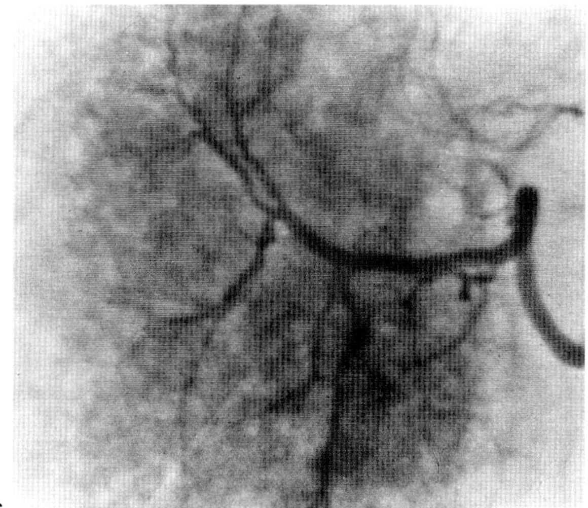

1980). Calcifications in a variety of patterns may be present in up to 25 % of cases (Teefey et al. 1986, Kunstlinger et al. 1980). Bolus injection followed by dynamic CT scanning (Fig. 4.4.3) is useful for the detection of isodense tumor, involvement of the portal vein and inferior vena cava, as well as for the demonstration of arteriovenous shunts and vascular pools (Hosoki 1982, Kunstlinger et al. 1980). Signs of portal vein involvement (Fig. 4.4.4) include increased diameter of the vessel, hypodensity, nonvisualization of a lobar portal vein, periportal hypervascularization, arterioportal shunting and differences in lobar attenuation (Mathieu et al. 1984). Biliary duct dilation occurs as a result of obstruction of the bile duct system by the tumor.

Compared to ultrasonography, CT is the best modality for showing lymph node involvement (Teefey et al. 1986). The findings on CT in hepatocellular carcinoma are not specific and may mimic other benign and malignant liver conditions (Kunstlinger et al. 1980).

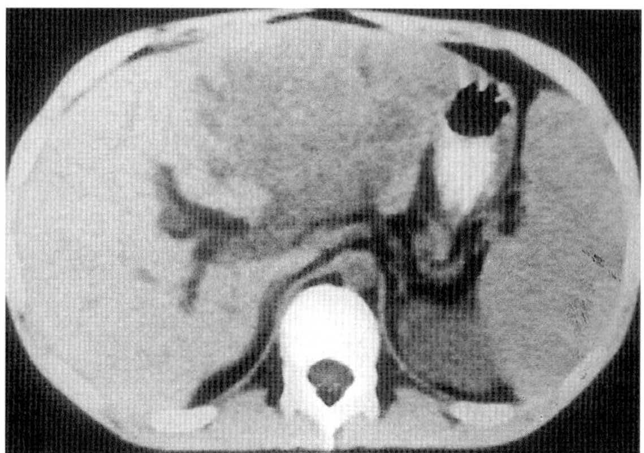

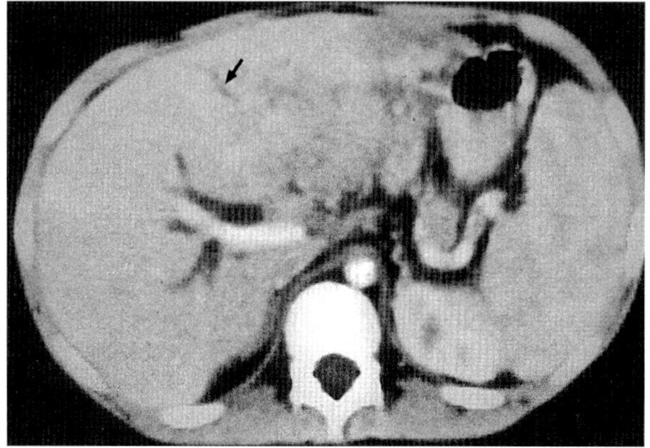

Fig. 4.4.**3** **Primary hepatocellular carcinoma;** large solitary tumor mass in the left liver lobe with necrosis.
a Contrast-enhanced CT: nodular isodense mass with multiple hypodense areas and a hypervascular rim
b MRI: tumor mass in the left liver lobe with low signal on SET
c Selective angiography of the left hepatic artery: extensive encasement and tumor "blush"

Fig. 4.4.**4** **Primary hepatocellular carcinoma**
a Precontrast scan. Hypodense tumor occupying the left liver lobe. Dilated intrahepatic bile ducts in the right liver lobe
b Dynamic CT scan during bolus injection shows the involvement of the left lobar portal vein and dilated bile ducts of the left liver lobe better (arrow)

Metastasis

The detection of liver metastases depends on the size of the lesions, the vascularity, and the examination technique used. The overall reported accuracy of CT ranges from 80%–90% (Alderson et al. 1983, Lundstedt et al. 1987, Miller et al. 1987). Metastases present as round or oval hypodense lesions and should be differentiated from focal fatty infiltration (Halvorsen et al. 1982). Focal fatty infiltration is non-spherical in configuration, does not show mass effect, and has a density close to that of water. Radionuclide liver-spleen scan will show a defect in case of metastasis and uptake, if fatty infiltration is present. Metastases can be necrotic or contain cystic components, and may mimic benign cystic neoplasm, abscesses or chronic hematoma (Barnes et al. 1981). Secondary diffuse involvement of the liver by lymphoma (Fig. 4.4.**15**) remains undetected on CT, and the overall sensitivity of CT for the detection of hepatic lymphoma has been reported to be as low as 57% (Zornoza and Grinaldi 1981).

Differential Diagnosis of Malignant Hepatic Tumors

Benign liver cysts are of water density and may be either solitary or multiple (Fig. 4.4.**5**). These cysts have a smooth wall with or without septations, and show no contrast enhancement. The differential diagnosis of a simple cyst includes cystadenoma, metastases of primary leiomyosarcoma or carcinoma of the colon, ovary or testis, melanoma, lymphangioma, abscess, chronic hematoma and pseudocyst (Barnes et al. 1981, Federle et al. 1981). Echinococcal cysts are unilocular or multilocular. The presence of calcifications and daughter cysts within the cyst wall are typical findings of hydatid disease.

Cavernous hemangiomas (Fig. 4.4.**6**) represent the most frequent benign solid liver masses. Typical features of cavernous hemangioma on CT are: a) diminished density on precontrast scan; b) early peripheral enhancement after contrast injection; c) progressive opacification from periphery to center; d) a delay of at least 3 min before total opacification; e) isodense appearance, with or without a hypodense cleft on delayed-scan images (Ashida et al. 1987). There is an 86% chance that a lesion with this typical appearance is actually a hemangioma (Freeny and Marks 1986).

Focal nodular hyperplasia (FNH) (Fig. 4.4.**16**) and hepatic adenoma (HA) (Fig. 4.4.**7**) are less frequent. These solid tumors are hypodense or isodense on precontrast scans. After contrast enhancement, they may become isodense, following initial hyperdensity during the arterial phase. A central scar of fibrous tissue is often present in

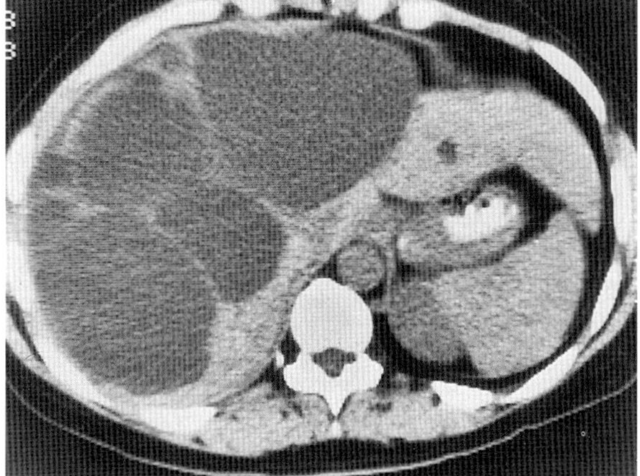
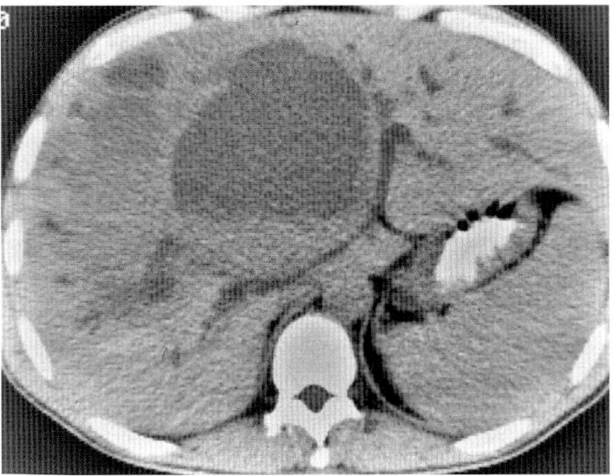

Fig. 4.4.**5 a** **Multiple benign liver cysts** in the right and left liver lobes
b **Multiple malignant liver cysts** in the right liver lobe. Note the irregular inner contour of the large cyst. Diagnosis: hemangioendothelioma

FNH. However, not all FNHs have a central scar, and a cavernous hemangioma may exhibit a cleft with similar appearance (Ashida et al. 1987, Fishman et al. 1982). HA is associated with long-term use of oral contraceptives. Patients often present with acute upper abdominal pain due to spontaneous hemorrhage and sometimes rupture and hemoperitoneum. During the acute phase, areas of high density within the tumor, representing fresh blood, can be noted. Hypodense areas in the central part of HA are due to necrosis or old blood (Fig. 4.4.**7**). FNH is not encapsulated, whereas HA is surrounded by a capsule consisting of hepatocytes with large fat vacuoles. This capsule of HA can be seen on CT as a ring of low fat density (Angres et al. 1980). Spontaneous regression of HA over a period of two years after discontinuation of oral contraceptives has been observed (Penkava et al. 1981). Radionuclide liver scan is helpful in differentiating FNH and HA because of the defect shown in HA and the usual uptake in the region of FNH (Federle et al. 1981).

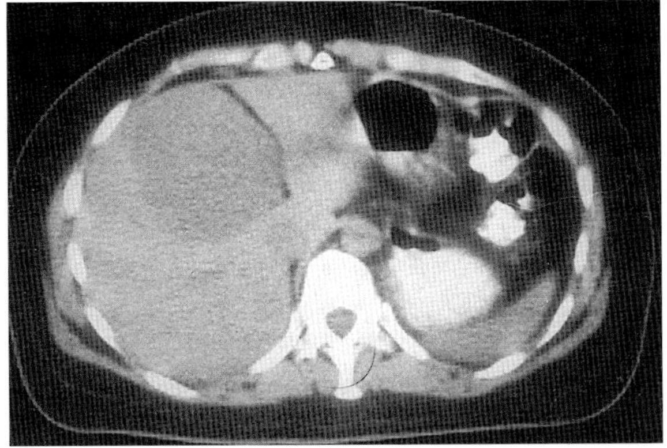

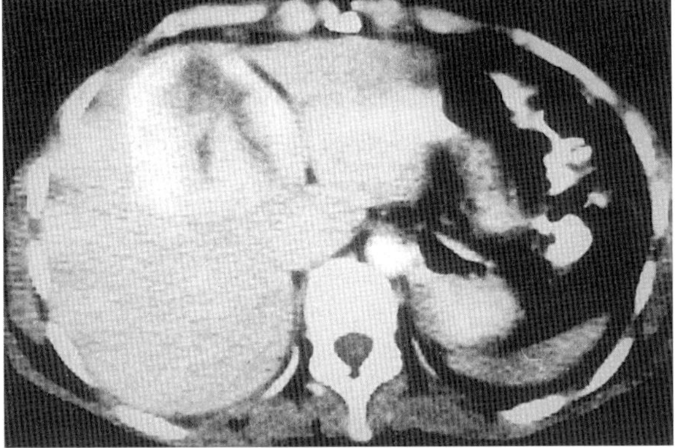

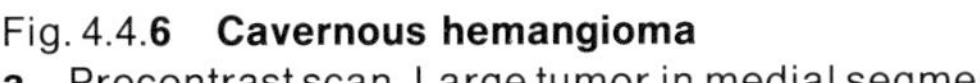

Fig. 4.4.**6** **Cavernous hemangioma**
a Precontrast scan. Large tumor in medial segment of left liver lobe
b Dynamic scan during bolus injection shows typical peripheral enhancement

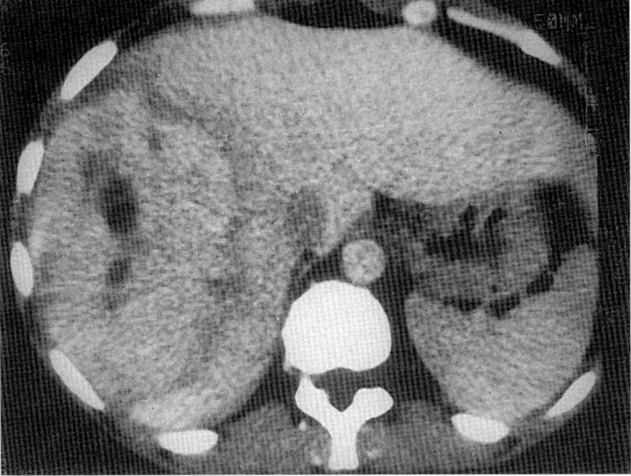

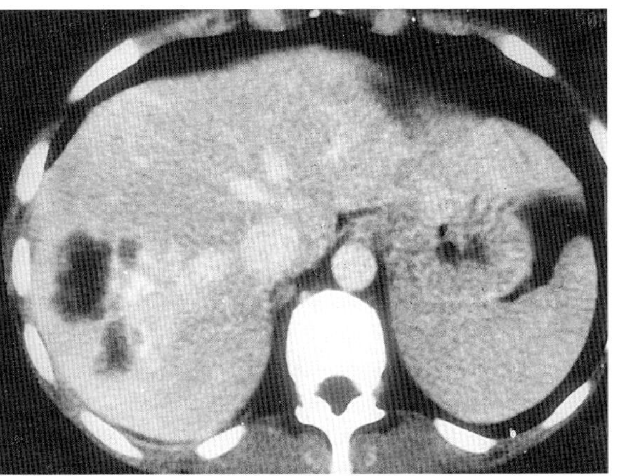

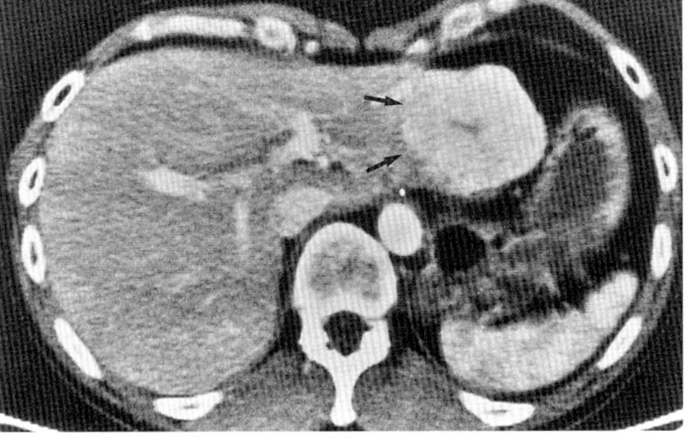

Fig. 4.4.**7** **Hepatic adenoma**
a Large enhancing tumor with peripheral hypodense rim and central necrosis due to previous episode of bleeding
b Five months later, after discontinuation of oral contraceptives, the tumor has decreased in size. Because of contra-indication to surgery neither laparotomy or biopsy were performed. The patient has been well during a follow-up of two years, with no clinical evidence of malignancy
c Dynamic CT: hyperdense, hypervascular round mass at left liver lobe with central necrosis (arrows)

Biliary Tract Tumors

Gallbladder Carcinoma

A symptomatic patient with gallbladder carcinoma usually suffers from advanced-stage disease. The most common finding is a mass replacing the gallbladder (Itai et al. 1980, Weiner et al. 1984). After contrast injection, gallbladder carcinoma tends to show strong enhancement (Itai 1980). Irregular thickening of the gallbladder wall and an intraluminal mass are signs of gallbladder carcinoma in less advanced disease. Direct spread to the liver is noted as a low-density area adjacent to the gallbladder (Fig. 4.4.**8a**). Tumor extension into the extrahepatic duct has been observed in 7% (Weiner et al. 1984). Gallstones are present in over 50% of cases. A porcelain gallbladder may be present in 25%, and should raise the suspicion of gallbladder carcinoma (Fig. 4.4.**8b**). Dilated intra- or extrahepatic bile ducts are a frequent finding (up to 50%), due to direct tumor extension into the bile ducts or compression by liver or lymph node

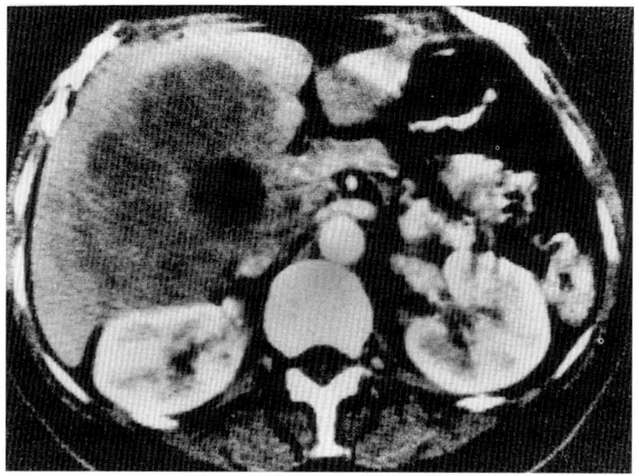

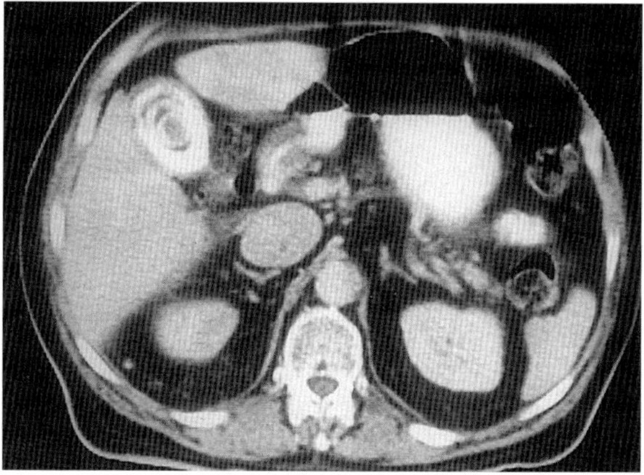

Fig. 4.4.**8 a**   **Contrast-enhanced CT:** nodular, hypodense well-delineated mass around gallbladder. Diagnosis: gallbladder carcinoma with extensive invasion into the liver parenchyma
b   **Porcelain gallbladder** and gallstones in asymptomatic patient. Note thickened wall. Gallbladder carcinoma should be excluded

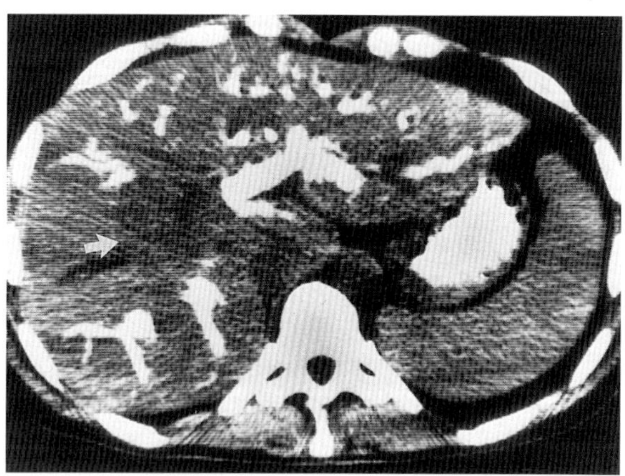

Fig. 4.4.**9**   **Hypodense mass at liver hilum.** Note obstruction of the intrahepatic dilated bile ducts of the right and left liver lobes, with stasis of contrast (introduced two days before via ERCP). Diagnosis: malignant Klatskin tumor

metastases. Metastatic lymph nodes around the distal common bile duct and pancreas may mimic pancreatic carcinoma (Weiner et al. 1984). The differential diagnosis includes acute or chronic cholecystitis, cholangiocarcinoma, liver tumor, and adenoma or polyp of the gallbladder, as well as intraluminal clot (Thorsen et al. 1984).

Cholangiocarcinoma

Primary biliary duct carcinoma presents as a hypodense or isodense mass compared to the liver. Cholangiocarcinoma tends to show less enhancement than gallbladder carcinoma (Thorsen et al. 1984). Intra- or extrahepatic biliary dilation is present in the majority of cases. Intrahepatic cholangiocarcinomas can be large tumors at the time of diagnosis, and difficult to differentiate from hepatocellular carcinoma. Some 26 % of cholangiocarcinomas are located at the junction of the right and left intrahepatic duct (Thorsen et al. 1984). These Klatskin tumors, as well as those arising in the distal hepatic or common bile duct, may be only 1–2 cm in diameter when detected in the jaundiced patient (Fig. 4.4.**9**). Rapid dynamic scanning immediately after a bolus injection is useful for better delineation of the tumor, portal vein and bile ducts. Gross lobar liver atrophy has been described as a finding in 19 % of patients with hilar cholangiocarcinoma (Klatskin tumor) (Carr et al. 1985).

Multiple benign bile duct hamartomas should be included in the differential diagnosis in patients with focal liver defects on CT and no clinical evidence of malignancy (Eisenberg et al. 1986). A choledochal cyst of moderate size should be considered as a possible diagnosis in patients with normal intrahepatic ducts and dilated common bile duct (Araki et al. 1980).

Pancreas

Normal Anatomy

Landmarks for the localization of the pancreas are the splenic vein and the confluence with the superior mesenteric vein. The head of the pancreas is positioned immediately anterior to the inferior vena cava, in close relation with the portal vein and duodenum. The uncinate process is the part of the head of the pancreas which extends posterior to the superior mesenteric vein. The common bile duct runs posteriorly within the head of the pancreas. The pancreatic duct is not usually seen on routine 10 mm precontrast CT scans. A thin fat plane between the splenic vein and the corpus and tail of the pancreas may mimic the pancreatic duct on precontrast scans. The tail of the pancreas extends anterior to the splenic vein into the hilum of the spleen. The size of the pancreas varies with the age of the patient. The contour of the pancreas is slightly lobulated and usually well outlined by surrounding peripancreatic fat. In elderly patients, fatty replacement of the pancreas may be noted.

Technical Considerations

Patient preparation for CT of the pancreas is the same as for any CT of the upper abdomen, with the exceptation that special care should be taken to obtain adequate opacification of the stomach and duodenum by means of orally administered contrast material. The only exception to this rule are those patients who are suspected of having biliary obstruction due to common bile duct stones. These patients should initially be examined without administration of oral contrast agent. The CT examination begins with a screening of the pancreas with 10 mm collimation with or without intravenous injection of contrast. The advantage of immediate contrast injection and drip infusion is the better delineation of vascular structures from adjacent pancreas. When a tumor is suspected on the initial scan, or should be excluded, further dynamic scans are obtained after bolus contrast injection and thin 5 mm collimation.

Pancreatic Carcinoma

A mass originating within the pancreas should raise the suspicion of pancreatic carcinoma. A small carcinoma, less than 1–2 cm in size, may remain undetected on CT even if meticulous dynamic scan technique with 5 mm collimation is used. Ampullary carcinomas (Fig. 4.4.**10**) in particular tend to be missed on CT, since these tumors give rise to the clinical symptoms of obstructive jaundice at an early stage, while the tumor is small (Baron et al. 1982). A dilated distal common bile duct and dilated main pancreatic duct can complicate the search for a small hypodense carcinoma on the contrast-enhanced scan (Fig. 4.4.**11**, 4.4.**13**). The loss of normal lobulation of the surface of the pancreas is a useful sign in locating the site of a small carcinoma. A pancreatic tumor should be considered unresectable in the presence of an irregular contour, signs of involvement of large arteries and veins, enlarged lymph nodes and liver metastases (Itai et al. 1982a). An irregular contour is indicative of infiltrative growth into surrounding structures (Fig. 4.4.**12a**). A thickened celiac axis or superior mesenteric artery (Fig. 4.4.**13**) correlates

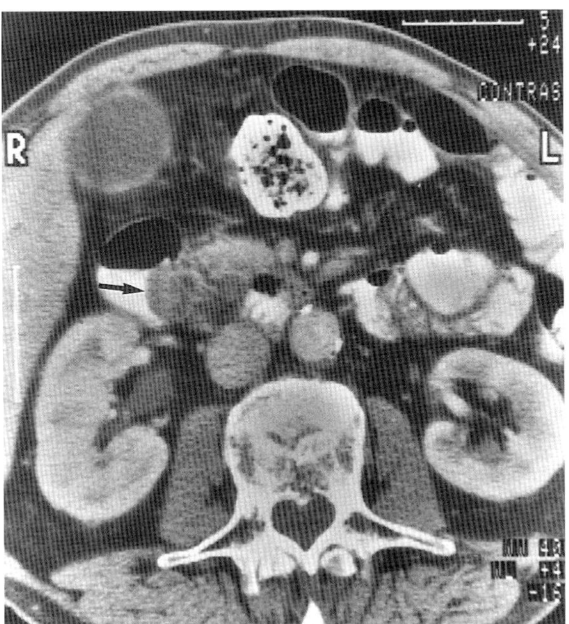

Fig. 4.4.**10** **Small round isodense lesion at the head of the pancreas,** protruding into the contrast-filled duodenum (arrow). Diagnosis: ampullary carcinoma

with tumor extension beyond the pancreatic pseudocapsule (Megibow et al. 1981). The presence of collateral vessels indicates tumor extension into the splenic, superior mesenteric or portal vein. Atrophy of the caudal portion of the pancreas has been described in both resectable and unresectable carcinoma (Itai et al. 1982a). Cyst formation has been reported in 8 % of proven pancreatic carcinomas (Itai et al. 1982b). These retention cysts have a similar appearance on CT to pseudocysts due to pancreatitis. Differentiation between pancreatic carcinoma and pancreatitis on CT can be difficult (Fig. 4.4.**12a**, **b**) or impossible without biopsy, since pancreatitis may be localized and present as a mass, or can occur secondary to a pre-existing carcinoma.

Cystadenoma and cystadenocarcinoma (Fig. 4.4.**13c**) present as frequently large multilocular cystic tumors. The diagnosis of papillary carcinoma should be considered in cases of a partially cystic mass (Kim et al. 1985). Papillary carcinoma presents as a large solid mass with cystic degeneration, often in young patients. Single or multiple metastases to the pancreas of primary kidney, breast or uterine malignancies, as well as melanoma, present as solid pancreatic masses and should be differentiated from pancreatic carcinoma (Rumancik et al. 1984). Pleomorphic carcinoma of the pancreas usually appears as a large mass with extensive metastatic lymph node metastases, and may mimic lymphoma (Wolfman et al. 1985).

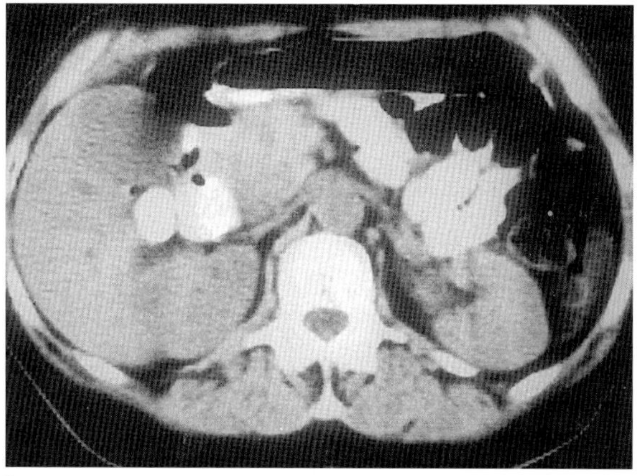

a

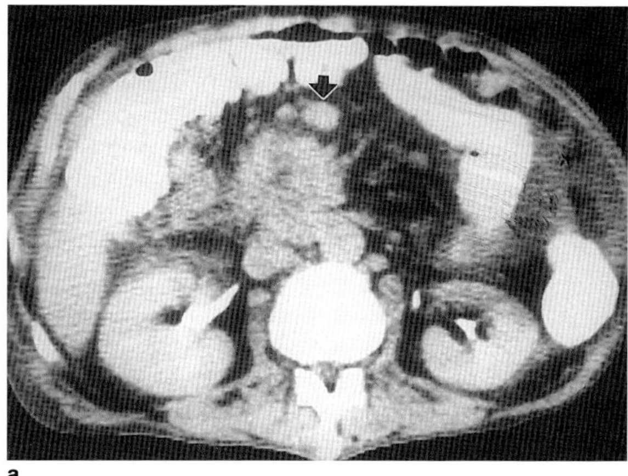

a

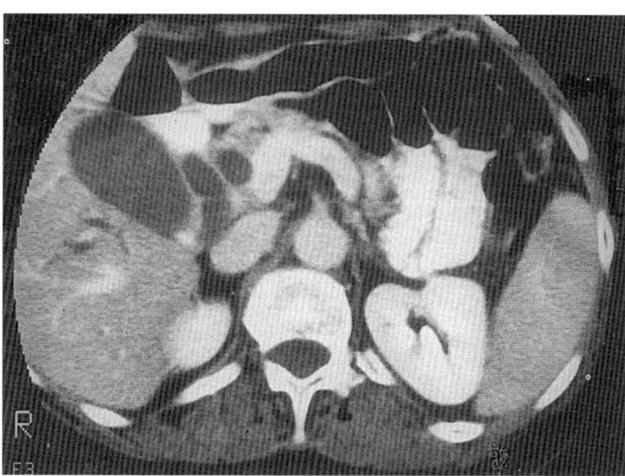

b

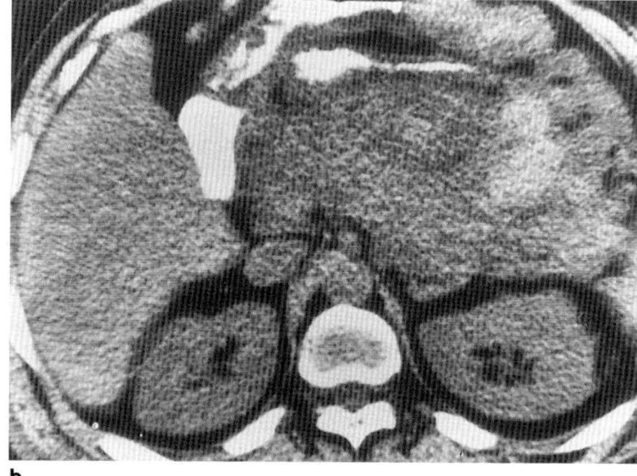

b

Fig. 4.4.12   Pancreatic carcinoma
a Irregular contour due to infiltration of the peripancreatic fat. Note mesenteric lymph node metastasis (arrow)
b Irregular isodense mass at pancreatic corpus region with areas of focal hypodensity (representing necrosis) and hyperdensity (representing hemorrhage). Diagnosis: hemorrhagic necrotizing pancreatitis

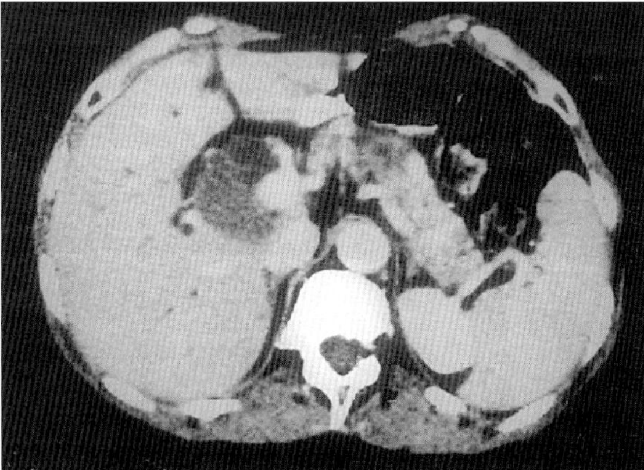

c

Fig. 4.4.11   Carcinoma of the head of the pancreas
a Precontrast scan. Large mass of the head of the pancreas. Fat plane between tumor and inferior vena cava intact
b Dynamic scan during bolus injection. Note dilated intrahepatic ducts, and dilated cystic and common bile duct
c Dynamic scan during bolus injection and thin 5 mm collimation shows normal-sized main pancreatic duct

Islet Cell Tumors

Islet cell tumors of the pancreas can be divided into two groups: **non-functioning and functioning islet cell tumors**. Non-functioning islet cell tumors are readily diagnosed on CT (96–100%) since they present as a large mass measuring up to 20 cm in diameter (Eelkema et al. 1984, Stark et al. 1984). Non-functioning islet cell tumors are difficult to differentiate from ductal adenocarcinoma (Fig. 4.4.14). Dilation of the common bile duct and pancreatic duct, atrophy of the caudal part as well as hepatic and lymph node metastasis, are also frequent findings in non-functioning islet cell tumors. Features that are to some extent typical for non-functioning islet cell tumor include calcifications, enhancement after contrast administration,

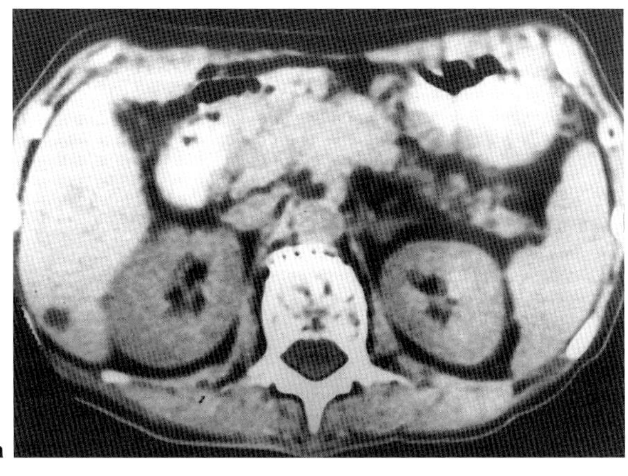

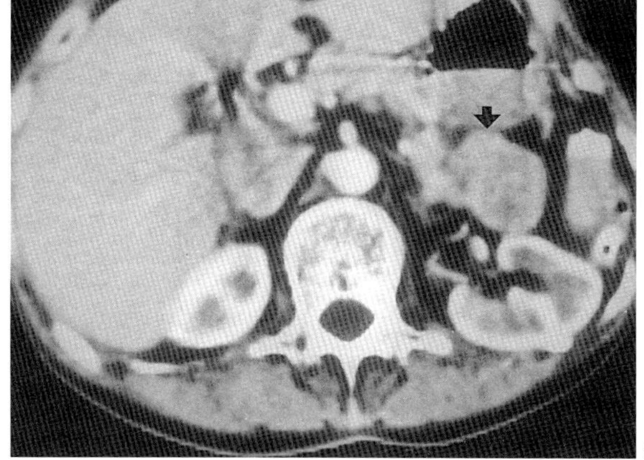

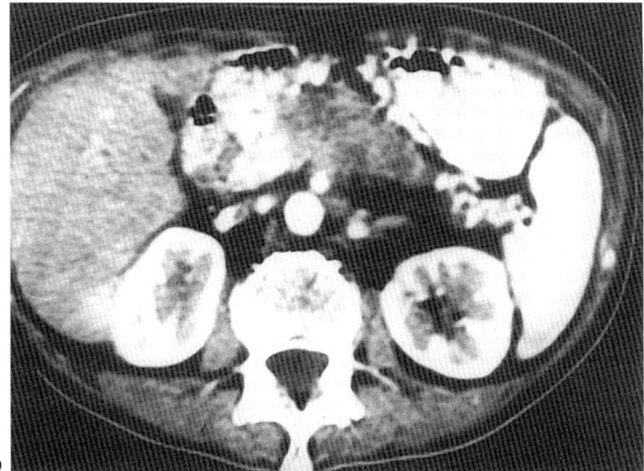

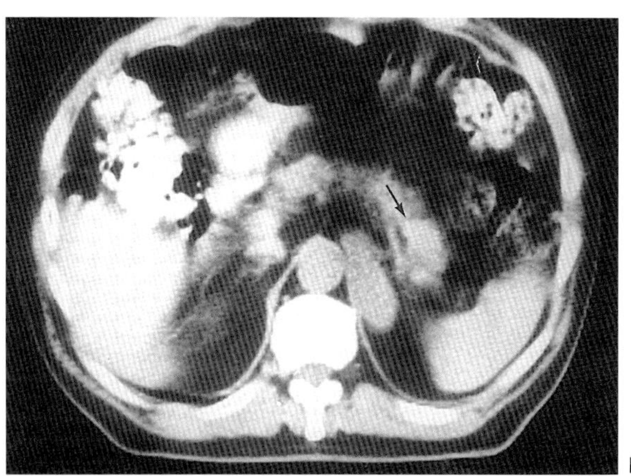

Fig. 4.4.**14 a** **Non-functioning islet cell tumor** in the tail of the pancreas (arrow)

b **Functioning islet cell tumor** in the tail of the pancreas. Gastrinoma in a patient with multiple endocrine adenomatosis (MEA I) syndrome. Note the associated left adrenal tumor. Gastrinoma shows enhancement after contrast injection (arrow)

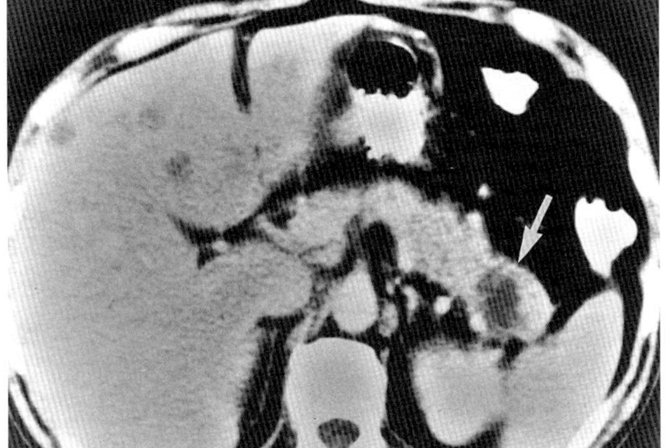

Fig. 4.4.**13** **Pancreatic carcinoma**

a Precontrast scan showing irregular posterior contour of the pancreas and liver metastases

b Dynamic CT during bolus injection shows enhancement of the lumen of the superior mesenteric artery and thickened wall

c Contrast-enhanced CT: irregularly delineated hypodense mass at the tail of the pancreas (arrow). Diagnosis: cystadenocarcinoma of the tail of the pancreas. Compare the patient's ultrasound examination: Fig. 4.2.**16**

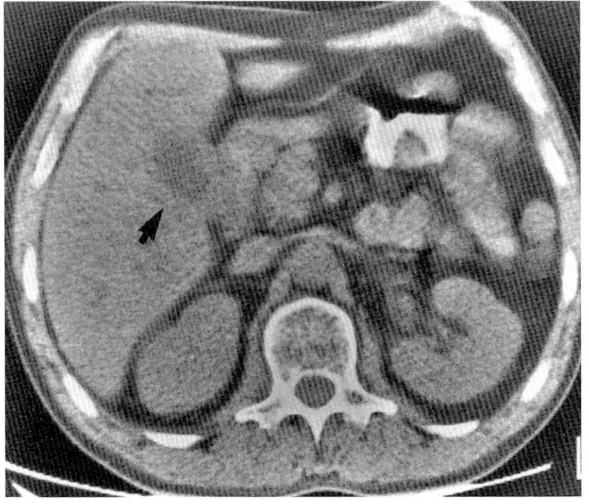

Fig. 4.4.**15** Small, hypodense, well-delineated mass (arrow) in isodense liver parenchyma. Diagnosis: non-Hodgkin lymphoma of the liver

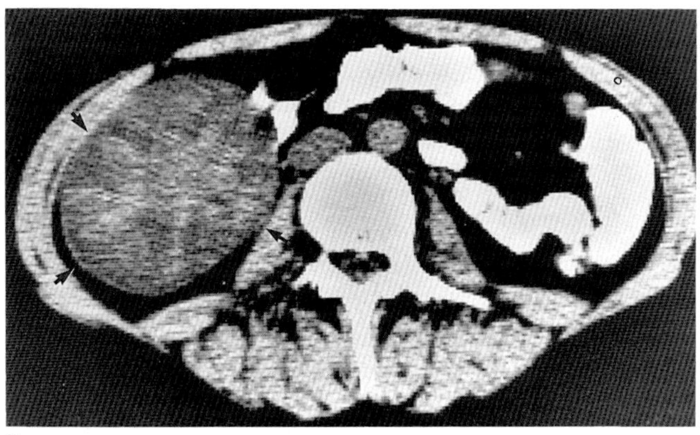

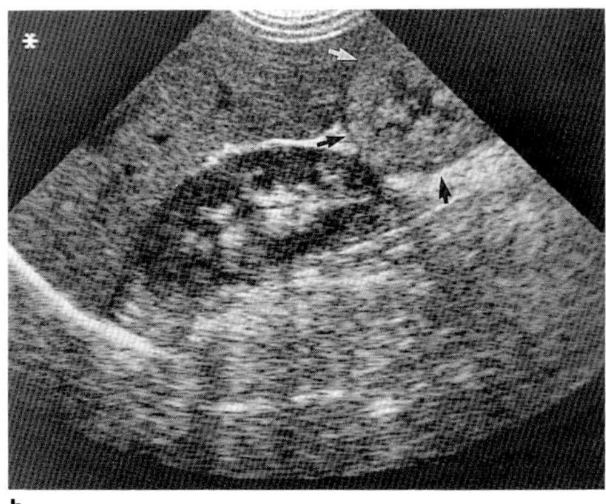

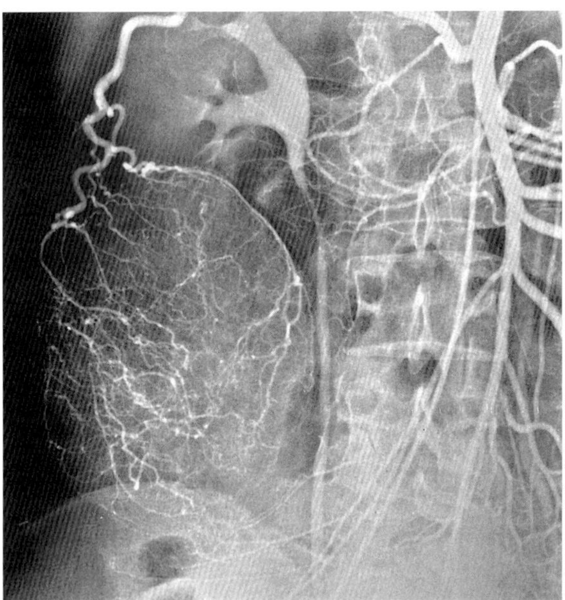

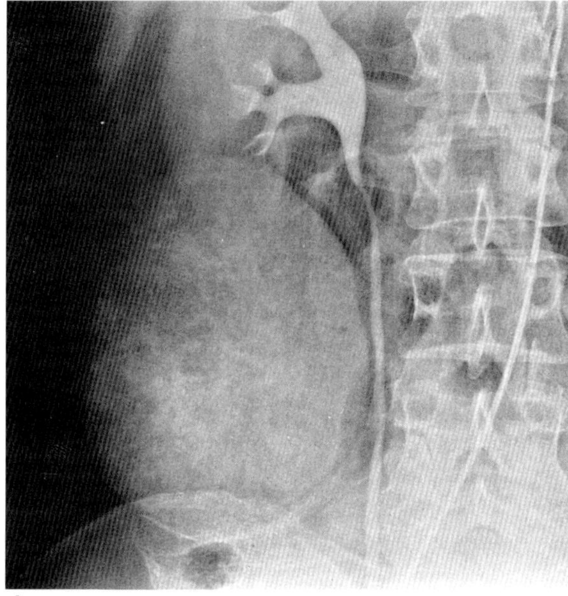

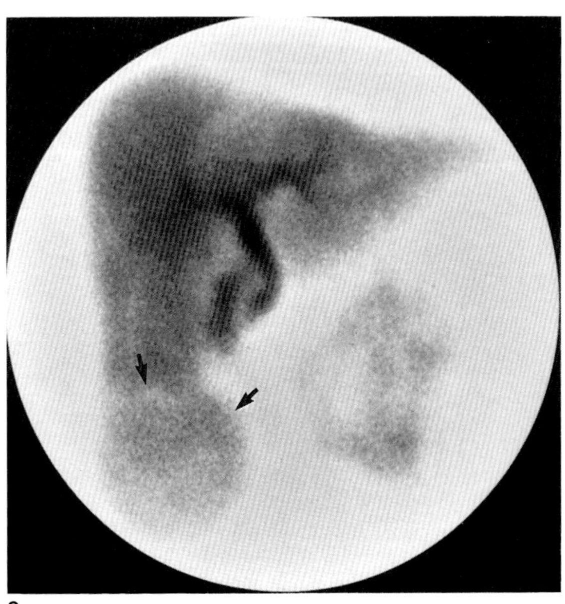

Fig. 4.4.**16**   **Focal nodular hyperplasia of right liver lobe**
a   CT: smooth-edged, round, isodense mass with diffuse hypo- and hyperdense areas in the right liver lobe (arrows)
b   US: hyperechogenic round mass with hypo- and hyperechogenic structures (arrows)
c, d   Angiography: selective catheterization of SMA. Arterial (**c**) and venous (**d**) phase. Hypervascular round structure at the right liver lobe. The main feeding vessel originates from the SMA
e   Nuclear scintigraphy: round structure (arrows) with diminished uptake in the right liver lobe

and absence of involvement of the mesenteric or celiac artery (Eelkema et al. 1984).

The detection of functioning islet cell tumors on CT is strongly dependent on the size and localization of the tumor. Gastrinomas less than 1 cm in diameter are prone to be missed on CT, whereas 83–95% of tumors larger than 3 cm will be detected (Wank et al. 1987). CT is less successful in the detection of extrapancreatic gastrinomas than in the detection of tumors of pancreatic origin (Rossi et al. 1985, Wank et al. 1987). Insulinomas, which are often very small, can be localized in approximately 50%, and gastrinomas in 75% of cases (Stark et al. 1984). In a series of 16 small islet cell tumors measuring 7–20 mm in diameter, CT detected 7 tumors (Günther et al. 1983). Functioning islet cell tumors do enhance after contrast administration, and dynamic contrast-enhanced CT scan is mandatory to facilitate the detection of these frequently small tumors (Fig. 4.4.**14b**). False-positive scans may result from tortuous splenic vessels or bowel loops. In the search for islet cell tumors, CT should be considered as a primary imaging modality, prior to angiography.

References

Alderson PO, et al. Computed tomography, ultrasound and scintigraphy of the liver in patients with colon or breast carcinoma: a prospective comparison. Radiology 1983; 149: 225.

Angres G, et al. Unusual ring in liver cell adenoma. AJR 1980; 135: 172.

Araki T, et al. CT of choledochal cyst. AJR 1980; 135: 729.

Ashida C, et al. Computed tomography of hepatic cavenous hemangioma. J Comput Assist Tomogr 1987; 11: 455.

Barnes PA, et al. Pitfalls in the diagnosis of hepatic cysts by computed tomography. Radiology 1981; 141: 129.

Baron RL, et al. A prospective comparison of the evaluation of biliary obstruction using compared tomography and ultrasonography. Radiology 1982; 145: 91.

Bernardino ME, et al. Delayed hepatic CT scanning: increased confidence and improved detection of hepatic metastases. Radiology 1986; 159: 71.

Bressler EL, et al. Hypervascular hepatic metastases: CT evaluation. Radiology 1987; 162: 49.

Carr DH, et al. Computed tomography of hilar cholangiocarcinoma: a new sign. AJR 1985; 145: 53.

Eelkema EA, et al. CT features of nonfunctioning islet cell carcinoma. AJR 1984; 143: 943.

Eisenberg D, et al. CT and sonography of multiple bile-duct hamartomas simulating malignant liver disease (case report). AJR 1986; 147: 279.

Federle MP, et al. Cystic hepatic neoplasms: complementary roles of CT and sonography. AJR 1981; 136: 345.

Fishman EK, et al. Computed tomography of benign hepatic tumors. J Comput Assist Tomogr 1982; 6: 472.

Foley WD, et al. Contrast enhancement technique for dynamic hepatic computed tomographic scanning. Radiology 1983; 147: 797.

Freeny PC, Marks MM. Computed arteriography of the liver. Radiology 1983; 148: 193.

Freeny PC, Marks WM. Patterns of contrast enhancement of benign and malignant hepatic neoplasms during bolus dynamic and delayed CT. Radiology 1986; 160: 613.

Günther RW, et al. Islet-cell tumors: detection of small lesions with computed tomography and ultrasound. Radiology 1983; 148: 485.

Halvorsen RA, et al. CT appearance of focal fatty infiltration of the liver. AJR 1982; 139: 277.

Hosoki T. Dynamic computed tomography of hepatocellular carcinoma. AJR 1982; 139: 1099.

Itai Y, et al. Computed tomography of gallbladder carcinoma. Radiology 1980; 137: 13.

Itai Y, et al. Pancreatic cysts caused by carcinoma of the pancreas: a pittfall in the diagnosis of pancreatic carcinoma. J Comput Assist Tomogr 1982a; 6: 772.

Itai Y, et al. Computed tomographic appearance of resectable pancreatic carcinoma. Radiology 1982b; 143: 719.

Kim, SY, et al. Papillary carcinoma of the pancreas: findings by US and CT. Radiology 1985; 154: 338.

Kunstlinger F, et al. Computed tomography of hepatocellular carcinoma. AJR 1980; 134: 431.

Lundstedt C, et al. Site and number of liver tumors recorded at angiography and computed tomography compared with the findings at laparotomy and of resected liver specimens. Acta Radiol 1987; 28: 153.

Lüning M, et al. CT diagnosis of hepatic adenoma. Eur J Radiol 1987; 7: 30.

Mathieu D, et al. Portal vein involvement in hepatocellular carcinoma: dynamic CT features. Radiology 1984; 152: 127.

Megibow AJ, et al. Thickening of the celiac axis and/or superior mesenteric artery: a sign of pancreatic carcinoma on computed tomography. Radiology 1981; 141: 449.

Miller DL, et al. Hepatic metastasis detection: comparison of three CT contrast enhancement methods. Radiology 1987; 165: 785.

Penkava RR, et al. Spontaneous resolution of oral-contraceptive-associated liver tumor. J Comput Assist Tomogr 1981; 5: 102.

Rossi P, et al. CT of functioning tumors of the pancreas. AJR 1985; 144: 57.

Rumancik WM, et al. Metastatic disease to the pancreas: evaluation by computed tomography. J Comput Assist Tomogr 1984; 8: 829.

Stark DD, et al. CT of pancreatic islet cell tumors. Radiology 1984; 150: 491.

Teefey SA, et al. Computed tomography and ultrasonography of hepatoma. Clin Radiol 1986; 37: 339.

Thorsen MK, et al. Primary biliary carcinoma: CT evaluation. Radiology 1984; 152: 479.

Wank SA, et al. Prospective study of the ability of computed axial tomography to localize gastrinomas in patients with Zollinger-Ellison syndrome. Gastroenterology 1987; 92: 905.

Weiner SN, et al. Sonography and computed tomography in the diagnosis of carcinoma of the gallbladder. AJR 1984; 142: 735.

Wolfman NT, et al. Pleomorphic carcinoma of the pancreas: computed-tomographic, sonographic, and pathologic findings. Radiology 1985; 154: 329.

Zeman RL, et al. Hepatic imaging: current status. Radiol Clin North Am 1985; 23: 473.

Zornoza J, Grinaldi S. Computed tomography in hepatic lymphoma. Radiology 1981; 138: 405.

4.5 Magnetic Resonance Imaging (MRI) in Hepatobiliary and Pancreatic Malignancies

L. Engelholm, D. Mathieu, C. Segebarth, J.M. Bigot, J. de Toeuf, and M. Zalcman

Introduction

Magnetic resonance imaging (MRI) demonstrates the liver and pancreas well and makes it possible to perform measurements of T1 and T2 relaxation times independently of one another. MRI has several advantages: direct multidirectional imaging capability, high-contrast sensitivity, and the ability to visualize hepatic structures without radiation and intravenous iodine contrast media.

The results of MRI have currently, in the liver, reached a high quality for the liver, and are competitive with computed tomography (CT) and ultrasonography (US). However, in contrast with the results in neuroradiology and the pelvis, the image quality obtained in the upper abdomen is subject to many sources of artefacts and degradation. Respiratory motion, cardiac or vascular pulsations, flow phenomena, peristaltic motion, and gross patient motion during the period of acquisition all contribute to the image degradation that may be observed.

Moreover, in hepatobiliary and pancreatic malignancies, MRI must be compared with other techniques such as US, CT and endoscopic retrograde cholangiopancreatography (ERCP). MRI has the ability to demonstrate dilatation of the biliary tree throughout its entire extent. However, the use of MRI for this particular purpose is relatively limited.

Normal Liver and Pancreas

On MRI, the normal liver and pancreas are visualized as homogeneous structure of intermediate signal intensity. MRI can define, without the use of contrast medium, vascular structures such as the aorta, the suprahepatic veins and arteries, the inferior vena cava, and the portal vein. The posterior portion of the pancreas is often well defined by the splenic vein. The anatomical segmentation of the liver is precisely defined. Sagittal or frontal slices may, in addition, analyze the suprahepatic or portal veins better. The normal bile ducts can be recognized on MR images. The pancreatic duct is only occasionally demonstrated by MRI, when the measurements are performed with body coils (Anacker et al. 1984, Davis et al. 1984, Haaga 1984a, Stark et al. 1984), and the normal Wirsung's duct is almost never visualized. However, with surface coils and thin slices, the normal pancreatic duct was seen as a linear dark structure with relatively low intensity on T1-weighted images in 5 cases out of 8 (Simeone et al. 1985).

MRI Techniques

MRI examination techniques for the liver and pancreas include the general preparation of the patient and MRI technical modalities.

General Preparation of the Patient

Hypotonia associated with gastric air distension reduces the gastric or duodenal motility, the artefacts associated with intestinal peristalsis, and enhances visualization of the pancreas (Weinreb et al. 1984b). Substances which opacify the digestive tract may be used, such as ammonium ferrite citrate (Wesbey et al. 1985), ferrite preparations (Hahn et al. 1987), or perfluorate derivates.

Liver

The slices are most often performed in the transverse plane, but sagittal or frontal planes are sometimes useful for the study of vessels or complex situations (Haaga 1984a, Hricak et al. 1985, Mathieu et al. 1988, Ros et al. 1986). The detection of liver tumors using MRI depends on good anatomic resolution and high cancer/liver contrast. Contrast between the liver and intrahepatic tumors is usually determined by T1 and T2 relaxation times of the normal liver and tumor tissue. For clinical purposes, use of both T1- and T2-weighted sequences for liver imaging are useful (Ferrucci 1986). Through analysis of the data from both types of pulse sequences, attempts to characterize lesions may be made: fat, hemorrhage, simple cysts, and fibrosis may be identified (Kressel 1988).

MRI Technical Modalities

Spin-echo sequences. Spin-echo (SE) with short TE/TR times gives T1-weighted images with excellent spatial resolution, offering good anatomic study of the liver, a good signal-to-noise ratio for magnetic fields inferior to T1, and fewer artefacts than T2-weighted images with long TE/TR (Stark et al. 1986c). Particularly short TR, short TE technique (TE 16/TR 250) is a powerful method of reducing motion artefacts and can be combined with signal averaging to suppress artefacts further, improve the signal-to-noise ratio, and maximize the best anatomic resolution (Ferrucci 1986). Interme-

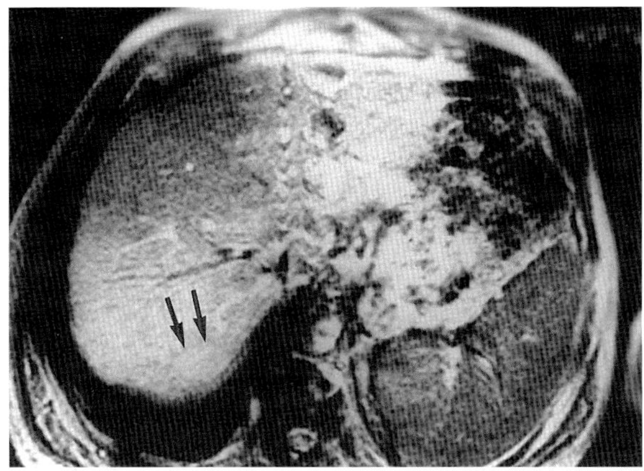

Fig. 4.5.**1**   **Fast imaging without gadolinium.** T2-weighted images SE α = 20°/54−16 msec. At the posterior portion of the right liver lobe, an ovular focal liver lesion with a slightly enhanced signal (arrows)

diate, less T1-weighted sequences (TE 30/TR 500) give a lower tumor-to-liver contrast.

T2-weighted information, obtained with long TE and TR, provides confirmation of lesion detection, often has a good contrast resolution, and is particularly useful for tissue characterization and differential diagnosis of space-occupying lesions (Demas et al. 1985, Foley et al. 1987, Glazer et al. 1986, Heiken et al. 1985, Moss et al. 1984). Multi-echo technique has often increased diagnostic success (Feinberg et al. 1985, Stark et al. 1986c).

Other MRI technical modalities (inversion recovery sequences, opposed phase technique, fast sequences, optimal pulse sequences, etc.) are beyond the scope of the present chapter and will therefore not be discussed.

Contrast Material Enhancement

The use of paramagnetic contrast agents may influence the relaxation times of the tumors or the normal liver, and intensify contrast in MRI images. Paramagnetic contrast agents modify T1 and T2 relaxation times (Brasch et al. 1984, Weinmann et al. 1984) (Figs. 4.5.**1**, 4.5.**2**). Gadolinium diethylene triamine pentaacetic acid (Gd-DTPA) (Fig. 4.5.**2**) is the most-used contrast agent (Carr et al. 1984, Curati et al. 1988, Hamm et al. 1987, Mano et al. 1987, Ohtomo et al. 1987, Runge et al. 1984). This agent is nearly identical pharmacokinetically to iodinated urographic contrast agents (Saini et al. 1986). The behavior of tumors with regard to the contrast media, such as vascularity and necrosis, must also be taken into consideration. Tumors have been found to be hypointense and hyperintense (Hamm et al. 1987). Tumors are mostly hypo-intense compared with the surrounding hepatic tissue during the dynamic examination immediately after administration of the contrast medium, and then show a comparatively high signal enhancement in later applied pulse sequences (Hamm et al. 1987). Hyperintense tumors show a rapid and very strong initial enhancement, followed by a constant level of signal intensity, and these hyperintense lesions present less contrast in the first 3 min after injection than in the precontrast images (Hamm et al. 1987).

Ferrite, an iron oxide that localizes within the reticuloendothelial system, is another contrast agent (Renshaw et al. 1986, Saini et al. 1987, Tsang et al. 1988, Weissleder et al. 1987). After IV injection, there is a powerful shortening of T2 relaxation time in the normal liver. On T2-weighted images, hepatic tumors are better detected: they appear more bright than the normal liver, related to

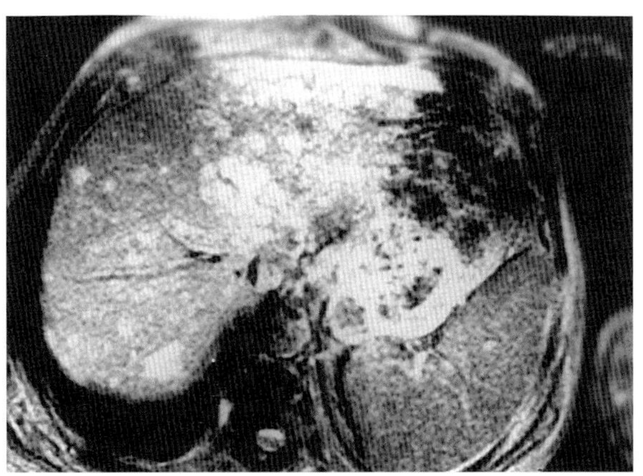

a

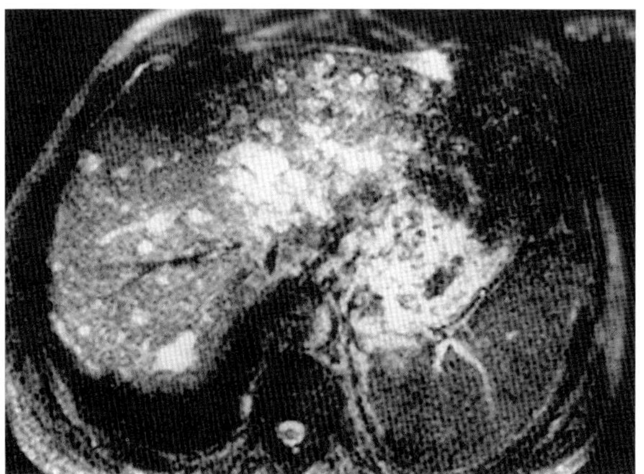

b

Fig. 4.5.**2**   **Fast imaging using gadolinium diethylene triamine pentaacetic acid** (Gd-DTPA). There are numerous other lesions in both liver lobes
a   First echo
b   Second echo

the diminution of the liver signal adjacent to the tumor (Saini et al. 1987, Weissleder et al. 1987).

With some improvements, contrast enhancement techniques will become essential in MRI of the liver.

Pancreas

The technical parameters in pulse sequences employed in the pancreas are similar to those in the liver. The use of more than one sequence is essential for adequate representation of the anatomical structures and evaluation of the pathology. There is no single optimal sequence. Pathological features not visible with one sequence may be detected by another sequence. The combination of several sequences allows MRI to approach or define the nature of pathological pancreatic structures.

T1-weighted pictures define fat planes well, provide superior anatomic detail, and have short acquisition times. T2-weighted sequences differentiate the liquid or solid nature of a pancreatic lesion better, but often produce more artefacts, especially at high field strength.

Multiple echos are useful. Multiple echo technique is interesting in differentiating the liquid or solid nature of a pancreatic enlargement, or in detecting necrotic areas in a tumor.

Pathology

MRI Features of Malignant Liver and Biliary Tumors

Primary liver tumors. Morphological MRI patterns of tumors are similar to those of CT: variable contour sharpness, size, location and local vascular displacement. The signal intensity of primary hepatic tumors, compared with normal liver, varies depending upon the MRI parameters and pulse sequences used to obtain the image. Most solid tumors possess increased intracellular water and therefore show prolongation of T1 and T2 relaxation time. They are dark on T1-weighted and brighter on T2-weighted sequences. Lipomas or hemorrhagic lesions may present a relatively enhanced signal on T1-weighted images. Tumors with central liquefaction necrosis or rich vascularization acquire the characteristics of fluids, and may show varying degrees of homogeneous persistence of a bright signal on late-echo images. Such cases may mimic hemangiomas or cysts.

Hepatocellular Carcinomas. Several authors (Ebara et al. 1986, Itai et al. 1986, Itoh et al. 1987, Vermess et al. 1985), have described MRI findings in hepatocellular carcinomas (HCC) (Figs. 4.5.**3**, 4.5.**4**) and proposed some specific morphologic findings.

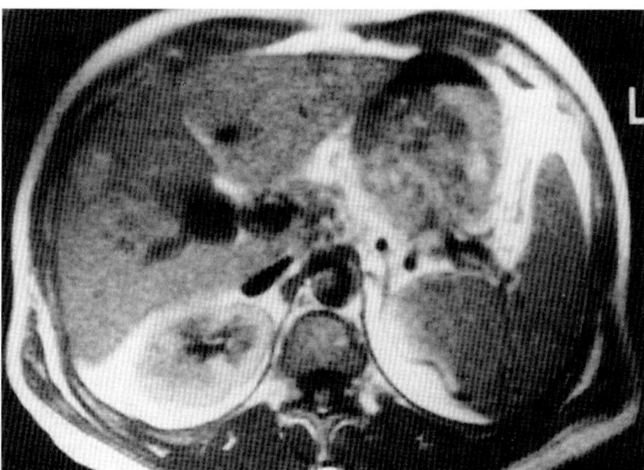

Fig. 4.5.**3** **Hepatocellular carcinoma.** T1-weighted spin-echo (TE 21 msec, TR 510 msec). A small, well-defined tumor with a slightly increased signal intensity compared to that of the normal liver

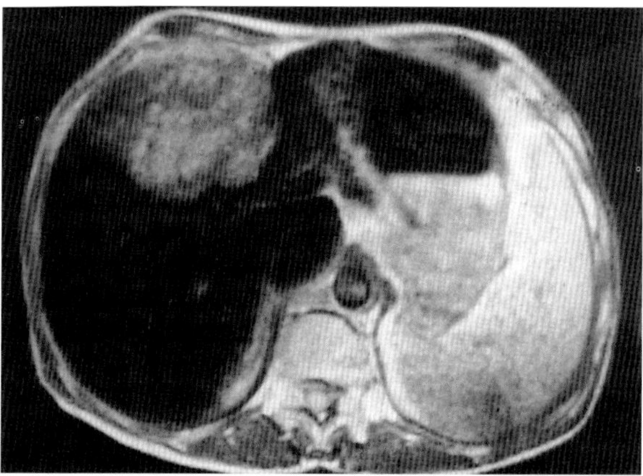

Fig. 4.5.**4** **Hepatocellular carcinoma,** hemochromatosis. A spin-echo image (TE 50 msec, TR 1050 msec). A heterogeneous anterior tumor presenting a relatively more intense signal than the non-involved dark liver. The low signal in the hemochromatosis liver is related to the shortened T1 values

MRI was of particular value in demonstrating internal architecture such as septa or non-homogeneity within hepatomas (Ebara et al. 1986, Itoh et al. 1987, Moss et al. 1984), in displaying the margins of tumors, and in depicting the relationship of the hepatic vasculature to the malignancy (Moss et al. 1984). Liver cirrhosis was suggested in many cases by changes in size and shape of individual segments of the liver (Itai et al. 1986). A variety of intensity patterns of hepatoma are described. Several authors have described, in HCC as in most hepatic tumors, a low signal on T1-weighted images and a high signal on T2-weighted images (Moss et al. 1984, Ohtomo et al. 1985a, Ohtomo et al. 1987). Relaxation times do not permit differentiation between hepatomas and metastases (Ebara et al. 1986, Foley et al. 1987).

Itoh et al. (1987) found almost half (28/58) of the tumors in their series to be hyperintense or isotense on T1-weighted SE (600/25) images, and considered this appearance of HCC on T1-weighted images one of the important characteristics for differentiation of HCC from other tumors (Fig. 4.5.**4**). This must be contrasted to metastatic tumors, which nearly all, show low intensity on T1-weighted images. On T2-weighted images, 56 of 58 cases were seen as high intensity and none were seen as low intensity. This feature of HCC closely resembles that of metastatic tumors and HCC cannot be differentiated from metastatic liver tumors on the basis of signal intensity on T2-weighted images.

Specific morphologic features of hepatocellular carcinoma are: a capsule surrounding the tumor, and mosaic patterns and tumor thrombi in the major portal veins or the inferior vena cava (Ebara et al. 1986, Itai et al. 1986, Itoh et al. 1987). Detection of metastases is important for preoperative evaluation.

Pseudocapsule. In primary hepatomas, a distinctive low-density peripheral rim may surround the tumor on T1-weighted (Ebara et al. 1986) or T2-weighted (Itoh et al. 1987) images.

Mosaic pattern. Intratumoral fibrous septa may be seen as low-intensity areas on T1-weighted SE (Itoh et al. 1987) or inversion recovery (Ebara et al. 1986) images.

Tumoral thrombi. Tumor thrombus that occurs frequently in hepatoma may be well demonstrated in major portal branches and in hepatic veins by MRI (Ebara et al. 1986, Grenier et al. 1984, Itoh et al. 1987, Ohtomo et al. 1985b). Tumor thrombus was diagnosed when high-intensity areas occupied the whole or the periphery of the portal trunk, its main branches or the inferior vena cava on the first echo image, and was suggested by the absence of large central veins.

Other abnormalities of intrahepatic vessels such as effacement, decrease in number, distortion, compression, and displacement, were also easily noted on MRI (Itai et al. 1986) and revealed the extent of tumor to varying degrees. All of these findings were demonstrated by MRI, but the frequency was lower than by US and dynamic CT in Itai's experience (Itai et al. 1986). Itoh et al (1987) detected all of the pseudocapsules depicted by CT, and detected additional cases with MRI. However, intratumoral septa were demonstrated in 3 cases, whereas CT showed them in 7 cases. Lymph node metastases and tumor thrombi in the portal vein were observed by both techniques, but MRI or CT were sometimes complementary (Itoh et al. 1987).

Metastases. Hepatic metastases usually appear as masses with a greater intensity than normal liver

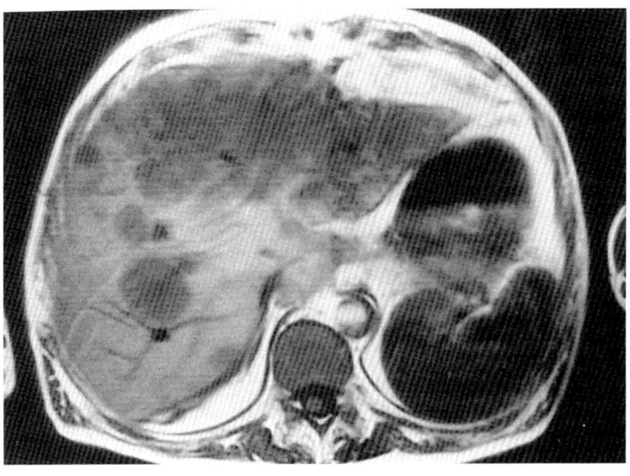

Fig. 4.5.**5** **Hepatic metastases.** A spin-echo T1-weighted image (TE 21 msec, TR 450 msec). A large metastatic infiltration of the left liver lobe and several round metastases are seen in the right liver. The relative signal intensity of the metastases is lower than in the normal liver

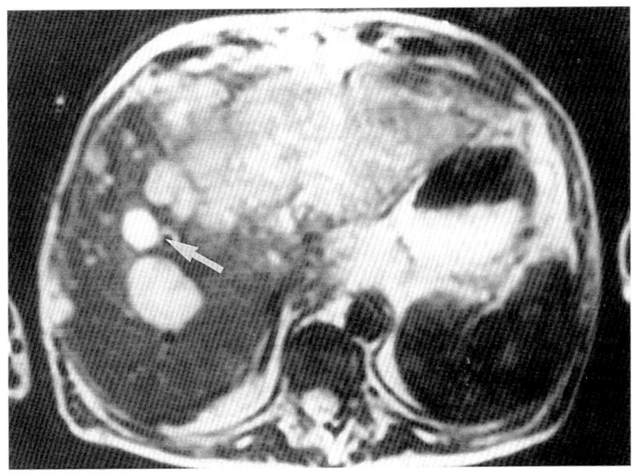

Fig. 4.5.**6** **Hepatic metastases.** A spin-echo T2-weighted image (TE 100 msec, TR 1400 msec). The relative signal intensity of the metastases is higher than in the normal liver. Some of the metastases are atypical, presenting a relatively high signal (arrow) similar to that in angiomas or cysts

on SE T2-weighted images, and with low intensity on SE T1-weighted (Figs. 4.5.**5**, 4.5.**6**) or inversion-recovery MRI (Moss et al. 1984). Metastatic lesions are characterized by prologation of T1 and T2 relaxation times. These values are, however, generally not as large as with hemangiomas or benign cysts. Thus, metastatic lesions, although showing some enhancement on T2-weighted images, do not demonstrate the same magnitude of enhancement as observed with cysts or hemangiomas.

There is considerable variation in the morphologic pattern of the signal intensity that may be observed with metastases. The lesions may be well defined and homogeneous. On T2-weighted images, hepatic metastases may show diffuse enhancement, centrally increased signal enhancement upon necrosis, or characteristic bright peripheral halo surrounding a low-density or isotense nodule (Ferrucci 1986). This peripheral halo was present in approximately one-fourth of the lesions, and was never observed in benign lesions such as cysts or hemangiomas (Ferrucci 1986).

Other signs indicating metastasis are: on T1-weighted pulse sequences, a low signal intensity mass containing a central lower signal intensity area; on T2-weighted sequences, a mass with a central high intensity region surrounded by a rim of tissue whose signal intensity is less than that of the central area (target sign).

Some metastases are atypical, and present a high signal (Fig. 4.5.**6**) on T2-weighted images, the signal being high on successive echos. Very vascularized lesions may simulate hemangiomas. This hypersignal has been described in metastases of endocrine tumors and gastric tumors, especially leiomyosarcoma or colloid cancer. Complete necrosed lesions may present a low signal on T1-weighted images and a bright signal on T2-weighted images mimicking cystic lesions.

Lymphomas. Hepatic lymphomatous involvement may be diffuse or localized. These lesions are equally well detected by both CT and MRI (Weinreb et al. 1984). Diffuse hepatic lymphoma can be detected by conventional MRI techniques, as the T1 and T2 relaxation times of infiltrated liver are increased by 41–45% over normal (Weissleder et al. 1987). With ferrite contrast medium injection, focal lesions are better visualized, but the diffuse forms are not detected (Weissleder et al. 1987).

Biliary tumors. MRI in the biliary tract has not received much attention in the literature, probably due to the high value of ERCP, US and CT. MRI can be useful for the study of the biliary tract, however, with frontal or sagittal slices, according to the craniocaudal development.

Dilated biliary ducts have a relatively low signal compared to the liver and pancreas on T1-weighted images, and a high signal on T2-weighted images (Dooms et al. 1986a), and two imaging sequences are recommended to obtain reliable demonstration of dilated bile ducts (Dooms et al. 1986a). At the level of the hepatic hilus, MRI provides excellent visualization of the vessels. The dilated common bile ducts are imaged with a lower signal intensity than the surrounding fat, and located anterior to the main portal vein. The optimal contrast between hepatic duct and surrounding fat is obtained using a short TR and TE (Dooms et al. 1986a).

Gallbladder cancer. The diagnosis of gallbladder cancer is based upon irregular wall thickening or liver invasion. Differential diagnosis with chronic cholecystitis associated with gallstones is difficult. Rossmann et al. (1987) suggest utilization of MRI when US or CT shows thickening of the gallbladder wall without any signs of acute cholecytitis or any other well known signs.

Cholangiocarcinoma. In cholangiocarcinoma, MRI and CT are particularly useful to evaluate operability, to research intrahepatic extension of the lesion, vascular involvement, hepatic metastases or local lymph nodes. Dooms et al. (1986b) reported the various MRI signs in a series of 9 cholangiocarcinomas as: local tumor signs, biliary dilatation and its extension in the liver. Cholangiocarcinomas were identified as soft-tissue masses. The T1 and T2 relaxation times of the cholangiocarcinomas were longer than those of normal liver. For T1 relaxation times, the same range for all masses was observed. Dilatation of the intrahepatic bile ducts was demonstrated by MRI in all cases. Displacement or invasion of the portal vein or the hepatic arterial branches in the region of the cholangiocarcinoma was demonstrated in 4 out of 9 patients. Occasionally, tumor extension into the gallbladder, invasion of the tumor into the surrounding liver tissue, hepatic metastases and regional lymphadenopathy was found (Dooms et al. 1986b). Differential diagnosis with biliary and peribiliary inflammatory processes is difficult.

Differential Diagnosis

MRI screening for liver cancer, as opposed to the frequent benign lesions, requires some tissue specificity to be clinically useful. Indeed, as much as 10% of the adult population possess either a benign hepatic hemangioma or a simple liver cyst (Ferrucci 1986).

On T1-weighted screening sequences, all space-occupying liver lesions (tumor, abscess, hemangioma, cyst) give a similar low-signal, dark appearance with few identifying features, except in some hepatomas, lipomas or hematomas. Small tumors and hemangiomas produce a similar dark lesion on T1 images. On T2 images, both tumors and hemangiomas appear bright. Hemangiomas have a contrast-to-noise ratio quantitatively larger than in liver cancer (Itai et al. 1985, Stark et al. 1985). In angiomas, heavily T2-weighted spin-echo pulse sequences have been found by several groups to give a highly reliable MRI appearance (Glazer 1988, Itai et al. 1985, Ohtomo et al. 1985a, Stark et al. 1985). Typically, and as distinct from solid cancers, the homogeneous, dense, bright signal with sharp margins persists on heavily T2-weighted delayed-echo images, whereas tumors fill in and become blurred. Malignant liver neoplasms tend to have a heterogeneous appearance with poorly defined margins, and are not as intense as hemangiomas on T2-SE weighted images (Stark et al. 1985). Metastases secondary to the colon have a less elevated signal than hemangiomas on T2-weighted sequences (Bree et al. 1987, Foley et al. 1987).

Moss et al. (1984) initially suggested that morphologically, and on the basis of T1 and T2 times, primary and metastatic liver cancers are generally indistinguishable from each other. Actually, MRI features can characterize some focal lesions: hemangiomas, focal nodular hyperplasia, encapsulated hepatoma, and hematomas. Some signal and morphologic patterns may also suggest metastatic disease (Higer and Bielke 1986).

A Comparison of MRI and CT

Advantages and disadvantages. CT and MRI show primary and metastatic hepatic tumors with comparable clarity. CT is better in demonstrating calcified foci within tumors, and can assess vascularity (vascular tumoral pattern in hepatoma, or rim enhancement typical of metastasis) following intravenous bolus injection of contrast medium. MRI displays more clearly the internal structure and the content of hepatic tumors and their relationship to vessels by its ability to display hepatic venous and portal anatomy without the use of contrast agents. Direct coronal and sagittal MRI can improve the localization of lesions prior to surgery. Surgical clips do not affect MRI scanning, but produce streak artefacts in CT.

Sensitivity. Clinical evaluation of the liver with MRI is a topic of controversy. Initial published reports on the use of MR for detection of liver lesions have been pessimistic (Doyle et al. 1982, Haaga 1984b). Other authors, however, are convinced that with appropriate techniques, MRI already has sufficient sensitivity and specificity to displace CT as the primary screening method for liver disease (Ferrucci 1986).

CT is currently an accepted standard for liver imaging due of its ability to show liver metastases with greater sensitivity and specificity than either sonography or radionuclide scanning. The apparent usefulness of MRI in selected hepatic disorders such as hemochromatosis (Fig. 4.5.4), portal hypertension, or the Budd-Chiari syndrome, is well established, but the major question concerns the efficacy of MRI versus CT in the detection of focal hepatic lesions, particularly metastases, and whether MRI can be effective as a primary screening technique for liver cancer detection (Bernardino 1987, Ferrucci 1986). Comparisons of MRI and CT have produced inconsistent results. Most comparative studies have been concerned with conventional,

non-enhanced MRI, and only a few (Nelson et al. 1988) compare CT with MRI performed with contrast agents and fast acquisition sequences. Some studies have found CT to be superior to MRI (Glazer et al. 1986, Nelson et al. 1988), others have found MRI to be comparable to CT, and others still have found MRI to be superior to CT (Curati et al. 1988, Reinig et al. 1987b, Vermess et al. 1985). Several groups have reported the accuracy of detection of metastases or tumors with MRI to be similar to that of CT (Doyle et al. 1982, Haaga 1984b, Heiken et al. 1985, Margulis et al. 1983, Moss et al. 1984).

MRI Features of Pancreatic Tumors

MRI signs in pancreatic tumors are morphologic or relative signal intensity abnormalities. Usually, the same type of morphologic findings are observed on MRI as on CT (Engelholm et al. 1987, 1988, Haaga 1984a, Jenkins et al. 1987, Simeone et al. 1985, Stark et al. 1984, 1986a). The MRI signs can be local morphologic changes related to the enlarged size or structure of the tumor. Other signs are due to extrapancreatic invasion or to biliary and pancreatic duct narrowing with obstruction.

In most tumors, there is significant enlargement beyond the normal pancreatic size (Fig. 4.5.8). The margins of the tumor may be quite well defined but are often blurred or distorted (Fig. 4.5.8) by some irregularity (Anacker et al. 1984, Engelholm et al. 1987, 1988, Haaga 1984a, Jenkins et al. 1987, Smith et al. 1982, Stark et al. 1984). Other morphologic features are biliary or pancreatic duct dilation (Anacker et al. 1984, Davis et al. 1984, Jenkins et al. 1987, Smith et al. 1982) due to obstruction of these ducts by the tumor. The dilated ducts are observed as a linear dark structure

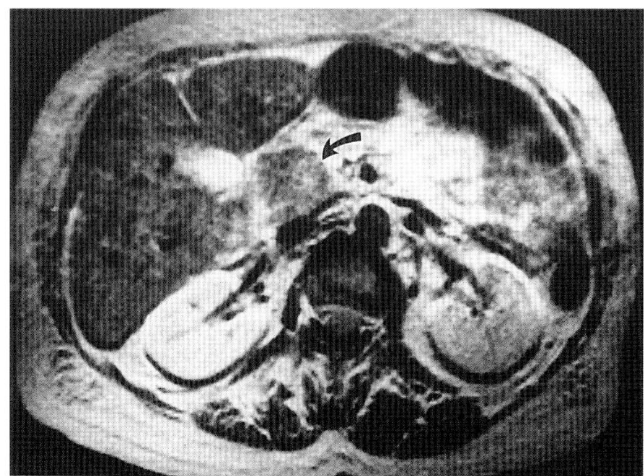

Fig. 4.5.7 **Malignant tumor of the pancreatic head.** T2-weighted spin-echo image (TE 100 msec, TR 1800 msec): The head is of normal size. There is focal, relatively enhanced signal intensity in the tumor area (arrow)

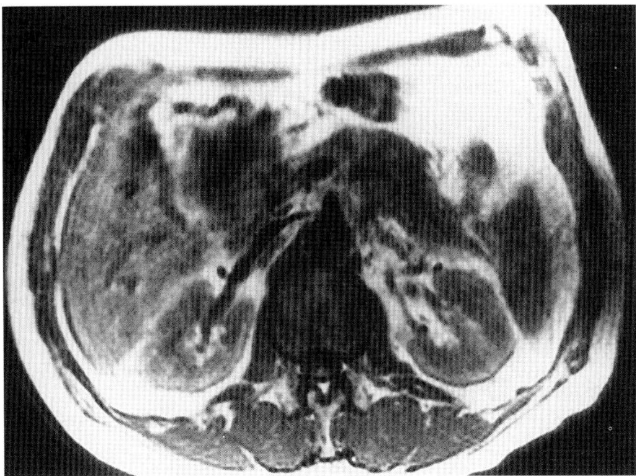

Fig. 4.5.**8 Malignant pancreatic tumor.** T1-weighted spin-echo image (TE 30 msec, TR 550 msec): The body and tail of the pancreas are enlarged, with posterior invasion and partial obliteration of the splenic vein

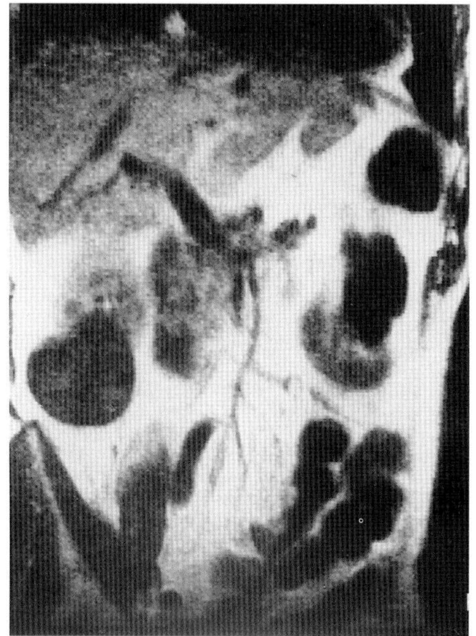

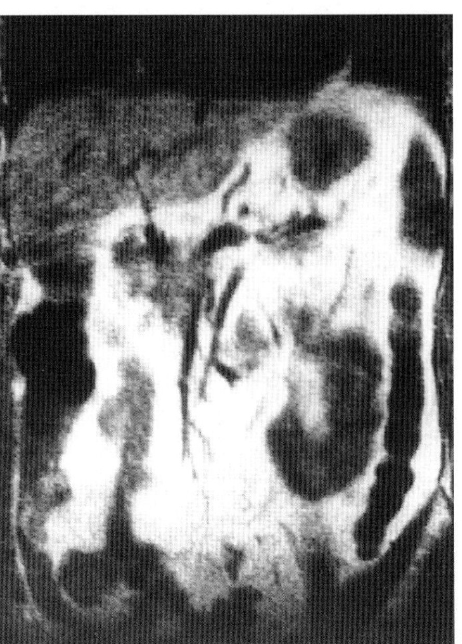

Fig. 4.5.**9 A malignant pancreatic tumor with vascular involvement.** Contiguous spin-echo T1-weighted frontal slices (TE 30 msec, TR 550 msec) in a tumor of the pancreatic head. Narrowing of the portal vein (**a**) and of the splenic vein (**b**) can be seen in the area of the splenoportal confluence

with relatively low intensity on T1-weighted images, and as relatively high intensity structures on T2-weighted images. But for identification of pancreatic duct dilatation, CT is superior to MRI (Anacker et al. 1984, Haaga 1984a).

Extrapancreatic tumoral development and infiltration of adjacent structures are accurately identified by MRI (Anacker et al. 1984, Engelholm et al. 1987, 1988, Stark et al. 1984, 1986a), but cannot be distinguished from inflammatory adhesions. Hepatic metastases (Anacker et al. 1984, Jenkins et al. 1987, Smith et al. 1982), enlarged lymph nodes, or posterior tumor invasion (Figs. 4.5.**8**, 4.5.**9**) may often obliterate the fat planes surrounding the vessels, such as the superior mesenteric artery. Early retroperitoneal invasion is better demonstrated with surface coils. Simeone et al. (1985) report a case which was not visualized with body coils or CT as disruption of the high-intensity retroperitoneal fat.

Vascular complications may be extrinsic compression, stenosis or thrombosis affecting the splenic vein, portal or inferior mesenteric veins, and less frequently the inferior vena cava. MRI can demonstrate vascular or perivascular invasion (Haaga 1984a) (Figs. 4.5.**8**, 4.5.**9**). Invasion of the perivascular fat by dense tumoral tissue is, as with CT, an indication of inoperability. Posterior perivascular invasions are particularly well demonstrated on SE T1-weighted images, which enhance the relative intensity of fat.

MRI is a valuable method of diagnosing venous thrombosis and collaterals, extrinsic compression, or venous stasis, without the use of contrast medium. The thrombosis may involve the portal (Hricak et al. 1985, Ohtomo et al. 1985b, Torres et al. 1987, Williams et al. 1985, Zirinsky et al. 1988), superior mesenteric (Zirinsky et al. 1988), inferior mesenteric (Williams et al. 1985), or splenic veins (Kneeland et al. 1984, Zirinsky et al. 1988). The diagnosis of portal venous thrombosis of the superior mesenteric or splenic veins may be based upon non-visualization of the vein and demonstration of collaterals (Hricak et al. 1985, Williams et al. 1985), or on identification of the intraluminal thrombus (Hricak et al. 1985, Torres et al. 1987, Zirinsky et al. 1988). The presence of collaterals suggests occlusion (Williams et al. 1985). These collaterals, venous derivations, are seen as multiple tubular structures giving few or no signals and localized in the areas characteristic for these abnormalities (Ohtomo et al. 1986b, Ros et al. 1986, Williams et al. 1985, Zirinsky et al. 1988). Collateral vessels in portal vein thrombosis occur most frequently at the porta hepatis (Zirinsky et al. 1988).

The relative signal intensity of the pancreatic tumor is described in the literature in various ways. There may be no difference between the normal and the abnormal pancreas (Davis et al. 1984, Engelholm et al. 1987, 1988, Haaga 1984a, Jenkins et al. 1987, Schmidt et al. 1985, Stark et al. 1984, Tscholakoff et al. 1987), non-homogeneous signal intensity (Anacker et al. 1984), or signal intensity differences between an adenocarcinoma and normal pancreatic tissue (Bydder and Young 1985, Engelholm et al. 1987, 1988, Haaga 1984a, Schmidt et al. 1985, Simeone et al. 1985, Tscholakoff et al. 1987). The local changes may involve focal enhancement of the relative signal intensity in the tumoral area (Engelholm et al. 1987, 1988, Haaga 1984a, Stark et al. 1984). The relative signal intensity of the pancreatic tumor may vary according to the different pulse sequences used. Surface coils are more precise for detecting or defining an abnormal intensity area in an enlarged pancreas (Simeone et al. 1985).

Endocrine Tumors

Endocrine tumors can be demonstrated by morphologic and intensity criteria (Stark et al. 1984). Islet cell carcinomas have occasionally been described. The relative intensity of the tumor is enhanced compared to the normal pancreas on T2-weighted sequences (Stark et al. 1984, Tscholakoff et al. 1987).

Lymphomas

Lymphomas of the pancreatic area cannot be differentiated from pancreatic tissue either by CT or by MRI (Tscholakoff et al. 1987). Both techniques demonstrate enlarged retroperitoneal lymph nodes, suggesting the diagnosis of lymphoma.

A Comparison of MRI, CT and ERCP

There is no clear superiority for MRI compared to CT in tumors with body coils (Engelholm 1987, 1988, Haaga 1984a, Tscholakoff et al. 1987), except when CT artefacts are apparently related to metallic surgical clips or endoscopic prostheses (Engelholm et al. 1987, 1988, Jenkins et al. 1987).

Some advantages in MRI are reported. It may provide a diagnosis missed by CT (Steiner and Bydder 1984). MRI was useful in assessing the extent in neoplastic disease: fat planes are demonstrated better by MRI (Stark et al. 1984). Tumoral extension, detection of metastases, and lymph nodes were better detected by MRI than by CT (Tscholakoff et al. 1987). MRI is reported to be superior to CT in demonstrating vascular patency or occlusion by an adjacent tumor (Stark et al. 1984). The advantages of MRI in the visualization of vascular abnormalities are: the possibility of visualizing vessels without the use of iodine contrast medium, and of performing frontal or sagittal slices which may give information complementary to CT. MRI proved to be a valuable non-invasive method for the diagnosis of portal venous thrombosis (Zirinsky et al. 1988), and is superior to CT and sonography.

Other authors (Engelholm et al. 1987, Haaga 1984a, Jenkins et al. 1987) report that MRI gives less information than CT, which provides better spatial resolution. We found MRI to be clearly inferior to CT. In a series of 29 cases, MRI has provided a diagnosis of cancer in 65.5%, when CT was successful in 93.1% (Engelholm et al. 1987).

For pancreatic tumors, ERCP is superior to MRI and CT. MRI does not permit differential diagnosis between cancer and pancreatitis, as CT does (Simeone et al. 1985, Tscholakoff et al. 1987). For operable cancer of the pancreas MRI and CT have little value, ERCP being superior. The main reason for the failure of MRI and CT is the fact that these techniques are used in patients in whom the disease is already at an advanced stage.

References

Anacker H, Rupp N, Reiser M. Magnetic resonance (MR) in the diagnosis of pancreatic disease. Eur J Radiol 1984; 4: 265–269.

Bernardino ME. Focal hepatic mass screening: MR imaging or CT scanning? Radiology 1987; 162: 282–283.

Brasch RC, Weinmann HJ, Wesbey GE. Contrast-enhanced NMR imaging: animal studies using gadolinium-DTPA complex. AJR 1984; 142: 619–624.

Bree RL, Schwab RE, Glazer GM, Fink-Benett D. The varied appearances of hepatic cavernous hemangioma with sonography, CT, MRI and scintigraphy. Radiographics 1987; 6: 1153–1174.

Bydder IR, Young IR. MR imaging: clinical use of the inversion recovery sequence. J Comput Assist Tomogr 1985; 9: 459–475.

Carr DH, Brown J, Bydder GM et al. Gadolinium-DTPA as a contrast agent in MRI: initial clinical experience in 20 patients. AJR 1984; 143: 215–224.

Curati WL, Halevy A, Gibson RN, Carr DH, Blumgart LH, Steiner RE. Ultrasound, CT, and MRI comparison in primary and secondary tumors of the liver. Gastrointest Radiol 1988; 13: 123–128.

Davis PL, Moss AA, Goldberg HI, Stark DS, Margulis AR. Nuclear magnetic resonance of the liver and pancreas. Radiographics 1984; 4: 159–169.

Demas BE, Hricak H, Goldberg HI, Margulis AR. Magnetic resonance imaging diagnosis of hepatic metastases in the presence of negative CT studies. J Clin Gastroenterol 1985; 7: 553–560.

Dooms GC, Fisher MR, Higgins CB, Hricak H, Goldberg HI, Margulis AR. MR imaging of the dilated biliary tract. Radiology 1986a; 158: 337–341.

Dooms GC, Kerlan RK Jr, Hricak H, Wall SD, Margulis AR. Cholangiocarcinoma: imaging by MR. Radiology 1986b; 159: 89–94.

Doyle FH, Pennock JM, Banks LM et al. Nuclear magnetic resonance (NMR) imaging of the liver: initial experience. AJR 1982; 138: 193–200.

Ebara M, Ohto M, Watanabe Y et al. Diagnosis of small hepatocellular carcinoma: correlation of MR imaging and tumor histologic studies. Radiology 1986; 159: 371–377.

Engelholm L, De Toeuf J, Zalcman M et al. Tomographie computée et resonance magnétique dans le cancer du pancréas: comparison avec la cholangio-wirsungographie. Acta Gastroenterol Belg 1987; 50: 195–210.

Engelholm L, Segebarth C, De Toeuf J, Zalcman M. IRM du pancreas. In: Vasile N, ed. IRM corps entier. Paris: Vigot, 1988: 219–235.

Feinberg DA, Mills CM, Posin JP et al. Multiple spin-echo magnetic resonance imaging. Radiology 1985; 155: 437–442.

Ferrucci JT. MR imaging of the liver. AJR 1986; 147: 1103–1116.

Foley WD, Kneeland JB, Cates JD et al. Contrast optimization for the detection of focal hepatic lesions by MR imaging at 1.5 T. AJR 1987; 149: 1155–1160.

Glazer GM. MR imaging of the liver, kidneys and adrenal glands. Radiology 1988; 166: 303–312.

Glazer GM, Aisen AM, Francis IR, Gross BH, Gyves JW, Ensminger WD. Evaluation of focal hepatic masses: a comparative study of MRI and CT. Gastrointest Radiol 1986; 11: 263–268.

Grenier P, Menu Y, Desbleds MT, Guilbeau JC, Lorphelin, Nahum H. L'imagerie par résonance magnétique (IRM) dans l'exploration des masses hépatiques. J Radiol 1984; 65: 819–827.

Haaga JR. Magnetic resonance imaging of the pancreas. Radiol Clin N Am 1984a; 22: 869–877.

Haaga JR. Magnetic resonance imaging of the liver. Radiol Clin N Am 1984b; 22: 879–890.

Hahn PF, Stark DD, Saini S, Lewis JM, Wittenberg J, Ferrucci JT. Ferrite particles for bowel contrast in MR imaging: design issues and feasibility studies. Radiology 1987; 164: 37–41.

Hamm B, Wolf KJ, Felix R. Conventional and rapid MR imaging of the liver with Gd-DTPA. Radiology 1987; 164: 313–320.

Heiken JP, Lee JKT, Glazer HS, Ling D. Hepatic metastases studied with MR and CT. Radiology 1985; 156: 423–427.

Higer HP, Bielke G. Gewebecharakterisierung mit T1, T2 und Protonendichte: Traum und Wirklichkeit. RöFo 1986; 144: 597–605.

Hricak H, Amparo E, Fisher MR, Crooks L, Higgins CB. Abdominal venous system: assessment using MR. Radiology 1985; 156: 415–422.

Itai Y, Ohtomo K, Furui S, Yamauchi T, Minami M, Yashiro N. Noninvasive diagnosis of small cavernous hemangioma of the liver: advantage of MRI. AJR 1985; 145: 1195–1199.

Itai Y, Ohtomo K, Furui S, Minami M, Yoshikawa K, Yashiro N. MR imaging of hepatocellular carcinomas. J Comput Assist Tomogr 1986; 10: 963–968.

Itoh K, Nishimura K, Togashi K et al. Hepatocellular carcinoma: MR imaging. Radiology 1987; 164: 21–25.

Jenkins JPR, Braganza JM, Hickey S, Isherwood I, Machin M. Quantitative tissue characterisation in pancreatic disease using magnetic resonance imaging. Br J Radiol 1987; 60: 333–341.

Kneeland JB, Auh YH, Zirinsky K, Rubenstein W, Kazam E. MR, CT, and ultrasonographic demonstration of splenic vein thrombosis. J Comput Assist Tomogr 1984; 8: 1199–1200.

Kressel HY. Strategies for magnetic resonance imaging of focal liver disease. Radiol Clin N Am 1988; 26: 607–615.

Mano I, Yoshida H, Nakabayashi K, Yashiro N, Iio M. Fast spin echo-imaging with suspended respiration: gadolinium enhanced MR imaging of liver tumors. J Comput Assist Tomogr 1987; 11: 173–180.

Margulis AR. Overview: current status of clinical magnetic resonance imaging. Radiographics 1984; 4: 76–96.

Margulis AR, Moss AA, Crooks LE, Kaufman L. Nuclear magnetic resonance in the diagnosis of tumors of the liver. Semin Roentgenol 1983; 18: 123–126.

Mathieu D, Anglade MC, Guinet C, Cauquil P, Roche A, Vasile N. IRM du foie. In Vasile N, ed. IRM corps entier. Paris: Vigot, 1988: 171–218.

Moss AA, Goldberg HI, Stark DB et al. Hepatic tumors: magnetic resonance and CT appearance. Radiology 1984; 150: 141–147.

Nelson RC, Chezmar JL, Steinberg HV et al. Focal hepatic lesions: detection by dynamic and delayed computed tomography versus short TE/TR spin echo and fast field echo magnetic resonance imaging. Gastrointest Radiol 1988, 13: 115–122.

Ohtomo K, Itai Y, Furui S, Yashro N, Yoshikawa K, Iio M. Hepatic tumors: differentiation by transverse relaxation time (T2) of magnetic resonance imaging. Radiology 1985a; 155: 421–423.

Ohtomo K, Itai Y, Furui S, Yoshikawa K, Yashiro N, Iio M. MR imaging of portal vein thrombosis in hepatocellular carcinoma. J Comput Assist Tomogr 1985b; 9: 328–329.

Ohtomo K, Itai Y, Iio M. Magnetic resonance imaging (MRI) of the liver. Magn Reson Annu 1986a; 2: 197–212.

Ohtomo K, Itai Y, Makita K et al. Portosystemic collaterals on MR imaging. J Comput Assist Tomogr 1986b; 10: 751–755.

Ohtomo K, Itai Y, Kohki Y, et al. Hepatic tumors: dynamic MR imaging. Radiology 1987; 163: 27–31.

Reinig JW, Dwyer AJ, Miller DL et al. Liver metastasis detection: comparative sensitivities of MR imaging and CT scanning. Radiology 1987b; 162: 43–47.

Renshaw PF, Owen CS, McLaughlin AG, et al. Ferromagnetic contrast agentia new approach. Magn Reson Med 1986; 3: 217–225.

Ros PR, Viamonte M, Soila K, Sheldon JJ, Tobias J, Cohen B. Demonstration of cavernomatous transformation of the portal vein by magnetic resonance imaging. Gastrointest Radiol 1986; 11: 90–92.

Rossmann MD, Friedman AC, Radecki PD, Caroline DF. MR imaging of gallbladder carcinoma. AJR 1987; 148: 143–144.

Runge VM, Clanton JA, Herzer WA, et al. Intravascular contrast agents suitable for magnetic resonance imaging. Radiology 1984; 153: 171–176.

Rupp N, Reiser M, Stetter E. The diagnostic value of morphology and relaxation times in NMR imaging of the body. Eur J Radiol 1983; 3: 68–76.

Saini S, Stark DD, Hahn PF, Wittenberg GJ, Brady TJ, Ferrucci JT Jr. Ferrite particles: a supermagnetic MR contrast agent for the enhanced detection of liver carcinoma. Radiology 1987; 162: 217–222.

Schmidt HC, Tscholakoff D, Hricak H, Higgins CB. MR image contrast and relaxation times of solid tumors in the chest, abdomen and pelvis. J Comput Assist Tomogr 1985; 9: 738–748.

Simeone JF, Edelman RR, Stark DD et al. Surface coil MR imaging of abdominal viscera, III: the pancreas. Radiology 1985; 157: 437–441.

Smith W, Reid A, Hutchinson JMS, Mallard JR. Nuclear magnetic resonance imaging of the pancreas. Radiology 1982; 142: 677–680.

Stark DD, Moss AA, Goldberg HI, Davis PL, Federle MP. Magnetic resonance and CT of the normal and diseased pancreas: a comparative study. Radiology 1984; 150: 153–162.

Stark DD, Felder RC, Wittenberg J, et al. Magnetic resonance imaging of cavernous hemangioma of the liver: tissue specific characterization. AJR 1985; 145: 213–220.

Stark DD, Moss AA, Goldberg HI. Nuclear magnetic resonance of the liver, spleen, and pancreas. Cardiovasc Intervent Radiol 1986a; 8: 329–341.

Stark DD, Wittenberg J, Middleton MJ, Ferrucci JT Jr. Liver metastases: detection by phase-contrast MR imaging. Radiology 1986b; 158: 327–332.

Stark DD, Wittenberg J, Edelman RR et al. Detection of hepatic metastases: analysis of pulse sequence performance in MR imaging. Radiology 1986c; 159: 365–370.

Stark DD, Hendrick RE, Hahn PF, Ferrucci JT Jr. Motion artifact reduction with fast spin-echo imaging. Radiology 1987a; 164: 183–191.

Stark DD, Wittenberg J, Butch RJ, Ferrucci JT Jr. Hepatic metastases: randomized, controlled comparison of detection with MR imaging and CT. Radiology 1987b; 165: 399–406.

Steiner RE, Bydder GN. Nuclear magnetic resonance in gastroenterology. Clin Gastroenterol 1984; 13: 265–279.

Torres WE, Gaylord GM, Whitmire L, Chuang VP, Bernardino ME. The correlation between MR and angiography in portal hypertension. AJR 1987; 148: 1109–1112.

Tsang Y, Stark DD, Chen MC, Weissleder R, Wittenberg J, Ferrucci JT. Hepatic micrometastases in the rat: ferrite-enhanced MR imaging. Radiology 1988; 167: 21–24.

Tscholakoff D, Hricak H, Thoeni R, Winkler ML, Margulis AR. MR imaging in the diagnosis of pancreatic disease. AJR 1987; 148: 703–709.

Uhlenbrock D, Borsch G, Beyer HK, et al. Erste Erfahrungen mit MR bei Lebertumoren. RöFo 1985; 143: 200–207.

Vermess M, Leung AWL, Bydder GM, et al. MR imaging of the liver in primary hepatocellular carcinoma. J Comput Assist Tomogr 1985; 9: 749–754.

Weinmann HJ, Brasch RC, Press WR, Wesbey GE. Characteristics of gadolinium-DTPA complex: a potential NMR contrast agent. AJR 1984; 142: 619–624.

Weinreb JC, Brateman L, Maravilla KR. Magnetic resonance imaging of hepatic lymphoma. AJR 1984a; 143: 1211–1214.

Weinreb JC, Maravilla KR, Redman HC, Nunnally R. Improved MR imaging of the upper abdomen with glucagon and gas. J Comput Assist Tomogr 1984b; 8: 835–838.

Weissleder R, Stark DD, Compton CC, Wittenberg J, Ferrucci JT. Ferrite-enhanced MR imaging of hepatic lymphoma: an experimental study in rats. AJR 1987; 149: 1161–1165.

Wesbey GE, Brasch RC, Goldberg HI, Engelstad BL. Dilute oral iron solutions as gastrointestinal contrast agents for magnetic resonance imaging: initial clinical experience. Magn Reson Imaging 1985; 3: 57–64.

Williams DM, Cho KJ, Aisen A, Eckhauser FE. Portal hypertension evaluated by MR imaging. Radiology 1985; 157: 703–706.

Zirinsky K, Markisz JA, Rubenstein WA et al. MR imaging of portal venous thrombosis: correlation with CT and sonography. AJR 1988; 150: 283–288.

4.6 Endoscopic Retrograde Cholangiopancreatography (ERCP)

K. Huibregtse, G. N. J. Tytgat

Introduction

Duodenoscopy and endoscopic cannulation of the papilla of Vater with visualization of the biliary tree and pancreatic duct was first described in 1968 (McCune et al.). Many enthusiastic reports on ERCP appeared from all over the world in the early 1970s. In a few years, ERCP became one of the most reliable methods of diagnosing biliary and pancreatic disorders. A vast literature on the subject is now available, and extensive review articles have appeared (Classen 1977, Classen and Phillip 1988, Cotton 1977, Kasugai 1975, Ohto et al. 1978).

The development and refinement of other diagnostic methods, such as ultrasonography, computer tomography and endoscopic ultrasound, have so far not affected the important place of ERCP in diagnosing biliopancreatic diseases. On the contrary, therapeutic procedures following cannulation of the papilla have been developed, such as endoscopic papillotomy and biliary drainage procedures, making ERCP an even more indispensable method.

Instruments

ERCP is a combined endoscopic and radiological method. A high-performance radiographic instrument with a TV image-intensifier system is required for optimal radiological diagnosis, but also to avoid complications through inadvertent overfilling of the pancreatic duct. Side-viewing endoscopes are used in patients with an intact stomach. These endoscopes are now available for diagnostic purposes with instrumentation channels of 2.8 or 3.7 mm. For therapeutic purposes, endoscopes are available with instrumentation channels of 4.2 and 5.5 mm (Olympus, Fujinon and Pentax). Cannulation of the papilla of Vater may be easier using a forward-viewing endoscope in same patients who have undergone a Billroth II resection (Osnes et al. 1986).

A whole variety of cannulation catheters is now commercially available, facilitating cannulation of the papilla for different anatomic specifications. In practice, however, only two or three different catheters are used by experienced endoscopists. We prefer catheters with a metal ball tip or a metal cone tip. The metal tip can easily be seen on the TV monitor and, without contrast injection, the catheter tip can be moved in the desired direction. The ball-tip catheter takes a 0.035 inch guide wire, which subsequently allows insertion of rather stiff

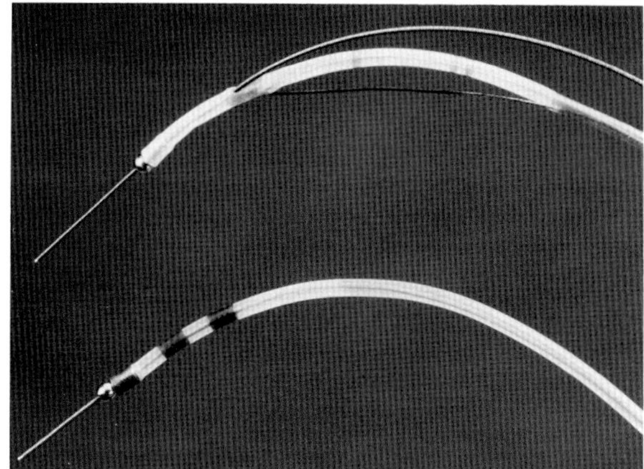

Fig. 4.6.**1**   **Metal ball tip catheter**, which takes a 0.035 inch guide wire. A papillotome can be inserted over the guidewire (Wilson Cook Med. Inc., Winston Salem, NC, USA)

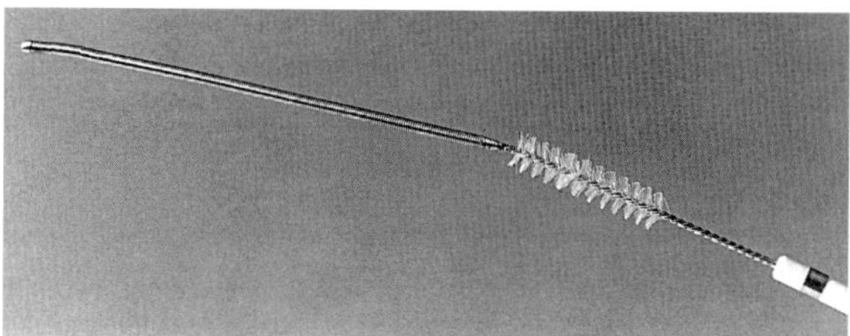

Fig. 4.6.**2**   **Cytology brush** for asymmetric, irregular strictures (Wilson Cook Med. Inc., Winston Salem, NC, USA)

cytology brushes, papillotomes or biliary drainage catheters (Fig. 4.6.**1**). A standard biopsy forceps is used for tissue sampling. A cytology brush mounted on a 2.5 m long guide wire with a 3 cm flexible tip can be used to pass through irregular strictures for sampling cytological specimen. This brush is advanced through a Teflon 7 Fr catheter with a metal ring at the tip (Fig. 4.6.**2**). Water soluble contrast materials are used, usually at a concentration of 60 %. Lower concentrations may be desirable for detecting small gallstones.

Procedure

The investigation and its potential risks are carefully explained to the patient. Further information on possible therapeutic procedures must be given to those patients in whom these procedures can be expected to be necessary following the diagnostic ERCP. Written consent is now required in many countries.

In most centres, intravenous sedation with diazepam or midazolam is given. The pharynx is anesthetized with a lidocaine spray. Fentanyl or meperidine can be added in individual cases. Relaxation of the duodenum can be obtained by administration of hyoscine butylbromide or glucagon. Relaxation of the sphincter of Oddi by ceruletide or glycerol nitrate has been reported to make cannulation easier, but most experienced endoscopists do not use such drugs. The technique of ERCP has not substantially changed since its introduction and is extensively described in the literature (Cotton 1977).

Cannulation of the papilla should only be attempted when the endoscope is straightened along the lesser curve of the stomach to bring the papilla into the center of the field of view. The orientation of the catheter tip can be changed by moving the elevator bridge, by moving the tip of the endoscope, or by advancing or withdrawing the endoscope. It may sometimes be helpful to bend the tip of the catheter in an acute curve, twisted to the left. Forceful pushing of the catheter into the papilla should be avoided in order to avoid trauma of this delicate structure. Trauma-induced edema will make subsequent cannulation more difficult and increases the risk of acute pancreatitis.

Radiography

A plain X-ray should be taken before the procedure, with the patient flat on his back, to make sure that the field is not obscured by old contrast material and to establish or rule out soft tissue shadows or calcifications. Radiographs are usually taken with the patient in the prone position during cannulation and injection of contrast material. Overviews are taken of the ductular systems and spot films of any abnormal or suspicious findings. The motor function of the papilla is best studied with the patient in the supine position after removal of the endoscope. Delayed films of the biliary tract are mandatory to demonstrate or rule out small concrements. The constant attendance of a radiologist is desirable and should improve the quality of the radiographic examination. For readily obvious reasons, this appears impossible in many endoscopy units.

Indications and Contra-Indications

The indications for ERCP can be divided into five main groups, and are listed in Table 4.6.1. Indications for ERCP have changed since its introduc-

Table 4.6.1 Indications for ERCP

I   Suspected biliary disorders
   a) jaundice or cholestasis
   b) post-cholecystectomy complaints
   c) post-biliary surgery complaints
   d) acute cholangitis
   e) acute biliary pancreatitis
   f) confirmation of disorders, demonstrated by other imaging techniques

II   Suspected pancreatic disorders
   a) obstructive jaundice
   b) upper abdominal pain
   c) increased serum amylase
   d) recent onset of diabetes mellitus
   e) unexplained weight loss
   f) steatorrhoea
   g) gastric varices
   h) ascites or pleura effusion
   i) confirmation of disorders, demonstrated by other imaging techniques

III   Prior to therapeutic endoscopic procedures
   a) endoscopic papillotomy
   b) endoscopic biliary drainage
   c) endoscopic pancreatic drainage
   d) balloon dilation of strictures

IV   Preoperative mapping
   a) chronic pancreatitis
   b) pancreas pseudocysts

V   Additional procedures
   a) collection of pure pancreatic juice or bile
   b) manometry of the sphincter of Oddi

tion, because the procedure proved to be less aggressive than originally believed and because other refined imaging techniques have become available. Cholangitis and acute pancreatitis have been contra-indications for many years. Nowadays cholangitis and acute biliary pancreatitis are formal indications for emergency ERCP, provided that an endoscopic therapeutic procedure can follow at the same session if this proves to be necessary or desirable. Ultrasonography has become the standard screening technique for patients with a suspected pancreatic disorder. ERCP is indicated in patients with chronic pancreatitis only when ultrasonography is ambiguous or when preoperative mapping is required (Dyrszka and Sanghavi 1983). The main contra-indications for ERCP are suspected abnormalities which carry an increased risk of infection, i.e. biliary strictures and pancreatic pseudocysts. An ERCP should only by performed in these situations when a drainage procedure can follow immediately after the diagnostic procedure. Antibiotic treatment should be started at once in case of inadvertent filling of an obstructed biliary or pancreatic ductal system, especially if adequate biliary drainage cannot be guaranteed.

Success Rate

The papilla is identified endoscopically in 98–99% of cases by experienced endoscopists. Difficulties in finding the papilla may arise in the case of large papillary tumors, duodenal stenosis, edematous folds due to acute pancreatitis, or when the papilla is located inside a diverticulum. In Billroth II patients, the success rate decreases to 60–85%. A long or kinked afferent loop may prevent the endoscope from being advanced to the area of the papilla. The success rate of cannulation depends on the experience and persistence of the investigator, but also on the underlying disease (Ohto et al. 1978). It is well known that cannulation of the common bile duct is easier in patients with gallstone disease than in patients with a distal common bile duct which is displaced or compressed by a pancreatic tumor.

Selective cholangiography is successful in only 90–95% of cases, even for skilled endoscopists. The success rate of pancreatography lies in the same order of magnitude in most larger series. Incision of the roof of the papilla with a diathermy knife can increase the success rate of cannulation of the common bile duct. This technique is, however, more aggressive and carries a higher risk, which justifies its use only in the setting of a therapeutic procedure and not for purely diagnostic purposes.

Complications

Acute pancreatitis is the most frequent complication of a diagnostic ERCP procedure (Table 4.6.**2**) (Bilbao et al. 1976, Rösch 1981). A slight rise of amylase is observed in 40–75% of cases (Hannigan et al. 1985, Okuno et al. 1985). This hyperamylasemia is not accompanied by clinical symptoms, and usually subsides in 1 to 2 days. A clinically obvious acute pancreatitis post-ERCP occurs in 0.7 to 7.4% of patients. Severe necrotizing pancreatitis is seen in 0.1% of patients. Overfilling of the pancreatic duct with contrast material, and induction of parenchymal contrast extravasation (paren-

Table 4.6.**2** **Complications of ERCP** (Rösch 1981)

Pancreatitis	0.7–7.4%
Cholangitis	0.6–0.8%
Abscess of pancreas	0.5–1.3%
Side-effects of drugs	0.1–0.6%
Injury to gastrointestinal tract	0.07–0.4%
Mortality	0.001–0.8%

chymography) are claimed to be the main causative factors in the development of acute pancreatitis. Trauma and subsequent edema of the papilla is in all probability an important causative factor as well. Repeated attempts at cannulation, or repeated pancreatic duct cannulation and filling, constitute the main risk factors. Acute pancreatitis has been observed in patients even after unsuccessful cannulation attempts of the pancreatic duct. Cholangitis was the most frequent and severe complication until biliary drainage procedures became possible. Cholangitis develops when the outflow of bile (and contrast material) is delayed or blocked by a biliary obstruction.

The causative pathogens are, in general, gram-negative bacteria, such as *Escherichia coli* and *Klebsiella* (Helm et al. 1984). Endoscopes and ancillary equipment can now be easily disinfected, and should be disinfected before every examination. It should no longer be possible for *Pseudomonas aeruginosa*, once the terror of endoscopists and endoscopy nurses, to be cultured from endoscopes or subsequently from patients with post-ERCP cholangitis. The best way preventing cholangitis is to create an unhindered bile flow immediately. This can be achieved by endoscopic sphincterotomy and stone extraction, or by an endoscopic biliary drainage procedure. Systemic antibiotics should be instituted at once in case of failure to clear obstructions from the biliary tree.

Infection of a pancreatic pseudocyst, with subsequent pancreatic abscess formation, should be a rare complication. Ultrasonography detects the greater majority of pseudocysts. ERCP should not be performed on these patients unless preoperative visualization of the pancreatic duct is desirable or mandatory for surgical planning. Side-effects of drugs, such as respiratory arrest, occur particularly in elderly and frail patients.

Endoscopic abnormalities

The distal stomach and pylorus can readily be inspected during passage of the duodenoscope towards the papilla. Impression of the antrum, displacement of the pylorus, and a duodenal stenosis may indicate the presence of a periampullary tumor. Pancreatic cancers may grow into the duodenal wall, and biopsies from any duodenal wall abnormality may reveal the malignancy. The growth of pancreatic cancers is usually seen proximally to a normal-looking papilla.

The minor papilla, if present, is located 1–2 cm proximal to the major papilla. Most duodenal diverticula are located in the descending part of the duodenum, near the papilla of Vater. Cannulation of a papilla in a diverticulum or in the

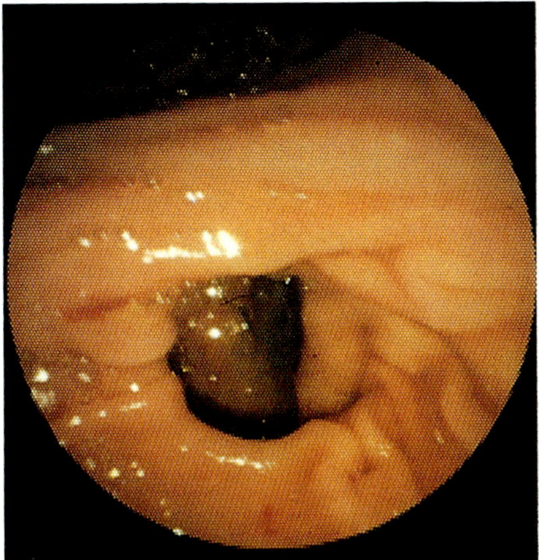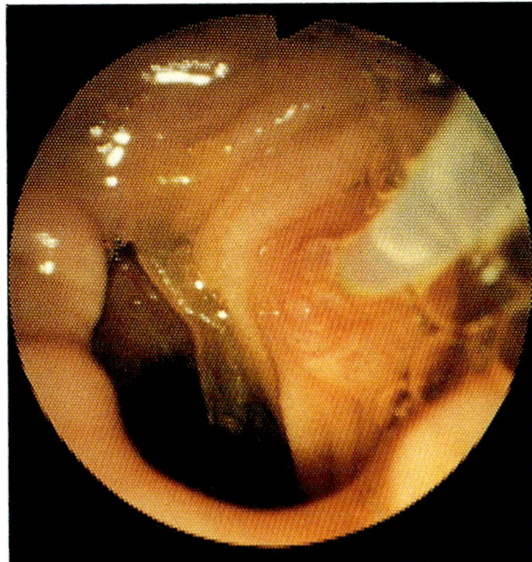

Fig. 4.6.**3** **Left:** the papilla is inside the mouth of a diverticulum. **Right:** the papilla is turned outside the diverticulum and is cannulated

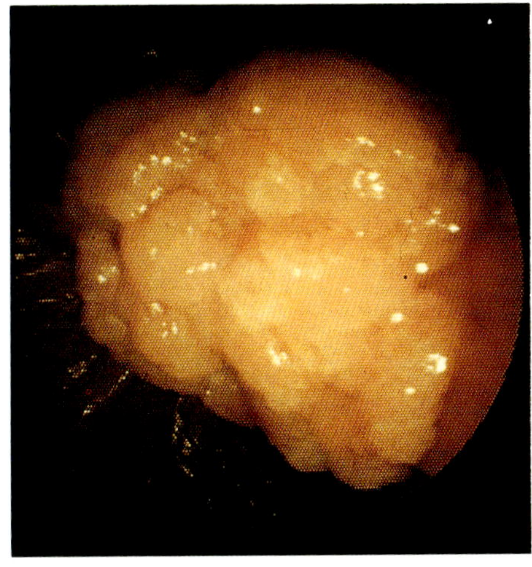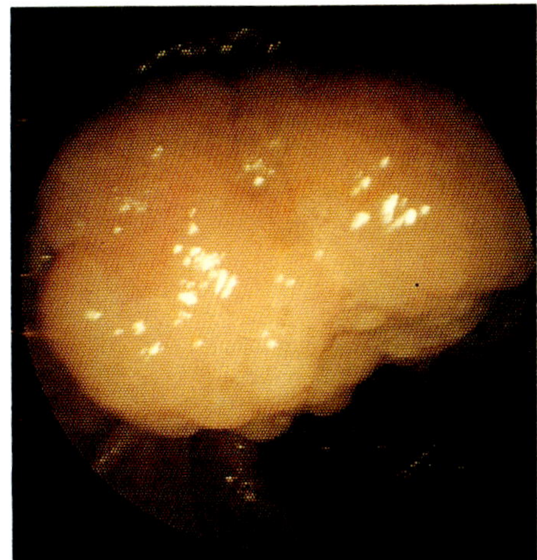

Fig. 4.6.**4** **A polypous, fleshy carcinoma** of the ampulla of Vater

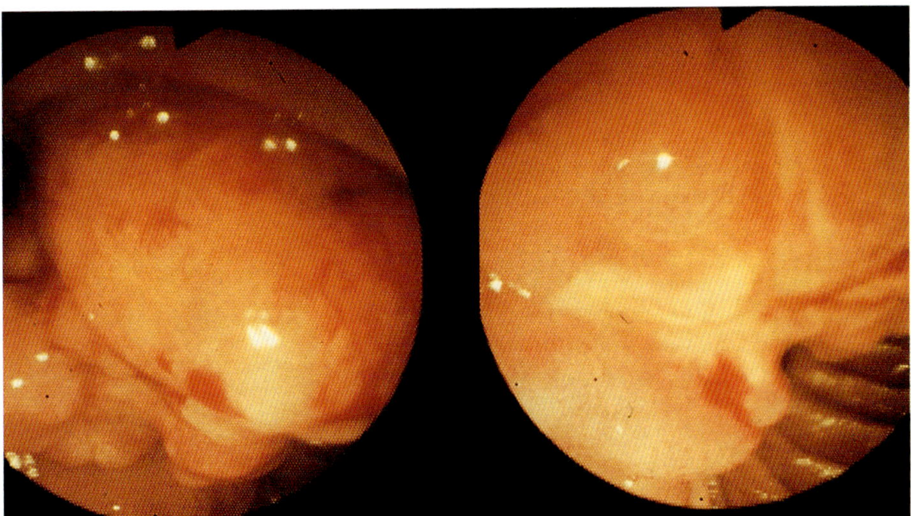

Fig. 4.6.**5** **A periampullary tumor. Right:** the papilla still has a normal-looking orifice

mouth of a diverticulum is more demanding (Fig. 4.6.**3**). Peripapillary diverticula are associated with an increased incidence of gallstones. The papilla and its region must be examined carefully prior to attempts at cannulation. Recent stone passage can be suspected when the orifice of the papilla is patent and surrounded by red, edematous edges. A parapapillary fistula due to spontaneous stone perforation or fausse route during surgical bougienage should be looked for (Tanaka and Ikeda 1983). A bulging papilla may be caused by an impacted stone or an ampullary tumor. Endoscopic papillotomy is generally necessary to make the final diagnosis. Carcinomas of the ampulla of Vater may be seen as fleshy, friable exophytic growths at the site of the papilla (Fig. 4.6.**4**). Cannulation of these tumors may be difficult, because bleeding upon touching the tumor with the cannula or endoscope will obscure the field. Carcinomas may also be seen as large ulcerative lesions surrounding the area of the papilla (Fig. 4.6.**5**). A bulging papilla, covered with normal duodenal mucosa, is found when the tumor arises from inside the ampulla. Histologic proof of malignancy can be obtained in only 85 % of cases, even when large snare biopsies are taken after the tumor has been exposed by endoscopic sphincterotomy (Bourgeois et al. 1984).

Cholangiography

The biliary tree is filled with contrast until the intrahepatic bile ducts, the cystic duct and the gallbladder are opacified and appropriate films can be taken. The outflow of contrast through the papilla is slow. The endoscope can be removed after opacification of the biliary tree, and a complete, detailed examination can be made with the patient in various positions. Delayed films must be taken so that small gallstones are not overlooked. The cystic duct can be considered occluded when gallbladder filling does not take place after complete filling of the intrahepatic bile ducts and after changing the position of the patient.

Air is occasionally injected with the contrast material. This must be avoided as much as possible, because air bubbles can be mistaken for gallstones. Air bubbles can be differentiated from gallstones by changing the position of the patient. Air bubbles tend to move proximally, and gallstones distally, with the patient in the upright position. A normal cholangiogram shows a common bile duct of not more than 9 mm in diameter. The common bile duct is wider in patients after cholecystectomy (Meier et al. 1984, Montefusco et al. 1984, Niederau et al. 1984, O'Connor et al. 1985). The cystic duct implantation may be found over the entire length of the common bile duct from the bifurcation up to the

area of the papilla. A slight narrowing of the common hepatic duct at the site of the confluence is occasionally seen. Just distal to the bifurcation vessels there may be an impression of the common hepatic duct, especially with the patient in the prone position. The intrapancreatic portion of the distal common bile duct may show a tubular narrowing. The anatomy of the intrahepatic biliary tree is very variable (Heloury et al. 1985). In general, the hepatic tree is considered normal when there is nice arborization, with smooth tapering and smooth lining of the branches. The gallbladder and cystic duct may also show various anatomical variations. Additional examination of the gallbladder after ERCP can be performed using drugs to study gallbladder motility.

Cholelithiasis

Gallstones may be found in all parts of the biliary tract (Figs. 4.6.**6**, 4.6.**7**). Gallstones vary in number, size and shape. Stones with an irregular shape are mostly composed of sludge, and small stones are mostly solid. Cholangiography has been shown to be indispensable in the investigation of patients with complications of gallstones and gallstone surgery. Gallstones may perforate through the bile

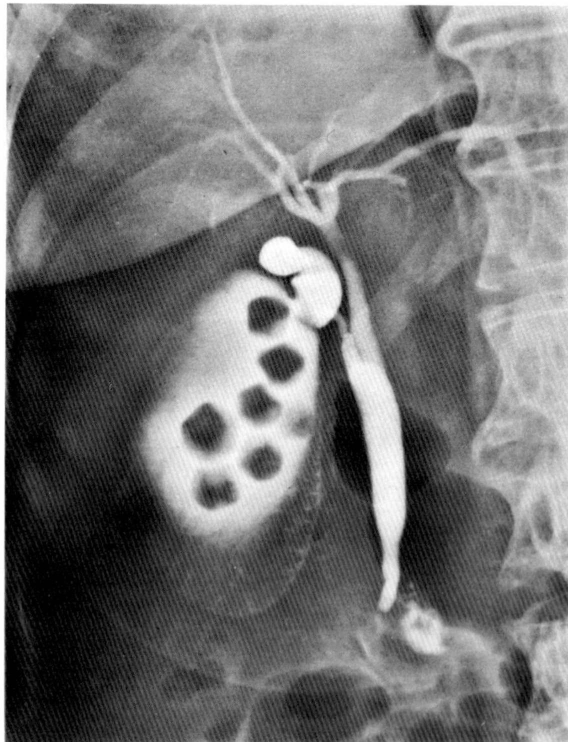

Fig. 4.6.**6 Gallbladder stones.** Normal intra- and extra-hepatic bile ducts

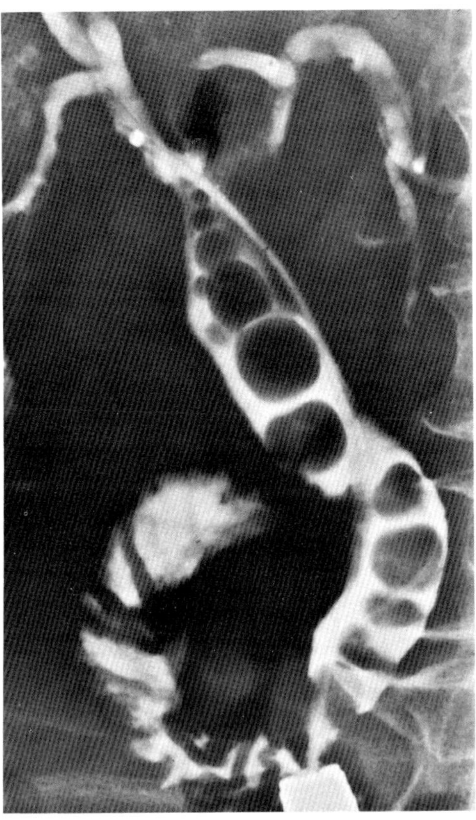

Fig. 4.6.**7**   **Multiple large gallstones in the common bile duct.** Patient with Billroth II gastrectomy

duct into the duodenum or pancreatic duct, leaving a fistula. Gallbladder fistulas may be detected after gallbladder stone migration and occasionally gallstone ileus. Impacted gallstones may give rise to inflammation and secondary stricturing of the bile duct. A gallstone impacted in the cystic duct with surrounding inflammation can give rise to an irregular stenosis of the common bile duct (Fig. 4.6.**8**). The stenosis of the bile duct in this so-called Mirizzi syndrome can mimic a malignant stricture (Cruz et al. 1983). Postoperative biliary strictures occur in 0.2 to 0.25 % of patients following biliary surgery (Fig. 4.6.**9**). These strictures are short and smooth, unless they are the result of extensive oversewing of a traumatized bile duct. Dilated ducts, proximal to the narrowed area are found in less than 50 % of patients (Huibregtse et al. 1986). In general differential diagnosis with a malignant stricture poses no problems. Also postoperative bile leaks or fistulas can be visualized via ERCP (Nelson 1984) (Fig. 4.6.**10**). The factors responsible for ongoing leakage are mostly a distal impacted stone or distal obstruction, which can also be easily demonstrated by ERCP. In a minority, closure of a fistula is retarded or prevented because of motor activity at the level of the sphincter of Oddi.

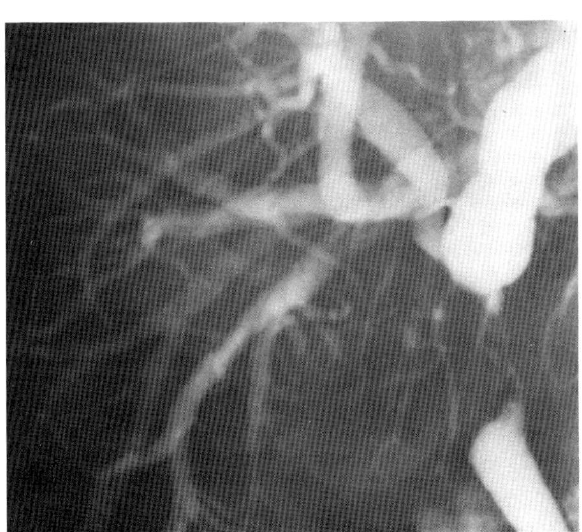

Fig. 4.6.**8**   **An impacted stone in the cystic duct** causes an irregular bile duct stricture (Mirizzi syndrome)

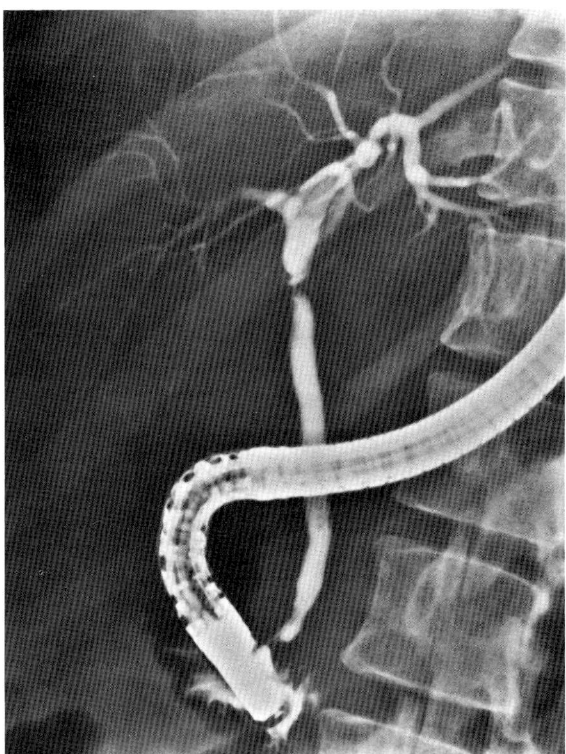

Fig. 4.6.**9**   **Characteristic postsurgical bile duct stricture**

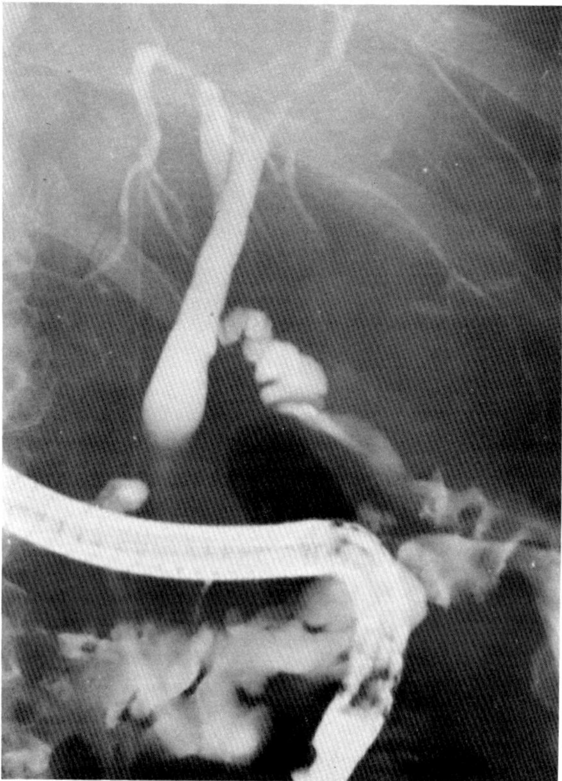

Fig. 4.6.**10   Postoperative leakage** from the cystic duct stump

Malignant Bile Duct Strictures

Bile duct carcinoma may develop at any level of the biliary tree (Benjamin 1982, Geenen 1983, Hadjis et al. 1985, Janes et al. 1982). However, most bile duct carcinomas are located at the confluence, or in the common hepatic duct. Concentric strictures, usually accompanied with "shouldering" are characteristic for cholangiocarcinoma. Intrahepatic bile duct dilation proximal to a tumor at the site of the confluence is seen in about 40–50% of the cases. Bile duct dilation is more prominent and present in nearly all patients when the stricture is located more distally. Hilar cholangiocarcinoma may be restricted to the subhilar common hepatic duct (type I) (Fig. 4.6.**11**), may be localised at the hilum, obstructing the free communication between the right and left intrahepatic systems (type II) (Fig. 4.6.**12**) or may extend into the liver affecting 2nd or 3rd order ducts (type III) (Fig. 4.6.**13**).

Filling of the intrahepatic bile ducts with contrast material may be difficult, even after deep cannulation in the case of firm, long strictures. Opacification may, however, become possible by wedging the diagnostic cannula with the help of a guide wire in the stricture (Fig. 4.6.**14**). High-pressure injection of contrast will then opacify the entire intrahepatic biliary system in virtually all cases.

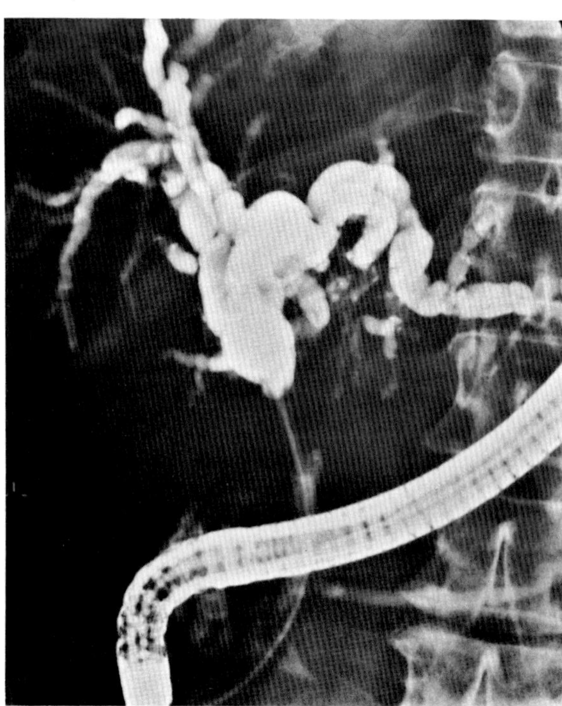

Fig. 4.6.**11   Cholangiocarcinoma** (Type I)

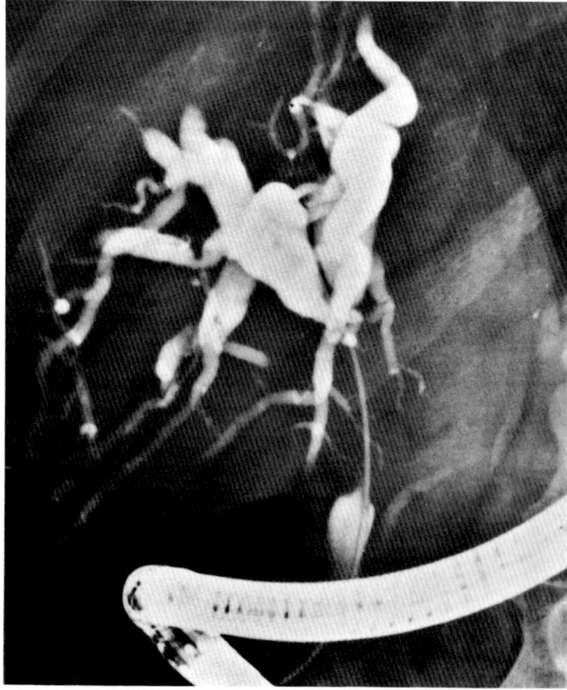

Fig. 4.6.**12 Cholangiocarcinoma at the bifurcation** (Type II)

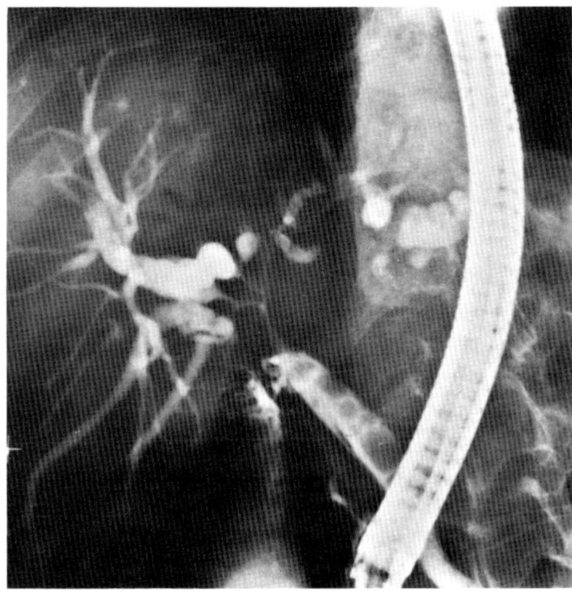

Fig. 4.6.**13**   Type III bile duct tumor at the site of the confluence

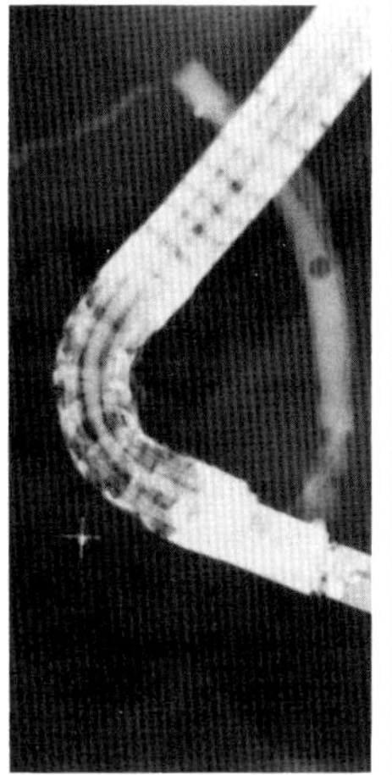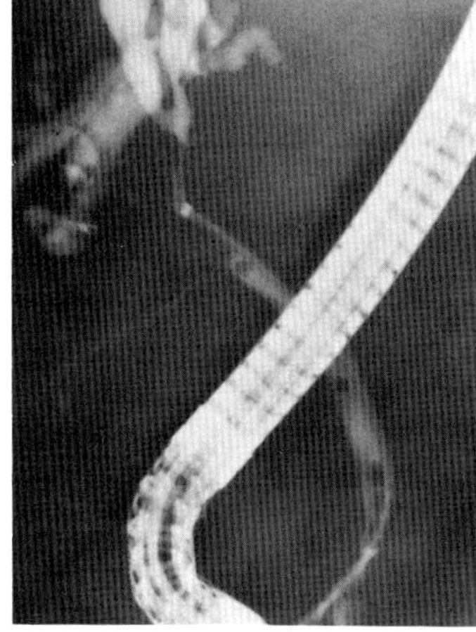

Fig. 4.6.**14**   **Left:** no filling of intrahepatic biliary tree. **Right:** the intrahepatic bile ducts are filled after wedging the catheter in the stricture

Differentiation between cholangiocarcinomas and primary sclerosing cholangitis may be difficult. Furthermore, the two diseases may coexist. Brush cytology or biopsy may be helpful when it shows malignant cells, but negative results do not rule out malignancy (Danzygier et al. 1983, Seifert et al. 1980). Our first experiences with the new cytology brush are very promising. Identical bile duct abnormalities have been described after irradiation (Martenson et al. 1986), local chemotherapy (Haq et al. 1986), and in the acquired immunodeficiency

syndrome (Roulot et al. 1987, Schneiderman et al. 1987).

Carcinoma of the gallbladder may cause obstructive jaundice by compression or growth into the common hepatic duct. Cholangiography shows a tapering or irregular stricture of the common hepatic duct, which is characteristically deviated from its normal position. A Mirizzi syndrome may give an identical picture and can be confused with malignancy. Gallbladder cancer may also spread into the bifurcation of the liver, involving right and left hepatic ducts. Carcinoma of the pancreas can produce obstruction of the intrapancreatic or suprapancreatic portion of the common bile duct (Fig. 4.6.**15**). The shape of the obstruction may be tapered, rounded, square or convex. The common bile duct frequently deviates medially, and the dilated proximal part of the bile duct may show a horizontal course. Occasionally, narrowing at the bifurcation is seen, due to metastatic disease.

Chronic pancreatitis gives rise to common bile duct obstruction in about 25 % of cases. Common bile duct strictures due to pancreatitis are mostly longer, smoothly delineated and incomplete in comparison to strictures produced by pancreatic cancer (Fig. 4.6.**16**). Usually, the ERCP catheter can easily be advanced through a stricture caused by chronic pancreatitis, in contrast to a stricture caused by pancreatic cancer. Pancreatography is

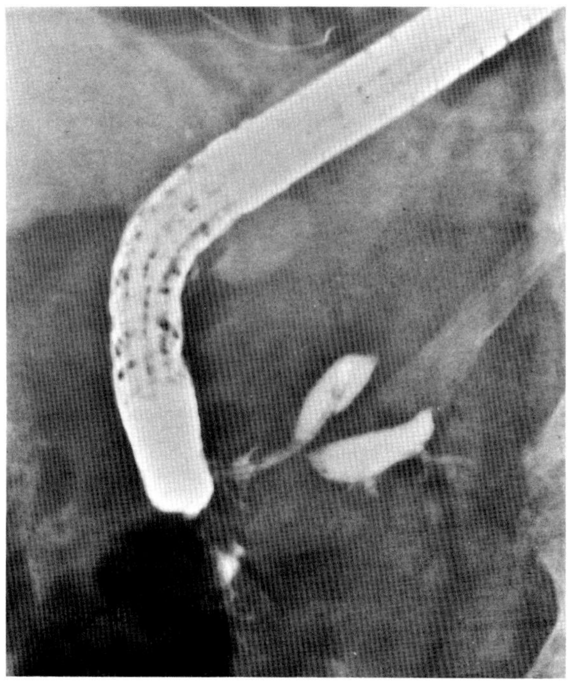

Fig. 4.6.**15**   **Both the common bile duct and the pancreatic duct show a stricture** in a patient with a pancreatic carcinoma (double duct sign)

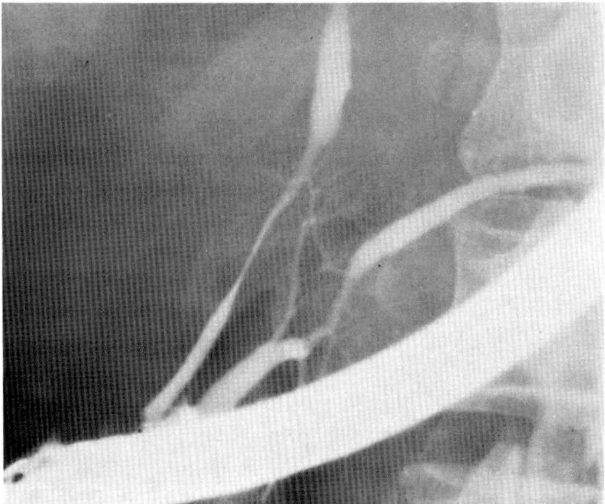

Fig. 4.6.**16**   **Pancreatic duct abnormalities** suggestive of chronic pancreatitis. The common bile duct shows a smooth narrowing

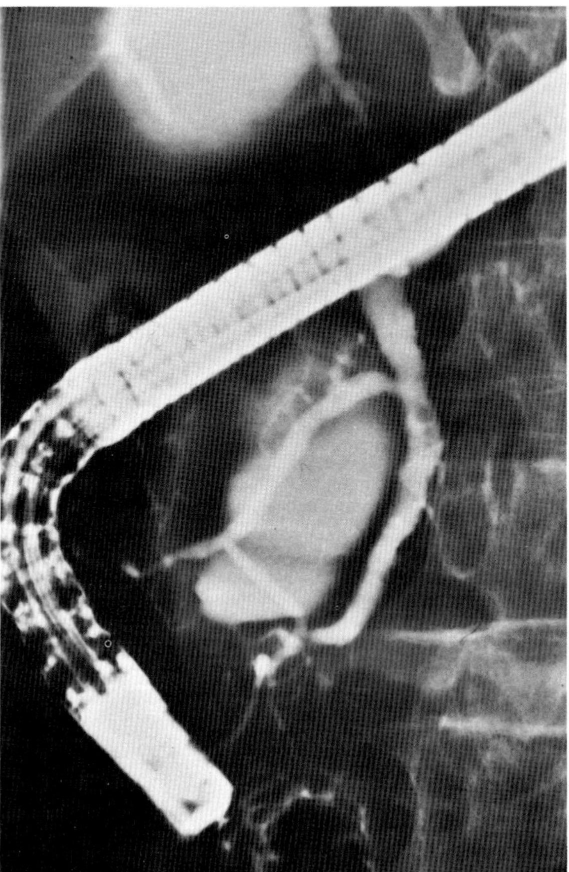

Fig. 4.6.**17**   **A carcinoma of the ampulla of Vater** with a highly dilated common bile duct. The pancreatic duct is not dilated, because outflow is guaranteed via the Santorini duct

generally helpful in making the differential diagnosis. It must, however, be borne in mind that pancreatic cancer occasionally develops in patients with chronic pancreatitis. Brush cytology of the bile duct is less helpful in such circumstances, because the pancreatic tumor has not yet invaded the common bile duct wall transmurally when jaundice develops. Distal common bile duct carcinoma may be indistinguishable from invading pancreatic cancer. A normal pancreatogram and a normal topography of the distal common bile duct however favor a cholangiocarcinoma. Metastatic disease in or around the head of the pancreas gives pictures identical to those seen in primary pancreatic cancer.

Periampullary Carcinomas

Cancer of the ampulla of Vater generally obstructs both the distal common bile duct and the pancreatic duct. The characteristic findings are a dilated bile duct and a dilated pancreatic duct together with a short irregular stricture at the site of the papilla. Shouldering of the obstructed common bile duct is frequently seen (Gmelin and Weiss 1981). Pancreatic duct dilation is absent when Santorini's duct and the minor papilla are patent (Fig. 4.6.**17**).

Other Malignancies

Intrahepatic metastases are best detected with ultrasonography. Intrahepatic duct displacement or amputation may be seen on cholangiography. Furthermore, interruption of intrahepatic bile ducts may be present. Cholangiographic findings of multiple intrahepatic metastases may be similar to those in macronodular liver cirrhosis. Lymphadenopathy due to lymph node metastasis or lymphoma produces rounded impressions in the bile duct wall.

Sclerosing Cholangitis

Sclerosing cholangitis generally gives abnormalities in both the intra- and extrahepatic biliary tree (La Russo et al. 1984, Li-Yeng and Goldberg 1984) (Fig. 4.6.**18**). However, occasionally only a local stricture is present, causing differential diagnostic difficulties with cholangiocarcinoma. Mostly, multiple strictures and dilations of varying length are seen, giving the characteristic picture of beading. Furthermore, diverticular outpouchings of the extrahepatic ducts are specific for sclerosing cholangitis (Fig. 4.6.**19**). Sclerosing cholangitis may be indistinguishable from a diffusely spreading form of cholangiocarcinoma (Fig. 4.6.**20**). Pancrea-

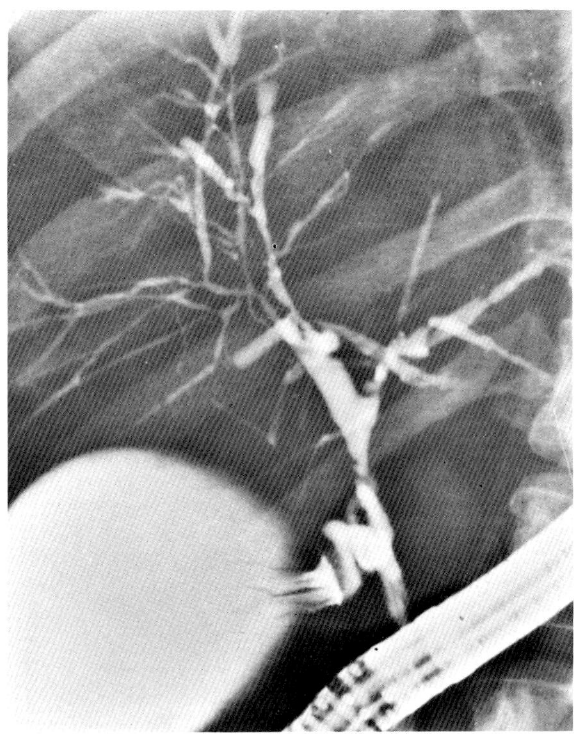

Fig. 4.6.**18** **Diffuse abnormalities of sclerosing cholangitis**

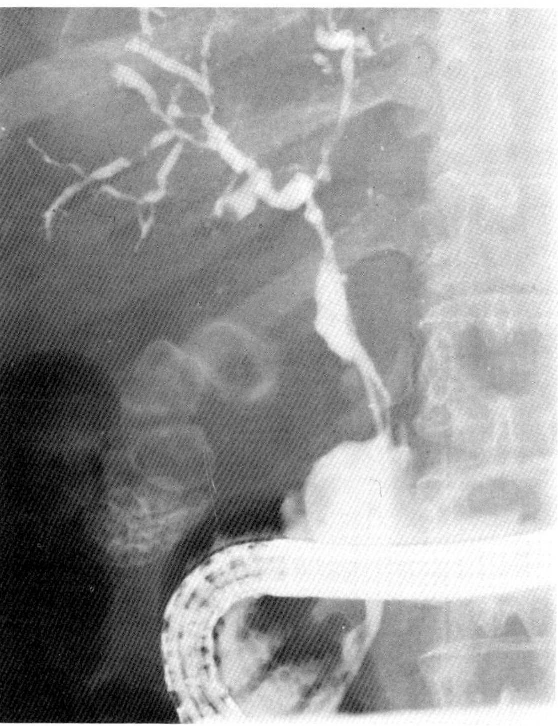

Fig. 4.6.**20** **Diffuse abnormalities** of diffusely spreading cholangiocarcinoma

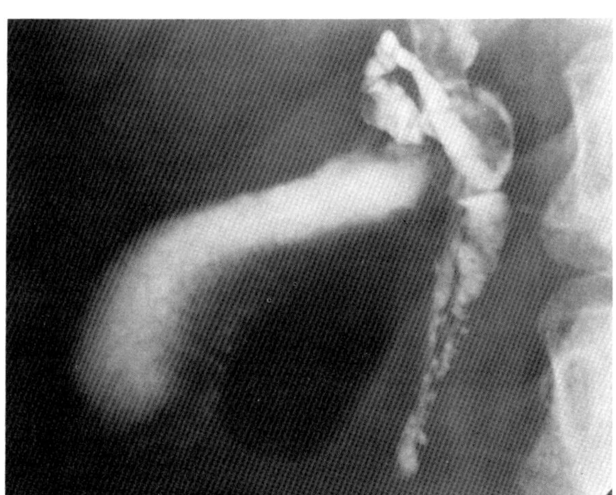

Fig. 4.6.**19** **Characteristic diverticular outpouchings** in primary sclerosing cholangitis

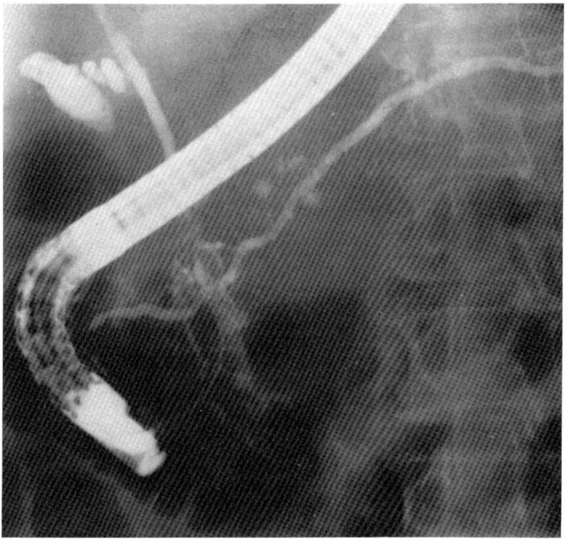

Fig. 4.6.**21** **Pancreas divisum** and signs of chronic pancreatitis in a patient with primary sclerosing cholangitis

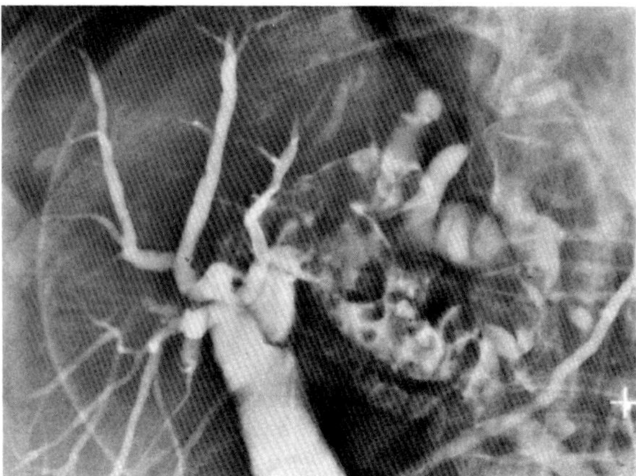

Fig. 4.6.**22   Intrahepatic bile duct cyst**, filled with concrements (Caroli disease)

tography shows irregularities of the ductal system in about 20 % of patients with sclerosing cholangitis (Kozarek 1988, Montefusco et al. 1984) (Fig. 4.6.**21**).

Rare Cholangiographic Findings

Choledochal cysts and Caroli's disease are rare diseases (Fig. 4.6.**22**). Cholangiography is useful in the preoperative assessment and in detecting complications like gallstones, abscesses and cholangiocarcinoma (Dayton et al. 1983). Cholangiocarcinoma develops in 7 % of patients with Caroli's disease and in 4 % of patients with choledochal cysts.

Abscesses secondary to bile duct obstructions may be seen on cholangiography when they communicate with the biliary tree. Urgent biliary drainage must be considered (Fig. 4.6.**23**). Echinococcus cysts may also communicate with the biliary tree and give characteristic findings. Daughter cysts may be seen in the bile duct as filling defects. These cysts can be removed after endoscopic papillotomy (Cottone et al. 1978).

A paucity of intrahepatic bile ducts is seen in liver cirrhosis and in the vanishing bile duct syndrome after liver transplantation. Macronodular liver cirrhosis can produce deviation and bile duct rarefaction. Furthermore, the bile ducts may show a kinking course due to shrinking of the liver.

Worms and foreign bodies are extreme rarities, and can be removed after endoscopic papillotomy.

Manometry of the Sphincter of Oddi

A triple lumen catheter introduced into the papilla is connected to an electromechanical pressure

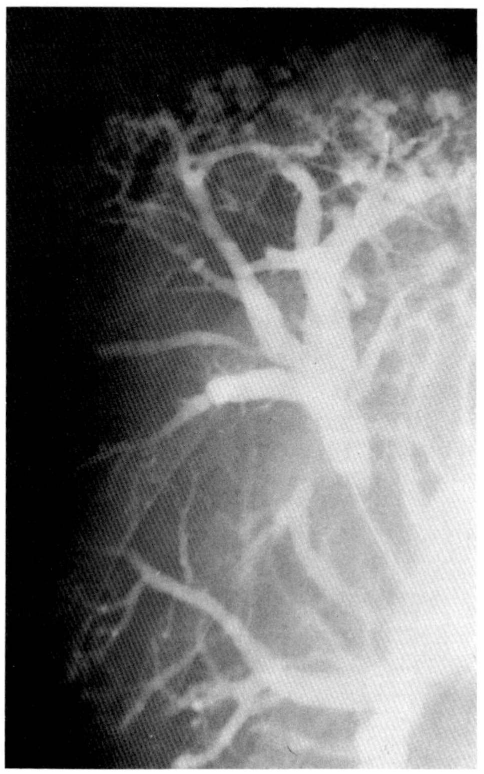

Fig. 4.6.**23   Multiple intrahepatic abscesses**

transducer to record pressure changes. With this method it is possible to analyze the bilio duodenal pressure difference, the frequency and amplitude of the contractions of the sphincter of Oddi, and the direction of propagation of the contraction waves. The normal bilio duodenal pressure difference is 9.6 mmHg, the frequency of the contractions is 5 per min, and the mean amplitude of the contractions is 100 mmHg (De Masi Corazziari et al. 1984, Poralla et al. 1985, Tanaka and Ikeda 1983). Biliary dyskinesia, benign papillary stenosis and cholelithiasis are the diseases extensively studied with manometry of the sphincter of Oddi. Manometry can be helpful in one clinical setting: it may indicate those patients with biliary dyskinesia who are going to benefit from endoscopic papillotomy.

Pancreatography

The pancreatic duct should be filled with contrast under fluoroscopic control until the tail and the first-order side branches are visualized. Further filling, and parenchymography in particular, should be avoided, to avoid the risk of acute pancreatitis. The pancreatic duct empties rapidly, and X-ray pictures should be taken at once, while the endoscope and the catheter are still in situ.

The Normal Pancreatogram

The normal pancreas is situated in the retroperitoneum and crosses the second lumbar vertebra. The course of the main pancreatic duct may be compared with the form of a pistol. The mean length of the pancreatic duct is about 20 cm. The width of the duct gradually decreases from head to tail. The mean diameters of the duct are 4 mm in the head, 3 mm in the corpus and 2 mm in the tail (Classen et al. 1973). Above the age of 40, the width of the main pancreatic duct increases significantly. Two major side branches in the pancreatic head can be observed. One leads to the uncinate process (ramus capitis inferior). The other connects the main pancreatic duct with the minor papilla (Santorini's duct). The major characteristics of normality are: a smooth lining of the pancreatic duct, absence of caliber changes, and tiny regular side branches. The shape of the pancreas varies considerably, and pancreatic duct deviations without indentation or derangement of the side branches are common and generally have low diagnostic significance.

Proper interpretation of a pancreatogram is complicated, because of the many congenital ductal anomalies, the commonest one resulting from incomplete fusion of the dorsal and ventral anlage. Cannulation of the main papilla may then result in opacification of only a small ventral portion (Fig. 4.6.**24**). Delineation of the remainder of the pancreas then requires opacification of Santorini's duct via the accessory or minor papilla. This anomaly (pancreas divisum) is seen in 4 to 6% of patients in ERCP studies. The question of whether the pancreas divisum predisposes to pancreatic diseases is still controversial (Cotton and Williams 1980, Delhaye et al. 1985). A rare anomaly is the annular pancreas, which may be shown by ERCP.

Chronic Pancreatitis

The ductular abnormalities in chronic pancreatitis range from normal to severe destruction. Chronic pancreatitis may be divided into 3 stages, according to the intensity of these changes (Fig. 4.6.**25**). In the first stage, minor irregularities of the small ducts are present as a result of inflammation and shrinkage. In the second stage, irregularities and minor caliber changes of the main duct, and more pronounced alterations of the side branches, are present. In the third stage, the entire ductal system is abnormal.

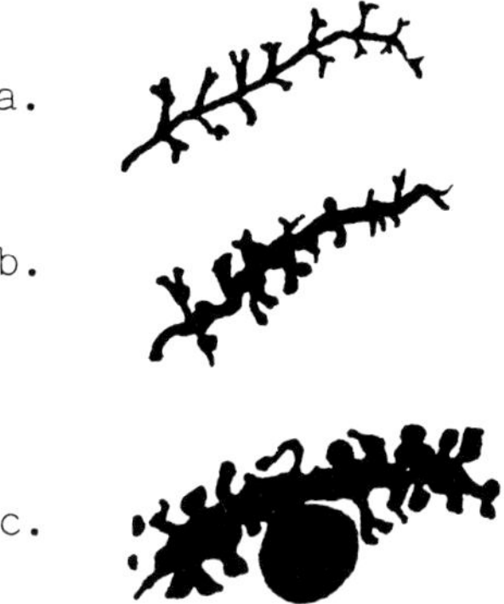

Fig. 4.6.**25** **Three stages of chronic pancreatitis:** a) first stage; b) second stage; c) third stage

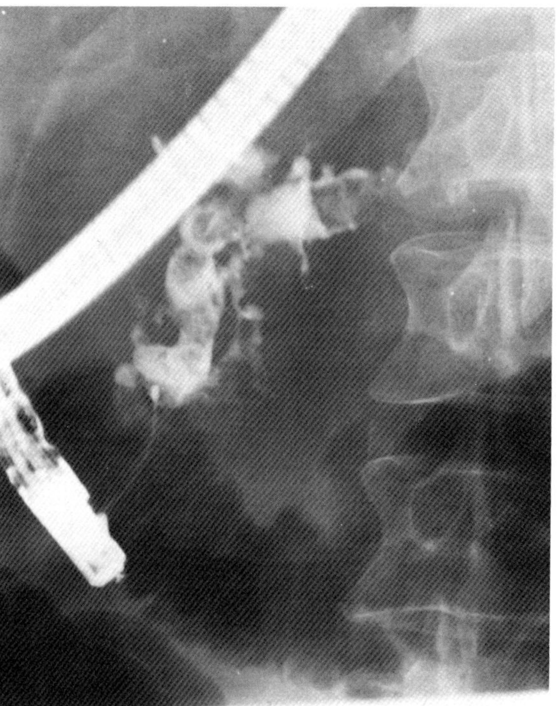

Fig. 4.6.**26** **Dilated pancreatic duct** filled with calcified protein plugs. Complete obstruction in the corpus of the pancreas

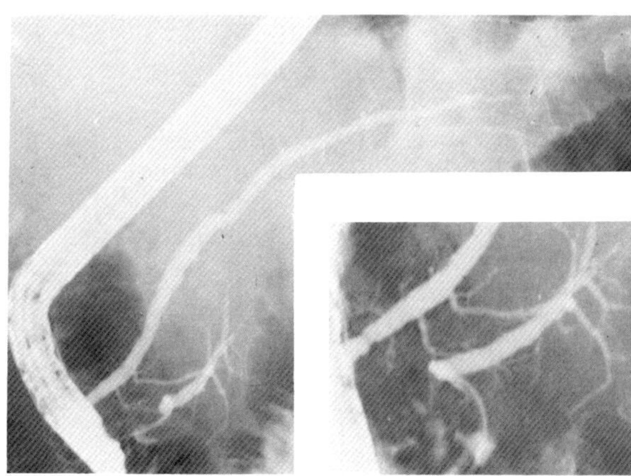

Fig. 4.6.**24** **Partially fused pancreatic duct.** The dorsal duct is connected via tiny side branches with the ventral duct

Table 4.6.3   Classification of pancreatograms in chronic pancreatitis (Axon et al. 1984)

Pancrea-togram	Side branches	Main duct
Normal	Normal	Normal
Equivocal	Less than 3 abnormal	Normal
Abnormal:		
Mild	More than 3 abnormal	Normal
Moderate	More than 3 abnormal	Abnormal
Marked	More than 3 abnormal	Abnormal plus one or more of: large cavity obstruction filling defects severe dilation severe irregularity

Changes may be diffuse (whole gland) or local (one-third or less involved of head, body or tail)

The main duct shows areas of dilation and stenosis. The side branches may be cystically dilated. Caliber changes with multiple strictures and dilations give the characteristic "chain of lakes" or "chain of pearls" appearance. Intraductular filling defects and calcifications may also be present (Fig. 4.6.**26**). In most patients, a combination of these findings are seen.

Several classifications of ductular changes in chronic pancreatitis have been presented. A new classification was suggested during an international workshop in March 1983 (Axon et al. 1984). The workshop suggested that the pancreatogram in chronic pancreatitis should be divided into normal,

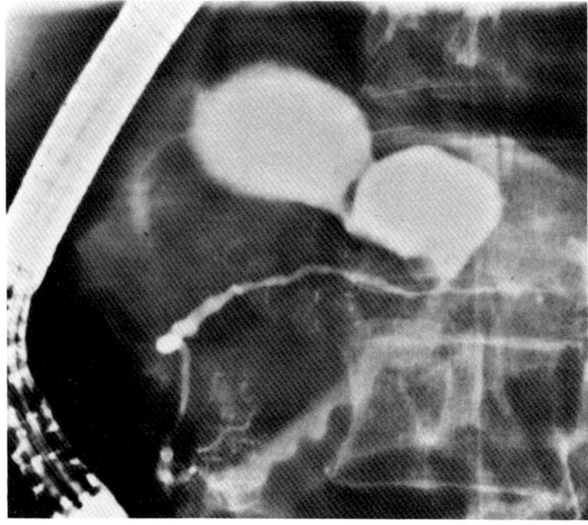

Fig. 4.6.**27**   **Irregularities of the main pancreatic duct** and filling of two large pseudocysts

equivocal, mild, moderate and severe alterations, which are either diffuse or localized (Table 4.6.**3**). Normal or equivocal duct changes are seen when only one or two side branches are affected. In mild ductular changes, three or more side branches are altered; the main duct, however, is normal. Moderate ductular changes display additional irregularities of the main duct. Severe chronic pancreatitis is diagnosed if the pancreatogram exhibits, in addition to moderate changes, one or more of the following findings: large cavities, obstruction, intraductular filling defect, mild dilation, or irregularity of the main pancreatic duct (Fig. 4.6.**27**).

This classification makes good correlation between different investigators, or groups of investigators, possible, and allows their documentation to be compared.

Pancreatic Carcinoma

The pancreatographic image of pancreatic carcinoma may be divided into 5 major types (Fig. 4.6.**28**): a) stenosis with prestenotic dilation; b) complete obstruction; c) tapering type (cf. Fig. 4.6.**29**); d) side branch deviation; e) cavity formation. These changes are not pathognomonic, but they are more often found in carcinoma than in chronic pancreatitis.

A normal pancreatogram may be found in 2.5 to 12.5% of cases with pancreatic carcinoma. The majority of pancreatic tumors are located in the head of the pancreas, and affect the common bile duct as well. The abnormalities of the distal common bile duct are very helpful in improving overall diagnostic accuracy (Plumley et al. 1982).

Cytological investigations of endoscopically collected pure pancreatic juice, or brush cytology of the pancreatic duct and common bile duct, may prove the malignant nature of the stricture. The results of cytology in pancreatic cancer vary between 40% and 87%.

Concluding Remarks

ERCP has contributed much to our knowledge of hepatobiliopancreatic diseases. It has become the method of choice in the diagnosis of some of these diseases through its unique combination of endoscopy and radiology. Therapeutic endoscopic papillotomy and endoscopic biliary and pancreatic drainage procedures are an extension of the diagnostic endoscopic procedure. Future development will make endoscopy and endoscopic treatment possible inside the biliary and pancreatic ducts with a "baby" endoscope, which can be inserted into the

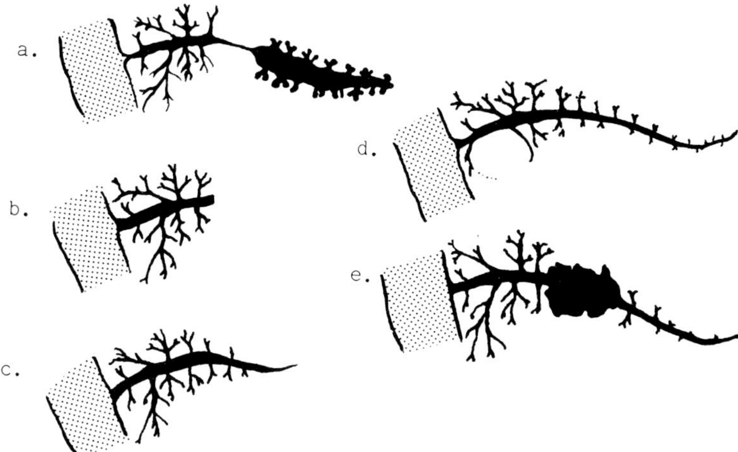

Fig. 4.6.**28** **Major types of pancreatic carcinoma**

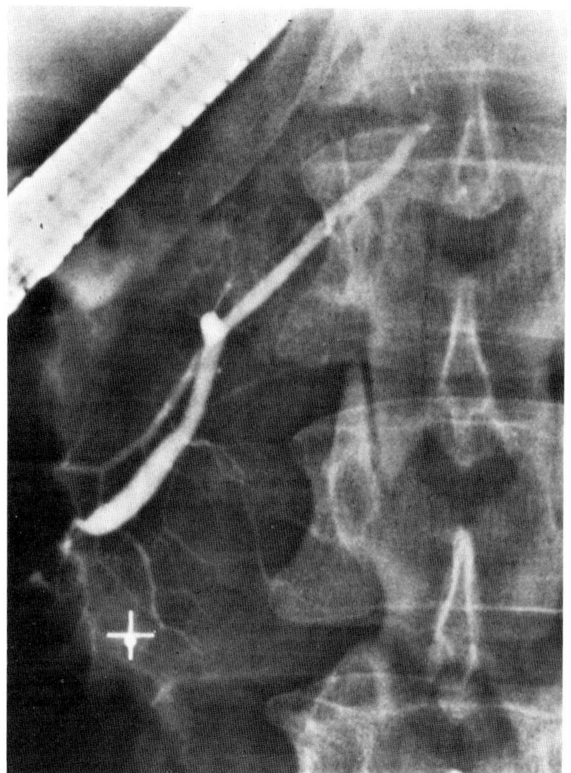

Fig. 4.6.**29** **Carcinoma in the corpus of the pancreas.** Tapering type

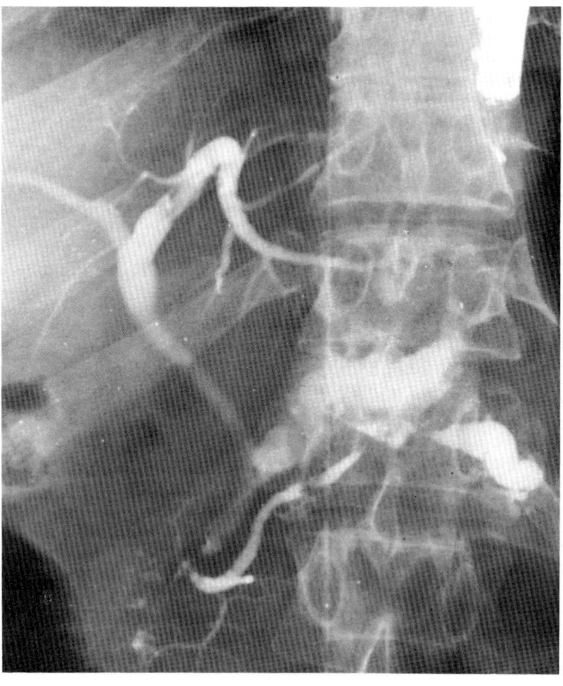

Fig. 4.6.**30** **Cystadenocarcinoma** of the pancreas

ducts to carry out various procedures under direct endoscopic vision (Kozarek 1988). Up till now, the main drawback of these instruments is their fragility and the tiny size of the instrumentation channel. The further development of very small chips will in all probability solve these problems.

References

Axon ATR, Classen M, Cotton PB, et al. Pancreatography in chronic pancreatitis: international definitions. International Workshop, Kings College, Cambridge, 23–25th March. Gut 1984; 25: 1107–1112.

Benjamin IS. The obstructed biliary tract. In: Blumgart LH, ed. The biliary tract. Edinburgh: Churchill Livingstone, 1982: chapter 10, 157.

Bilbao MK, Dotter CT, Lee RG, Katon RM. Complications of endoscopic retrograde cholangiopancreatography (ERCP): a study of 1000 cases. Gastroenterology 1976; 70: 314–320.

Bourgeois N, Dunham F, Verhest A, Cremer M. Endoscopic biopsies of the papilla of Vater at the time of endoscopic sphincterotomy: difficulties in interpretation. Gastrointest Endosc 1984; 30: 163–166.

Classen M. Endoscopic retrograde cholangiopancreatography (ERCP). In: Bianchi L, Gerok W, Sickinger K, eds. Liver and bile. MTP Press, Lancaster, 1977: 235–241.

Classen M, Phillip J. Endoscopic retrograde choledochopancreatography. In: Blumgart LH, ed. Surgery of the liver and biliary tract. Edinburgh: Churchill Livingstone, 1988: 257–275.

Classen M, Hellwig H, Rösch W. Anatomy of the pancreatic duct: a duodenoscopic-radiological study. Endoscopy 1973; 5: 14–17.

Cotton PB. Progress report ERCP. Gut 1977; 18: 316–341.

Cotton PB. Congenital anomaly of pancreas divisum as a cause of obstructive pain and pancreatitis. Gut 1980; 21: 105–114.

Cotton PB, Williams CB, eds. Practical gastrointestinal endoscopy. Blackwell: Oxford, 1980: 55–76.

Cottone M, Amuso M, Cotton P. Endoscopic retrograde cholangiography in hepatic hydatid disease. Br J Surg 1978; 66: 107.

Cruz FO, Barriga P, Tocornal J, Burhenne HJ. Radiology of the Mirizzi syndrome: diagnostic importance of the transhepatic cholangiogram. Gastrointest Radiol 1983; 8: 249–253.

Danzygier H, Phillip J, Hagenmüller F, et al. Forceps biopsy of human bile ducts: light and electron microscopical findings, clinical significance. Gastroenterology 1983; 84: 1132.

Dayton MT, Longmire WP, Tompkins RK. Caroli's disease: a premalignant condition? Am J Surg 1983; 145: 41–48.

Delhaye M, Engelholm L, Cremer M. Pancreas divisum: congenital anatomic variant or anomaly. Gastroenterology 1985; 89: 951–958.

De Masi Corazziari E, Habib FI, Fontana B, Gatti V, Fegiz GF, Torsoli A. Manometric study of the sphincter of Oddi in patients with and without common bile duct stones. Gut 1984; 25: 275–278.

Dyrszka H, Sanghavi B. Hepatic hydatid disease: findings on endoscopic retrograde cholangiography. Gastrointest Endosc 1983; 29: 248–249.

Gebhardt C, Riemann JF, Lux G. The importance of ERCP for the surgical tactic in haemorrhagic necrotizing pancreatitis (preliminary report). Endoscopy 1983; 15: 55–58.

Geenen JE. Sphincter of Oddi manometry. Clin Gastroenterol 1983; 12 (suppl 1): 108–114.

Gibson RN, Yeung E, Thompson JN, et al. Radiological evaluation of bile duct obstruction: level, cause and tumour resectability. Radiology 1986; 160: 43–47.

Gmelin E, Weiss HD. Tumours in the region of the papilla of Vater. Eur J Radiol 1981; 1: 301–306.

Goodman AJ, Neoptolemos JP, Carr-Locke DL, Finlay DBL, Fossard DP. Detection of gall stones after acute pancreatitis. Gut 1985; 26: 642–645.

Hadjis NS, Collier NA, Blumgart LH. Malignant masquerade at the hilum of the liver. Br J Surg 1985; 72: 659–661.

Hannigan BF, Keeling PWN, Stavin B, Thompson RPH. Hyperamylasemia after ERCP with ionic and non-ionic contrast media. Gastrointest Endosc 1985; 31: 109–110.

Haq MM, Valdes LG, Peterson DF, Gourley WK. Fibrosis of extrahepatic biliary system after continuous hepatic artery infusion of floxuridine through an implantable pump (infusaid pump). Cancer 1986; 57: 1281–1283.

Helm EB, Bauernfeind A, Frech K, Hagenmüller F. Pseudomonas-Septikämie nach endoskopischen Eingriffen am Gallengangsystem. Dtsch Med Wochenschr 1984; 109: 698–701.

Heloury Y, Leborgne J, Rogez JM, Robert R, Lehur PA, Pannier M, Barbin JY. Radiological anatomy of the bile ducts based on intraoperative investigation in 250 cases. Anat Clin 1985; 7: 93–102.

Huibregtse K, Katon RM, Tytgat GNJ. Endoscopic treatment of postoperative biliary strictures. Endoscopy 1986; 18: 133–137.

Janes JO, Laughlin CL, Goldberger LE, Berk RN. Differential features of some unusual biliary tumors. Gastrointest Radiol 1982; 7: 341–348.

Kasugai T. Recent advances in the endoscopic retrograde cholangiopancreatography. Digestion 1975; 13: 76–99.

Kozarek RA. Direct cholangioscopy and pancreatoscopy at time of endoscopic retrograde cholangiopancreatography. Am J Gastroenterol 1988; 83: 55–57.

Lankisch PG, Creutzfeldt W. Exokrine Pankreasinsuffizienz bei primär sklerosierender Cholangitis. Z Gastroenterol 1987; 25: 174–181.

La Russo NF, Wiesner RH, Ludwig J, MacCarty RL. Primary sclerosing cholangitis. N Engl J Med 1984; 310: 899–903.

Li-Yeng C, Goldberg HI. Sclerosing cholangitis: broad spectrum of radiographic features. Gastrointest Radiol 1984; 9: 39–47.

McCune WS, Shorb PE, Moscowitz H. Endoscopic cannulation of the ampulla of Vater: a preliminary report. Ann Surg 1968; 167: 752.

Martenson JA, Gunderson LL, Buskirk SJ et al. Hepatic duct stricture after radical radiation therapy for biliary cancer: recurrence or fibrosis? Mayo Clin Proc 1986; 61: 530–536.

Meier P, Ansel H, Silvis S, Vennes J. Comparison of ultrasound and ERCP measurements of bile duct size. Gastroenterology 1984; 87: 615.

Montefusco PP, Geiss AC, Bronzo RL, Randall S, Kahn E, McKinley MJ. Sclerosing cholangitis, chronic pancreatitis and Sjögren's syndrome: a syndrome complex. Am J. Surg 1984; 147: 822–826.

Mueller PR, Ferrucci JT, Simeone J, et al. Postcholecystectomy bile duct dilatation: myth of reality? AJR 1981; 136: 355–358.

Nelson AM. Demonstration of a traumatic biliary fistula by ERCP. Gastointest Endosc 1984; 30: 315–316.

Niederau C, Sonnenberg A, Müller J. Comparison of the extrahepatic bile duct size measured by ultrasound and by different radiographic methods. Gastroenterology 1984; 87: 615–621.

O'Connor HJ, Bartlett RJ, Hamilton I et al. Bile duct calibere: the discrepancy between ultrasonic and retrograde cholangiographic measurement in the post-cholecystectomy patient. Clin Radiol 1985; 36: 507–510.

Ohto M, Ono T, Tsuchiya Y, Saisho H, eds. Cholangiography and pancreatography. Tokyo: Igaku-Shoin, 1978.

Okuno M, Himeno S, Kurakawa M et al. Changes in serum levels of pancreatic isoamylase, lipase, trysin and elastase 1 h after endoscopic retrograde pancreatography. Hepatogastroenterology 1985; 32: 87–90.

Osnes M, Rosseland AR, Aabakken L. Endoscopic retrograde cholangiography and endoscopic papillotomy in patients with a previous Billroth-II resection. Gut 1986; 27: 1193–1198.

Plumley TF, Rohrmann CA, Freeny PC, et al. Double duct sign: reassessed significance in ERCP. AJR 1982; 138: 31–35.

Poralla T, Staritz M, Manns M, Klose K, Hommel G, Meyer zum Büschenfelde KH. Age and sex dependency of bile duct diameter and bile duct pressure: an ERC manometry study. Z Gastroenterol 1985; 23: 235–239.

Rösch W. Report on a symposium '10 years of ERCP': diagnostic and therapeutic aspects. E.S.G.E. Newsletter 1981; 15: 8–9.

Roulot D, Valla D, Brun-Vezinet F et al. Cholangitis in the acquired immunodeficiency syndrome, report of two cases and review of the literature. Gut 1987; 28: 1653–1660.

Schneiderman DJ, Cello JP, Laing FC. Papillary stenosis and sclerosing cholangitis in the acquired immunodeficiency syndrome. Ann Intern Med 1987; 106: 546–549.

Seifert E, Urakami Y, Elster K. Duodenoscopic guided biopsy of the biliary and pancreatic duct. Endoscopy 1980; 9: 154.

Tanaka M, Ikeda S. Parapapillary choledochoduodenal fistula: an analysis of 83 consecutive patients diagnosed at ERCP. Gastrointest Endosc 1983; 29: 88–89.

Toouli J, Geenen JE, Hogan WJ, Doods WJ, Arndorfer RC. Sphincter of Oddi motor activity: a comparison between patients with common bile duct stones and controls. Gastroenterology 1982; 82: 111–117.

4.7   Ultrasound-Guided Percutaneous Transhepatic Cholangiography and Drainage in Malignant Biliary Disease

J. S. Laméris

Introduction

Although percutaneous transhepatic cholangiography (PTC) dates back to 1937, it was only after the introduction of the Chiba needle in 1968 that this diagnostic method was more widely accepted (Okuda 1980). For years, PTC was the only way to visualize the bile duct system. The accepted technique for this procedure was a right lateral puncture in the midaxillary line, usually in the 9th intercostal space. The direction of the needle in the right lobe of the liver depended on the relation between liver, lung and vertebral column and was guided by fluoroscopy. Injection of contrast medium was done while the Chiba needle was slowly withdrawn.

Although the success rate of imaging dilated bile ducts was as high as 98 %, the complication rate was not negligible, and varied between 3 and 10 % (Harbin et al. 1980). Major complications were bile leakage, intraperitoneal hemorrhage, pneumothorax and septicemia. In many institutions, this diagnostic method was, even after the introduction of the Chiba needle, only considered safe when laparotomy was undertaken directly afterwards.

In the early 1960s, Glenn and Arner showed that intraperitoneal bile leakage could be prevented by temporarily leaving a catheter for *external* drainage in place (Arner et al. 1962, Glenn et al. 1962). Molnar and Stockum (1974) described a procedure for *internal* bile drainage. A teflon tube with multiple side-holes above and below the level of the stenotic area was able to drain the bile directly into the duodenum (Fig. 4.7.1).

Percutaneous transhepatic biliary drainage was generally performed as a two-step procedure. After fine-needle percutaneous transhepatic cholangiography, one of the main bile ducts was punctured with an 18 gauge needle with a preloaded catheter under fluoroscopic control. Then, with methods used for angiography (Seldinger technique), a catheter was introduced into the bile duct.

Nowadays diagnostic PTC has lost much of its importance. Bile duct dilation is easily recognized with non-invasive methods such as ultrasound (US) and computed tomography (CT). In the majority of patients with obstructive jaundice, the cause of the bile duct obstruction will become clear with these imaging techniques. The endoscopic approach to the biliary system has a comparable success rate in imaging the bile duct system, but circumvents complications due to the transperitoneal and transhepatic route used for PTC. Further refinements in technique and equipment, and especially the use of ultrasound-guided puncture for PTC, have led to a shift in emphasis from diagnostic to therapeutic aims.

The use of ultrasound has the advantage of puncturing a selected dilated bile duct. It reduces the number of punctures needed for effective visualizing and drainage of the biliary system, and avoids complications such as bleeding or pneumothorax (Makuuci et al. 1980, Laméris et al. 1985). Bile leakage and septicemia due to the pressure rise in the biliary system after contrast injection are avoided to a great extent when the one-step ultrasound-guided drainage method is used.

Method

Patient Preparation

Antibiotic prophylaxis is started 24 h beforehand, and continued for 24 h afterwards; parenteral ampicillin and gentamicin are recommended. Bleeding and clotting times should be corrected when indicated. Local anesthesia and systemic sedatives and analgetics should be given in adequate amounts. An intravenous cannula is necessary for rapid administration of fluids in case of hypotension or septic shock. The skin of the upper abdomen and the lower thoracic region is prepared, allowing flexibility in the choice of the puncture site. The ultrasound transducer is wrapped in a sterile sleeve. Commercially available sterile gel is used as coupling agent for skin contact.

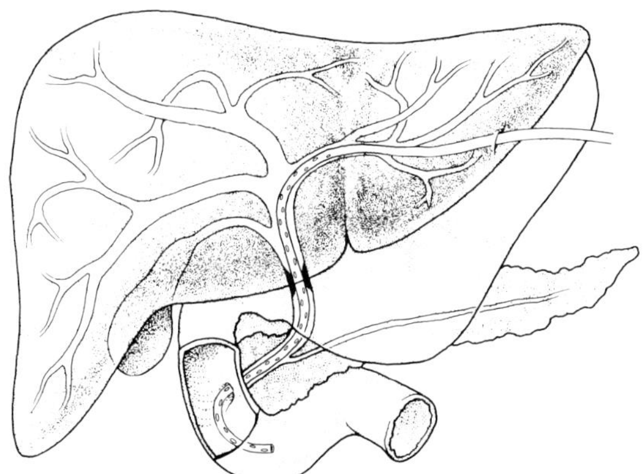

Fig. 4.7.1   **Internal drainage** by means of a multiple side-hole catheter

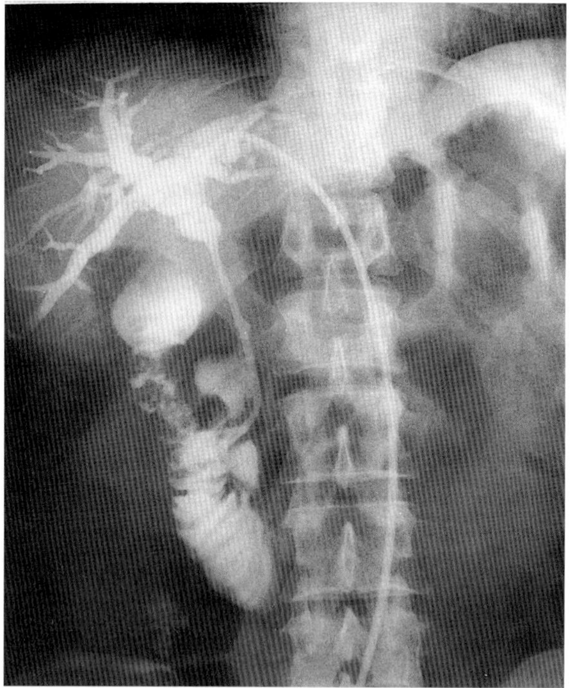

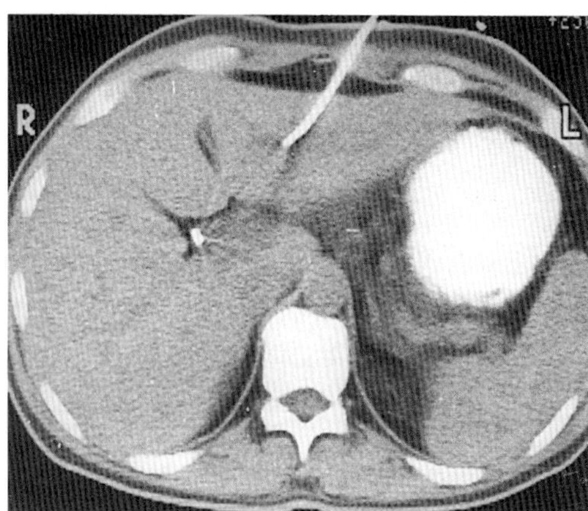

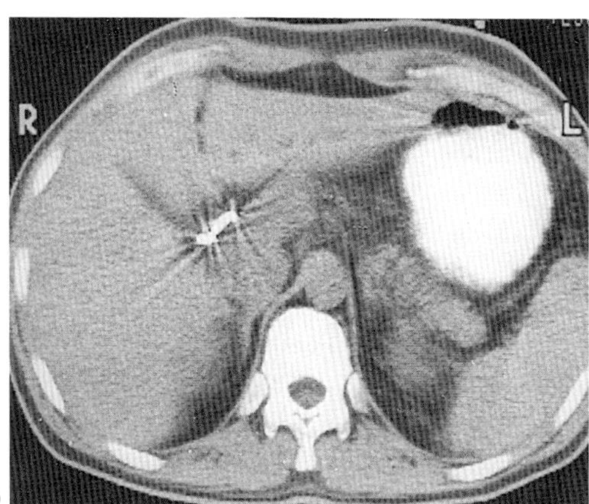

Fig. 4.7.**2   Percutaneous transhepatic biliary drainage** in a patient with pancreatic carcinoma. The anterior approach to the left lobe bile ducts is shown on **a** cholangiography and **b** CT-scan

The Puncture Site

With ultrasound guidance, there is no longer any preference for the traditional right lateral intercostal approach. The initial puncture route is chosen in such a way that the introduction of a guide wire and a catheter will subsequently be possible. This means that the angle between the puncture route and the bile duct should not be too steep. For several reasons an anterior approach to the left lobe bile ducts is advantageous (Fig. 4.7.**2**). It avoids the risk of a transpleural puncture. In addition, an anteriorly placed catheter appears to give less discomfort to the patient. Dislodgment of the catheter and buckling of the catheter in the space between the liver and the abdominal wall will occur less frequently when the catheter is positioned in the left liver lobe than with right-sided intercostal catheters. A possible explanation is that respiratory movement between the right lobe of the liver and the adjacent abdominal wall is greater than between the left lobe and the anterior abdominal wall (Laméris et al. 1985).

However, when the biliary obstruction is located at the confluence of the left and right hepatic ducts, or whenever the left lobe bile ducts are poorly visualized by ultrasound, a right lateral, preferably subcostal approach is indicated.

The true extension of the pleural space, especially in sick and older patients, is not indicated by the level of the air-filled lung parenchyma as seen on fluoroscopy or ultrasound. The collapsed pleural space can reach as far as the 9th or 10th costa. Traversing the collapsed pleural space with a catheter can lead to hemorrhage, pleura effusion and empyema, and should therefore be avoided (Dawson et al. 1983, Mueller et al. 1982, Neff et al. 1984). In these cases, ultrasound guidance facilitates a right subcostal puncture.

Puncture Technique

The 22 gauge needle is inserted with the patient holding his breath. Bending of the needle due to movements between the transducer and the skin is prevented by guiding the fine needle through the transducer and the skin with a short, stiff 18 gauge needle. The correct position of the needle tip within the bile duct is confirmed by the discharge of bile after removing the stylet. A thin guide wire (0.046 cm) is then introduced through the 22 gauge needle. This action is observed by ultrasound. The small guide wire serves as guidance for an 18 gauge needle with a preloaded teflon sheath. With this needle point inside the bile duct, the teflon sheath will easily follow the guide wire (Fig. 4.7.**3**).

After aspiration of bile, a water-soluble contrast agent is injected into the bile system. Fluoroscopy and radiography in several positions are

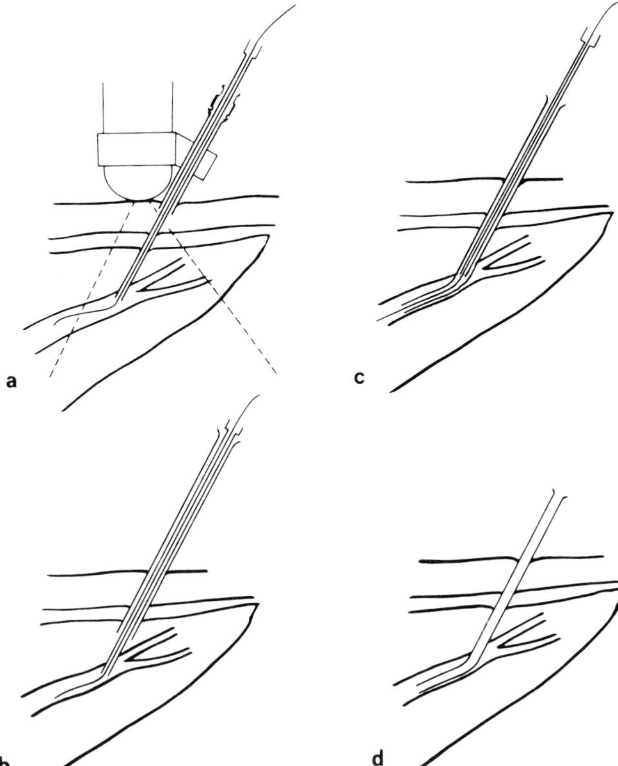

Fig. 4.7.3   Technique of ultrasound-guided biliary drainage

a Initial puncture with a 22 gauge needle. The needle is directed through the skin by a short 18 gauge needle. A 0.046 cm guide wire is introduced into the bile duct

b An 18 gauge needle with a pre-loaded Teflon sheath is introduced over the guide wire

c With the needle point inside the bile duct, the Teflon sheath is pushed into the bile duct.

d The situation after removal of the 18 gauge needle and the guide wire. The catheter allows introduction of a thicker guide wire and subsequent placement of larger catheters

used to document the correct position of the catheter and to define the nature of the bile duct obstruction. Whenever signs of cholangitis are present, the procedure is stopped after a pigtail catheter has been left for *external* drainage. Bile is cultured for specific antibiotic treatment.

External drainage should be prolonged until the clinical situation of the patient has stabilized. When infection is not present, attempts are made to pass the obstruction. Torque control guide wires are very helpful in these manipulations. When the stenosis is passed, *internal* drainage can be achieved by introducing a multiple side-hole catheter. If attempts to pass the stenosis fail, a second attempt after several days of drainage will often be successful. The explanation is that, once the prestenotic dilation has diminished, the lumen of the bile duct will be better matched to the stenotic part. This facilitates the transversal of the stenosis with a guide wire and the subsequent passage of a catheter.

Catheter Materials

Initial drainage catheters are usually made of polyethylene and are 8–10 Fr in size. Long-term drainage catheters should be made of soft non-kinking biocompatible materials, such as polyurethane, percuflex etc. A pigtail shape is preferred for external drainage. Internal drainage

catheters should have side-holes proximally and distally to the stenotic area. Individual adaptations to the length of the prestenotic bile duct, the length of the stenosis and the poststenotic tract are best carried out by using straight or slightly curved catheters and cutting in side-holes manually. Side-holes are cut in the pre- and poststenotic tract, but not in bends or in the region of the obstruction. In this way, kinking of the catheter or tumor overgrowth in the catheter lumen is prevented.

Since intraparenchymal side-holes can cause severe bleeding, the intraductal position of the prestenotic side-holes must be controlled fluoroscopically by marking the distance to the first side-hole on a guide wire before insertion. Multiple side-hole catheters should have a stiff inner tubing in order to prevent buckling of the catheter during the introduction. Long-term drainage catheters should have a minimum size of 12 Fr.

Maintenance

Several devices have been developed to fix the catheter to the skin; a simple suture is probably still the safest solution. Much, however, depends on the patient's ability to take care of the catheter. Irrigation of the catheter is performed daily with installation of approximately 20 ml of normal saline solution. Internal drainage catheters should not be aspirated, otherwise small bowel contents may contaminate the biliary system, or even block the catheter. Catheter exchange is usually done every three months, or more frequently if necessary. It should be explained to patients and their physicians whenever there are signs of catheter malfunction (leakage, cholangitis), quick correction is of great importance.

The Biliary Endoprosthesis

An internal drainage catheter can be replaced percutaneously with an endoprosthesis (Dooley et al. 1981, Burcharth et al. 1981, Gouma et al. 1983, Lammer and Neumayer 1986). The advantages of drainage by endoprosthesis compared to catheter drainage are obvious. There is no need for incessant care for the catheter, and patients are not constantly confronted with their illness. Blockage of a catheter, however, is easier to correct than a blocked endoprosthesis. In patients for whom inability to pass the stenosis was the reason for failed endoscopic drainage, a blocked percutaneously placed endoprosthesis can be exchanged endoscopically.

Repeating the percutaneous procedure in order to replace a blocked endoprosthesis will often make severe demands on the patient's condition. Whenever it is known that the papillary region cannot be reached by endoscope, it is wise to consider carefully the placement of an endoprosthesis. The patient's own attitude towards the presence of a catheter and, because blockage occurs most frequently three months after insertion, his life expectancy are of importance. The technique for percutaneous insertion of an endoprosthesis is illustrated in Figure 4.7.**4**.

First, the catheter is removed over a guide wire. A catheter with an outer diameter that corresponds with the inner diameter of the endoprosthesis is then inserted. This catheter serves as a guide for the endoprosthesis. The endoprosthesis is pushed forwards with a stiff catheter of the same diameter as the endoprosthesis. A suture is looped through the proximal end of the prosthesis to allow it to be pulled back should it be pushed too far. If left and right catheters are replaced simultaneously, the suture enables one endoprosthesis to be maintained in a stable position while the other is inserted. Once the endoprosthesis is in place, the suture is removed then the guide wire, the catheter and finally the pusher catheter.

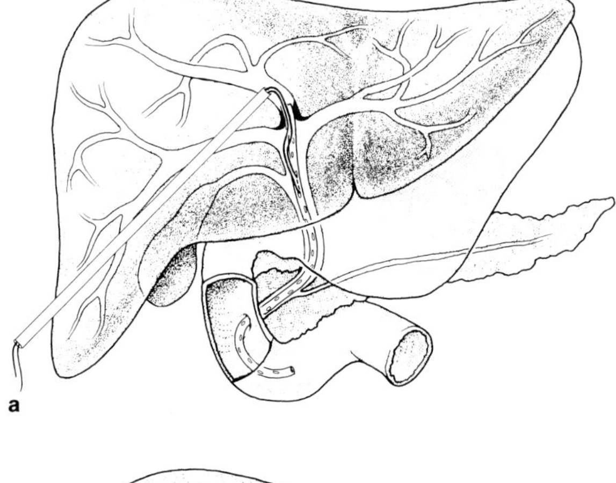

a

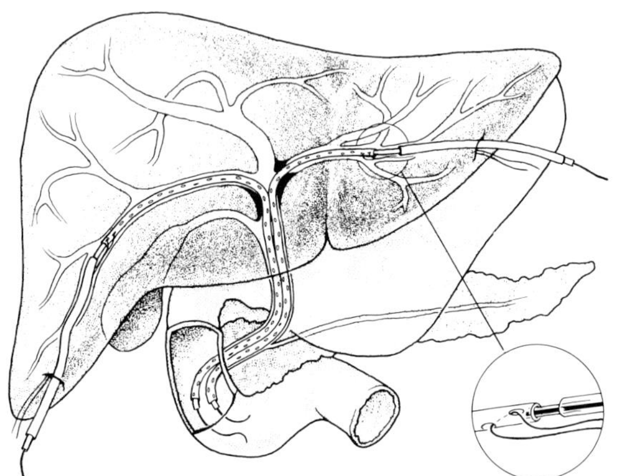

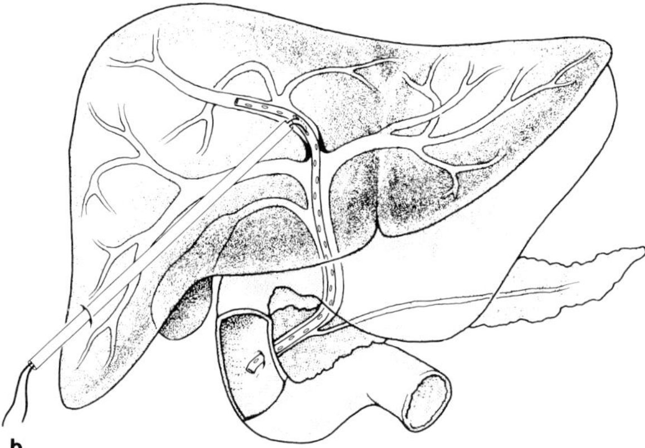

b

Fig. 4.7.**4**   **Percutaneous instalment of an endoprosthesis.** The catheter has been replaced by a guide wire and a catheter with an outer diameter that corresponds with the inner diameter of the endoprosthesis. A suture is looped through the proximal end of the prosthesis to allow it to be pulled back, should it be pushed to far. Once the endoprosthesis is in place, first the suture, then the guide wire, the catheter and finally the pusher catheter are removed

Fig. 4.7.**5**   **Technique of proximal placement of a percutaneous endoprosthesis**
a   The endoprosthesis is pushed entirely into the bile duct system. The suture is looped through two side-holes at the middle part of the endoprosthesis. The suture has been passed through the pusher catheter
b   Pulling the suture will result in a proximal position of the endoprosthesis

Adequate length in the prestenotic part of the endoprosthesis is important for its function. In patients with perihilar obstructions, it is unfortunately not always possible to enter the bile duct system peripherally. In particular, the dorsocranial part of the right lobe ducts are often punctured just above the stenosis. Owman and Lunderquist (1983) described a method of proximal placement for a percutaneous endoprosthesis (Fig. 4.7.**5**). Instead of attaching the suture at the proximal end of the endoprosthesis, it is looped through two side-holes at the middle part. The suture is drawn through the pusher catheter in order to prevent cutting into the liver parenchyma during retraction. When the endoprosthesis has been pushed entirely into the bile duct, and only the proximal part is lying prestenotically, the guide wire and catheter are removed. The suture is then slowly retracted. With the pusher catheter, the endoprosthesis is forced to follow the bile duct towards its more proximal part. The pusher catheter is removed after the suture has been pulled out.

The length of the endoprosthesis and the position of the side-holes are best adapted to the patient's individual circumstances. The diameter should be no less than 10 Fr. The optimum moment of insertion of the endoprosthesis is after approximately one week of catheter drainage. Otherwise, bloodclots and debris will cause early clogging of the prosthesis. The procedure can be done on an out-patient basis.

Biopsy of Obstructive Lesions

Pathologic examination of aspirated bile is a simple method of examining the histopathological nature of the stenosis (Muro 1983). Since the presence of a catheter through the stenosis leads to a higher amount of cells in the bile, results are better in patients with internal drainage catheters than with external drainage catheters. Although the yield of bile cytology is low, it will give a correct diagnosis in only about 30 % of patients. Due to its simplicity and lack of false-positive outcomes, however, it has still a place. Percutaneous fine-needle biopsies are suited for mass-like lesions seen on CT or US examination (Hancke et al. 1975, Ferrucci et al. 1980). The presence of the catheter in the stenosis can also provide a target for biopsy under fluoroscopic control. This method can be used for extraductal lesions. For primary ductal lesions with intraductal tumor extension, however, it is better to use the internal drainage catheter as conduit for an intraluminal biopsy. The catheter should be replaced with two guide wires, one to preserve the tract through the stenosis, the other to guide an introducer sheath for the biopsy procedure.

Intraluminal cytological biopsy can be done with brushes that are pushed to and from the lesion, and with fine-needle biopsies (Mendez et al. 1980, Elyaderani and Gabriele 1980, Cropper and Gold 1983, Cohan et al. 1986). Histological specimens are obtained by introducing a grasping forceps.

Clinical Applications

Introduction

Ultrasound-guided puncture has facilitated percutaneous procedures in the obstructed biliary system in such a manner that PTC without drainage should be considered obsolete. Probably the only indication left for PTC without drainage is imaging the subtotal stenosed biliodigestive anastomosis in patients who present with recurrent cholangitis and who are under consideration for surgical correction. Our own experience with more than 350 patients who underwent ultrasound-guided PTC and drainage started in 1980. Despite the introduction of endoscopic drainage procedures, the number of percutaneous procedures has not decreased. Still there has been a gradual change in patient material. Endoscopic drainage has been very successful in patients with distally located common bile duct stenosis. For percutaneous procedures, the emphasis is on patients with perihilar obstructions and postsurgical patients.

A major indication for percutaneous drainage is palliation in patients with malignant jaundice. Other indications are percutaneous treatment of benign disorders such as cholangitis, bile duct stones and balloon dilation of benign strictures. Discussion of the latter indications, however, is not within the scope of this chapter.

Percutaneous drainage can be performed on patients with malignant jaundice as a pre-operative measure or for palliation. Wound healing, resistance to infection and blood coagulation are negatively influenced by raised bilirubin levels. Yet the benefits of preoperative percutaneous drainage were not obvious in controlled studies (Hatfield et al. 1982, McPherson et al. 1982), and the infectious complications of preoperative drainage may even jeopardize the outcome of the definitive operation.

In our institution, preoperative drainage is only considered in patients with cholangitis. Nowadays one of the most frequent causes of cholangitis in patients with malignant biliary obstruction is a foregoing endoscopic retrograde cholangiopancreatography (ERCP) without drainage.

Curative surgery is not possible in the vast majority of patients presenting with a malignant biliary obstruction (Buckwalter et al. 1965, Rossi et

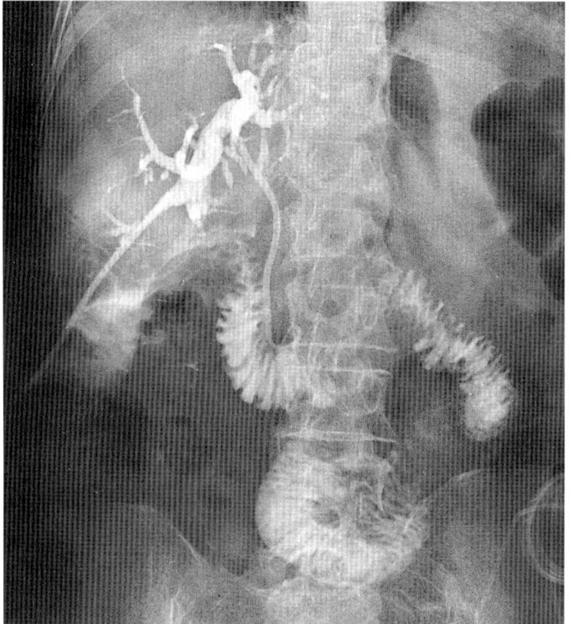

a

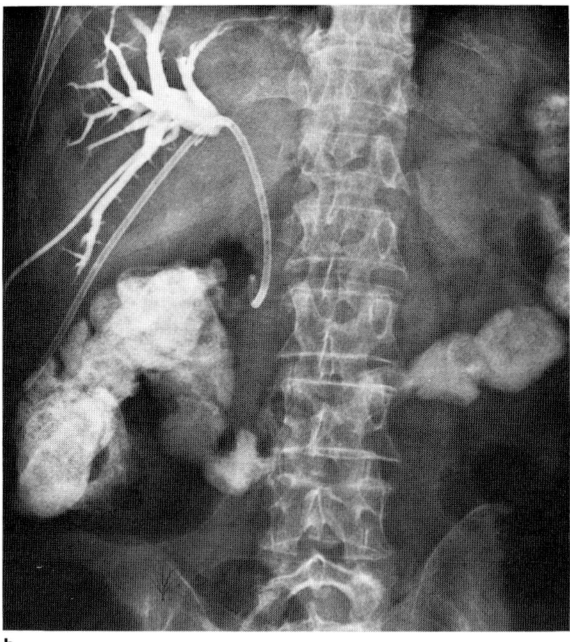

b

c

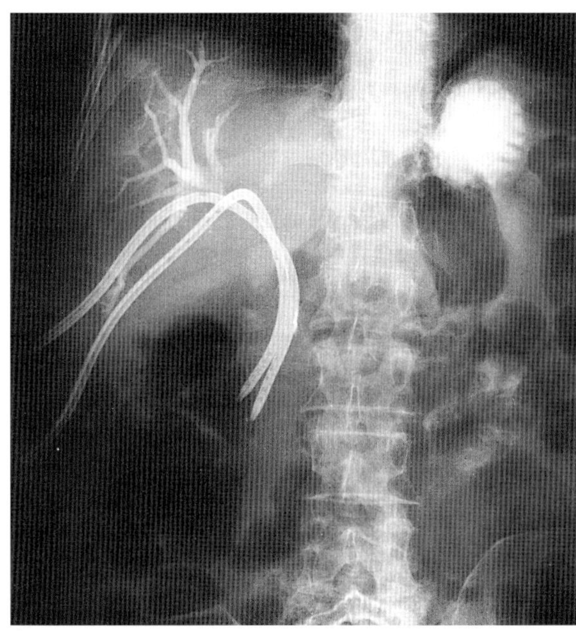

d

Fig. 4.7.6 Work-up in a 66-year old female with perihilar biliary obstruction

a   Right-sided subcostal catheter placement: incomplete drainage of right lobe bile duct; complete drainage of the left lobe

b   Additional drainage of the right lobe

c   Intraluminal forceps biopsy showed cholangio-carcinoma

d   Placement of two 10 Fr catheters suited for intraluminal irradiation (iridium 192)

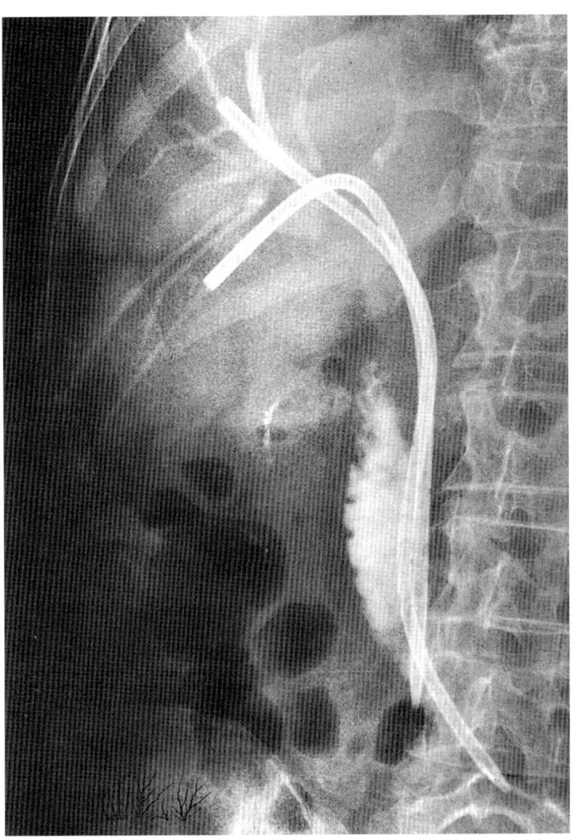

e Replacement of the catheters by two 12 Fr endoprostheses using the technique described in Fig. 4.7.**5**.

al. 1985). Palliative treatment to relieve jaundice is therefore necessary. The complexity, results and complications of biliary drainage in malignant jaundice, however, depend to a large extent on the site of the stenosis (Laméris et al. 1987). Patients with mid- or distal common bile duct obstructions who can be treated with one catheter or endoprosthesis, should therefore be distinguished from patients with perihilar obstruction, who often need separate drainage of both liver lobes.

Mid- or Distal Obstruction

The most common causes of mid- and distal common bile duct obstruction are periampullary and pancreatic carcinoma and primary cholangiocarcinoma. Periductal lymph node metastasis can also cause obstruction below the level of bifurcation. A leading feature of this group of patients is that one catheter or endoprosthesis is sufficient for complete drainage. Decrease in bilirubin levels after catheter placement is seen in over 90 % of patients. Internal drainage can be achieved in 70–80 % (Gouma et al. 1983, Ferrucci et al. 1980, Clark et al. 1981). However, since endoscopic drainage has even better results, i.e. a higher percentage of internal drainage, the percutaneous

technique should be considered as an alternative after a failed endoscopic drainage. In our experience, inability to pass the stenosis with the endoscopic approach has no predictive value for the chances with the percutaneous technique; even in these patients, 70 % will have successful percutaneous internal drainage (Laméris et al. 1987).

Perihilar Obstructions

Tumor infiltration of the porta hepatis results in obstruction of the left and right hepatic ducts. The most common causes of this are metastatic disease, gallbladder carcinoma and cholangiocarcinoma (Klatskin tumor) (Klatskin 1965). Obstruction of branches of the hepatic ducts due to tumor infiltration seems to occur more frequently on the right side, due to an anatomical difference between the right and the left hepatic duct: on the right side, the smaller ducts enter the main one in close proximity to the hilum, whereas there is a larger segment of main duct without branches on the left side. Careful US and CT examination of the liver to discover these segmental occlusions should precede any percutaneous drainage procedure (Gibney et al. 1987). If more than two catheters are needed for complete drainage of the right lobe, patients seldom benefit from the drainage, due to catheter problems and cholangitis. In these cases, single drainage of the left lobe should be considered. Although we have never seen bilirubin levels return to normal, drainage of the left lobe was sufficient, in most cases, to treat pruritus.

Occlusion of the segmental ducts can also occur in the post-drainage phase. This will nearly always lead to severe septic complications. Local intraluminal radiotherapy with iridium 192 wires is recommended to prevent these complications by stopping local tumor spread (Fletcher et al. 1981, Karani et al. 1985). Whereas in patients with mid- or distal common bile duct stenosis there is a preference for endoscopic drainage, this is not straightforward for patients with perihilar obstructions. The success rate of endoscopic drainage in these patients is significantly lower, at the expense of more complications than in patients with stenosis below the level of the bifurcation (Laméris et al. 1987). The main complication is cholangitis due to inadequate or failed drainage. The results of percutaneous drainage are also less good if the obstruction is located in the perihilar region. Although normal levels of bilirubin can be achieved in 80 % of these patients, complete internal drainage is only possible in 50–60 % of patients (Laméris et al. 1987).

Reasons for performing percutaneous drainage as a primary method may be, for example, that cholangitis after failed endoscopic drainage increases the risk of complications with percutaneous manipulations. Collapsed bile ducts and the presence of one endoscopic endoprosthesis can hamper a successful outcome for percutaneous drainage in perihilar disease. Moreover, the success of endoscopic drainage is not adversely effected by preceding percutaneous drainage. Another reason for performing catheter drainage is the possibility of treating patients with cholangiocarcinoma with intraluminal radiotherapy with iridium 192 wires (Fig. 4.7.**6**).

Contra-Indications

Patients with extensive metastatic disease or tumor spread throughout the liver respond poorly to drainage procedures, show a higher complication rate and should therefore be excluded. Ascites may complicate percutaneous drainage in several ways. Drainage of infected bile in the presence of ascites will always cause peritonitis and should therefore be considered as an absolute contra-indication. Leakage of ascitic fluid along the drainage catheter is another problem. Ascites that comes into being during long-term drainage seldom causes leakage, thanks to a firm tract to the liver. Internal catheter drainage in patients with ascites is often difficult due to high intra-abdominal pressure. Another reason for the failure of internal catheter drainage can be bowel loop occlusions, often due to metastatic disease.

Complications of Percutaneous Catheter Drainage

Complications related to the puncture itself, such as hemorrhage, portobiliary fistulas or pneumothorax, occur in 8–24% of cases with the former "blind" method (Mueller et al. 1982, Carrosco et al. 1984, Hamlin et al. 1986), but are seldom seen with the ultrasound-guided method (Makuuci et al. 1980, Laméris et al. 1985, 1987). In the case of cholangitis, a major indication for percutaneous drainage, septic complications do occur in about 10% of the patients, despite all precautionary measures. The septic complications vary from mild bacteremia to severe, even lethal, septic shock and can only be reduced by limiting manipulations within the infected bile duct system.

The most significant complication associated with percutaneous drainage, however, is sepsis related to catheter occlusion or dislodgement (Cohan et al. 1986). Almost every patient on long-term catheter drainage will live through one or more episodes of cholangitis. The first sign of catheter malfunction is often bile leakage along the catheter. The patient and his physician should be aware of this and react immediately. Routinely exchanging the catheter at two- to three-month intervals helps to prevent these problems. Severe,

almost untreatable, cholangitis caused by segmental occlusions of the intrahepatic bile ducts due to further tumor growth may develop at a late stage of perihilar disease.

Alternative Percutaneous Methods

Percutaneous Cholecystography and Cholecystostomy

Percutaneous puncture of the gallbladder was first described by Burckhardt and Mueller (1921). Their aim was to delineate the bile ducts by injection of contrast material into the gallbladder. They foresaw the possibilities of influencing acute cholecystitis and of dissolving gallstones. In order to prevent intraperitoneal bile leakage, they advocated a transhepatic puncture route. Nowadays, percutaneous puncture of the gallbladder is used for diagnostic purposes, for drainage in acute cholecystitis, for drainage in malignant biliary obstruction and for stone dissolution and removal (Laméris et al. 1984, Van Sonnenberg et al. 1986).

The puncture technique is the same as that described for PTC. The initial puncture is performed with ultrasound guidance with a 22 gauge needle. Drainage catheters can be placed using the Seldinger technique. A transhepatic route to the bare area of the gallbladder is used to prevent bile leakage.

In patients with malignant obstructive jaundice, percutaneous cholecystography and drainage is useful if the obstruction is below the level of the cystic duct. It is applied after failed percutaneous transhepatic biliary procedures and, since it is a simple procedure that can be performed entirely under ultrasound control, in critically ill septic patients as a bedside procedure.

Percutaneous gallbladder drainage for malignant biliary obstruction should be considered as a temporizing measure. Subsequent procedures are required to effect permanent long-term management.

Percutaneous Transjejunal Procedures

Roux-en-Y biliary jejunal anastomoses can be constructed in such a way that a segment is attached under the abdominal wall. This part of the Roux-en-Y anastomosis is marked with metal clips, and can also be identified by ultrasound examination. Percutaneous puncture and catheterization of the fixed loop is then possible. Catheters can be manipulated through the jejunal loop, through the anastomosis into the bile ducts (Russell et al. 1986, Maroney and Ring 1987). This technique can be applied for (repeated) dilation of benign strictures and for placement of long-term stents in patients with a recurrent malignant obstruction.

Conclusions

Ultrasound-guided percutaneous transhepatic biliary drainage is safe and effective in decompressing the biliary system. In patients with malignant obstructive disease, the procedure can be applied, in some cases, to improve the patient's condition prior to surgery, and in non-resectable malignant disease for long-term palliation. The pros and cons of any palliative measure chosen in these patients should be weighed carefully against each other in each individual case. In real terms, this means that in patients with mid- or distal common bile duct stenosis, percutaneous drainage should be considered only after failed endoscopic drainage, whereas in perihilar obstruction it can be applied as the first drainage method. Close co-operation between endoscopist and radiologist should be the foundation of effective palliative treatment in these complex patients.

References

Arner O, Hagberg S, Seldinger SI. Percutaneous transhepatic cholangiography: puncture of dilated and non dilated bile ducts under roentgen television control. Surgery 1962; 52: 561–571.

Buckwalter, JA, Lawton RL, Tidrick RT. Bypass operations for neoplastic biliary tract obstruction. Am J Surg 1965; 109: 100–106.

Burcharth F, Efsen F, Christiansen LA, et al. Non surgical internal biliary drainage by endoprosthesis. Surg Gynecol Obstet 1981; 153: 857–860.

Burckhardt H, Mueller W. Versuche über die Punktion der Gallenblase und ihre Röntgendarstellung. Dtsch Z Chir 1921; 161: 168.

Carrosco CH, Zornoza J, Bechtel WJ. Malignant biliary obstruction: complications of percutaneous biliary drainage. Radiology 1984; 152: 343–346.

Clark RA, Mitchell SE, Colley DP, Alexander E. Percutaneous catheter biliary decompression. AJR 1981; 137: 503–509.

Cohan RH, Illescas FF, Braun SD. Fine needle aspiration biopsy in malignant obstructive jaundice. Gastrointest Radiol 1986; 11(2): 145–150.

Cohan RJ, Illescas FF, Saeed M, Perlmutt LM, Braun SD, Newman GE, Dunnick NR. Infectious complications of percutaneous biliary drainage. Invest Radiol 1986; 21: 705–709.

Cropper LD, Gold RE. Simplified brush biopsy of bile ducts. Radiology 1983; 148: 307.

Dawson SL, Neff CC, Mueller PR, et al. Fatal hemorrhage after inadvertent transpleural biliary drainage. AJR 1983; 141: 33–343.

Dooley JS, Dick R, Irving D, Olney J, Sherlock S. Relief of bileduct obstruction by the percutaneous transhepatic insertion of an endoprosthesis. Clin Radiol 1981; 32: 163–172.

Eggermont AM, Laméris JS, Jeekel J. Ultrasound-guided percutaneous transhepatic cholecystostomy for acute acalculous cholecystitis. Arch Surg 1985; 120: 1354–1356.

Elyaderani M, Gabriele OF. Brush and forceps biopsy of biliary ducts via percutaneous transhepatic catheterization. Radiology 1980; 135: 777–778.

Ferrucci JT, Mueller PR, Harbin WP. Percutaneous transhepatic biliary drainage. Radiology 1980; 135: 1–13.

Ferrucci JT, Wittenberg J, Mueller PR, et al. Diagnosis of abdominal malignancy by radiologic fine needle biopsy. AJR 1980; 134: 323–330.

Fletcher MS, Brinkley D, Dawson JL, Numerley H, Wheeler PG, Williams R. Treatment of high bile duct carcinoma by internal radiotherapy with iridium-192 wire. Lancet 1981; 172–174.

Gibney RG, Cooperberg PL, Scudamore CH, Nagy AG. Segmental biliary obstruction: false-negative diagnosis with direct cholangiography without US guidance. Radiology 1987; 164: 27–30.

Glenn F, Evans JA, Mujahed Z, Thorbjarnason B. Percutaneous transhepatic cholangiography. Ann Surg 1962; 156: 451–462.

Gouma DJ, Wesdorp RIC, Oosterbroek RJ, Soeters PB, Greep JM. Percutaneous transhepatic drainage and insertion of an endoprosthesis for obstructive jaundice. Am J Surg 1983; 145: 763–767.

Hamlin JA, Friedman M, Stein MG, Bray JF. Percutaneous biliary drainage: complications of 118 consecutive catheterizations. Radiology 1986; 158: 199–202.

Hancke S, Holm HH, Koch F. Ultrasonically guided percutaneous fine needle biopsy of the pancreas. Surg Gynecol Obstet 1975; 140: 361–364.

Harbin WP, Mueller PR, Ferrucci JT. Transhepatic cholangiography: complications and use patterns of the fine needle technique. Radiology 1980; 135: 15–22.

Hatfield AR, Tobias R, Terblanche J, Girdwood AH, Fataar S, Harries-Jones R, Kernoff L, Marks IN. Preoperative external biliary drainage in obstructive jaundice: a prospective controlled clinical trial. Lancet 1982; ii: 896–899.

Karani J, Fletcher M, Brinkley D, Dawson JL, Williams R, Munnerley H. Internal biliary drainage and local radiotherapy with Iridium-192 wire in treatment of hilar cholangiocarcinoma. Clin Radiol 1985; 36: 603–606.

Klatskin G. Adenocarcinoma of the hepatic duct at its bifurcation within the porta hepatis: an unusual tumour with distinctive clinical and pathological features. Am J Med 1965; 38: 241–256.

Laméris JS, Jeekel J, Havelaar IJ, van Seyen AJ. Percutaneous transhepatic cholecystostomy. RöFo 1984; 142: 80–82.

Laméris JS, Obertop H, Jeekel J. Biliary drainage by ultrasound guided puncture of the left hepatic duct. Clin Radiol 1985; 36: 269–274.

Laméris JS, Stoker J, Dees J, Nix GAJJ, van Blankenstein M, Jeekel J. Non-surgical palliative treatment of patients with malignant biliary obstruction: the place of endoscopic and percutaneous drainage. Clin Radiol 1987; 38: 603–608.

Lammer J, Neumayer K. Biliary drainage endoprostheses: experience with 201 placements. Radiology 1986; 159: 625–629.

McPherson GAD, Benjamin IS, Habib NA, Bowley NB, Blumgart LH. Percutaneous transhepatic drainage in obstructive jaundice: advantages and problems. Br J Surg 1982; 69: 261–264.

Makuuci M, Bandai Y, Ito T, Watanabe G, et al. Ultrasonically guided percutaneous transhepatic bile drainage: a single-step procedure without cholangiography. Radiology 1980; 136: 165–169.

Maroney TP, Ring EJ. Percutaneous transjejunal catheterization of Roux-en-Y biliary-jejunal anastomoses. Radiology 1987; 164: 151–153.

Mendez G, Russell E, Levi JU, Koolpe J, Cohen M. Percutaneous brush biopsy and internal drainage of biliary tree through endoprosthesis. AJR 1980; 134: 653–659.

Molnar W, Stockum AE. Relief of obstructive jaundice through percutaneous transhepatic catheter: a new therapeutic method. AJR 1974; 122: 346–367.

Mueller PR, van Sonnenberg E, Ferrucci JT. Percutaneous biliary drainage: technical and catheter related problems in 200 procedures. AJR 1982; 138: 17–32.

Muro A. Bile cytology: a routine addition to percutaneous biliary drainage. Radiology 1983; 149: 846.

Neff CC, Mueller PR, Ferrucci JT, Dawson SL, Wittenberg J, Simeone JF, Butch RJ. Serious complications following transgression of the pleural space in drainage procedures. Radiology 1984; 152: 335.

Okuda K. Thin needle percutaneous transhepatic cholangiography: a historical review. Endoscopy 1980; 12: 2.

Owman T, Lunderquist A. Sling retraction for proximal placement of percutaneous transhepatic biliary endoprosthesis. Radiology 1983; 146: 228–229.

Rossi RL, Heiss FW, Beckmann CF, Braasch JW. Management of cancer of the bile duct. Surg Clin North Am 1985; 65: 59–78.

Russell E, Yrizarry JM, Huber JS, Nunez D Jr, Hutson DG, Schiff E, Rajender Reddy K, Jeffers LJ, Williams A. Percutaneous transjejunal biliary dilatation: alternate management for benign strictures. Radiology 1986; 159: 209–214.

Shaver RW, Hawkins IF Jr, Soong J. Percutaneous cholecystostomy. AJR 1982; 138: 1133–1136.

Van Sonnenberg E, Wittich GR, Casola G, Princenthal RA, Hofmann AF, Keightley A, Wing VW. Diagnostic and therapeutic percutaneous gallbladder procedures. Radiology 1986; 160: 23–26.

4.8   Percutaneous Transhepatic Biliary Drainage (PTBD)

J. Weber

We differentiate between temporary or permanent *catheter drainage* (internal, external or combined internal and external biliary drainage) and permanent internal bile drainage via a tract *endoprosthe-* *ses.* All drainage measures are developed from percutaneous transhepatic cholangiography (PTC) (Figs. 4.8.**1**, 4.8.**2**, 4.8.**3**).

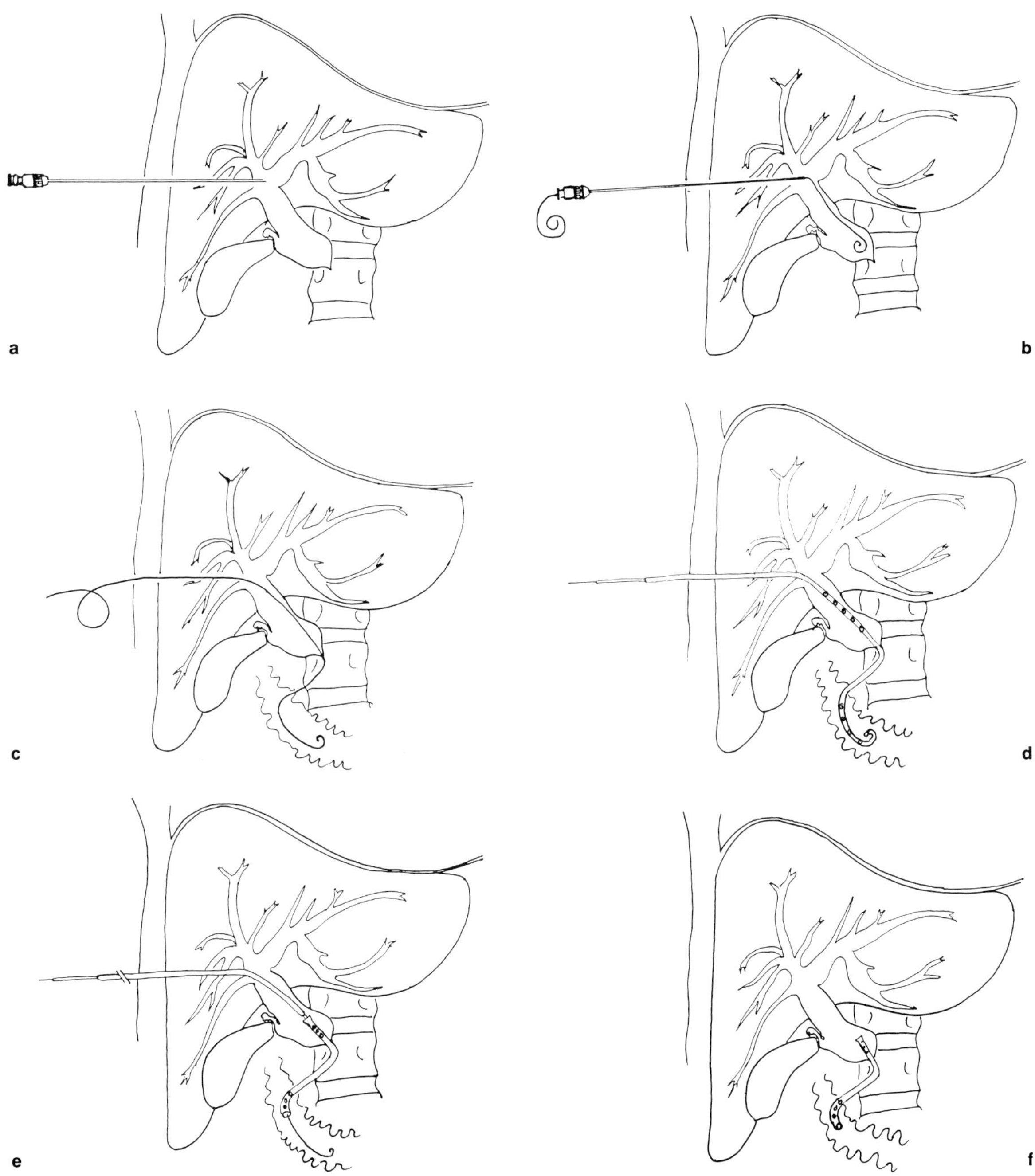

Fig. 4.8.**1   Steps in PTC and PTBD.** (After Dooley et al., Clin Radiol 1981; 32: 163)
a   Diagnostic PTC

b–d Biliary duct drainage (PTBD) with external or combined external-internal catheter drainage
e, f Internal drainage via an endoprosthesis

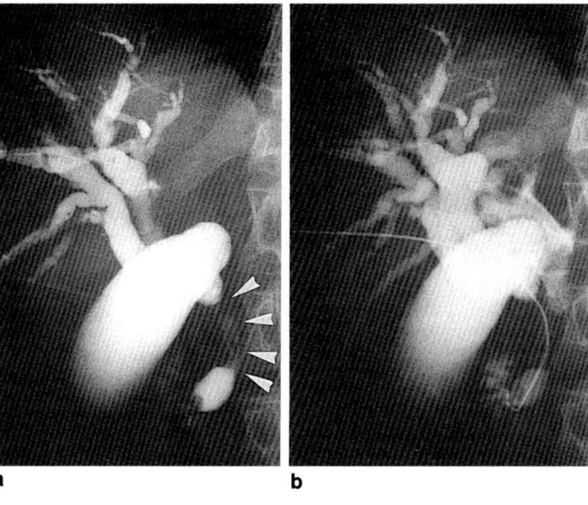

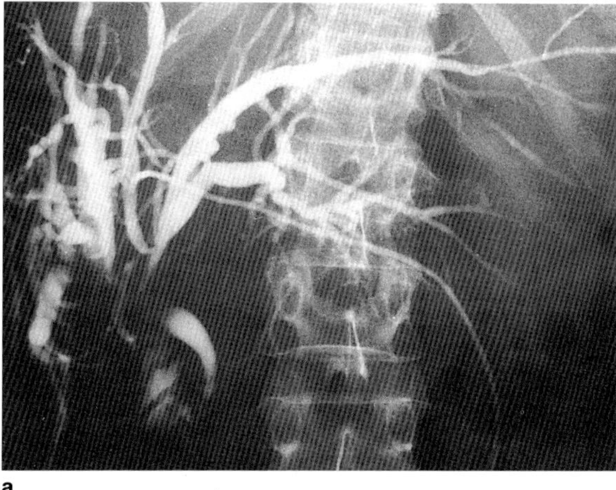

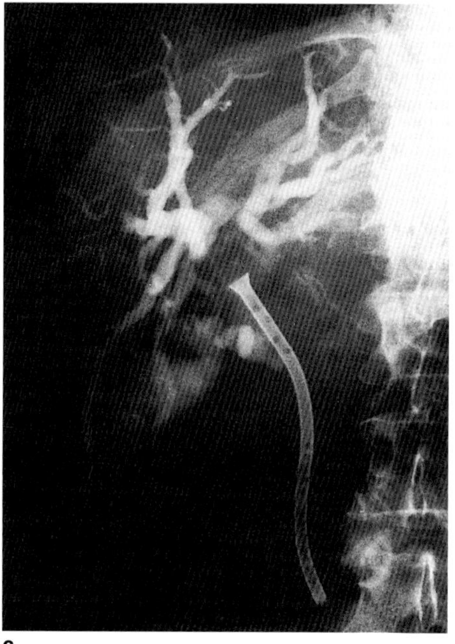

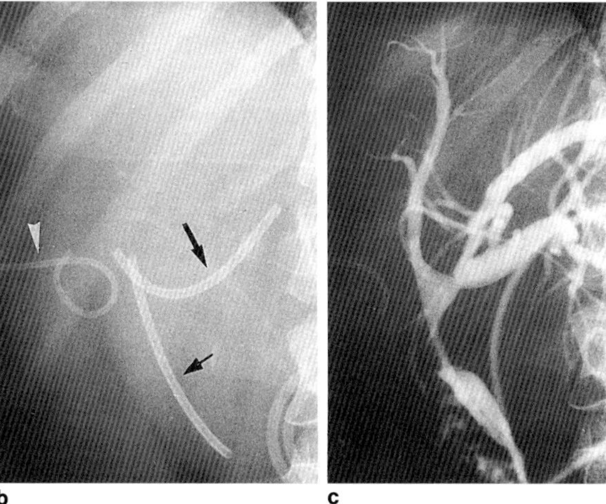

Fig. 4.8.3   PTC and PTBD from the left side
a   Following PTC and partial bile duct enhancement from the right side, the intrahepatic biliary system is punctured and drained from the left
b, c   In a cholangiocarcinoma obstructing all major hepatic bile ducts individually at the level of the porta hepatis, a left-sided internal drainage was carried out (arrow), and another bridging intrahepatic stent was placed (heavy arrow). A right-sided temporary external catheter drainage (arrow head) was later removed

Fig. 4.8.2   PTC and PTBD from the right side
a   Extrahepatic bile duct stenosis from cholangiocarcinoma, diagnosed by PTC
b   Bypass with a J guide wire
c   Internal drainage with a 10 Fr Lunderquist-Owman endoprosthesis draining directly into the duodenum

To diminish the risks of PTC, it is worthwhile planning the diagnostic and therapeutic measures together. Otherwise there is the danger of bile fistulation (including infected bile) through the puncture fistula canal to below the liver capsule or into the abdominal cavity, with subsequent danger of biliary peritonitis. The method used in biliary drainage is determined from the findings documented in cholangiography. If the stenosis can be passed with a guide wire without major technical problems or difficulties for the patient, passage using a drainage catheter is usually also successful (with or without bougie dilation), so that combined internal and external bile drainage can be brought about *at once* (Figs. 4.8.**2**, 4.8.**3**). In high-level, *and in* very firm, high-grade stenosis or biliary obstruction (especially where there are demands on space in the porta hepatis), an *external* catheter drainage of the dammed-up bile is often the only therapeutic measure possible in the first passage (Fig. 4.8.**4**).

Apart from the usual 5–12 Fr catheters, home-made stents from angiographic catheter materials, or individual alterations of the side-holes needed for draining the bile are useful. In central stenosis of the main intrahepatic canals of the hepatic duct, as is frequently the case with growing cholangiocarcinoma in the porta hepatis, multiple drainage may be necessary to relieve the left and right lobes of the liver (Fig. 4.8.5). 5–7 Fr catheters, with a relatively thin lumen, are suitable for *external* biliary drainage as a temporary measure and sometimes as a permanent one. The major problems are due to suitable positioning of the catheter tip and side-holes, and the best possible fixation.

Various commercially available catheter systems, such as the pigtail catheter (Fig. 4.8.**6a**), Günther nephrostomy catheter (Fig. 4.8.**6b**) or Sachs biliary drain (Fig. 4.8.**6c**) are introduced via an angiographic guide wire or Lunderquist guide wire (which has a stiff shaft and flexible tip). They should be fixed in position at the skin exit site with sutures or skin-friendly sticking plaster. Drainage bags that can be worn by out-patients or fixed to the body or thigh collect the daily production of bile in whole or in part. The catheters have to be irrigated daily, the drainage bags changed, and the fistula canal regularly dressed. Antibiotic protection has to be aimed as precisely as possible at the bacteriological spectrum established. Loss of fluid and minerals (especially calium) has to be calculated with regular laboratory tests, as is also the case for the „normalization" of the total bilirubin and liver transaminases. The application of a *two-stage procedure* when changing an external catheter drainage to an internal biliary drainage (with a catheter or endoprosthesis) serves to avoid serious complications. The main complication is the danger of bleeding from the fistula canal (Passariello et al. 1985, Rupp and Weiss 1980). So long as the latter has not yet been partly organized by granulation tissue, tears in the neighboring vessels in the early organization phase during catheter changing and

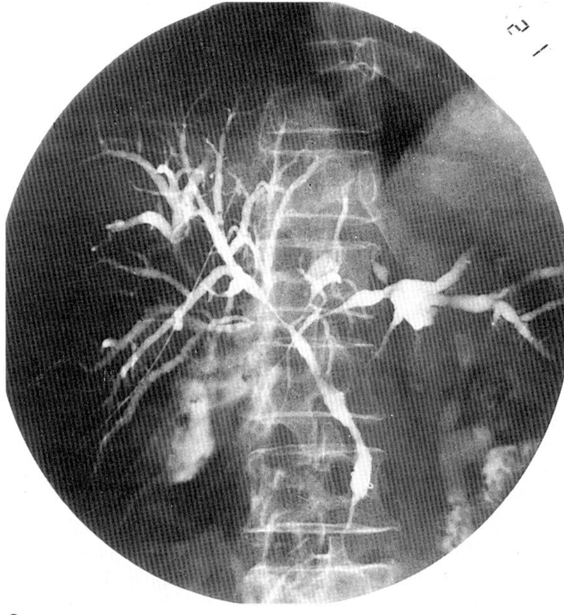

a

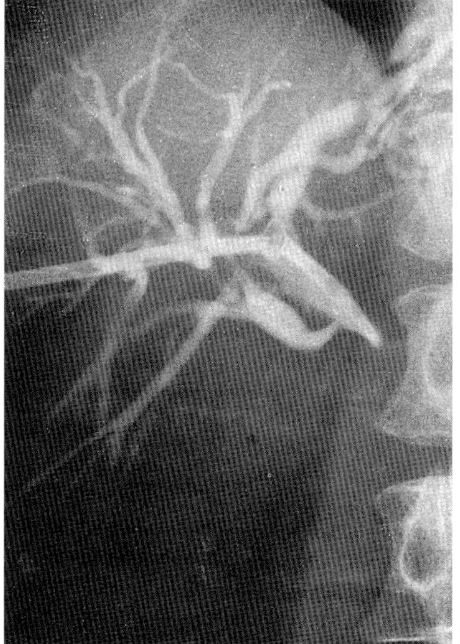

b

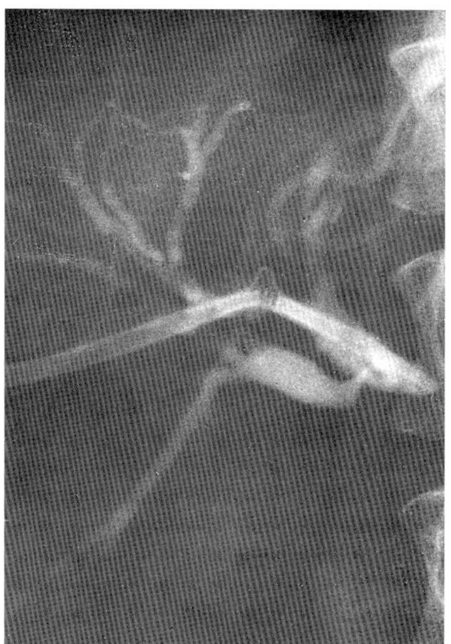

c

Fig. 4.8.4 PTC and external catheter drainage
a Cholangiocarcinoma stenosing all intrahepatic bile ducts subtotally, as proven by PTC from the right

b, c Catheter drainage was carried out, clearing only the right part of the liver. A 12 Fr Sachs biliary drain was fixed by itself inside the biliary duct

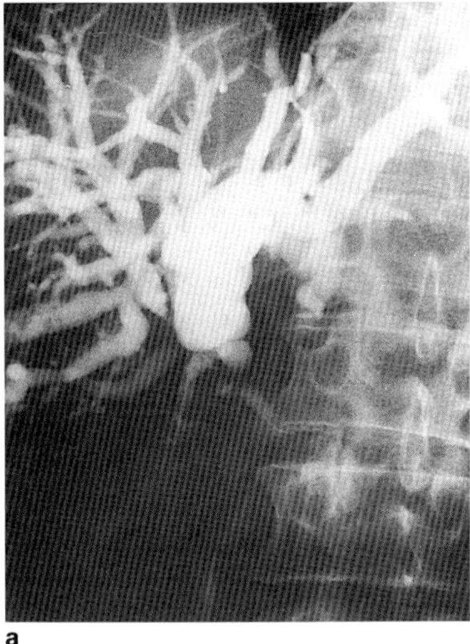
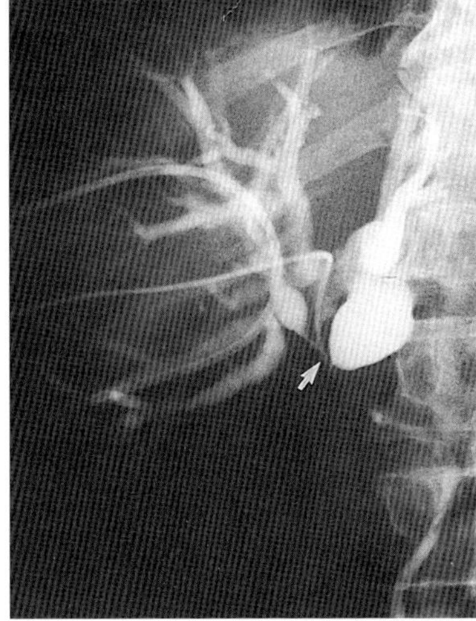
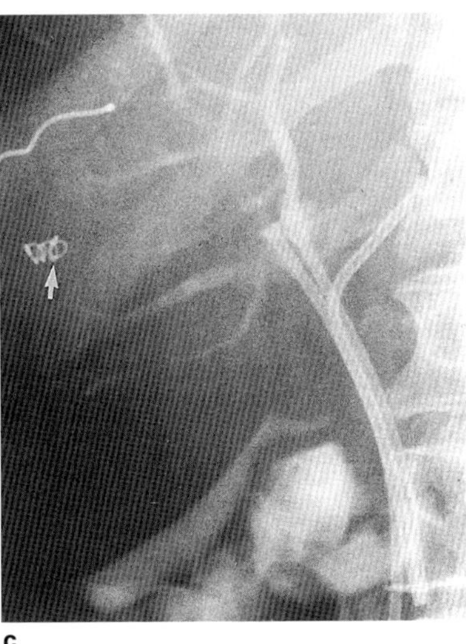

a   b   c

Fig. 4.8.5   Multiple drainage through 3 endoprostheses
a, b A 41-year-old patient with cholangiocarcinoma that has grown into the porta hepatis with stenosis of the main branch of the hepatic duct (arrow). 3 home-made 8 Fr endoprostheses were inserted to give complete internal palliative drainage (2 prostheses from the right, 1 prosthesis from the left)
c Fistulas from previous catheter drainage were closed with Gianturco coils (arrow) (Weber 1985)

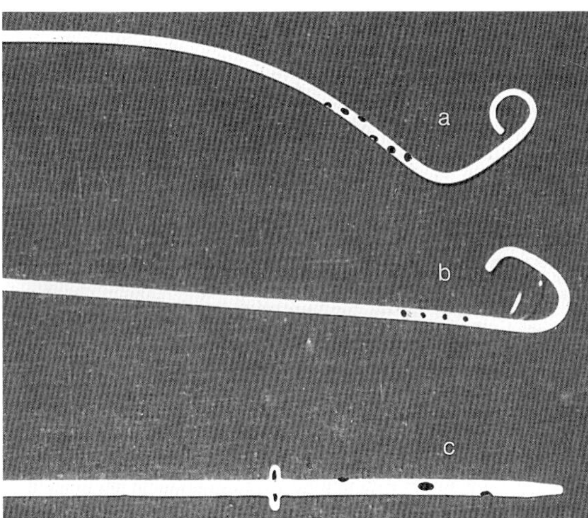

Fig. 4.8.6   Catheters for biliary drainage (PTBD)
a *Pigtail Catheter* (8 Fr) for external or combined internal and external drainage
b *Günther Nephrostomy Catheter* (7 Fr) for external biliary drainage. The hook-shaped catheter tip is fixed with nylon sutures
c *Sachs Biliary Drain* (12 Fr) for external or combined internal and external drainage. Fixation in the biliary canals is achieved with a spring mechanism

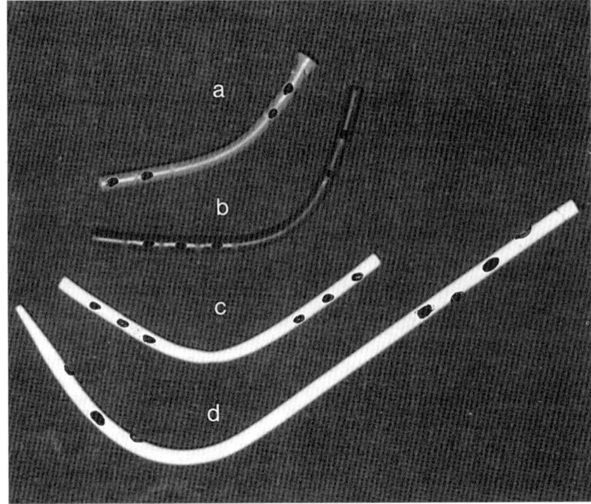

Fig. 4.8.7   Prostheses for biliary drainage (PTBD)
a–c *Lunderquist-Owman Endoprostheses* (8 Fr) with or without flattened end for fixation proximal to the stenosis
d *Carey-Coons Soft Stent* (12 Fr), 20 cm long prostheses made of relatively soft material with large side perforations for the drainage of long stenoses

bougie dilation, as well as the application of large-bore endoprostheses (12 Fr) (Figs. 4.8.**7**, 4.8.**8**) can scarcely be avoided.

On the other hand, complications can also appear in the two-stage process, with the catheter slipping, the drainage being pulled out, infection of the fistula canal, etc. This indicates that the *interval* between PTC with combined external drainage and permanent drainage should be kept as short as possible. For this reason, we usually carry out a biliary prosthesis within 8 days if the bilirubin values are regressing significantly, and we do not wait for complete normalization of the bilirubin and transaminases (Fig. 4.8.**9**).

The concept of replacing a temporary catheter drainage against an endoprosthesis guiding to internal biliary drainage is based on the fact that this can mean a considerable improvement in the quality of life for the patient, within the framework of *palliation* (Passariello et al. 1985, Riemann 1984, Weber and Höver 1987). But it requires an uncomplicated, continuous internal bile drainage through broad-caliber endoprostheses that remain fully functional within the average life expectancy of tumor patients (about 7 months) (Oleaga and Ring 1981, Passariello et al. 1985). It is seldom possible to carry out an exchange by endoscopy in cases of premature endoprosthesis blockage, and a percutaneous recanalization is almost always impossible. On the other hand, this can often be compensated for by parallel insertion of a *second* endoprosthesis (Fig. 4.8.**10**). Combined internal and external biliary tract drainage generally permits a trouble-free exchange of catheters, but the problems of wound dressing, pain, etc. are difficult to surmount for the majority of patients (Weber and Höver 1986, 1987).

The curative possibilities of *local radiation therapy* through the drainage catheter following the afterloading principle (Koch et al. 1986) can be integrated into the concept of a two-stage process in percutaneous transhepatic biliary drainage (Itami et al. 1986). After PTC and PTBD through a sufficiently large drainage catheter that has passed the tumor stenosis, a relatively high-dose irradiation can be carried out with the help of a wire-shape iridium source. Individual doses of 10–20 Gy in succession or fractionally distributed over time until a total dose of between 25 and 50 Gy has been applied (Itami et al. 1986, Koester 1984) (Fig. 4.8.**11**). The radioactive source is introduced with an appropriate application instrument (in an inner safety catheter previously introduced into the drainage catheter) under radiographic control, so that radiation source acts directly on the tumor. The total radiation load on the neighboring liver tissue can be significantly reduced according to the square-of-distance law (Fig. 4.8.**11 c**).

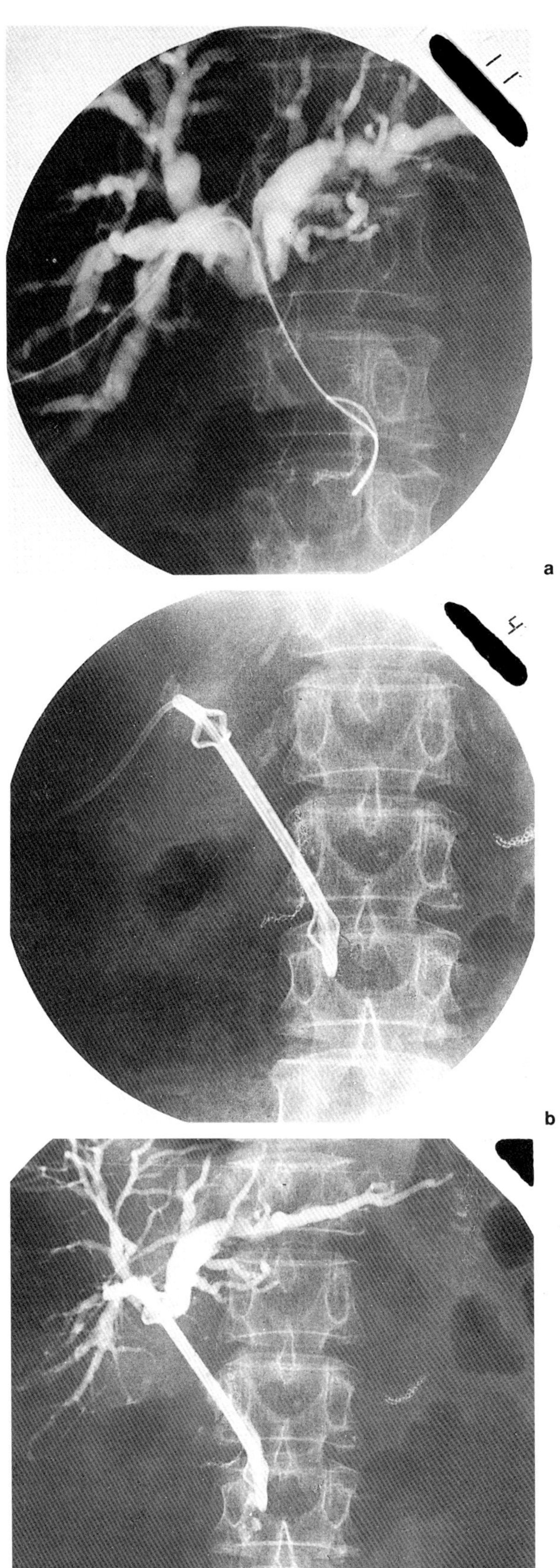

Fig. 4.8.**8**   **Large bore endoprosthesis** ▶
a In a patient with cholangiocarcinoma causing stenosis at the level of the hepatic duct below the porta hepatis, the guide wire has passed the stenosis
b A 12 Fr double mushrom endoprosthesis was placed, and external drainage was maintained for 3 days for safety
c The endoprosthesis was removed afterwards, leading to complete internal biliary drainage

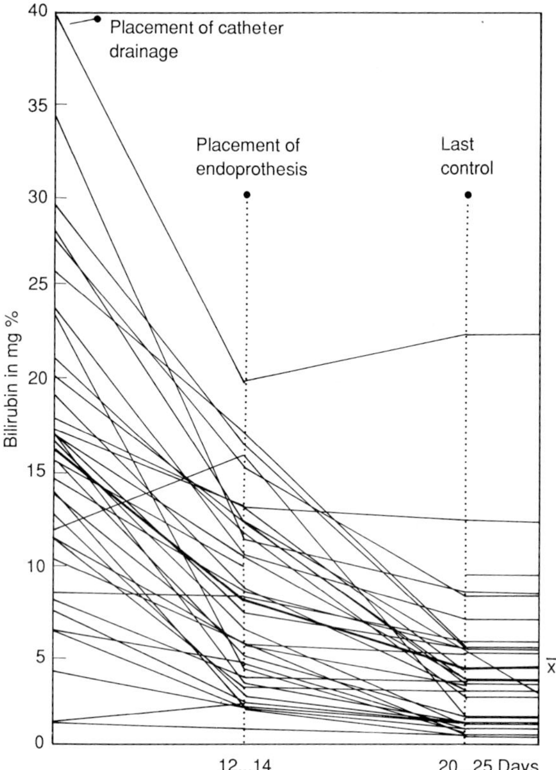

Fig. 4.8.**9   Sinking bilirubin values** as a parameter for changing a combined internal and external catheter drainage to an internal biliary drainage by endoprosthesis; n = 37. (From Weber and Höver 1985)

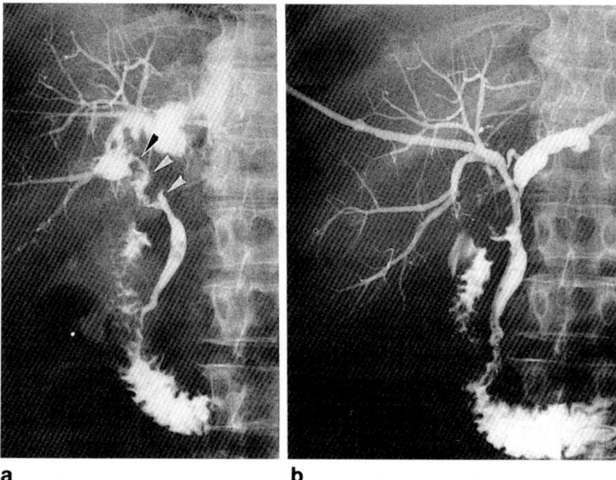

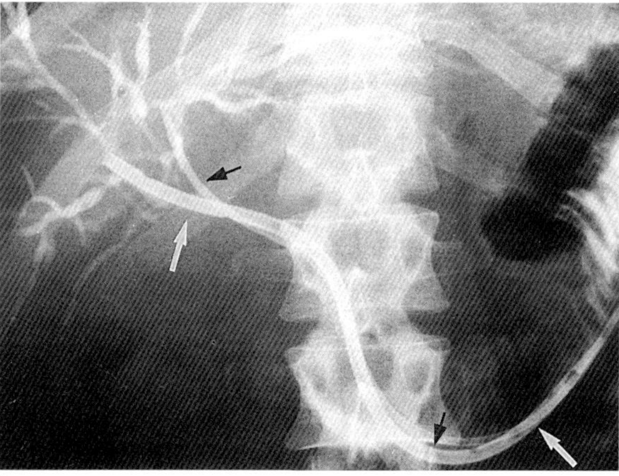

Fig. 4.8.**10   Substitution of non-functioning stent**
a   In a patient with cholangiocarcinoma on the level of the porta hepatis and inside the liver, internal biliary drainage was carried out with a right-sided transhepatic approach
b   External biliary catheter decompression was applied for 8 days
c   A 7 Fr home-made endoprosthesis (small arrows) proved insufficiency for internal drainage and was supported by another large-bore stent: A 12 Fr Carey-Coons soft biliary stent (large arrows) was placed a week later by means of a right-sided PTC/PTBD

This method is particularly suitable for direct irradiation of *cholangiocarcinomas* in the biliary canals at the porta hepatis and in the extrahepatic biliary duct system. In the literature, and among our own patient population however, only preliminary, if encouraging, reports are available (Itami et al. 1986, Koch et al. 1986, Koester 1984).

Complications and Technical Problems with PTBD

Our personal experience shows 6,1 % of minor bleeding with catheter drainage, and 7,7 % of serious *bleeding* (hematoma development and tamponade) (Fig. 4.8.**12**). With biliary canal endoprosthesis, 6,1 % minor bleeding and 3,8 % serious bleeding can be expected. *Fistulas* (mainly due to infected bile) are to be expected in 3,8 % with catheter drainage and in 1,5 % with biliary canal endoprosthesis (Fig. 4.8.**13**). Serious *infection* was seen in 7,7 % with catheter drainage and in 2,3 % with endoprosthesis. The total complication rate was about 23 %, and 22 % connected with all drainage measures. At 29,5 % external bile, cath-

eter drainage showed a significantly higher complication rate than combined with internal and external catheter drainage (20 %). With endoprostheses there were 16 % complications (Weber 1985, Weber and Höver 1985, 1986, 1987) (Table 4.8.**1**).

The definition of complications varies a great deal in the radiology and endoscopy literature. The result is that literature comparison leaves many questions open. According to Riemann (1984), the total complication rate in transhepatic biliary drainage is 22,6 %. Passariello (1985) differentiates between 10,2 % of minor and 19,9 % of serious complications due to percutaneous transhepatic

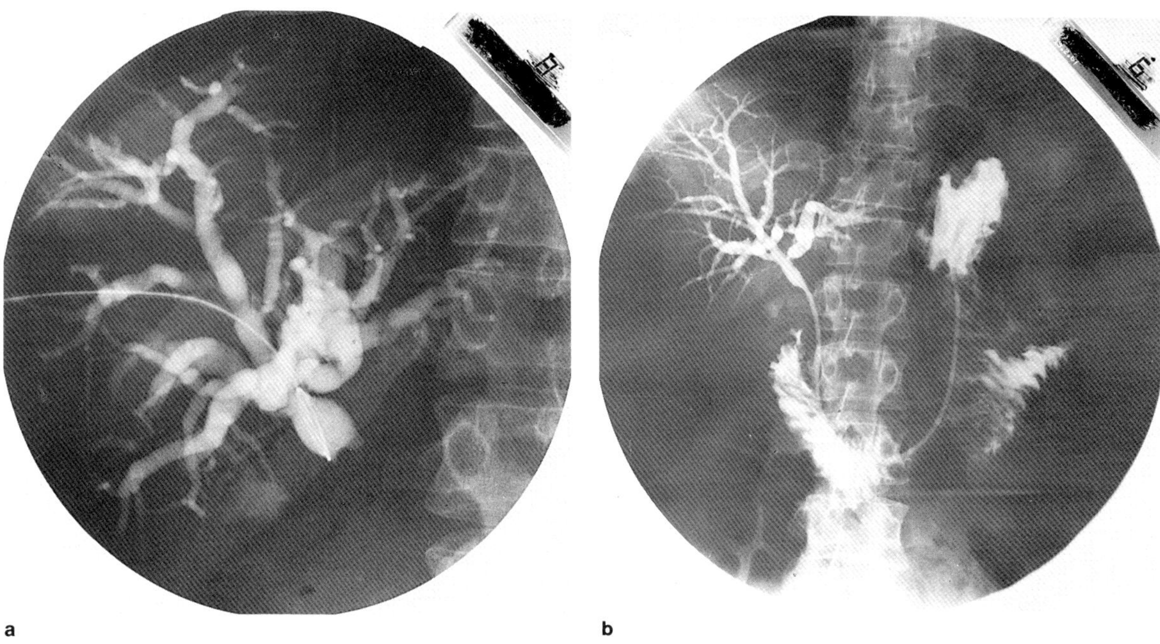

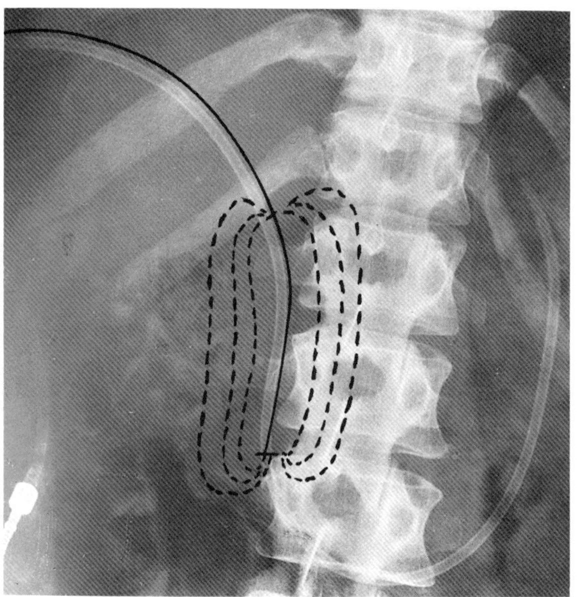

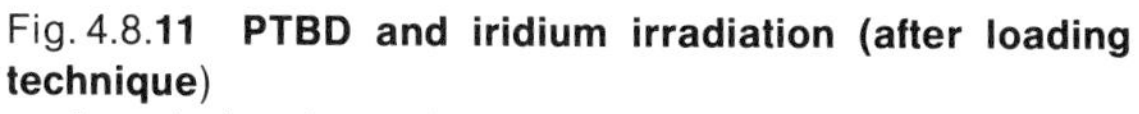

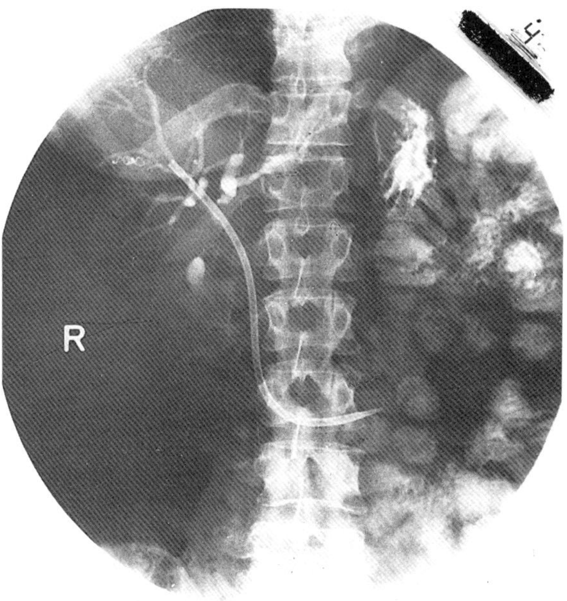

Fig. 4.8.11 PTBD and iridium irradiation (after loading technique)

a In a cholangiocarcinoma with biliary canal obstruction, a combined internal and external 12 Fr catheter drainage is placed

b, c Through the drainage catheter fractionated ^{192}Ir irradiation follows for 10 days, with a total dose of 50 Gy (Prof. K. Hübener, Dept. of Radiotherapy, University Clinic, Eppendorf, Hamburg)

d The drainage catheter is later replaced by a biliary canal endoprosthesis

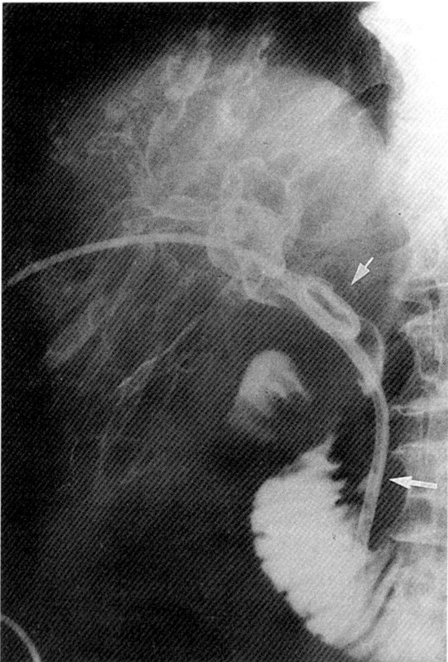

Fig. 4.8.**12   PTBD complications. Massive bleeding** into the biliary tract immediately after positioning of a biliary canal endoprosthesis following PTC. Massive bleeding with tamponade of the biliary tract is frequent, but can be controlled by plugging the transhepatic fistula canal. With NaCl irrigation the coagulate rapidly dissolves (Weber 1985)

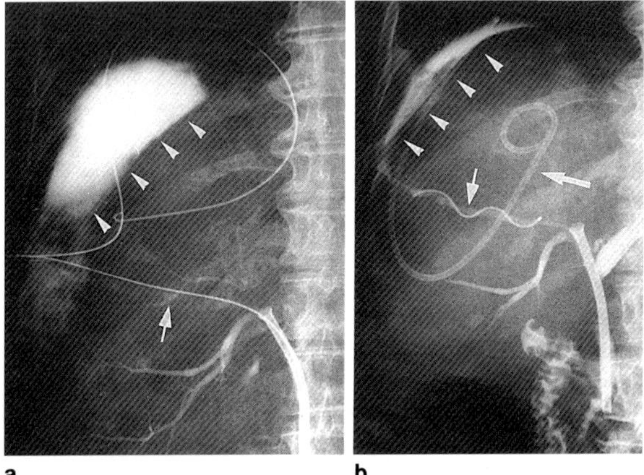

a   b

Fig. 4.8.**13   PTBD complications: biliary fistula** and subphrenic abscess.

a Following the 24 h placement of an external catheter drainage, infected subphrenic bile leakage has caused an abscess (arrow heads)

b The transhepatic fistula was reentered using a 10 Fr "lost" endoprosthesis, and then was blocked with a Gianturco coil (small arrow). Percutaneous catheter drainage of the abscess (large arrow) cleared the subphrenic space within 5 days (arrow heads).

Table 4.8.**1   PTBD complications in 73 patients** (80 interventions, 125 drainage procedures: 77 catheter drainages and 48 endoprostheses)

Complications	PTC	Catheter drainage	Endopros- thesis	Total
Serious bleeding	2	9	7	18 (14.4%)
Uncontrollable biliary fistulas	–	7	–	7 (5.6%)
Abscess	–	4	–	4 (3.2%)
Peritonitis	–	1	1	2 (1.6%)
Pleural empyema	–	1	–	1 (0.8%)
Septicemia	–	2	–	2 (1.6%)
Mortality	–	4	1	5/73 (6.8%) 5/12 (4.0%)

methods. In endoscopic biliary canal drainage and prosthesis, the average complication rate is 24% according to Kühner et al. (1984), 27% according to Wurbs and Gebhardt (1982) and 26,3% according to Hagenmueller (1984), although they could be reduced to about 10% with increasing experience (Hagenmueller and Soehendra 1983). The latter, however, also applies to the radiologic transhepatic method. For this method, the total mortality is placed at 1,4% to 7,7% (Burchardt 1978, Passariello et al. 1985, Pereiras et al. 1978, Riemann 1984, Rupp and Weiss 1980, Weber and Höver 1985), and for endoscopic drainage at 1,1% to 7,9% (Hagenmueller and Soehendra 1983, Huibregtse et al. 1981, Kuehner et al. 1984, Soehendra and Reynders-Frederix 1979). It seems that there are no major differences in risk between the transhepatic and endoscopic methods. All these figures are valid for *early* complications. Currently, the literature offers no clear statements on *late* complications in prostheses displacement or blockage (Fig. 4.8.**14**), although individual observations have been made with large-bore endoprostheses (Hoevels and Ihse 1979, Oleaga and Ring 1981). In the majority of cases, an obstructed bile duct endoprosthesis can be bypassed, using the transhepatic route to push a new one (Fig. 4.8.**10b**). The same strategy may be used in patients in whom an occluded endoscopic stent cannot be replaced (Fig. 4.8.**15b**).

From our point of view, however, preference is to be given to the endoscopic method independently of the caliber and size of the endoprosthesis, provided that this is possible on the basis of the anatomic conditions previously described (and can be carried out with sufficient technical expertise). This, however, narrows the spectrum of percutaneous transhepatic drainage additionally by increasing technically difficult cases (e.g. after Billroth II and Roux's anastomosis or similar contraindications to the endoscopic method) (Fig. 4.8.**15**).

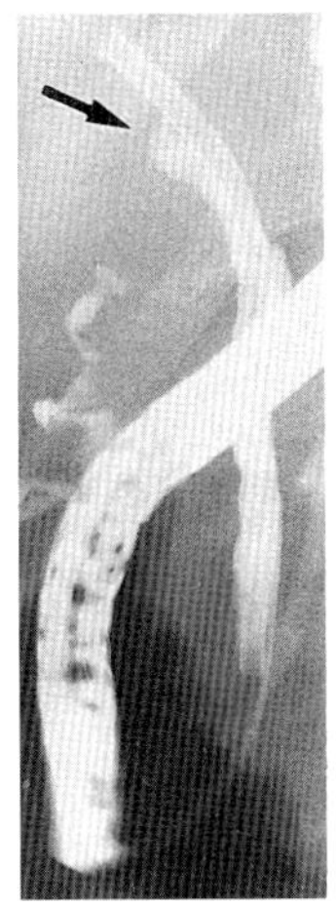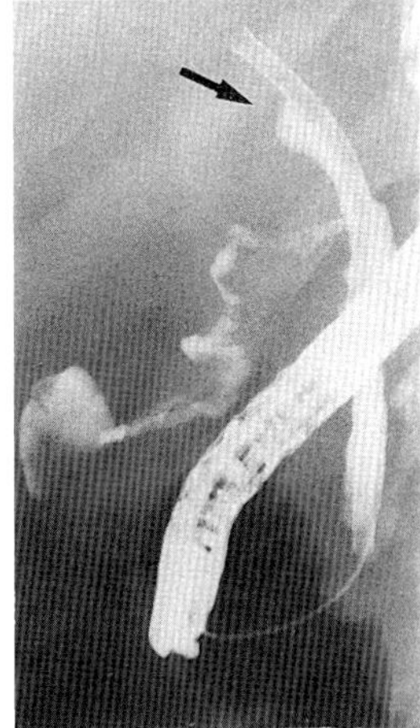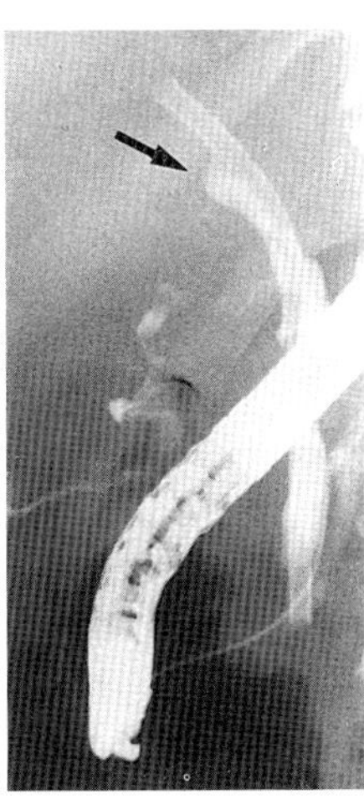

Fig. 4.8.14 PTBD complications: prosthesis obstruction. Even with the use of large-bore endoprostheses draining directly into the duodenum, prosthesis obstruction can occur at a very early stage owing to intestinal contents and/or ascending infection. The obstruction can be shown by ERPC, but the prosthesis can usually not be recanalized. Arrows: retrograde filling of the bile duct up to the stenosis

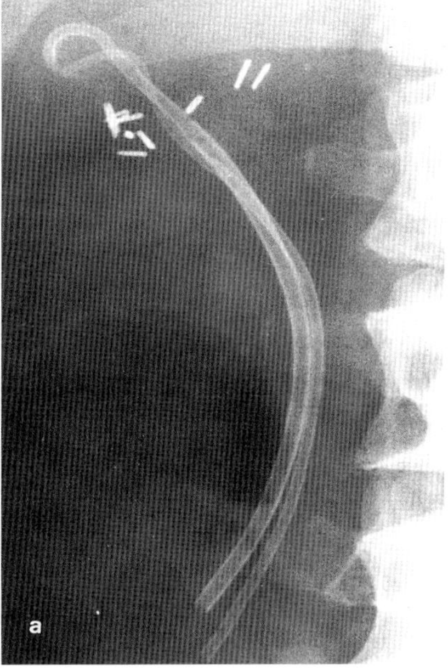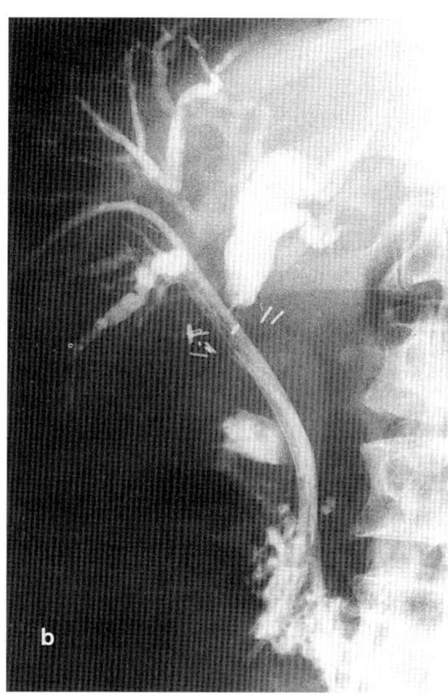

Fig. 4.8.15 Bypassing an obstructed surgical endoprosthesis
a In a patient with cholangiocarcinoma an endoprosthesis was placed surgically. However, it obstructed 10 weeks later, causing recurrent jaundice
b A combined external-internal catheter-drainage was carried out using the transhepatic route

The localization, character and number of the stenoses also may influence technical difficulties in PTBD and their consequences according to complication rate, as in the endoscopic method (Table 4.8.2). A combination of diagnostic PTC and therapeutic biliary drainage (temporary or permanent) within *one* investigative process is always advisable to reduce the risks of PTC. On principle, *multiple drainage* in high, intrahepatic biliary obstruction is technically possible (Figs. 4.8.4, 4.8.5), but the indication is very critical, and should be seen from the point of view of *palliation* in order to achieve the best possible balance between risks, complications and therapeutic palliative gain for the patient (Weber and Höver 1986, 1987). Persistent cholestasis in a smaller liver lobe (e.g. the left

hepatic lobe), involving up to a third of the parenchyma, is acceptable from this point of view (Fig. 4.8.**4b, c**). In a two-stage process offering intermittent iridium radiation therapy (afterloading principle), particularly *close coordination* between the radiologist responsible for drainage and the radiation therapist is needed. Antibiotic protective measures to combat infection are useful. We advise against simultaneous cytostatic therapy. A combination of localized iridium irridation and conventional radiotherapy is possible, and application of the fractionated total dose is recommended. At the same time it is important to avoid displacement and loxal infection of the percutaneous for long-lasting catheter in place. We consider a change to *internal* biliary drainage using a stent later on as

Table 4.8.2   Localization of biliary tract stenoses and obstructions in 74 patients. Etiology and types of PTBD in 130 drainage procedures

	Obstructive jaundice		External biliary drainage	Internal biliary drainage	Trans-hepatic prosthesis
a	Cholangiocarcinoma	17			
	Pancreas carcinoma	–			
	Metastases	6			
	Total	23 (17.7%)	11	6	6
b	Cholangiocarcinoma	16			
	Pancreas carcinoma	3			
	Metastases	13			
	Total	32 (24.6%)	11	8	13
c	Cholangiocarcinoma	8			
	Pancreas carcinoma	7			
	Metastases, lymphoma	7			
	Stones, stenoses	–			
	Total	22 (16.9%)	7	6	9
d	Cholangiocarcinoma	6			
	Pancreas carcinoma	23			
	Metastases, lymphoma	17			
	Papilla tumors	–			
	Stones, stenoses	7			
	Total	53 (40.8%)	15	16	22
Total interventions 84	Total drainage procedures	130 (100%)	44 (33.8%)	36 (27.7%)	50 (38.5%)

long as there are no long-term therapy results that ensure a chance of cure. A later endoscopic removal of the biliary endoprosthesis can be kept in mind. Considering the difficulty (and in most cases the impossibility) of applying iridium irradiation via the nasobiliary endoscopic route, percutaneous transhepatic afterloading irradiation in suitable cases is much simpler to carry out. It also seems to us to be less invasive against the surgical approach by enterostomy.

In summary, since the introduction of biliary catheter drainage and endoprostheses in the mid-1970s, the *palliative* approach to malignant biliary duct stenosis causing obstructive jaundice has changed considerably. While the average mortality with pure surgical methods (biliodigestive anastomosis) was 25% (Ott and Gelfand 1981); intra-operative catheter relief of the blocked and infected biliary tract was able to reduce the operative risk to 4–16% (Takada 1976, Denning 1981, both cited in Weber and Höver 1985, 1987). The palliative possibilities of endoscopic or percutaneous biliary tract drainage have partly been able to replace the operative method, which involved a high recurrence of obstruction in the anastomosed biliary canals and recurrence of jaundice. In combination with iridium irradiation on the afterloading principle, PTBD has been able to open up new *curative* prospects in malignant obstructive jaundice. Catheter drainage and biliary tract endoprostheses have to be matched to local conditions when a choice is being made between endoscopic or percutaneous transhepatic access. Technical practicability and the reduction of complications are equally influenced by the level of experience of the endoscopist and the interventional radiologist. Close interdisciplinary cooperation between the abdominal surgeon, the endoscopist and the radiologist is indispensable in establishing the indication, the implementation of drainage measures, and aftercare.

References

Ariyama J, Shirakabe H, Ohashi K, et al. Experience with percutaneous transhepatic cholangiography using the Japanese needle. Gastrointest Radiol 1978; 2: 359.

Atkinson MM, Happey MG, Smiddy FG. New methods for diagnostic and research: percutaneous transhepatic cholangiography. Gut 1960; 1: 357.

Baron RL, Stanley RJ, Lee JKT, Koehler HE, Melson A, Balfe DM, Weyman PJ. A prospective comparison of the evaluation of biliary obstruction using computed tomography and ultrasonography. Radiology 1982; 145: 91.

Burcharth F. A new endoprosthesis for nonoperative intubation of the biliary tract in malignant obstructive jaundice. Surg Gynecol Obstet 1978; 146: 76.

Castaneda-Zuniga WR, Tadavarthy SM, Laerum F, Amplatz K. Anterior approach for biliary duct drainage. Radiology 1981; 139: 746.

Ferrucci JT, Mueller PR, Harbin WP. Percutaneous transhepatic biliary drainage: technique, results and applications. Radiology 1980; 135: 1.

Hagenmueller F. Results of endoscopic biliduodenal drainage in malignant bile duct stenosis. In: Classen M, Geenen JE, Kaway K, eds. Non-surgical biliary drainage. Berlin: Springer, 1984: 94–104.

Hagenmueller F, Sohendra N. Non-surgical biliary drainage. Clin Gastroenterol 1983; 12 (suppl 1): 297–316.

Hoevels J, Ihse, I. Percutaneous transhepatic insertion of a permanent endoprosthesis in obstructive lesions of the extrahepatic bile ducts. Gastrointest Radiol 1979; 4: 367.

Hoevels J, Lunderquist A, Ihse I. Perkutane transhepatische Intubation der Gallengänge zur kombinierten inneren und äußeren Drainage bei extrahepatischer Cholestase. RöFo 1978; 129: 533.

Huibregtse K, Haverkamp HJ, Tytgat GN. Transpapillary positioning of a large 3.2 mm biliary endoprosthesis. Endoscopy 1981; 13: 217.

Itami J, Saegusa K, Tsuchiya Y, Mamiya T, et al. Intrakavitäre High-dose-rate-Afterloading-Bestrahlung beim inoperablen malignen Gallengangsverschluß. In: Itami J, ed. Intrakavitäre Radiotherapie des Gallengangsmalignoms. Strahlentherapie und Onkologie 1986; 162: 105–110.

Koch K, Schumacher W, Krumhaar D, et al. Iridium afterloading technique: basic principles and effects. Tumordiagn Ther 1986; 7 (suppl): 36–38.

Koenigsberg M, Wiener SN, Walzer A. The accuracy of sonography in the differential diagnosis of obstructive jaundice: a comparison with cholangiography. Radiology 1979; 133: 157.

Koester R. Percutaneous transhepatic drainage: technique, results, and special applications. In: Baert AL, et al., eds. Frontiers in European radiology; vol 4. Berlin: Springer 1984.

Kuehner W, Frimberger E, Stoelzle L, et al. Transpapilläre biliäre Drainagen. Z Gastroenterol 1984; 22: 57.

Molnar W, Stockum AE. Transhepatic dilatation of choledochoenterostomy strictures. Radiology 1978; 129: 59.

Nickols DA, MacCarty RL, Gaffey TA. Cholangiographic evaluation of bile duct carcinoma. AJR 1983; 141: 1291.

Okuda K, Tanikawa K, Emura T, et al. Non-surgical percutaneous transhepatic cholangiography: diagnostic significance in medial problems of the liver. Dig Dis 1974; 19: 21.

Oleaga JA, Ring EJ. Interventional biliary radiology. In: Ring EJ, McLean GK, eds. Interventional radiology: principles and techniques. Boston: Little Brown, 1981.

Ott DJ, Gelfand DW. Complications of gastrointestinal-radiologic procedures, II: complications related to biliary tract studies. Gastrointest Radiol 1981; 6: 47.

Passariello R, Pavone P, Rossi P, et al. Percutaneous biliary drainage in neoplastic jaundice: statistical data from a computerized multicentric study. Acta Radiol 1985.

Pereiras RV, Rheingold OJ, Hutson D, Mejia J, Viamonte M, et al. Relief of malignant obstructive jaundice by percutaneous insertion of a permanent prosthesis in the biliary tree. Ann Intern Med 1978; 89: 589.

Riemann JF. Extrahepatische Cholestase: Transhepatische Drainagen. Z Gastroenterol 1984; 22: 64.

Rupp N, Weiss H-D. Perkutan eingebrachte Gallengangsprothesen als Primärmaßnahme bei Verschlußikterus. RöFo 1980; 133: 279.

Soehendra N, Reynders-Frederix V. Palliative Gallengangsdrainage. Eine neue Methode zur endoskopischen Einführung eines inneren Drains. Dtsch Med Wochenschr 1979; 104: 206.

Weber J. Die Verwendung von Gianturco-Spiralen bei der perkutanen transhepatischen Gallengangsdrainage. RöFo 1985; 143: 459.

Weber J, Höver S. Technische Probleme der perkutanen transhepatischen Gallengangsdrainage. RöFo 1985; 143: 534.

Weber J, Höver S. Perkutane transhepatische Gallengangsdrainage (PTD/P) per Katheter und Endoprothese: Ergebnisse und Komplikationen bei 130 Eingriffen. In: Barthelheimer A, Ossenberg F-W, Schreiber HW, Seifert G, eds. Therapie in der Diskussion. München: Pflaum, 1986.

Weber J, Höver S. Technische Probleme und Komplikationen bei der perkutanen transhepatischen Gallengangsdrainage. Radiol Diagn (Berl) 1987; 28: 555.

Wurbs D, Gebhardt J. Endoskopische Diagnostik und Therapie bei Gallenerkrankungen. Chirurg 1982; 53: 751.

4.9 Angiography in the Preoperative Staging of Hepatobiliary and Pancreatic Malignancies

K. H. Schuur, J. W. A. J. Reeders

Introduction

Owing to the increase in diagnostic modalities – ultrasound (US), endoscopic ultrasonography (EUS), computed tomography (CT), and magnetic resonance imaging (MRI) – angiography has lost a great deal of its importance in the evaluation of diseases of the pancreas and liver. Formerly, angiography was the method of choice for evaluating space-occupying lesions in the upper abdomen. Since US, CT and MRI are now available in many hospitals, the number of angiographic procedures for space-occupying lesions in the pancreas and liver has been dramatically reduced. Previously, the angiographer had to answer the question: "Is there a malignancy?" Today, the question is: "There is a malignancy, is it resectable?" (Mukai et al. 1987a). Along with several other factors influencing the patient's operability and resectability such as general condition, presence of associated diseases, lymph node metastases, malignant ascites etc., angiography plays an important role in answering this question. The present chapter deals with the problem of how to use angiography to assess the resectability of a malignancy in the region of the pancreas and liver.

Normal Arterial Anatomy

Since knowledge of vascular anatomy is necessary to study the pathological situation, a review of the normal vascular supply of the liver and pancreas will be given here (Lunderquist 1965, 1967). Blood supply to the upper abdominal organs originates from the celiac axis and the superior mesenteric artery, both arising on the ventral wall of the abdominal aorta at the level of the 12th thoracic – 1st lumbar vertebra. In most cases, the celiac axis divides into three branches (Fig. 4.9.1): the splenic artery (supplying the spleen), the left gastric artery (for vascularization of the gastric fundus and distal esophagus) and the common hepatic artery. The latter gives off the gastroduodenal artery (see below), and continues as the proper hepatic artery. This vessel supplies the liver, dividing into a left hepatic artery (for the left lobe) and a right hepatic artery (for the right lobe). The gallbladder is supplied by the cystic artery, arising from the right hepatic artery.

Arterial supply to the pancreas is provided by several arteries (Fig. 4.9.2). The gastroduodenal artery gives off two branches for vascularization of

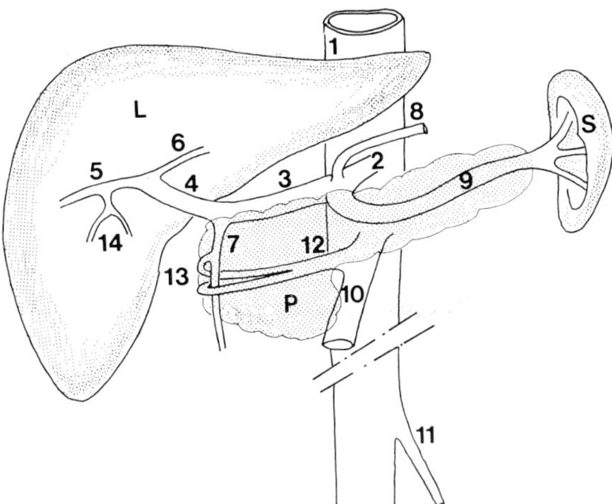

Fig. 4.9.1 **Normal arterial anatomy of the upper abdomen**
 1 Abdominal aorta
 2 Celiac axis
 3 Common hepatic artery
 4 Proper hepatic artery
 5 Right hepatic artery
 6 Left hepatic artery
 7 Gastroduodenal artery
 8 Left gastric artery
 9 Splenic artery
10 Superior mesenteric artery
11 Inferior mesenteric artery
12 Inferior pancreaticoduodenal artery
13 Anterior and posterior superior pancreaticoduodenal arteries
14 Cystic artery
L Liver
S Spleen
P Pancreas

the head of the pancreas: the posterior and anterior superior pancreaticoduodenal arteries. They pass the pancreatic head ventrally and dorsally. They fuse and form a communication with the superior mesenteric artery: the inferior pancreaticoduodenal artery. This pathway is an important collateral route between the celiac axis and the superior mesenteric artery. In normal cases, flow in the gastroduodenal artery is in the caudal direction, but this flow can be reversed in pathological conditions such as cirrhosis of the liver, stenosis or occlusion of the celiac axis or the common hepatic artery, arteriovenous shunts in the liver, or hepatic tumors demanding large amounts of blood.

The body of the pancreas is supplied by the dorsal pancreatic artery, arising from the celiac axis near its trifurcation. This vessel also gives off a branch to the uncinate process. Usually, it gives rise to the transverse pancreatic artery that runs through the tail of the pancreas. The main supply to

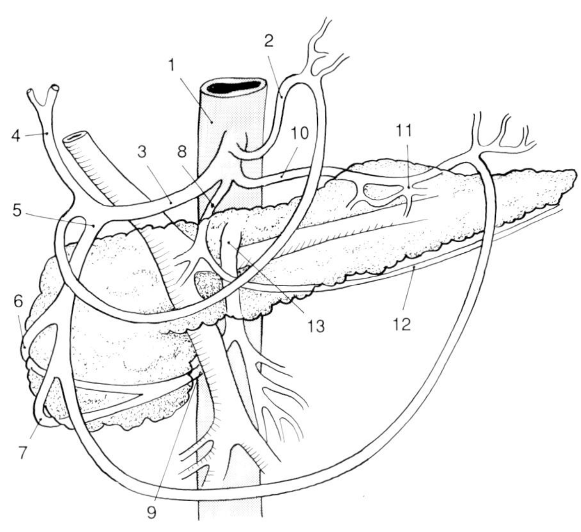

Fig. 4.9.**2a Arterial blood supply of the pancreas** (after Lunderquist 1965)

 1 Abdominal aorta
 2 Celiac axis
 3 Common hepatic artery
 4 Proper hepatic artery
 5 Gastroduodenal artery
 6 Posterior superior pancreaticoduodenal artery
 7 Anterior superior pancreaticoduodenal artery
 8 Dorsal pancreatic artery
 9 Inferior pancreaticoduodenal artery
10 Splenic artery
11 Pancreatica magna artery
12 Transverse pancreatic artery
13 Superior mesenteric artery

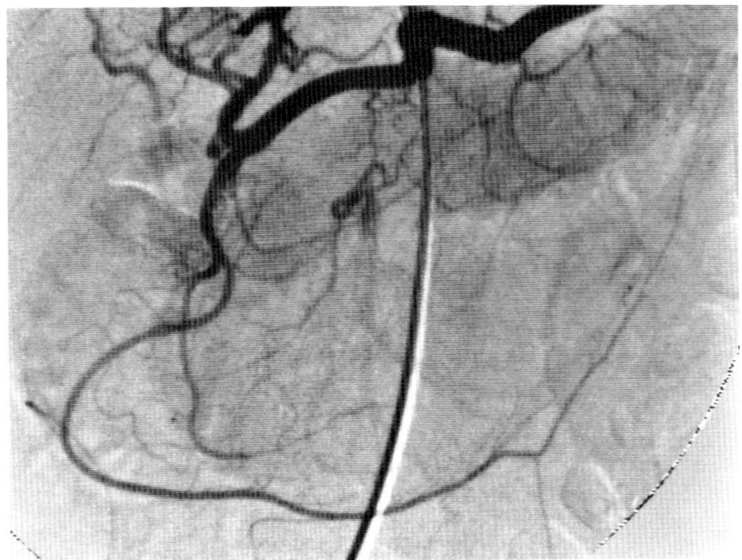

2b DSA: Normal pancreatic vascularization after selective catheterization of the celiac trunk. The ventral pancreatic arcades originate from the gastroduodenal artery. The dorsal pancreatic arcades originate from the splenic artery.

Fig. 4.9.**3 The most frequent anatomical variants in the arterial supply of the liver** (after Lunderquist 1965, 1967)

 1 Left gastric artery (LGA)
 2 Splenic artery
 3 Common hepatic artery (CHA)
 4 Superior mesenteric artery (SMA)
 5 Proper hepatic artery
 6 Right hepatic artery (RHA)
 7 Left hepatic artery (LHA)
 8 Gastroduodenal artery

a: normal situation. **b**: RHA arising from SMA. **c**: CHA arising from SMA. **d**: LHA arising from LGA. **e**: common trunk. **f**: separate origins

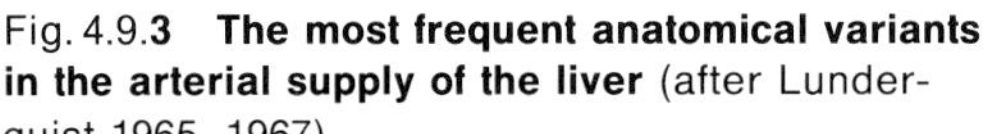

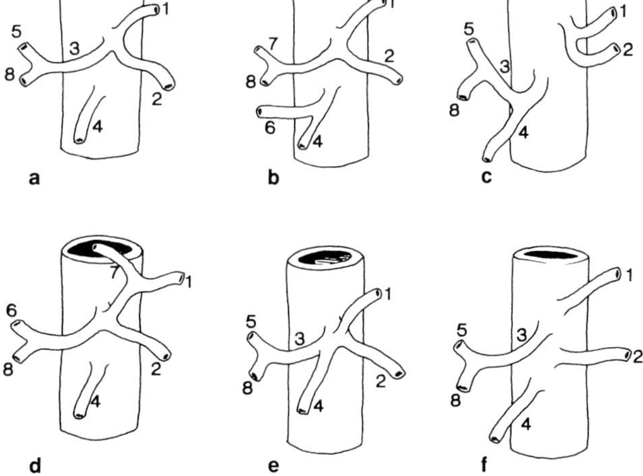

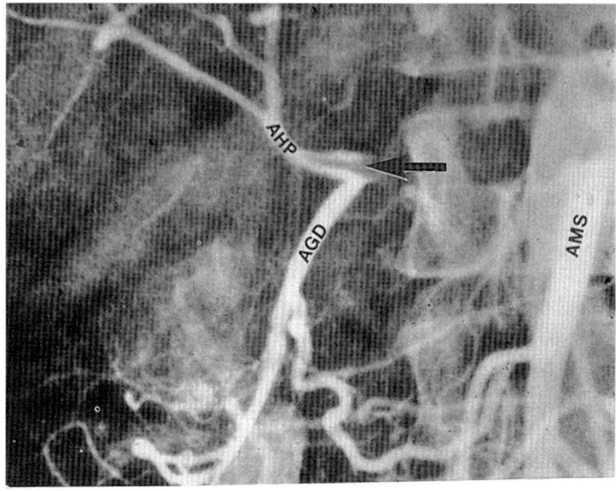

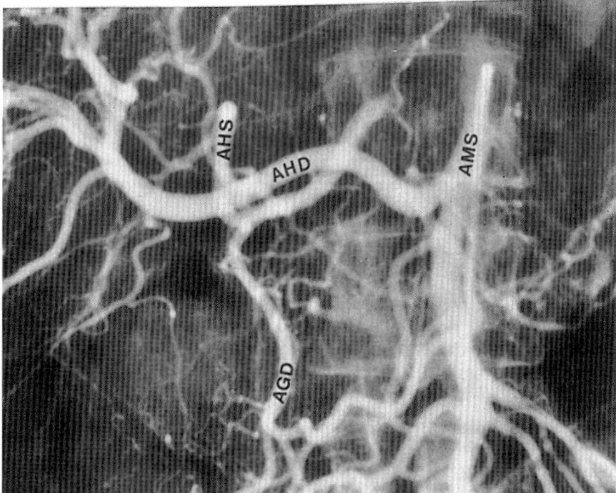

Fig. 4.9.**4   The most common arterial anatomic variant.**
The right hepatic artery (AHD) arises from the superior
mesenteric artery (AMS). The left hepatic artery (AHS)
arises from the celiac axis. AHP = proper hepatic artery;
AGD = gastroduodenal artery. Steal from AMS to AHP
(arrow)

the body and tail of the pancreas arises from the
splenic artery: the pancreatica magna artery. Branches from this artery communicate with the transverse pancreatic artery. In addition, there are
several smaller branches arising from the splenic
artery and supplying the pancreas.

Knowledge of anatomical variants is essential,
especially in preoperative evaluation of hepatic and
pancreatic malignancies. Arterial variants occur in
about 15% of all cases. A survey of the most
frequent anatomical variants is given schematically
in Figure 4.9.**3**. In a study of 64 cirrhotic patients,
however, we found variants in about 50% of cases
(Schuur 1983). The most common arterial anatomic variant is the right hepatic artery, arising
from the superior mesenteric artery (Fig. 4.9.**4**).
This situation occurs in about 20–50% of all
variants. Other variants are:

- The common hepatic artery, arising from the
  superior mesenteric artery (14%).
- The left hepatic artery, arising from the left
  gastric artery (17%).
- The left hepatic artery, arising proximally to the
  gastroduodenal artery (10%). In these cases,
  there is no proper hepatic artery.
- A common trunk (hepatic artery, splenic artery,
  left gastric artery, superior mesenteric artery)
  (3%).
- Arteries arising directly from the aorta (1%).

Normal Venous Anatomy

Only the larger veins are discussed here, as they are
important in cases of pancreatic or hepatic tumors.
The splenic vein and the superior mesenteric vein
fuse at the level of L1–L2 on the right side, forming
the portal vein (Fig. 4.9.**5**). These three veins are
very important in patients with malignancies of the
liver or pancreas. The splenic vein runs along the
upper posterior border of the pancreas, and can
easily be invaded by tumor growth. The superior
mesenteric vein is surrounded by the head and
uncinate process of the pancreas, and can be
invaded by tumor growth in this part of the
pancreas.
Malignancies of the liver may grow into the main
portal vein, and tumor (thrombi) from the splenic
and superior mesenteric vein may proceed into the
portal vein. Thus, evaluation of the patency of these

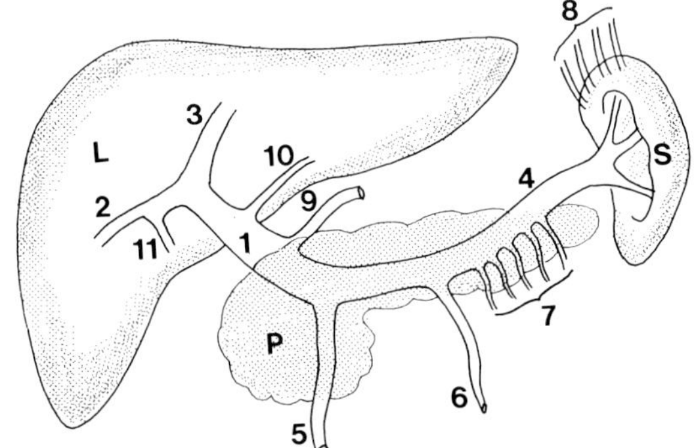

Fig. 4.9.**5   Normal venous anatomy of the upper abdomen**
1 Portal vein
2 Right portal branch
3 Left portal branch
4 Splenic vein
5 Superior mesenteric vein
6 Inferior mesenteric vein
7 Pancreatic veins
8 Short gastric veins
9 Left gastric vein
10 Right gastric vein
11 Cystic vein
L   Liver
S   Spleen
P   Pancreas

veins is necessary before planning an operation. As an anatomic variant, the inferior mesenteric vein, which normally enters the splenic vein, may also enter the portal vein at the fusion point of the splenic and superior mesenteric veins.

Angiographic Technique

In order to obtain an impression of the gross vascular anatomy of the upper abdomen, we prefer to make a midstream aortogram. In this way, obstructions of the larger arteries can already be seen (Fig. 4.9.6). Moreover, an overall impression is gained of the situation of the abdominal aorta, giving an idea of the amount of atherosclerotic plaques. This can be important if liver transplantation is a therapeutic possibility.

Midstream aortography. For this we use a 5 or 6 Fr pigtail catheter with multiple side-holes. The catheter is positioned at the level of the 12th thoracic vertebra, and an injection of 50 ml of water-soluble contrast medium (350 mg I/ml) with a flow of 25 ml per second is given by automatic injection. Imaging is performed every half second for 4 seconds and every second for the next 4 seconds. In normal cases, the portal vein should therefore be visible on the last pictures.

Selective injections. For pre-operative evaluation only, superselective catheterization of small arteries of the pancreas is not necessary. Initially, injections into the celiac axis and splenic artery, or both, *and* the superior mesenteric artery are sufficient. For catheterization of both arteries, a cobra head 6 Fr catheter can be used. In order to obtain

good and adequate opacification of the splenic, mesenteric and portal veins, a dose of 60 ml of contrast should be injected into the corresponding arteries, with a flow of 6–10 ml per second. Pictures should be made over a sufficiently long period, especially if portal obstruction is present or suspected. Most of the time an estimate of the flow velocity may be obtained by referring to the aortogram. In certain cases, pictures have to be made for 20–30 seconds after injecting the contrast medium. If visualization of the venous system alone, which is the indicator for resectability of the tumor mass of the pancreas, is needed, then we prefer to make the first picture just before the start of the injection to allow photographic subtraction, and the second picture at the end of the injection. This may last 10 seconds. The following pictures can then be made at intervals of 2–3 seconds. Highly informative pictures can be obtained by injecting simultaneously into the splenic artery and the superior mesenteric artery. This can be carried out using a Y-connector (Fig. 4.9.7). The technique is extremely informative, especially if there is any doubt about the patency of the portal vein (flow effects; see below) and/or ingrowth of the tumor mass into the confluence of the splenic vein and superior mesenteric vein.

DSA technique. If there is a normal or slightly decreased flow rate in the portal venous system, we prefer to use the digital subtraction angiography (DSA) technique. Injection of the same amounts of contrast medium provides excellent visualization of the veins. However, if the flow time is prolonged, DSA may be insufficient or even impossible owing to patient movements and respiration artefacts (Hoevels et al. 1987).

Pharmaco-angiography. Improvement of visualization of the venous system can also be obtained via intra-arterial administration of drugs. Tolazoline (Priscol®) is the most commonly used drug (Freeny 1983). It is a vasodilating drug, and is administered in a dose of 20–50 mg intra-arterially, 30–60 seconds prior to contrast injection. It has a slightly hypotensive effect which lasts for about 15 min. For this reason, it should not be used in patients with coronary artery disease, cerebrovascular insufficiency and myocardial infarction (Friedman et al. 1987).

For the evaluation of liver malignancies, injection into the common or proper artery is sufficient. An injection of about 30 ml of contrast agent can be used, with a flow rate of 8–10 ml per second. If separate evaluation of each liver lobe is needed, injection into the left and right hepatic arteries separately is necessary. In these cases, a lower injection rate of about 4–8 ml per second should be given. Images should be made every half second for 4 seconds, and every second for the next 4–8 seconds.

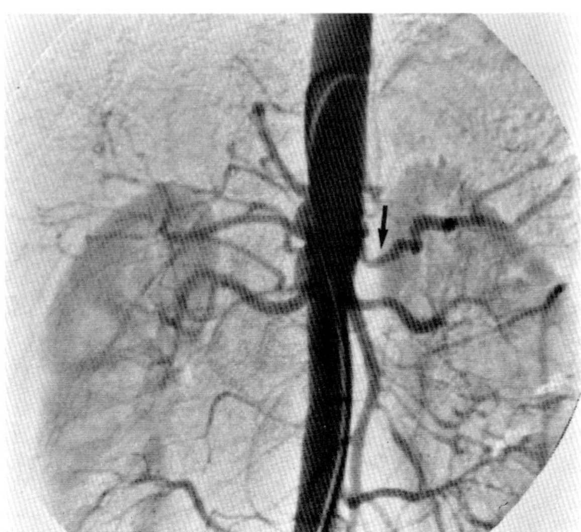

Fig. 4.9.6 Midstream aortography. A large malignant mass at the corpus of pancreas with vaso-invasive ingrowth into the splenic artery (encasement: see arrow) near the origin of the celiac trunk

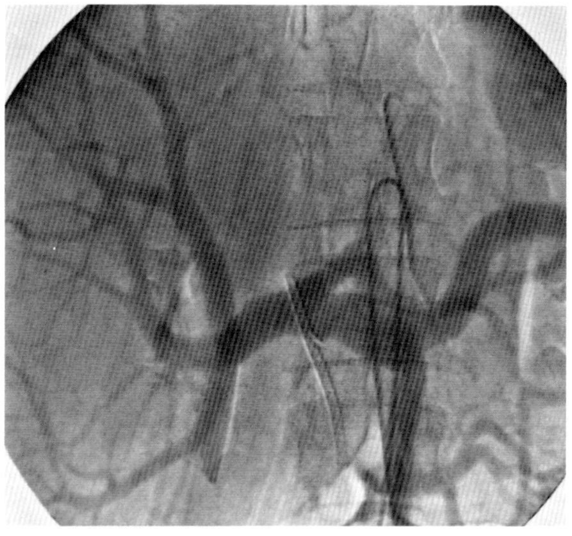

a

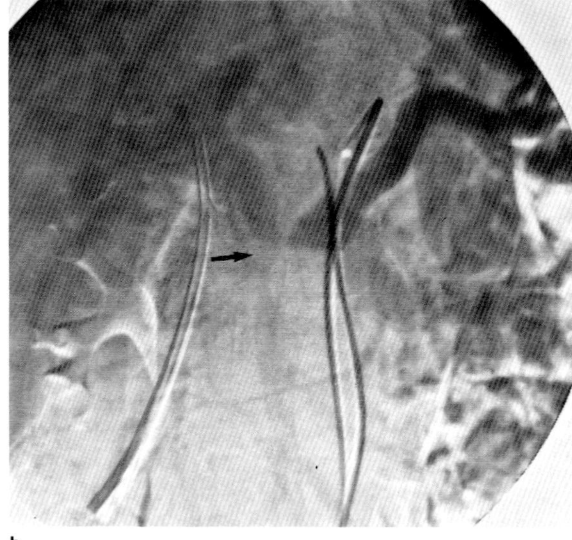

b

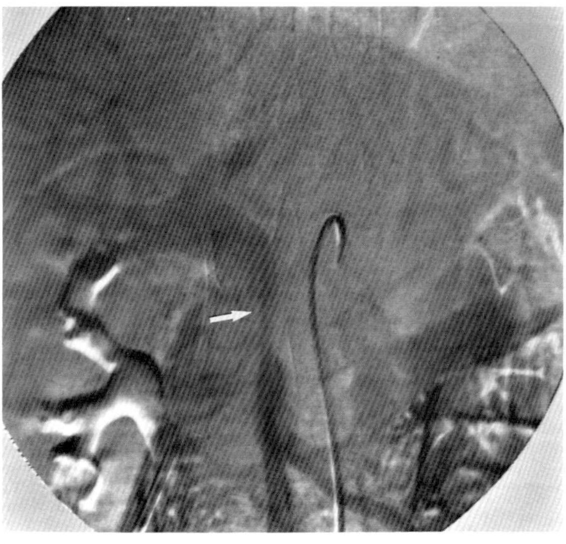

c

Fig. 4.9.**7   DSA: Late-phase arteriography. a** Normal venous flow pattern of the splenic vein, superior mesenteric vein and portal venous system after simultaneous injection of contrast agent into the celiac trunk and superior mesenteric artery. Note the two catheters.

b, c   Separate injections into the celiac trunk and superior mesenteric artery. A large malignant tumor mass at the junction of the pancreatic head and corpus, with vaso-invasive ingrowth into the confluence of the splenic vein and superior mesenteric vein. Note the extensive narrowing of the superior mesenteric vein (arrow). The abnormalities are not as well delineated as they are with simultaneous injection (**a**).

For angiographic detection of liver metastases, the infusion technique may be useful. In this case 50 ml of contrast agent is injected into the common hepatic artery or proper hepatic artery with a flow rate of 5 ml per second. Pictures are taken over a period of 40 seconds. As blood supply to the metastases is provided by hepatic artery branches, contrast agent in normal liver tissue is "washed out" by portal venous flow. This technique is especially useful in visualizing lesions in the left liver lobe (Takashima and Matsui 1980, Flannigan et al. 1983).

Angiographic Staging of Liver Malignancies

In patients with known primary or secondary hepatic malignancies and without other contra-indications to operation, a few questions have to be cleared up before surgical intervention can be performed. First, there is the problem of whether the tumor is located in the right or left lobe or in both lobes. If other imaging modalities have demonstrated a well-defined mass in one or both liver lobes, angiography is of no further help. However, if there is any doubt about the exact location and spread of the tumor, angiography may be very useful. As a rule, injections into the common or proper hepatic artery provide sufficient information. If not, separate injections into both hepatic arteries have to be done.

Secondly, the radiologist has to answer the question of whether the portal vein is patent and free of tumor. To answer this, injections have to be made into the splenic, hepatic and superior mesenteric arteries. As liver tumors are vascularized by

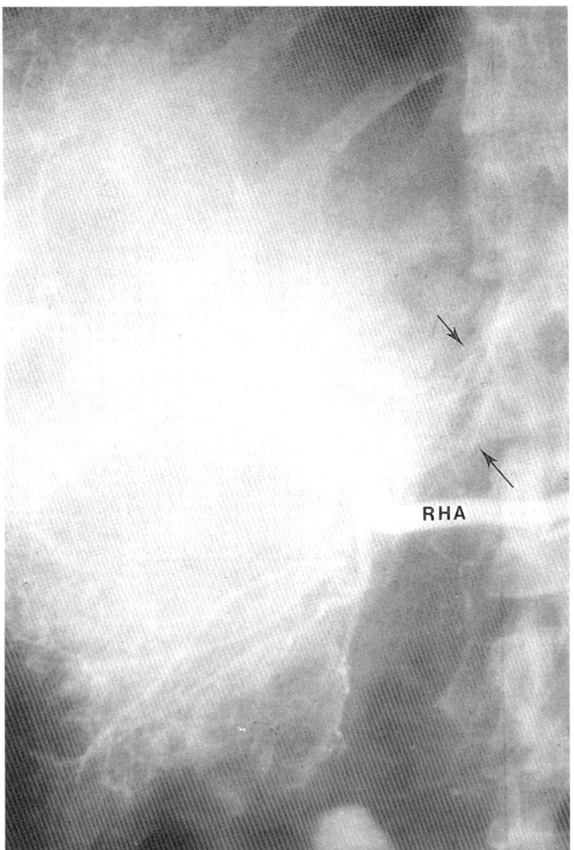

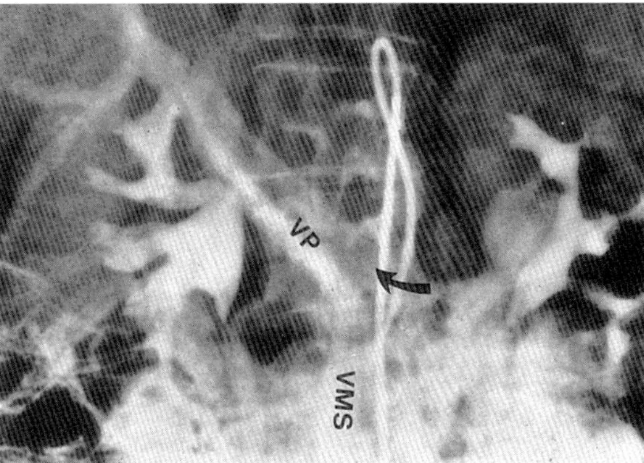

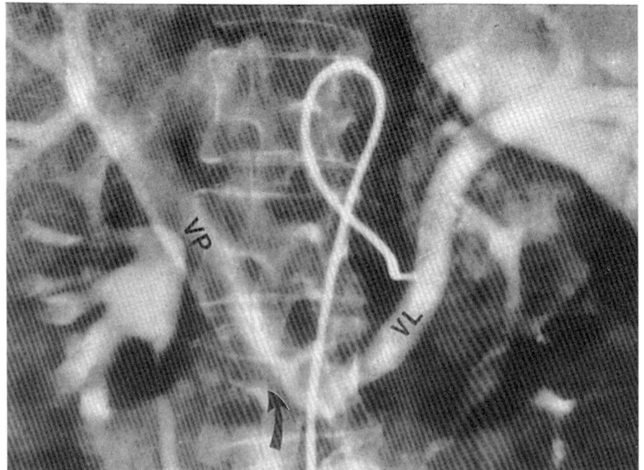

Fig. 4.9.**8** **Large hepatocellular carcinoma.** Injection into the right hepatic artery (arising from the superior mesenteric artery: "thread and streaks sign," indicating tumor growth into the portal vein (arrows) and excessive staining of the contrast medium in the liver parenchyma

Fig. 4.9.**9** **Flow effects in the portal vein**
a SMA injection, venous phase. Visualization of the superior mesenteric vein (VMS) and the portal vein (VP). Filling defect in the portal vein due to inflow of blood from the splenic vein (arrow)
b Splenic artery injection, venous phase. Visualisation of the splenic vein (VL) and the portal vein (VP). Inflow effect from VMS (arrow)

the hepatic artery, tumor invasion into the portal vein can already be seen on hepatic artery injection. Tumor thrombus in the portal vein can be observed as very thin, straight-running arteries, located over the portal vein tract. This is called the "thread and streaks sign" (Fig. 4.9.**8**) (Okuda et al. 1975). The portal vein itself is, of course, visualized in the venous phase of splenic and superior mesenteric artery injections. In normal cases, layering of the contrast agent can be seen in the portal vein owing to inflow of non-opacified blood from the other (non-injected) organ. It is essential to recognize this situation, and it should not be misinterpreted as a partial portal thrombosis (Fig. 4.9.**9**). In normal cases, the portal vein has a straight shape without curves. If a curved portal vein is seen, one should be alert to tumor in the liver hilum.

In the case of total portal stenosis or thrombosis, collateral veins occur, surrounding the original portal vein. Collateral veins may also occur at other locations, and follow the same routes as seen in portal hypertension. Portocaval anastomoses are drawn schematically in Figures 4.9.**10** and 4.9.**11**. These anastomoses can be divided into normal portal veins with reversed flow (short gastric veins, left gastric vein, superior and inferior mesenteric veins), on the one hand, and communicating collaterals (umbilical vein, splenocaval shunts, retroperitoneal communications, intrahepatic portovenous shunts) on the other.

Thirdly, there is the question of whether the large liver arteries are encased or even occluded by tumor growth. As hepatic arteries show fewer atherosclerotic changes compared with other vessels, one should always be aware of encasement if irregularities are present. Steal of blood from the superior mesenteric artery via the gastroduodenal artery into the hepatic artery can be a symptom of hepatic artery stenosis. Of course, this situation should be differentiated from stenosis at the origin

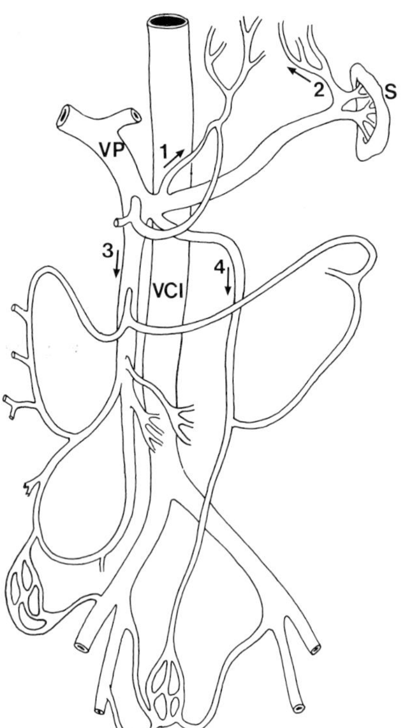

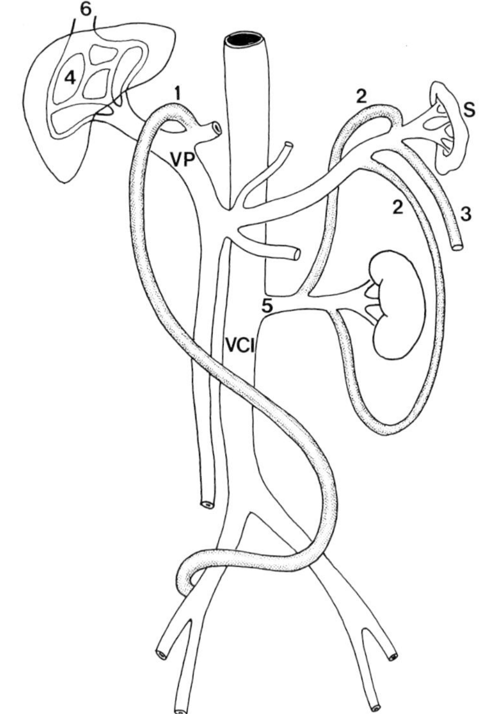

Fig. 4.9.**10**   **Portocaval anastomoses**. Reversed flow in normal portal veins
1   Left gastric vein
2   Short gastric veins
3   Superior mesenteric vein
4   Inferior mesenteric vein
VP Portal vein
VCI Inferior vena cava

Fig. 4.9.**11**   **Communicating collaterals**
1   Umbilical vein
2   Splenorenal shunts
3   Retroperitoneal veins from the spleen
4   Intrahepatic portovenous shunts
5   Left renal vein
6   Hepatic vein
VP Portal vein
VCI Inferior vena cava

of the celiac axis, owing to the diaphragmatic crura (Fig. 4.9.**12**). Steal of blood can also be observed in the case of increased arterial liver flow, as seen in arteriovenous malformations or shunts (trauma!), and in large hepatic tumors (Fig. 4.9.**9**). As there is an inverse proportion between the arterial and portal supply to the liver, obstruction of portal venous inflow due to tumor invasion may lead to an increase in arterial flow and steal from the superior mesenteric arteries.

If a surgeon wishes to operate on a patient with a malignancy in the region of the junction of the left and right bile ducts (Klatskin tumor), it is essential that he is informed on the status of the arteries at the bifurcation of the hepatic artery. Invasion of tumor into this artery makes surgical removal difficult or even impossible (Fig. 4.9.**13**, 4.9.**14**). This is not the case in pancreatic head carcinoma. Tumor invasion into the gastroduodenal artery (Fig. 4.9.**15**) does not necessarily mean surgical inoperability, unless the veins are also involved in the tumor process.

The key questions in liver resections can be summarized as follows (Mukai et al. 1987 b):

1. Will there be enough functioning liver tissue left after resection? (cave cirrhosis)
2. Will there be sufficient vascular and biliary anastomoses left to supply the remaining liver tissue?

Many surgeons like to be informed prior to operation about the status of the vascular system, the degree of atherosclerosis, and the exact angiographic liver anatomy. This applies particularly in cases where liver transplantation is at issue.

Angiographic Staging of Pancreatic Malignancies

In preoperative assessment of pancreatic tumor resectability, angiography is the method of choice, as visualization of the vascular bed around the pancreas is necessary (Jahn et al. 1984). Pancreatic tumors may grow into both the arteries and the veins and give rise to encasement of vessels and thrombosis. The splenic vein, superior mesenteric vein and portal vein are normally visible in the venous phase of celiac or superior mesenteric artery

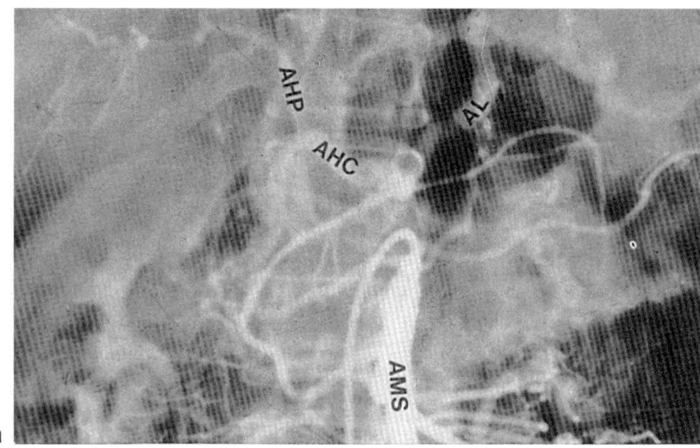

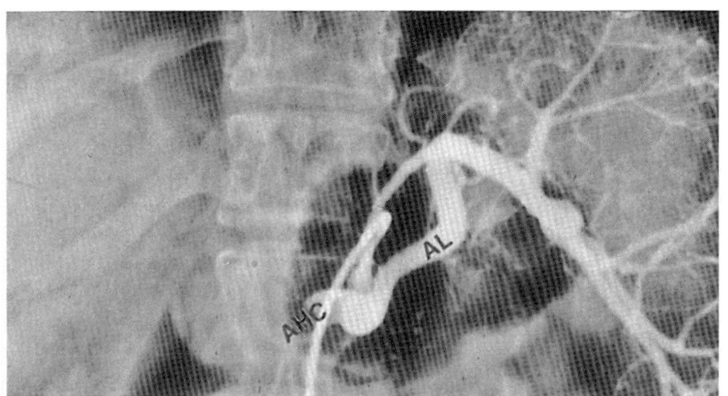

Fig. 4.9.12   Steal effect
a SMA injection. Steal to the common hepatic artery (AHC) and the splenic artery (AL). AHP = proper hepatic artery
b Celiac axis injection. Only the proximal part of the common hepatic artery (AHC) is visualized. AL = splenic artery

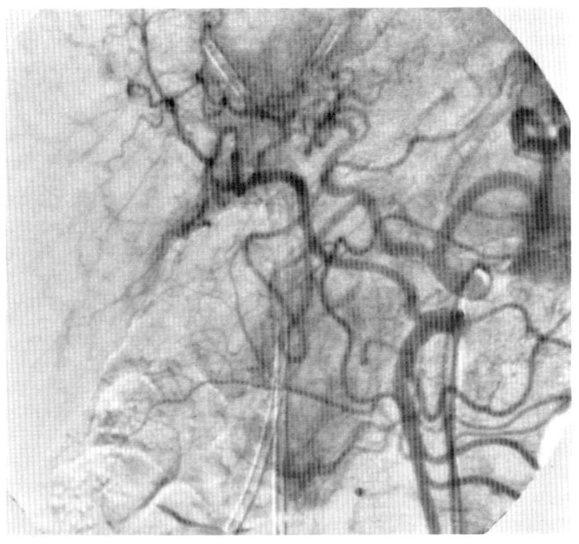

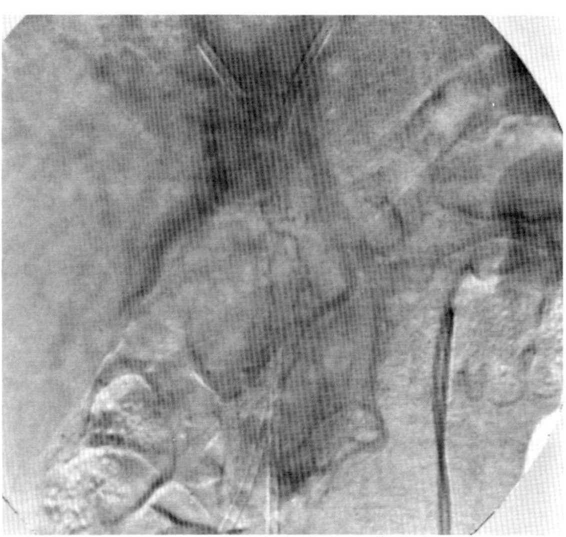

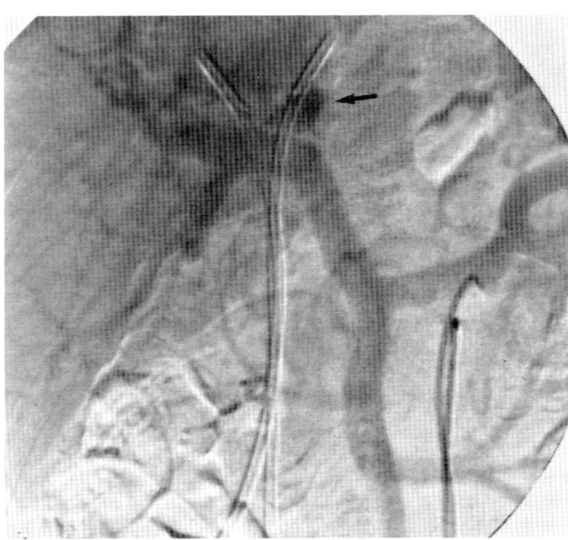

Fig. 4.9.13   Klatskin tumor
DSA:
a Selective arteriography of the celiac trunk and superior mesenteric artery shows extensive encasement of the left and right hepatic arteries in the arterial phase
b tumor "blush" in the late arterial – early venous phase
c Simultaneous injection of contrast medium into the celiac trunk and superior mesenteric artery via a Y-connector shows obstruction of the left portal vein (arrow)

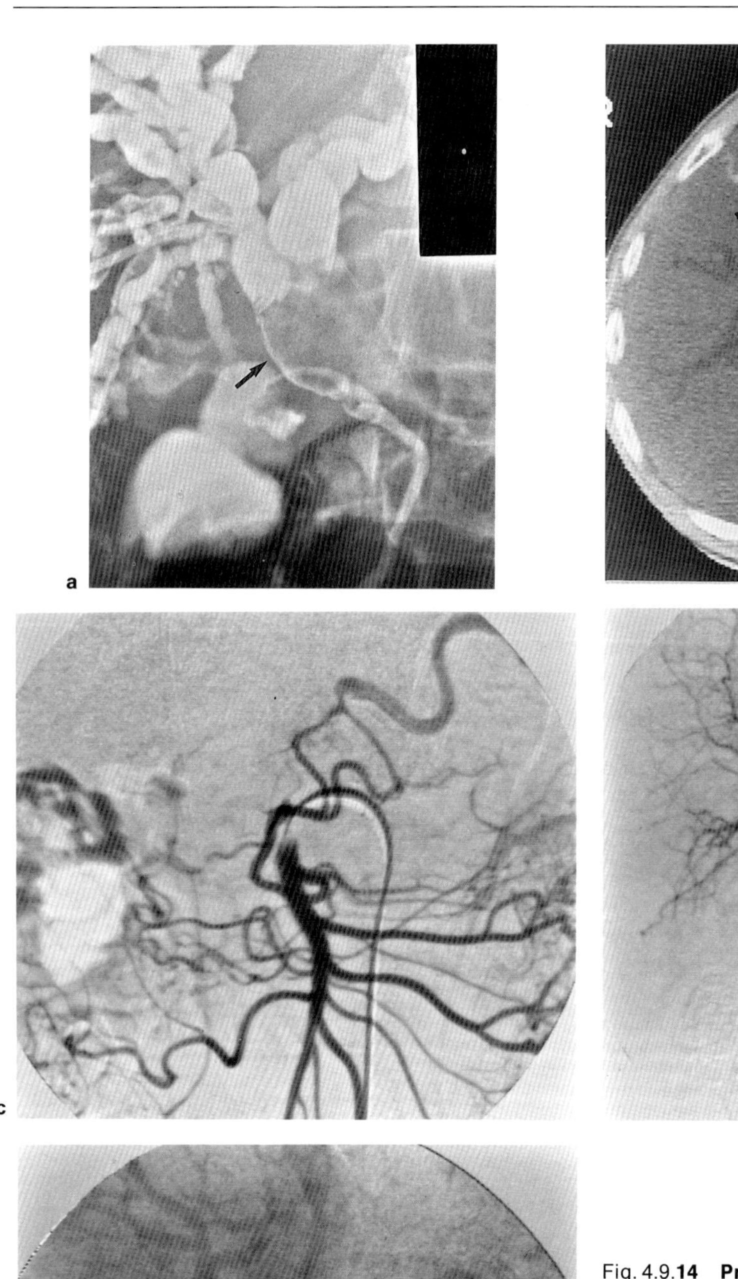
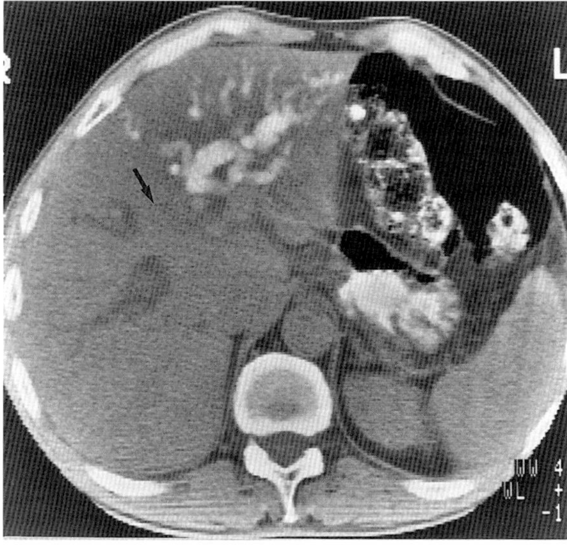
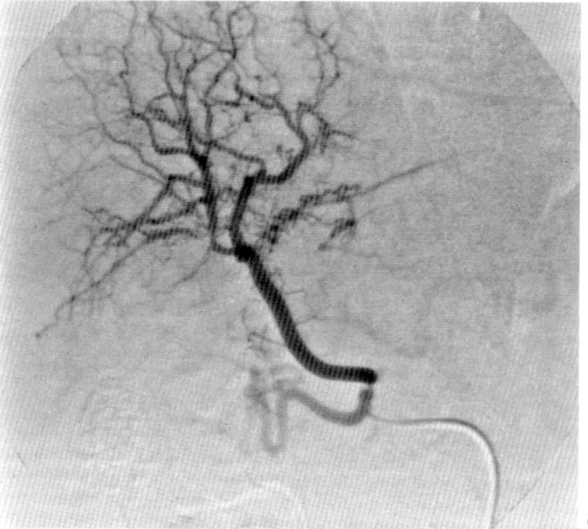
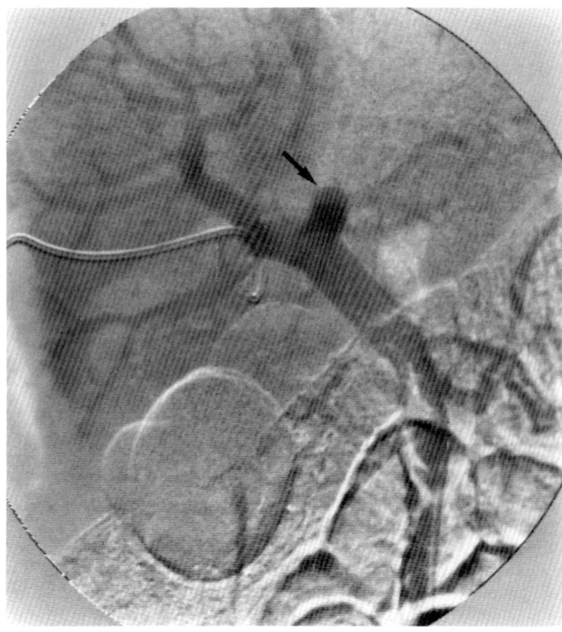

Fig. 4.9.**14** **Primary cholangiocarcinoma** with extensive tumor infiltration into the bifurcation

a ERCP: A mass at the proximal common bile duct (arrow), causing dilation of both intrahepatic biliary systems

b CT. An isodense tumor mass at the liver hilum, totally obstructing the left intrahepatic bile system (contrast stasis due to earlier ERCP). There is still adequate drainage of the right intrahepatic system

c DSA: Selective catheterization of the superior mesenteric artery shows filling of the celiac trunk via collateral circulation of the gastroduodenal artery

d DSA: Selective catheterization of a branch of the superior mesenteric artery shows extensive encasement of the right hepatic artery, originating from the superior mesenteric artery, due to tumor growth

e DSA: Late-phase arteriography via selective catheterization of the SMA shows, however, normal venous flow in the superior mesenteric vein, and right and left (arrow) portal system.

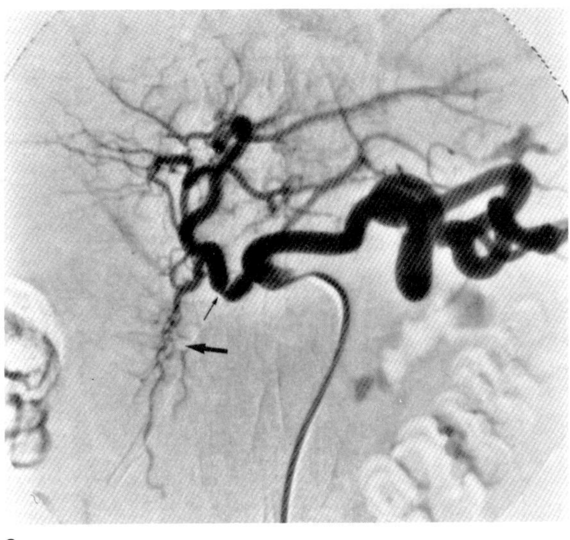

a

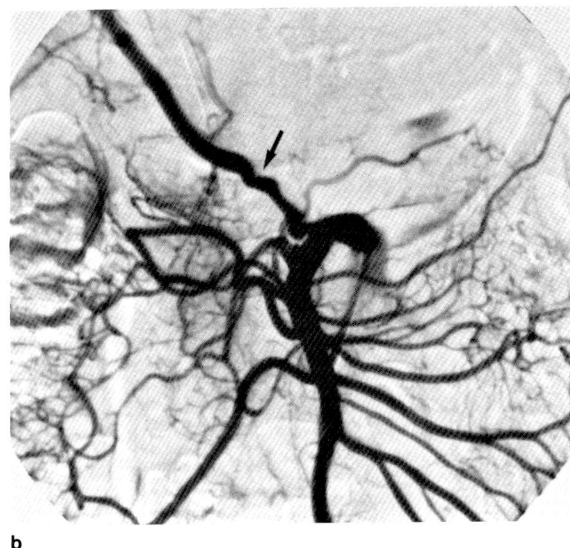

b

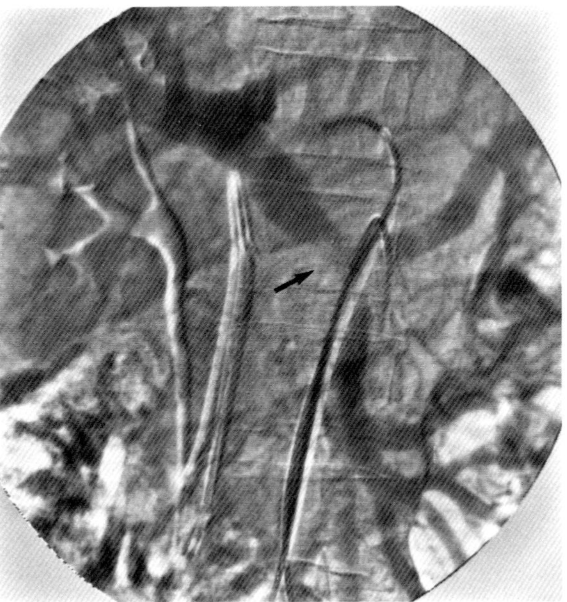

c

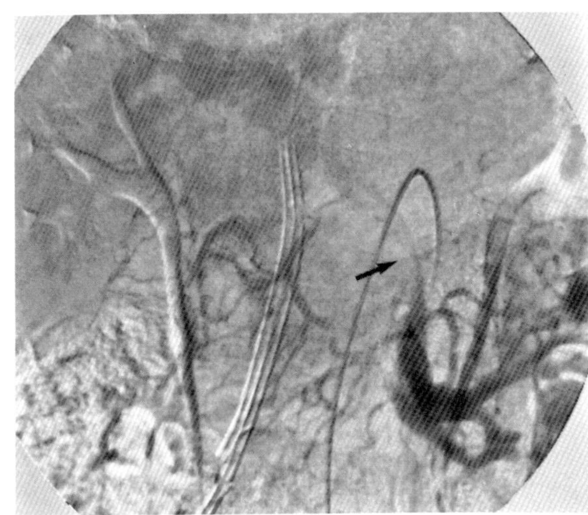

d

Fig. 4.9.**15 Pancreatic carcinoma**
DSA:
a Selective arteriography of the celiac trunk. Encasement of the gastroduodenal artery (arrow)
b Selective arteriography of the superior mesenteric artery. Slight encasement of the right hepatic artery, originating from the superior mesenteric artery (arrow)

c/d Late-phase arteriography (selective arteriography of the celiac trunk and superior mesenteric artery). Simultaneous injection via a Y-connector into both systems shows encasement and compression of the confluence of the splenic vein and superior mesenteric vein
Note multiple collaterals due to impaired venous flow (d) in the very late venous phase.

injection as well-filled, clearly defined vessels. If a part of this venous system does not opacify well, pathology due to compression is to be expected. As can be seen in ultrasound, the veins can easily be occluded by local compression. To avoid misdiagnosis, compression of the upper abdomen, as sometimes used routinely in DSA of the abdomen, should for this reason not be used in these patients.

Encasement of arteries can be observed during injections into the splenic and superior mesenteric arteries; encasement of veins can be seen during the venous phase of these injections. Tumors of the head and body of the pancreas will encase the hepatic superior mesenteric arteries and the gastroduodenal artery (Figs. 4.9.**15**, 4.9.**16**). Encasement of the superior mesenteric vein may proceed into

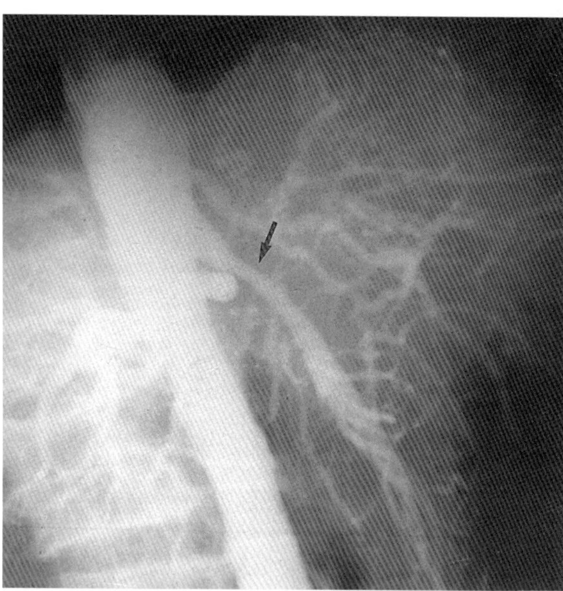

Fig. 4.9.**16** **Carcinoma of the head of the pancreas.** Encasement of the superior mesenteric artery (arrow), shown on a lateral aortogram

the portal vein (Suzuki et al. 1981). A tumor with encasement or thrombosis at this location is often unresectable (Fig. 4.9.**15**). If the tumor is located in the pancreatic body or tail, or both, pathology will be seen in the splenic artery and vein (Fig. 4.9.**6**). As many surgeons perform resections of this part of the pancreas together with a splenectomy, local encasement of the splenic artery or vein does not necessarily mean that the patient cannot be operated on for technical reasons.

Owing to their thinner walls, veins are affected more readily than arteries. The fact should also be borne in mind that the splenic artery shows more atherosclerotic changes compared to the hepatic arteries. The venous phase can be helpful in these cases, as a patent splenic vein in relation to an irregular splenic artery is most likely attributable to atherosclerosis. Visualization of smaller intrapancreatic arteries and veins is not necessary for the purposes of surgical resection.

References

Flannigan BD, et al. Intra-arterial digital subtraction angiography: comparison with conventional arteriography. Radiology 1983; 148: 17–21.

Freeny PC. Angiography of hepatic neoplasms. Semin Roentgenol 1983; 18: 114–122.

Friedman AC et al. Angiography of pancreatic neoplasms. In: Friedman AC, Radiology of the liver, biliary tract, pancreas and spleen. Baltimore: Williams and Wilkins, 1987: 814–835.

Hoevels J, et al. Intraarterielle DSA versus konventionelle Angiographie zur Resektabilitätsbeurteilung des Pankreas- und periampullären Karzinoms. RöFo 1987; 146: 291–294.

Jahn SZ et al. Comparison of CT and angiography in assessing resectability of pancreatic carcinoma. AJR 1984; 142: 525–529.

Lunderquist A. Angiography in carcinoma of the pancreas. Acta Radiol (Stockh) 1965; 235 (suppl).

Lunderquist A. Arterial segmental supply of the liver. Acta Radiol (Stockh) 1967; 272 (suppl).

Mukai JK, et al. Imaging of surgically relevant hepatic vascular and segmental anatomy, part 1. AJR 1987a; 149: 287–292.

Mukai JK, et al. Imaging of surgically relevant hepatic vascular and segmental anatomy, part 2. AJR 1987b; 149: 293–297.

Okuda K, et al. Demonstration of growing casts of hepatocellular carcinoma in the portal vein by celiac angiography: the thread and streaks sign. Radiology 1975; 117: 303–309.

Schuur KH. Angiografie bij levercirrose. Thesis, Groningen 1983.

Suzuki T, et al. Manifestations of carcinoma of the uncinate process by means of superior mesenteric arteriography. Surg Gynecol Obstet 1981; 152: 163–170.

Takashima T, Matsui O. Infusion hepatic angiography in the detection of small hepatocellular carcinomas. Radiology 1980; 136: 321–325.

4.10 Nuclear Medicine in Biliary and Pancreatic Malignancies

E.A. van Royen

Introduction

The development of ultrasonography (US), computed tomography (CT) and nuclear magnetic resonance imaging (MRI), has changed the indications for nuclear medicine as a diagnostic tool for the evaluation of malignant tumors. However, nuclear medicine maintains its unique ability to visualize the function and metabolism of living tissues in health and disease by the application of radiolabeled biochemical substances. No other technique is currently available which can do this at the same level of sensitivity and safety without interfering with normal function (Paans et al. 1985).

Monoclonal Antibodies: Diagnostic and Therapeutic Management

The development of the technique of preparing highly specific monoclonal antibodies against a wide variety of antigens is of special interest for nuclear medicine. Since most monoclonal antibodies can be labeled by radionuclides suitable for external imaging by the gamma camera without loss of specificity, quite a lot of studies have been initiated into "immunoscintigraphy" in oncology.

This concept is based on the existence of tumor-specific antigens not shared with normal cells. The use of polyclonal radiolabeled antibodies against carcinoembryonic antigen (CEA) was proposed some years ago as a technique for the detection of gastro-intestinal cancer (Goldenberg et al. 1978). Other antigens have also been tried, but scanning by these antibodies generally turned out to lack sufficient sensitivity and specificity for useful clinical applications (Mack et al. 1980). Monoclonal antibodies are of potentially greater value due to their higher purity and specificity. However, the same restraints underlie the basic concept: the tumor antigen must be specific, present outside the cell membrane, and accessible via the peripheral blood circulation. Moreover, labeling of the antibody by radionuclides such as technetium 99, iodine 123 or 131, or indium 111 should not affect its binding to the antigen. Cross-reactivity with normal tissue and residence time within the blood circulation should be minimal in order to obtain sufficient contrast between target and background.

The localization of tumors by immunoscintigraphy employing monoclonal antibodies has now been reported for colorectal cancer (Smedley et al. 1983), breast cancer (Rainsbury et al. 1983), malignant melanoma (Larson et al. 1983), ovarian cancer (Epenetos et al. 1982), and cutaneous malignant lymphoma (Carrasquillo et al. 1986). Of special interest is the development of monoclonal antibodies against the carbohydrate antigen 19-9 (CA 19-9) in pancreatic cancer.

No nuclear medicine procedures exist today which have been proved to be useful in the clinical investigation of pancreatic malignancy. Scintigraphy with selenium 75 methionine is obsolete due to the development of ultrasound, X-ray computed tomography and endoscopic retrograde cannulation of the pancreatic duct.

In pancreas transplantation, the viability of blood flow through the graft may be assessed by ^{99}Tc-labeled hexamethylpropyleneamine (^{99}TcHMPAO), a newly-developed lipophilic blood flow tracer, as shown by Teule et al. (1987). Recently, a monoclonal antibody has been developed against the carbohydrate antigen 19-9 (CA 19-9). This antigen, which has been identified as a sialytated lacto-N fucopentoase II, an oligosaccharide related to the Lewis blood group antigen, has been proposed as a sensitive serum tumor marker in pancreatic cancer (Haglund et al. 1986 b, Steinberg et al. 1986). Although the antibody was obtained from mice immunized with a human colorectal cancer cell line, and initially developed to detect colorectal adenocarcinoma, the highest levels of CA 19-9 are found in pancreatic adenocarcinoma. But adenocarcinoma of the stomach, hepatobiliary tree and colon will also evoke this tumor marker. The immunohistochemistry of pancreatic tumors has demonstrated that the CA 19-9 antigen is predominantly found in the apical border of cells lining the lumina of malignant glands, and in the mucus inside the lumina. Poorly differentiated adenocarcinomas showed less uptake of CA 19-9 antibody, while in anaplastic carcinoma, almost no staining was found (Haglund et al. 1986 a). Radiolabeled CA 19-9 antibody is available, and gamma camera studies to visualize gastro-intestinal tumors externally have been performed (Bares et al. 1987), but data as to the utility of this procedure in pancreatic cancer are lacking.

We performed a pilot study on the feasibility of external gamma-camera imaging of tumors of the pancreas and choledochal ducts with ^{131}I-labeled monoclonal CA 19-9 antibody. Uptake was demonstrable by the gamma camera in only one out of nine patients, in a Klatskin tumor prior to surgery (Fig. 4.10.1). In general, target to non-target activity ratios were too low for external imaging. Since studies were performed 2–3 days before surgery, tissue specimens could also be studied by gamma

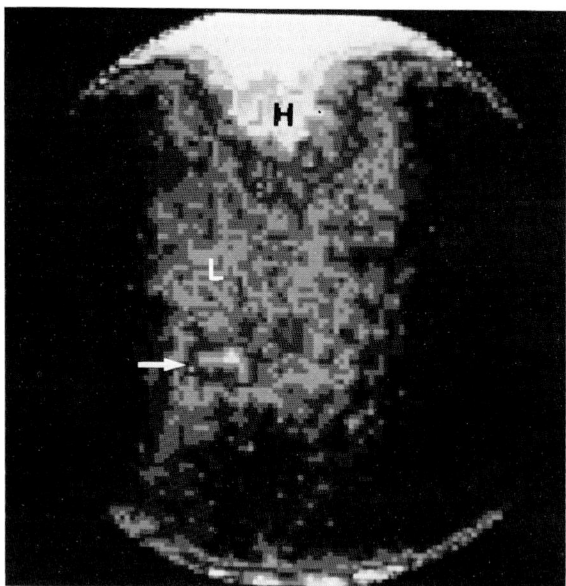

Fig. 4.10.**1   Uptake of** [131]**I-labeled monoclonal CA 19-9 antibody in a Klatskin tumor** (arrow). Other structures seen are the heart (H) and liver (L)

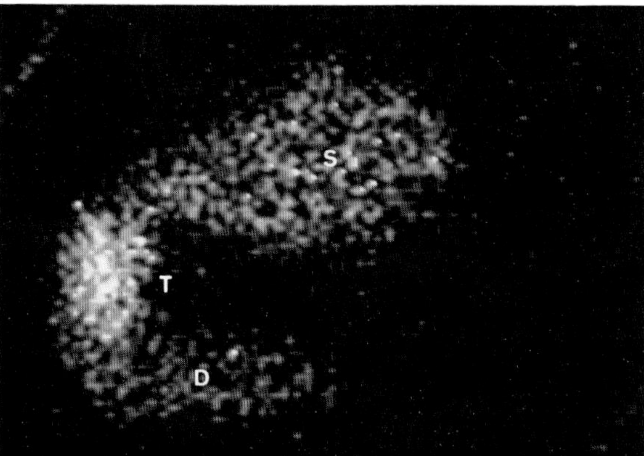

Fig. 4.10.**2   Uptake of** [131]**I-labeled monoclonal CA 19-9 antibody in pancreatic cancer.** Antibody was injected 2 days before surgery. The surgical specimen was imaged on a gamma camera showing slight uptake in the stomach (S) and duodenum (D), and high uptake in the tumor area (T)

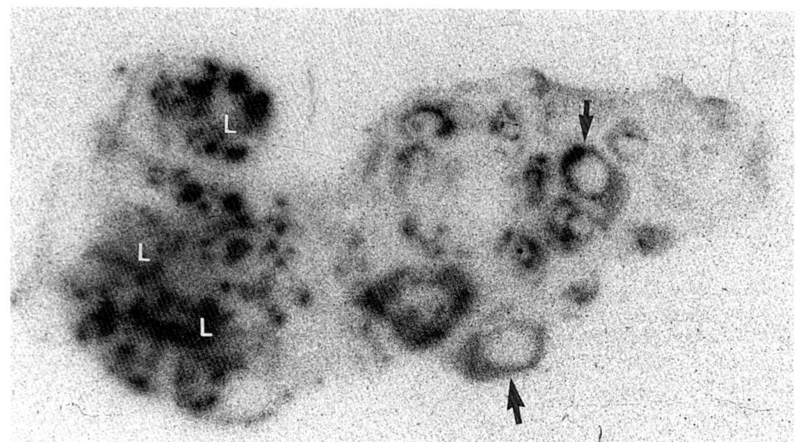

a

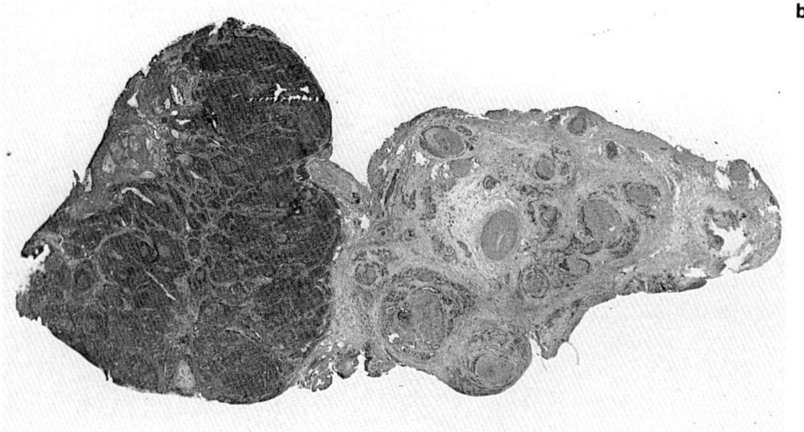

b

Fig. 4.10.**3**
a   Autoradiography of a surgical specimen of pancreatic cancer. ^{131}I-labeled CA 19-9 antibody was injected 2 days before surgery. Autoradiography shows antibody uptake in a lymph node (L) and circular uptake around nerves (arrow), representing tumor infiltration of the perineurium
b   Hematoxylin eosin staining of the same preparation

camera, autoradiography and gamma counting. In all 5 patients suffering from adenocarcinoma of the head of the pancreas, the surgical specimen obtained during a Whipple procedure clearly demonstrated increased uptake in the tumor area (Fig. 4.10.2). Autoradiography also showed increased uptake in tumor cells (Fig. 4.10.3).

Nuclear Medicine Therapy

If a radiolabeled agent is specifically taken up by a tumor, it may be used not only for diagnostic but also for therapeutic purposes. Particularly if α- or β-particle-emitting radionuclides are employed which deliver most of their radiation energy to tissues within the millimeter to centimeter range, extremely high local doses may be administered with little or no systemic effect. The classical example is ^{131}I therapy in thyroid carcinoma; the administration of 30 mCi may result in doses ranging from 50000 to 250000 rads, depending on the uptake in the target tissue. These doses cannot be achieved by external radiotherapy.

Liver metastases are rare in thyroid cancer. Of greater interest here is the therapy of metastatic carcinoid and malignant pheochromocytoma, which often spreads to the liver, using ^{131}I metaiodobenzylguanidine (^{131}IMIBG). ^{131}IMIBG is an analogue of a biogene amine precursor which accumulates in the neurosecretory storage granules of the chromaffin cells. Apart from scintigraphic localization of pheochromocytoma, radionuclide therapy of liver metastases of malignant pheochromocytoma was reported by Sisson et al. (1984). Liver metastases of carcinoid may also be treated palliatively by ^{131}IMIBG, since this tumor arises from enterochromaffin cells (Hoefnagel et al. 1987). Figure 4.10.4 shows the uptake of ^{131}IMIBG in liver metastases of carcinoid. After treatment with a single 200 mCi dose, which had little or no side effects, good palliation was obtained with a sub-

stantial decrease of flushes, diarrhea and pain. In patients suffering from liver metastases receiving regional chemotherapy, the perfusion pattern may be monitored by the injection of ^{99}Tc-labeled microspheres via the arterial catheter. Proper placement of the arterial catheter can be checked to obtain optimal flow distribution. Aberrant hepatic arterial anatomy resulting in incomplete perfusion is quite often found (Yang et al. 1982).

References

Bares R, Fass J, Weiller G, Truong S, Beull U, Stirner H, Schumpelick V. Planar vs. SPECT radioimmunoscintigraphy: clinical experience with Tc-99m, In-111, and I-131 labelled monoclonal antibodies (MAB) against CEA and/or CA 19-9. Nucl Med 1987; 26 (abstract): 24.

Carrasquillo JA, Bunn PA, Keeman AM, Reydnolds JC, Schroff RW, Foon KA, et al. Radioimmuno detection of cutaneous T-cell lymphoma with III In-labeled T 101 monoclonal antibody. N Engl J Med 1986; 315: 673–680.

Epenetos AA, Mather S, Granowska M. Targeting of iodine-123 labelled monoclonal antibodies to ovary, breast and gastrointestinal tumours. Lancet 1982; ii: 999–1004.

Goldenberg DM, DeLand F, Kim E. Use of radiolabeled antibodies to carcinoembryonic antigen for the detection and localization of diverse cancers by external photoscanning. N Engl J Med 1978; 298: 1384–1388.

Haglund C, Lindgren J, Roberts PJ, Nordling S. Gastrointestinal cancer-associated antigen CA 19-9 in histological specimens of pancreatic tumours and pancreatitis. Br J Cancer 1986a; 53: 189–195.

Haglund C, Roberts PJ, Kuusela P, Scheinin TM, Makela O, Jalanko H. Evaluation of CA 19-9 as a serum tumour marker in pancreatic cancer. Br J Cancer 1986b; 53: 197–202.

Hoefnagel CA, den Hartog Jager FCA, Taal BG, Abeling NGGM, Engelsman EE. The role of I-131-MIBG in the diagnosis and therapy of carcinoids. Eur J Nucl Med 1987; 13: 187–191.

Larson S, Brown JP, Wright PW, Carrasquillo JA, Hellstrom I, Hellstrom KE. Imaging of melanoma with I-131 labeled monoclonal antibodies. J Nucl Med 1983; 24: 123–128.

Mack JP, Carrel S, Formi M, Ritschard J, Donath A, Alberto P. Tumour localization of radiolabeled antibodies against carcinoembryonic antigen in patients with carcinoma: a critical evaluation. N Engl J Med 1980; 303: 5–10.

Paans AMJ, Vaalburg W, Woldring MG. A comparison of the sensitivity of PET and NMR for in vivo quantitative metabolic imaging. Eur J Nucl Med 1985; 11: 73–75.

Rainsbury RM, Ott RJ, Westwood JH. Localisation of metastatic breast carcinoma by a monoclonal antibody chelate labelled with Indium-111. Lancet 1983; ii: 934–938.

Sisson JC, Shapiro B, Beierwaltes WH, Glowniak JV, Nakajo M, Magner TJ, et al. Radiopharmaceutical treatment of malignant pheochromocytoma. J Nucl Med 1984; 25: 197–206.

Smedley HM, Finan P, Lennox ES. Localisation of metastatic carcinoma by a radiolabeled monoclonal antibody. Br J Cancer 1983; 47: 253–259.

Steinberg WM, Gelfland R, Anderson KK, Glenn J, Kurtziman SH, Sindelar WF, Toskes PP. Comparison of the sensitivity and specificity of the CA 19-9 and carcinoembryonic antigen assays in detecting cancer of the pancreas. Gastroenterology 1986; 90: 343–349.

Teule GJJ, Leunissen K, van der Linden ES, van Hooff J, Kootstra G, Heidendal GAK. Quantitative assessment of graft perfusion in combined kidney and pancreas-spleen transplantation: a potential application of Tc HMPAO. Nucl Med 1987; 26, P 220 (abstract).

Yang PJ, Thrall JH, Ensminger WD, Niederhuber JE, Gyves JW, Tuseau M, et al. Perfusion scintigraphy (Tc-99m MAA) during surgery for placement of chemotherapy catheter in hepatic cancer: concise communication. J Nucl Med 1982; 23: 1066–1069.

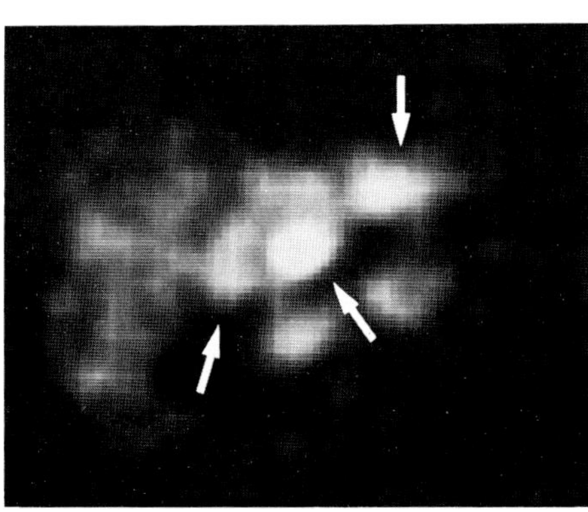

Fig. 4.10.4 ^{131}I metaiodobenzylguanidine uptake in liver metastases of carcinoid (arrows)

4.11 Scintigraphic Studies in the Diagnostic Differentiation of Primary and Secondary Liver Tumors

R. Montz and H.-W. Müller-Gärtner

Abbreviations

FNH	Focal nodular hyperplasia
HA	Hemangioma
HCC	Hepatocellular carcinoma
IDA	Iminodiacetic acid derivatives
RES	Reticuloendothelial system
RMAB	Radiolabeled monoclonal antibodies
SPET	Single-photon emission tomography

Numerous radiopharmaceuticals have been employed in the scintigraphic detection and diagnostic differentiation of liver tumors. The underlying aim is to differentiate these tumors in vivo on the basis of their different functional characteristics. ^{99m}Tc-labeled colloids, for example, are able to image the reticuloendothelial system (RES) of the liver, viz. the function of Kupffer cells. ^{99m}Tc-labeled iminodiacetic acid derivatives (IDA) provide succeessful visualization of the hepatobiliary system. ^{99m}Tc-labeled red blood cells image the blood pool, and gallium-67 accumulates in various malignant and benign tumors, possibly by binding a ^{67}Ga-transferrin complex to transferrin receptors. The recent introduction of radiolabeled monoclonal antibodies (RMAB) has broadened the spectrum of in vivo diagnosis in liver pathology. However, a single tracer with 100% sensitivity or specificity for any of the various liver tumors is at present not available.

The numerous reports in the literature on scintigraphic results in liver tumors are frequently unsuitable for comparison, due to methodological differences. The use of a variety of radiotracers and differing techniques, each applied to a restricted number of patients, makes definitive statements on the clinical validity of these procedures difficult. The present article reviews the state of the art in

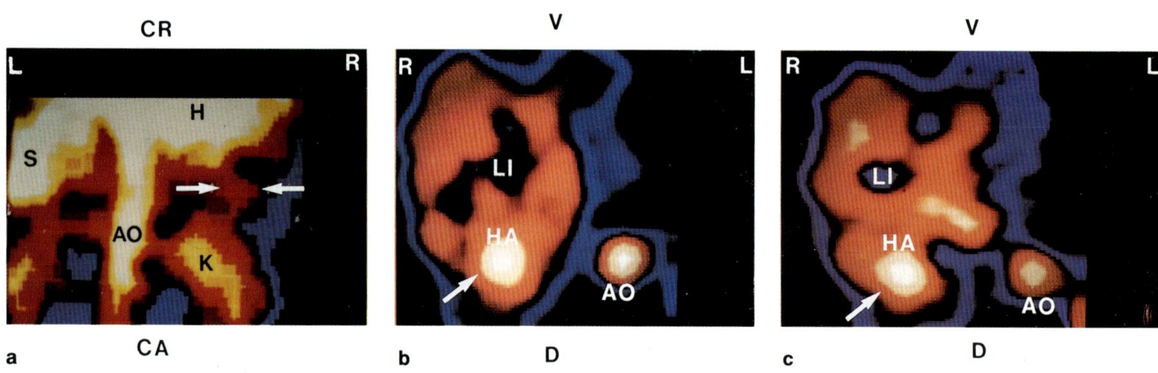

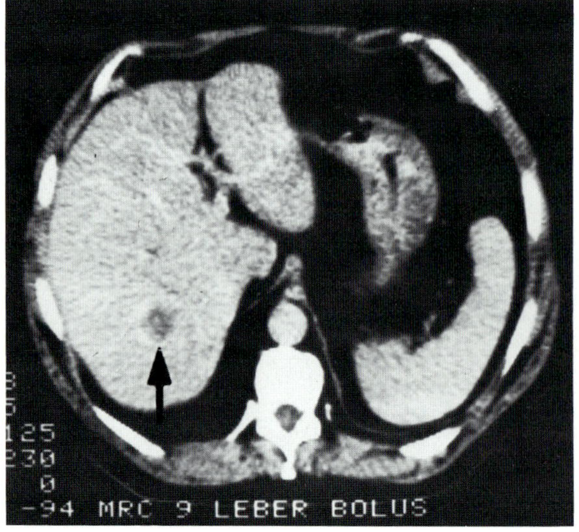

d

Fig. 4.11.1 ^{99m}**Tc-labeled red blood cell scintigraphy and computed tomography of a cavernous hemangioma**

a Planar scintigraphy from posterior: perfusion scintigraphy, 40–50 s post-injection. Normal perfusion of the hemangioma (arrows) compared with the surrounding normal liver tissue. S = spleen; AO = aorta; H = heart; K = kidney;   R = right;   L = left;   CR = cranial; CA = caudal

b, c Transverse section of single-photon emission tomography: acquisition time, 15-20 min (**b**) and 120–130 min (**c**) post-injection. The blood pool of the hemangioma (HA) is significantly increased when compared with the surrounding normal liver tissue (LI). Normal perfusion with increased blood pool is referred to as inflow/blood pool mismatch. AO = aorta; R = right; L = left; V = ventral; D = dorsal

d Computed tomography: transverse section of the liver corresponding to the anatomical level of **b** and **c**. The diameter of the hemangioma (arrow) is 1.2 cm. (Courtesy of Prof. Dr. E. Bücheler, Department of Radiology, University of Hamburg, Federal Republic of Germany)

liver scintigraphy, and points to open questions in this challenging field of clinical science.

Characteristic Results

Cavernous hemangiomas, the most frequent benign liver tumors (prevalence in autopsies up to 7%), show reduced or normal perfusion in comparison with the surrounding liver tissue scintigraphically, but reveal an increased blood pool on delayed scans (Fig. 4.11.**1**). This constellation will be referred to as inflow/blood pool mismatch in this context.

Focal nodular hyperplasias (FNHs) of the liver, and regenerative nodules in cirrhotic livers, show hyperperfusion in the arterial phase, IDA uptake and retention, and colloid accumulation by Kupffer cells, being part of the RES (Fig. 4.11.**2**).

Hepatocellular adenomas show faint perfusion, no colloid phagocytosis, but some uptake and marked retention of IDA.

Hepatocellular carcinomas (HCCs) reveal hyperperfusion in the arterial phase, some IDA uptake, absence of colloid uptake, accumulation of gallium-67 and or RMAB against alphafetoprotein, and sometimes accumulation of bone-seeking agents.

Liver metastases are presented as cold areas in scintigrams of the hepatobiliary system, liver RES and blood pool (Fig. 4.11.**3**). They accumulate RMAB directed against antigens in cases where tumor cells elicit antigen expression (Fig. 4.11.**4**).

Exceptions

Hemangiomas

Cavernous hemangiomas and capillary hemangiomas or hemangioendotheliomas in children, despite a diameter equal to or exceeding 2 cm for planar imaging and 1 cm for single-photon emission tomography (SPET), have been reported as escaping detection by late blood pool scintigraphy in 8 out of 154 investigated patients, corresponding to a false-negative rate of 5% (Brecht-Krauss et al.

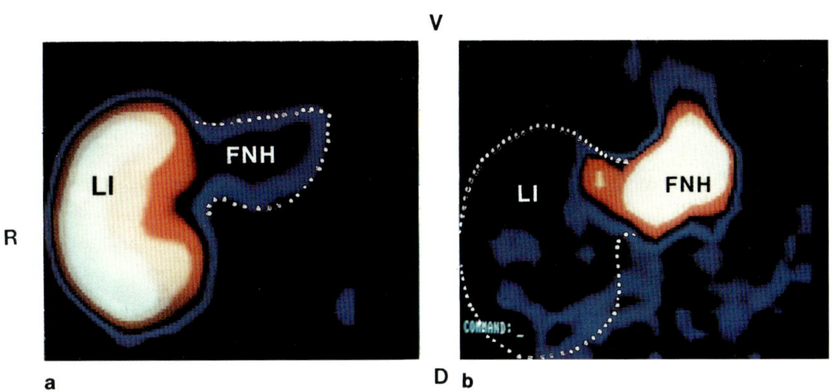

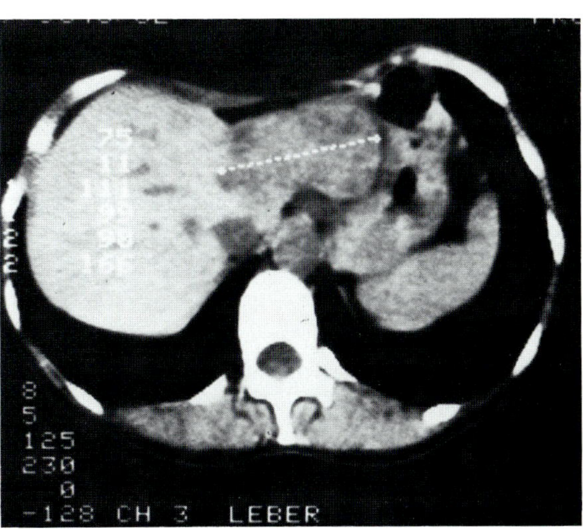

Fig. 4.11.2   Multitracer scintigraphy and computed tomography in focal nodular hyperplasia

a, b Single-photon emission tomography, transverse sections. The focal nodular hyperplasia (FNH) exhibits weak phagocytic activity of the reticuloendothelial system (**a**, ^{99m}Tc colloid) and significantly increased IDA retention (**b**) compared with normal liver tissue (LI). Arterial perfusion of FNH proved to be significantly increased (not shown). R = right; L = left; V = ventral; D = dorsal

c Computed tomography: transverse section of the liver corresponding to the anatomical level of **a** and **b**. The focal nodular hyperplasia is indicated by a broken line. (Courtesy of Prof. Dr. E. Bücheler, Department of Radiology, University of Hamburg, Federal Republic of Germany)

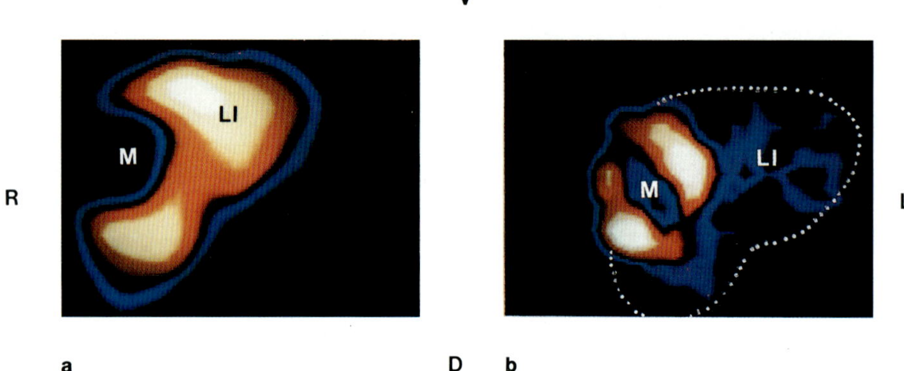

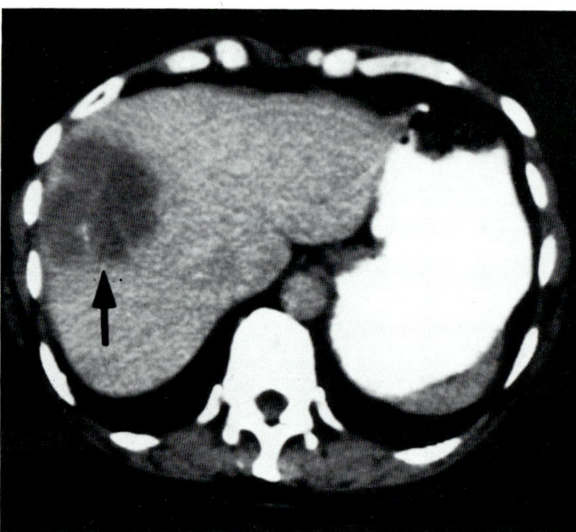

Fig. 4.11.3 Multitracer scintigraphy (single-photon emission tomography) and computed tomography in a liver metastasis. R = right; L = left; V = ventral; D = dorsal
a Transverse section. Absence of phagocytic activity, e.g. absence of the reticuloendothelial system (^{99m}Tc colloid) in the metastasis (M) of a colon carcinoma, but regular and homogeneous function of the reticuloendothelial system in normal liver tissue (LI)
b Transverse section. Absence of iminodiacetic acid (IDA) uptake *within* the metastasis (M) but IDA retention in the normal liver tissue *adjacent* to the metastasis ("rim sign")
c Computed tomography: transverse section of the liver corresponding to the anatomical level of **a** and **b**. The metastasis is indicated by the arrow. (Courtesy of Prof. Dr. E. Bücheler, Department of Radiology, University of Hamburg, Federal Republic of Germany)

1986, Brodsky et al. 1987, Engel et al. 1983, Front et al. 1984, Miller 1987, Moinuddin et al. 1985, Rabinowitz et al. 1984). This can possibly be explained through advanced fibrosis.

In six out of the above mentioned 154 patients, HAs have been reported to be hyperperfused. But this does not appear to apply to the arterial phase of perfusion, and this is likely to be a distinctive feature of HA in contrast to FNH or HCC. The latter may also show increased blood pool and hyperperfusion (no inflow/blood pool mismatch), but this is – in contrast to HA – due to an increased perfusion in the arterial phase on the basis of dilated hepatic arteries (Miller 1987, Rabinowitz et al. 1984).

In this context, hypervascularized liver metastases should also be taken into consideration, but they have not yet been investigated in a sufficient number of cases. However, an inflow/blood pool mismatch is unlikely to be demonstrable in these metastases.

Focal Nodular Hyperplasias

In 8 out of 76 investigated cases, FNH did not show hyperfusion (Heintz et al. 1986, Schild et al. 1987). Colloid uptake was absent in 13.6 % of 169 investigated FNHs (Schild et al. 1987). Hepatobiliary activity of FNHs was not detected in 4 out of 36 patients (Schild et al. 1987); "trapping" or retention of IDA was not observed in 4 out of 66 patients (Heintz et al. 1986, Schild et al. 1987).

Hepatocellular Adenomas

Previous reports on the absence of Kupffer cells in adenomas now appear to be inconsistent. Hepatocellular adenomas contain Kupffer cells (Lubbers et al. 1987). However, only 3 out of 13 such tumors accumulated radiocolloid (Lubbers et al. 1987). The lack of colloid uptake in the remaining cases may possibly be due to hypoperfusion.

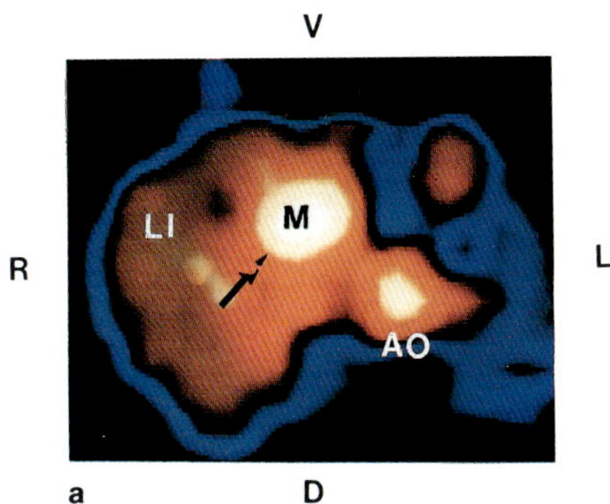

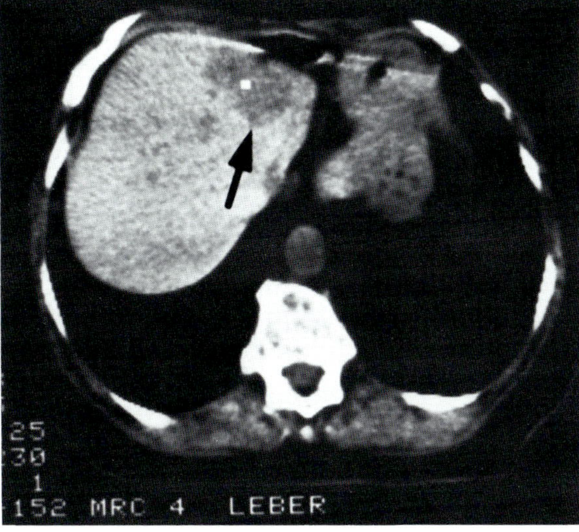

b

Fig. 4.11.4 Scintigraphy with radiolabeled monoclonal carcinoembryonic antigen (CEA) antibodies and computed tomography: hepatic metastasis of a colon carcinoma

a Single-photon emission tomography. The liver metastasis (M) clearly shows enhanced CEA antibody binding (24 h after intravenous injection) when compared with the surrounding normal liver tissue (LI). AO = aorta; R = right; L = left; V = ventral; D = dorsal. Phagocytic activity in the reticuloendothelial system was absent in this metastasis, as revealed by ^{99m}Tc colloid scintigraphy (not shown)

b Computed tomography: transverse section of the liver corresponding to the anatomical level of **a**. The metastasis is indicated by an arrow. (Courtesy of Prof. Dr. E. Bücheler, Department of Radiology, University of Hamburg, Federal Republic of Germany)

Hepatocellular Carcinomas

The scintigraphic patterns of HCC appear to be rather variable. Only hyperperfusion in the arterial phase can be regarded as a common characteristic of HCC, but this is not a specific sign at all. In addition, about 90% of HCCs show uptake of gallium-67 equal to or higher than normal liver tissue. However, regenerative liver nodules, FNHs and hepatocellular adenomas, some liver metastases, lymphomas and abscesses have similarly high levels of gallium-67 uptake (Cornelius and Atterbury 1984). Imaging of alphafetoprotein-excreting HCCs has been made possible through immunoscintigraphy with RMAB, but non-specific accumulation in normal liver also occurs. Occasionally, accumulation of bone-seeking radiopharmaceuticals has been observed in HCCs, but this also applies to liver metastases, cholangiosarcomas and cavernous HAs (Burkhalter et al. 1986).

Liver metastases

Breast cancer metastases to the liver were observed to take up ^{99m}Tc-IDA on the basis of planar scintigraphy in 3 patients (Hasegawa et al. 1986, Vincent and Renner 1984). However, it should be noted that such findings with planar scintigraphy may be due to segmental bile duct obstruction or dilation (Hasegawa et al. 1986) as well as to perifocal IDA retention (Fig. 4.11.**3**), described as "rim-sign" (Hasegawa et al. 1986, Remedios et al. 1986, Savitch et al. 1983).

Multitracer Scintigraphy

The aim of non-invasive differentiation of liver lesions, especially solitary ones, is to select those tumors requiring surgical intervention from benign tumors which do not. The former are hepatocellular carcinomas, adenomas and solitary metastases, the latter are hemangiomas and focal nodular hyperplasias, as well as regenerative nodules in cirrhotic livers. Diagnostic procedures which claim to be able to rule out malignancy must reveal unequivocal results. High specificity must therefore be aimed for. However, none of the morphological or functional in vivo imaging methods such as ultrasound, computed tomography, magnetic resonance or liver scintigraphy fulfils this requirement. Scintigraphic procedures using several tracers may certainly improve diagnostic reliability. Several proposals have been made.

Perfusion imaging by sequential scintigraphy following bolus injection of a radiopharmaceutical is generally considered to be mandatory, and usually represents the first step in all liver studies. Lee and Shapiro (1983) proposed the combination of ^{99m}Tc-labeled sulfur colloid, ^{99m}Tc-labeled IDA and gallium-67. An absence of sulfur colloid uptake in combination with gallium-67 avidity and hyperperfusion was considered to be indicative of HCC (Lee et al. 1985). Delayed hepatobiliary imaging may improve the specificity in diagnosing HCC, because 26 out of 49 HCCs were found to retain activity (Hasegawa et al. 1986).

Much greater difficulty is involved in the goal of ruling out malignancy. Creutzig et al. (1984b) reported on the combined application of delayed blood pool and hepatobiliary scintigraphy, with additional perfusion imaging. The differential indication for or against surgery was correctly achieved in 79 out of 81 (Creutzig et al. 1984b) and 139 out of 147 patients (Heintz et al. 1986) respectively. Biersack et al. (1980) and Tanasescu et al. (1984) reported on the successful combination of perfusion, colloid and IDA scintigraphy in the diagnosis of FNH.

Our own experience is still confined to a limited number of patients in a prospective study. We are making use of perfusion imaging in combination with early (5–20 min after injection) and late (2 h) tomography of the blood pool or IDA, or both, followed by SPET of the RES. If judged necessary, complementary investigations such as immuno-SPET are performed in addition. The differentiation between HA, FNH, HCC and liver metastasis was correct in 26 out of 30 investigated patients, as verified by surgery. In 3 patients the scintigraphic diagnosis was inconclusive. In one patient, the "rim-sign" in the adjacent normal liver tissue of a liver metastasis (Fig. 4.11.3) was erroneously taken to be indicative of HCC.

Conclusions

The wide spectrum of radiopharmaceuticals for scintigraphic studies of liver lesions (Table 4.11.1) is an opportunity for medical science to establish reliable, non-invasive in vivo methods of differentiating between benign and malignant liver tumors.

As will now be obvious, SPET is essential, because its superiority over planar scintigraphy of the liver is well documented (Brodsky et al. 1987, Kudo et al. 1986). Some conflicting results, as reported from planar studies, may thus be avoided. Our recommendations for multitracer scintigraphy are summarized in Table 4.11.2.

In view of the many uncertainties resulting from past literature, prospective studies, ideally conducted in different centers, are now needed. Nevertheless, a review of the literature with special attention to the studies carried out by Creutzig et al. (1984a, 1984b) provides us with a reasonable degree of confidence that unequivocal scintigraphic

Table 4.11.1 Scintigraphic diagnostic procedures providing optimal differentiation between different focal liver diseases. This synopsis is based on currently available literature (characteristic results including frequency of exceptions). + + = good potential for differentiation, + = moderate potential for differentiation, (+) = questionable potential for differentiation

Differential diagnosis	Perfusion	Blood pool	IDA	Colloid	RMAB	Gallium-67
CHA/MET		+ +			+ +	+
CHA/FNH	+	+ +	+ +	+ +		
CHA/HAD		+ +	+			
CHA/HCC	(+)	(+)	(+)		+	+
MET/FNH	(+)		+ +	+ +	+ +	
MET/HAD			+ +			
MET/HCC			(+)		+	
FNH/HAD	+			(+)		
FNH/HCC			(+)	+	+	+
HAD/HCC	+					+

(For CHA/HCC, the Perfusion (+) and Blood pool (+) entries are linked by the annotation "mismatch + +".)

CHA = cavernous hemangioma, MET = liver metastasis, FNH = focal nodular hyperplasia, HAD = hepatocellular adenoma, HCC = hepatocellular carcinoma, IDA = iminodiacetic acid derivatives (hepatobiliary agents), RMAB = radiolabeled monoclonal antibodies

Table 4.11.2 Recommended scintigraphic diagnostic procedure for multitracer scintigraphy for the differentiation of solid liver tumors. Planar scintigraphy should be performed in the immediate vicinity of the lesion

Diagnosis	Perfusion	Blood pool 2 h p.i.		Hepatobiliary System 5–20 min 2 h p.i.		RES	RMAB
	PLSC	PLSC	SPET	SPET	SPET	SPET	SPET
Predominant suspicion							
Hemangioma	×	×	×			×	
Metastases	×					×	×
Focal nodular hyperplasia	×			×	×	×	
Hepatocellular carcinoma/ adenoma	×	×	×	×	×	×	(×)

RES = reticuloendothelial system, RMAB = radiolabeled monoclonal antibodies specific for the suspected primary tumor, PLSC = Planar scintigraphy, SPET = single photon emission tomography

Table 4.11.3 Characteristic results of multitracer scintigraphy for hemangioma, focal nodular hyperplasia, and liver metastases. Equal to (↔), more (↑), or less (↓) than normal liver activity; ○ = zero activity

Diagnosis	Perfusion	Blood pool 2 h p.i.		Hepatobiliary System 5–20 min p.i. 2 h p.i.		Phagocyt. RES	RMAB
	planar	planar	SPET	SPET	SPET	SPET	SPET
Hemangioma	↔↓	↑	↑	○	○	○	
Focal nodular hyperplasia	↑	↔↑	↔↑	↕↔	↑	↕↔	
Liver metastases	↕↔	↔↓	↔↓	○	○	○	↑

results revealing the characteristics of HA, FNH or immunoscintigraphically positive liver metastases (Table 4.11.3) are accurate. Otherwise scintigraphic in vivo diagnoses of liver tumors should be regarded with reservation. This is the scientific field in liver scintigraphy on which future research should be focussed.

References

Bergmann J-F, Lumbroso J-D, Manil L, Saccavini J-C, Rougier P, Assicot M, Mathieu A, Bellet D, Bohuon C. Radiolabelled monoclonal antibodies against alpha-fetoprotein for in vivo localization of human hepatocellular carcinoma by immunoscintigraphy. Eur J Nucl Med 1987; 13: 385–390.

Biersack HJ, Thelen M, Torres JF, Lackner K, Winkler CG. Focal nodular hyperplasia of the liver as established by 99m-Tc-sulfur colloid and HIDA scintigraphy. Radiology 1980; 137: 187–190.

Brecht-Krauss D, König K-P, Adam WE. Wertigkeit und Stellenwert der Blutpool-Szintigraphie bei Leberhämangiomen. Nuklearmedizin 1986; 25: 114–116.

Brodsky RI, Friedman AC, Maurer AH, Radecki PD, Caroline DF. Hepatic cavernous HA: diagnosis with 99m-Tc-labelled red cells and single-photon emission CT. AJR 1987; 148: 125–129.

Burkhalter JL, Morano JU, Patel BR. Accumulation of Technetium-99m MDP in a cavernous hemangioma of the liver. Clin Nucl Med 1986; 11: 498–500.

Cornelius EA, Atterbury CE. Problems in the imaging diagnosis of hepatoma. Clin Nucl Med 1984; 9: 30–38.

Creutzig H, Glatz KF, Müller S, Schober O, Brölsch C, Neuhaus P, Lang W. Classification of liver tumors by radionuclide imaging. J Nucl Med 1984a; 25: 402.

Creutzig H, Brölsch C, Glatz K, Neuhaus P, Müller S, Schober O, Lang W, Hundeshagen H, Pichlmayr R. Nuklearmedizinische Differentialdiagnostik intrahepatischer Raumforderungen. Dtsch Med Wochenschr 1984b; 109: 861–863.

Engel MA, Marks DS, Sandler MA, Shetty P. Differentiation of focal intrahepatic lesions with 99m-Tc red blood cell imaging. Radiology 1983; 146: 777–782.

Front D, Israel O, Groshar D, Weininger J. Technetium-99m-labelled red blood cell imaging. Semin Nucl Med 1984; 14: 226–250.

Hasegawa Y, Nakano S, Ibuka K, Hashizume T, Noguchi A, Sasaki Y, Imaoka S, Fujita M, Kawamoto S, Kasugai H, Tanaka S, Kojima J, Ishigami S. Specific diagnosis of hepatocellular carcinoma by delayed hepatobiliary imaging. Cancer 1986; 57: 230–236.

Heintz P, Glatz KF, Schwarzrock R, Schober O, Neuhaus P, Creutzig H. Szintigraphischer Nachweis eines metastasierenden hepatozellulären Karzinoms. RöFo 1986; 144: 111–113.

Kudo M, Hirasa M, Takakuwa H, Ibuki Y, Fujimi K, Miyamura M, Tomita S, Komori H, Todo A, Kitaura Y, Ikebuko K, Torizuka K. Small hepatocellular carcinomas in chronic liver disease: detection with SPECT. Radiology 1986; 159: 697–703.

Lee VW, Shapiro JH. Specific diagnosis of hepatoma using 99m-Tc-HIDA and other radionuclides. Eur J Nucl Med 1983; 8: 191–195.

Lee VW, O'Brien MJ, Morris PM, Devereux DF, Shapiro JH. The specific diagnosis of hepatocellular carcinoma by scintigraphy: multiple radiotracer approach. Cancer 1985; 56: 25–36.

Lubbers PR, Ros PR, Goodman ZD, Ishak KG. Accumulation of Technetium-99m sulfur colloid by hepatocellular adenoma: scintigraphic-pathologic correlation. AJR 1987; 148: 1105–1108.

Miller JH. Technetium-99m-labelled red blood cells in the evaluation of hemangiomas of the liver in infants and children. J Nucl Med 1987; 28: 1412–1418.

Moinuddin M, Allison JR, Montgomery JH, Rockett JF, McMurray JM. Scintigraphic diagnosis of hepatic hemangioma: its role in the management of hepatic mass lesions. AJR 1985; 145: 223–228.

Montz R, Klapdor R, Rothe B, Heller M. Immunoscintigraphy and radioimmunotherapy in patients with pancreatic carcinoma. Nuklearmedizin 1986; 25: 239–244.

Munz DL. Immunszintigraphie mit monoklonalen Antikörpern. Dtsch Med Wochenschr 1987; 112: 649–654.

Pirovino M, Triller J, Steffen R. Die fokale Hyperplasie der Leber. Schweiz Med Wochenschr 1987; 117: 1165–1173.

Rabinowitz SA, McKusick KA, Strauss HW. 99m-Tc red blood cell scintigraphy in evaluating focal liver lesions. AJR 1984; 143: 63–68.

Remedios PA, Colletti PM, Ralls PW. Hepatic amebic abscess: cholescintigraphic rim enhancement. Radiology 1986; 160: 395–398.

Savitch I, Kew MC, Paterson A, Esser JD, Levin J. Uptake of Tc-99m di-isopropyliminodiacetic acid by hepatocellular carcinoma: concise communication. J Nucl Med 1983; 24: 1119–1122.

Schild H, Kreitner K-F, Thelen M, Grönninger J, Weber M, Börner N, Störkel J, Eißner D. Fokal-noduläre Hyperplasie der Leber bei 930 Patienten. RöFo 1987; 147: 612–618.

Tanasescu D, Brachman M, Rigby J, Yadegar J, Ramanna L, Waxman A. Scintigraphic triad in focal nodular hyperplasia. Am J Gastroenterol 1984; 79: 61–64.

Vincent LM, Renner JB. Uptake of hepatobiliary agents by hepatocellular carcinoma. AJR 1984; 143: 1119–1120.

4.12 Laboratory Investigations in Hepatobiliary and Pancreatic Malignancies: the Role of Tumor Markers

G. Klose and W. Schmiegel

Interest in the evaluation of tumor markers in gastrointestinal malignancies has resulted from their potential for early detection of malignant growth with improvement of survival. Tumor-associated markers are usually substances produced either by the tumor or by secondarily induced metabolic markers. Among various laboratory parameters of limited clinical significance (enzymes and isoenzymes, tissue polypeptide antigen (TPA), β-2-microglobulin, ferritin, fibronectin and α-1-antitrypsin), the characteristic feature of some malignant tumors – the synthesisis and secretion of products, usually glycoproteins, stemming from the cell membrane – represented an advance in the diagnosis and management of hepatobiliary and pancreatic cancer. Several oncofetal antigens normally present during fetal life occur at low concentrations in adults, and may circulate in high concentrations in intra-abdominal malignancies (Table 4.12.1). Although no tumor-*specific* antigen has yet been demonstrated, the development of monoclonal antibodies of precisely defined specificity may improve the possibilities of discriminating, not only between cancer and normal tissue, but also between cancer and non-malignant growth and inflammatory conditions.

This article is an attempt to review the clinical usefulness of oncofetal and mucin antigens in screening, diagnosis, staging, prognosis and follow-up of hepatobiliary and pancreatic malignancies.

Oncofetal Antigens

AFP

Alphafetoprotein (AFP), a glycoprotein of approximately 72 kDa, was first described in experimental liver tumors in mice (Abelev et al. 1963). The finding of elevated levels of AFP in a patient with primary liver cancer (Tatarinow 1964), strongly emphasized the potential value of fetal proteins as tumor markers.

Table 4.12.1 Properties and usefulness of tumor-associated antigens in hepatobiliary and pancreatic malignancies

Marker	Upper normal limit	Properties (molecular weight)	Occurence in malignancy (sensitivity)*	Non-malignant conditions associated with elevated plasma levels
AFP	10 ng/ml	Glycoprotein, 72 kDa	Hepatocellular carcinoma (70–90%) Cholangiocarcinoma (10%)	Hepatitis, cirrhosis, biliary tract obstruction, alcoholic liver disease
CEA	5 ng/ml	Glycoprotein, 180 kDa	Colorectal carcinoma (30–70%) Gastric cancer, pancreatic cancer, lung and breast cancer	Smoking, liver disease (obstructive jaundice, hepatitis, alcohol). Bowel diseases, peptic ulcer, pancreatitis, renal failure, fibro-cystic breast disease
CA 19-9	37 U/ml	Mucin-bound, sialoganglioside	Pancreatic cancer (72–79%), biliary cancer (67–73%), gastric cancer (42–62%), colorectal cancer (19–41%), non-gastric, hepatocellular breast, lung, renal, prostatic, ovarian cancer, lymphomas	Benign biliary diseases, benign pancreatic diseases
CA 125	35 U/ml	Mucin-type glycoprotein	Ovarian cancer (80%), other gynecological malignancies, pancreatic cancer (60%), other gastrointestinal malignancies	Benign pancreatic and liver disease
DUPAN-2	150 U/ml	Mucin-like glycoprotein	Pancreatic and biliary tract cancer (70%)	Benign hepatobiliary diseases (hepatitis, cholelithiasis)

* A test's sensitivity depends on the cut-off point and the stage of disease. The greater the sensitivity achieved by lowering the cut-off point, the lower the specificity of the assay in distinguishing normal from diseased. The earlier the stage of cancer, the less likely a tumor marker assay is to detect it

Cut-off levels of serum assays, sensitivity and specificity. Most healthy adults have a serum AFP concentration of less than 10 ng/ml. Serum AFP concentrations between normal and 100 ng/ml may occur in patients with non-malignant liver disease. AFP levels over 500 ng/ml are normally diagnostic for hepatocellular carcinoma (HCC) (Warnes and Smith 1987). The frequency of AFP elevation in HCC, however, varies in different series from 30–90% (Alpert 1976).

CEA

Carcinoembryonic antigen (CEA) was first isolated from primary colonic adenocarcinomas (Gold and Freedman 1965). Initially, CEA was thought to be expressed exclusively in cancers of the gastrointestinal tract. Elevated CEA levels, however, may occur in many cancers, including non-gastrointestinal tumors and various benign conditions (Shively and Beatty 1985). CEA is a member of a complex family of glycoproteins, and has a molecular weight of approximately 180 kDa (Gold et al. 1970, Hammarström et al. 1975, Hammarström 1985).

Cut-off levels of serum assays, sensitivity and specificity. CEA can be detected as a normal serum protein, especially in smokers, and the distribution of the plasma levels of CEA for normal and disease populations overlap. 97% of the healthy non-smoking population have CEA concentrations between 0 and 5 ng/ml. Elevated levels of plasma CEA are seen in patients with a wide range of non-malignant gastrointestinal diseases, including liver disease, peptic ulcer, diverticular disease, pancreatitis and inflammatory bowel disease (Shively and Beatty 1985). Since the antigen is eliminated mainly by the liver, liver insufficiency is a frequent cause of increased values (Begent 1984). CEA levels may be diagnostic for colonic cancer, but are seldom sufficiently sensitive to detect localized cancer (Zamcheck and Martin 1981). Elevated values of CEA are found in patients with a variety of cancers, including paticularily those of the gastrointestinal tract, but also in ovary, lung and breast cancer (De Young and Ashman 1978, Hammarström 1985).

CEA-like antigens. CEA shows cross-reactivity with closely-related molecules. The first substance immunologically cross-reactive with CEA was named non-specific cross-reacting antigen (NCA) (van Kleist et al. 1972). In order of molecular weight, NCA-160, NCA-95, NCA-55, low molecular weight CEA, normal fetal antigen (NFA-1) and biliary glycoprotein 1 (BGP-1) have been described (Buchegger et al. 1984, Hammarström 1985). CEA-like antigens occur in cancerous tissues as well as in normal and fetal tissues.

CA 19-9

CA 19-9 was described as gastrointestinal cancer-associated antigen, defined by a mouse monoclonal antibody raised against a human colonic carcinoma cell line (Koprowski et al. 1979). The CA 19-9 antigen occurs in man in fetal tissues as well as in normal adult pancreas, stomach, gallbladder and bile duct (Atkinson et al. 1982, Arends et al. 1983, Dietel et al. 1986). Elevated serum levels of CA 19-9 are found in patients with pancreatic, biliary and gastric cancer (Heptner et al. 1985). The antigen determinant of CA 19-9, carried by sialogangliosides and mucins, is derived from Lewis A blood group substance (Magnani et al. 1982). About 5% of the population lacking the encoding gene ($Le^{(-a-b)}$) are therefore unable to synthesize the CA 19-9 antigen.

Cut-off levels of serum assays, sensitivity and specificity. 0.6% of the normal population may have values greater than 37 U/ml (Del Villano et al. 1983). CA 19-9 is highly valued for its clinical usefulness as an antigen related to pancreatic cancers (72–79%), whereas elevated levels occur less frequently in biliary cancer (67–75%), gastric cancer (42–62%) and in colorectal cancer (19–41%) (Haglund et al. 1986c).

CA 50

CA 50 was found as a carcinoma-associated antigen by a monoclonal antibody (C 50) against colorectal carcinoma cells (Lindholm et al. 1983). CA 50 immunoreactive material is associated with mucin-type glycoproteins of high molecular weight. CA 50 appears to have a somewhat broader carbohydrate-binding specificity than CA 19-9, and can react with tumor antigens from individuals who are Lewis-negative (Hammarström 1985).

Cut-off levels of serum assays, sensitivity and specificity. 17 U/ml is considered the upper limit of the normal range (Holmgren et al. 1984). Elevated values of the CA 50 antigen have been found in various gastrointestinal cancers and in benign, pancreatic, biliary and liver diseases (Holmgren et al. 1984, Bruhn 1986). Although CA 50 is sensitive to the existence of adenocarcinomas in the colorectum, pancreas, and stomach and to lymphomas, an increase of CA 50 antigen levels in many inflammatory conditions has to be considered (Bruhn et al. 1985).

CA 125

This antigen was detected by monoclonal antibody OC 125, originally raised against an ovarian cystadenocarcinoma cell line (Bast et al. 1981). The CA 125 antigen has also been demonstrated in non-gynecological tumors, including pancreatic carcinomas, and in normal tissues such as the normal pancreas (Dietel et al. 1986). CA 125 appears to be associated with a high molecular weight mucin-like glycoprotein (Bast et al. 1983).

Cut-off levels of serum assays, sensitivity and specificity. A cut-off level of 35 U/ml had a 99% confidence level in a normal population (Bast et al. 1983). Elevated CA 125 levels have been found in patients with various gastrointestinal cancers, i.e. pancreatic cancer (59–60%) and colorectal carcinomas (20%) (Bast et al. 1983, Klapdor et al. 1984a). Benign gastrointestinal diseases such as pancreatitis (38%), peritonitis (75%), hepatitis (23%), and liver cirrhosis (64%) may also be associated with elevated CA 125 serum levels.

DUPAN-2

DUPAN-2 is a high molecular weight mucin-like glycoprotein defined by a murine monoclonal antibody against a pancreatic ductal adenocarcinoma cell line (Metzgar et al. 1984). The DUPAN-2 epitope has been shown to be non-cross-reactive with CEA and CA 19-9 (Lan et al. 1985).

Cut-off levels of serum assay, sensitivity and specificity. Less than 150 U/ml are found in 99% of healthy subjects. A cut-off level of 400 U/ml is suggested as useful in differentiating pancreatic cancers and biliary tract cancers from benign diseases such as hepatitis and cholelithiasis.

POA

Pancreatic oncofetal antigen (POA) is defined by antibodies against extracts of human fetal pancreas (Banwo et al. 1974). PAO is inferior to CA 19-9 and CEA, and does not permit differential diagnosis between benign and malignant pancreatic disease (Schmiegel et al. 1985a).

PSTI, TATI

Pancreatic secretory trypsin inhibitor (PSTI) is a polypeptide secreted by pancreatic acinar cells together with zymogens (von Fritz et al. 1967). Tumor-associated trypsin inhibitor (TATI) is believed to be identical or at least closely related to PSTI. Elevated serum levels have been reported in acute and relapsing pancreatitis as well as in various cancers (Eddeland 1978).

Clinical Usefulness

Hepatobiliary Malignancies

Screening. Screening for HCC may be valuable in high-risk groups such as patients with cirrhosis, hepatitis B-markers or hemochromatosis (Warnes and Smith 1987). The cut-off point at which AFP levels become diagnostic for HCC is controversial, however. Whether the fucosylated AFP variant improves sensitivity and specificity (Aoyagi et al. 1985) remains to be determined.

Diagnosis. Patients with hepatobiliary malignancies other than HCC may have high serum levels of CA 19-9 (Gupta et al. 1983) or CEA (Shively and Beatty 1985), but none has proved to be clinically relevant for easier detection of "early" localized tumors.

Staging and prognosis. Since correlations between tumor volume and plasma levels of tumor markers exist, it is apparent that the higher the levels at the time of diagnosis, the more advanced the clinical stage. Coexisting conditions such as biliary obstruction, however, may contribute to the limited value for *staging* of tumor markers so far due to lack of specificity.

Pancreatic cancer

Screening. The sensitivities and specificities of the tumor-associated antigens are too low for screening purposes in *asymptomatic* individuals.

Diagnosis. More than 70%, and usually less than 80%, of patients with adenocarcinoma of the pancreas have elevated CA 19-9 serum levels (Del Villano et al. 1983, Haglund et al. 1986a, Schmiegel et al. 1985). Elevated CA 50 levels were found in more than 71% of patients with pancreatic cancer (Paganuzzi et al. 1985). CA 19-9 and CA 50 have higher sensitivities than CEA for the diagnosis of pancreatic cancer (Haglund et al. 1986b). A combination of the CA 19-9 and CA 50 tests gave no further diagnostic improvement because of the similarity of the two antigens. The CA 125 test is not sensitive enough for the diagnosis of pancreatic cancer. DUPAN-2 may be a further aid in the diagnosis of pancreatic cancer. High levels of DUPAN-2, however, are of limited specificity for malignant neoplasm in neighboring organs, i.e. pancreas, biliary tract and liver. In conclusion, therefore CA 19-9 and CA 50 seem to be useful in addition to other diagnostic methods in symptomatic patients in whom there is a suspicion of pancreatic cancer.

Endocrine and other unusual pancreatic tumors are beyond the scope of this article.

Staging and prognosis. The highest values for CA 19-9 and CA 50 were found in patients with advanced carcinoma (Sakahara et al. 1986, Habib et al. 1986). Elevated tumor-associated antigen levels have been found in the pancreatic ductal fluid (Schmiegel et al. 1985a), but the diagnostic potential is limited by a lack of specificity. CA 19-9 and CA 50 may be helpful in monitoring surgically resected patients with pancreatic cancer (Kapdor et al. 1984b). Whether this information leads to more effective treatment remains to be determined.

Summary and Conclusion

Evidence exists for the clinical usefulness of tumor-associated antigens in hepatobiliary and pancreatic malignancies. AFP currently represents the closest approach to the ideal of a tumor marker for the screening and diagnosis of primary liver cancer. The sensitivity and specificity of tumor markers in detecting secondary liver cancer depends on the origin of the cancer. CA 19-9 and CA 50 have higher diagnostic sensitivity and specificity for pancreatic cancer than CEA. Repeated testing over time will improve diagnostic efficacy. Although the sensitivity and specificity of CA 19-9 and CA 50 are too low for the *screening* of an asymptomatic population, the assay may be promising in the follow-up of radically operated patients with pancreatic cancer. New markers such as DUPAN-2 may be promising for the diagnosis of pancreatic cancer, but their superiority to other markers still has to be established in longer series.

References

Abelev GI, Perova SD, Khramkova NI, Postnikova ZA, Irlin IS. Production of embryonal d-globulin by transplantable mouse hepatomas. Transplantation 1963; 1: 174–180.

Alpert E. Human alpha-fetoprotein (AFP): development biology and clinical significance. Prog Liver Dis 1976; 5: 337–349.

Aoyagi Y, Isemura M, Suzuki Y. Fucosylated alpha-fetoprotein as marker of early hepatocellular carcinoma. Lancet 1985; 1353.

Arends JW, Verstynen C, Bosman FT, Hilgers J, Steplewski Z. Distribution of monoclonal antibody-defined monosialoganglioside in normal and cancerous human tissues: an immunoperoxidase study. Hybridoma 1983; 2: 219–229.

Atkinson BF, Ernst CS, Herlyn M, Steplewski Z, Sears HF, Koprowski H. Gastrointestinal cancer-associated antigen in immunoperoxidase assay. Cancer Res 1982; 42: 4820–4823.

Banwo O, Versey J, Hobbs JR. New oncofetal antigen for human pancreas. Lancet 1974; i: 643–645.

Bast RC Jr, Feeney M, Lazarus H, Nadler LM, Colvin RB, Knapp RC. Reactivity of a monoclonal antibody with human ovarian carcinoma. J Clin Invest 1981; 68: 1331–1337.

Bast RC Jr, Klug TL, St John E, Jenison E, Niloff JM, Lazarus H, Berkowitz RS, Leavitt T, Griffiths CT, Parker L, Zurawski VR Jr, Knapp RC. A radioimmunoassay using a monoclonal antibody to monitor the course of epithelial ovarian cancer. N Engl J Med. 1983; 309: 883–887.

Begent RHJ. The value of carcinoembryonic antigen measurement in clinical practice. Ann Clin Biochem 1984; 21: 231–238.

Bruhn HD. CA 50 in serum of patients with carcinoma. Dtsch Med Wochenschr 1986; 111: 1267–1272.

Bruhn HD, Everding A, Joos B, Hedderich J. Clinical experience with the carbohydrate antigen CA 50 in the serum of carcinoma patients. In: Holmgren J, ed. Tumor marker antigens. Lund: Studentenliteratur, 1985: 94–105.

Buchegger F, Schreyer M, Carrel S, Mach J-P. Monoclonal antibodies identify a CEA crossreacting antigen of 95 kD (NCA 95) distinct in antigenicity and tissue distribution from the previously described NCA of 55 kD. Int J Cancer 1984; 33: 643–649.

Del Villano BC, Brennan S, Brock P, Bucher C, Liu V, McClure M, Rake B, Space S, Westrick B, Schoemaker H, Zurawski VR Jr. Radioimmunometric assay for a monoclonal antibody-defined tumor marker, CA 19-9. Clin Chem 1983; 29: 549–552.

De Young NJ, Ashman LK. Physiochemical and immunochemical properties of carcinoembryonic antigen (CEA) from different tumour sources. Aust J Exp Biol Med Sci 1978; 56: 321–331.

Dietel, M, Arps, H, Klapdor, R, Müller-Hagen S, Sieck M, Hoffmann L Antigen detection by the monoclonal antibodies CA 19-9 and CA 125 in normal and tumor tissue and patients sera. J. Cancer Res Clin Oncol 1986; 111: 257–265.

Gold, P, Freedman SO. Demonstration of tumor-specific antigens in human colonic carcinomata by immunological tolerance and absorption techniques. J Exp Med 1965; 121: 439–462.

Gold, P, Krupey, J, Ansari H. Position of the carcinoembryonic antigen of the human digestive system in ultrastructure of tumor cell surface. J. Natl Cancer Inst 1970; 45: 219–225.

Gupta, MK, Arciaga, R, Bocci C. Measurement of a monoclonal-antibody-defined antigen (CA 19-9) in the sera of patients with malignant and nonmalignant diseases: comparison with carcinoembryonic antigen. Cancer 1983; 56: 277–283.

Habib NA, Hershman MJ, Haberland F, Papp L, Wood CB, Williamson RCN. The use of CA 50 radioimmunoassay in differentiating benign and malignant pancreatic disease. Br J Cancer 1986; 53: 697–699.

Haglund C, Lindgren J, Roberts PJ, Nordling S. Gastrointestinal cancer-associated antigen CA 19-9 in histological specimens of pancreatic tumours and pancreatitis. Br J Cancer 1986a; 53: 189–195.

Haglund C, Roberts PJ, Kuusela, P, Jalanko, H. Tumor markers in pancreatic cancer. Scand J Gastroenterol 1986b; 21 (suppl 126): 75–78.

Haglund C, Roberts PJ, Kuusela P, Scheinin TM, Mäkelä O, Jalanko H. Evaluation of CA 19-9 as a serum tumour marker in pancreatic cancer. Br J Cancer 1986c; 53: 197–202.

Haglund C, Huhtala M-L, Halila H, Nordling S, Roberts PJ, Scheinin TM, Stenman U-H. Tumour-associated trypsin inhibitor (TATI), in patients with pancreatic cancer, pancreatitis and benign biliary disease. Br J Cancer 1986d; 54: 297–304.

Hammarström S. Chemistry and immunology of CEA, CA 19-9 and CA 50. In: Holmgren J, ed. Tumor marker antigens. Lund: Studentlitteratur, 1985: 34–51.

Hammarström S, Engvall E, Johansson BG, Svensson S, Sundblad G, Goldstein IJ. Nature of the tumor-associated determinant(s) of carcinoembryonic antigen. Proc Natl Acad Sci USA 1975; 72: 1528–1532.

Heptner G, Domschke S, Schneider MU, Domschke W. The place of tumour-associated antigen CA 19-9 in the differential diagnosis of pancreatic disease. Dtsch Med Wochenschr 1985; 110: 624–628.

Holmgren J, Lindholm L, Persson B, Lagergard T, Nilsson O, Svennerholm L, Rudenstam C-M, Unsgaard B, Yngvason F, Pettersson S, Kilander AF. Detection by monoclonal antibody of carbohydrate antigen CA 50 in serum of patients with carcinoma. Br Med J 1984; 288: 1479–1482.

Klapdor R, Lehmann U, Bahlo M, Schmiegel W, Guthoff A, Schreiber HW, Greten H. CA 19-9 and CEA in the follow-up of exocrine pancreatic cancer disease. Gastroenterology 1984a; 86: 1137.

Klapdor R, Klapdor U, Bahlo M, Dallek M, Kremer B, van Ackeren H, Schreiber HW, Greten H. CA 12-5 bei Karzinomen des Verdauungstraktes. Dtsch Med Wochenschr 1984b; 109: 1949–1954.

Koprowski H, Steplewski Z, Mitchell K, Herlyn D, Fuhrer P. Colorectal carcinoma antigens detected by hybridoma antibodies. Somatic Cell Mol Genet 1979; 5: 957–972.

Lan MS, Finn OJ, Fernstein PD, Metzgar RS. Isolation and properties of a human pancreatic adenocarcinoma-associated antigen DU-PAN-2. Cancer Res 1985; 45: 305–310.

Lindholm L, Holmgren J, Svennerholm L, Fredman P, Nilsson O, Persson B, Myrvold H, Lagergard T. Monoclonal antibodies against gastrointestinal tumour-associated antigens isolated as monosialogangliosides. Int Arch Allergy Appl Immunol 1983; 71: 178–181.

Magnani JL, Nilsson B, Brockhaus M, Zopf D, Stepelewski Z, Koprowski H, Ginsburg V. A monoclonal antibody-defined antigen associated with gastrointestinal cancer is a ganglioside containing sialylated lacto-N-fucopentaose II. J Biol Chem 1982; 257: 14365–14369.

Metzgar RS, Rodriguez M, Finn OS, Lan MS, Daasch UN, Fernstein PD, Meyers WC, Sindelar WF, Sandler RS, Seigler HF. Detection of a pancreatic cancer associated antigen (DU-PAN-2 antigen) in serum and ascites of patients with adenocarcinoma. Proc Natl Acad Sci USA 1984; 5242–5246.

Paganuzzi M, Marroni P, Boccardo F, Valenti G, Ferrara GB, Cerri E, Secco GB. Clinical evaluation of CA 50 in sera of patients with different tumors. In: Holmgren J, ed. Tumor marker antigens. Lund: Studentlitteratur, 1985: 134–145.

Sakahara H, Endo K, Nakajima K, Nakashima T, Koizumi M, Ohta H, Hidaka A, Kohno S, Nakano Y, Naito A, Suzuki T, Torizuka K. Serum CA 19-9 concentrations and computed tomography findings in patients with pancreatic carcinoma. Cancer 1986; 57: 1324–1326.

Schmiegel WH, Eberl W, Kreiker C, Kalthoff H, Bützow GH, Jessen K, Klapdor R, Soehendra N, Wargenau M, Classen M, Greten H, Thiele H-G. Multiparametric tumor marker (CA 19-9, CEA, AFP, POA) analyses of pancreatic juices and sera in pancreatic diseases. Hepatogastroenterology 1985a; 32: 141–145.

Schmiegel WH, Kreiker C, Eberl W, Arndt R, Classen M, Greten H, Jessen K, Kalthoff H, Soehendra N, Thiele H-G. Monoclonal antibody defines CA 19-9 in pancreatic juices and sera. Gut 1985b; 26: 456–460.

Shively JE, Beatty JD. CEA-related antigens: molecular biology and clinical significance. Crit Rev Oncol Hematol 1985; 2: 355–399.

Steinberg WM, Glenn J, Kurtzman S, Sindelar WF. A new assay to diagnose and monitor therapy of pancreatic cancer. Clin Res 1984; 32: 286A.

Steinberg WM, Gelfand R, Anderson KK, Glenn J, Kurtzman SH, Sindelar WF, Toskes PP. Comparison of the sensitivity and specificity of the CA 19-9 and carcinoembryonic antigen assays in detecting cancer of the pancreas. Gastroenterology 1986; 90: 343–349.

Tatarinow YS. Detection of embryo specific α-globulin in serum of a patient with primary liver cancer. Vopr Med Khim 1964; 10: 90.

Von Fritz H, Hüller I, Wiedemann M. Werle E. Über Proteaseinhibitoren, V: Zur Chemie und Physiologie der spezifischen Trypsininhibitoren aus den Bauchspeicheldrüsen von Rind, Hund, Schwein und Mensch. Hoppe Seylers Z Physiol Chem 1967; 348: 405–418.

Von Kleist S, Chavanel G, Burtin P. Identification of an antigen from normal human tissue that crossreacts with the carcinoembryonic antigen. Proc Natl Acad Sci USA 1972; 69: 2492–2494.

Warnes TW, Smith A. Tumor markers in diagnosis and management. Clin Gastroenterol 1987; 1 (suppl 1): 63–88.

Zamcheck N, Martin EW. Factors controlling the circulating CEA levels in pancreatic cancer: some clinical correlations. Cancer 1981; 47: 1620–1627.

5 Preoperative Considerations

5.1 Anesthesia for Major Hepatobiliary and Pancreatic Malignancies

N. Moerman, W. W. A. Zuurmond and A. E. M. Floor

Introduction

The incidence and severity of hepatic damage during anesthesia cannot as yet be precisely monitored. However, liver function may be impaired by several factors during anesthesia (Strunin and Davies 1983), arising from anesthetic management, the surgery itself and the underlying disease.

Preoperative Assessment

Well-planned anesthesia is based upon good preoperative assessment. The outcome of the operation is determined to a great extent by the patient's physical fitness. Every effort to improve the state of health before the operation must be made. In patients undergoing major hepatobiliary surgery, the normal preoperative evaluation includes not only assessment of cardio-pulmonary and renal function, but also investigations related to the liver. The most important factors are the patient's physical and mental state, liver function reserve and clotting status. Questions regarding the patient's medical history, previous incidences of jaundice or hepatitis, increased bleeding tendency, reactions to previous anesthesia, current drug therapy, alcohol and drug abuse should be made. It is only in the advanced stages of liver disease that significant abnormalities are found in the patient's physical and mental condition. Indeed, in this situation several organ systems may be involved, such as the brain, kidneys and vascular system.

Essential laboratory tests includes liver function tests, plasma protein levels, clotting profile, hemoglobin, hematocrit, electrolytes, creatinine and urea (Chopra and Griffin 1985). Patients scheduled for major hepatic bile surgery may have normal liver function tests. In the case of preoperative extrahepatic obstruction, an endoprosthesis can be placed to improve bile drainage. In cirrhotic patients, liver damage is largely irreversible. Severe liver disease is always accompanied by disturbed liver function tests.

To grade the severity of liver disease, Pugh et al. (1973) described a classification system based on three laboratory tests (bilirubin, albumin and prothrombin) and two clinical observations (encephalopathy grade and ascites). Each of these parameters may score 1, 2 or 3 points for increasing abnormality. Patients with a low score (5–6 points) are considered to have a good level of operation risk and patients with high scores (10–15 points) have a poor level of operation risk.

Coagulation

Hemostatic abnormalities are common in liver disease. For this reason it is important to be informed about the patient's clotting status. In liver failure, there is a deficiency of the coagulation factors fibrinogen and vitamin K-dependent factors II, VII, IX and X. Clotting defects may be aggravated by thrombocytopenia and qualitative platelet disturbances. Antithrombin III synthesis is also lowered, and this leads to increased fibrinolysis. Vitamin K deficiency is common in biliary obstruction, and the synthesis of vitamin K-dependent clotting factors is reduced.

Because bleeding is the most frequent complication in liver surgery, efforts must be made to correct or improve any clotting deficiency. Preoperative treatment can be started with vitamin K, 2×10 mg daily. Sometimes two or three days are needed for correction. In emergency situations, correction can be achieved by means of fresh frozen plasma or clotting-factor concentration (II, VII, IX, X), and if necessary with concentrated platelet transfusion.

Preoperative Visit

The preoperative visit is an essential part of good patient care. Patients faced with this type of operation can be very ill. Most of them are aware of the seriousness of the operation and know about the postoperative intensive care period. The anesthetist plays an important role in reducing the patient's anxiety by dealing with his fears and anxieties for the coming operation and anesthesia. Explanations of what anesthesia means and some information about the postoperative period, to the extent that the patient is interested and able to understand, may not only reduce preoperative anxiety but are also important for postoperative well-being.

Visiting the patient gives the anesthetist the opportunity to obtain information about venous accessibility. Good running venous lines can be lifesaving during the operation. Central lines are important, as they can be used not only for cardiac monitoring but also become crucial in case of massive transfusions. Putting in these lines the day before saves time on the day of operation. If an epidural block is planned, the anatomy of the patient's spine is also important. Anatomical disorders may hinder an epidural block. Advance information about possible problems reduces problems on the day of the operation.

Anesthetic Considerations

Liver Blood Flow and Anesthesia

The liver belongs to the splanchnic organs along with the gallbladder, spleen, pancreas and digestive tract. The blood flow through these organs is the splanchnic blood flow, which is directly related to perfusion pressure and inversely proportional to the resistance in the splanchnic area (Strunin and Davies 1986). Total liver blood flow is about 25% of the cardiac output. The portal vein supplies 70% of liver blood flow, but can supply only half of the oxygen demand. The other 50% of oxygen comes from the hepatic artery, which supplies 30% of the liver perfusion. Blood drains from the liver via the hepatic veins into the inferior vena cava.

During the operation and anesthesia, a number of factors may influence liver blood flow. All anesthetic techniques (general or regional) decrease hepatic blood flow. During spinal and epidural anesthesia, the liver blood flow parallels the reduction in arterial blood pressure. The same is true when halothane, enflurane or isoflurane are used. Although studies in animals have shown an increase in hepatic artery blood flow during isoflurane anesthesia, the total hepatic blood flow (hepatic arterial flow plus portal flow) decreases. Positive pressure ventilation increases vascular resistance in the splanchnic area and thereby decreases liver blood flow. Oxygen and carbon dioxide are important; both hypoxia and hypercarbia may cause an increase in sympathetic nervous activity and a fall in splanchnic blood flow and liver perfusion. Normocapnic ventilation will probably cause the least interruption in hepatic blood flow.

All anesthetic agents influence liver blood flow. However, surgical intervention itself is often the most relevant factor producing a decrease in the liver blood flow (Gelman 1976).

Massive Blood Loss and Clotting Defects

During liver surgery, especially in liver resections, shunt operations or reinterventions, massive blood loss is common. The anesthetist is responsible for arranging large-bore intravenous cannulae. Autotransfusion equipment can be helpful. There must be a well-organized blood bank. Perioperative clotting defects, caused either by the preoperative condition of the patient or by massive blood loss, make it necessary for the anesthetist to be closely informed about the clotting status. Prompt laboratory service during the operation is essential.

Temperature

The patient's temperature during the operation may decrease considerably during prolonged surgery. This is a common problem during this type of operation because of the extent of the operation field, contact of the bowels and viscera with theater air, and massive intravenous fluid and blood administration. To solve this problem, it is essential that a heating mattress is used, that theater temperature is sufficiently increased, that the bowels are wrapped to prevent transpiration, and that the infusion fluids and blood are warmed to body temperature. In addition, warming and humidification of the inspired gases helps to prevent further cooling. The anesthetist must monitor body temperature. In spite of all these measures, it nevertheless sometimes happens that a decrease in body temperature cannot be prevented. Postoperative patient management should include the correction of temperature to normal values, this being one of the contributing factors in postoperative controlled ventilation.

Hypotension

Hypotension may occur during anesthesia and operation for hepatobiliary surgery. Besides massive blood loss, other factors may be involved, such as:

- Surgical manipulations resulting in acute obstruction of the inferior vena cava blood flow. Temporary clamping of the inferior vena cava is sometimes unavoidable for surgical reasons.
- Apparent or insidious infection at the start of the operation may induce hypotension due either to septicemia or to circulating endotoxins.
- Resecting more than 30% of the liver parenchyma may result in a decrease of the portal outflow tract, causing transient portal hypertension and acute peripheral hypovolemia (Stone 1975, Stone et al. 1969).
- Unexpected hypotension may occur following air or tumor embolism. The anesthetist should be aware of this complication during incision and surgery of the inferior vena cava. Hiccuping at this stage of surgery can be fatal.

Impaired Liver Function and Drug Metabolism

Impaired liver function may influence the pharmacokinetics of anesthetic drugs. Elimination of anesthetics by the liver may be impaired by:

- the underlying preoperative liver disease
- deterioration of liver function perioperatively due to altered hepatic blood flow during anesthesia and surgery
- loss of liver parenchyma due to the surgical intervention (Zoli et al. 1986).

In addition, a low plasma protein level may result in an increased free fraction of the anesthetic drugs.

Hepatotoxicity of Anesthetic Agents

During major hepatobiliary surgery, drugs suspected of hepatotoxicity must be avoided. Most anesthetic drugs can be used safely. Nevertheless, some anesthetics are still controversial. The halogenated hydrocarbons halothane, enflurane and isoflurane have been administered to patients scheduled for this type of operation. From a theoretical point of view with regard to volatile anesthetics, isoflurane should be preferred, being the anesthetic with the lowest level ($< 1\%$) of biodegradation (Brown and Gandolfi 1987, Stricker and Spoelstra 1985). Harmful effects of the prolonged administration of nitrous oxide are questionable. Bowel distension during long operations might be another reason for avoiding nitrous oxide.

Perioperative Pain Management

Anesthesia for major hepatobiliary surgery should include the opioids fentanyl, sufentanil or alfentanil either by bolus injection or continuous infusion. Special attention has to be paid to patients with advanced stages of liver disease. Enhanced sensitivity and prolonged action may be expected.

Postoperatively, especially after upper abdominal surgery, patients may suffer from severe pain. Pain relief is necessary not only for humanitarian but also for therapeutic reasons. Abdominal wounds tend to impair respiration by inhibition of deep breathing, coughing and sputum clearance. Atelectasis, perfusion inequality, shunting of venous blood, and a decrease of functional residual capacity can occur. Following insufficient postoperative pain relief, pulmonary complications are therefore likely to occur.

Anesthetic technique can be an important factor in preventing postoperative pain. The anesthetist has to plan his dosage scheme during the operation, avoiding the administration of opioid antagonists on the one hand, and on the other, respiratory depression caused by the opioids themselves. Postoperative controlled ventilation should sometimes be preferred to the more unstable condition of early extubation. Good preoperative information can decrease the analgesic demand postoperatively. Neither drugs nor regional anesthetic techniques can relieve postoperative pain without the attention from doctors and nurses which the operated patient requires. Opioids should be administered intramuscularly or intravenously in adequate doses and at suitable intervals. Respiratory parameters should be controlled intensively. Continuous administration of opioids either in the recovery room, in intensive care or in the general ward, where close observation and monitoring is assured, should be considered.

"Combined anesthesia", general and epidural with catheter, is an elegant technique for major hepatobiliary surgery. The segmental spread of 4–8 ml bupivacaine 0.25–0.5% with adrenalin 1 : 200000, instilled epidurally at one spinal level below the center of incision (e.g. T 7–8 for subcostal incision) results in pain relief with little sympathetic or motor block (Torda 1983). During anesthesia, the patient's need for opioids and relaxation is less, and after the operation, pain relief can be achieved by epidurally administered local anesthetics, opioids, or a mixture of both. This results in early extubation and mobilization of a pain-free patient. Instilling epidural opioids demands close observation of respiratory parameters, and parenteral administration of opioids is forbidden. Of course, coagulation defects may occur perioperatively, and careful consideration of this must be taken into account when an epidural block is thought to be of value. Each patient should be considered individually.

Hypnotics

Impaired liver function may result in prolonged action of hypnotics. Benzodiazepines (diazepam or midazolam), barbiturates (thiopentone or methohexitone), etomidate or propofol can be used safely as the induction agent, taking into account the considerations mentioned above.

To prevent prolonged administration of nitrous oxide, a continuous infusion of hypnotics might be preferred. Benzodiazepines and barbiturates could accumulate, however, resulting in a prolongation of the recovery period. Etomidate decreases cortisol levels during continuous administration for a longer period. Applications for the promising new hypnotic drug propofol during anesthesia for major hepatobiliary surgery are not yet known.

Relaxation

Dundee and Gray (1953) described "resistence to curare" in patients with liver disease. This phenomenon has also been described for other nondepolarizing neuromuscular blocking drugs, such as pancuronium. Increased distribution volume may be an explanation. Westra et al. (1981) observed a delay in the onset of paralysis. Total clearance of pancuronium is particularly decreased in obstructive jaundice. Larger doses of pancuronium are therefore needed to achieve an effective blood concentration. However, this results in a longer duration of action. Vecuronium is also mainly cleared from the plasma by the liver, and relies on biliary excretion, so that its effects are possibly prolonged in liver disease (Miller 1986).

Atracurium is metabolized in a completely different way (Ward and Neil 1983). A nonenzymatic breakdown in plasma by the Hofmann reaction makes its metabolism independent of liver and renal function. From a theoretical point of view, atracurium seems to be the muscle relaxant of choice in patients with liver disease, although the toxic effects of its metabolites have not been fully determined (Chapple et al. 1987).

Monitoring

As major bleeding is one of the main problems during this type of operation, intensive cardiovascular monitoring is essential. Besides routine measurement of heart rate, arterial blood pressure and electrocardiogram, central venous pressure monitoring is recommended. Indeed, in case of severe cardiac or pulmonary disease, it is necessary to use a pulmonary artery catheter to obtain information about pulmonary arterial pressure, pulmonary capillary wedge pressure and cardiac output. Furthermore, the central venous pressure or pulmonary artery pressure line can be used for the aspiration of air should embolism occur. An indwelling arterial catheter allows continuous arterial blood pressure measurement and regular arterial blood sampling. Blood gases, acid-base balance, hemoglobin, hematocrit, serum electrolytes, blood glucose and clotting status can thus be finely controlled.

For optimal ventilation, end tidal expiratory carbon dioxide measurement is necessary. Pulse oximetry is now recommended for continuous measurement of oxygen saturation. During anesthesia, proper measurement of muscle relaxation should be performed using a relaxograph. For temperature control, a thermistor probe is placed in the esophagus via the nasal route. Urine production should be controlled, and bladder catheterization is necessary.

References

Brown BR, Gandolfi AJ. Adverse effects of volatile anaesthetics. Br J Anaesth 1987; 59: 14–23.

Chapple DJ, Miller AA, Ward JB, Wheatly PL. Cardiovascular and neurological effects of laudanosine. Studies in mice and rats, and in conscious and anaesthetized dogs. Br J Anaesth 1987; 59: 218–225.

Chopra S, Griffin PH. Laboratory tests and diagnostic procedures in evaluation of liver disease. Am J Med 1985; 79: 221–230.

Dundee JW, Gray TC. Resistance to d-tubocurarine chloride in the presence of liver disease. Lancet 1953; ii: 16–17.

Gelman SI. Disturbances in hepatic blood flow during anaesthesia and surgery. Arch Surg 1976; 111: 881–883.

Miller RD. Pharmacokinetics of atracurium and other neuromuscular blocking agents in normal patients and those with renal or hepatic dysfunction. Br J Anaesth 1986; 58: 11 S–13 S.

Pugh RNH, Murray-Lyan IM, Dawson JL, Pietroni MC, Williams R. Transection of the oesophagus for bleeding oesophageal varices. Br J Anaesth 1973; 60: 646–649.

Stone HH. Major hepatic resections in children. J Pediatr Surg 1975; 10: 127–134.

Stone HH, Long WD, Smith RB. Physiologic considerations in major hepatic resections. Am J Surg 1969; 78: 117–84.

Stricker BHC, Spoelstra P, eds. Drug induced hepatic injury I. Amsterdam: Elsevier, 1985.

Strunin L, Davies JM. The liver and anaesthesia. Can Anaesth Soc J 1983; 30: 208–217.

Strunin L, Davies JM. Effects of anaesthetics in liver circulation. In: Altura BM, ed. Cardiovascular actions of anaesthetic drugs used in anaesthesia; vol 2. Basel: Karger, 1986: 162–178.

Torda TT. Management of acute and postoperative pain. Int Anesthesiol Clin 1983; 21: 27–46.

Ward S, Neil EAM. Pharmacokinetics of atracurium in acute hepatic failure (with acute renal failure). Br J Anaesth 1983; 55: 1169.

Westra P, Vermeer GA, de Lange AR, Scuf AHJ, Meyer DKF, Wesseling H. Hepatic and renal disposition of pancuronium and gallamine in patients with extrahepatic cholestasis. Br J Anaesth 1981; 53: 331–338.

Zoli M, Marchesini G, Melli A, et al. Evaluation of liver volume and liver function following hepatic resection in man. Liver 1986; 6: 286–291.

5.2 Preoperative Evaluation and Management of Patients with Hepatobiliary and Pancreatic Malignancies

R. A. F. M. Chamuleau

Introduction

Adequate preoperative investigation is an essential part of the management of any patient about to undergo surgery. Hepatobiliary and pancreatic surgery is not an exception to this rule. On the contrary, surgeons have approached jaundiced patients with justifiable trepidation for almost a century, because they seem to be predisposed to innumerable postoperative complications (Allison 1988).

Operations on patients with hepatobiliary disease present four particular dangers: hepatic insufficiency, hemorrhage, infection and renal failure. In addition to the routine aspects of preoperative investigation, therefore, special attention should be paid to these.

General Aspects

The general preoperative examination of the patient with hepatobiliary or pancreatic malignancy is the same as for any other abdominal surgery. Since a detailed inventory of such a general assessment is beyond the scope of this chapter, the reader is referred for details to Kammerer and Gross (1983).

A few general points should be emphasized. As a rule, preoperative assessment of the cardiovascular and respiratory system is required. Antihypertensive therapy should be continued up to the time of surgery, and the anesthetist should be informed. Patients with pulmonary problems will require preoperative physiotherapy and, if necessary, bronchodilators. Sputum should be cultured, and if infection is present, antibiotic treatment should be instituted. Insulin-dependent diabetics should receive continuous intravenous infusion of glucose with short-acting insulin, based on a regular estimation of blood glucose. In patients with non-insulin-dependent diabetes, the antidiabetic drug should be stopped preoperatively.

Specific Aspects

Assessment of Liver Function

Surgical intervention in patients with liver disease carries considerable risks (Gill et al. 1983). It is importance to assess the functional capacity of the liver preoperatively, even more so if partial liver resection is involved. Pre-existing liver cirrhosis

Table 5.2.1 **Modified Child Classification**. After Pugh et al. (1973)

Parameter	Score		
	1	2	3
Serum bilirubin (mg/100 ml)	1–2	2–3	> 3
Albumin (g/l)	> 35	28–35	< 28
Prothrombin time (seconds prolonged)	1–4	4–6	> 6
Encephalopathy (grade)	–	1–2	3–4
Ascites	absent	slight	moderate

Group designation: A = 5–6 points; B = 7–9 points, C = 10–15 points

carries a high mortality rate, but is not an absolute contra-indication. A vast experience in liver resection for primary hepatocellular carcinoma in cirrhotics has been obtained, particularly in Asia (Nagasue et al. 1986, Nagao et al. 1987).

The functional capacity of the liver as a whole can be assessed by the classic Child-Turcotte classification, modified by Pugh et al. (1973); see Table 5.2.1. Child C patients carry a high risk, and should not be subjected to major liver resection. If the need is felt for a further specification of liver function in order to predict postoperative morbidity and mortality, the hepatic biotransformation capacity for endogenous and exogenous toxic substances and hepatic protein synthetic capacity may be of paramount importance.

Biotransformation capacity depends mainly on the mixed function oxidase system, which can be tested by antipyrine (McPherson 1982), aminopyrine (Gill et al. 1983, Villeneuve et al. 1986) or caffeine (Renner et al. 1984) clearance. McPherson et al. (1982) showed that in jaundiced patients, antipyrine half-life did not correlate with standard biochemical liver function tests, but correlated positively with the postoperative half-life of endogenous bilirubin, and inversely with the hepatic cytochrome P-450 content of intraoperative liver biopsies. In their series, four out of six patients with an antipyrine half-life of more than 20 died. Jaundiced patients with an initial antipyrine half-life exceeding 15 h showed significant improvement after drainage. This suggests that antipyrine half-life may be an aid in the selection of high-risk patients with obstructive jaundice for biliary drainage preceding definitive surgery.

Since the aminopyrine breath test and caffeine clearance both test the cytochrome P-450 system, comparable predictive value can be expected. An aminopyrine breath test of less than 2.3% is associated with extremely high postoperative mortality in cirrhotics undergoing surgery, while those patients with normal aminopyrine breath test values tolerate elective surgery well (Gill et al. 1983). As a rule, a proper estimation of the protein-synthetic capacity of the liver is difficult to obtain in the clinical situation. Plasma concentrations of albumin, cholinesterase, vitamin K-dependent coagulation factors, etc., provide some indication. However, these do not strictly reflect synthetic capacity, since they not only depend on synthetic capacity but also on the biological half-life, the availability of precursors, breakdown, or consumption. Dynamic measurements of labeled amino acid precursors for specific proteins are reliable tests for synthetic capacity, but are usually time-consuming and a burden to the patient.

Clowes et al. (1984) have proposed the use of the central plasma clearance of amino acids (CPCR-AA) as a measure of hepatic protein-synthetic capacity. They demonstrated a fair correlation between CPCR-AA in vivo and protein-synthetic capacity measured in vitro in liver biopsies of the same patients. In 35 cirrhotic patients undergoing major surgery, a fair correlation between the preoperative CPCR-AA and survival was found. They concluded that if the preoperative CPCR-AA did not approach a value of about 200 ml/min/m^2, patients with cirrhosis were prone to die postoperatively due to overwhelming infection and multisystem organ failure. A disadvantage of the CPCR-AA test is the prerequisite that the cardiac output must be measured, usually invasively using thermodilution with a Swan–Ganz catheter. Prospective studies are awaited before the use of the CPCR-AA can be recommended.

Many other liver function tests (quantitative and semiquantitative; Table 5.2.2) have been developed. Only a minority have practical implications for clinical judgment and management. Computer-assisted multivariance analysis of multiple tests have been evaluated without any dramatic improvement in decision-making (Solberg et al. 1976, Hamilton 1977). It is postulated in any case that prognosis of surgical hepatobiliary patients depends on the (remaining) functional mass of the liver after surgery (Zoli et al. 1986).

The ability of the liver to cope with infection (synthesis of acute-phase proteins, Kupffer cell activity) and to regenerate after partial resection plays an essential role in the prognosis (see the section on immune status below). A prospective study in which these parameters are correlated with prognosis in comparison with the classic Child–Turcotte classification is in progress in our hospital.

Table 5.2.2   Quantitative and semi-quantitative liver function tests

Test	Significance
Serum albumin, clotting factors, cholinesterase	Protein synthesis
Arterial ammonia, plasma amino acid, maximal rate of urea synthesis	Amino acid metabolism Ammonia detoxification
Glucose, galactose, cholesterol, lipoprotein, triglyceride, bile acid	Carbohydrate metabolism Lipid and bile acid metabolism
BSP, ICG, antipyrine, aminopyrine, caffeine	Biotransformation, cytochrome P-450, liver flow
Rectal/Oral NH$_3$ loading	Portosystemic shunting
Endotoxinemia, gamma-globulin	Kupffer cell function
EEG, evoked response, psychomotor tests	Hepatic encephalopathy

BSP: bromsulfophthalein; ICG: indocyanine green; EEG: electroencephalogram

A quite different problem in the evaluation of hepatic reserve in jaundiced patients and patients undergoing major liver resection is the predictability of the development of hepatic encephalopathy (HE) postoperatively. It is well known that the incidence of HE is related to the amount of functional liver mass and the extent of portosystemic shunting. The latter can be assessed by an ammonium loading test as described by Gips et al. (1973) or by the bioavailability of sorbitol (Cavanna et al. 1987). Subclinical HE should be a warning sign in cirrhotic patients before surgery is considered. Psychomotor tests (Gill et al. 1986), electroencephalogram spectral analysis (van der Rijt et al. 1984) and evoked response measurements (Tarter et al. 1987) can be indicative. If subclinical HE is present, it contributes to the balance of potential risks and benefits of surgery. In the postoperative phase, protein restriction can be necessary in order to prevent hyperammonemia.

Coagulation Profile

Clotting abnormalities are often encountered in patients undergoing hepatobiliary surgery, for various reasons:

Hepatocellular dysfunction. The prothrombin time is often prolonged in patients with severe liver disease, reflecting low levels of clotting factors I, II, V, VII, IX, X, XI and XII, whose production is dependent on normal liver function. Furthermore, normal liver function plays an important role in the deactivation of activated factors and clotting inhibitors.

Vitamin K deficiency due to malnutrition or malabsorption caused by intestinal bile acid deficiency in cholestatic patients.

Preoperative consumption and loss of platelets and clotting factors, not sufficiently compensated for transfusion.

Preoperative assessment of the coagulation capacity includes: full blood count, testing of the extrinsic (prothrombin time), and intrinsic clotting system (activated partial thromboplastin time) and thrombin time. A bleeding time is useful if thrombopenia is present or thrombocytopathy is expected (uremia, recent use of salicylate etc). Measurement of specific clotting factors is only indicated if coagulation defects were found in the screening tests mentioned above. If considerable deficiency is present, the question of whether this will be reversible postoperatively must be answered. Temporary correction is always possible with vitamin K, fresh frozen plasma, antithrombin 3, purified clotting factors and platelet suspensions, but defects pointing to irreversible hepatocellular dysfunction should be taken into account when assessing the balance of acceptable surgical risks.

If coagulation has to be monitored very closely during major surgery, the accelerated clotting time (ACT) (Whitwham and Morgan 1988) or the thromboelastogram can be useful. An increase in ACT indicates a reduction of fibrinogen, activation of the clotting system, or failure of the liver to deactivate the clotting factors or inhibitors of coagulation. None of these tests is really superior to another, and the choice depends entirely on the experience and facilities of the surgical department in question.

Immune Status

The stress of physical injury presents a major challenge to the body's metabolism and to the host immunological defense (Blackburn and Menkes 1983). It provokes an immediate, non-specific response which will initiate wound healing and prevent infection. Since the incidence of infective complications postoperatively, especially in the jaundiced patient, is rather high (Edwards and Blumgart 1987), pleas have been made to determine the immune status in patients before surgery (Jeppsson et al. 1986). Immediate host defense, involving neutrophil activity, immunoglobulin synthesis and complement activation, prevents microbial invasion and colonization. Assessment of the immune status includes: total lymphocyte count, mixed leucocyte response, immunoglobulin levels and phagocytic capacity, complement levels, lym-

phokine production and delayed hypersensitivity skin testing. There is some evidence that anergy to various skin test antigens has a predictive value for the development of sepsis, but caution in the interpretation is needed (Jeppsson et al. 1988). Evidence that either one single test or a combination of tests can predict the incidence and severity of postoperative infection is lacking.

Defense against bacterial invasion is also dependent on nutritional status, hepatic protein-synthetic capacity, and functional capacity of the macrophage system (reticuloendothelial system). There is good evidence that problems such as diffuse intravascular coagulation, acute respiratory distress syndrome, and hypotension postoperatively, are not only caused by gram-negative septicemia, but also by circulating endotoxins, not always prevented by adequate antibiotic therapy.

Future developments in this field could be passive immunization of the patient with anti-lipopolysaccharide antibodies preferably of monoclonal origin (Baumgartner et al. 1985). The optimal moment to administer this immunotherapy depends on early and reliable detection of endotoxinemia. We take adequate antibiotic therapy for granted. The administration of antibiotics should be started preferably at least 24 h before the operation if a history of recent cholangitis is present, or bacterial contamination of the biliary tree is very likely. Prevention of endotoxinemia is not an easy task. Preoperative bowel decontamination did not affect the outcome in the jaundiced patient (Hunt et al. 1982). Preoperative *external* drainage (McPherson et al. 1984, Hatfield et al. 1982) of the patient with biliary obstruction is probably not helpful, since binding of endotoxins in the bowel lumen by bile acids is impaired. Preoperative *internal* drainage may have a better outcome. However, from a theoretical point of view, the advantage of internal bile drainage could be counteracted by insertion of microorganisms into the bile ducts by the endoprosthesis. A well-designed prospective study in this respect is therefore urgently needed.

Renal Function

Two aspects of liver and kidney function in patients with hepatobiliary and pancreatic malignancy are of relevance to the surgeon: a) obstructive jaundice and renal failure, and b) liver insufficiency and functional renal failure, concerning a wide spectrum varying from increased sodium retention to full-blown renal failure, the so-called hepatorenal syndrome (HRS) (Allison 1988).

Obstructive jaundice and renal failure. Despite improvements in intensive care, acute renal failure (ARF) in the jaundiced patient continues to be a significant problem associated with a high mortality rate (Pitt et al. 1981, Blaney et al. 1983, Armstrong et al. 1984, Allison 1988). The exact pathophysiology is still speculative: a combination of renal vasoconstriction, tubular obstruction, impaired glomerular filtration, and black-leakage of filtrate across damaged tubular cells caused by endogenous nephrotoxins (bilirubin, endotoxin, bile acid, etc.) plays a role (Allison 1988). Since the relation between liver insufficiency or cholestatic jaundice and renal failure is well known, the question arises, which patients are particularly at risk?

Statistical evaluation of risk factors measured in large numbers of patients has revealed no special parameter. The following factors may play a role: high plasma bilirubin (> 200 μmol/l, hematocrit $< 30\%$, and albumin < 30 g/l) (Jeppsson et al. 1986), but a specific predictor has not been found. In any case, preoperative management to try to prevent ARF postoperatively should include correction of hypovolemia, hypoalbuminemia and anemia. Known infections should be treated, especially cholangitis. Aminoglycosides should be used very carefully because of their potential nephrotoxicity.

Liver insufficiency and functional renal failure. Renal failure is quite common in liver cirrhosis. Wilkinson et al. (1975) reported an incidence of $50-75\%$. The spectrum varies from impaired sodium excretion to full-blown HRS. HRS should be differentiated from prerenal oliguria and acute tubular necrosis. Prerenal oliguria responds to volume expansion, either well-sustained or unsustained by dopamine. The exact pathophysiology of HRS is still unknown. One essential aspect is vascular instability, with active cortical vasoconstriction (Epstein et al. 1970).

Those at risk are usually suffering from cirrhosis with portal hypertension, jaundice, and hypoalbuminemia, and most of them have moderate to severe ascites. Impaired renal function is often missed, since a sense of false security may be obtained by a normal serum creatinine concentration. Impaired ability to excrete a given sodium load is an early sign of incipient functional renal failure in cirrhotics. Early assessment of the sodium balance can warn the surgeon and internist in making their decision about the risks of major surgery.

Nutritional State

Patients requiring hepatic surgery are at risk preoperatively due to malnutrition, malabsorption, or hepatic dysfunction. The liver plays a central role in the control of carbohydrate, protein and fat metabolism, and stores vitamins. Maintenance of nor-

moglycemia is essential for normal body function. Although an adult liver is able to store only about 70 g of glycogen (less than is required to supply the brain for a day), patients scheduled for liver surgery should receive 1000 ml 10% glucose the evening and the morning before the operation (Jeppsson et al. 1986).

Fat intolerance in jaundiced patients often leads to the prescription of low-fat diets by the clinician, resulting in the patient losing body weight. However, jaundiced patients are able to tolerate parenteral fat suppletion very well, and this is advocated preoperatively if nutritional supplementation is needed. Even cirrhotic patients usually tolerate reasonable amounts of protein (50 g/day) without signs of hepatic encephalopathy. Indication for specific sources of nutritional protein (vegetable protein) or branched-chain amino acids are still controversial (Morgan and Levine 1986). Subclinical vitamin deficiencies may occur in malnourished patients or those with alcoholic liver disease, and should be restored preoperatively by multivitamin therapy, which is cheap and harmless (Morgan and Levine 1986).

Primary and secondary liver tumors can cause abdominal pain, anorexia and weight loss. Dietary history, body weight, body height and skin fold thickness measurements are useful to identify malnutrition. More sophisticated parameters are total body nitrogen or total body potassium measurement, or both, as an index of body cell mass (Goode and Hawkins 1977). Visceral protein status can be assessed by serum albumin ($T^1/_2 = 12$ days), transferrin ($T^1/_2 = 8$ days) or thyroxine-binding prealbumin (TBPA) ($T^1/_2 = 2$ days). Jeppsson et al. (1986) showed that in jaundiced patients, prediction of operative mortality was possible using preoperative TBPA measurement.

Risk factors in hepatobiliary surgery are summarized in Table 5.2.3. However, evaluation of the individual patient undergoing surgery remains particularly difficult. Studying 8 nutritional factors and using linear discriminant analysis, Jeppson et al. (1986) found total body potassium and TBPA to be of greatest help in identifying patients at risk from either major complications or death. Correction of the nutritional state of the patient with hepatobiliary or pancreatic malignancy is of great

Table 5.2.3 Specific risk factors in hepatobiliary surgery. After Jeppson et al. (1986).

Malignancy	Bacterial infection
Diabetes mellitus	Jaundice (Bilirubin > 200 μmol/l)
Liver cirrhosis	Malnutrition
Renal insufficiency	Weight loss $> 10\%$

importance preoperatively, and should be started at an early stage.

Conclusion

Apart from the general preoperative management routine in any major abdominal surgery, patients with hepatobiliary and pancreatic malignancy (HPB) present various specific problems: increased risk of hepatic insufficiency, impaired coagulation, infectious complications and renal failure. The HPB patient is often malnourished due to malabsorption, malnutrition, or both. Insulin-dependent diabetes mellitus in the pancreatic patient is managed in the conventional way. As a consequence, the overall prognosis is closely related to these risk factors.

With regard to liver function, prognostic value can be attributed to the (modified) Child classification for cirrhotic patients, and major surgery on patients in the Child C group should be an exception. A combination of an elimination test (antipyrine, aminopyrine, caffeine) and protein-synthetic capacity measurement (vitamin K-dependent clotting factors, plasma cholinesterase activity) is indicative for hepatic reserve capacity in pre- and post-liver resection patients.

Measures to control malnourishment and volume depletion are important to diminish the risk of postoperative infection and renal failure. Preoperative glycogen loading of the liver by glucose infusion can be advised. Screening of the clotting profile is essential to anticipate bleeding problems. Hemorrhagic diathesis can be prevented by an adequate supply of fresh frozen plasma, purified clotting factors and antithrombin 3. Management of infectious complications is based on early culturing of body fluids and adequate antibiotic therapy. Preoperative drainage of the jaundiced patient is still controversial. Prospective studies in this respect are needed.

Close cooperation between the surgeon, the internist and the anesthetist guarantees the best outcome for the patient.

References

Allison MEM. The kidney and the liver. Pre- and postoperative factors. In: Blumgart LH, ed. Surgery of the liver and biliary tract. Edinburgh: Churchill Livingstone, 1988: 405–421.

Armstrong CP, Dixon JM, Taylor TV, Davies GC. Surgical experience of deeply jaundiced patients with bile duct obstruction. Brit J Surg 1984; 71: 234–238.

Baumgartner JD, Glauser MP, McCutchan JA, et al. Prevention of gram-negative shock and death in surgical patients by antibody to endotoxin core glycolipid. Lancet 1985; ii: 59–63.

Blackburn GL, Menkes E. Surgical immunology. In: Chandra RJ, ed. Primary and secondary immunodeficiency disorders. Edinburgh: Churchill Livingstone, 1983: 263–271.

Blaney SL, Fearon KCH, Gilmour WH, Osborne DH, Carter DC. Prediction of risk in biliary surgery. Brit J Surg 1983; 70: 535–538.

Cavanna A, Molino G, Ballare M, Torchio M, et al. Non-invasive evaluation of portal-systemic shunting in man by D-sorbitol bioavailability. J Hepatol 1987; 5: 154–161.

Clowes GHA, McDermott WW, Williams LF, et al. Amino acid clearance and prognosis in surgical patients with cirrhosis. Surgery 1984; 96: 675–684.

Edwards WH, Blumgart LH. Liver resection in malignant disease. Semin Surg Oncol 1987; 3: 1–11.

Epstein M, Berk DP, Hollenberg NK, Adams DG, Chalmers TC, Abrams HL, et al. Renal failure in the patient with cirrhosis: the role of active vasoconstriction. Am J Med 1970; 49: 175–185.

Gill RA, Goodman MW, Golfus GR, Onstad GR, Bubrick MP. Aminopyrine breath test predicts surgical risk for patients with liver disease. Ann Surg 1983; 198-6: 701–704.

Gips CH, Qué GS, Wibbens Alberts M. The arterial ammonia curve after oral and intraduodenal loading with ammonium acetate. Neth J Med 1973; 16: 14–17.

Goode AW, Hawkins T. The use of 40K counting and its relationship to other estimates of lean body mass. In: Advances in parenteral nutrition. MTP Press, Lancaster 1977.

Hamilton M. A simple discriminant function for hepatic disease. J Clin Pathol 1977; 30: 454–459.

Hatfield ARW, Ter Blanche J, Sataar S, Kernoff L, Tobias R, Girdwood AH, et al. Preoperative external biliary drainage in obstructive jaundice. Lancet 1982; ii: 896–899.

Hunt DR, Allison MEM, Prentice CRM, Blumgart LH. Endotoxemia, disturbance of coagulation, and obstructive jaundice. Am J Surg 1982; 144: 325–329.

Jeppsson B, Halliday AW, Blumgart LH, Bengmark S. Pre- and postoperative nutrition in liver surgery. In: Bengmark S, Blumgart LH, eds. Liver surgery. Edinburgh: Churchill Livingstone, 1986: 166–181.

Kammerer WS, Gross RJ, eds. Medical consultation, role of the internist on surgical, obstetric and psychiatric services. Baltimore: Williams and Wilkins, 1983.

McPherson GAD, Benjamin IS, Boobis AR, Brodie MJ, Hampden C, Blumgart LH. Antipyrine elimination as a dynamic test of hepatic functional integrity in obstructive jaundice. Gut 1982; 23: 734–738.

McPherson GAD, Benjamin IS, Hodgson HJF, Bowley NB, Allison DJ, Blumgart LH. Preoperative percutaneous transhepatic biliary drainage: the results of a controlled trial. Brit J Surg 1984; 71: 371–375.

Morgan MY, Levine JA. Nutritional management of patients with liver disease. J Clin Nutr Gastroenterol 1986; 1: 303–314.

Nagao T, Inque S, Goto S et al. Hepatic resection for hepatocellular carcinoma. Ann Surg 1987; 205: 33–40.

Nagasue N, Yukaya H, Ogawa Y, et al. Clinical experience with 118 hepatic resections for hepatocellular carcinoma. Surgery 1986; 99: 694–701.

Pitt HA, Cameron JL, Posties RG, Gadacz TR. Factors affecting mortality in biliary tract surgery. Am J Surg 1981; 141: 66–72.

Pitt HA, Gomes AS, Lois JF, Mann LL, Deutsch LS, Longmire WP. Does preoperative percutaneous biliary drainage reduce operative risk or increase hospital costs? Ann Surg 1985; 201: 545–553.

Pugh RNH, Murray-Lyon IM, Danson JL, Pietroni MC, Williams R. Transsection of esophagus for bleeding varices. Br J Surg 1973; 60: 646.

Renner E, Wietholtz H, Huguenin P, et al. Caffeïne: a model compound for measuring liver function. Hepatology 1984; 4: 38–46.

Solberg HE, Skrede S, Elgjo K, Blomhoff JP, Gjone E. Classification of liver diseases by clinical chemical laboratory results and cluster analysis. Scand J Clin Lab Invest, 1976; 36: 81–85.

Van der Rijt CCD, Schalm SW, de Groot GH, de Vlieger M. Objective measurement of hepatic encephalopathy by means of automated EEG analysis. Electroencephalogr Clin Neurophysiol 1984; 57: 423–426.

Tarter RE, Sclabassi RJ, Sandford SL, Hays AL, Carra JP, van Thiel DH. Relationship between hepatic injury status and event related potentials. Clin Electroencephalogr 1987; 18: 15–19.

Villeneuve JP, Infante-Rivard C, Ampelas M, et al. Prognostic value of the aminopyrine breath test in cirrhotic patients. Hepatology 1986; 6: 928–931.

Whitwham JG, Morgan M. Anesthesia for major hepatobiliary surgery. In: Blumgart LH, ed. Surgery of the liver and biliary tract. Edinburgh: Churchill Livingstone, 1988: 437–451.

Wilkinson SP, Hirst D, Portman B, Williams R. Pathogenesis of renal failure in cirrhosis and fulminant hepatic failure. Postgrad Med J 1975; 51: 503–505.

Zoli M, Marchesini G, Melli A, et al. Evaluation of liver volume and liver function following hepatic resection in man. Liver 1986; 6: 286–291.

5.3   Hemostasis, Blood Coagulation and Fibrinolysis in Liver Disease

M. Levi, A.W.A. Lensing, and J.W. ten Cate

Role of the Liver in Normal Hemostasis

The liver is the major production site of (non-immunoglobulin) protein, and of most plasma coagulation factors. There is substantial evidence that fibrinogen and factors II, V, VII, VIII:C, IX, X, XI, XII, and XIII, and the coagulation inhibitors antithrombin III, proteins C and S, and the components of the fibrinolytic system, plasminogen and α-2-antiplasmin respectively, are all synthesized by the liver. In addition, it has become clear that the liver contributes to coagulation and its control by removing activated clotting factors from the circulation (Mannucci and Forman 1982) (Table 5.3.1).

Production of Coagulation Components

Of all the plasma coagulation factors, factors II, VII, IX, and X are dependent on vitamin K for synthesis. Vitamin K is required for the γ-carboxylation of precursor molecules within the hepatocytes. In addition, fibrinogen and factors V and VIII:C are also produced within the liver. The liver is the sole source of plasma fibrinogen with a steady state synthetic rate of 1.7 to 5.0 g/day and with synthetic potential of up to a possible 20-fold increase in production rate. Platelet fibrinogen may not be solely derived from the liver, since normal fibrinogen in platelets of patients with abnormal plasma fibrinogen has been described. The biosynthesis of factor V has been demonstrated in a human hepatocellular carcinoma cell line, confirming other indirect evidence that the liver is the major source of plasma factor V. Recent liver perfusion studies have tended to favor the liver as the source of factor VIII:C. Severe hepatic failure, however, does not lead to factor VIII deficiency, and several observations suggest that another cell type, present in several organs, may be the real location of factor VIII synthesis. Recent studies suggest that factor VIII synthesis may occur in hepatic sinusoidal endothelial cells. The vitamin K-dependent coagulation inhibitors protein C and protein S, and the non-vitamin K-dependent coagulation inhibitor antithrombin III, are also synthesized by the liver.

With regard to the fibrinolytic system, plasminogen, the inactive precursor of plasmin, is thought to be synthesized by liver cells. Granulocytes, particularly the eosinophils, are known to contain plasminogen, and the possibility that these cells manufacture the protein has not been ruled

Table 5.3.**1**   **The clotting cascade.** Solid lines indicate direct activation of precursor zymogen to enzyme; interrupted lines show paths of inhibition

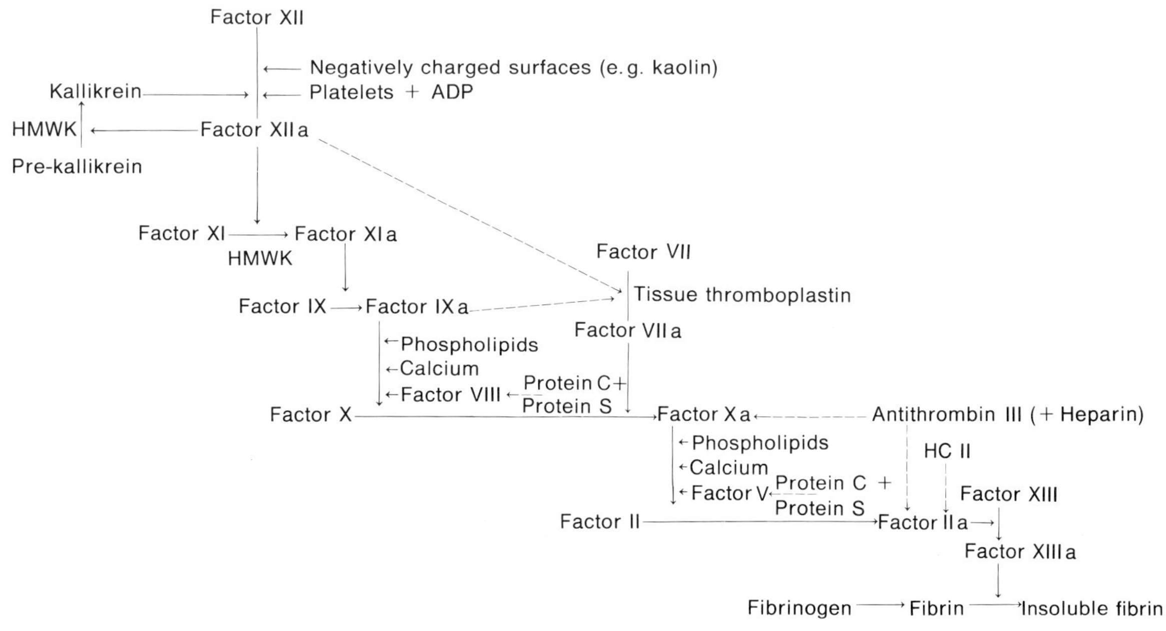

ADP: adenosine diphosphate; HC: heparin cofactor; HMWK: high molecular weight kinninogen

out. It appears that α-2-antiplasmin is also synthesized by the liver, and is homologous with other proteolytic inhibitors of hepatic origin.

Hepatic Clearance of Activated Coagulation Components

There is evidence to suggest that the normal liver contributes to coagulation homeostasis by removing active clotting factors from the circulation (Deykin 1966). It has been shown that intravascular coagulation was less intense when blood thromboplastin was injected into the portal circulation than when the same thromboplastin was injected into the peripheral circulation (Spaet et al. 1961). These experiments also indicated that thromboplastin was removed from the circulation by the hepatic reticuloendothelial system. Later reports have indicated that the normal liver is capable of removing activated clotting factors from the circulation. It has been demonstrated that perfusion of serum through the liver reduces the levels of activated factors, while unactivated factors are not affected. It seems clear that the normal liver is capable of clearing the circulating blood of clot-promoting proteins that might otherwise cause continuing coagulation. Evidence has also been presented to show that the normal liver rapidly clears plasminogen activator from the circulation, by a mechanism which is as yet not explained.

Hemostasis in Liver Disease

Hemostatic abnormalities in liver disease comprise a large spectrum of defects: decreased synthesis of coagulation factors, impaired clearance of activated coagulation factors by the liver, dysfibrinogenemia, quantitative and qualitative platelet abnormalities, vitamin K-dependent clotting factor deficiency, accelerated fibrinolysis, and disseminated intravascular coagulation. Hemostatic abnormalities often share common characteristics in patients with acute toxic or infectious hepatitis, chronic liver disease, biliary obstruction and other liver diseases. Those of relevance to hepatobiliary and pancreatic malignancy will be discussed here.

Chronic Hepatocellular Disease

Although the majority of patients with chronic liver disease demonstrate coagulation abnormalities, clinically severe coagulation disorders are rare. Several clotting factors and inhibitors are inadequately synthesized; thrombocytopenia, thrombocytopathy, and dysfibrinogenemia may also occur.

Thrombocytopenia and Thrombocytopathy in Cirrhosis of the Liver

Thrombocytopenia in liver cirrhosis may be mild to moderate. It is caused by increased platelet pooling in the spleen due to congestive splenomegaly and enhanced sequestration of platelets at the site of incompletely endothelialized sinusoids of the regenerating liver, resulting in decreased platelet survival (Toghill et al. 1977). Other mechanisms may be operative in patients with alcoholic liver disease, such as folic acid deficiency, mostly due to inadequate dietary intake, and direct toxic effects of ethanol on megakaryocytes and circulating platelets (Cowan 1980). Platelet function abnormalities are often seen in patients with chronic liver disease. An inhibitory effect of fibrinogen degradation products (FDPs) on platelets seems unlikely, as plasma FDP levels and platelet dysfunction do not correlate. Various pathogenic explanations for these platelet defects similar to those described in acute hepatic failure have been considered: 1) a reduction in the number of the larger and more hemostatically active platelets; 2) an alteration in cholesterol:phospholipid ratios, associated with reduced availability of arachidonic acid; 3) a decrease in total platelet adenine nucleotides, associated with an increased adenosine triphosphate:adenosine diphosphate (ATP:ADP) ratio (Rubin et al. 1977). In patients with alcoholic liver cirrhosis, additional factors may be considered, e.g. direct toxic effects of ethanol on platelets.

Coagulation Protein and Fibrinolysis Abnormalities in Chronic Liver Disease

Clotting factors and clotting inhibitors are inadequately synthesized because of progressive loss of liver parenchymal cells in chronic liver disease (Rapaport et al. 1960). Plasma fibrinogen is normal or even increased in the majority of patients with stable chronic liver disease, but mild to moderate hypofibrinogenemia is occasionally seen. The hypofibrinogenemia could be caused by impaired synthesis, enhanced consumption – disseminated intravascular coagulation (DIC) – or due to pooling into extravascular spaces (ascites) (Michell 1975). Dysfibrinogenemia is common in liver cirrhosis, but whether this disorder contributes to abnormal bleeding is unclear. Accelerated fibrinolysis – as measured by the euglobulin clot lysis time and a hyperfibrinolytic state – is observed in chronic liver disease, and is probably due to increased levels of plasminogen activators in plasma due to impaired hepatic clearance and decreased levels of α-2-antiplasmin and histidine-rich glycoprotein. This enhanced fibrinolysis could also be explained as a mechanism secondary to DIC (Tytgat et al. 1968).

Disseminated Intravascular Coagulation in Chronic Liver Disease

Low-grade DIC often occurs in patients with chronic severe liver disease. Shortened fibrinogen survival disposes towards DIC, and this can be prolonged towards normal by the administration of heparin or human antithrombin III concentrate (Schipper and ten Cate 1982). As pathogenic pathways for DIC, the same mechanisms as described in acute liver disease are to be considered. Release of thromboplastic substances from necrotic hepatocytes into the circulation, and liberation of intestine-derived endotoxins into the portal system, in particular, may play an important role in the initiation of DIC, which can be facilitated by impaired clearance of activated clotting factors by the liver and reduced levels of coagulation inhibitors such as antithrombin III and protein C. However, the antithrombin III deficiency in cirrhosis appears to be due more to impaired synthesis and accelerated transcapillary flux than to intravascular consumption (Knot et al. 1984).

Cholestasis

Biliary tract obstruction caused by neoplasms or stones may rarely result in impaired absorption of vitamin K and subsequent coagulation abnormalities. More prolonged obstruction causes a decrease in factors II, VII, IX and X. Moreover, fibrinolysis may be impaired, partly due to a decrease in the level of protein C (Dioguardi et al. 1973).

Neoplastic Liver Disease

Coagulation abnormalities in patients with neoplastic liver disease are comparable to those in patients with chronic liver disease, with the exception that in patients with neoplastic liver disease, plasma fibrinogen is almost always elevated.

An association between hepatoma and dysfibrinogenemia also exists, with defective fibrin polymerization and hypersialated fibrinogen. It is not clear whether the abnormal fibrinogen is produced by cirrhotic hepatocytes or hepatoma cells. Liver tumors can cause hemostatic problems due to changes in the vascular pattern in the organ. Hepatocellular carcinoma almost always develops in cirrhotic livers in which vessels and sinusoids are embedded in fibrotic tissue, so that contraction, as a physiological response to injury, is hampered (van der Watt et al. 1977).

Intrahepatic Portal Vein Thrombosis and Intrahepatic Hemorrhage

Intrahepatic portal vein thrombosis, or Budd–Chiari syndrome, may be associated with drug ingestion (especially use of oral contraceptives) as well as with underlying diseases such as vena caval web or septum, hepatic tumors, hypercoagulability, myeloproliferative disorders (polycythemia vera) or thrombosis of the hepatic veins or the inferior vena cava. The Budd–Chiari syndrome has a very poor prognosis (Ecker et al. 1966). As with intrahepatic thrombosis, hemorrhage into the liver has been reported in a group of patients exposed to anabolic steroids or oral contraceptives. Intrahepatic hemorrhage may occur in addition to intrahepatic microvascular thrombosis, as for example in ecclampsia of pregnancy.

Hemostatic Problems in Surgical Procedures on the Liver

Hemostatic problems have been encountered in specific surgical procedures of the liver such as portosystemic shunts, hepatic resection, liver transplants and peritoneovenous shunts.

Portocaval shunt surgery for portal hypertension may be complicated by excessive bleeding and exacerbation of pre-existing hemostatic abnormalities, particularly accelerated fibrinolysis. Low fibrinogen levels and marked spontaneous fibrinolytic activity are present in cirrhotic patients, with clotting abnormalities during shunt procedures (Grossi et al. 1962).

Extensive liver resection, either for trauma or for tumor, has been associated with a variety of hemostatic abnormalities. Major resection is accompanied with a transient decrease in vitamin K-dependent clotting factors and an increase in plasma fibrinogen concentration. Elevated levels of FDP have been reported (Iwatsuki et al. 1983).

Acute and often severe hemostatic disorders can follow liver transplantation. The most critical period is the brief anhepatic phase that occurs during the surgical procedure or the period directly thereafter. The acute coagulopathy is probably due to the temporary failure to remove activated coagulation factors and fibrinolytic activators that are released into the circulation during surgical trauma. The state of preservation of the transplanted organ closely corresponds to the severity and duration of the hemostatic disorders. If the transplanted liver is damaged, the coagulopathy persists and may become worse. However, when the graft is in good condition, the coagulation abnormalities resolve rapidly. Hepatic transplant rejection is accompanied with low-grade DIC, and is therefore similar to the situation encountered in renal rejection. The features most frequently encountered are an increase in serum FDP and thrombocytopenia. Immune-mediated injury of the vascular endothelium induced by transplant rejection, and release of procoagulant substances from the ischemically damaged hepatocyte, may be responsible for further activation of disseminated intravascular coagulation (Knot et al. 1989). Peritoneovenous (or Le Veen) shunt insertion causing reinfusion of ascitic fluid may cause DIC and occasionally serious bleeding, due to cellular and soluble procoagulants in the ascitic fluid. Removing most of the ascitic fluid from the peritoneal cavity before insertion of the shunt can reduce the risk of DIC substantially.

Coagulation Tests in Hepatic Disease

The coagulation defect in liver disease is complex, involving many stages in the coagulation mechanism and thus potentially affecting all global coagulation and hemostatic tests. Thrombocytopenia and platelet dysfunction are revealed by platelet count and bleeding time tests. Reduction in the levels of all coagulation factors are reflected by a prolonged activated partial thromboplastin time (APTT) and prothrombin time (PT). A marked prolongation of the PT is restricted to extensive hepatocellular injury only. The PT may be prolonged even when the APTT is still normal, due to a selective decrease of factor VII synthesis, the most sensitive coagulation factor in liver disease because of its short half-life. In addition, vitamin K deficiency does not in general affect the APTT while it prolongs the PT. Thus, a prolonged PT may be explained by two mechanisms, easily differentiated by the ability of the liver to utilize parenteral vitamin K. Obstructive jaundice results in reduced vitamin K absorption from the gastrointestinal tract, and may be associated with an increase in PT due to a deficiency of vitamin K-dependent factors. This can be corrected by parenteral vitamin K administration. In the case of extensive parenchymal damage, the liver utilization of parenteral vitamin K is defective, and correction of the PT will not occur. The thrombin time may be prolonged due to hypofibrinogenemia or dysfibrinogenemia when concurrent heparin administration or paraproteinemia are excluded. The fibrinolytic system is likewise liver-dependent, so that liver disease will affect plasminogen and α-2-antiplasmin plasma concentrations. The fibrinolytic parameters may also be influenced by an enhanced fibrinolytic state in liver disease, which can be observed in decreased levels of fibrinogen and plasminogen. DIC in liver disease may occur as described above, and will result in prolonged APTT and PT, decreased platelet count, raised FDPs and decreased antithrombin III, fibrinogen and plasminogen concentrations (Biland et al. 1978, Christensen et al. 1985). The Normotest, which reflects any reduction of vitamin K-dependent factors (except factor IX) has in the past been considered a more sensitive test compared to PT in liver disease, but is not now thought to be superior to PT.

Management of the Coagulation Defect in Liver Disease

Although it may be difficult to determine the underlying hemostatic defects, the therapeutic strategy must be adapted to the specific clinical circumstances and the pathophysiological disorder. Patients who are not bleeding, in spite of a deficiency in coagulation factors and abnormal coagulation tests, need no special treatment. Treatment is indicated depending on the clinical circumstances (e.g. bleeding) or prophylactically before liver biopsy or surgery. Correction of the hemostatic defect must be accompanied by general supportive measures and more specific clinical interventions, such as sclerotherapy of bleeding esophageal varices.

Vitamin K (10 mg s.c. or i.v.) will achieve maximal correction of the PT within 24 h. Abnormality of PT persisting beyond this period indicates hepatocellular dysfunction.

Fresh frozen plasma (FFP) contains all coagulation factors and inhibitors present in blood and thus theoretically represents the most appropriate product for the correction of multiple defects found in liver disease. A disadvantage of the use of FFP in correcting the coagulation factor deficiency is the requirement of large amounts of plasma, with the subsequent problem of fluid overload. This problem can be overcome by exchange transfusion in combination with transfusion of FFP. An approach of this sort only has a temporary effect, but may be appropriate during a life-threatening period of hemostatic failure. The effects of FFP last for a few hours. In patients undergoing surgery, repeated administration of FFP will be necessary to obtain hemostatic improvement (Mannucci et al. 1976).

Another therapeutic strategy is represented by **prothrombin complex concentrates** (PCC), which contain variable concentrations of factor II, VII, IX and X. Despite potential benefits, there are serious limitations to their use (Blatt et al. 1981). An increase in the incidence of thromboembolic events and perhaps even DIC has been associated with the administration of PCC. PCC contains variable amounts of activated coagulation factors (II a, X a, VII a, IX a) which cannot be adequately neutralized in patients with liver disease due to the reduced plasma concentration of antithrombin III and impaired hepatic clearance. Moreover, some coagulation factors that are decreased in liver disease are not present in significant amounts in PCC (such as factor V). Stopping the bleeding and correcting the coagulation tests may thus not be accomplished by infusion of PCC alone. Lastly, despite increased sensitivity of techniques for detection of the hepatitis virus and careful screening of all pooled plasma, the risk of transmitting HIV or, in particular, non-A non-B hepatitis is still present, although this risk is markedly reduced or even eliminated with heat-treated concentrates. Contamination through activated coagulation factors may soon be reduced by improved fractionation techniques and in vitro testing for spontaneous thrombin generation. The risk of thromboembolism may also be diminished by the concomitant administration of FFP to increase the levels of antithrombin III or by human antithrombin III concentrate. The simultaneous infusion of FFP may also correct the coagulation factors that are deficient but not present in PCC (such as factor V). Maximal correction is obtained by the combination of FFP and PCC and is achieved within 15 min, enabling a liver biopsy to be carried out (Mannucci et al. 1976). However, taking into account the potential complications and the lack of evidence for clinical effectiveness in the control of bleeding, PCC cannot generally be recommended in patients with liver disease.

Platelet transfusions may be considered in patients with marked thrombocytopenia and serious bleeding. However, platelet concentrates may be ineffective due to rapid removal of the platelets by the enlarged spleen in liver cirrhosis. In patients with bleeding, or the risk of bleeding in the case of liver biopsy, thrombocytopenia is an obvious hazard. However, when a correctly performed and standardized bleeding time reveals normal values, platelet transfusion is not required. When the bleeding time is prolonged, platelets have to be transfused.

Heparin treatment has been considered in patients with liver disease to counteract the concurrent low-grade DIC (Gazzard et al. 1974). Esophageal varices and other gastrointestinal lesions often complicate liver disease, and the heparin-enhanced risk of bleeding must be considered with extreme care. Moreover, the results of heparin treatment are variable, and its clinical efficacy has not been proved in a controlled clinical study. Heparin treatment of patients with a severe coagulation disorder of hepatic origin may be indicated in the case of thromboembolic complications. Alternative treatment with a caval vein filter to prevent pulmonary embolism should be seriously considered.

Human **antithrombin III concentrates** have been effectively used in patients with liver cirrhosis and DIC, and in fulminant hepatitis or acute fatty liver of pregnancy. However, prevention of DIC by administering antithrombin III concentrates following Le Veen shunt insertion was not successful (Büller and ten Cate 1983). Adequately controlled trials have not yet been performed, and its use should be limited to the treatment of severe DIC and bleeding.

Desmopressin has been introduced as a new therapeutic approach in recent years. Desmopressin (i.v.) produces a substantial increase in the plasma concentration of factor VIII:C and factor VIII:WF (von Willebrand factor), and is used in the treatment of patients with von Willebrand's disease and with mild or moderate hemophilia A. Desmopressin shortens bleeding in patients with a variety of bleeding disorders, and is effectively used in these patients for prophylaxis and treatment of bleeding. Infusion of desmopressin in cirrhotic patients induces a variable shortening of the prolonged bleeding time and of APTT, and an increase of factors VIII:C, VIII:WF, XI and XII (Levi et al. 1988). The efficacy of desmopressin in cirrhotic patients with bleeding has never been described, and the clinical relevance of its use therefore remains to be established.

Fibrinolytic inhibitors such as ε-aminocaproic acid and tranexamic acid may inhibit a hyperfibrinolytic state. However, controlled clinical studies have not yet been carried out either in stable cirrhotic patients or in bleeding patients with liver disease.

References

Biland L, Duckert F, Prisender S, Nyman D. Quantitative estimation of coagulation factors in liver disease: the diagnostic and prognostic value of factor XIII, factor V, and plasminogen. Thromb Haemost 1978; 39: 646.

Blatt PM, White GC, Kindgon HS. Use of prothrombin complex concentrates in acquired coagulopathies. In: Lusher JM, Barnhart MI, eds. Acquired disorders in children: abnormalities of hemostasis. New York: Masson, 1981: 127.

Büller HR, ten Cate JW. Antithrombin III infusion in patients undergoing peritoneovenous shunt operation: failure in the prevention of DIC. Thromb Haemostas 1983; 49: 128–131.

Christensen E, Schlichting P, Fauerholdt L, et al., and the Copenhagen Study Group for Liver Disease. Changes of laboratory variables with time in cirrhosis: prognostic and therapeutic significance. Hepatology 1985; 5: 843.

Cowan DH. Effect of alcoholism on hemostasis. Semin Hematol 1980; 17: 137.

Deykin D. The role of liver in serum induced hypercoagulability. J Clin Invest 1966; 45: 256–263.

Dioguardi N, Mari D, Del Ninno E, Mannucci PM. Fibrinolysis in cholestatic jaundice. Br Med J 1973; ii: 778.

Ecker JA, McKittrick JE, Failing RM. Thrombosis of the hepatic veins: the Budd–Chiari syndrome. Am J Gastroenterol 1966; 45: 429–443.

Gazzard BG, Clarke R, Bori-Kakchanyavat Y, Williams R. A controlled trial of heparin therapy in the coagulation defect of paracetamol induced hepatic necrosis. Gut 1974; 15: 89.

Grossi CE, Rousselot LM, Panke WF. Coagulation defects in patients with cirrhosis of the liver undergoing porta-systemic shunts. Am J Surg 1962; 104: 512.

Harmon DC, Demirjian Z, Ellman L, Fischer JE. Disseminated intravascular coagulation with the peritoneovenous shunt. Ann Intern Med 1979; 90: 774.

Iwatsuki S, Shaw BW, Starzl TE. Experience with 150 liver resections. Ann Surg 1983; 197: 247.

Knot E, ten Cate JW, Drijfhout HR, et al. Antithrombin III metabolism in patients with liver disease. J Clin Pathol 1984; 37: 523.

Knot EAR, Porte RJ, Terpstra OT, et al. Coagulation and fibrinolysis in the first human auxiliary partial liver transplantation in Rotterdam. Fibrinolysis 1989 (in press).

Levi M, Agnelli G, Longetti M, et al. DDAVP and haemostasis in chronic liver disease. Fibrinolysis 1988; 2: 74.

Mannucci PM, Forman SP. Hemostasis and liver disease. In: Colman RW, et al., eds. Hemostasis and thrombosis: basic principles and clinical practice. Philadelphia: Lippincott, 1982.

Mannucci PM, Franchi F, Dioguardi N. Correction of abnormal coagulation in chronic liver disease by combined use of fresh-frozen plasma and prothrombin complex concentrates. Lancet 1976; ii: 542.

Michell RH: Inositol phospholipids and cell surface receptor function. Biochim Biophys Acta 1975; 415: 81.

Rapaport SI, Ames SB, Mikkelsen S, Goodman JR. Plasma clotting factors in chronic hepatocellular disease. N Engl J Med 1960; 263: 278.

Rubin MH, Weston MJ, Bullock G, et al. Abnormal platelet function and ultrastructure in fulminant hepatic failure. Q J Med 1977; 46: 339.

Schipper HG, ten Cate JW. Antithrombin III transfusion in patients with hepatic cirrhosis. Br J Haematol 1982; 52: 25.

Spaet H, Horowitz HI, Franklin DZ, et al. Reticuloendothelial clearance of blood thromboplastin by rats. Blood 1961; 17: 196.

Toghill PJ, Green S, Ferguson R. Platelet dynamics in chronic liver disease with special reference to the role of the spleen. J Clin Pathol 1977; 30: 367.

Tytgat GN, Collen D, de Vreker RR, Verstraete M. Investigations on the fibrinolytic system in liver cirrhosis. Acta Haematol 1968; 40: 265.

Tytgat GN, Collen D, Verstraete M. Metabolism of fibrinogen in cirrhosis of the liver. J Clin Invest 1971; 50: 1690.

Van der Watt JA, Gomperts ED, Kew MC. Hemostatic factors in primary hepatocellular cancer. Cancer 1977; 40: 1593.

6 Surgical Management of Malignant Tumors of the Liver

6.1 Expectations and Possibilities of Liver Resection in the Management of Hepatocellular Carcinoma

T. K. Choi and J. Wong

Hepatocellular carcinoma (HCC) is one of the most common malignant neoplasms in the world. Its incidence varies greatly according to geographical location, and is at its highest in sub-Saharan Africa. The annual age-standardized rate in Mozambique is 103.8 per 100 000 males. The rate is about 30 per 100 000 for Chinese males in Southeast Asia. Southeast Asian males of other ethnic groups, and Japanese males, have a lower incidence, at 6–15 per 100 000. For the rest of the world, the incidence is still lower, between 2 and 5 per 100 000 population (Linsell and Higginson 1976, Menck and Henderson 1982).

Since the early 1970s, screening programs have been in progress in China, Japan and Taiwan to discover HCC at an early stage. These programs cover entire populations (Shanghai Group 1979, Tang et al. 1980), or high risk individuals (Shinagawa et al. 1984, Heyward et al. 1985, Sheu et al. 1985, Lee et al. 1986). Most of the patients identified as harboring HCCs are asymptomatic, and many of the tumors are less than 5 cm in diameter. The resectability, operative mortality and prognosis for small tumors differ from those for larger tumors, which are usually found in patients presenting with symptoms. These two catagories of HCC (large and small) will therefore be discussed separately.

Expectations and Possibilities of Liver Resection for Large (Symptomatic) Tumors

The analysis of the results of the screening programs mentioned, and clinical pathological studies of small and subclinical HCC (Chen et al. 1982, Tang et al. 1982, Nagasue et al. 1984, Okuda et al. 1977), shed light on the natural history of this tumor. It is now known that for most tumors, the growth is relentless and exponential, terminating in the death of the patient. The duration from the first detectable rise in the serum alpha-fetoprotein level to a subclinical tumor of 4 cm in diameter is about 10 months. In about 4 more months, the tumor will enlarge to 9 cm in diameter, and it is at this stage that patients start to have symptoms. Death occurs another four months later (Tang et al. 1982, Nagasue et al. 1984). Thus, by the time a patient seeks a doctor's advice because of symptoms, the tumor is large and the patient's condition is rapidly deteriorating. Moreover, in most reports from Asia, the proportion of patients with liver cirrhosis is as high as 85% (Lee et al. 1982). Resection may be impossible in some patients not because of the advanced staging of the tumor, but because of the advanced cirrhotic state, often in combination with its strategic location. The rate of resection for patients presenting with symptoms is thus low, between 9% and 27% (Lee et al. 1982, Okuda 1980, Ong and Chan 1976, Liver Cancer Study Group of Japan 1984). The rate is higher in reports from Western countries (Fortner et al. 1978, Lim and Bongard 1984), probably because of the lower

Table 6.1.1 Survival after resection of hepatocellular carcinoma

Authors	n	Operative mortality (%)	Survival (%)				
			1 yr	2 yr	3 yr	4 yr	5 yr
+* Lin (1976)	118	11.8	35.0	24.4	20.0	–	19.0
+ Lee et al. (1982)	165	20.0	45.0	30.0	20.0	–	20.0
+* Wu et al. (1980)	181	8.8	55.9	36.8	38.9	–	16.0
Lee et al. (1986)	47	–	76.0	–	–	8.0	–
Lim and Bongard (1984)	22	36.0	35.7	–	–	–	–
Li et al. (1985)	100	11.4	–	–	34.1	–	23.5
* Nagao et al. (1987)	94	19.0	73.0	–	42.0	–	25.0
Liver Cancer Study Group of Japan (1984)	243	–	56.0	35.0	–	–	–
+ Foster (1970)	296	24.0	–	33.3	–	–	14.0
	Asian	24.0	–	23.0	–	–	6.0
	Non-Asian	22.0	–	59.0	–	–	36.0
+ Fortner et al. (1978)	42	16.7	85.0	–	50.0	–	37.0
+* Adson and Weiland (1981)	60	6.7	–	–	65.0	–	36.0
+ Iwatsuki et al. (1983)	43	9.3	77.8	59.5	55.7	–	46.0
Thompson et al. (1983)	26	26.9	–	–	–	–	38.0

+ A small number of other primary liver tumors included
* operative death excluded in calculating percentage survival

incidence of liver cirrhosis (Foster 1970). For large tumors, the operations performed are right or left hepatic lobectomy, extended right hepatectomy (right trisegmentectomy), or left trisegmentectomy (Starzl et al. 1982). For tumors involving the left lateral segment, a left lateral segment resection may suffice. A resection margin of 3 cm of normal liver beyond the area involved (by the main tumor or by satellite nodules) is considered sufficient. The margin may be reduced to 1 cm if obtaining a larger margin will lead to additional loss of limited functional liver parenchyma in cirrhotic patients (Liver Cancer Study Group of Japan 1984, Kanematsu et al. 1984). However, the site of the tumor may preclude the preservation of an intact segment or lobe of the liver.

The results of liver resection are shown in Table 6.1.1. The most frequent complications encountered were postoperative intra-abdominal hemorrhage, gastrointestinal bleeding, liver failure, subphrenic abscesses, pleural effusion, and bile leakage. The operative mortality ranged from 6.7% to 36%. The common causes of death were liver failure, intra-abdominal hemorrhage, and sepsis from subphrenic or intra-abdominal abscesses.

The presence of liver cirrhosis greatly influences operative mortality. Virtually all patients developing liver failure have some degree of liver cirrhosis. Hemorrhage during or after the operative procedure also occurs more frequently in cirrhosis due to defective coagulation. Nagasue et al. (1986) showed that in their series of 118 liver resections, 32 out of 33 complications and all the operative deaths occurred in the group with liver cirrhosis.

The postoperative survival of Asian patients is worse than that of non-Asian patients. For Asian patients, the one-year survival rate ranges from 35% to 50%, the two-year survival rate is between 24% and 36%, and the five-year survival rate ranges from less than 10% to 25% (Table 6.1.1). The postoperative survival of Western patients is 77 to 85% for one year and 37 to 46% for five years (Table 6.1.1). Thus, the survival of Asian patients is poor even after a successful resection. This may also be a reflection of the high incidence of liver cirrhosis. An analysis of the cause of late death in a combined Japanese study (Liver Cancer Study Group of Japan 1984) showed that residual or recurrent HCC was directly responsible for death in 34% of the patients, liver failure was the cause in 34%, and gastrointestinal bleeding from esophageal varices or other sources was the cause in 18% of the patients. The incidence of liver cirrhosis in this study was 45%, indicating that surgical series are biased in selecting patients with non-cirrhotic livers. This and another study (Nagasue et al. 1986) also emphasized that the survival of non-cirrhotics after liver resection is much better than that of cirrhotics and is on a par with that of non-Asian patients.

Expectations and Possibilities of Liver Resection for Small (Asymptomatic) Tumors

The screening of high-risk individuals or populations with a high annual incidence of HCC has

Table 6.1.2   Survival after resection of small hepatocellular carcinoma

Authors	n	Operative mortality (%)	Survival (%) 1 yr	2 yr	3 yr	4 yr	5 yr
Tang et al. (1982)	+ 66	–	79.1	67.8	61.6	55.5	–
Hsu et al. (1985)	49	8.2	81.6	77.6	–	–	–
* Kanematsu et al. (1984)	32	12.5	85.0	70.0	–	–	22.0
Lee et al. (1986)	62	3.0	92.0	–	44.0	–	–

+ All cases diagnosed by mass survey and treated by resection, including some tumors greater than 5 cm in diameter
* Operative death excluded in calculating survival

detected tumors at an early stage. The serum alpha-fetoprotein level, high resolution real-time ultrasonography, or both, are employed for screening. Suspicious nodules are usually aspirated under ultrasound or computed tomography guidance for cytological confirmation (Tatsuta et al. 1984, Ajdukiewicz et al. 1985). Screening tests are repeated every three to four months. Not all asymptomatic HCCs are small. Only about 50% of those discovered at initial screening are less than 5 cm in diameter (Sheu et al. 1985). The tumors discovered on subsequent screening of the same individuals are usually small. Approximately 25% of small HCCs are accompanied by satellite nodules. The number of satellite nodules is usually less than five, and they are situated around the main tumor (Chen et al. 1982, Okuda et al. 1977, Hsu et al. 1985).

Approximately 60% of asymptomatic HCCs are resectable (Shanghai Group 1979). Limited resection is carried out for small HCCs; segmentectomy or subsegmentectomy usually suffice. Enucleation with a small margin of uninvolved liver is acceptable if the liver is severely cirrhotic and the tumor is uninodular (Kanematsu et al. 1984). The results of resection are shown in Table 6.1.2. The operative mortality was between 3% and 12.5%. The one-year survival rate was over 80%, and the four-year survival rate was 44% to 55%. As all these reports are confined to Asian patients, compared with large tumors in a similar population, it appears that the prognosis after resection is much better when the tumors are discovered early and are small. The improvement in survival may in part be due to the higher proportion of functional liver parenchyma remaining after resection. The chance of patients dying from liver failure or other complications related to liver cirrhosis is less.

Liver Resection in Patients with Cirrhosis

Cirrhosis presents a special problem in patients undergoing liver resection (Kanematsu et al. 1984, Kinami et al. 1986, Bismuth et al. 1986). Patients with cirrhosis have a higher chance of succumbing to operative complications and developing postoperative liver failure. Besides the usual panel of blood tests, the indocyanine green (ICG) or bromosulfophthalein retention tests are useful in evaluating the liver function of patients preoperatively. The indocyanine green retention test has been combined with the measurement of the proportion of functional liver parenchyma to be resected, to predict whether a patient will survive the resective procedure (Okamoto et al. 1984). For patients with an ICG_{15min} retention of greater than 30%, resections other than the enucleation of small tumors are not advisable. If the ICG_{15min} retention is between 15% and 30%, major resection should not be performed unless the amount of uninvolved parenchyma resected is less than 40%. Enucleation of tumors with a margin of 1 cm or less has been shown to be accompanied by an acceptable operative mortality as well as survival in patients with small HCCs and liver cirrhosis (Kanematsu et al. 1984). The majority of small tumors are encapsulated, and vascular invasion is less common (Chen et al. 1982, Hsu et al. 1985). Penetration through the capsule, if it occurs, is only limited to a short distance in the pericapsular parenchyma. Enucleation with a 1 cm margin is theoretically an adequate operation for such tumors, and should be performed whenever possible in cirrhotic patients.

In conclusion, for advanced HCC, the results of resection are poor and survival severely limited. Further major improvement on the operative mortality may not be expected, as it has probably reached the lower limit. Modern pre- and postoperative care, anesthetic techniques and antibiotics have decreased, but not eliminated, the number of deaths due to intraoperative blood loss, coagulopathy and postoperative infection. Late deaths are usually caused by local recurrence, multicentricity, liver failure, or other consequences of cirrhosis. On the other hand, the radicality of the resection is limited by the segmental arrangements of the blood supply and the degree of cirrhosis. There is no foreseeable solution to the cirrhotic condition. Thus it is not realistic to expect improvement on long-term survival. Liver transplantation has been performed on patients with HCC (Iwatsuki et al. 1985), and this procedure merits more evaluation because the cirrhotic condition is also treated, but the development of metastatic disease is unpredictable. In spite of the generally unfavorable outcome, surgical resection should still be performed if possible, because it offers the only hope of cure for the patient. The prognosis of small HCC is good. The main obstacle is the low yield of the screening programs. Further research into the risk factors of developing HCC is worthwhile.

References

Adson MA, Weiland LH. Resection of primary solid hepatic tumours. Am J Surg 1981; 141: 18–21.

Ajdukiewicz A, Crowden A, Hudson E, Pyne C. Liver aspiration in the diagnosis of hepatocellular carcinoma in Gambia. J Clin Pathol 1985; 38: 185–192.

Bismuth H, Houssin D, Ornowski J, Meriggi F. Liver resections in cirrhotic patients: a Western experience. World J Surg 1986; 10: 311–317.

Chen DS, Sheu JC, Sung JL, et al. Small hepatocellular carcinoma: a clinicopathological study in thirteen patients. Gastroenterology 1982; 83: 1109–1119.

Fortner JG, Kim DK, Maclean BJ, et al. Major hepatic resection for neoplasia: personal experience in 108 patients. Ann Surg 1978; 188: 363–369.

Foster JH. Survival after liver resection for cancer. Cancer 1970; 26: 493–502.

Heyward WL, Lanier AP, McMahon BJ, Fitzgerald MA, Kilkenny S, Paprocki TR. Early detection of primary hepatocellular carcinoma: screening for primary hepatocellular carcinoma among persons infected with hepatitis B virus. JAMA 1985; 254: 3052–3054.

Hsu HC, Sheu JC, Lui YH, et al. Prognostic histological features of resected small hepatocellular carcinoma (HCC) in Taiwan. Cancer 1985; 56: 672–680.

Iwatsuki S, Shaw BW, Starzl TE. Experience with 150 liver resections. Ann Surg 1983; 197: 247–253.

Iwatsuki S, Gordon RD, Shaw BW, Starzl TE. Role of liver transplantation in cancer therapy. Ann Surg 1985; 202: 401–407.

Kanematsu T, Takenaka K, Matsumata T, Furnita T, Sugimachi K, Inokuchi K. Limited hepatic resection effective for selected cirrhotic patients with primary liver cancer. Ann Surg 1984; 199: 51–56.

Kinami Y, Takashima S, Miyazaki I. Hepatic resection for hepatocellular carcinoma associated with liver cirrhosis. World J Surg 1986; 10: 294–301.

Lee CS, Sung JL, Hwang LY, et al. Surgical treatment of 109 patients with symptomatic and asymptomatic hepatocellular carcinoma. Surgery 1986; 99: 481–490.

Lee NW, Wong J, Ong GB. The surgical management of primary carcinoma of the liver. World J Surg 1982; 6: 66–75.

Li GC, Wang CE, Zhu SL, et al. Hepatectomy for primary liver cancer in 114 cases. Chin Med J 1985; 98: 377–383.

Lim RC, Bongard FS. Hepatocellular carcinoma. Arch Surg 1984; 119: 637–642.

Lin TY. Recent advances in technique of hepatic lobectomy and results of surgical treatment for primary carcinoma of the liver. Prog Liver Dis 1976; 5: 668–682.

Linsell CA, Higginson J. The geographic pathology of liver cell cancer. In: Cameron HM, Linsell CA, Warwick GP, eds. Liver cell cancer. Amsterdam: Elsevier, 1976: 1.

Liver Cancer Study Group of Japan. Primary liver cancer in Japan. Cancer 1984; 54: 1747–1755.

Menck HR, Henderson BE. Cancer incidence patterns in the Pacific Basin. In: National Cancer Institute; Monograph 62. U.S. Department of Health and Human Sciences, 1982: 101–120.

Nagao T, Gota S, Kawano N, et al. Hepatic resection for hepatocellular carcinoma: clinical features and long-term prognosis. Ann Surg 1987; 205: 33–40.

Nagasue N, Yukaya H, Hamada T, Hirose S, Kanashima R, Inokuchi K. The natural history of hepatocellular carcinoma: a study of 100 untreated cases. Cancer 1984; 54: 1461–1465.

Nagasue N, Yukaya H, Ogawa Y, Sasaki Y, Chang YC, Niimi K. Clinical experience with 118 hepatic resections for hepatocellular carcinoma. Surgery 1986; 99: 694–702.

Okamoto E, Kyo A, Yamanaka N, Tanaka N, Kuwata K. Prediction of the safe limits of hepatectomy by combined volumetric and functional measurements in patients with impaired liver function. Surgery 1984; 95: 586–591.

Okuda K. Primary liver cancers in Japan. Cancer 1980; 45: 2663–2672.

Okuda K, Nakashima T, Obata T, Kubo Y. Clinicopathological studies of minute hepatocellular carcinoma. Gastroenterology 1977; 73: 109–115.

Ong GB, Chan KW. Primary carcinoma of the liver. Surg Gynecol Obstet 1976; 143: 31–36.

Shanghai Coordinating Group for Research on Liver Cancer. Diagnosis and treatment of primary hepatocellular carcinoma in early stage. Chin Med J 1979; 92: 801–806.

Sheu JC, Sung JL, Chen DS. Early detection of hepatocellular carcinoma by real-time ultrasonography. Cancer 1985; 56: 660–666.

Shinagawa T, Ohto M, Kimura K, et al. Diagnosis and clinical features of small hepatocellular carcinoma with emphasis on utility of real-time ultrasonography. Gastroenterology 1984; 86: 495–502.

Starzl TE, Iwatsuki S, Shaw BW, et al. Left hepatic trisegmentectomy. Surg Gynecol Obstet 1982; 155: 21–27.

Tang ZY, Yang BH, Tang CL, Yu YQ, Lin ZY, Weng HZ. Evaluation of population screening for hepatocellular carcinoma. Chin Med J 1980; 93: 795–799.

Tang ZY, Ying YY, Gu TJ. Hepatocellular carcinoma: changing concepts in recent years. Prog Liver Dis 1982; 8: 637–647.

Tatsuta M, Yamamoto R, Kasugai H, et al. Cytohistologic diagnosis of neoplasms of the liver by ultrasonically guided fine-needle aspiration biopsy. Cancer 1984; 54: 1682–1686.

Thompson HH, Tompkins RK, Longmire WP. Major Hepatic resection: a 25-year experience. Ann Surg 1983; 197: 375–387.

Wu M, Chen H, Zhang X, Yao X, Yang J. Primary hepatic carcinoma resection over 18 years. Chin Med J 1980; 93: 723–728.

6.2   Expectations and Possibilities of Liver Resection in the Management of Secondary Liver Tumors

G. Gozzetti and Alighieri Mazziotti

In the majority of Western departments of surgery, liver metastases are the most common indication for hepatic resection (Table 6.2.1). The liver is a frequent site for metastases of tumors arising from the colon and rectum (25%), stomach (20%) and pancreas (49%). Surgical treatment embraces mostly metastases from colorectal tumors, and endocrine tumors of the digestive tract, the latter having the best survival rates after hepatic resection (Wanebo 1982). More rarely, resections have been performed for metastases from other primary tumors which have spread to the liver via the systemic blood stream, such as tumors in the breast, kidneys, or leiomyosarcoma. Reported results, however, are poor. Metastases from colorectal tumors are found in 20–25% of patients at the time of surgery for the primary tumor. In another 30% of patients, metastatic spread occurs at different times after surgery. Liver resection is possible in about 10% of patients with metastases (Table 6.2.1). Of these, only 30% will achieve long-term cure.

In this chapter, we focus on some of the problems involved in hepatic resections from colorectal cancer, including pre- and intraoperative diagnosis, technical procedures, long-term outcome and prognostic factors, in an attempt to establish selection criteria for patients suitable for surgical treatment.

Pre- and Intraoperative Diagnostic Possibilities

Ultrasound is the most widespread screening examination for liver metastases, and has been in routine use in our hospital for the past ten years. In the overwhelming majority of our patients undergoing liver resections for metastases, diagnosis was made during follow-up ultrasound in patients with colorectal cancer. Laboratory tests have proved less reliable, and carcinoembryonic antigen determination has a specificity under 60% (Kemeny 1982). Diagnostic ultrasound has become increasingly important in recent years since the development of linear probes which display real-time images of the organ explored. The sensitiveness and accuracy of ultrasound imaging is discussed elsewhere in this book. Ultrasonography is the basic imaging technique and the least expensive; it can detect lesions as small as 1–2 cm in diameter (Fig. 6.2.1).

The accuracy of imaging techniques was investigated by Gunven et al. (1985) in a group of patients with liver metastases who subsequently underwent laparotomy and intraoperative echography. 31 patients with colorectal tumors were

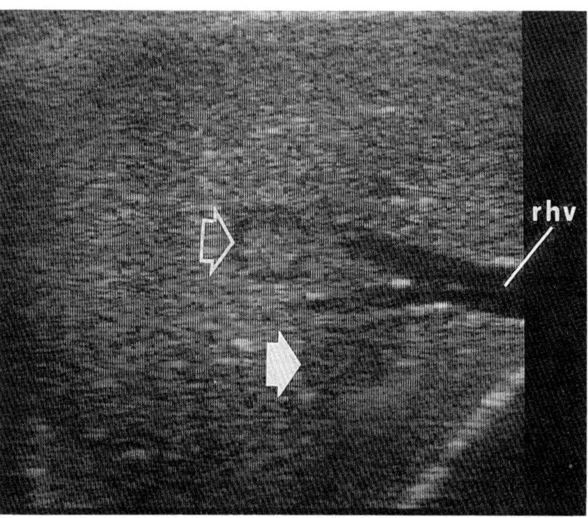

Fig. 6.2.1   **Small liver metastases from rectal carcinoma detected by real-time ultrasonography.** The hollow arrow indicates a 2 cm target lesion; the white arrow indicates a smaller hypoechoic metastasis near the right hepatic vein (rhv). (By courtesy of Dr. L. Bolondi, Department of Medicine, University of Bologna)

Table 6.2.1   **Liver resections:** indications, operative mortality and resectability rate

		(30-Day) operative mortality		Resectability rate (%)
Metastases	60	1	(1.6%)	14
Hepatocarcinomas				
non-cirrhotic	22	1	(4.5%)	44
cirrhotic	33	4	(12.1%)	36.6
Benign tumors	9	0		8.5
Hydatic cysts	11	0		11.4
Hilar cholangiocarcinoma	8	0		25

examined by angiography, computed tomography (CT), and real-time ultrasound using 3.5 MHz probes. Intraoperative echography was performed with higher-frequency probes from 5 to 7.5 MHz. Angiography failed to detect lesions under 1 cm and allowed diagnosis in 31 % of lesions between 1 and 2 cm in size and in 90 % of larger masses. CT displayed less than 50 % of the 1 cm lesions, about half of the lesions between 1 and 2 cm, and 97 % of the larger masses. Preoperative ultrasound showed suspect signs of a lesion under 1 cm in size in 9 % of cases, and displayed 40 % of lesions between 1 and 2 cm in size and 90 % of larger masses. Five metastases over 2 cm were not shown by ultrasound, since they were located in the posterior liver segments, which are blind areas for echographic exploration.

Intraoperative ultrasound has made an important step forwards in the diagnosis of intrahepatic lesions. High-frequency probes can be used, as there is less tissue to pass through. This improves the resolution capacity, with a greater possibility of detecting lesions 4–5 mm in diameter (Fig. 6.2.**2**). Ultrasound has been in routine use in our liver surgery department for over 4 years (Gozzetti et al. 1986a, 1986b, 1988). A prospective study was carried out on a group of patients after laparotomy with a diagnosis of intrahepatic tumor, who were investigated before surgery by ultrasound, CT and angiography, and during surgery by ultrasound. The results of this study of 26 patients with non-cirrhotic livers are reported in Table 6.2.**2**. Intraoperative ultrasound revealed 95.4 % of lesions, as against 84.1 % in preoperative ultrasound, 65.9 % in angiography, and 77.2 % in CT. Only two tiny metastases just beneath the capsule were not displayed. Intraoperative ultrasound revealed only 50 % of lesions under 1 cm, and metastases over 3 cm located in liver segments VII and VIII were missed on two occasions. Another prospective study is currently underway in our department to assess the importance of intraoperative ultrasound in detecting occult liver metastases following surgery for primary digestive tract tumors. Of the 68 patients examined up to now, all of whom underwent preoperative ultrasound, in-

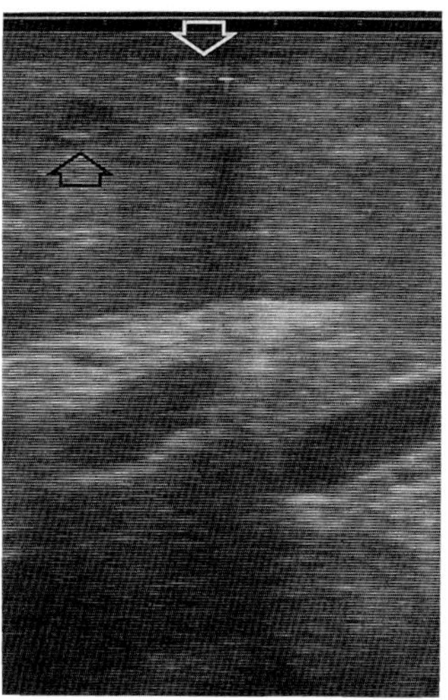

Fig. 6.2.**2   Small intrahepatic lesions detected by intraoperative ultrasonography.** A 4 mm isoechogenic metastasis (white arrow) and thrombus in a peripheral portal branch (black arrow) in the left lobe, in a patient with a main tumor in the lateral segments of the right lobe.

traoperative ultrasound revealed nine lesions which were not palpable during surgery or detected by ultrasound beforehand. In 3 patients, the lesions were small nodules from 0.4 to 1 cm (Figs. 6.2.**2**, 6.2.**3**), and in 2 cases larger metastases were located in the bare area of the liver (Fig. 6.2.**3d**). In most cases this information enabled us to change the surgical strategy and avoid a fruitless major resection. Similar results on the importance of intraoperative ultrasound in surgery of the digestive tract or pancreatic tumors have been reported by Boldrini et al. (1987) and Castaing et al. (1986).

A further advantage of intraoperative ultrasound is the possibility of studying the relations between the lesion and the intrahepatic vessels, to prevent accidental damage to the main vascular trunks during resection and extend the margins of the resection in cases of vascular infiltration. Ultrasound exploration also displays the exact location of the tumor and its distance from vascular struc-

Table 6.2.**2   Results of pre- and intraoperative diagnosis of liver metastases.** Comparison between CT scan, angiography, and pre- and intraoperative ultrasonography in 26 patients

Size	No. of lesions	Computed tomography	Angiography	Preoperative ultrasound	Intraoperative ultrasound	Nonpalpable lesions
< 1 cm	6	3	1	3	4	3
1–3 cm	11	6	4	8	11	2
> 3 cm	27	25	24	26	27	–
Total	44	34 (77.2 %)	29 (65.9 %)	37 (84.1 %)	42 (95.4 %)	

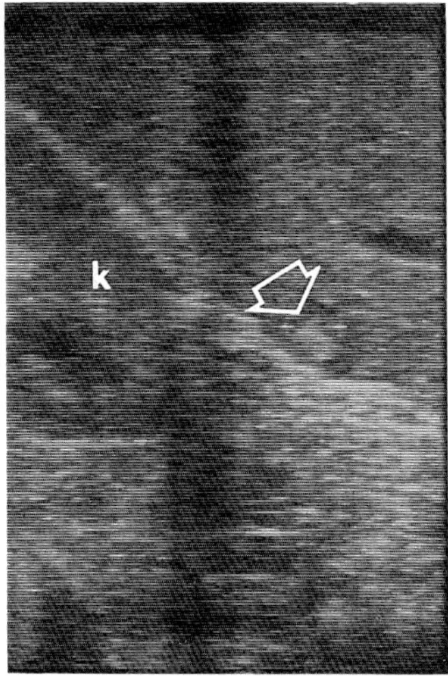
a

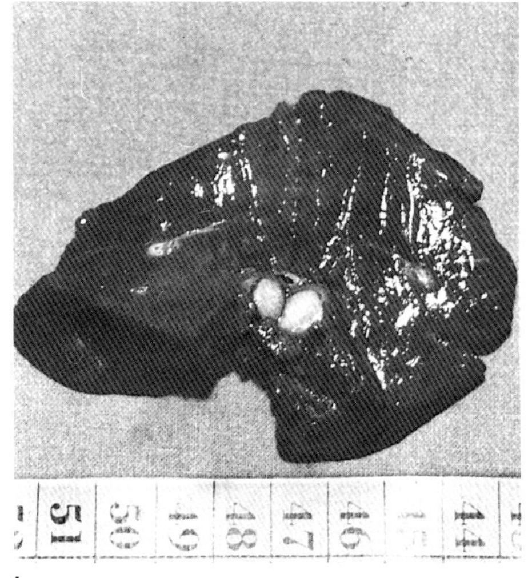
b

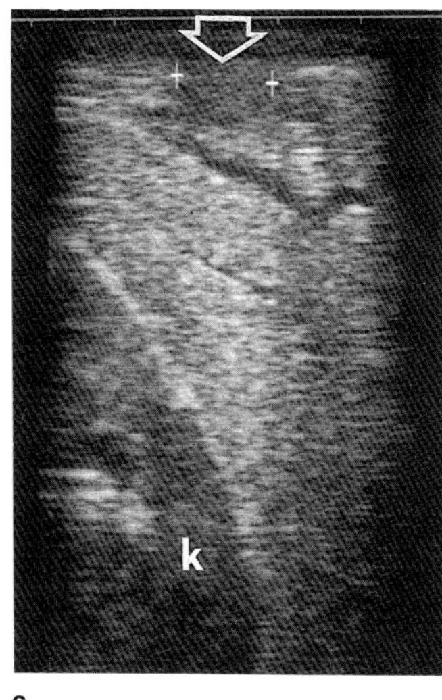
c

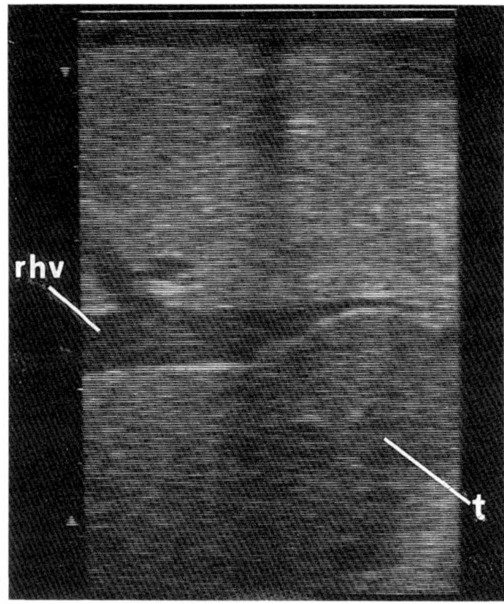
d

Fig. 6.2.**3** **Occult hepatic metastases revealed by intraoperative ultrasonography** during surgery for digestive tract tumor.
a 6 mm hyperechogenic metastases with peripheral halo (arrow) sited in the bare area of segment 7 (k = kidney)
b The lesion has been removed with a wedge resection
c Hypoechogenic 1 cm metastasis (arrow), in a patient with pancreatic carcinoma. The planned pancreatic resection was avoided thanks to the discovery of the hepatic lesion (k = kidney)
d A large isoechogenic metastasis in the 7th segment, which escaped detection during preoperative ultrasonography as it was hidden by the ribs. Note the compression of the right hepatic vein (rhv). The lesion became palpable only after the section of the right triangular ligament

tures such as the vena cava (Fig. 6.2.**4**), and, furthermore, demonstrates the relations between lesions and liver segments to allow segmental resections.

Resection Techniques

Hepatic resections are increasingly common in a number of surgical departments, and have an acceptable operative mortality rate of around 5 % in elective surgery and non-cirrhotic livers (Adson 1987, August et al. 1985, Cady and McDermott 1985, Ekberg et al. 1987, Gennari et al. 1986, Iwatsuki et al. 1986, Logan et al. 1982, Nordlinger et al. 1987). Controlled hepatectomy involves ligation of the peduncular vessels before parenchymal resection. Preliminary clamping of the suprahepatic vein is a critical point in the procedure, and many surgeons recommend ligation and transection of the vein before proceeding in parenchymal transection. This technique is indicated in right or left formal hepatectomy, and allows good control of hemostasis during the resection. In segmental resections, the glissonian peduncles cannot be clamped prior to excision, as they run right through the liver. In these cases we adopt a transparenchymal technique, ligating the vascular peduncles within the liver during resection. Clamping of the peduncle is recommended for this procedure, as it reduces blood loss during the operation. Clamping can be prolonged for as long as 50 min (Huguet et al. 1978), although the normal time required for metastatic resections is less than 30 min. Our recent experience with tumors in cirrhosis has demonstrated that even the cirrhotic liver tolerated clamp-

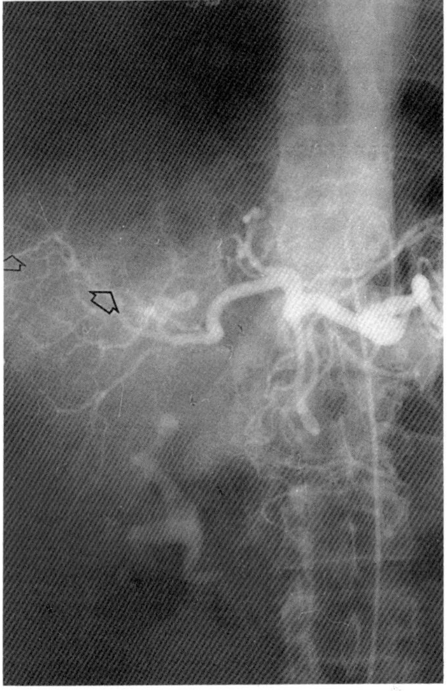

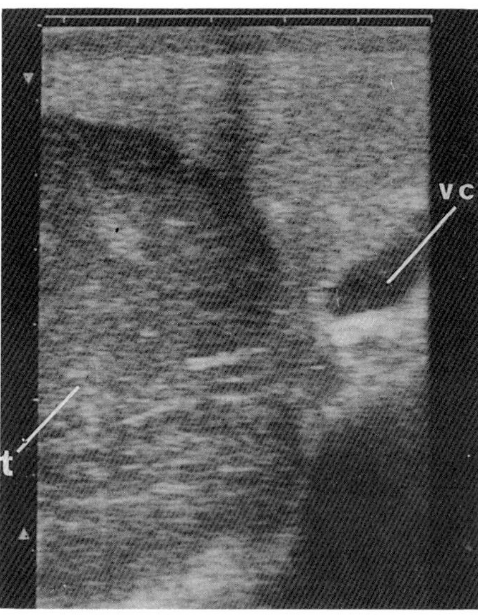

Fig. 6.2.**4 Relationship between tumor and intrahepatic vessels**, shown by intraoperative ultrasonography.
a A huge hypovascular metastasis of the right lobe
b Intraoperative ultrasound demonstrates a gap between the tumor (t) and the vena cava (vc), thus permitting the liver resection.

ing of the peduncle during resection without adverse effects (Gozzetti et al. 1988). Important technical precautions which can be taken to avoid postoperative complications are thorough hemostasis and biliostasis of the resected surface, and prevention of ischemia or parenchymal necrosis, which may occur when full-thickness sutures are used or when part of the residual liver becomes devascularized secondary to inadequate resection because of fear of bleeding.

Which would be the most suitable resection for metastases: anatomical hepatectomy, local wedge or segmental resection? At present, general confusion exists about the extent of resection. However, no difference has been noted between major and segmental resections in terms of long-term survival (Adson 1987, Ekberg et al. 1987). Extended hepatectomies have shown a poorer outcome compared with wedge resections or standard hepatectomies, which is probably due to the larger size of the tumor resected (Hughes et al. 1986, Iwatsuki et al. 1986). The choice of resection is dependent on the extent and location of the tumor. Local excision with a margin of at least 1–2 cm from the lesion is adequate for small metastases, especially those located on the liver surface or detected during surgery for the primary tumor. Segmental resections are indicated for deeper parenchymal tumors confined to a single or two adjacent hepatic segments. Intraoperative ultrasound is a guideline for the resection procedure, as it displays the exact location of the lesion and its relations with the intrahepatic vascular peduncles, and rules out the presence of other nodules. Formal hepatectomy is indicated for multiple lesions confined to one lobe, giant metastases or lesions close to a major vascular peduncle, and central hepatic lesions.

Timing of the Metastasis: Synchronous and Metachronous

It is generally held that liver metastases present at the time of surgery for the primary intestinal tumor can only be resected if they are small, or located in the left lobe or on the liver surface, accessible by the incision used for the colectomy. In our experience, out of 185 patients with synchronous hepatic metastases, 19 (10.2%) underwent hepatic resection at the time of primary surgery: one had a left hepatectomy, 4 had a left lateral lobectomy, 2 had a right hepatectomy, and 12 had a wedge resection or segmentectomy. This did not affect mortality, and only one patient had to undergo further surgery for a subphrenic abscess.

When metastases are large, or located in the posterior liver segments, and thus require major hepatectomy, resection should be postponed for a few months to reduce the operative risk and exclude those patients with invasive primary cancer or widespread intra- and extrahepatic metastases. A number of series report no differences between the survival rates of patients operated for synchronous or metachronous metastases (Adson 1987, Cady and McDermott 1985, Ekberg et al. 1987). According to Iwatsuki (1986), the time of onset of metastases – 1, 2 or 3 years after colectomy – did not affect the patient's prognosis. Other series state that synchronous metastases indicate a worse prognosis than those appearing 12 to 18 months after surgery (Hughes et al. 1986, Logan et al. 1982).

Results

In our series, 60 patients underwent hepatic resection for liver metastases; in 45 cases, the primary tumor was a colorectal cancer, in 3 a digestive apudoma, and in the remaining cases an extradigestive neoplasia (kidney, adrenal, breast, etc.). A major hepatectomy was performed in 28 cases, a left or segmental lobectomy in 24, and a wedge resection in 8. One patient died within 30 days of surgery due to hemorrhage from a duodenal ulcer (operative mortality = 1.6%). One patient had a subphrenic abscess which required a surgical drainage. 16 patients died within two years from tumor recurrence; 12 cases had intrahepatic relapse, and 4 had peritoneal carcinosis with ascites. These short survival times involved patients with more than 4 liver metastases (4 cases), with large tumors (2 cases) or patients with inadequate resection margins (5 cases); in 5, recurrence was at the site of the primary colorectal tumor. Actuarial survival at 3 years in hepatic resections for colorectal metastases is 30%. All patients who underwent resections for metastases from endocrine or digestive tract tumors are alive without signs of recurrence three years after surgery. Patients operated on for metastases from primary tumors of the breast, kidney or other digestive tract cancers, died within two years after surgery (Fig. 6.2.5).

Results of Collective Series: Determinants of Prognosis

All series reported in the literature have the drawbacks of retrospective studies, as there are at present no randomized series which compare surgical treatment with the natural history of the disease. The data are often difficult to assess, since earlier series do not include several factors affecting the prognosis, and report variables which preclude accurate statistical analysis. Clinical reports generally involve a limited number of patients, and few exceed 50 cases. Survival rates are usually actuarial. Many of these series include large and small metastases alike, often omitting grading of the primary tumor, or other important factors such as the state of the lymph nodes, and the type of resection (with or without an adequate margin of healthy tissue). However, an analysis of the major series offers some guidelines for patient selection and indication for the most suitable treatment. An overall analysis of the most recent series (Table 6.2.3) shows that hepatic resection is beneficial in roughly 1/4 of cases operated on, while actuarial survival at 5 years varies from 18 to 42%. Numerous prognostic determinants have been identified in literature series, some of which are compared in Table 6.2.3. The major factors responsible are the size and number of metastases, the grading of the primary tumor, and whether the metastases are synchronous or metachronous.

Primary tumor. The site of the primary tumor is of no prognostic importance for Adson (1987), while others have reported a higher mortality rate and local recurrence if the primary tumor was located in the rectum (Bozzetti et al. 1987). Staging of the primary tumor according to Dukes' criteria has been evaluated by different authors. Some found no relation to prognosis (August et al. 1985, Logan et al. 1982, Nordlinger et al. 1987), while others noted that the locoregional stage of the primary tumor is an important determinant of survival following hepatic resection (Adson 1987, Fortner et al. 1984a, Hughes et al. 1986, Iwatsuki et al. 1986). Grading of tumor differentiation, a direct sign of neoplastic biology, is not usually reported in published series.

Metastasis. The size and number of metastases are of biological importance, since larger metastases or multiple lesions have a longer evolution and hence a greater possibility of producing recurrent metastases in the liver. These lesions also have technical significance, since the greater the size or

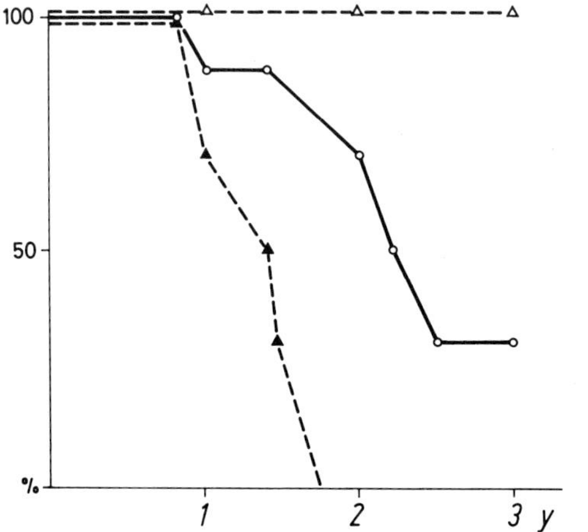

Fig. 6.2.**5 Survival curve after liver resection for metastasis.** Interrupted line, blank triangle: metastases from endocrine tumors. Continuous line: colorectal cancers. Interrupted line, dark triangle: extradigestive tumors.

Table 6.2.3   Factors influencing prognosis after liver resection for metastases. From collective series

Author(s) (year)	No. of patients	Operative mortality (%)	5-year survival (%)	Stage of primary tumor	Size of metastases	No. of metastases	Resective margin	Extra-hepatic metastases	Synchronous vs. metachronous
Logan et al. (1982)	19	5.3	–	NO	NO	YES	–	–	YES
Fortner et al. (1984a)	65	7	40	YES	–	–	–	–	NO
August et al. (1985)	33	0	[53]*	NO	NO	YES	YES	–	NO
Cady and McDermott (1985)	23	0	–	–	–	YES	YES	–	–
Hughes et al. (1986)	859	–	33	YES	YES	YES	YES	YES	YES
Iwatsuki et al. (1986)	60	0	45	YES	YES	YES	–	–	NO
Adson (1987)	141	2.8	23	YES	NO	NO	–	YES	–
Bozzetti et al. (1987)	48	2.1	35	NO	YES	YES	–	–	NO
Ekberg et al. (1987)	72	5.6	16	NO	YES	YES	YES	YES	NO
Nordlinger et al. (1987)	80	5	25	NO	NO	NO	–	–	NO

* 4 years

number of the metastases, the lower the chances of a satisfactory resection from an anatomical standpoint. The results of different series are comparable, and show no differences between metastases over or under 5 cm, while the most unfavorable results are reported for large tumors (Table 6.2.**3**). Most authors report survival rates limited by the number of lesions, and more than 3 metastases are now thought to contra-indicate resection. Despite this, recent reports from the Mayo Clinic failed to notice worse trends for multiple metastases in comparison with single ones (Adson 1987).

Patterns of Recurrence

The liver is the most common site of recurrence following resection for hepatic metastases, and roughly a quarter of cases present an isolated intrahepatic recurrence (Ekberg et al. 1987, Hughes et al. 1986, Nordlinger et al. 1987). Several recent studies have made a critical analysis of recurrence factors. Ekberg et al. (1987) examined a retrospective series of 68 hepatic resections, Hughes et al. (1986) made a multicentric retrospective study on 607 patients, while Bozzetti et al. (1987) evaluated 45 cases. Hepatic recurrence is found in over 60 % of patients, and in 30 % of them isolated recurrent tumors are found. Lung metastases are less common, and occur much later. Around 10 % of patients have a 25 % incidence of initial recurrence at the site of intestinal anastomosis. In over 30 % of patients, recurrence is detected within a year after surgery. Ekberg's and Hughes' studies agree on the factors influencing recurrence. The key factor is the resection margin in relation to the macroscopic limits of the tumor: a resection margin of less than 10 mm gives rise to a high rate of recurrence. Another factor affecting prognosis is the presence of lymph node metastases in the abdomen or hepatic peduncle which, even when removed along with matched liver lesions, have been shown to limit survival significantly. This factor was emphasized in Hughes' extensive review, as well as in previous reports (Adson 1987, Ekberg et al. 1987, Fortner et al. 1984a). Finally, the bilobal location of hepatic metastases has often been noted in relation to recurrence.

The Role of Alternative Surgical Management: Hepatic Artery Infusion

Intrahepatic arterial chemotherapy became popular in the early 1980s with the widespread use of the implantable pump or port, which allowed safe, reliable access, easily acceptable for the patient, for a continuous or discontinuous delivery of chemotherapeutic agents. The rationale for this technique is based on the high concentration of drugs in the liver and metastases delivered by the arterial blood supply, the greater effect of antiblastic drugs administered in slow continuous infusion, and the elective hepatic extraction of anti-cancer drugs which reduce systemic side effects. 5-Fluorouracil (5-FU) and fluorodeoxyuridine (FUDR) are the most widely used agents. The best response is achieved when different drugs are combined. In our experience, the most effective combination is 5-FU and 4-epidoxorubicin, with an average survival of 16 months (20 in responders and 11 in non-responders) and a 5-month average response period (Rossi et al. 1987). A high rate of response to treatment was reported in the first non-randomized series in the literature, and this was followed by widespread application of the method, with over 5000 implantations to date. Initially optimistic results were subsequently reappraised in later studies, especially as regards the real benefits in terms of long-term survival. The highest percentages of response depend on patient selection, the best being reported for patients with no more than 30% of liver involvement (Fortner 1984b). There have also been increasingly frequent reports of negative effects on the liver after continuous infusion of chemotherapeutic agents, including chemical hepatitis and sclerosing cholangitis.

Balch and Levin (1987) recently reviewed several randomized studies, some still in progress, comparing continuous intra-arterial infusion with intravenous FUDR chemotherapy. Available results include those of the Memorial Sloane Kettering Cancer Center of New York and the Northern Californian Oncology Group. Both of these studies showed a higher response rate for the group using intra-arterial chemotherapy, but no clear difference in terms of survival. Symptomatic patients are the only ones to gain effective palliation and constitute a clear-cut group for whom intra-arterial chemotherapy can be recommended. In cases of diffuse asymptomatic metastases, drug management is still in the experimental stage. A recent non-randomized series reported that intra-arterial chemotherapy was combined with partial or total removal of liver metastases (Hodgson et al. 1986).

The average survival time of patients with chemotherapy only was 6 months, the group of patients with tumor resections combined with pump infusions showing better results in terms of long-term survival. Indeed, even in the presence of bilobal metastases, there was an average survival of 60% for 24 months, suggesting that the more radical the treatment in addition to chemotherapy, the better the results. In our series, two cases of hepatic resection for multiple bilobal metastases received intra-arterial pump chemotherapy and both patients are alive without signs of recurrence three years after surgery.

Conclusions

Given our limited knowledge of the biology of metastatic tumors, surgical resection remains the only form of treatment available for liver metastases. Selected patients can be referred for surgery, considering the current low operative risk for hepatectomy. A critical analysis of literature reports offers some guidelines for surgical treatment: technical measures such as free section margins reduce postoperative recurrence, which is mostly intra-hepatic. Intraoperative ultrasound is a useful adjunct to detect occult lesions and display relations between the lesions and the intrahepatic vessels for a safer and more radical surgical resec-

tion. Between 25% and 35% of patients operated, depending on the selection criteria used, remain free of disease in a follow-up period of 5 years. The best results can be expected in patients with a single metastasis from a colorectal tumor and radical resection of the primary carcinoma. Surgical treatment can also be considered in cases of multiple metastases in one lobe, and occasionally bilobar lesions, even when one large metastasis is localized in one lobe and a second small lesion in the other. Multiple metastases in both lobes are not suitable for surgical resection, and no other forms of treatment have proved beneficial up to now, including regional intra-arterial chemotherapy. The role of adjuvant, systemic or intra-arterial chemotherapy in combination with hepatic resection has yet to be established.

References

Adson MA. Resection of liver metastases: when is it worthwhile? World J Surg 1987; 11: 511–520.

August DA, Sugarbaker PH, Ottow RT, Gianola FJ, Schneider PD. Hepatic resection of colorectal metastases: influence of clinical factors and adjuvant intraperitoneal 5-fluorouracil via Tenckhoff catheter on survival. Ann Surg 1985; 201: 210–218.

Balch CM, Levin B. Regional and systemic chemotherapy for colorectal metastases to the liver. World J Surg 1987; 11: 521–526.

Bengmark S, Jonsson PE. Surgical treatment of liver metastases. In: Weiss L, Gilbert H, Hall GK, eds. Liver metastases. Boston: Medical Publishers, 1982: 294–321.

Boldrini G, De Gaetano AM, Giovannini I, Castagneto M, Casagrande C, Castiglioni G. The systematic use of operative ultrasound for detection of liver metastases during colorectal surgery. World J Surg 1987; 11: 622–627.

Bozzetti F, Bignami P, Morabito A, Doci R, Gennari L. Patterns of failure following surgical resection of colorectal cancer liver metastases. Ann Surg 1987; 205: 264–269.

Cady B, McDermott WV. Major hepatic resection for metachronous metastases from colon cancer. Ann Surg 1985; 201: 204–209.

Castaing D, Emond J, Kunstlinger F, Bismuth H. Utility of operative ultrasound in the surgical management of liver tumors. Ann Surg 1986; 204: 600–605.

Ekberg H, Tranberg K-G, Andersson R et al. Pattern of recurrence in liver resection of colorectal secondaries. World J Surg 1987; 11: 541–547.

Fortner JG, Maj JSS, Golbey RB, Cox EB, Maclean BJ. Multivariate analysis of a personal series of 247 consecutive patients with liver metastases from colorectal cancer, I: treatment by hepatic resection. Ann Surg 1984a; 199: 306–315.

Fortner JG, Silva JS, Cox EB, Golbey RB, Gallowitz H, Maclean BJ. Multivariate analysis of a personal series of 247 patients with liver metastases from colorectal cancer, II: treatment by intrahepatic chemotherapy. Ann Surg 1984b; 199: 317–324.

Gennari M, Doci R, Bignami P, Bozzetti F. Surgical treatment of hepatic metastases from colorectal cancer. Ann Surg 1986; 203: 49–54.

Gozzetti G, Mazziotti A, Bolondi L. Ecografia Intra-operatorio in Chirurgia Epato-biliare e Pancreatica. Milano: Masson, 1986a.

Gozzetti G, Mazziotti A, Bolondi L, et al. Intraoperative ultrasonography in surgery for liver tumors. Surgery 1986b; 99: 573–579.

Gozzetti G, Mazziotti A, Cavallari A, et al. Clinical experience of hepatic resections for hepatocellular carcinoma in patients with cirrhosis. Surg Gynecol Obstet 1988; 166: 503–510.

Gunven P, Makuuchi M, Takayasu K, Mariyama N, Yamasaki S, Hasegawa H. Preoperative imaging of liver metastases: comparison of angiography, CT scan, and ultrasonography. Ann Surg 1985; 202: 573–579.

Hodgson WJB, Mittelman A, Katz S, et al. Treatment of colorectal hepatic metastases by intrahepatic chemotherapy alone or as an adjuvant to complete or partial removal of metastatic disease. Ann Surg 1986; 203: 420–425.

Hughes KS, Simon R, Songhorabodi S, et al. Resection of the liver for colorectal carcinoma metastases: a multi-institutional study of patterns of recurrence. Surgery 1986; 100: 278–284.

Huguet C, Nordlinger B, Bloch P, Courad J. Tolerance of the human liver to prolonged normothermic ischemia: a biological study of 20 patients submitted to extensive hepatectomy. Arch Surg 1978; 113: 1448–1451.

Iwatsuki S, Esquivel CO, Gordon RD, Starzl TE. Liver resection for metastatic colorectal cancer. Surgery 1986; 100: 804–808.

Kemeny MM, Sugarbaker PH, Smith TJ, et al. A prospective analysis of laboratory tests and imaging studies to detect hepatic lesions. Ann Surg 1982; 195: 163–167.

Logan SE, Meier SJ, Ramming KP, Morton DL, Longmire WP. Hepatic resection of metastatic colorectal carcinoma. Arch Surg 1982; 117: 25–28.

Nordlinger B, Parc R, Delva E, Quilichini M-A, Hannoun L, Huguet C. Hepatic resection for colorectal liver metastases. Ann Surg 1987; 205: 256–263.

Rossi AP, Casadio M, Piana E, et al. Regional chemotherapy of liver metastases from colorectal cancer. Proc ECCO 1987; 4: 170.

Wanebo HJ. Surgical resection of liver metastases. In: Weiss L, Gilbert H, Hall GK, eds. Liver metastases. Boston: Medical Publishers, 1982: 322–336.

6.3 Hepatic Resections for Metastatic Tumors

S. Iwatsuki and T. E. Starzl

The most common malignant neoplasm of the liver by far is metastatic tumor. Edmonson and Peters (1982) reported that among 7299 autopsies of extrahepatic primary malignancies, 38% of them had metastases to the liver, and they found that the five most common primary malignancies which had spread to the liver were bronchogenic, colonic, pancreatic, mammary and gastric cancer.

Although hepatic metastasis is a common event in the course of various malignant neoplasms, hepatic resection is uncommon. By the time the hepatic metastases are found, malignant tumors have usually already spread to extrahepatic sites. As an example, only 5–10% of patients who developed hepatic metastasis from colorectal cancer are candidates for hepatic resection, which comprises the largest number of patients for this operation (Wagner et al. 1984, Wood et al. 1976). As a rule, once hepatic metastasis is established, the disease is far advanced and the prognosis is extremely poor.

Over the years the authors have treated 118 patients with hepatic metastases of various malignant neoplasms by hepatic resection. The experience is summarized in this chapter.

Case Materials and Methods

Over the last 20 years, a total of 400 patients have been treated by subtotal hepatic resection at our institution. 108 of these patients received surgery at the University of Colorado Health Sciences Center before 1981, and since 1981 the remaining 292 patients were operated upon at the University Health Center of Pittsburgh. 181 patients had histologically benign hepatic lesions and the remaining 219 patients had histologically malignant hepatic neoplasms. Of the 219 hepatic malignancies, 101 were primary hepatic malignancies and 118 were metastatic tumors (Table 6.3.1).

The most common metastatic tumor treated by hepatic resection was colorectal cancer (86 patients), followed by adrenal cancer and renal cancer (5 patients each) and by carcinoid tumor, breast cancer and leiomyosarcoma (4 patients

Table 6.3.1 Indications of 400 hepatic resections

Primary hepatic malignancy	101 patients
Secondary hepatic malignancy	118 patients
Histologically benign hepatic lesion	181 patients

Table 6.3.2 Histology of 118 secondary hepatic malignancies

	No. of patients
Colorectal cancer	86
Adrenal cancer	5
Renal cancer	5
Carcinoid tumor	4
Breast cancer	4
Leiomyosarcoma of GI tract	4
Ovarian cancer	2
Melanoma	2
Glycagonoma (pancreas)	1
Squamous cell cancer of cervix	1
Medullary carcinoma of thyroid	1
Spindle cell sarcoma of intestine	1
Endometrial sarcoma of uterus	1
Ewing's sarcoma	1
Total	118

each). The origins of all metastatic hepatic malignancies are listed in Table 6.3.2.

The survival rates were calculated as of November 15, 1987 by the Kaplan–Meier method. Statistical comparisons were made by the Breslow and Mantel–Cox methods. The difference was considered as significant when the p value was less than 0.05.

Our operative techniques have been described in detail elsewhere (Starzl et al. 1975, 1980, 1982). The extent of hepatic resections was classified into the following six types: right and left trisegmentectomy, right and left lobectomy, left lateral segmentectomy, and non-anatomical local excision or wedge resection. Right trisegmentectomy is the removal of the entire right lobe plus the medial segment of the left lobe. Extended right lobectomy, which removes a part of the medial segment with the right lobe, was classified as right lobectomy in this report. Left trisegmentectomy is the removal of the entire left lobe plus the anterior segment of the right lobe. Extended left lobectomy was classified as left lobectomy. The extent of resection by various techniques is depicted in Figure 6.3.1.

Results

Operative Mortality

All deaths within a month of hepatic resection were counted as operative deaths. There was, however, no operative death for metastatic liver tumors after 40 right trisegmentectomies, 5 left trisegmentectomies, 38 right lobectomies, 16 left lobectomies,

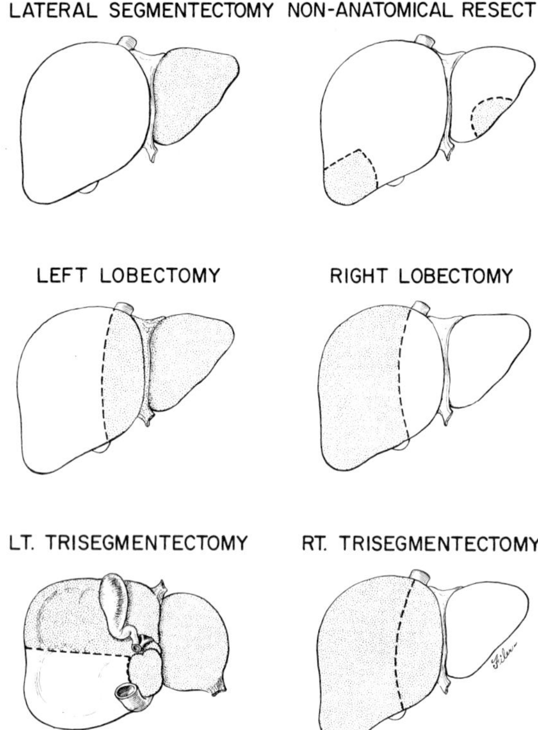

Fig. 6.3.**1**   **Six kinds of hepatic resection**

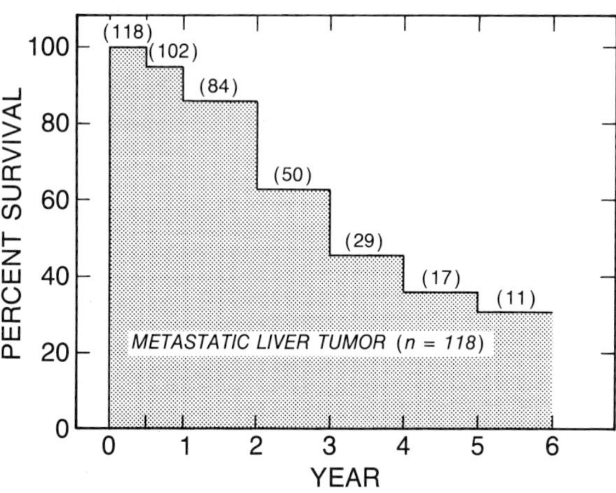

Fig. 6.3.**2**   **Actuarial survival rates** of 118 patients with various hepatic metastases after hepatic resection

12 left lateral segmentectomies and 7 non-anatomical, wedge resections. The operative mortality was zero percent after 118 liver resections.

Survival Rates

The overall survival rates of 118 patients with metastatic liver tumors were 86 % at 1 year, 63 % at 2 years, 46 % at 3 years, 36 % at 4 years and 31 % at 5 years after hepatic resection (Figure 6.3.**2**). The survival rates of patients with hepatic metastases from colorectal cancer were significantly higher than those of patients with metastases from malignancies other than colorectal cancer (*p* less than 0.05), as shown in Figure 6.3.**3**. 1–5 year survival rates of the former were 90 %, 70 %, 50 %, 38 % and 38 %, respectively, and those of the latter were 73 %, 42 %, 33 %, 28 % and 16 %, respectively.

Causes of Death

A total of 56 deaths were confirmed as of November 15, 1987. All but two patients died with recurrence of malignant tumors. One of the two patients died suddenly at home in the second postoperative month, and another patient died from liver failure in the third month. The majority of the recurrences were intra-abdominal, inside and outside the remaining liver, followed by lung, bone and brain metastases.

Five-Year Survivors

Among the 36 patients who had had hepatic resection more than 5 years ago, 11 patients lived more than 5 years (actual 5-year survival rate of 31 %). 9 of the 11 patients had had hepatic resection for metastatic colorectal cancer, one patient having metastasis from neuroblastoma of the right adrenal gland and another patient having metastatic carcinoid tumor of the ileum. 3 of the 5-year survivors had had right trisegmentectomy, 3 had had right lobectomy, and 4 had had left lateral segmentectomy.

Discussion

None of the 118 patients with hepatic metastases died within a month after hepatic resection, but 8 of the 101 patients with primary hepatic malignancy and 4 of the 101 patients with histologically benign hepatic lesions dies within a month of the operation (Table 6.3.**3**). 5 of the 8 deaths among patients with primary hepatic malignancy occurred in the patients with cirrhosis. 2 of the 4 deaths among patients with histologically benign lesions occurred in hepatic trauma, one in fungal abscess, and another in misdiagnosed hepatoma in the cirrhotic liver. 8 of the 12 operative deaths were after trisegmentectomies, 3 were after right lobectomy and one after a wedge resection. The operative mortality rate of 3 % (12 out of 400 patients) in our series and those of others (Fortner et al. 1981, Lin et al. 1987, Thompson et al. 1983, Tsuzuki et al. 1984) clearly indicates that hepatic resection can now be performed quite safely if the liver is not cirrhotic. The lower operative mortality among patients with metastatic tumors in our series and those of others (Adson et al. 1987, August et al. 1985, Fortner et al.

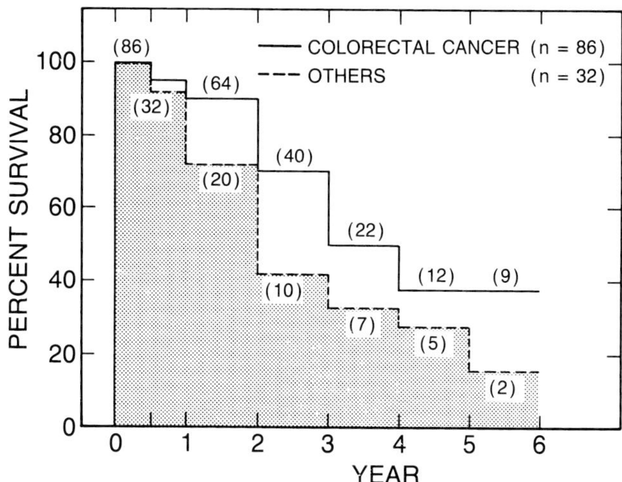

Fig. 6.3.**3 Actuarial survival rates** of 86 patients with hepatic metastases from colorectal cancer were significantly better than those of 32 patients with metastases from other than colorectal cancer after hepatic resection. Solid line: colorectal cancer; broken line: others

Table 6.3.3 Operative mortality (deaths within a month)

	Right trisegmentectomy	Left trisegmentectomy	Right Lobectomy	Left Lobectomy	Left lateral Segmentectomy	Local Excision	Total
Primary malignancy	4 of 47	2 of 8	1 of 16	0 of 17	0 of 3	1 of 10	8 of 101
Secondary malignancy	0 of 40	0 of 5	0 of 38	0 of 16	0 of 12	0 of 7	0 of 118
Benign Lesion	2 of 32	0 of 2	2 of 55	0 of 14	0 of 8	0 of 70	4 of 181
Total	6 of 119	2 of 15	3 of 109	0 of 47	0 of 23	1 of 87	12 of 400

1984, Nordlinger et al. 1987) may reflect the fact that the remaining part of the liver is usually normal in secondary hepatic malignancy.

The survival rates after hepatic resection for metastatic colorectal cancer in this report (90% at 1 year, 50% at 3 years, and 38% at 5 years) are slightly better than those obtained by others (Starzl et al. 1975, 1980, 1982, Thompson et al. 1983), but the differences are probably not statistically significant. In our first report (Iwatsuki et al. 1983) the 5-year actuarial survival rate was 57%, and in the second report (Iwatsuki et al. 1986) it was 46%. In this report, the 5-year actuarial survival rate has decreased further to 38%, and the 5-year actual survival rate was 31%. This decline in the survival rate is mainly due to the method of survival calculation (the method of Kaplan–Meier), but is also due to the fact that more advanced lesions were resected by trisegmentectomies during the last 5 years. The prognosis for metastatic lesions requiring trisegmentectomies was much worse than that of lesions which required lobectomies and lesser resections (Iwatsuki et al. 1986).

Median survival rates of patients who had had unresected solitary and multiple unilobar lesions were 21 and 15 months, respectively, according to the report from the Mayo Clinic (Edmondson and Peters 1982). In our experience, the median survival rate for unilobar lesions, the lesions which were removed by lobectomy or lesser resection, was more than 48 months, while that for bilobar lesions, the lesions which required trisegmentectomies, was more than 24 months (Wagner et al. 1984). This improved survival rate by hepatic resection clearly justifies our efforts whenever possible to remove all hepatic metastases from colorectal cancer.

Isolated hepatic metastases from malignant tumors other than colorectal cancer are rare, and the experience in hepatic resection for these non-colorectal metastases is quite limited. Our personal group of 32 such patients is the largest in the literature to our knowledge. A larger collection can only be found in the multi-institutional review by Foster (1978). Although it may not be meaningful to consider all metastases from various primary malignancies as a group, the survival rates after hepatic resection of metastases from non-colorectal cancer were significantly worse than those of colorectal cancer, as shown in Figure 6.3.3. The median survival rate of this group was 20 months.

However, 7 patients survived more than 3 years after hepatic resection; one patient with neuroblastoma of the adrenal gland and one patient with carcinoid tumor lived more than 7 years, one patient with leiomyosarcoma of the rectum, one patient with medullary carcinoma of the thyroid and endometrial sarcoma of the uterus lived more than 4 years, and one patient with leiomyosarcoma of the stomach and one patient with adenocarcinoma of the ovary lived more than 3 years.

In Foster's collective review (1978), 9 (13 %) of the 69 patients died postoperatively, but 19 patients lived more than 2 years, 8 of whom lived more than 5 years. Half of these long-term survivors had Wilms' tumor. The median survival rate for Wilms' tumor was 24 months, but that of other malignancies, such as melanoma, leiomyosarcoma, and cancers of the pancreas, stomach, uterus, ovary, kidney and breast, was less than 12 months. Based on these data, Foster concluded, 10 years ago, that hepatic resection of metastases from non-colorectal cancer should be discouraged. We have been in disagreement with his conclusion. In our experience there was no operative mortality after hepatic resection of metastatic tumors, and three-quarters of these patients were expected to live more than one year. It is unfortunate that the physical and psychological palliation achieved by this aggressive but safe operative approach cannot be expressed numerically. We will continue in our efforts to remove these otherwise untreatable malignant lesions surgically until a safer and more effective therapy can be established.

It is quite discouraging, though, to realize that nearly all of the deaths after successful removal of hepatic metastasis were caused directly or indirectly by recurrence of the primary malignancy. The recurrence most frequently occurred during the first couple of years after hepatic resection, but also recurred even after 5 years. There was usually enough time for adjuvant therapy. As major hepatic resection can now be performed with a minimum of risk, safer and more effective adjuvant chemotherapy and immunotherapy must be developed for further improvement in survival rates.

Acknowledgement

Research for this paper was supported by research grants from the Veterans' Administration and Project Grant No. AM 29961 from the National Institutes of Health, Bethesda, Maryland.

References

Adson MA, van Heerden JA, Adson MH, Wagner JS, Ilstrup DH. Resection of hepatic metastases from colorectal cancer. Arch Surg 1987; 119: 647–651.

August DA, Sugarbaker PH, Ottow RT. Hepatic resection of colorectal metastases. Ann Surg 1985; 201: 210–218.

Edmondson HA, Peters RL. Neoplasms of the liver. In: Schiff L, Schiff ER, eds. Diseases of the liver. 5th ed. Philadelphia: Lippincott, 1982: 1101–1157.

Fortner JG, Maclean BJ, Kim DK, et al. The seventies evolution in liver surgery for cancer. Cancer 1981; 47: 2162–2166.

Fortner JG, Silva JS, Golbey RB, Cox EB, Maclean BJ. Multivariate analysis of a personal series of 247 consecutive patients with liver metastases from colorectal cancer, I: treatment by hepatic resection. Ann Surg 1984; 199: 306–316.

Foster JH. Survival after liver resection for secondary tumors. Am J Surg 1978; 135: 389–394.

Iwatsuki S, Shaw BW Jr, Starzl TE. Experience with 150 liver resections. Ann Surg 1983; 197: 247–253.

Iwatsuki S, Esquivel CO, Gordon RD, Starzl TE. Liver resection for metastatic colorectal cancer. Surgery 1986; 100: 804–810.

Lin TY, Lee CS, Chen KU, Chen CC. Role of surgery in the treatment of primary carcinoma of the liver: a 31-year experience. Br J Surg 1987; 74: 839–842.

Nordlinger B, Parc R, Delva E, Quilichini M, Hannoun L, Huguet C. Hepatic resection for colorectal liver metastases. Ann Surg 1987; 205: 256–263.

Starzl TE, Bell RH, Beart RW, Putnam CW. Hepatic trisegmentectomy and other liver resections. Surg Gynecol Obstet 1975; 141: 429–437.

Starzl TE, Koep LJ, Weil R III, Lilly JR, Putnam CW, Aldrete JA. Right trisegmentectomy for hepatic neoplasms. Surg Gynecol Obstet 1980; 150: 208–214.

Starzl TE, Iwatsuki S, Shaw BW Jr, et al. Left hepatic trisegmentectomy. Surg Gynecol Obstet 1982; 155: 21–27.

Thompson HH, Tomkins RK, Longmire WP Jr. Major hepatic resection: a 25-year experience. Ann Surg 1983; 197: 375–388.

Tsuzuki T, Ogata Y, Iida S, Shimazu M. Hepatic resection in 125 patients. Arch Surg 1984; 119: 1025–1032.

Wagner JS, Adson MA, van Heerden JA, Adson MH, Ilstrup DM. The natural history of hepatic metastases from colorectal cancer. Ann Surg 1984; 199: 502–508.

Wood CB, Gillis CR, Blumgart LH. A retrospective study of the natural history of patients with liver metastases from colorectal cancer. Clin Oncol 1976; 2: 285–288.

6.4 Surgical Techniques

B. Kremer and D. Henne-Bruns

The first successful liver resection was performed by Langenbruch in 1886 in Berlin. Since then several techniques have been developed for the resection of various sites and areas of the liver, based on the liver's segmental anatomical structure (Adson and van Heerden 1980, Bismuth 1982, Blumgart 1988, Couinauld 1954, Esser 1979b, Fortner et al. 1978, 1984, Foster and Berman 1977, Funovics and Fritsch 1983, Goldsmith and Woodburne 1957, Iwatsuki et al. 1983, Pichlmayr et al. 1984, Priesching 1986, Starzl et al. 1980, 1982, Stone 1977, Thompson et al. 1983, Tsuzuki et al. 1983, 1984). According to Couinauld (1954), all "anatomical" or "classical" types of hepatic resection are defined by the segmental structure of the liver (Bismuth 1982, Goldsmith and Woodburne 1957) (Fig. 6.4.**1**). Each segment is supplied by a separate branch of the arterial and portal triad and is drained by a segmental branch of the right, median or left hepatic veins.

Systematization of surgical procedures. By definition, there are four types of major resections: right and left hepatectomy and right and left lobectomy (Fig. 6.4.**2**). The plane of resection for a right or left hepatectomy lies between the left side of the gallbladder and the caval vein. In right hepatectomies segments V, VI, VII and VIII are therefore resected, in left hepatectomies segments I, II, III and IVa and b. Extended right hepatectomy (synonyms: right lobectomy, right trisegmentectomy) (Starzl et al. 1980) includes the resection of segments IVa and b, and left lateral segmentectomy (synonym: left lobectomy) comprises segments II and III. Extended left hepatectomy (synonym: left trisegmentectomy) (Starzl et al. 1982) is a rarely-performed operation extending a left hepatectomy to segments V and VIII. Smaller tumor masses can also be sufficiently resected by segmentectomies with the intention of cure, with 2–3 cm safety margins around the tumor (see Chapter 6.5 below).

Preoperative Diagnostic Procedures

Preoperative investigations should clarify the origin, extent and resectability of a liver tumor. In addition, any extrahepatic tumor manifestations should be evaluated (Esser 1979a, Foster and Berman 1977, Kremer and Henne-Bruns 1986, Mimura et al. 1986, Okamoto et al. 1984, Stone 1977, Thompson et al. 1983).

Ultrasound investigations of the liver are able to detect tumorous lesions larger than 1.5–2.0 cm. The extent of a tumor, and its relation to biliary or vascular structures such as the portal or caval vein, can be assessed. Additional information about the liver parenchyma (fibrosis, cirrhosis) or the enlargement of intra-abdominal lymph nodes can be obtained.

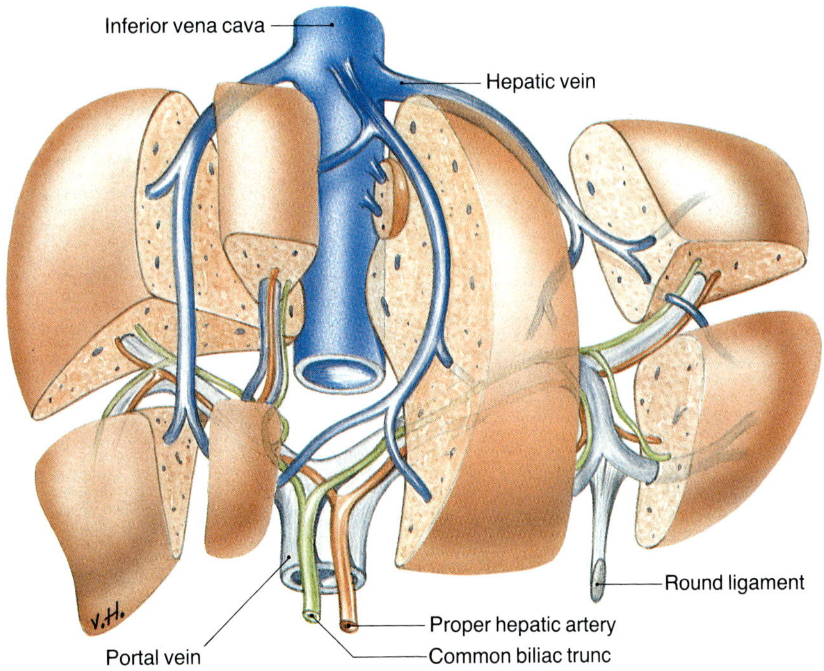

Fig. 6.4.**1 Segmental structure of the liver** according to Couinauld

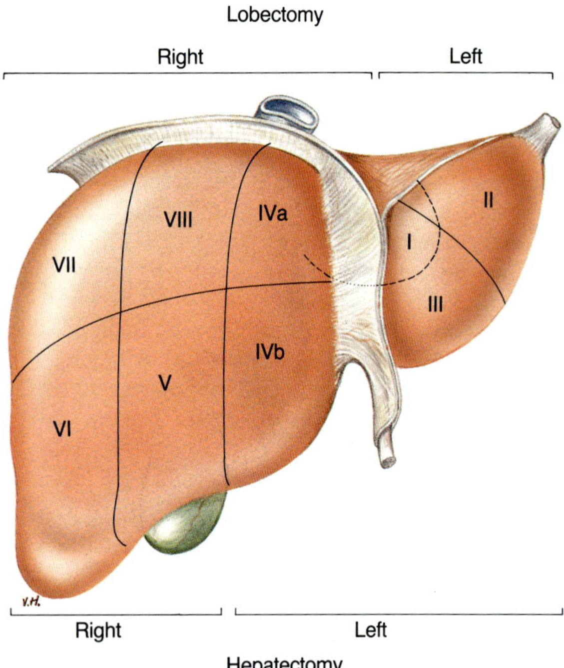

Fig. 6.4.**2 Systematization of surgical procedures** in hepatic resections

Intraoperative ultrasound investigations are able to detect tumorous lesions larger than 1 cm and therefore sometimes additional metastases. In addition, the relation of the tumor to the segmental structure can be identified.

Computerized tomography (CT scan) is a useful preoperative investigation demonstrating the extent of a tumor and its relation to intra- and extrahepatic structures. In addition, the structure and volume of the tumor-free parenchyma can be determined, thus allowing an assessment of risk and resectability.

With **sequential hepatic scintigraphy** techniques (^{99}Tc-HIDA, ^{99}Tc colloid and ^{99}Tc erythrocytes) primary and secondary liver malignancies can be differentiated. In benign hepatic neoplasias such as hemangioma or focal nodular hyperplasia (FNH) the diagnosis can also be established by this form of examination. Differentiation between liver adenoma and primary liver cell carcinoma is not possible, because both lesions arise from liver cells and therefore show a similar enhancement of the isotopes. However, since both constitute an absolute indication for liver resection, the preoperative differentiation is of minor importance. Elevated or normal α-1-fetoprotein generally provides additional information about the genesis.

Selective arteriography of the celiac trunk and superior mesenteric artery, combined with an indirect splenoportogram, provides information about the hepatic blood supply (e. g. whether there is an accessory right hepatic artery originating from the mesenteric artery), occlusion of the intrahepatic vessels and vascularity of the tumor. Variations of the hepatic blood supply are very common (up to 40%). They should be recognized preoperatively to avoid surgical complications. If the implantation of a catheter system for locoregional chemotherapy is planned as an additional or alternative treatment to the liver resection, the degree of vascularity of the tumor has to be evaluated, because intra-arterial chemotherapy can only be effective in hypervascularized lesions (about 30% of the metastases of colorectal carcinomas). Hyper- and hypovascularized lesions can be observed in the same liver. In patients with irresectable liver tumors in which disarterialization or chemoembolization of a liver lobe or segment is planned, indirect splenoportography has to exclude a portal vein thrombosis prior to this treatment, because otherwise a fatal hepatic necrosis may occur.

Cavography is a rarely indicated investigation in patients with large liver tumors. Even if a stenosis of the caval vein could be observed, this technique cannot differentiate between tumorous infiltration of the vein and a mere compression of the vessel by the tumor mass. Only exploration and extented mobilization can clarify the resectability (Blumgart 1988, Brölsch 1986, Launois et al. 1979).

Laparoscopy combined with biopsy is rarely indicated to establish an indication for liver resection, although cytology of a tumor mass may help to define alternative treatments, especially in high-risk patients.

In secondary liver tumors, preoperative investigations should search for further extrahepatic tumor manifestation, although extrahepatic lesions do not necessarily exclude patients from liver resection (e. g. solitary liver and lung mestastases of colorectal carcinomas, palliative resection in symptomatic patients) (Kremer and Henne-Bruns 1986, Neuhaus et al. 1986).

Positioning of the Patient for Hepatic Surgery

For all liver resections the patient has to be positioned slighty extended on his back. Both arms are spread out at right angles. Self-retractors fixed directly distal from the axilla to the table facilitate exposure, especially in large tumors or obese patients. The elevation of the right side is not necessary because adequate exposure can also be achieved after mobilization of the liver by tilting the table.

A transverse upper abdominal and median incision allows good exposure of the liver

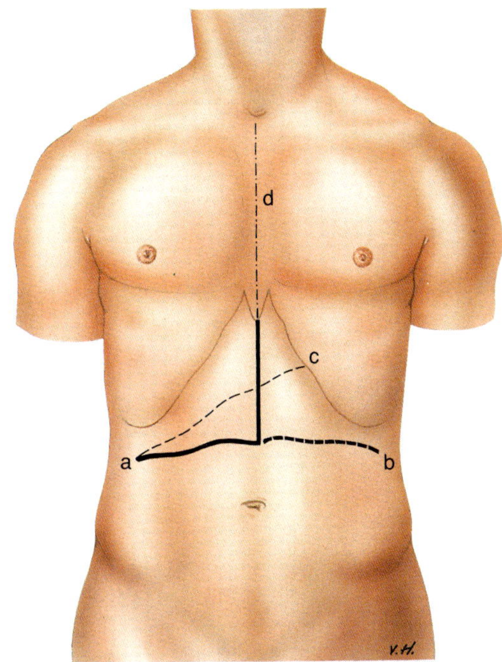

Fig. 6.4.**3 Approaches in hepatic surgery.** Transverse upper abdominal laparotomy with median extension always allows good exposure (a and b). In slim patients or peripherically located lesions, a median incision extended to the right (a) is sufficient

(Fig. 6.4.**3a** and **b**). The myocutaneous flaps arising from this approach are folded back around the costal arch and fixed with self-retractors. In slim patients with hepatic tumors located peripherally in the right or the left liver lobe, median upper abdominal laparotomy with transverse extension only to the right side may be sufficient (Fig. 6.4.**3a**). A thoraco-abdominal approach was never necessary in our experience, not even in liver transplantations. It should be avoided in order to reduce pulmonary complications originating from pleural effusions (Iwatsuki et al. 1983, Longmire and Tompkins 1981, Neuhaus et al. 1986, Pichlmayr et al. 1984, Priesching 1986, Starzl et al. 1980, Thompson et al. 1983, Tsuzuki et al. 1984).

Exploration of the Abdominal Cavity

After laparotomy, a careful exploration of the abdominal cavity is performed with attention to the following points:

- Pathological findings unrelated to the liver disease?
- Extrahepatic tumor manifestations?
- Resectability of the liver tumor?

All of these steps are an essential component of every abdominal operation, especially in patients with tumor disease. They therefore do not require any further description. The abdominal exploration can be impeded in patients who have had previous abdominal operations, due to multiple adhesions. But this is no reason to desist from a careful preparation of the abdominal cavity to allow palpatory exclusion of further malignant lesions.

The exploration of the lymph nodes begins with the dissection of the hepatoduodenal ligament and complete removal of the lymphatic tissue, which is examined histologically. If enlarged and suspicious lymph nodes are found, the specimens are examined intraoperatively by frozen sections. The dissection of the lymphatic tissue of the hepatoduodenal ligament should always include lymph nodes behind the portal vein and the common bile duct. Exploration of the lymph nodes along the hepatic artery up to the celiac trunk requires incision of the lesser omentum. After removal of this lymphatic tissue and rapid histological examination if required, the caudate lobe (segment I) can be explored and tumor involvement, with possible infiltration of the caval vein, can be appraised. Assessment of the resectability of large, centrally located liver tumors requires in addition the severance of the falciform, triangular and coronary ligaments (Fig. 6.4.**4**) (Adson et al. 1980, Bismuth 1982, Fortner et al. 1978, 1984, Funovics and Fritsch 1983, Iwatsuki et al. 1983, Lin 1979, Pichlmayr et al. 1984, Priesching 1986, Starzl et al. 1980, Thompson et al. 1983, Tsuzuki et al. 1984).

Right Hemihepatectomy

Mobilization of the liver. The dissection begins with the severing of the falciform ligament (Fig. 6.4.**4a**), continuing proximally up to the suprahepatic vena cava and incision of the peritoneal duplicature. It continues ventrally of the caval vein to the left and right side until the courses and orifices of the right, median and left hepatic veins are visible (Fig. 6.4.**5**). Following this the right liver lobe is mobilized. The peritoneal duplicature therefore has to be incised laterally between the right liver lobe and the diaphragm. The severing of the peritoneal duplicature then continues ventrally of the infrahepatic caval vein to the foramen of Winslow. After subsequently severing the right triangular ligament, the right liver lobe can be luxated forward and the organ can be rotated to the left, exposing the retrohepatic segment of the vena cava, which can now be explored (Fig. 6.4.**6a**). While dissecting the triangular ligament and the right peritoneal duplicature, attention has to be paid to the right adrenal gland, which sometimes adheres firmly to the

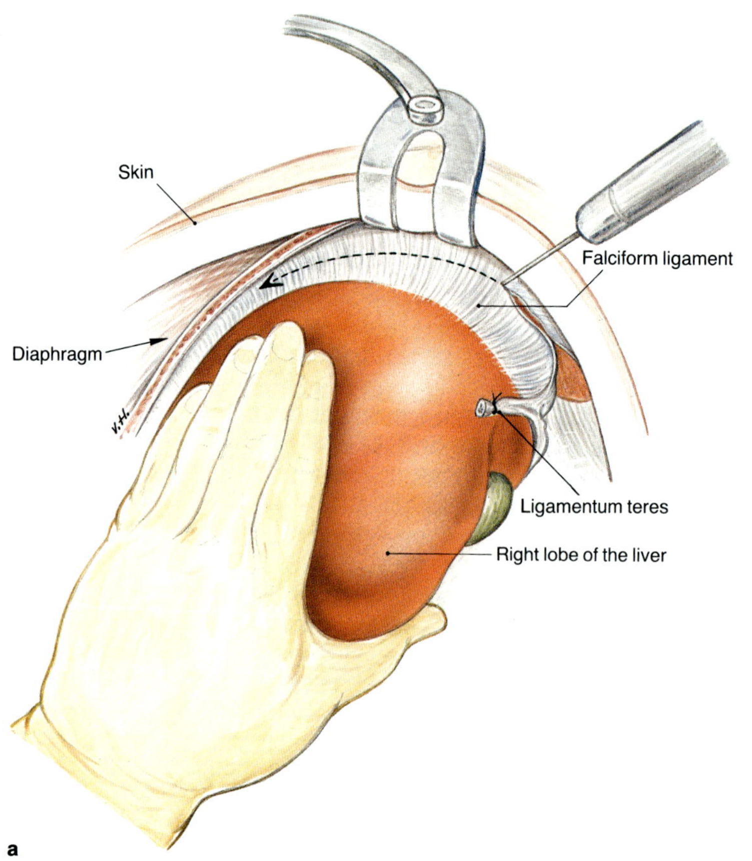

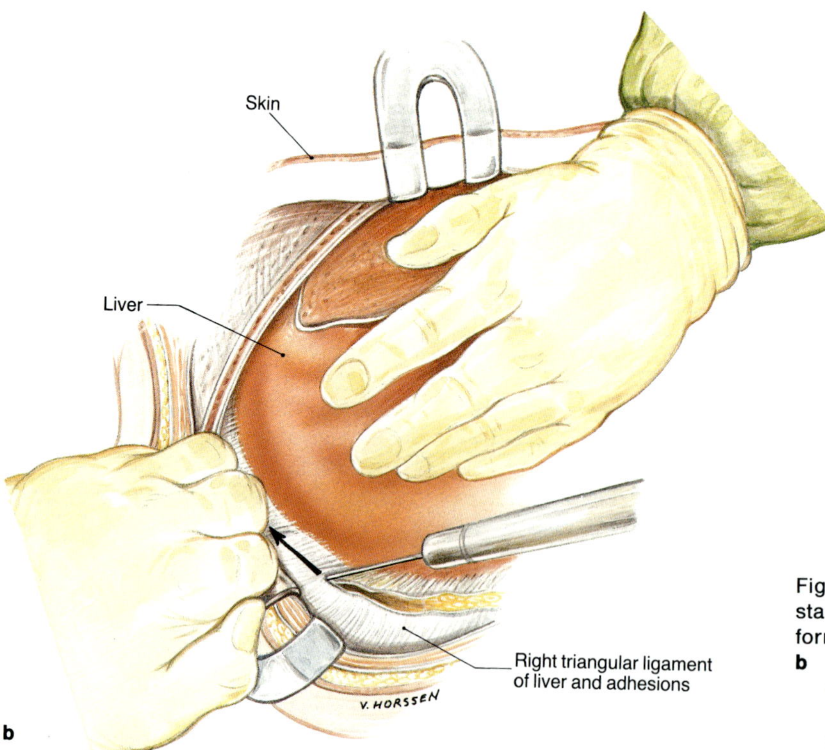

Fig. 6.4.4a Mobilization of the liver starts with the severing of the falciform ligament. Line of incision: -----
b Mobilization of the right liver is continued by transecting the right triangular and coronary ligaments, exposing the retroperitoneal surface of the right lobe

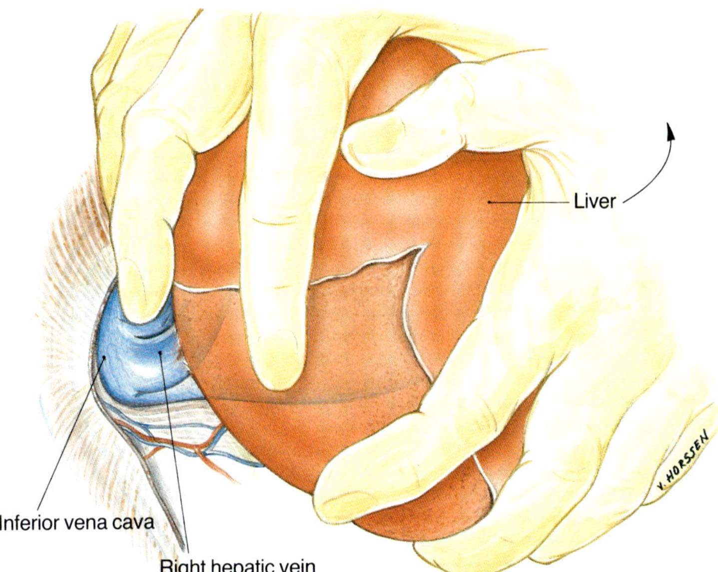

Fig. 6.4.**5 Severing the right triangular and coronary ligaments** allows exposure of the right hepatic vein and the right adrenal gland. The gland should be removed along with the tumor if the tumor is firmly adherent to it

posterior surface of the liver. In these cases the gland has to be carefully freed in order to avoid hemorrhages. If the tumor itself is firmly adherent to the adrenal gland, the gland should be removed with the tumor.

Preparation of the retrohepatic caval vein. Complete mobilization of the right liver lobe is followed by a good exposure of the retrohepatic caval vein. Smaller liver veins draining directly into the vena cava are visible. They are carefully dissected and severed between ligatures or clips (Fig. 6.4.**6b, c**). The dissection of the retrohepatic vena cava then continues proximally, exposing the opening of the right hepatic vein. If the ventral part of the suprahepatic vena cava is completely freed from connective tissue, the right hepatic vein can usually be snared (Fig. 6.4.**7**). In some cases the confluence of the right and median hepatic veins is located too distantly in the parenchyma. It may then be safer to isolate the right hepatic vein during the phase of parenchymal dissection. In such cases, or in large hepatic tumors, we prefer to loop the suprahepatic and infrahepatic vena cava in order to be able to occlude the vessel if necessary.

Dissection of the hepatoduodenal ligament. The dissection of the hepatoduodenal ligament with isolation of the common bile duct, hepatic artery and portal vein (Fig. 6.4.**8**) can either be performed directly after the abdominal exploration, combined with a lymph node dissection for staging reasons, or after mobilization of the liver. The plane of resection in right hepatectomy lies between the gallbladder bed, or just left of it, and the caval vein. A cholecystectomy therefore facilitates the overview. The cholecystectomy is usually carried out in a

retrograde fashion with severance of the cystic duct and the cystic artery between ligatures (Fig. 6.4.**9**). Afterwards the gallbladder is removed. Hemostasis in the gallbladder bed can be achieved quickly by sapphire coagulation. After transverse incision of the hilar serosa (Fig. 6.4.**8**) and severing of the perivascular lymph and nerve tissue, the choledochal and hepatic ducts and proper hepatic artery can be identified and snared. Difficult anatomical conditions sometimes require an initial resection of the left lateral lymph node group at the hepatoduodenal ligament, to expose the origin of the common hepatic artery, the proper hepatic artery and the gastroduodenal artery. Afterwards the arterial vessels can easily be followed to their division into a right and left branch.

The most frequent variation in the arterial blood supply to the liver consists of a right hepatic artery originating from the mesenteric artery (Fig. 6.4.**10**). This artery usually follows the choledochal duct at its dorsal, right lateral margin to the liver hilum and can easily be identified and snared if the common bile duct has been isolated and looped beforehand. Variations in the arterial blood supply of the liver should be known before the operation, and it should be kept in mind that the left hepatic artery may also originate from the left gastric artery, reaching the left liver lobe through the lesser omentum at the base of the umbilical fissure (Fig. 6.4.**10a**).

The exposure of the right and left hepatic ducts can be more difficult than the dissection of the arterial vessels, because the hepatic bifurcation is usually located more centrally in the liver hilus. After isolation of the right and left hepatic ducts,

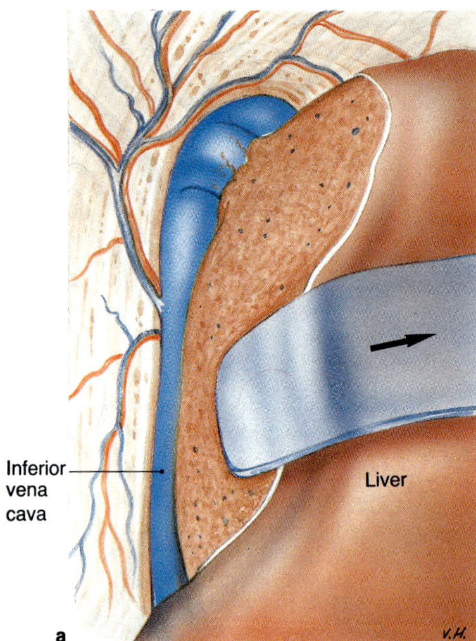

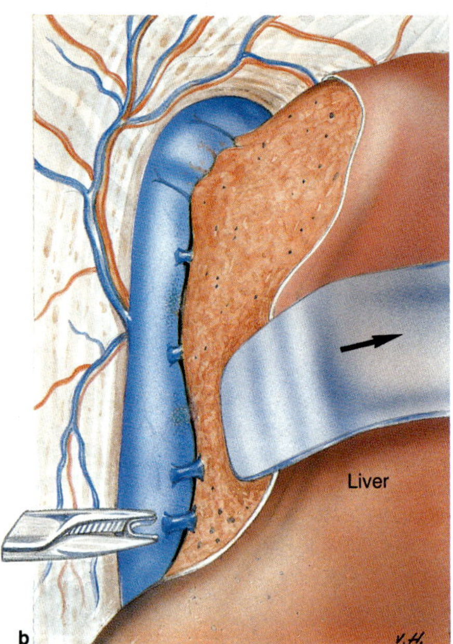

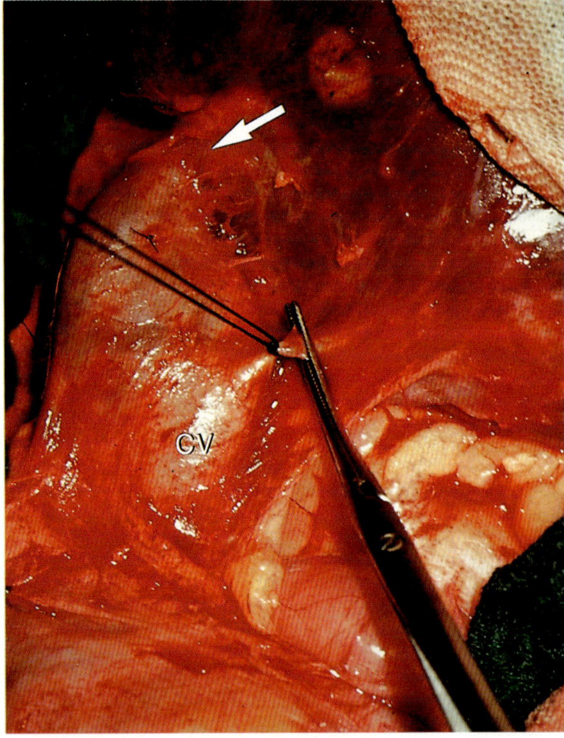

Fig. 6.4.6 a   Complete mobilization of the right liver lobe allows access to the retrohepatic vena cava

b   Exposure of the retrohepatic vena cava requires careful severance of the small hepatic veins directly entering segment IV

c   Intraoperative view of the exposed vena cava (CV). A hepatic vein of segment IV is ligated and clamped. The right hepatic vein is partially freed (arrow)

the right hepatic artery, which usually enters the liver dorsal to the hepatic duct, can be transected and tied with fine atraumatic suture material (4-0, 5-0) (Fig. 6.4.**11**). Pulling the proper hepatic artery to left lateral, and the common bile duct to right lateral, the portal vein can be exposed between the two structures. Nervous and lymphatic tissue around the portal vein is dissected and removed. The dissection of the portal vein and the right portal branch can also be carried out from the right lateral margin of the hepatoduodenal ligament, pulling the common bile duct and the hepatic artery to the left side (Fig. 6.4.**12**). The preparation at the portal vein continues centrally, exposing the division of the portal vein branches by placing a vessel loop around the right branch.

The next step of the operation is the severance of the right hepatic duct, closing the stumps with fine resorbable suture material (5-0) (Fig. 6.4.**11 a**). The right branch of the portal vein is now completely exposed and can be divided between two hemostatic clamps (Fig. 6.4.**12**). The peripheral stump is sutured with non-resorbable material (2-0, 3-0). The central stump is closed with a fine, vascular suture (4-0, 5-0), which must not constrict the portal vein. In addition, attention must be paid to ensure that a blind end is not left at the portal bifurcation, because this may cause a retrograde portal vein thrombosis. This complication may occur as a result of the 60 % reduced portal venous bed after right hemihepatectomy (Brölsch 1986, Mimura et al. 1986).

Resection of the liver parenchyma. Division of the right hepatic artery and portal vein is followed

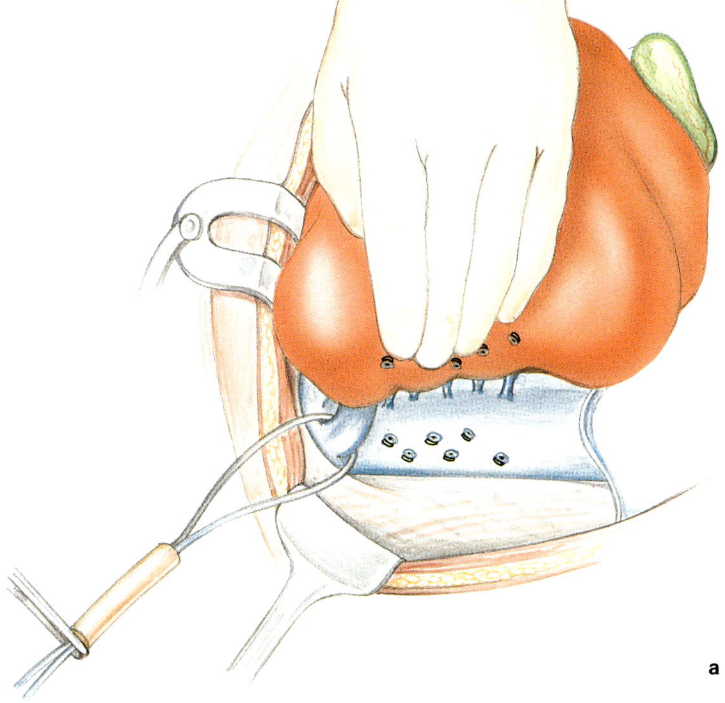

by a clearly visible demarcation of the devascularized liver parenchyma. Prior to resection, a tourniquet is placed around the remaining portal vein and hepatic artery, which is occluded (Pringle maneuver) during the resection phase (Esser 1979a, 1979b, Longmire and Tompkins 1981). In patients with normal liver function, a warm ischemic period of 45 min is tolerated by the liver. If it is expected that this interval will be significantly exceeded, a temporary reperfusion of the liver after 30 min of ischemia should be carried out for 10–15 min with slight compression of the resection surface. Afterwards the Pringle maneuver can be repeated for 30 min. Using this technique, we performed a trisegmentectomy on the left side with an overall warm ischemic period of 75 min and without any complications. Before severance of the hepatic parenchyma, the right hepatic vein can be divided between hemostatic clamps (Fig. 6.4.**13**), closing the stumps with vascular sutures (4-0). Technical problems at the hepatic vein may necessitate a temporary occlusion of the infra- and suprahepatic caval vein, which is usually tolerated by the patient. If the right hemihepatectomy is carried out step by step as described, the subsequent severing of the liver parenchyma can be performed without major bleeding (Lin 1973).

Prior to resection, the liver capsule is incised with diathermy from the left lateral margin of the gallbladder bed to the right hepatic vein (Fig. 6.4.**14**). The resection plane follows the inci-

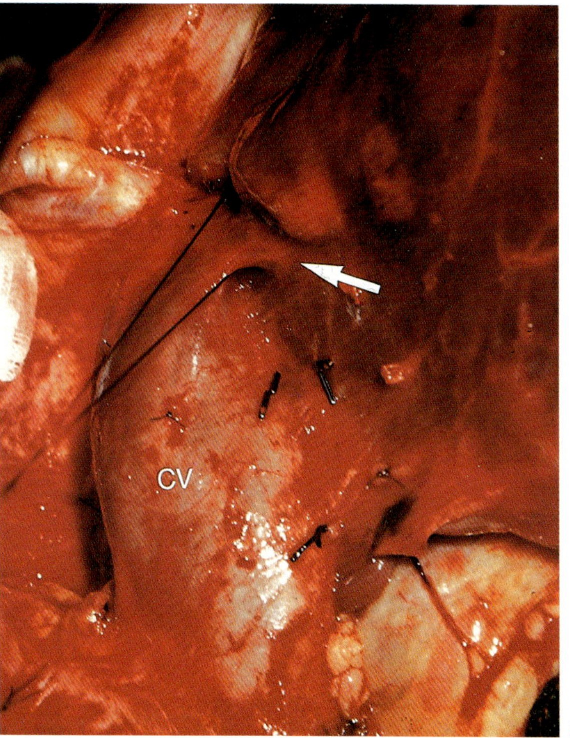

Fig. 6.4.**7a**   **Dissection of the retrohepatic caval segment** is continued from distal to proximal, exposing the right hepatic vein, which can now be looped
b   Intraoperative situation after dissection of the retrohepatic vena cava (CV). Segmental veins are clipped (titanium). The right hepatic vein is looped (arrow)

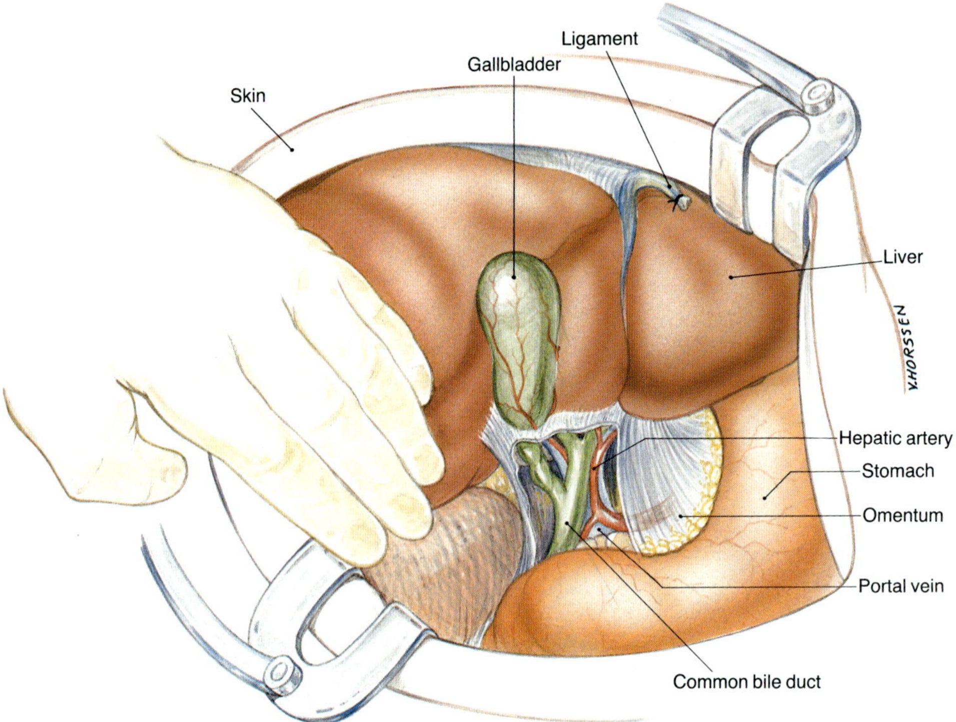

Fig. 6.4.**8**   **All structures of the hepatoduodenal ligament have to be identified** in anatomical hepatic resections

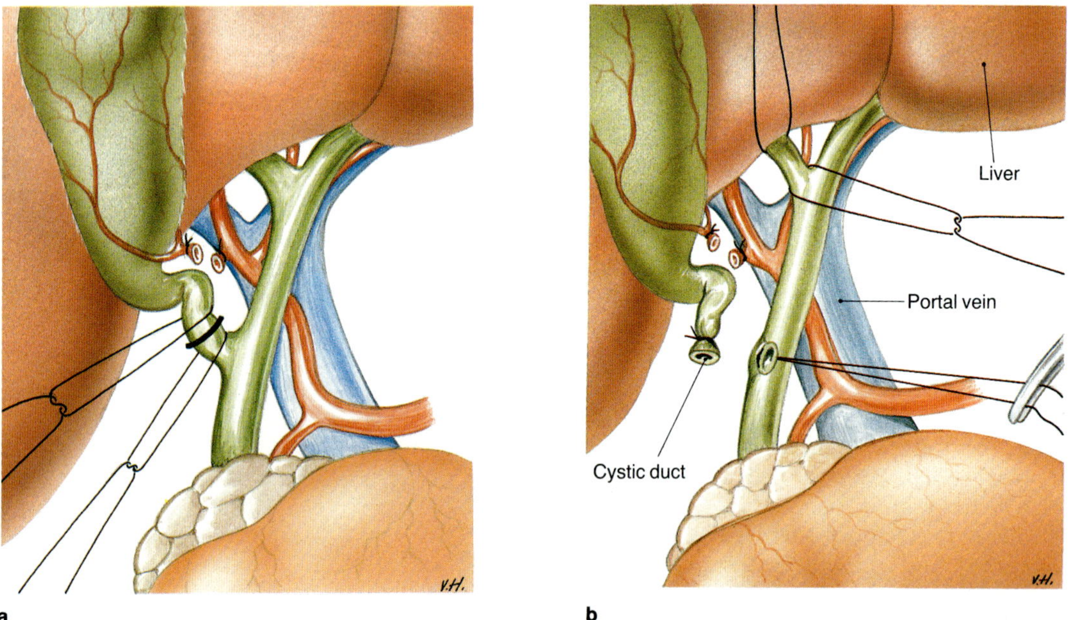

Fig. 6.4.**9**   **Prior to hemihepatectomy, carrying out cholecystectomy facilitates the approach to the central structures of the hepatoduodenal ligament.**
a   The cystic artery is divided
b   Division of the cystic duct and preparation of the right hepatic duct

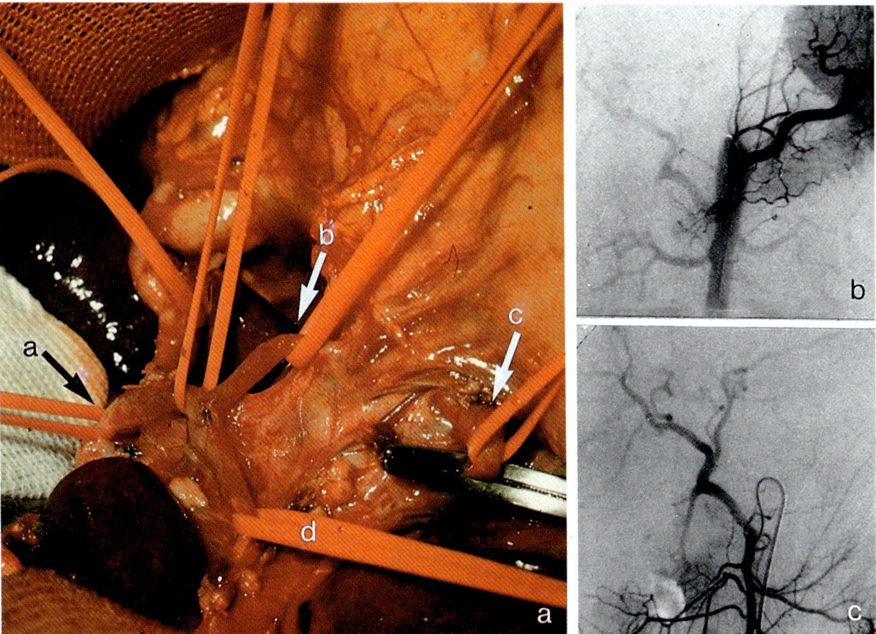

Fig. 6.4.**10** **Variations in the hepatic blood supply**
a Intraoperative situation showing most of the possible vascular variations at the hepatoduodenal ligament: the right hepatic artery (c) arises from the superior mesenteric artery, the left hepatic artery (a) originates from the left gastric artery, giving off a separate artery to segment IV (d) from which the gastroduodenal artery originates (b)
b Celiacography in a different patient, showing only the splenic artery and the left gastric artery arising from the celiac trunk
c Angiography of the superior mesenteric artery (same patient as in **b**). The common hepatic artery originates from the superior mesenteric artery

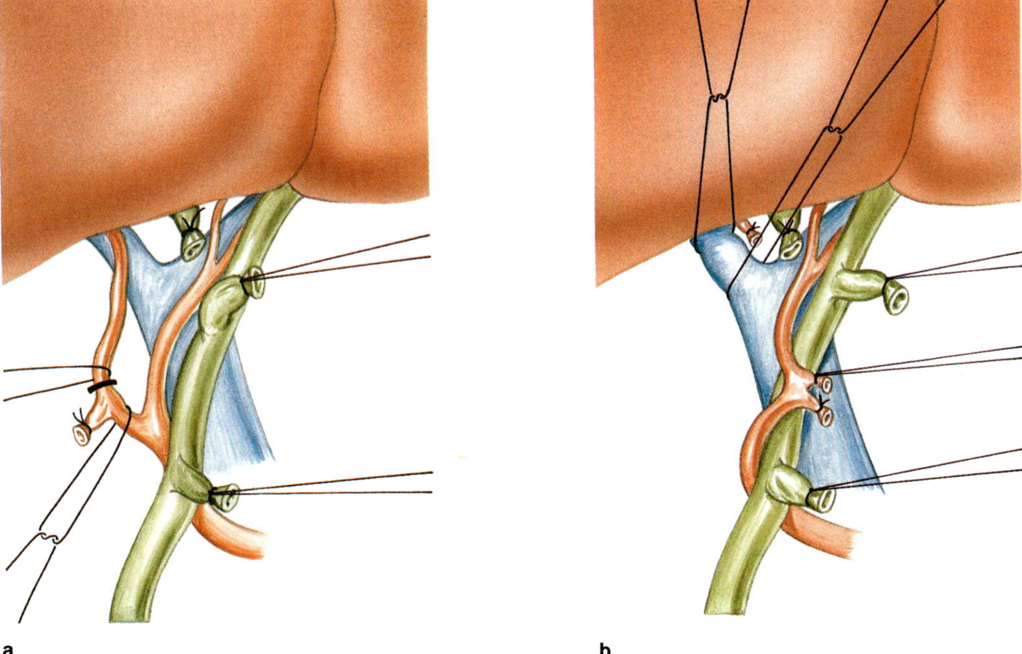

Fig. 6.4.**11** **Preparation of hilar structures**
a The right hepatic artery is looped, the right hepatic duct dissected
b After division of the right hepatic artery, the right portal branch is exposed and looped

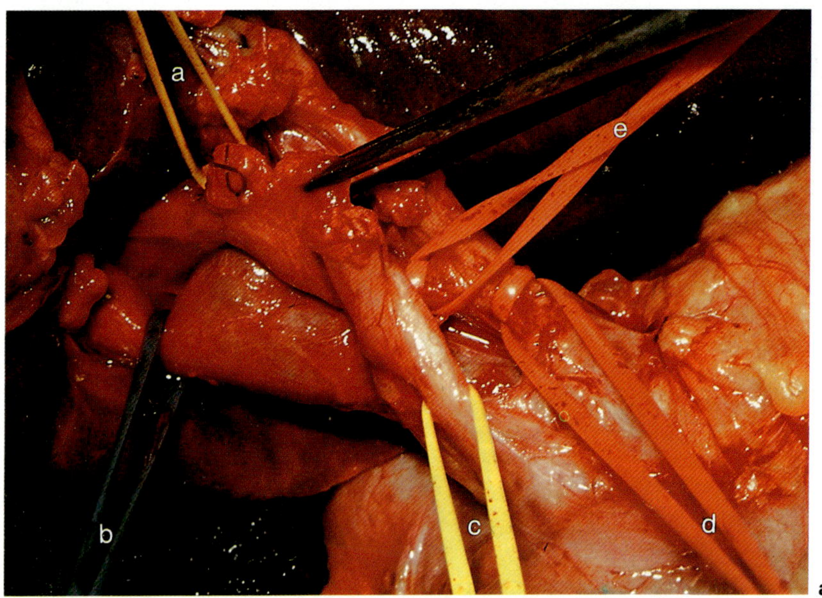

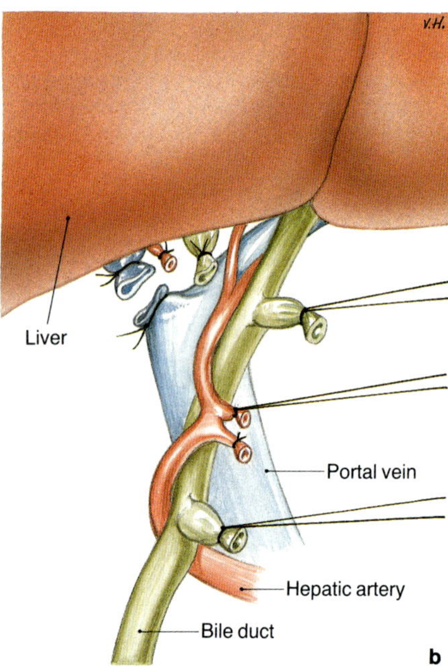

Fig. 6.4.12 Preparation of hilar structures

a (a) The left hepatic duct is looped. Traction of the right hepatic duct (forceps) and the common bile duct (c) to the left allows exposure of the right lateral margin of the portal vein and of the main right portal branch (b). The proper hepatic artery (d) and the right hepatic artery (e) are looped

b The right hepatic artery, bile duct and portal branch are dissected

sion dorsally to the retrohepatic vena cava (Fig. 6.4.16). The liver tissue is carefully pushed apart with scissors or a clamp. Vessels and bile ducts are grasped separately with fine clamps on the remaining left side of the liver, and ligatures are applied immediately, or after parenchymal severance has been completed, with absorbable suture material (2-0–4-0). Alternatively titanium clips can be used, but only for smaller vessels (Fig. 6.4.15). Steel clips should be avoided, since they cause artefacts in the CT scan investigations which are usually performed later in patient follow-up.

The use of an ultrasonic dissector for the severance of the liver parenchyma offers technical comfort but is more time-consuming. A reduction in blood loss cannot be achieved merely by using ultrasonic dissection. The aim in any kind of liver resection is to achieve a flat resection surface with carefully, separately ligated vessels and bile ducts (Fig. 6.4.17). Minor bleeding sites can be treated after releasing the arterial and portal blood flow by sutures or sapphire coagulation (Iwatsuki et al. 1983, Neuhaus et al. 1986, Pichlmayr et al. 1984, Starzl et al. 1982). If the resection surface is slightly concave, the margins of the liver capsule can sometimes be approximated by single interrupted sutures. Such sutures may only be applied if no disturbance to the parenchymal blood supply occurs. The resection surface can be covered with fibrin tissue-adhesive sealant or collagen fleece coated with fibrin tissue-adhesive sealant (Fig. 6.4.18). Using such techniques the rate of postoperative bile leakages was less than than 2%, and therefore a minor problem.

Drainage. The operation is completed by the introduction of soft drains (Penrose, "easy flow") which are placed subphrenically at the resection plane and usually removed 2–4 days after the operation.

Technical variations on the procedure described mainly affect the extent of hilar prepar-

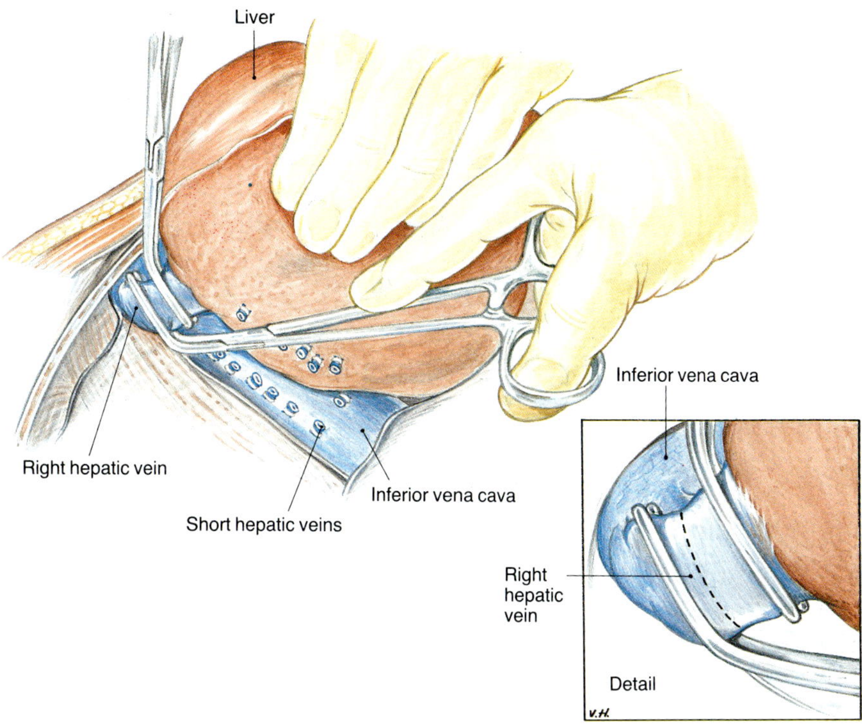

Fig. 6.4.**13** **The right hepatic vein can be severed between vascular clamps** after dissection of the right hepatic artery and right portal vein

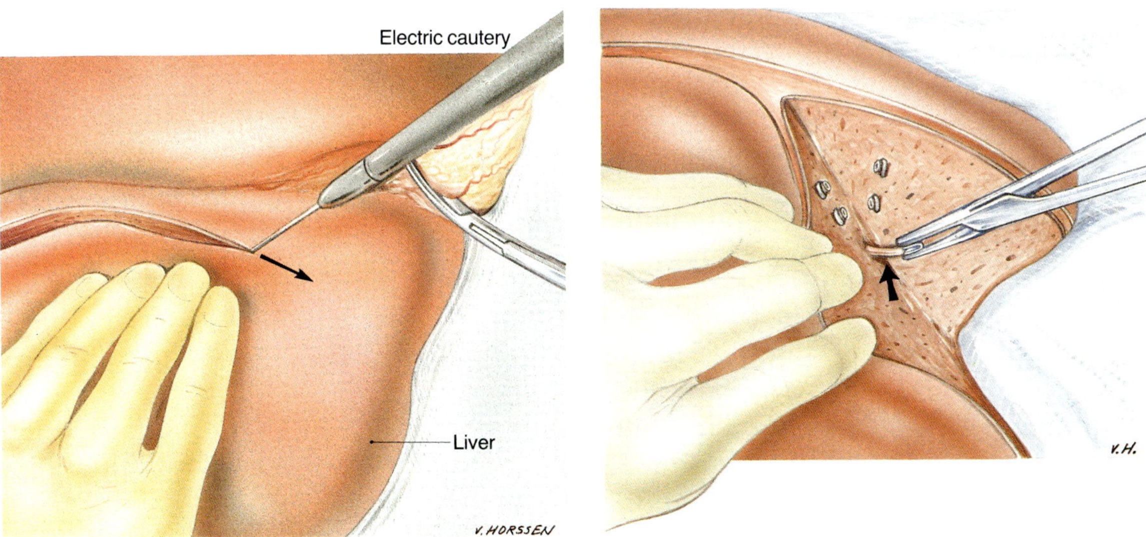

Fig. 6.4.**14** **The liver capsula is incised** (arrow) after occlusion of the hepatic blood supply by a Pringle maneuver

Fig. 6.4.**15** **Dissection of the liver parenchyma** proceeds in small steps. Vessels and bile ducts are clasped with clamps and ligated or clipped (arrow) during dissection

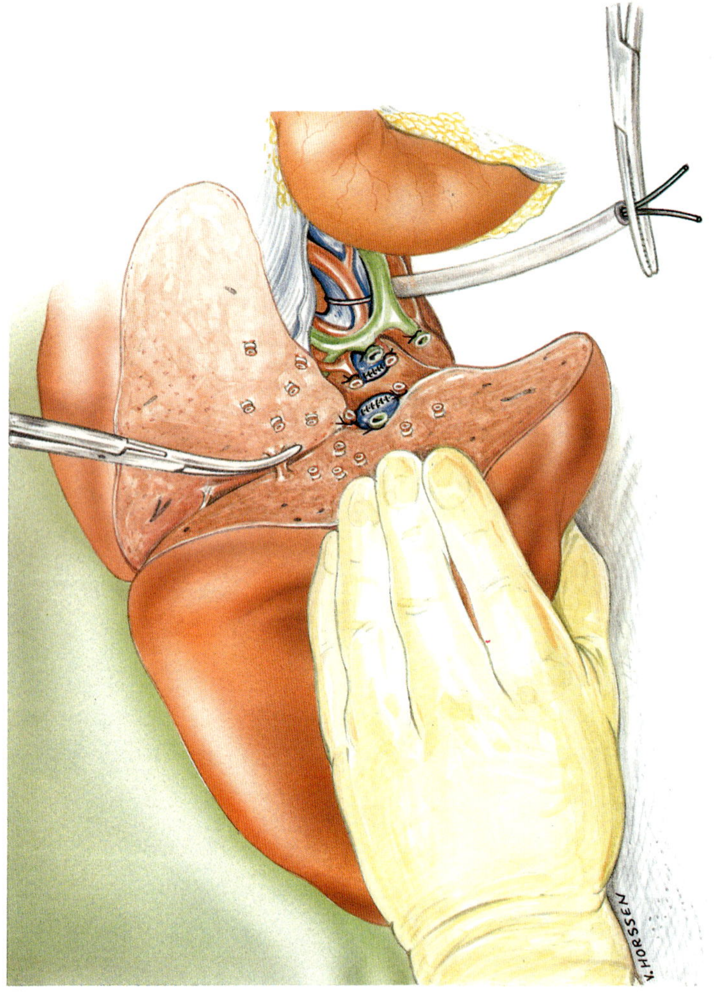

Fig. 6.4.**16** **The dissection plane follows the incision dorsally to the vena cava**

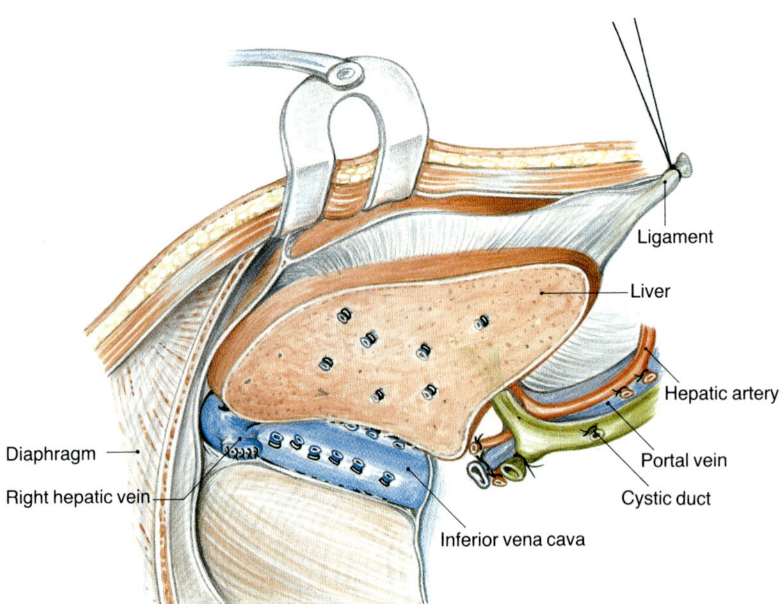

Fig. 6.4.**17** **The right hemihepatectomy is completed.** Note: the right hepatic vein is sutured; the resection surface is flat

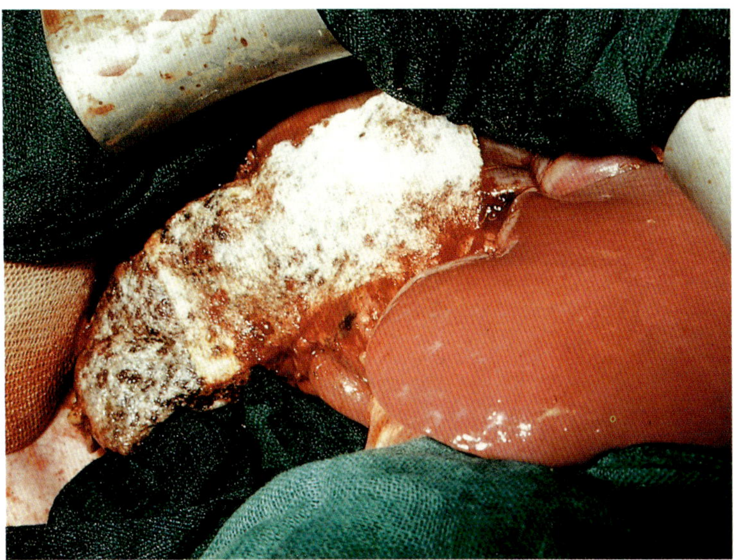

Fig. 6.4.**18   Intraoperative situation after resection of segments IV b, V, VI and VII.** The resection surface is covered by a fibrin-coated collagen fleece

ation. In tumors located peripherally from the hepatic hilus, the dissection of the right hepatic artery alone prior to resection may be sufficient. In these cases, the right portal branch and right bile duct are carefully exposed, clamped and suture-ligated during the parenchymal dissection following the Pringle maneuver (Esser 1979a, 1979b, Longmire 1981). Large or centrally located tumors sometimes require a "non-anatomical" procedure instead of a "strictly anatomical" resection technique (Kremer and Henne-Bruns 1986, Priesching 1986). The mobilization of the right liver lobe should always be carried out completely. Lack of mobilization is directly related to surgical complications, because hemorrhages at the hepatic veins or the hepatic hilus can only be treated if these structures have been previously exposed. Hemorrhages arising from an incidental partial resection of the hepatic or caval vein can be controlled if the vena cava has been looped with tourniquets supra- and infrahepatically prior to resection. While compressing the hole in the vein from dorsal with the left hand, it is possible to apply a vascular suture to the lesion.

Extended Right Hepatectomy (Right Trisegmentectomy)

Extended right hemihepatectomy meens removal of the entire right liver lobe (segments IV a and b, V – VIII) (Fig. 6.4.**19**). The resection line is marked by the falciform ligament and the umbilical fissure. Right lobectomy removes about 70–80% of the liver parenchyma and reduces the portal vascular bed by about 75% (Brölsch 1986). Even in patients with normal liver function, this operation includes the risk of postoperative hepatic failure. The technical details are analogous to those in right hepatectomy, with the following special features.

For an extended right hepatectomy, a transverse upper abdominal laparotomy with extension in the median up to the xiphoid (Fig. 6.4.**3a** and **b**) should always be used. Because the plan of resection is extended towards the left side of the liver compared to a right hepatectomy, the liver also has to be adequately mobilized. This means that the dissection of the retrohepatic caval vein also has to be extended to the left side. Not only hepatic veins draining directly from segment IV into the vena cava have to be severed, therefore, but also some hepatic veins arising from the caudate lobe, which itself is only exceptionally removed in extended right hepatectomies (Fig. 6.4.**20**). This extensive retrohepatic dissection combined, with the severing of the right and left triangular and coronary ligaments, allows exploration of the hepatic veins. In contrast to right hepatectomy, right lobectomy also requires the preparation of the median and left hepatic veins. It is important to evaluate the course of the median and left hepatic veins as well as their junction with the caval vein. Although the median vein can rarely be separated from the left hepatic vein, the identification of the site of opening into the vena cava is important to avoid accidental resection of the left vein and major hemorrhages.

After the hilar structures have been dissected, the right hepatic duct has to be divided and sutured with fine absorbable material (5-0). The course of the left hepatic duct has to be identified and the duct mobilized to the left in order to prevent injuries later on, during parenchymal severance. After this, the right hepatic artery and right portal vein are severed, as described above. The left hepatic artery

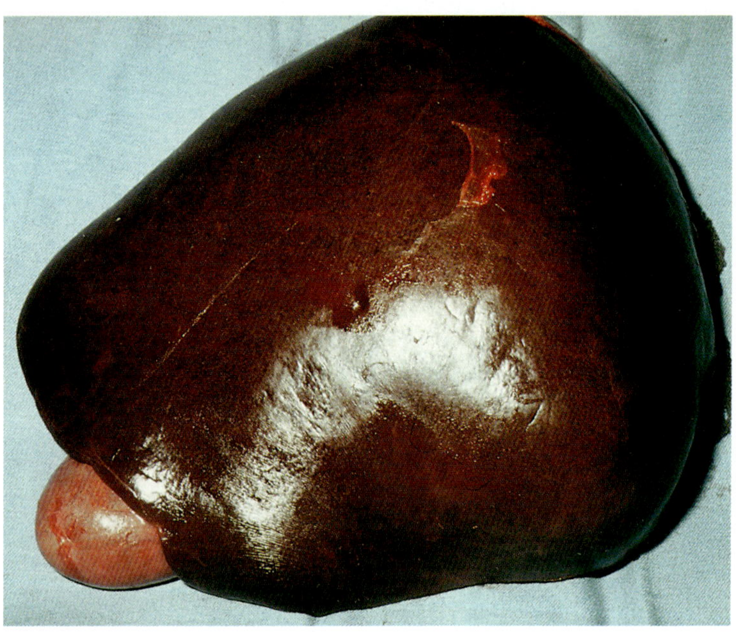

Fig. 6.4.**19   The entire right liver lobe is removed** in extended right hepatectomy

and the portal vein are dissected free far into the liver hilus in order to be able to resect segment IV without injuring these structures. To sever the parenchyma, the ligamentum teres is gripped with a clamp and drawn to proximal and forward. A parenchymal bridge frequently present between segments III and IV is transected by diathermy. Afterwards, the liver capsule is incised at the right side, parallel to the falciform ligament. After occlusion of the arterial and portal blood flow (Pringle maneuver), the right hepatic vein can be severed between clamps and suture-ligated. The parenchymal severance is carried out with the same technique described for hemihepatectomy. Caution must be used in severing the segmental portal branches supplying segment IV and arising reversely from the main left portal branch with a short segment. A dissection of the parenchyma directly through the umbilical fissure might leave the resection plane too far to the left, bringing a risk of accidental resection of the portal branches of segments II and III.

In most cases, the indication for an extended right hepatectomy is a large tumor of the right side not necessarily involving the caudate lobe (segment I), which can then be preserved (Fig. 6.4.**20a**). Tumors originating from segment IV and extending to the right, in which a segmental resection (segment IV) is impossible, usually require an extended right hepatectomy including segment I. Access to the caudate lobe in these cases is not difficult, because of mobilization of the right liver lobe (Fig. 6.4.**20b**) has already been carried out. In order to be able to occlude the supra- and infrahepatic caval veins, the left lobe has also already been mobilized. It is therefore no trouble to separate

the partially mobilized caudate lobe completely from the right side of the caval vein, and, in some additional steps, from the left side. The use of hemostatic titanium clips to sever veins opening directly from segment I into the vena cava offers a technical improvement in this phase of the operation. At least the retrohepatic caval segment is completely freed from the hepatic tissue up to the hepatic veins and a circular approach to the retrohepatic segment of the vena cava is possible. In the majority of cases no lumbar venous branches drain into this segment, but attention must be paid to the suprarenal veins.

The extended right hemihepatectomy (right trisegmentectomy) has three major technical pitfalls:

- Injury to the left bile duct, especially if the segmental bile duct from segment IV could not be identified during the hilar dissection;
- Injury to the arterial or portal blood supply of segments II and III during dissection of the parenchyma in the umbilical fissure, instead of remaining just to the right of this plane;
- Injury to the left hepatic vein due to resection of the median hepatic vein.

The occlusion of the arterial and portal blood flow should not exceed 30 min in extended right hemihepatectomy in order to avoid ischemic damage to residual parenchyma. The parenchymal bridge between the right and left liver lobes is relatively small, so that dissection should always be possible within this period of time. A single bolus of 500–1000 mg prednisone injected prior to releasing the arterial and portal blood flow may reduce the edema of the

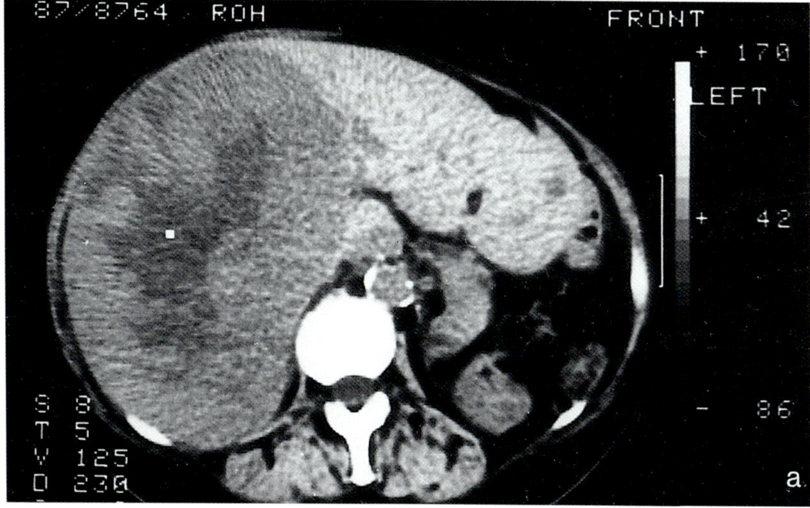

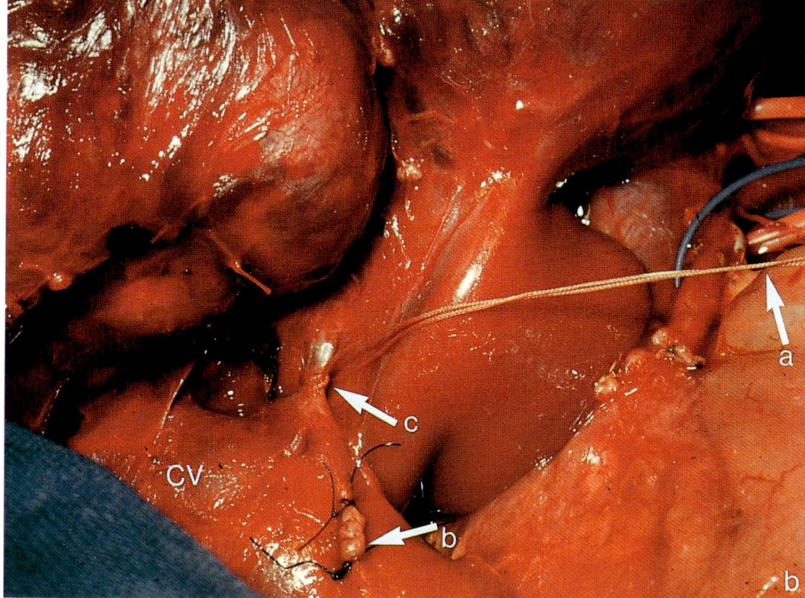

Fig. 6.4.**20** **Extended right hepatectomy**

a CT scan of a huge liver tumor involving the right lobe

b The size of the tumor requires an extended right hepatectomy including segment I. The hilar structures are prepared (a); the hepatic veins of segment IV (b) and segment I (c) are dissected.
CV = vena cava

residual parenchyma (segments II and III and occasionally also I) which invariably occurs.

The remaining resection surface is small compared to that following right hemihepatectomy, and hemostasis at the plane of resection should never be a problem. Penetrating sutures must be strictly avoided, because they may restrict the function of the residual parenchyma by disturbing the blood flow. Finally, application of collagen fleeces and fibrin glue should always achieve sufficient hemostasis (Fig. 6.4.**18**). Subphrenic insertion of soft drains (Penrose, "easy flow") is the last step in the operation prior to layer-by-layer closure of the laparotomy.

Potential Postoperative Problems

Using the technique described, 162 liver resections were performed between 1983 and 1987, with an overall mortality of 6.3 %, in 70 % of which cases death was due to postoperative liver failure. In these cases the functional capacity of the remaining parenchyma was overestimated (Kremer and Henne-Bruns 1986, Okamoto et al. 1984, Stone 1977). Reoperation was indicated in 3.7 % of the patients because of abscess formation or bleeding.

Summarizing our experience, the following symptoms or problems can be observed postoperatively after extended liver resection:

- Pleural effusions after right hepatectomy or extended right hepatectomy in about 30% of cases;
- Hyperbilirubinemia after extended hepatectomies (bilirubin 2.5–30 mg/dl) decreasing 3–7 days after the operation;
- Decrease of clotting factors V and VII to 30–50% of normal values.

Further technical problems and their intra- or postoperative management are described in Chapter 6.7 below.

Left Hepatectomy

The main indications for a left hepatectomy are primary or secondary malignancies of the liver predominantly located in the area of the falciform ligament. In cases in which the tumor growth involves segment IV, left hepatectomy has to be extended to segment VIII or segment V, or both (extended left hepatectomy) (Starzl et al. 1982). In most cases except Klatskin tumors (Bismuth 1982, Klatskin 1965, Launois et al. 1979, Tsuzuki et al. 1983; Chapter 8.1 below), the resection of a left-side hepatic tumor does not require simultaneous resection of the caudate lobe. The decision to undertake a combined resection with segment I must be made individually on the basis of the location and histological grading of the tumor.

Our preferred approach in patients with centrally-located large left-side hepatic tumors consists of a transverse upper abdominal laparotomy with a median extension to the xiphoid (Fig. 6.4.**3a** and **b**). Smaller tumor masses can be easily surgically inspected by a median laparotomy transversely extended to the right (Fig. 6.4.**3a**).

After exploration of the abdominal cavity for any pathological findings or extrahepatic tumor manifestations, the falciform ligament is dissected up to the hepatic veins. Further dissection of the left triangular and coronary ligaments allows identification of the left hepatic vein. Usually the dissection is begun by severing the fibrous appendix of the left lobe. The left phrenic vein empties into the left hepatic vein and therefore represents a structure which can guide the exposure of the left hepatic vein (Fig. 6.4.**21**). Incision of the peritoneal duplicature between the right liver lobe and the diaphragm from the left to the right shows the position of the right and median hepatic veins. Mobilization of the left lobe is completed by dissection of the lesser omentum. Attention must be paid to an atypical left hepatic artery originating from the left gastric artery or the celiac trunk, passing the lesser omentum at the base of the umbilical fissure (Fig. 6.4.**10a**).

In large tumors located close to the venous drainage (Fig. 6.4.**22**), the right liver lobe should be completely mobilized in order to be able to check the retrohepatic caval segment and the hepatic

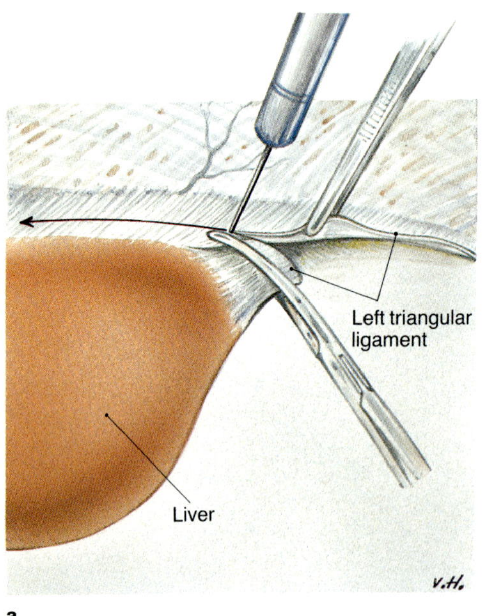

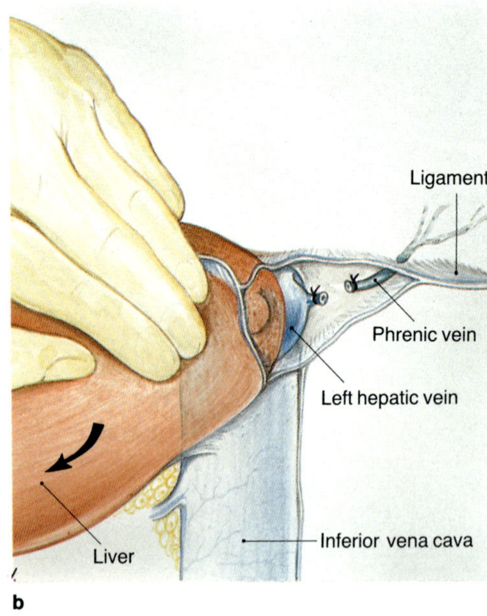

Fig. 6.4.**21**   **Left hepatectomy**
a   Mobilization of the left hepatic lobe, transection of the left triangular ligament
b   The left phrenic vein represents a guide structure for the left lateral margin of the left hepatic vein

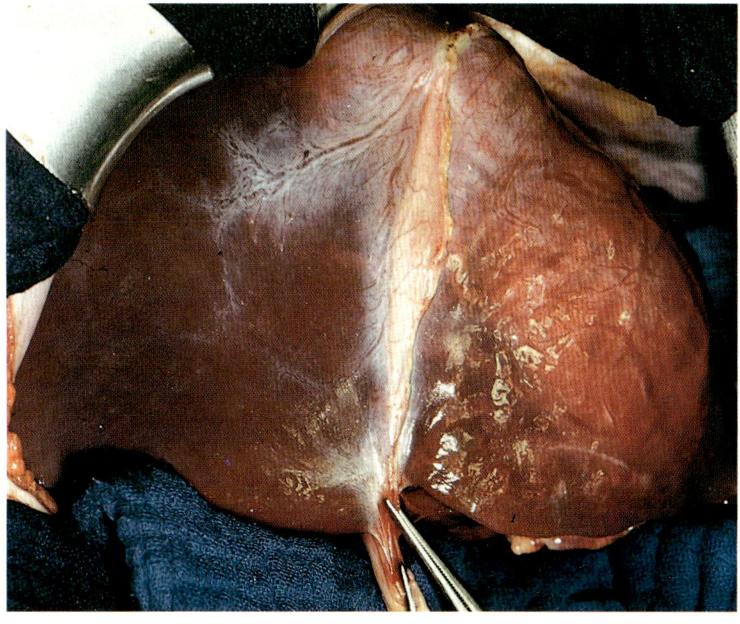

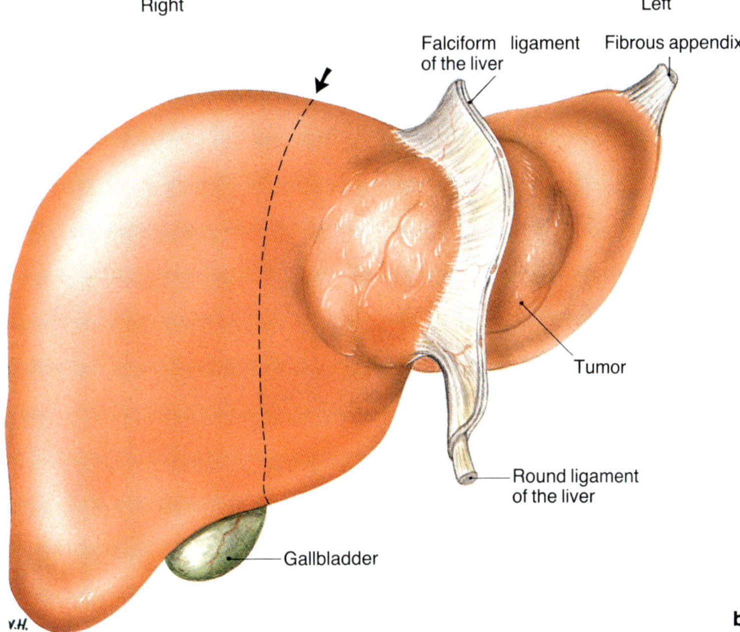

Fig. 6.4.22 Left hepatectomy

a Hepatocellular carcinoma involving the left lobe of the liver, reaching the left and median hepatic veins

b Resection plane in left hepatectomy

veins at all times (Figs. 6.4.**6a**, **b**, 6.4.**7**). In cases in which the tumor location requires a combined resection with the caudate lobe, mobilization of the right side offers an easy approach for the dissection of veins of segment I emptying directly into the retrohepatic caval segment (Fig. 6.4.**20**).

The subsequent phase of the operative procedure consists of the preparation and dissection of the hepatoduodenal ligament. Preparation starts at the base of the hepatoduodenal ligament with a transverse incision of the serosa. The perivascular lymph and nerve tissue is then dissected between small clamps and tied with fine ligatures. The use of diathermy in this phase is not advantageous, and can produce time-consuming multiple bleeding. After resection of the lymph node, invariably present, covering the common hepatic artery and the origin of the gastroduodenal artery, the preparation of the hilar structures follows the proper hepatic artery to the bifurcation of the right and left

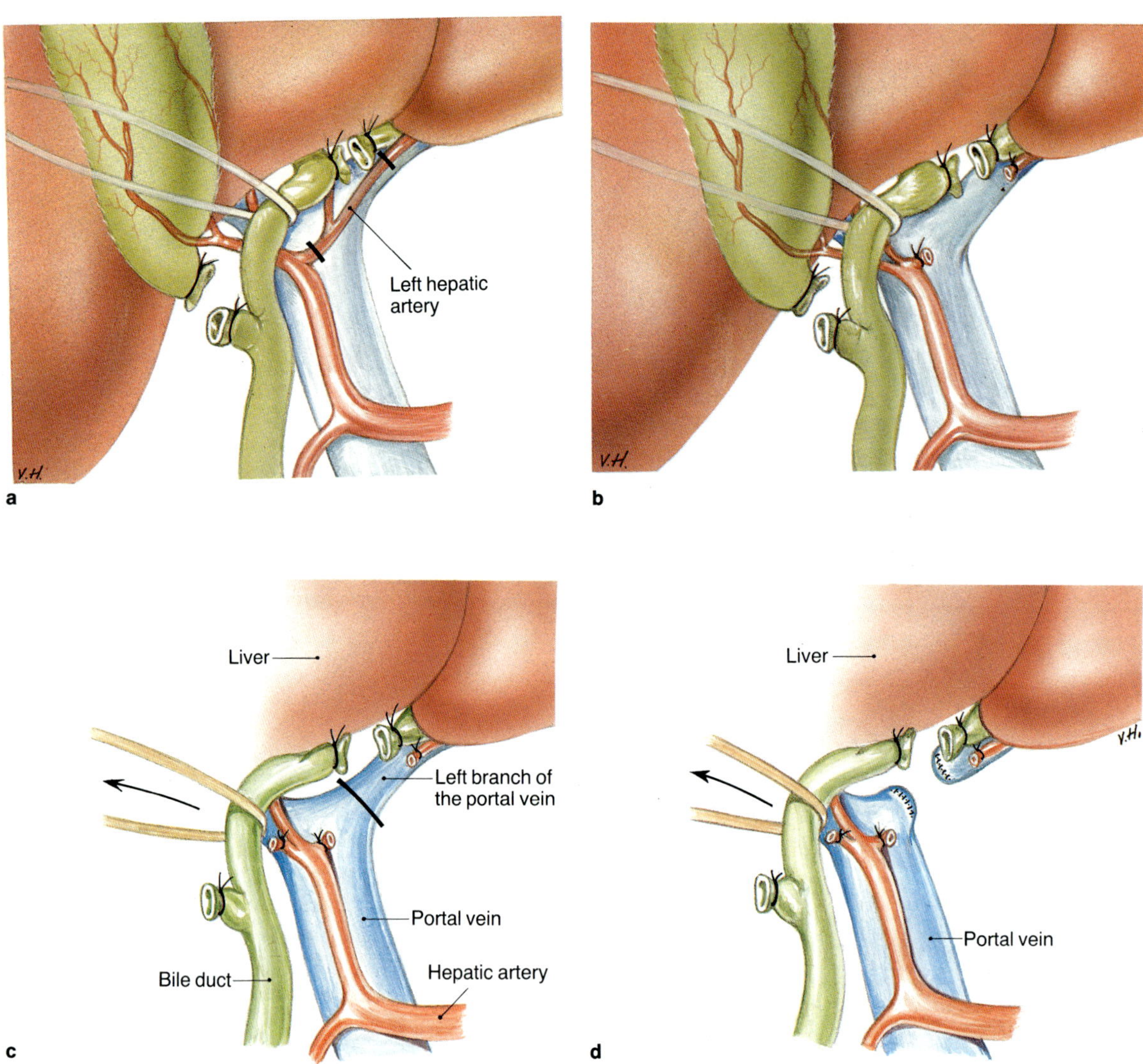

Fig. 6.4.23   Hilar dissection in left hepatectomy. (After *Priesching*)
a   Transection of the cystic and left hepatic duct, exposure of the left hepatic artery
b   Transection of the left hepatic artery
c   Transection of the left hepatic duct and artery allows exposure of the left branch of the portal vein
d   Transection of the left branch of the portal vein

hepatic arteries (Fig. 6.4.23). Usually the left hepatic artery branches after a short distance into two segmental arteries, one for segment IV and the other to the left lateral segments. For hilar preparation of the hepatoduodenal ligament previous cholecystectomy is beneficial. The cystic duct and cystic artery are dissected between ligatures and the gallbladder is removed retrogradely. Hemostasis of the hepatic bed can be carried out by sapphire coagulation. The hepatic duct and proper hepatic artery are then bridled. By drawing the hepatic artery to the left, and the bile duct to the right side, the portal vein can be exposed between the two structures (Fig. 6.4.24a). Severing of the left hepatic artery initially between fine suture-ligatures offers

an easier approach to the portal bifurcation and left portal branch (Fig. 6.4.24b). After dissection of perivascular lymph and nerve tissue, the left portal branch is looped.

The next step consists of the identification of the left hepatic duct. The bile duct bifurcation is located centrally at the hilus. The dissection therefore has to follow the left lateral margin of the hepatic duct very carefully to the left side of the liver hilus. The right hepatic artery usually crosses posterior to the hepatic duct. In difficult situations a probe inserted via the cystic stump can be helpful in identifying the hepatic ducts and avoiding damage to the right duct. After severing the left hepatic duct between fine resorbable sutures

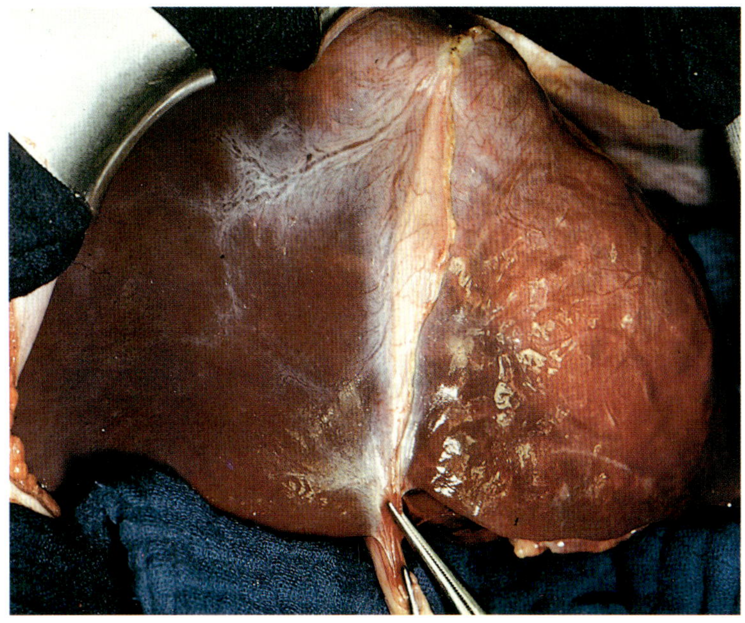

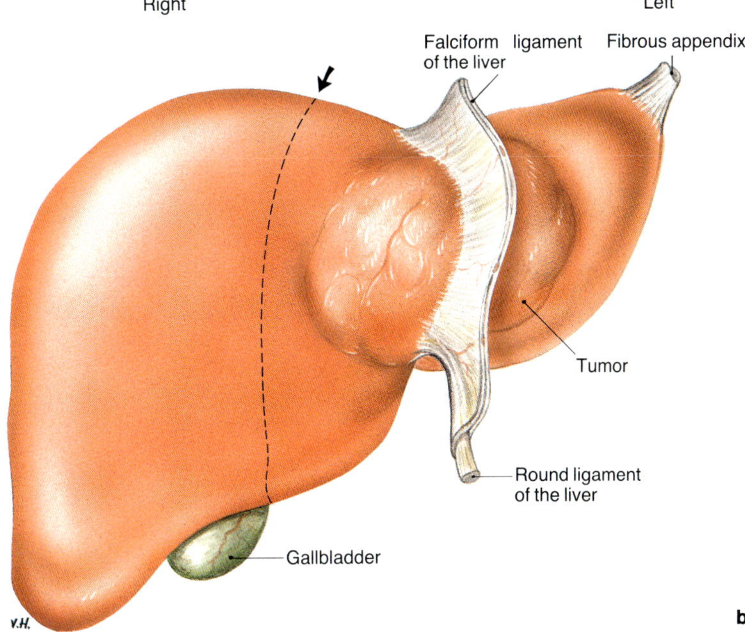

Fig. 6.4.22   Left hepatectomy
a Hepatocellular carcinoma involving the left lobe of the liver, reaching the left and median hepatic veins
b Resection plane in left hepatectomy

veins at all times (Figs. 6.4.**6a**, **b**, 6.4.**7**). In cases in which the tumor location requires a combined resection with the caudate lobe, mobilization of the right side offers an easy approach for the dissection of veins of segment I emptying directly into the retrohepatic caval segment (Fig. 6.4.**20**).

The subsequent phase of the operative procedure consists of the preparation and dissection of the hepatoduodenal ligament. Preparation starts at the base of the hepatoduodenal ligament with a transverse incision of the serosa. The perivascular lymph and nerve tissue is then dissected between small clamps and tied with fine ligatures. The use of diathermy in this phase is not advantageous, and can produce time-consuming multiple bleeding. After resection of the lymph node, invariably present, covering the common hepatic artery and the origin of the gastroduodenal artery, the preparation of the hilar structures follows the proper hepatic artery to the bifurcation of the right and left

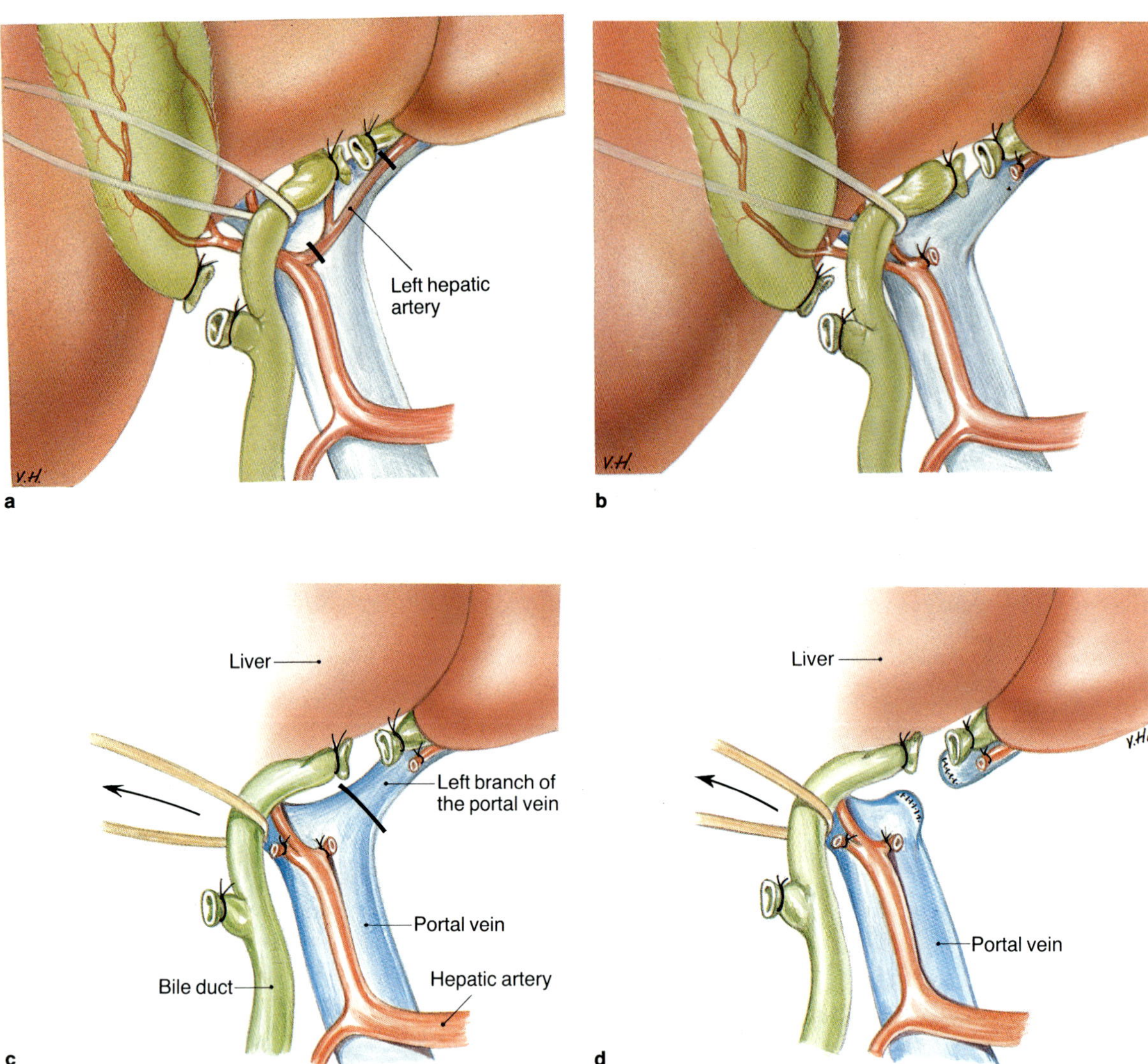

Fig. 6.4.23   Hilar dissection in left hepatectomy. (After *Priesching*)
a   Transection of the cystic and left hepatic duct, exposure of the left hepatic artery
b   Transection of the left hepatic artery
c   Transection of the left hepatic duct and artery allows exposure of the left branch of the portal vein
d   Transection of the left branch of the portal vein

hepatic arteries (Fig. 6.4.23). Usually the left hepatic artery branches after a short distance into two segmental arteries, one for segment IV and the other to the left lateral segments. For hilar preparation of the hepatoduodenal ligament previous cholecystectomy is beneficial. The cystic duct and cystic artery are dissected between ligatures and the gallbladder is removed retrogradely. Hemostasis of the hepatic bed can be carried out by sapphire coagulation. The hepatic duct and proper hepatic artery are then bridled. By drawing the hepatic artery to the left, and the bile duct to the right side, the portal vein can be exposed between the two structures (Fig. 6.4.**24a**). Severing of the left hepatic artery initially between fine suture-ligatures offers

an easier approach to the portal bifurcation and left portal branch (Fig. 6.4.**24b**). After dissection of perivascular lymph and nerve tissue, the left portal branch is looped.

The next step consists of the identification of the left hepatic duct. The bile duct bifurcation is located centrally at the hilus. The dissection therefore has to follow the left lateral margin of the hepatic duct very carefully to the left side of the liver hilus. The right hepatic artery usually crosses posterior to the hepatic duct. In difficult situations a probe inserted via the cystic stump can be helpful in identifying the hepatic ducts and avoiding damage to the right duct. After severing the left hepatic duct between fine resorbable sutures

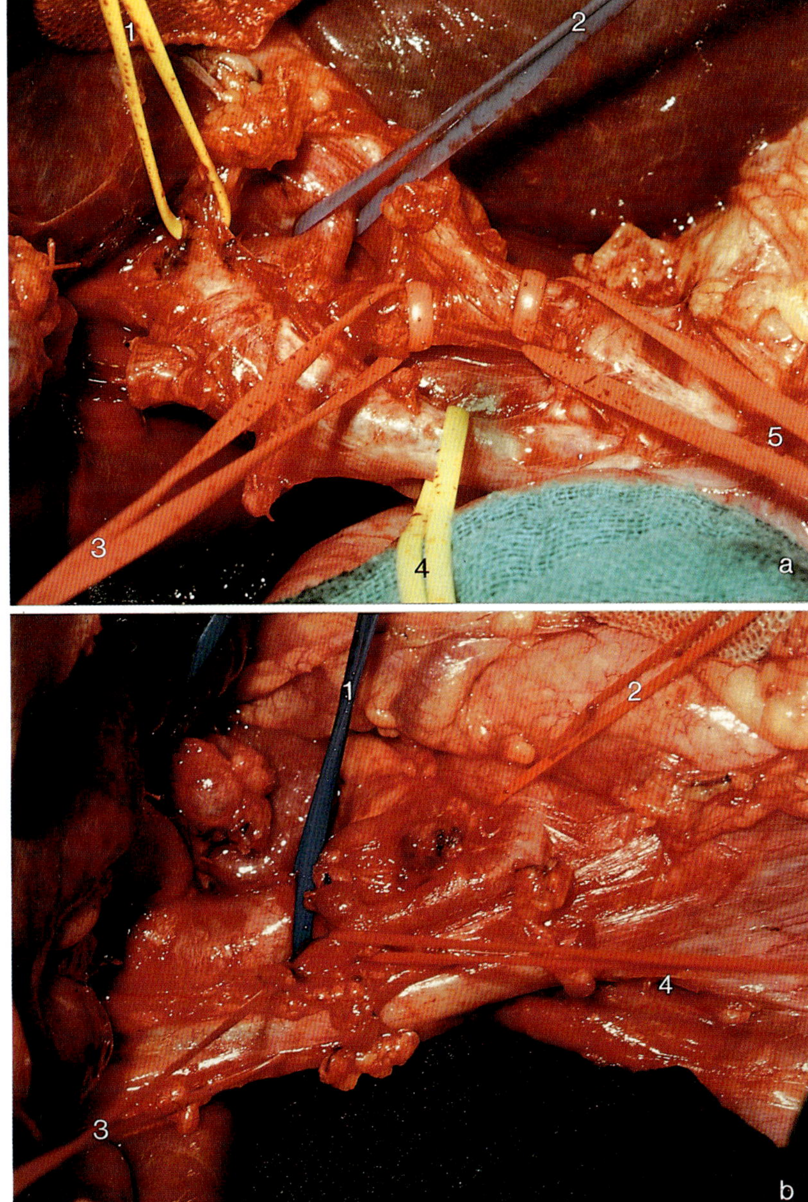

Fig. 6.4.**24** **Intraoperative exposure of hilar structures in left hepatectomy**

a 1 left hepatic duct; 2 left portal branch; 3 right hepatic artery; 4 common bile duct; 5 proper hepatic artery

b Situation after severing the left hepatic duct and left hepatic artery: 1 portal vein; 2 common hepatic artery; 3 hepatic duct; 4 right hepatic artery

(Fig. 6.4.**23a**) the left portal branch is dissected between vascular clamps. The peripheral stump is sutured with strong suture material (2-0, 3-0) whereas the central stump is oversewn by vascular suture (5-0, 4-0). Stenosis of the right portal branch and the formation of a blind end, which may be the origin of a portal venous thrombosis, have to be carefully avoided.

The resection plane for the transparenchymatous phase lies between the gallbladder bed and the hepatic venous outflow. In tumors located close to the hepatic veins it is safer to bridle the right hepatic vein in order to avoid damage to the venous drainage of that side. In contrast with right hepatectomy, the transection of the parenchyma in left hepatectomy does not proceed right on to the caval vein but changes direction a little to the left side, leaving some distance to the hilar structures of the right hepatic side and reaching the left lateral margin of the retrohepatic caval segment and the caudate lobe (Priesching 1986) (Fig. 6.4.**25**). If the caudate lobe is simultaneously resected, the dissection proceeds straight down to the caval vein (Fig. 6.4.**26**). During dissection of the parenchyma, the remaining blood flow to the right liver is occluded by a Pringle maneuver. The left hepatic vein and the left branches of the median hepatic vein are usually transsected between clamps at the

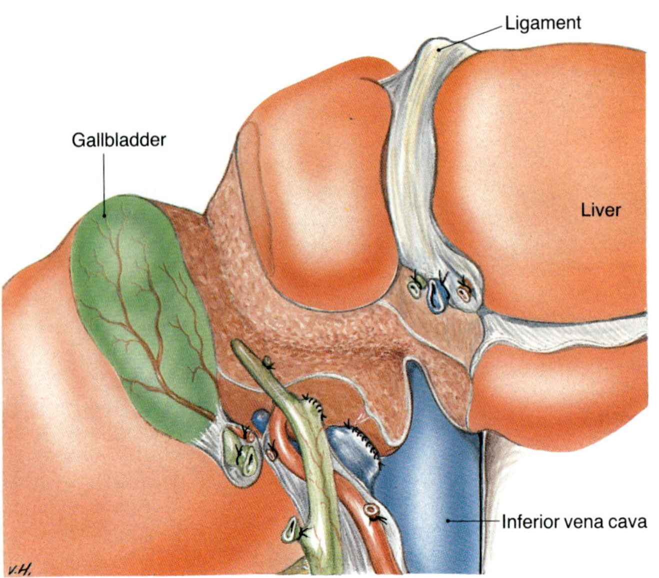

Fig. 6.4.**25**   **Resection plane of left hepatectomy** including segment I. (After *Priesching*)

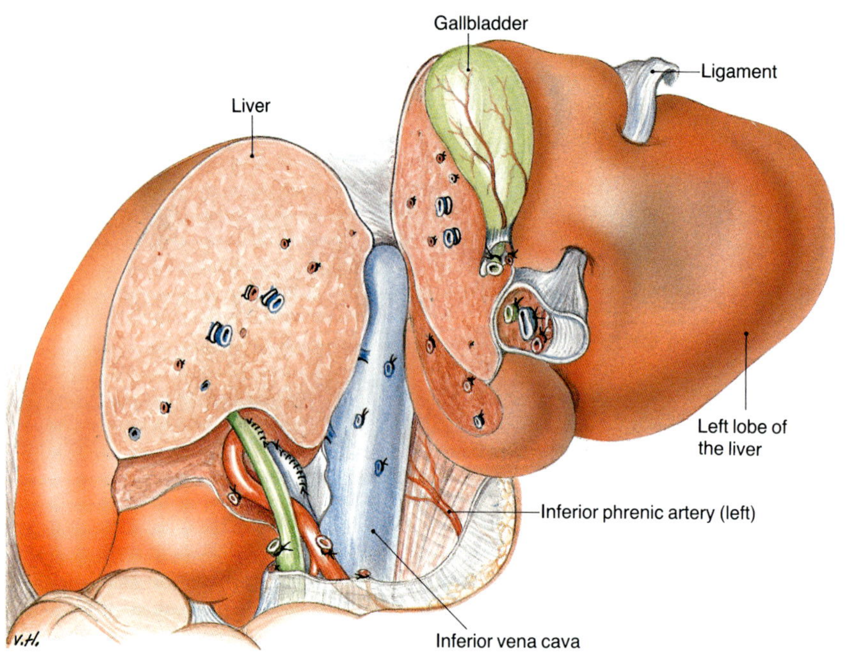

Fig. 6.4.**26**   **Completed transection of the parenchyma in left hepatectomy** including segment I, exposing the vena cava. (After *Priesching*)

end of the transparenchymatous phase of the operation (Fig. 6.4.**27**). The technique of transparenchymatous dissection and the different methods of handling the resection surface are identical to those described in detail for right hepatectomy.

Left Lateral Segmentectomy (Left Lobectomy)

This type of operation represents the left lateral bisegmentectomy of segments II and III. Most cases do not require separation and dissection of

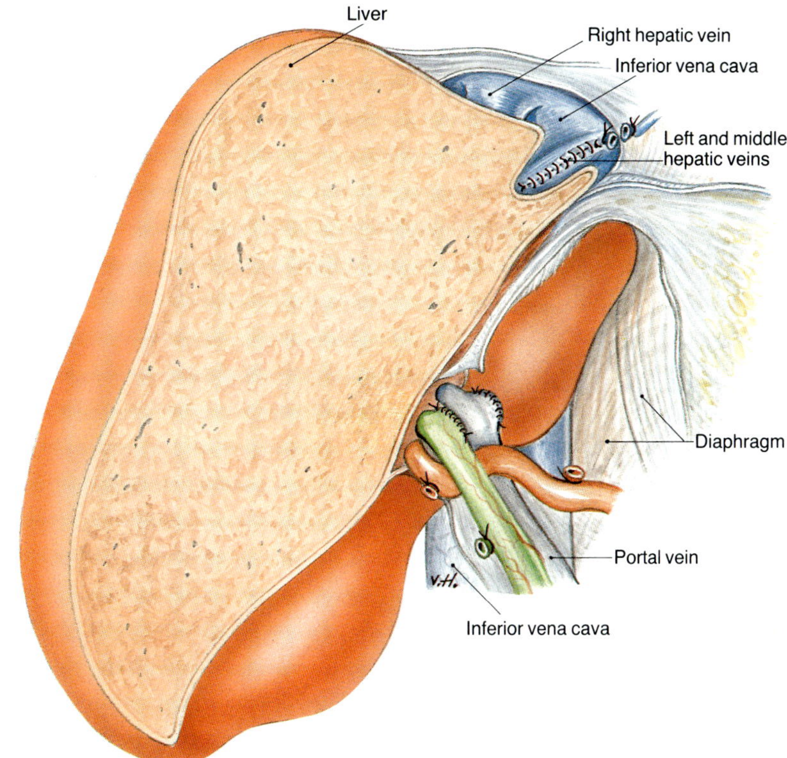

Fig. 6.4.**27** **Resection plane in left hepatectomy** after removal of the left side. The left hepatic vein is oversewn. (After *Priesching*)

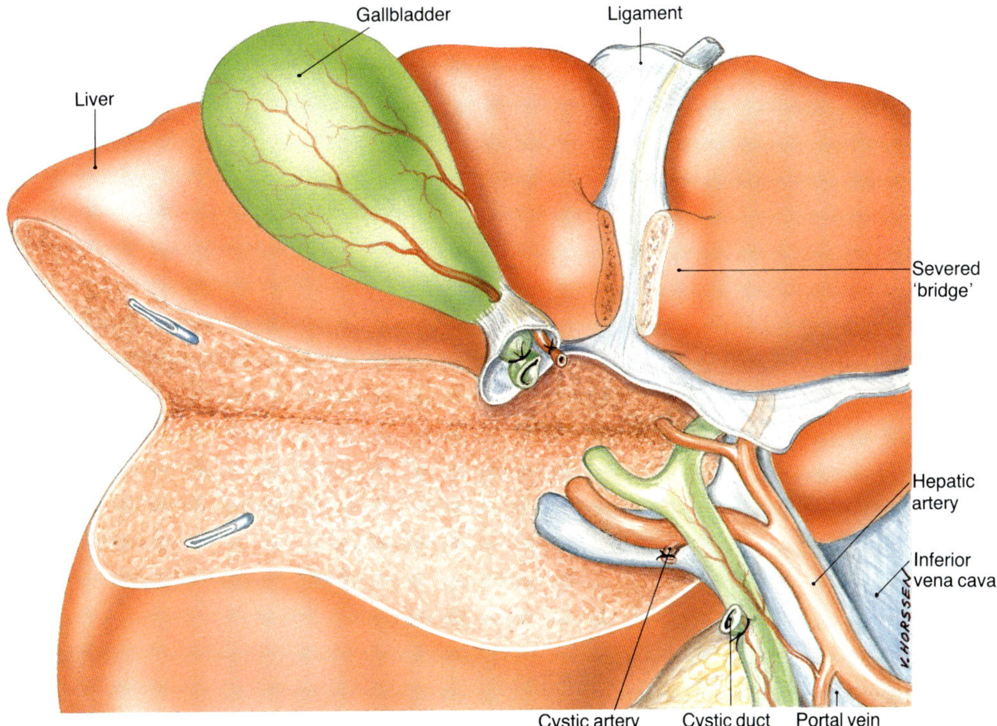

Fig. 6.4.**28** Resection plane in extended left hepatectomy

the hilar structures. Sometimes the left hepatic artery is dissected prior to the transection of the parenchyma. The left lobe is mobilized by transecting the falciform and left triangular ligaments, and the left hepatic vein is identified but divided later on during the transparenchymatous phase. Mobilization is completed by dissection of the lesser omentum. After occlusion of the hepatic blood supply by a Pringle maneuver, the hepatic capsule is incised left, parallel to the falciform ligament. The liver parenchyma is dissected as described. The left hepatic duct and the segmental portal branches to segments II and III can be easily identified and secured at the base of the parenchymatous dissection. Damage to the recurring portal branches to segment IV has to be avoided. The division of the left hepatic vein completes the removal of the left lateral segments. The small resection surface can be covered by the falciform ligament.

Extended Left Hepatectomy (Left Hepatic Trisegmentectomy)

A left hepatectomy extended to right anterior segments V and VIII represents a rarely indicated and rarely described operation (Blumgart 1988, Priesching 1986, Starzl et al. 1982). The plane of resection of an extended left hepatectomy lies on the right side of the gallbladder and reaches the right hepatic vein in a curved line. Sometimes there is an additional fissure on the posterior side of the right lobe between segments V and VI, which facilitates the right approach to the intrahepatic preparation and identification of the portal branches feeding segments VI, VII, V and VIII (Fig. 6.4.**28**). Depending on the size and location of the tumor, the decision has to be taken whether an additional resection of segment I is required.

The principal steps of the operation do not essentially differ in cases in which segment I is resected and those in which it is not. In all cases, this operation requires extensive mobilization of the whole liver and the ability to control all of the supplying and draining hepatic vessels at any time. The preparation of the hilar structures is identical to that described above for left hepatectomy. Complete mobilization of the right and left lobes, with placement of infrahepatic and suprahepatic tourniquets around the caval vein, is obligatory (Fig. 6.4.**29**). In addition, the right hepatic vein has to be isolated and looped to control hemorrhage by accidental injury to this vessel during the transparenchymatous phase. In most cases, access to the hepatic veins is limited due to the size and location of the tumor. It is therefore easier to turn the patient slightly to the left side and to start the parenchymatous dissection between segments V and VI after

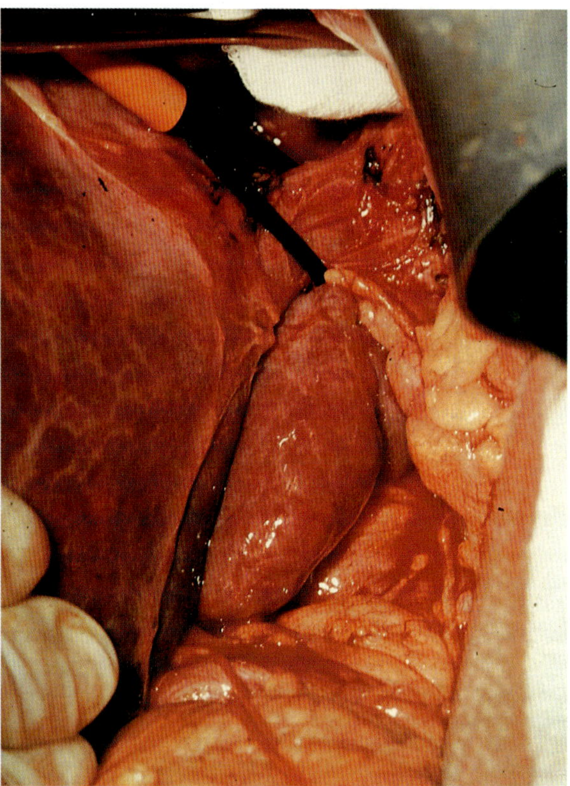

Fig. 6.4.**29   Extended left hepatectomy.** Notice the tourniquet around the suprahepatic vena cava

occlusion of the arterial and portal blood flow. By careful elevation of the tumor, the hepatic tissue is transected down to the hilar structures, exposing the anatomical spaces between segments V and VI and between segments VII and VIII (Figs. 6.4.**28**, 6.4.**30**). The potential tumor-free margin is limited by the course of the hilar structures to segments VI and VII and by the right hepatic vein. The step-by-step transection is concomitant with an increasing ability to turn the tumor and resected tissue to the left, allowing safer preparation of the right hepatic vein and its branches from segment VIII (Figs. 6.4.**30**, 6.4.**31**).

The indication for extended left hepatectomy is usually a huge tumor which will displace the right hepatic vein dorsally and to the right, leaving little space at the right hepatic and caval veins. Due to the tumor size, it can also be rather difficult to place a common clamp safely on the median and left hepatic veins before severance this being the last step of the transparenchymatous procedure (Fig. 6.4.**31**). Alternatively, the retrohepatic caval segment can be clamped out by occlusion of the infra- and suprahepatic tourniquets. In this case the stumps of the median and left hepatic veins can be oversewn without technical problems after removal

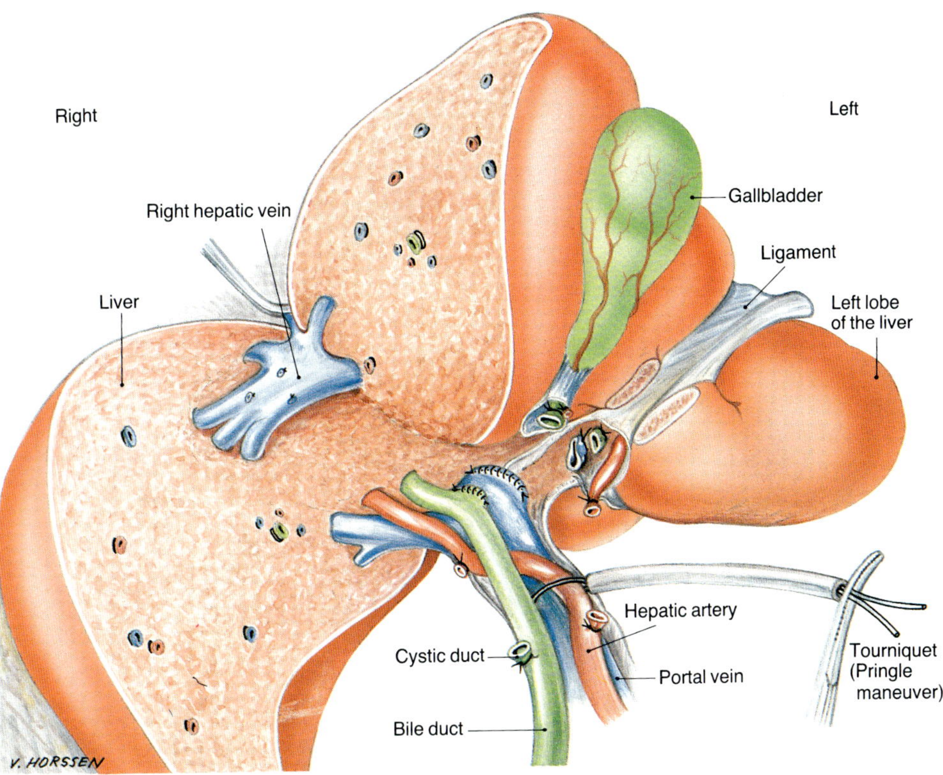

Fig. 6.4.**30** During advanced transection of the parenchyma in extended left hepatectomy, the tumor-bearing left side can be rotated to the left, allowing exposure of the right and middle hepatic veins

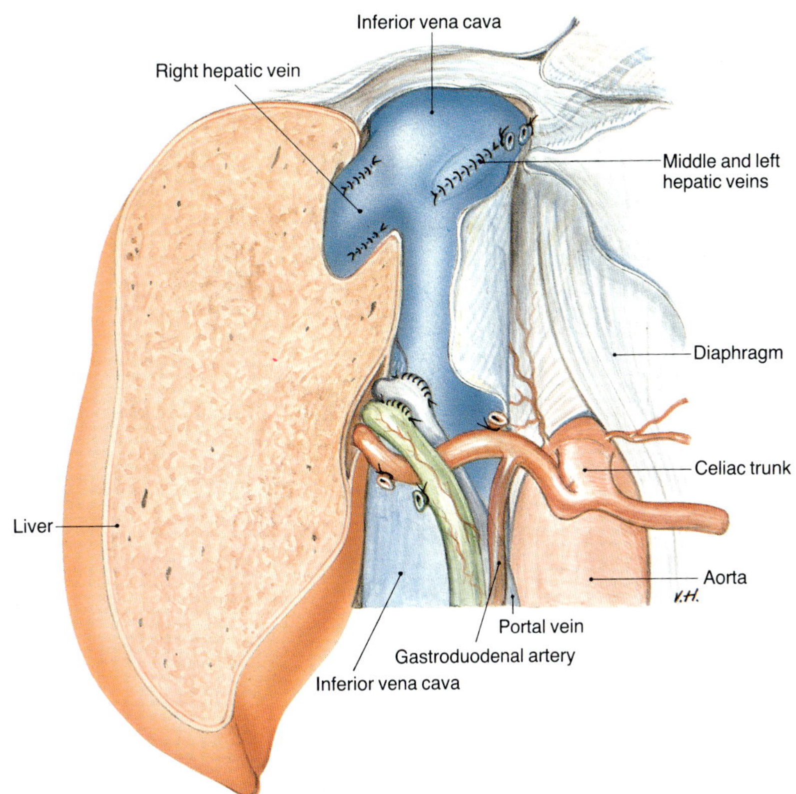

Fig. 6.4.**31 Resection plane after left extended hepatectomy.** The middle and left hepatic veins are oversewn

of the tumor. The treatment of the resection surface is identical to that for all other types of hepatic resection described above.

Potential pitfalls. There is no difference in the operative procedure between extended left hepatectomy and other types of hepatic resections. The specific technical problems of the operation result from huge tumor size and the tumor's central location, which compromise visibility during the most essential steps of the operation such as the hilar approach and the intraparenchymatous identification of the portal branches to segments VI, VII, V and VIII. Iatrogenic damage to portal branch V or VII and accidental resection of the right segmental hepatic ducts are therefore the predominant technical mishaps in the operation. Occlusion of the hepatoduodenal ligament and, if necessary, simultaneous clamping of the caval vein, allow the injured portal branch to be sutured. Accidental resection of the right hepatic duct requires a biliodigestive anastomosis with a Roux-en-Y jejunal segment. Injuries to the right hepatic vein can only be safely sutured in case of a prophylactic placement of supra- and infrahepatic caval tourniquets. Further technical problems can be caused by tumor infiltration of the median or left hepatic veins, or both. In these cases, placing of a clamp before transection may be followed by extensive bleeding caused by a rupture of the tumor-infiltrated venous segment. Such complications may require a patch graft of the vena cava underlining the importance of a potential control of the supplying and draining blood flow.

References

Adson MA, van Heerden J. Major hepatic resections for metastatic colorectal cancer. Ann Surg 1980; 191: 576.

Bismuth H. Surgical anatomy and anatomical surgery of the liver. World J Surg 1982; 6: 3.

Blumgart LM. Liver resection: liver and biliary tumors. In: Blumgart LM, ed. Surgery of the liver and biliary tract. Edinburgh: Churchill Livingstone, 1988: 1251.

Brölsch C. Chirurgische Behandlung von Lebererkrankungen. In: Bock HE, Gerok W, Hartmann F, Schuster HP, eds. Klinik der Gegenwart. München: Urban and Schwarzenberg, 1986: 492.

Couinauld C. Bases anatomiques des hépatectomies gauche et droite réglées: techniques qui en découlent. J Chir (Paris) 1954; 70: 933.

Esser G. Leberresektion bei Leberzirrhose. Chirurg 1979a; 50: 146.

Esser G. Zeit- und blutsparende Leberresektion. Chirurg 1979b; 50: 136.

Fortner JG, Kim DK, Maclean BJ. Major hepatic resections for neoplasia: personal experience in 108 patients. Ann Surg 1978; 188: 363.

Fortner JG, Silva JS, Golbey RB, Cox EB, Maclean BJ. Multivariate analysis of a personal series of 247 consecutive patients with liver metastases from colorectal cancer, I: treatment by hepatic resection. Ann Surg 1984; 199: 306.

Foster JH, Berman MM. Solid liver tumours. In: Major problems in clinical surgery; vol 22. Philadelphia: Saunders, 1977: 1.

Funovics J, Fritsch A. Leberresektionen bei primären Tumoren und Metastasen. In: Häring R, ed. Chirurgie der Leber. Weinheim: Edition Medizin, 1983.

Goldsmith NA, Woodburne RT. The surgical anatomy pertaining to liver resection. Surg Gynecol Obstet 1957; 105: 310.

Iwatsuki S, Shaw BW Jr, Starzl TE. Experience with 150 liver resections. Ann Surg 1983; 197: 247.

Klatskin G. Adenocarcinoma of the hepatic duct at its bifurcation with the porta hepatis: an unusual tumor with distinctive clinical and pathological features. Am J Med 1965; 38: 241.

Kremer B, Henne-Bruns D. Das postoperative Leberausfallkoma. Zentralbl Chir 1986; 111: 1166.

Launois B, Campion JP, Brissot P, Gosselin N. Carcinoma of the hepatic hilus: surgical management and the case for resection. Ann Surg 1979; 190: 151.

Lin T. Results in 107 hepatic lobectomies with a preliminary report on the use of a clamp to reduce blood loss. Ann Surg 1973; 177: 413.

Lin TY. Resectional therapy for primary malignant hepatic tumors. In: Murphy GP, ed. International Advances in surgical oncology; vol 2. New York: Liss, 1979: 25.

Longmire WP, Tompkins RK, eds. Manual of liver surgery. Berlin: Springer, 1981.

Mimura H, Takakura N, Ohno Y, Matsuda T, Kin H, Hamazaki K, Tsumura M, Toda S, Hiraki Y. Determination of the extent of feasible hepatic resection from hepatic blood flow. World J Surg 1986; 10 (2): 302.

Neuhaus P, Ringe B, Bechstein W, Pichlmayr R. Ergebnisse und Bedeutung der Resektion von Lebermetastasen colorektaler Tumoren. Langenbecks Arch Chir 1986; 369: 789.

Okamoto E, Kyo A, Yamanaka N, Tanaka N, Kuwata K. Prediction of the safe limits of hepatectomy by combined volumetric and functional measurements in patients with impaired hepatic function. Surgery 1984; 95: 586.

Pichlmayr R, Neuhaus P, Brölsch C. Die Chancen einer chirurgischen Behandlung von Lebertumoren. Verh Dtsch Krebs-Ges 1984; 5: 473.

Priesching A. Leberresektionen. München: Urban and Schwarzenberg, 1986.

Starzl T, Köp L, Weil R, Lilly JR, Putnam C, Aldrete A. Right trisegmentectomy for hepatic neoplasms. Surg Gynecol Obstet 1980; 150: 208.

Starzl T, Iwatsuki S, Shaw BW. Left hepatic trisegmentectomy. Surg Gynecol Obstet 1982; 155: 21.

Stone HH. Preoperative and postoperative care. Surg Clin North Am 1977; 57: 2.

Thompson HH, Tompkins RK, Longmire WP. Major hepatic resection: a 25-year experience. Ann Surg 1983; 197: 375.

Tsuzuki T, Okata Y, Iida S, et al. Carcinoma of the bifurcation of the hepatic ducts. Arch Surg 1983; 118: 1147.

Tsuzuki T, Ogata Y, Iida S, Shimazu M. Hepatic resection in 125 patients. Arch Surg 1984; 119: 1025.

6.5 Segment-Orientated Resection of the Liver: Rationale and Technique

J. Scheele

Introduction

During the last decade, liver resection has gained widespread acceptance. Two factors have promoted this increased popularity. Firstly, operative mortality and morbidity have been remarkably reduced, so that even major hepatic resection does not need to be regarded as heroic surgery. Secondly, the effectiveness of adequate tumor removal on prognosis has been sufficiently proved, in particular for primary malignancies and for metastases from colorectal carcinomas (Adson 1987, 1988, Ekberg et al. 1987, Fortner and Papachristou 1979, Hugnet and Moniel 1983, Okuda et al. 1984, Masselot and Leborgne 1978, Scheele 1988, Thompson et al. 1983).

Problems Experienced in Classical Resection Procedures

In addition to obvious surgical complications such as bleeding, biliary leakage and abscess formation, there are two contrasting aspects of traditional resection procedures which are of considerable importance in terms of the operative approach:

1. In the case of a non-cirrhotic healthy liver, a resection of up to 80 % can be tolerated and, thanks to the huge regenerative capacity, can be compensated for within a few weeks (Blumgart et al. 1971, Lin et al. 1979). However, such a favorable course of events cannot generally be taken for granted. It is likely that a reduction of the functional liver parenchyma by more than 50 % will cause temporary or possibly long-lasting liver failure, which may ultimately become fatal (Bismuth et al. 1982). This post-resectional hepatic reserve is of particular importance for common anatomical resections on the right lobe. It is less significant when the majority of the parenchyma in this area has been replaced by an extensive tumor mass. A compensatory hypertrophy of the non-affected left lobe has already occurred pre-operatively in most of these patients, and the loss of actual parenchyma as a result of the resection is very limited. A comparable resection because of multiple or unfavorably located smaller lesions, however, increases the risk of an acute liver failure considerably (Fig. 6.5.1).

2. In view of the significant physiological sequelae of an extensive functional hepatic reduction, "atypical" approaches have been recommended for resection of minor tumors of the right lobe, even recently (Brown et al. 1988). Palpation, however, often underestimates the intrahepatic extent of a growth, so that very small resection margins may frequently result. This aspect was analyzed in patients who had undergone liver resection for colorectal metastases at our hospital between 1960 and 1985. In contrast to the surgeon's intraoperative impression of having performed a radical procedure, histological examination revealed

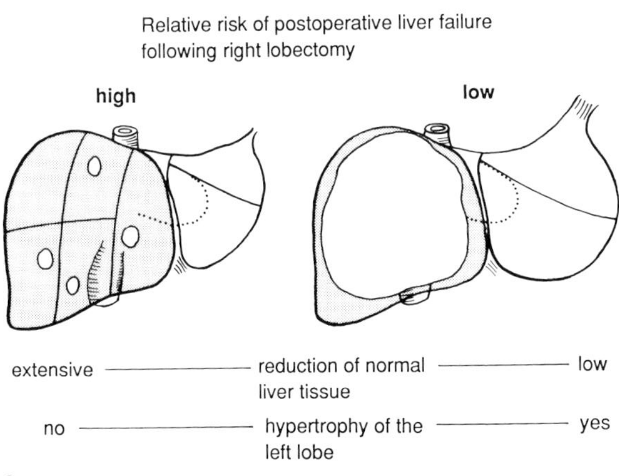

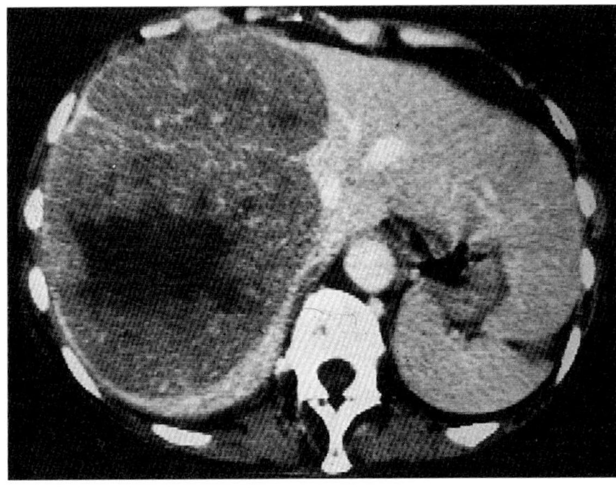

Fig. 6.5.1 **Risk of hepatic failure following right lobectomy**
a Impact of tumor type and distribution
b Compensatory hypertrophy of the left lobe extending to the splenic hilum in a patient with two bulky metastases from a small bowel sarcoma in segments VII and VIII

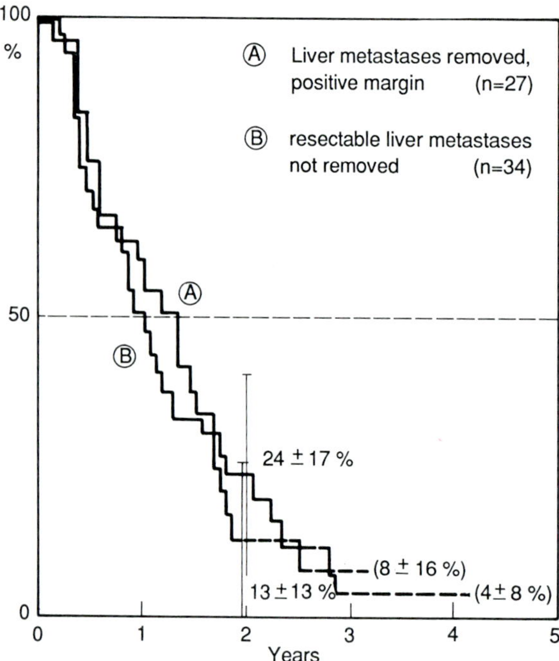

Fig. 6.5.**2** **Lack of prognostic benefit** following putative curative resection of colorectal liver metastases with positive margins compared to a historical group of untreated patients with resectable hepatic involvement (adapted from Gall and Scheele 1987)

tumor infiltration at the edge of the specimen in 35 % of the cases following wedge-shaped excision of small marginal tumors. No prognostic benefit could be demonstrated for this subgroup of patients who had all gross tumor removed but with positive margins remaining (Gall and Scheele 1987, Scheele 1988) (Fig. 6.5.**2**).

Aggressive surgical management of hepatic malignancies should therefore guarantee, on the one hand, a clear margin, and, on the other hand, preserve a maximum of non-involved liver parenchyma. I believe a segment-orientated approach often offers substantial advantages in the optimal achievement of both of these contrasting goals.

Principles of the Segment-Orientated Resection Technique

Anatomical Basis

From its anterior aspect, the liver appears to be divided into a major right lobe and a clearly smaller left lobe along the line of the falciform ligament and the insertion of the ligamentum teres. If the organ is removed and inspected from the posterior and inferior surface, a division into two similarly-sized portions is more evident, the boundary being

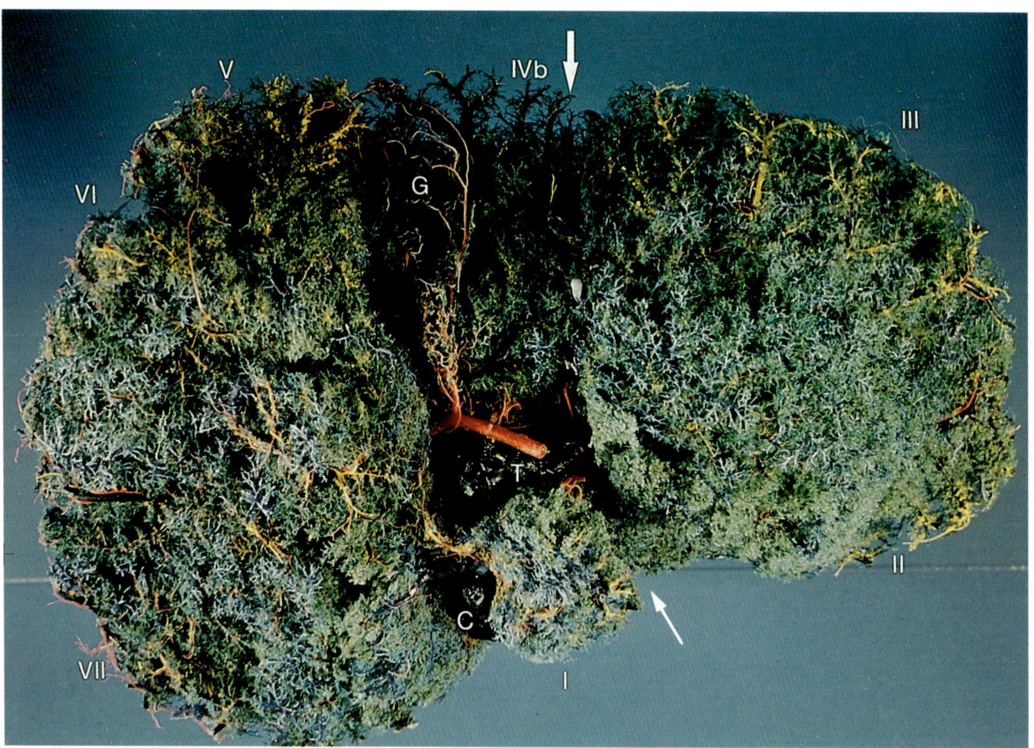

Fig. 6.5.**3** **Liver after injection** of hepatic artery (red), portal vein (green), bile duct (yellow), and hepatic veins (blue); posterior aspect with noticeable hypertrophy of the left lobe. C: vena cava; G: gallbladder; T: transverse portion of left portal vein; large arrow: umbilical fissure; small arrow: fissure of venous ligament

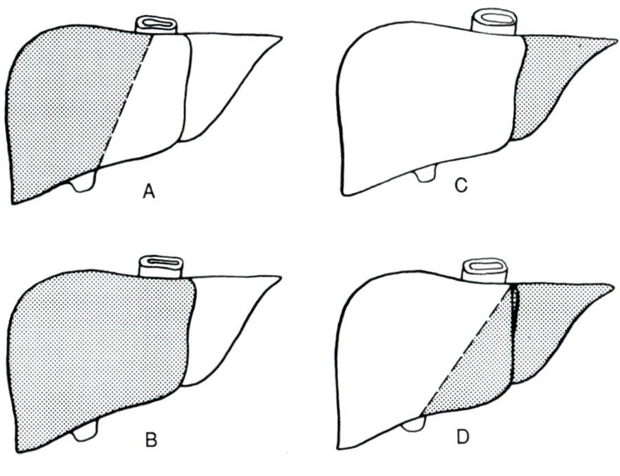

Fig. 6.5.**4   Common anatomical hepatic resections** (adapted from Bismuth (1982))

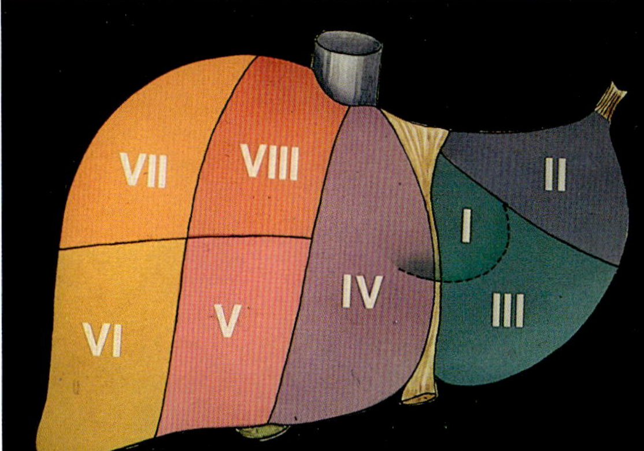

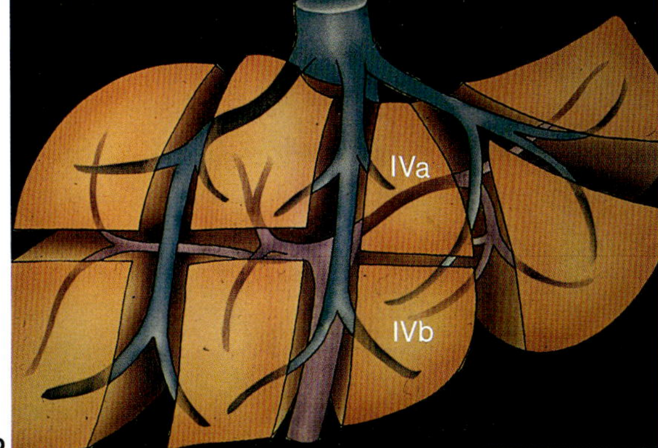

Fig. 6.5.**5   Segmental anatomy of the liver**
a   Classification according to Couinaud (1957)
b   Modification with subdivision of segments IVa and IVb; segment I is not indicated

formed by the inferior vena cava and the gall bladder (Fig. 6.5.**3**).

The two underlying intrahepatic planes, the left intersegmental plane and the main fissure (or Cantlie's line), respectively, represent the landmarks for classical anatomical hepatic resections. In contrast to the majority of English nomenclature usage (Starzl et al. 1975), but following Hobsley (1958) and Bismuth (1982), I propose that resections along the main fissure be defined as "hepatectomies," and those along the umbilical fissure as "lobectomies" (Fig. 6.5.**4**).

Segmentectomies are based on a further subdivision of the liver which is determined by the distribution of the portal triad. These three structures (hepatic artery, portal vein and bile duct) usually divide into a right and left trunk at the liver hilum. As a result, two functional liver halves are formed which abut at the main fissure, i.e. at the resection line for the two hepatectomies. The portal pedicles to the right half of the liver divide at their entrance to the organ into a posterior and an anterior branch, which after a further 1–2 cm lead into cranial and caudal branches (Fig. 6.5.**6b**). According to Couinaud (1957), the segments in the right lobe of the liver are defined by these third-order ramifications (Fig. 6.5.**5a**).

In the left half of the liver, there is a different distribution pattern for the hepatic artery and bile duct on the one hand, and the portal vein on the other. The latter first passes between the quadrate and caudate lobes, forming the transverse part (Figs. 6.5.**3**, 6.5.**5b**, 6.5.**6**). At the posterior end of the umbilical fissure, the portal vein curves anteriorly, becoming the umbilical part, and runs to the insertion of the round ligament. It branches to segment II at the posterior vertex between the transverse and umbilical parts before finally divid-

ing into the ramifications for segments III and IV (Figs. 6.5.**6**, 6.5.**8**). In contrast, the hepatic artery and bile duct both first divide into branches for segment IV and the anatomical left lobe which then demonstrate the cranial/caudal distribution as on the right hemiliver.

The caudate lobe is positioned between the hilar branching of the portal triad anteriorly, and the inferior vena cava posteriorly. It protrudes predominantly to the left side of the vena cava but also extends, as the caudate process, slightly to the right. The margins of the caudate process are difficult to define clearly, and the size varies from a very thin layer to a considerably developed portion of parenchyma. The arterial and portal venous supplies to segment I usually consist of three thin branches each, mostly from the region of the hilar bifurcation and the adjacent portions of the main trunks. The biliary drainage usually consists of only two small ducts (Mizumoto and Suzuki 1988). As a rule, the portal pedicles to the caudate process originate from the right pedicles and those to the caudate lobe from the left side or from the bifurcation area itself (Fig. 6.5.**6c**).

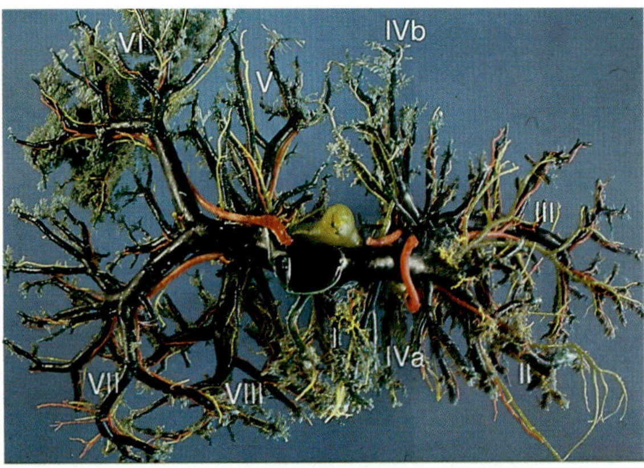

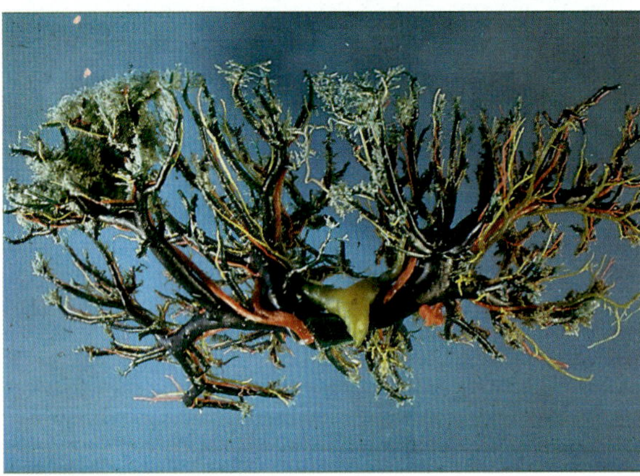

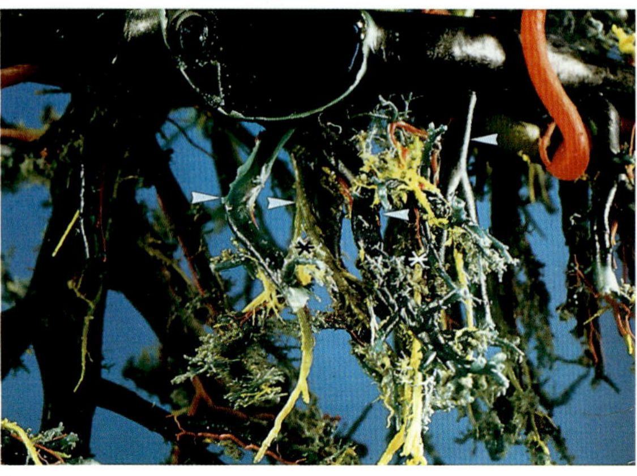

Fig. 6.5.**6   Corrosion cast of a human liver** after filling of the portal structures and subtotal removal of small tributaries. Numbers indicate segments

a   Posterior aspect demonstrating the difference in branching characteristics of lateral vs. medial segments

b   Caudal aspect showing the anteriorly and cranially directed arched branches to segments IVa and VIII, respectively

c   Close-up of segment I with four portal veins (small arrows) originating from the bifurcation area and the transverse portion of the left trunk, and two draining bile ducts (*)

The anatomical planes between the individual segments are not crossed by large branches of the portal pedicles, and therefore provide avascular borders which facilitate the surgical transection of the parenchyma (Fig. 6.5.**16**). Only the large hepatic veins have to be considered, which run just anteriorly of the main portal pedicles within these intersegmental boundaries and receive a few major side branches draining the respective neighboring segments (Fig. 6.5.**5b**). The final result is a fan-shaped interlocking of portal supply and venous drainage dovetailed into a complex spatial pattern. As a schematic aid to orientation, it may be stated that the segmental borders are defined on the body's longitudinal axis by the path of the main hepatic veins and on the transverse axis by the branching of the portal pedicles (Fig. 6.5.**5b**).

These structural principles of the segmental organization of the liver were elaborated in detail, using corrosion techniques, more than 30 years ago (Elias and Petty 1952, Goldsmith and Woodburne 1957, Healey and Schroy 1953, Hjortsjö 1951, Hobsky 1958), with some basic aspects beeing 100 years old (Cantlie 1898, Rex 1888). With regard to practical application, however, there are a number of less commonly known important anatomical features that need to be grasped before undertaking safe segmental resection.

Characteristics of Portal Branching

The portal pedicles leading to the peripheral segments II, III, VI and VII are characterized by a large main trunk, and, on the right side, by a peripheral arborization in addition (Fig. 6.5.**6a**). In contrast, the centrally-located segments IV, V and VIII show an early ramification, sometimes bush-like, often fan-shaped, aligned on the body's longitudinal axis. As well as minor branches radiating directly from the respective main trunk (Figs. 6.5.**6b**, 6.5.7), one or two arched branches are also found here which initially run anteriorly and then turn cranially, delivering side branches both caudally and cranially. Consequently, as a rule, in a central monosegmentectomy several portal pedicles at various depths in the parenchyma must be dealt with, while the anteriorly directed main trunk must be carefully preserved (Fig. 6.5.**22a**). Occasionally this type of ramification, with an arched main trunk delivering multiple portal branches caudally to segment VI before finally running upwards to feed segment VII, may also be found in the posterior sector of the right lobe.

Subdivision of Segment IV

It is not only the arterial inflow and bile drainage of segment IV which show some similarity to those of the "double segments" V and VIII, but also the

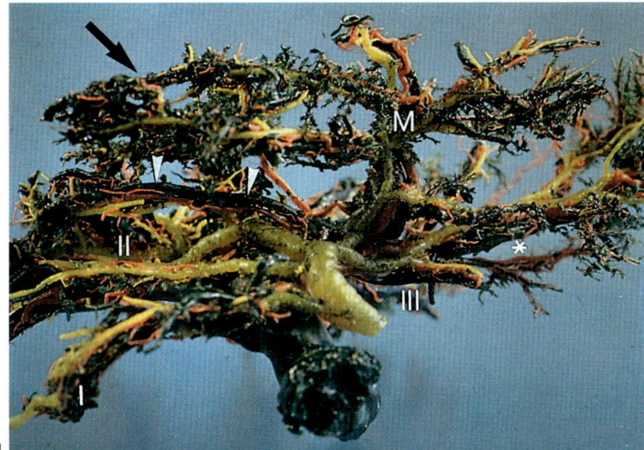

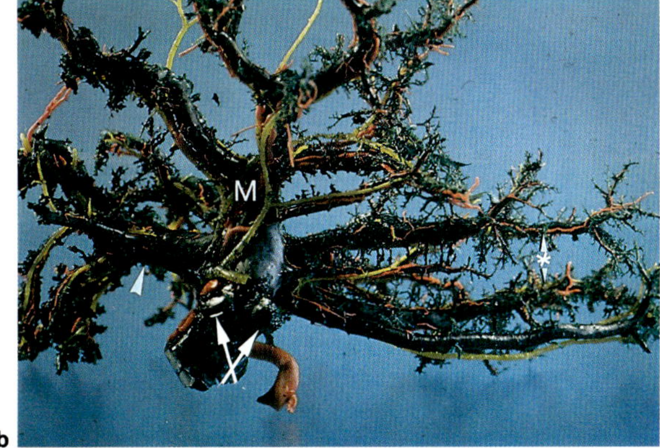

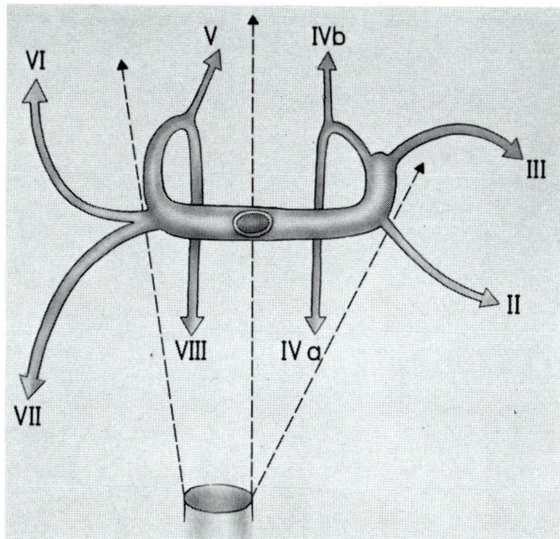

Fig. 6.5.**8**   **Scheme of portal venous distribution** in a posterior view, indicating an almost symmetrical basic structure of both halves of the liver

Fig. 6.5.**7**   **Comparison of portal triad distribution to segment IV and to the right anterior sector V/VIII**
a   Distribution to the left half of the liver. I, II, and III: pedicles to respective segments; M: anteriorly directed main trunk to segment IV; small arrows: cranially-originating branch to subsegment IVa; *: caudally-directed supplementary branches; large arrow: arched cranially-directed termination of the main pedicle
b   View of the double segment V/VIII from the right side after removal of the pedicles to the posterior sector. M: anteriorly-directed trunk with sequential branches in cranial and caudal directions; small arrow: early cranially-directed branches to segment VIII; *: early caudally-directed branches to segment V; large arrows: portal pedicle VI/VII

organization of the portal venous supply (Fig. 6.5.7). Short branches originate from the posterocranial part of segment IV shortly after the exit of the pedicle for segment II (Fig.6.5.**22b**) and extend from there to the left hepatic vein orifice (Sales et al. 1984). The further peripherally rising main portal pedicle is supplemented by a group of minor tributaries which mainly radiate caudally into the quadrate lobe (Figs. 6.5.**6b**, 6.5.**7a**). During its further course anteriorly, the main pedicle gives off two or three caudal branches prior to turning in the direction of the venous confluence in the form of 1 or 2 large, arching terminal branches (Elias and Petty 1942, Sales et al. 1984, Scheele 1989a) (Figs. 6.5.**7a**, 6.5.**22a**).

In some cases, the similarity of segment IV to the anterior right sector (segments V and VIII) (Fig. 6.5.**7b**) gives the impression of an almost symmetrical basic structure in both liver halves (Fig. 6.5.**8**). Although this might be the exception rather than the rule, it seems anatomically justified and surgically useful to subdivide segment IV along this anteriorly directed main portal pedicle into an apical and caudal section (Goldsmith and Woodburne 1957, Priesching 1986, Scheele 1989a). In keeping with a recently established nomenclature, I propose the classification of the smaller apical portion as segment IVa, and the clearly larger caudal portion or quadrate lobe as segment IVb (Fig. 6.5.**5b**).

Hepatic Venous Drainage

Besides the basic organization of the three major hepatic veins running along intersegmental planes (Fig. 6.5.**9a**), the venous drainage of the liver is characterized by a wide range of variations both in the extent of the respective flow territories and with the presence of additional veins draining directly into the vena cava. Atypical drainage of segment VI, which may be either via a predominant middle hepatic vein or via tributary retrohepatic veins, is of particular interest for surgical reasons. Retrohepatic veins can be found to some extent in the majority of cases and form the main venous drainage of segment VI in approximately 25% of cases (Masselot and Leborgne 1978, Scheele 1989a) (Figs. 6.5.**9b**, **c**). A dominant middle hepatic vein accounts for a similar proportion (Masselot and Leborgne 1978). If they are well developed, both of these variations allow a combined resection of

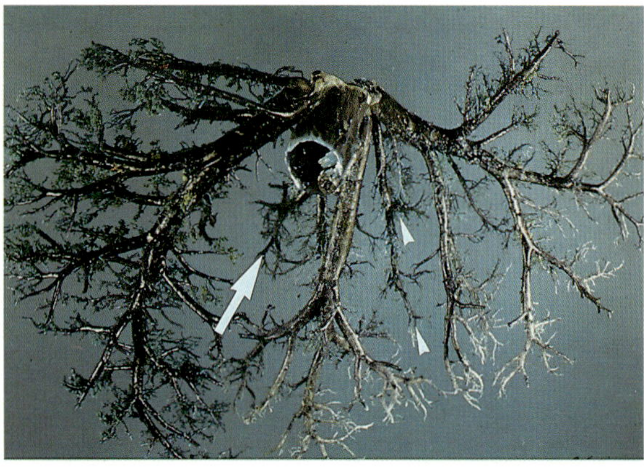

a

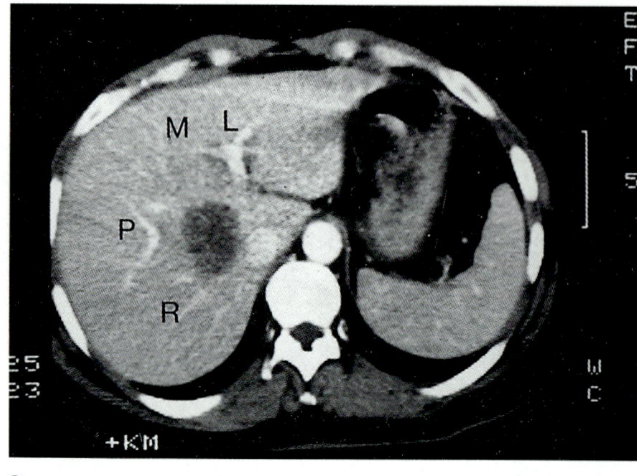

a

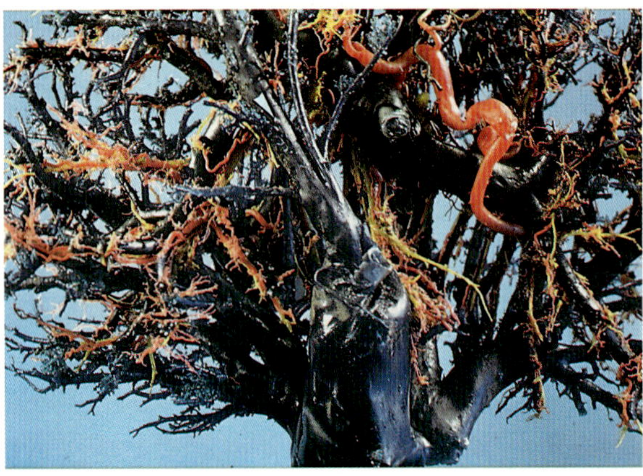

b

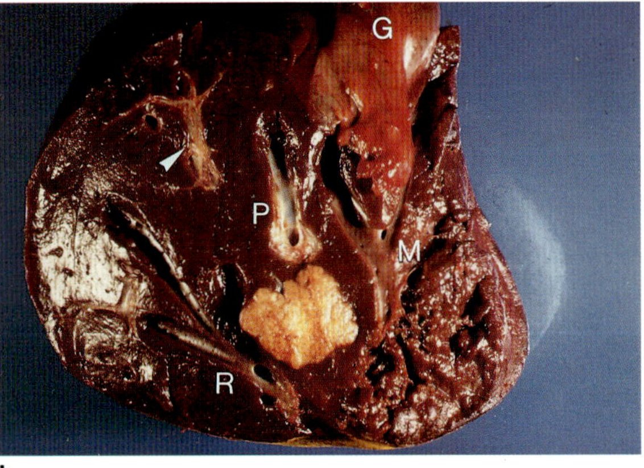

b

Fig. 6.5.10 Small solitary metastasis of segment VIII. R:
right hepatic vein; M: middle hepatic vein; L: left portal
pedicles; P: portal branching to segments VIII and V; G:
gallbladder; arrow: terminal portal branch to segment VI
- **a** CT scan demonstrating the vicinity of the tumor to the
  right hepatic vein and the anterior portal branching
- **b** Specimen confirming this tumor–anatomical relationship

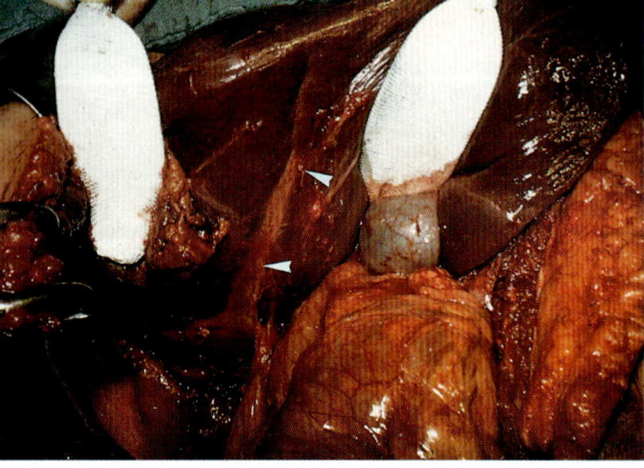

c

Fig. 6.5.9 Venous drainage of the liver
- **a** Standard distribution. Large arrow: short veins from
  the caudate lobe entering directly into the vena cava;
  small arrows: umbilical veins with the predominant
  branch terminating into the confluence of the middle
  and left hepatic veins
- **b** Inferior retrohepatic vein (arrow) draining segment VI
  and parts of segment V
- **c** Inferior retrohepatic vein in situ (arrows)

segments VII and VIII, including the ligation of the
right hepatic vein, without resultant venous congestion of segment VI (Andrus and Kaminsky 1986,
Makuuchi et al. 1987, Scheele 1989b) (Figs. 6.5.**33**,
6.5.**38**).

Equally important for a special group of
segmentectomies is the small umbilical vein, which
almost always runs alongside the falciform ligament between the middle and left hepatic veins
(Masselot and Leborgne 1978). In 70 % of cases it is
single, and usually flows into the terminal portion
of the left hepatic vein. Very rarely it drains into the
middle vein or directly into the angle formed by the
confluence of the middle and left hepatic veins
(Fig. 6.5.**9a**). The umbilical vein appears to be able
to drain at least parts of segment IVb after ligation
of the middle hepatic vein (Fig. 6.5.**35b**).

Oncological Rationale

The growth of both primary and metastatic liver tumors is generally limited to one segment (Goldsmith and Woodburne 1957) (Fig. 6.5.**10**). With the exception of less common diffuse infiltrating tumors, which in any case are almost never suitable for resection, and of some forms of cholangiocellular carcinoma, tumors remain restricted to their respective segment even after assuming huge proportions. Due to extensive growth the segment boundary is somewhat displaced by the tumor, but is very rarely transgressed (Fig. 6.5.**11**).

In addition to this direct continuous tumor growth, malignant liver tumors may also spread by discontinuous intra- and extrahepatic dissemination. Extrahepatic dissemination may be caused by retrograde lymphatic permeation, particularly to the hilar nodes, or by hematogenous distribution via the hepatic veins to distant organs. Both of these modes of dissemination generally exclude curative resection. Conversely, the prognostic importance of localized intrahepatic hematogenous spread is disputed (Ekberg et al. 1987, Masselot and Leborgne 1978, Scheele 1988). It is supposed to be based upon tumor invasion of a portal venous branch. With sudden increases in intrahepatic pressure (e. g. with coughing), tumor cells can be detached, and as a result of a temporary reversal of blood flow, they can be carried into an adjacent portal venous branch (Bismuth et al. 1987, Makuuchi et al. 1985, Nakashima and Kojiro 1987). In this way it is possible to account for step-by-step intrahepatic dissemination. This can range from satellite metastases in the immediate vicinity of a large mass, and therefore lying within the same segment, to involvement of the corresponding adjacent segment, or ultimately a complete liver lobe or bilateral spread (Fig. 6.5.**12**). With respect to the resection technique it is particularly important that the small satellite metastases, which are not usually noticed intraoperatively, lie in the same segment as the macroscopically identifiable main tumor mass.

Apart from the technical advantages provided by transection of the parenchyma along avascular planes, these two pathological aspects, that both continuous tumor expansion and early discontinuous intrahepatic spread remain within anatomical boundaries, represent the decisive oncological rationale for a segment-orientated approach in hepatic surgery.

Definition of Terms and Classification

The term "segmentectomy" has been used to describe types of resection which are to be established between the four classical anatomically defined resections and the smaller atypical procedures, with regard to their extent (Blumgart 1988).

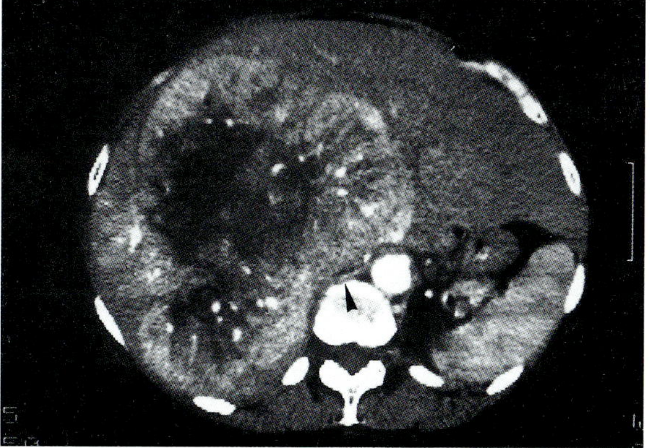

a

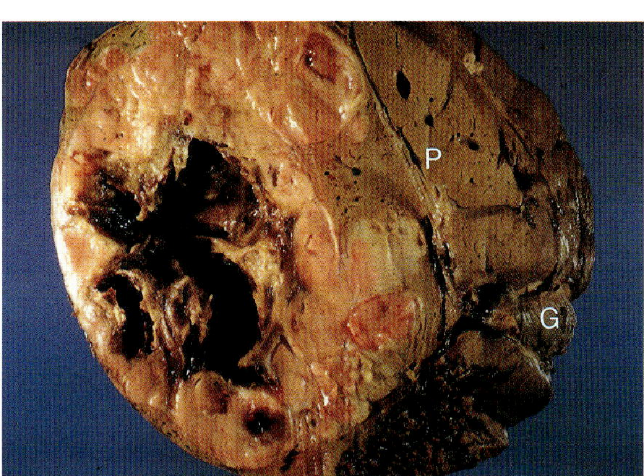

b

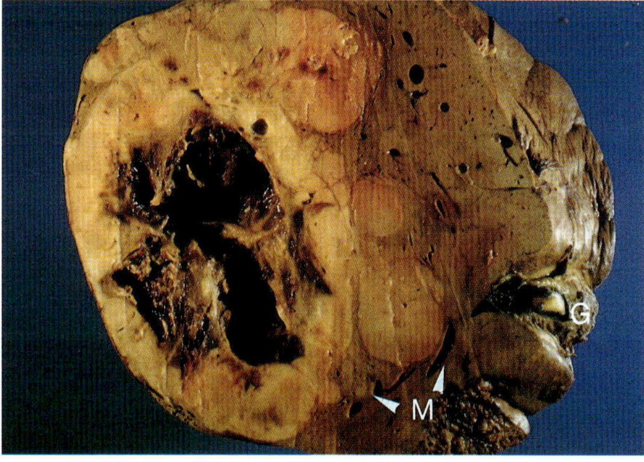

c

Fig. 6.5.**11 Large solitary metastasis of segment VII,** pushing segment VIII anteriorly and segments V and IV caudally. M: middle hepatic vein; P: portal branching to the posterior sector; G: gallbladder; arrow: vena cava
a CT scan showing the left lobe with no noticeable enlargement
b Posterior section of the specimen following right lobectomy. The level of posterior portal branching is pushed downward, but not transgressed by the tumor
c More anteriorly located section. The main fissure, indicated by the gallbladder and middle hepatic vein, is pushed to the left, but also not transgressed by the tumor

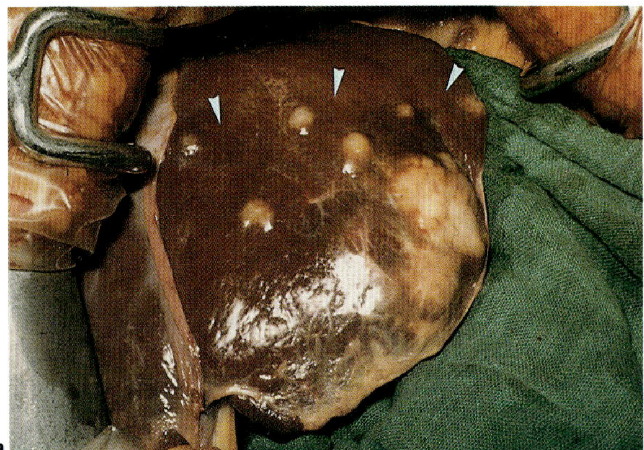

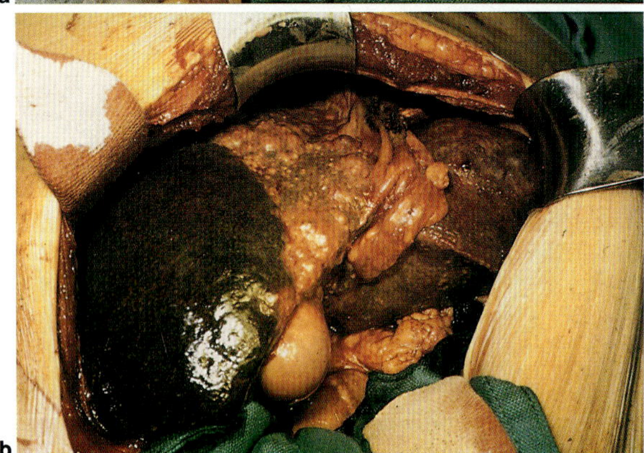

Fig. 6.5.**12 Step-by-step intrahepatic tumor dissemination**

a 4 cm colorectal liver metastasis of segment III with several satellite metastases confined to the same segment; color change following ligation of the portal pedicle III indicates the segmental border anteriorly (arrows)

b Fusion of multiple liver metastases from malignant melanoma confined to the left half of the liver; biliary obstruction due to hilar lymph node involvement

These types of definition have only limited application, and are hardly appropriate to give emphasis to the decisive criteria and advantages of a truly segment-orientated resection technique.

As it is understood in this chapter, a segment-orientated resection (SOR) is distinguished from the atypical procedures in that it is in principle orientated to the anatomical structure of the liver, not to the presumed extent of the pathological findings. Compared with the classical techniques of common hepatectomies and lobectomies, respectively, it is characterized by the transection line deviating at least partially from the main and umbilical fissure, respectively. From a practical point of view, this approach allows better adaptation of the procedure to the individual extent of the disease, particularly in the right hepatic lobe.

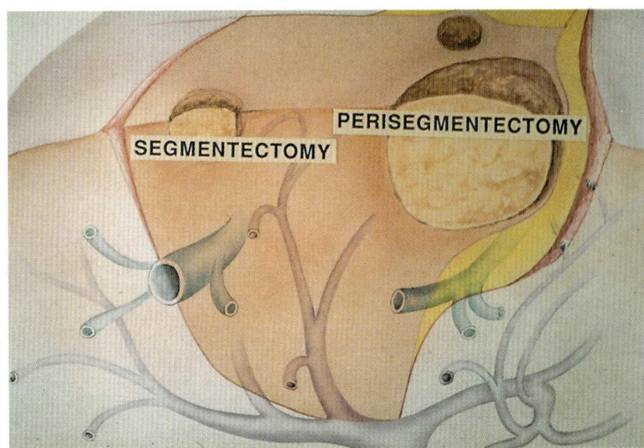

Fig. 6.5.**13 Principles of "segmentectomy" and "perisegmentectomy"**

Four main SOR-groups can be defined according to the extent of the intervention:

1. *Monosegmentectomies* constitute the complete removal of a single anatomical unit as defined above.

2. *Bi- and polysegmentectomies* involve the removal of multiple interconnected individual segments.

3. *SOR-modifications of classical resections* represent a subgroup of polysegmentectomies, of which the IVa (+ V – VIII) resection (a right lobectomy modified by preservation of the quadrate lobe) is of particular importance (Figs. 6.5.**17b**, 6.5.**35b**).

4. *Multiple segmentectomies* consist of simultaneous segmental resections carried out on different areas of the same liver.

Within the confines of these SOR approaches there are basically two different types of parenchyma transection: "segmentectomy" and "perisegmentectomy" (Fig. 6.5.**13**).

a) A true segmentectomy is suitable for the vast majority of situations and is technically simpler. The liver parenchyma is here separated as exactly as possible along the non-vascular boundary, a procedure which has been made considerably easier by the new "ultrasonic dissectors." The separation of the parenchyma proceeds very rapidly, since in most of the longitudinal planes there are only some large veins which run into the main trunks to be divided, and in the transverse part of the transection or along the umbilical fissure there are only a few portal trunks to ligate (Fig. 6.5.**16a**). This form of liver resection is ideally suited to benign lesions and for limited malignant tumors when pre- and intraoperative examinations show sufficient distance between the tumor surface and the envisaged resection planes (Figs. 6.5.**23**, 6.5.**30a**, 6.5.**33**).

b) Large or awkwardly positioned malignant tumors often lie close to the intrahepatic interfaces

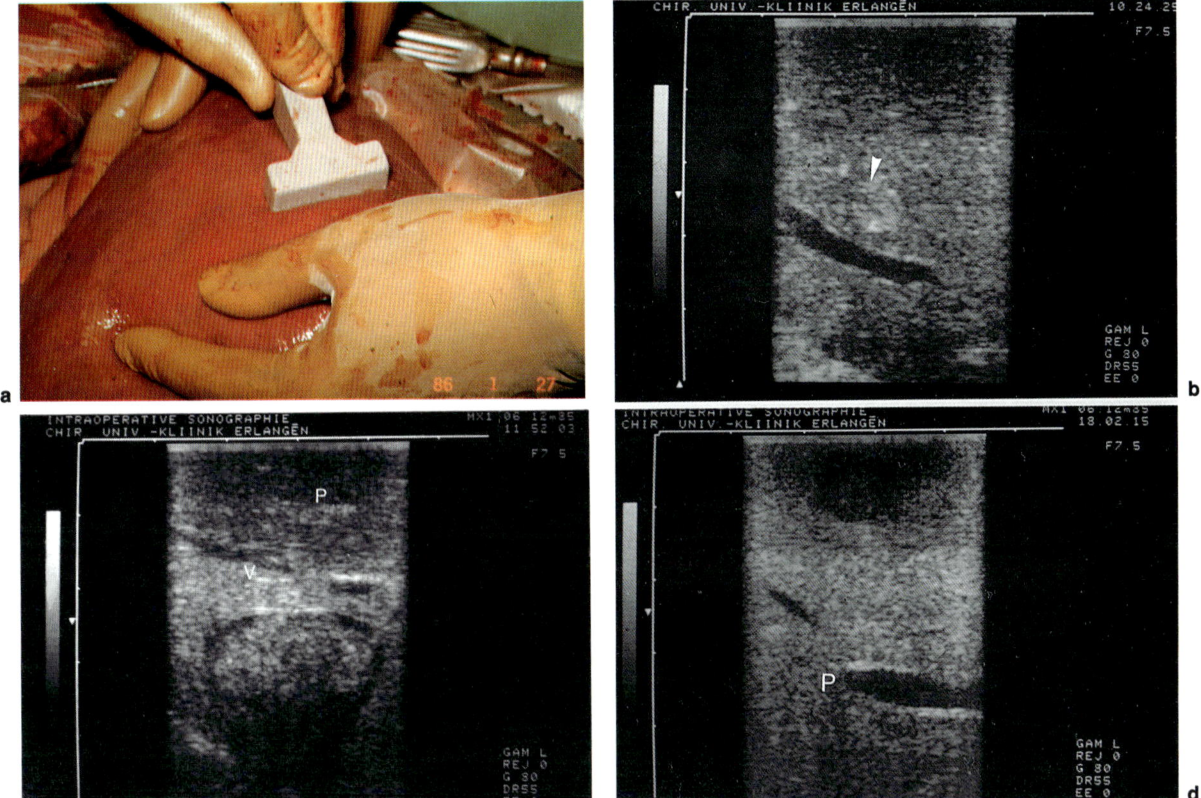

Fig. 6.5.14 Routine decision-making using intraoperative ultrasound. V: hepatic vein; P: portal pedicle
a   Re-imaging of the liver with simultaneous palpation
b   Small, previously undiscovered metastases in the vicinity of a hepatic venous branch
c   5 mm distance between a colorectal metastasis posteriorly located in segment VI and a peripheral branch of the right hepatic vein
d   Investigation of the same tumor with the ultrasonic probe placed at the inferior surface of the liver (i.e. scanning in anterior–superior direction) demonstrates a 2 cm distance from the portal pedicle VI

intended for the separation of the parenchyma. In this situation the resection line has to encroach slightly into the neighboring segment so that the oncological barrier function of the boundary is consciously used to guarantee radical tumor removal. This type of resection should be described as a "perisegmentectomy" (Figs. 6.5.**20**, 6.5.**30b–d**). Division of the parenchyma proceeds noticeably more slowly, due to the numerous small transverse portal pedicles which require individual ligation.

Technical Aids

Intraoperative Ultrasound

Intraoperative ultrasound has achieved a very high status in the field of hepatic resection for various reasons, including accurate definition of tumor extent, planning of the particular resection required and performance of the operation itself (Bismuth and Castaing 1987, Bismuth et al. 1987, Makuuchi et al. 1985, 1987).

In the case of malignant disease, a critical selection of patients suitable for resection still represents a fundamental problem. Intraoperative ultrasound as a supplement to the pre-operative diagnostic imaging permits a re-examination of the liver under direct vision, combined with simultaneous palpation. This offers superb sensitivity as regards the detection of smaller, previously undetected tumor nodules (Fig. 6.5.**14b**) and allows a well-directed biopsy of suspicious, more deeply located lesions. The ability to re-image during surgery is particularly important in patients with indurated, fibrotic or even cirrhotic parenchyma. Deep-lying lesions suspected as a result of the pre-operative diagnostic work-up are in these cases often no longer recognizable by palpation. Intraoperative ultrasound is therefore invaluable both in confirming the presence of the presumed lesion and also in localizing it precisely within the segmental hepatic architecture (Fig. 6.5.**15**).

A second reason for routine use of intraoperative ultrasound is its outstanding accuracy and

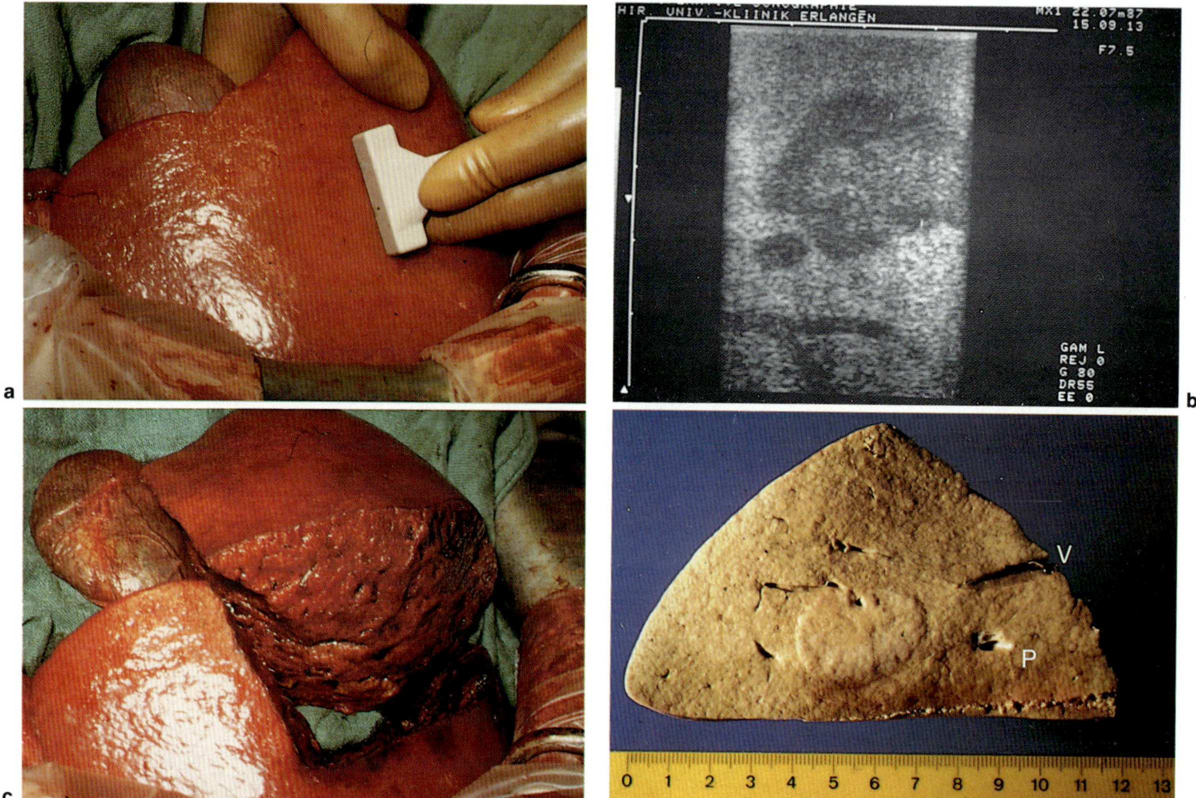

Fig. 6.5.**15   Intraoperative ultrasound during resection of a non-palpable colorectal metastasis** at the lateral edge of segment V, with mild liver cirrhosis present. V: hepatic vein; P: portal pedicle
a   Search for the lesion
b   Main lesion and small satellite tumor close to a branch of the right hepatic vein
c   Bisegmentectomy (V + VI) with cholecystectomy
d   Specimen demonstrating the intrahepatic tumor nodule surrounded by cirrhotic parenchyma

remarkable facilitation both of individualized resection planning and particularly of the performance of SOR procedures. The main venous trunks and the branching points of the portal pedicles can be quite easily defined; as a result, it is possible to judge the position of the intersegmental boundary zones. After confirming deep-seated reference points, the projection of the respective intersegmental plane can be estimated with a relatively small margin of error. For this purpose, it is assumed that the transverse boundaries between segments VI and VII or V and VIII run almost at a right angle to the longitudinal body axis onto the point of portal ramifications. Within the longitudinal segmental boundaries, the main fissure corresponds to the gallbladder bed and therefore lies approximately 30 degrees to the right of the liver when lying *in situ*, and between 0 and 15 degrees to the left after complete mobilization and supportive padding of the right lobe. The direction of the left intersegmental fissure is particularly easy to define, in view of the clear landmarks on the upper and lower surfaces; it runs somewhat sagit-

tally with the liver *in situ*. The right intersegmental fissure between the posterior and anterior sector is the most difficult to find. *In situ*, it lies almost in the frontal layer, or may be tilted backwards, whereas after mobilization and anterior displacement of the right lobe it runs at an angle of approximately 45 degrees to the vena cava (Bismuth 1982, Mukai et al. 1987a).

Ultrasound enables these orientating estimations of the segment boundaries at the liver surface to be made more precisely. The probe is focused on the intrahepatic reference structure, and is then turned so that the ultrasound beam is parallel to the estimated segment boundary. If the area is now scanned by moving the probe repeatedly backwards and forwards, a sudden reduction of the intrahepatic echoes often becomes noticeable. This is a strong indication of the avascular and ductless boundary area between adjacent segments.

In a similar way, evidence of anatomical variations can be established using intraoperative ultrasound. This is achieved by following the course of particular structures longitudinally with the probe. For example, a dominant middle hepatic vein running as far as segment VI, a large right retrohepatic vein, or a trifurcation of the portal vein can be demonstrated (Makuuchi et al. 1987).

Besides this detailed analysis of the individual anatomical organization, the intrahepatic extent of pathological findings and the distance to the simultaneously determined segment boundaries can be measured very accurately (Figs. 6.5.**14c**, **d**, 6.5.**15b**). By repeatedly checking the tumor–anatomical interrelationships, a reliable individual selection between atypical wedge excision, one of the SOR-procedures to be described in detail below, or an anatomical standard resection is facilitated. Also, a rational decision can be made as to whether the liver transection should be performed in the vascular-free boundary area or should encroach onto the adjacent segment.

Parenchyma Transection

Equally important for the performance of segment-orientated liver resections is a subtle technique for parenchyma transection. We have found the "ultrasonic dissectors," used in more than 300 liver resections since 1982 in our hospital, to be particularly suitable. They combine selective tissue-shattering using high-frequency mechanical vibration with an irrigation and constant aspiration of the debris created. Longitudinal mechanical oscillations at 23 and 26 kHz respectively, are generated either by a magnetostrictive transducer (CUSA) or by electrostrictive piezoceramics (NUSS). The oscillations then pass through the connecting body to a conical tip which acts as an amplifier. While the frequency is constant, the amplitude changes by up to 300 microns depending on the power input.

The mechanism of action is based on "cavitation," which may be explained as the poor ability of tissue to join the oscillations. Contacted cells are compressed by the outward movement of the tip but are not able to follow the backward movement. A low-pressure area is thus created which for physical reasons results in the transformation of fluid and dissolved gas to a gaseous state. As a consequence of mechanical damage as well as intracellular microbubble formation, the cell membranes rupture. The resulting fragmentation effect is proportional to the water content of the cells. This permits highly selective tissue removal depending on the power set (Andrus and Kaminsky 1986, Hodgson and DelGuercio 1984, Hodgson et al. 1988, Ottow et al. 1985).

In comparison with the conventional finger fracture technique or even with the crash method employing fine scissors or clamps, the use of this instrument allows a particularly exact preparation orientated to tumor extent and liver structure. The

exclusively axially-directed effect of the oscillatory energy fragments the liver parenchyma within a 1–2 mm wide layer and results in a thin layer of devitalized cells coating the raw surface (Okuda et al. 1984). Simultaneously, an irrigating saline spray suspends the fragments, which are then continuously aspirated to allow a constantly clear view. Small vessels and bile ducts within the resection area are preserved due to their high collagen and elastin and low water content. They can be dealt with individually either by electrocoagulation or by ligation (Fig. 6.5.**16a**). This leads to smooth, usually dry primary wounds.

In a non-cirrhotic liver, this selective tissue-shattering also allows wide exposure of important intrahepatic structures without direct injury to them (Fig. 6.5.**16b**). This is of particular value if a segment has to be preserved for reasons of postoperative hepatic capacity but a malignant tumor is lying very close to its portal pedicle.

Although in our experience the ultrasound dissector offers advantages for liver resection in general, it becomes essential for a sophisticated SOR-approach. As soon as the avascular boundary planes are reached, the tissue cutting proceeds easily and quickly, since there are almost no vessels or ducts crossing the site. By maintaining some tension on the wound, the liver gapes apart as if spontaneously at the ideal anatomical boundary. The instrument is, however, equally important in those areas where an extended perisegmental resection is being deliberately attempted for reasons of tumor extension. Because of the numerous portal structures to be cut, the dissection requires a great deal of time and multiple fine ligatures. Nevertheless, as opposed to conventional methods, particularly a somewhat roughly performed finger fracture technique, no lateral tears occur either in the resected or in the remaining liver, so that in the case of a malignant tumor, even when the margin of clearance is very small, a complete layer of intact liver parenchyma is maintained, thus fulfilling the prime criterion for a potentially curative surgical intervention.

Hemostasis

What was previously a major problem, controlling hemorrhage, has largely been solved by the anatomical approach and the method of parenchyma transection described above. Residual bleeding can be effectively eliminated either by infrared contact coagulation, which results in a superficial tissue necrosis 3–4 mm in depth (Fig. 6.5.**17a**) or using fibrinogen sealant (Guthy 1986, Scheele 1982). This biological two-component adhesive can be applied using a spray device or in combination with a

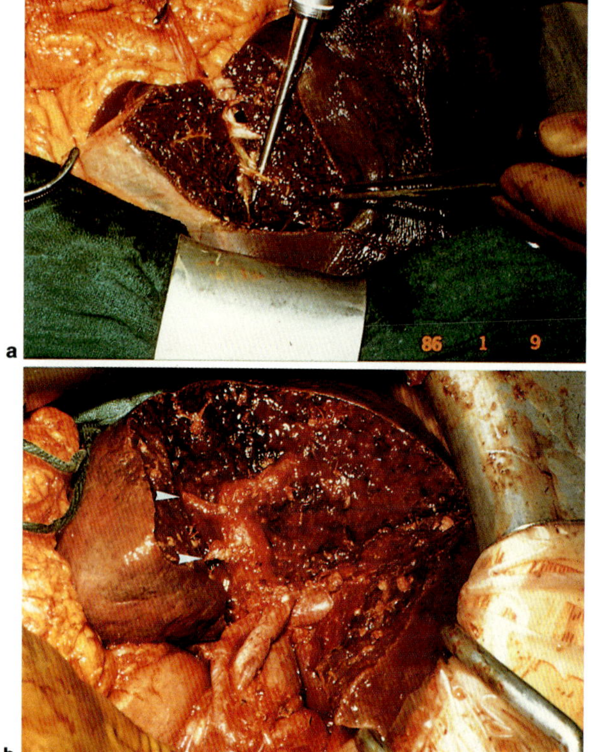
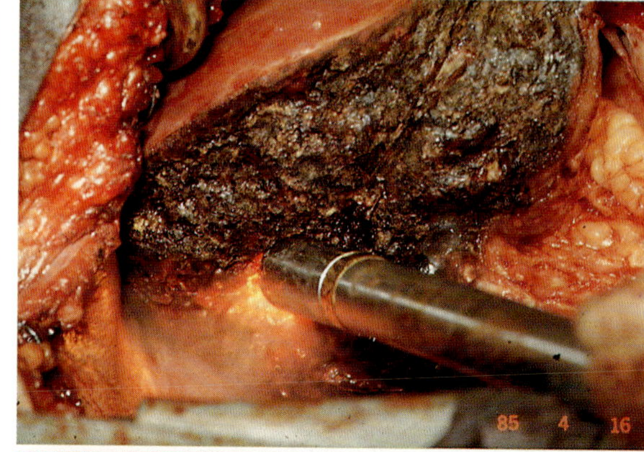
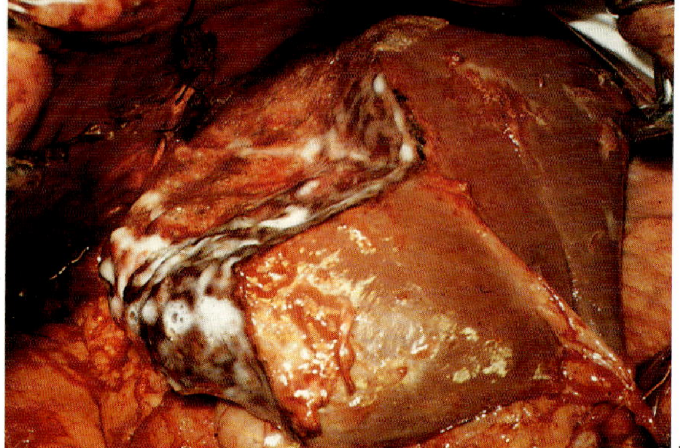
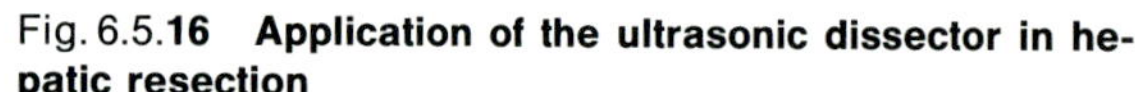

Fig. 6.5.**16   Application of the ultrasonic dissector in hepatic resection**

a   Complete exposure of the umbilical portion and the pedicles radiating to segment IV precisely along the intersegmental boundary in isolated IVb resection for a symptomatic focal nodular hyperplasia compressing the hilum

b   Segmentectomy (III–V) for a cholangiocarcinoma with mild cirrhosis present. Wide skeletonization of the anterior portal pedicle, preserving all branches to segment VIII and two smaller branches to the retained right third of segment V (arrows). The transverse part of the left portal vein is also completely exposed

Fig. 6.5.**17   Recent techniques of achieving reliable hemostasis**

a   Infrared contact coagulation after right hepatectomy

b   Fibrinogen adhesive following IVa (+ V–VIII) resection encroaching on segment II. Combination with collagen fleece and the venous confluence, spray technique caudally

collagen fleece (Fig. 6.5.**17b**). Due to the direct application of highly concentrated clotting factors, this method is effective even where reduced systemic coagulation capacity is present. Moreover, it offers particular advantages in the vicinity of important intrahepatic vascular structures, since its optimal tissue compatibility prevents any damage.

Surgical Strategy

The SOR approach cannot be viewed in isolation. Basically related to the classical anatomical procedures, it allows resections to be better adapted to individual requirements, especially in the right hepatic lobe. With regard to atypical resections, both their necessity and importance are reduced but not totally eliminated. The appropriate choice between the various operative procedures is made simpler by some basic rules.

Preoperative Imaging

Preoperative diagnostic imaging in itself should allow precise anatomical orientation. Ultrasound offers the advantage of a dynamic mode of examination with free choice of the sectional plane, but requires close cooperation between the surgeon and the ultrasonographer. Since it is possible to make a detailed strategic assessment only during the examination itself, the results, including diameters and distances of practical interest, should be entered on a segmental sketch (Fig. 6.5.**18a**). In borderline cases I have found a cooperative examination by the ultrasound expert and surgeon to be most useful. Computerized tomography (CT) and magnetic resonance imaging (MRI) offer the advantage of easier reinterpretation and orientation later on. Sections at the level of the venous confluence (Fig. 6.5.**18b**), the left and right portal branching (Fig. 6.5.**10a**) and at the level of the gallbladder and hepatoduodenal ligament are all indispensable basic requirements for detailed segmental orientation (Mukai et al. 1987a). With respect to CT scanning, a contrast study and suitable gradation (window 350–450) are essential to provide specific surgical information. MRI already offers a better depiction of the intrahepatic vessels (Fig. 6.5.**18c**) and the advantage of a free choice of sectional planes. The future application and value of substraction techniques or three-dimensional calculations are difficult to assess at the present time.

Intraoperative Reexamination

Adequate preoperative imaging usually allows provisional planning of the resection (Mukai et al. 1987b). The final decision regarding resectability and the choice of procedure, however, is not made until the laparotomy, particularly in the case of multiple malignant lesions. The advantages of routine intraoperative ultrasound at this point have already been pointed out. The examination should be made according to a fixed checklist (Bismuth 1987). After initial focusing on a known lesion and optimal adjustment of the instrument, the following examination sequence has proved its value in my experience: (1) search for further comparable lesions, (2) image the liver veins from right to left, (3) image the portal structures, starting at the hilum, first to the right and then to the left, and (4) conclusively establish the relationship between the lesions discovered and the intrahepatic boundaries.

Choice of Operation

There are several important factors in the differential indication of the various types of resection: number, size, position and type of the pathological lesions, extent of the parenchyma reduction required and, where applicable, already present compensatory hypertrophy of non-involved areas.

An important preliminary decision is centered on the presence of parenchymal disease. Where there is moderate or severe cirrhosis, which fortunately occurs less frequently in the West, the resection of more than 2 segments increases the risk of a functional liver failure drastically. In these patients the extent of resection should be limited in the case of marginal tumors to economical atypical

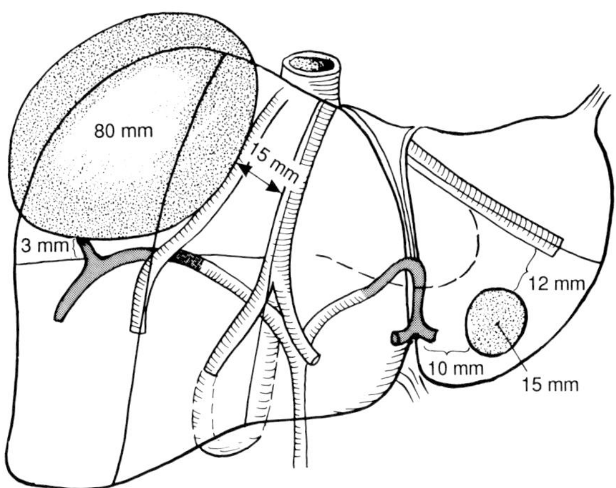

a

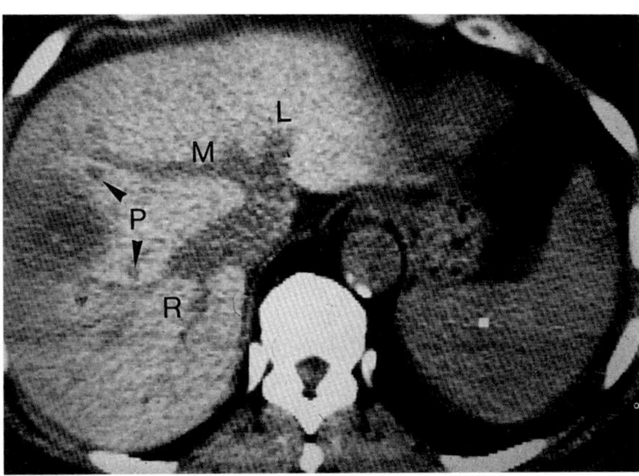

b

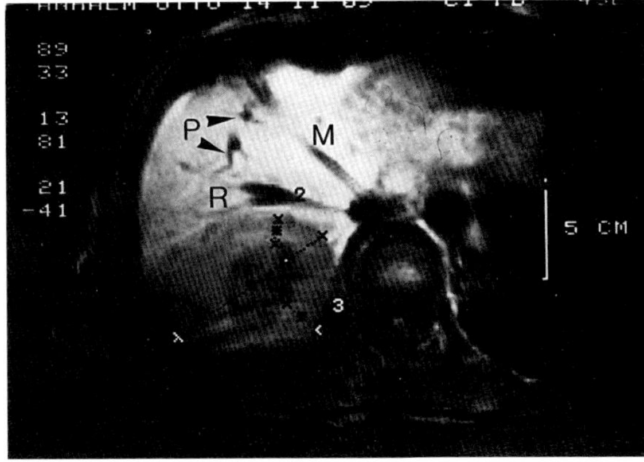

c

Fig. 6.5.**18** **Reliable preoperative imaging.** R: right hepatic vein; M: middle hepatic vein; L: left hepatic vein; P: portal pedicle to segment VIII
a Routine documentation of ultrasound findings
b CT scan at the level of the venous confluence showing a peripherally located colorectal metastasis from segment VIII, 1 cm from a right branch of the middle hepatic vein (see figure 6.5.**33**)
c MRI of a segment VII metastasis located close to the main trunk of the right hepatic vein

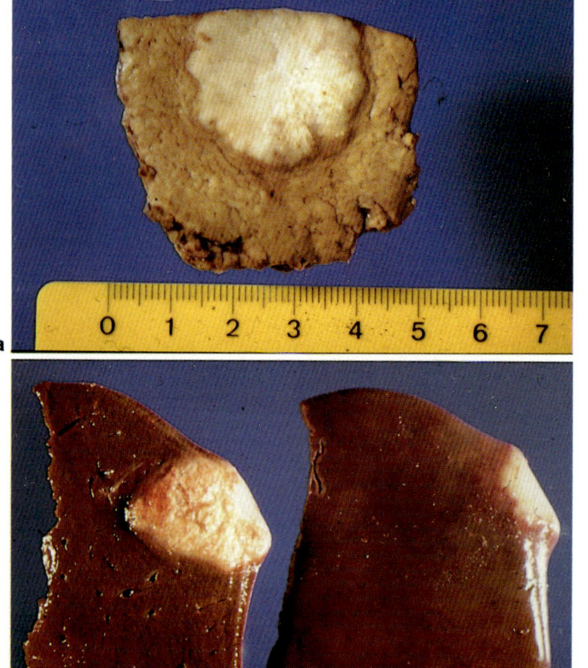
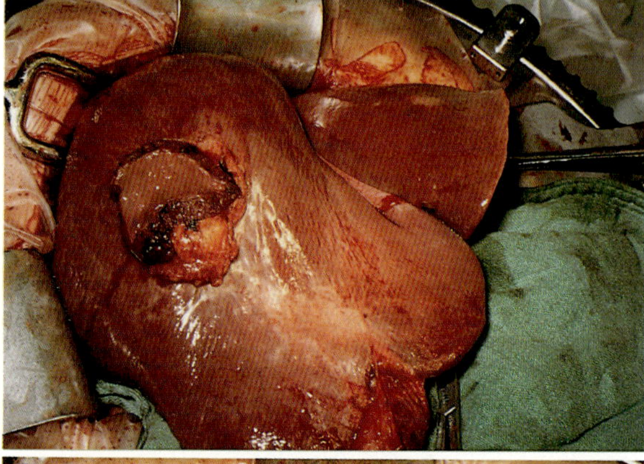
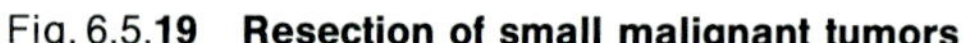
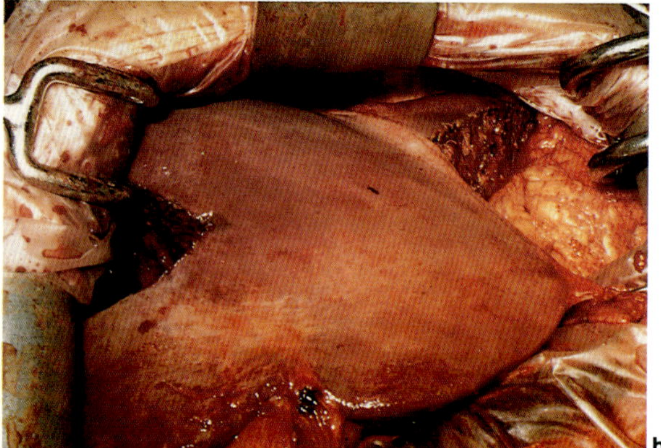

Fig. 6.5.19   Resection of small malignant tumors
a U-shaped local excision of a small hepatocellular carcinoma resulting in a clear margin greater than 5 mm
b Segmentectomy VII for a solitary colorectal metastasis. From the outside, the intrahepatic extension is likely to be underestimated

Fig. 6.5.20   Indication for segmentectomy on the left lobe
a Bilateral colorectal metastases involving segment VII (adherent part of the diaphragm excised) and segment III
b The left tumors are removed by monosegmentectomy III, preserving any resection eventually required at the right side. Here a perisegmentectomy VII is being performed

excisions with small margins, and in the case of an intrahepatic localization to a monosegmentectomy (Bismuth et al. 1982, 1987, Franco et al. 1985, Lee et al. 1985, Lin et al. 1979, Makuuchi et al. 1987, Okuda et al. 1984, Priesching 1986). Anatomical orientation, which is noticeably more difficult in a cirrhotic liver, can be made more precise by ultrasound-guided puncture of the respective portal vein and dye injection, with or without previous cannulation with small balloon catheters (Bismuth and Castaing 1987, Bismuth et al. 1987, Makuuchi et al. 1985, 1987).

There is still one indication for local excision in a non-cirrhotic liver: a subcapsular lesion, less than 3 cm in size, located at a sufficient distance from the major veins and the area of portal branching. However, this procedure should in no way underestimate the intrahepatic extent of a tumor. It should always be made in an arch or box shape, and never in a V-form (Fig. 6.5.19 a). In the case of malignant tumors of more than 2.5 cm in diameter, we prin-

cipally attempt a suitable anatomical resection, mainly on grounds of radicality (Fig. 6.5.19 b). This approach is also ideally suited to larger benign lesions because of its technical advantages during surgery.

The preference for an SOR alternative to an otherwise standard resection gains particular importance with respect to right lobectomy (Bismuth et al. 1982). Apart from individual examples with massive compensatory hypertrophy of the left lobe (Fig. 6.5.1 b), the preservation of a non-involved quadrate lobe (segment IV b) considerably reduces the risk of post-resectional hepatic failure (Figs. 6.5.17 b, 6.5.22 b, 6.5.35 b). A typical indication for this SOR [IV a + (V−VIII)], is presented by a metastasis of segment VIII lying close to the portal pedicle and the middle hepatic vein, since radical tumor removal is only guaranteed here by simultaneous resection of the subsegment IV a. A corresponding stepped SOR modification is also possible with respect to a right hepatectomy

(Fig. 6.5.**35 a**), but is only useful in very selected cases. As a rule it can be stated that such parenchyma-preserving SOR modifications are useful when 4 segments and more than 50 % of the functional parenchyma would otherwise have to be removed.

Operative Technique in SOR Procedures

In order to guarantee an optimum dry field, I carry out all resections under inflow occlusion (Pringle's maneuver). The hilar clamps are opened 1–2 min every 15–20 min in order to relieve portal venous congestion and the metabolic products collected in the splanchnic circulation. Before first clamping, 1 million units of aprotinin are given intravenously in order to block aggressive enzymatic activity (e. g. proteases, kinases).

Left Hepatic Lobe

The isolated resection of segments II or III is only considered in exceptional cases with simultaneous substantial right resection (Fig. 6.5.**20**). If possible, the portal pedicles should first be prepared and ligated. For segment III they are easily accessible at the base of the round ligament, whereas the branches leading to segment II are identifiable after lifting the left lobe and tracing the venous ligament in the cranial portion of the groove between the left and caudate lobes. The border between the two left segments is difficult to define without preliminary preparation of their portal pedicles. As opposed to the horizontally lying transverse boundaries of the right lobe, it tends to run from upper anterior to lower posterior.

Segment IV

Both the caudal subsegment IV b (Fig. 6.5.**21**) and the whole segment (Fig. 6.5.**22**) are technically easy to remove. On the right, the pale groove along the middle of the gallbladder bed and the large main trunk of the middle hepatic vein, identified by ultrasound, and on the left, the falciform and round ligaments, all serve as guiding landmarks. After division of the tissue bridge (Fig. 6.5.**21 b**) concealing the round ligament, the portal pedicles radiating from the umbilical portion are separated either directly from the liver underside as the first step, or from above after preliminary division of the parenchyma (Fig. 6.5.**16 a**). In the case of an isolated IV b resection, the large main branch which usually arises from the deepest point of the umbilical fissure must not be compromised. Its anteriorly directed course indicates the level of the transverse parenchymal transection (as it does in the converse case, i. e. during removal of the apical subsegment IV a while preserving IV b) (Fig. 6.5.**22**).

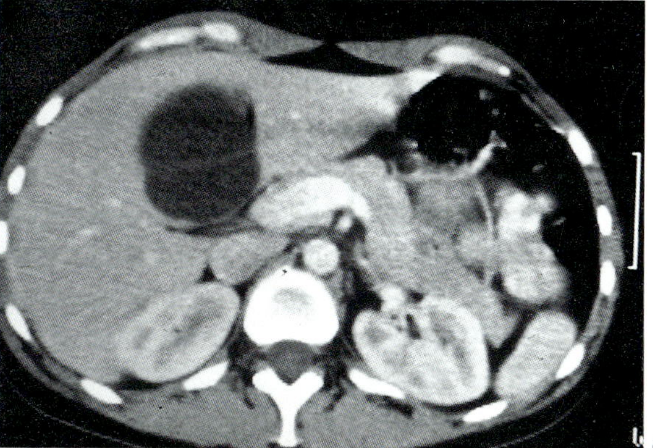

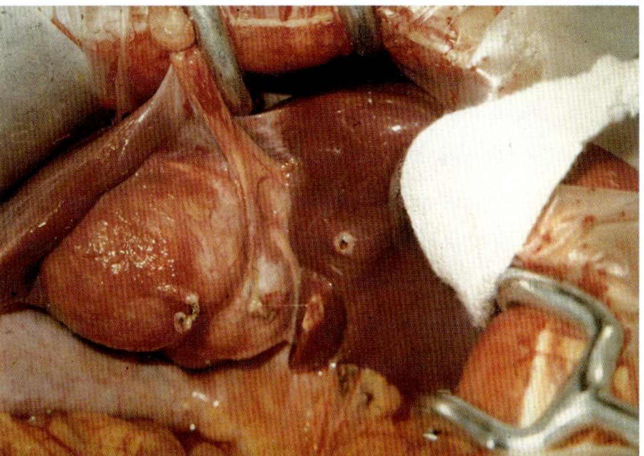

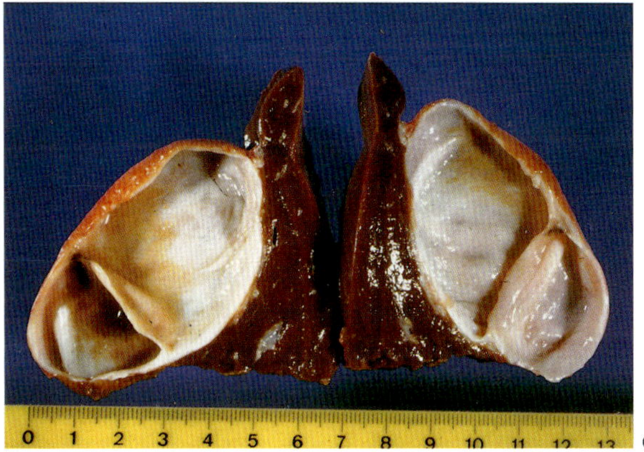

Fig. 6.5.**21** **Resection of segment IV b** for a symptomatic cyst extending close to the umbilical fissure **a** CT scan demonstrating a "double-bubble" cyst with compression of the hilum **b** Cyst in situ after dividing the tissue bridge concealing the round ligament **c** Specimen

If the whole of segment IV is resected, all portal pedicles running from the umbilical portion to the left are divided, whereas the middle hepatic vein is usually preserved (Fig. 6.5.**23**). Larger cranially-located malignant lesions, however, require a limited perisegmental extension (Fig. 6.5.**24**). If the middle hepatic vein must be ligated to achieve a clear margin, the umbilical vein should be preserved.

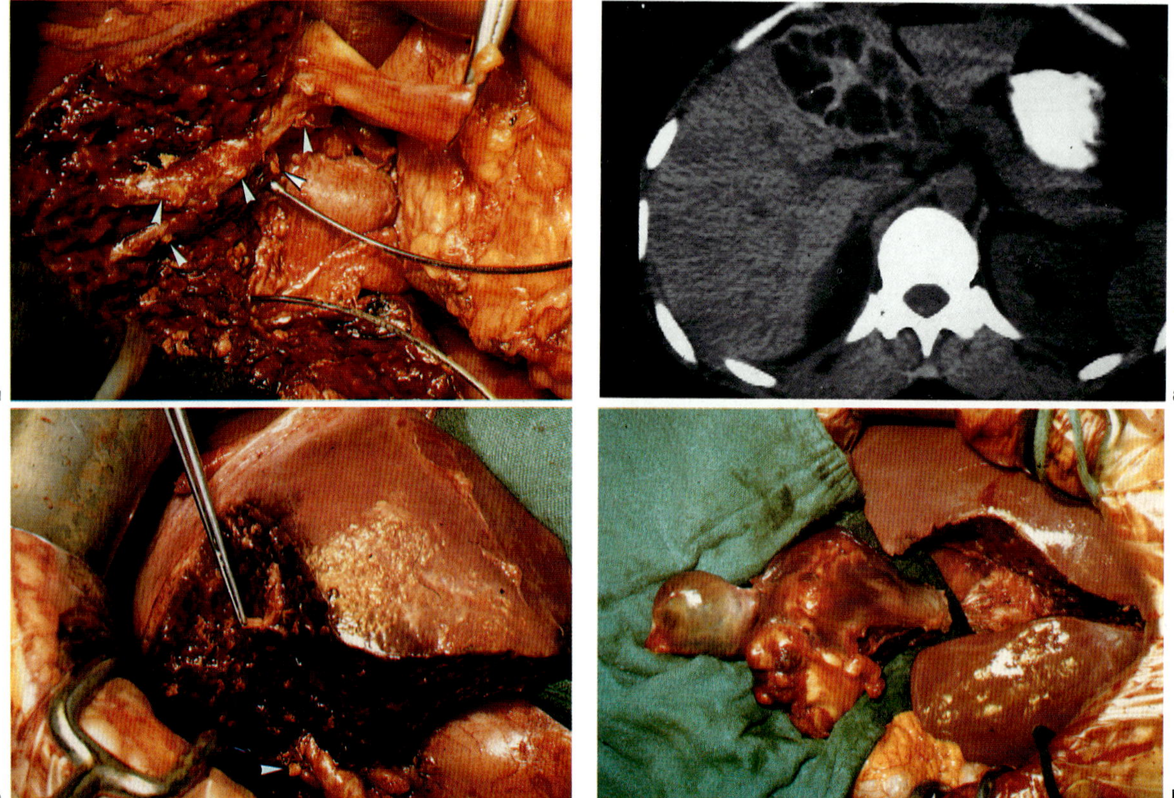

Fig. 6.5.**22** **Separate resection of subsegments IVa and IVb**, respectively **a** Bisegmentectomy (IVb + V) combined with hilar resection for gallbladder cancer involving the common bile duct. Two major arched portal venous branches running cranially to segment IVa are preserved, while caudally directed pedicles and side branches (arrows) are ligated. Bile ducts stented by curved metal probes **b** SOR [IVa + (V–VIII)] for two colorectal metastases in segments VI and VIII. The transverse portion of the left portal structure is exposed. A short proximally radiating branch to segment IVa (small arrow) and the main arched branch to segment IVa (forceps) are ligated, whereas the anteriorly-directed main trunk is preserved and appears at the transverse resection plane

Fig. 6.5.**23** **Complete segmentectomy IV and cholecystectomy** for hydatid cyst
a CT scan
b Post-resection defect and specimen

Caudal Area of the Right Hepatic Lobe

An SOR approach which is often useful is bisegmentectomy (IVb + V). In the case of moderately advanced hilar carcinoma it allows better removal en bloc of the hepatic duct bifurcation together with the affected liver parts than the isolated IVb segmentectomy proposed by others (Andrus and Kaminsky 1986, Bismuth et al. 1982) (Fig. 6.5.**25**). The intrahepatic bile ducts can be separated at various levels, depending on the extent of the tumor. This bisegmentectomy also provides optimal resection of locally infiltrating gallbladder carcinoma (Andrus and Kaminsky 1986, Köckerling et al. 1988, Scheele 1989b), and not only

because of the large margins of clearance. Since the venous drainage of the gallbladder opens directly into small portal venous branches supplying the two adjacent segments, the preferred area of limited hematogenous spread is also completely removed by this approach (Fig. 6.5.**26**). As far as the operative technique is concerned, the left resection line in this bisegmentectomy is defined in the same way as described for the isolated IVb resection. In addition to the anteriorly directed main pedicle for segment IV, the portal branching of the segments V/VIII serves as a second orientation point for the transverse boundary. The right boundary is more difficult to define, since the right hepatic vein has usually already branched considerably. For a rough estimation, the center between the gallbladder and the right liver edge may serve. However, tiny grooves or fissures on the liver underside are often indicators of the exact course (Figs. 6.5.**26a**, 6.5.**28**, 6.5.**29b**).

The additional extension to a (IVb + V + VI) resection is required in the case of large tumors,

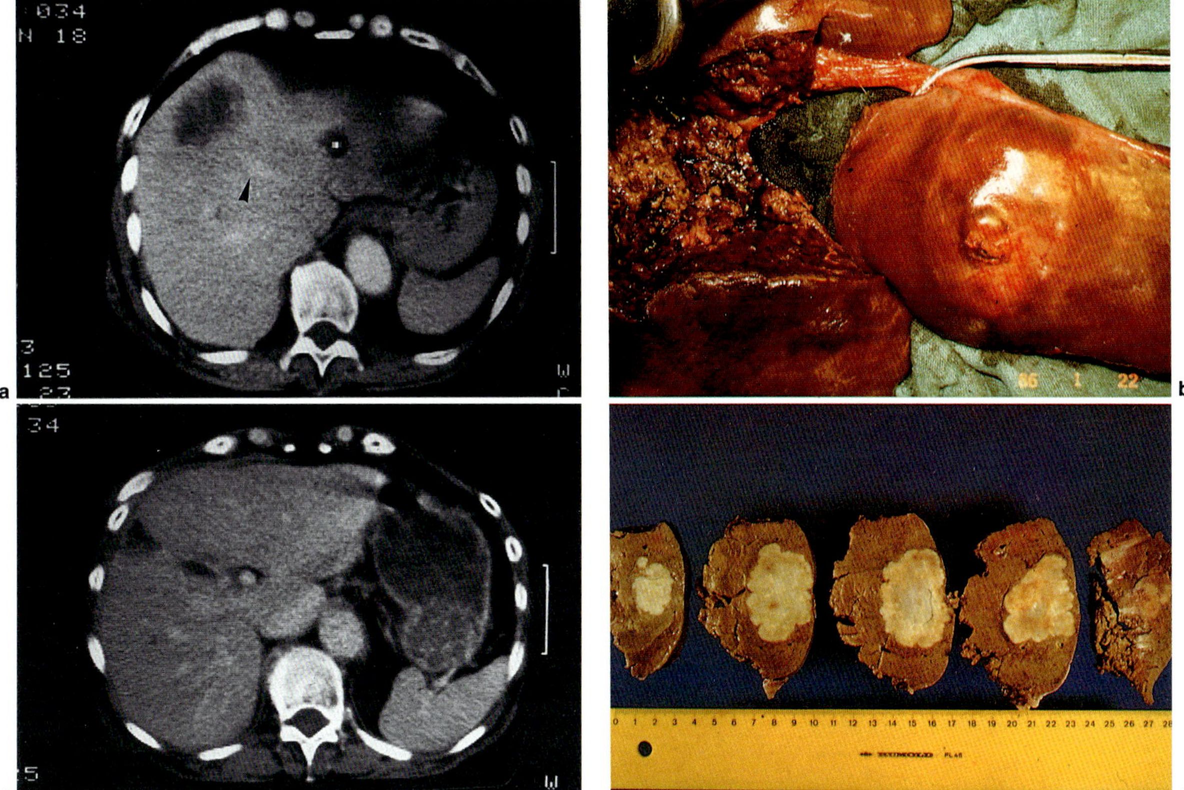

Fig. 6.5.**24** **Cranially-located colorectal metastasis of segment IV a, removed by perisegmentectomy IV**
a Preoperative CT scan showing the metastasis close to the trunk and a left side branch of the middle hepatic vein (arrow) and the main fissure. Benign cyst in the left lobe
b Radical resection encroaching on segment VIII, with ligation of the middle hepatic vein
c Postoperative CT scan with the two parts of the liver remnant in close contact
d Slices of the specimen demonstrate that the tumor is surrounded by a sufficient margin of clearance

for instance a gallbladder carcinoma infiltrating close to the V/VI boundary (Couinaud 1957) (Fig. 6.5.**27**). From the point of view of operative technique, this procedure is easier, since the transverse resection line is simply continued to the right edge of the liver, with ultrasound monitoring of the easily identifiable portal branching to VI/VII. In contrast to a bisegmentectomy (IV b + V), the right lobe should be mobilized for the additional removal of segment VI.

An isolated resection of segments V or VI, or their simultaneous removal, simply requires another combination of the resection lines already described (Figs. 6.5.**28**, 6.5.**29**).

Cranial Section of the Right Hepatic Lobe

The complete mobilization of the entire right lobe as far as the vena cava is an indispensable prerequisite for resections of the cranial right-sided segments. The main fissure along the middle hepatic vein and the boundary between subsegment IV a

and the left lobe are easy to determine. The latter can be identified by projecting the continuation of the falciform ligament over the pars affixa in the direction of the left vena cava edge or by focusing on the umbilical vein with ultrasound. The third longitudinal boundary between segments VII and VIII is less difficult to determine than its caudal continuation V/VI, since the terminal portion of the right hepatic vein can already be seen as a large main trunk. The transverse resection lines are determined under ultrasonic monitoring of the portal branching levels in the same way as described in caudal SOR procedures.

Isolated segment VII resection offers a most convenient radical removal of malignancies which are not sited too close to the vena cava (Fig. 6.5.**30**). There is usually a clearly defined portal pedicle together with 3 or 4 larger venous tributaries which run partly into the terminal portion of the right hepatic vein or enter directly into the vena cava. In order to stay within the intersegmental plane dorsally, consideration must be given to the fact that the boundary to segment VIII remains at a consid-

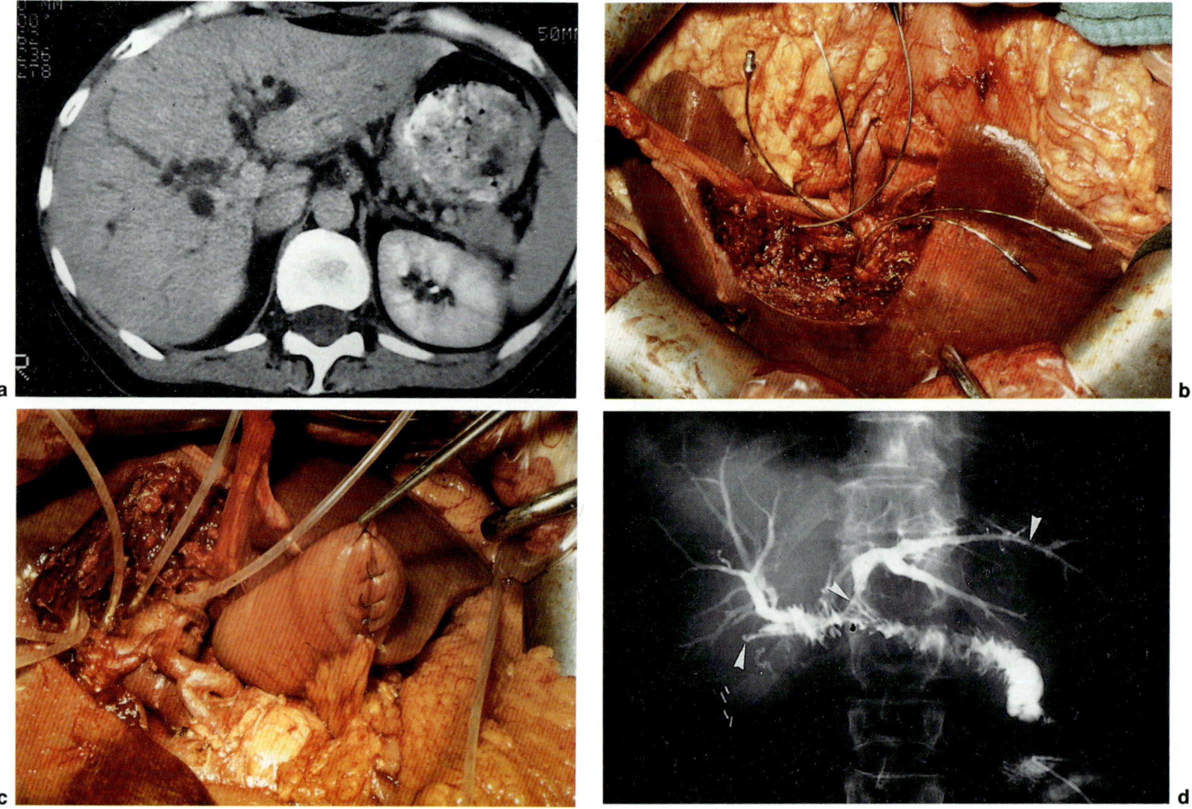

Fig. 6.5.25   Resection of a Klatskin tumor with a bisegmentectomy (IV + V)
a Preoperative CT scan demonstrating a localized tumor and dilation of the bile ducts on both sides
b Cannulation of 5 out of 7 separately divided ducts using curved probes for transhepatic catheter placement and subsequent individual anastomosis, technique of Neuhaus (1984)
c Silicon drains for temporary stenting of the anastomoses to a Roux-en-Y loop. Segment I is removed as well
d X-ray examination 10 days postoperatively before removing the last intraluminal drain (arrows)

erable angle, even after luxation of the right lobe and runs to the middle of the anterior surface of the vena cava. The parenchymal defect remaining at the end of an isolated monosegmentectomy in VII or VI can usually be completely closed without tension (Fig. 6.5.**31**).

The main indications for a monosegmentectomy in VIII are minor, centrally-situated solitary metastases and, in particular, small liver cell carcinomas in cirrhotic patients, since the traditional anatomically-based alternative would consist of a right hepatectomy (Franco et al. 1985) (Fig. 6.5.**32**).

Even in a non-cirrhotic liver, the complete removal of segment VIII technically presents the most demanding monosegmentectomy (Bismuth et al. 1982). As mentioned in connection with segment VII resection, there is a tendency to make an incomplete tissue removal in the dorsal direction because of a lack of anatomical orientation and the

hazards involved in damage to the major hepatic veins. Ideally, the fan-shaped confluence of the right hepatic vein on the right, the large anterior main portal trunk caudally, and the middle hepatic vein on the left, but no major area of the vena cava, should be exposed.

Tumors located in either segment VIII or VII which encroach upon the right hepatic vein can often be managed by a bisegmentectomy (VII + VIII), even with complete severing of the right hepatic vein (Andrus and Kaminsky 1986, Makuuchi et al. 1987) (Fig. 6.5.**33**). Provided that a retrohepatic vein (Fig. 6.5.**9**) or a dominant middle hepatic vein exists, venous drainage problems can be disregarded. However, even for 4 of our patients with no such vessels demonstrable, a follow-up resection only became necessary in one case because of a rapidly progressing congestion of segment VI. Immediate localization of a segment VIII tumor on the middle hepatic vein requires (IVa + VIII)

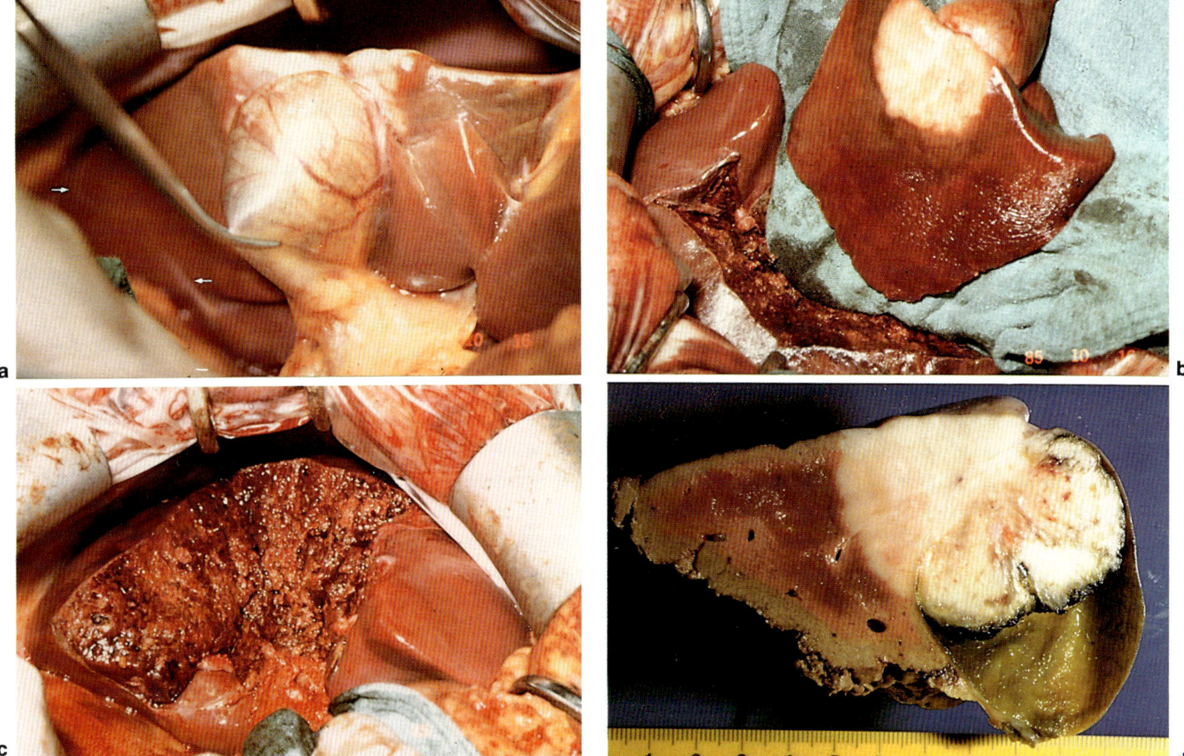

Fig. 6.5.26 Radical resection of gallbladder cancer infiltrating the liver (pT 3)
a Tumor of the fundus of the gallbladder directly invading both adjacent segments (arrow: boundary V/VI)
b En bloc resection using a bisegmentectomy (IV b + V)
c U-shaped parenchymal defect with exposure of the hilum
d Specimen with wide margin of clearance

bisegmentectomy. Despite ligation of the middle vein, sufficient blood drainage for segments IV b and V usually remains via the umbilical and the right hepatic veins, respectively (Fig. 6.5.**34**).

Segmentectomies Involving the Upper and Lower Right Lobe

A corresponding extension of the right hepatectomy to the subsegment IV a, resulting in a stepped resection plane, is to be recommended in dealing with metastases near to both the middle hepatic vein and the portal branching in segment VIII, or for multiple tumors with a corresponding pattern of distribution. This resection [IV a + (V–VIII)] may often replace the right lobectomy otherwise necessary and, by preserving the quadrate lobe, considerably reduces the hazard of post-resectional hepatic insufficiency (Figs. 6.5.**17 b**, 6.5.**22 b**, 6.5.**35 b**).

If the longitudinal resection planes are each shifted one segment to the right, the SOR (V–VIII) results. It consists of a comparable minus-variation of the right hepatectomy adequate for badly placed lesions in segment VII (Fig. 6.5.**35 a**). This modifi-

cation is technically more lavish than the [IV a + (V–VIII)] resection, and is less significant with regard to the postoperative functional reserve.

Apart from these variations, mention should also be made of the bisegmentectomy (VI + VII) and – the most common form of "segment-orientated" resection on the right lobe – right hepatectomy and lobectomy.

Segment I

Surgical access to the caudate lobe and process is difficult because of their concealed anatomical position between the hilum and the vena cava, and their somewhat obscure boundaries anteriorly and to the right. Particularly in its diseased state, however, this segment demonstrates the wide spectrum of classical resection and SOR techniques particularly clearly.

The isolated monosegmentectomy I, performed from the left, is suitable for small lesions lying in the left half of the caudate lobe, in particular for benign tumors (Bismuth et al. 1982). The parenchyma is not divided until after complete separation of the caudate lobe from the retroperitoneum and vena cava. Ideally, the cranial portion

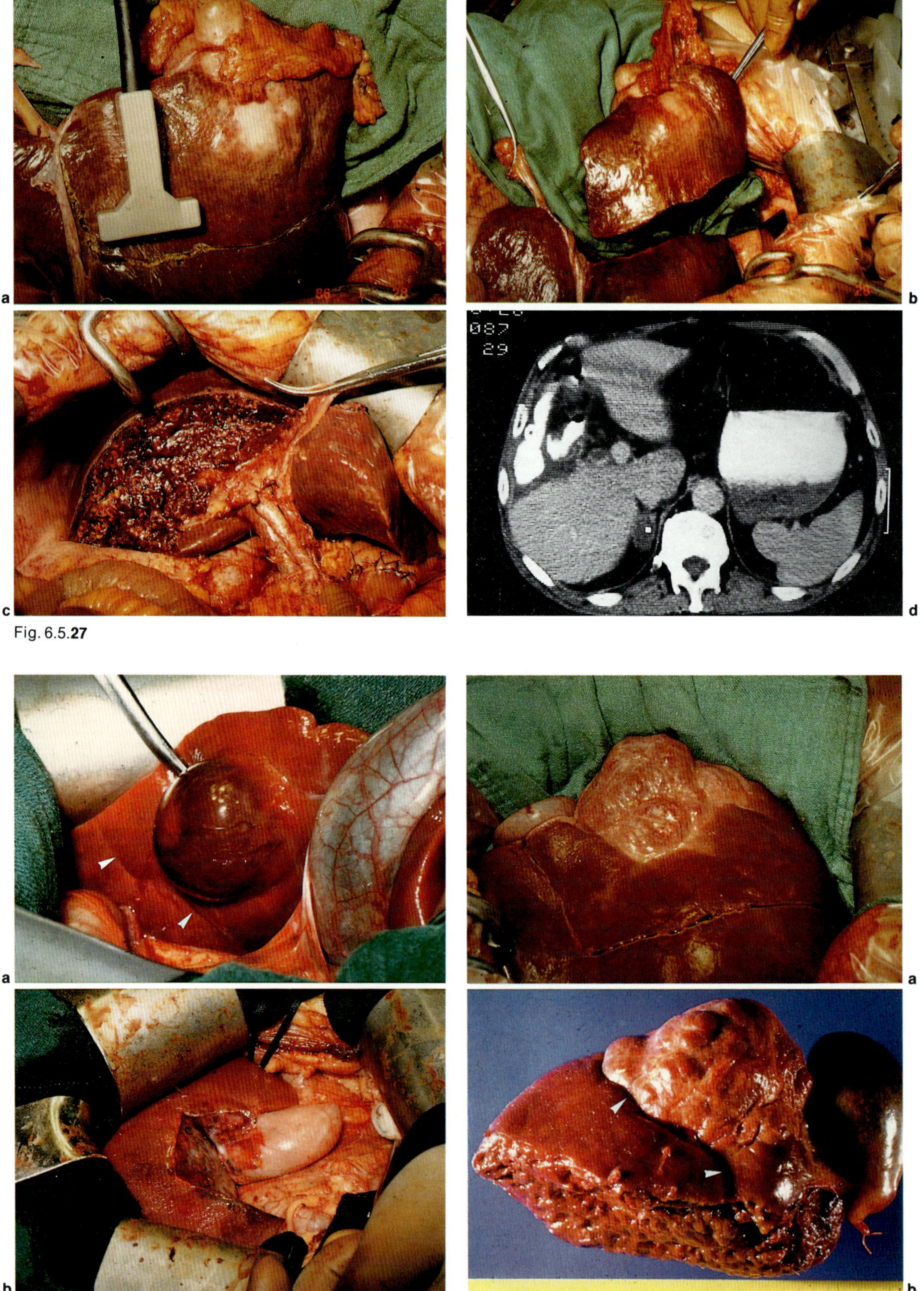

Fig. 6.5.**27**

Fig. 6.5.**28**

Fig. 6.5.**29**

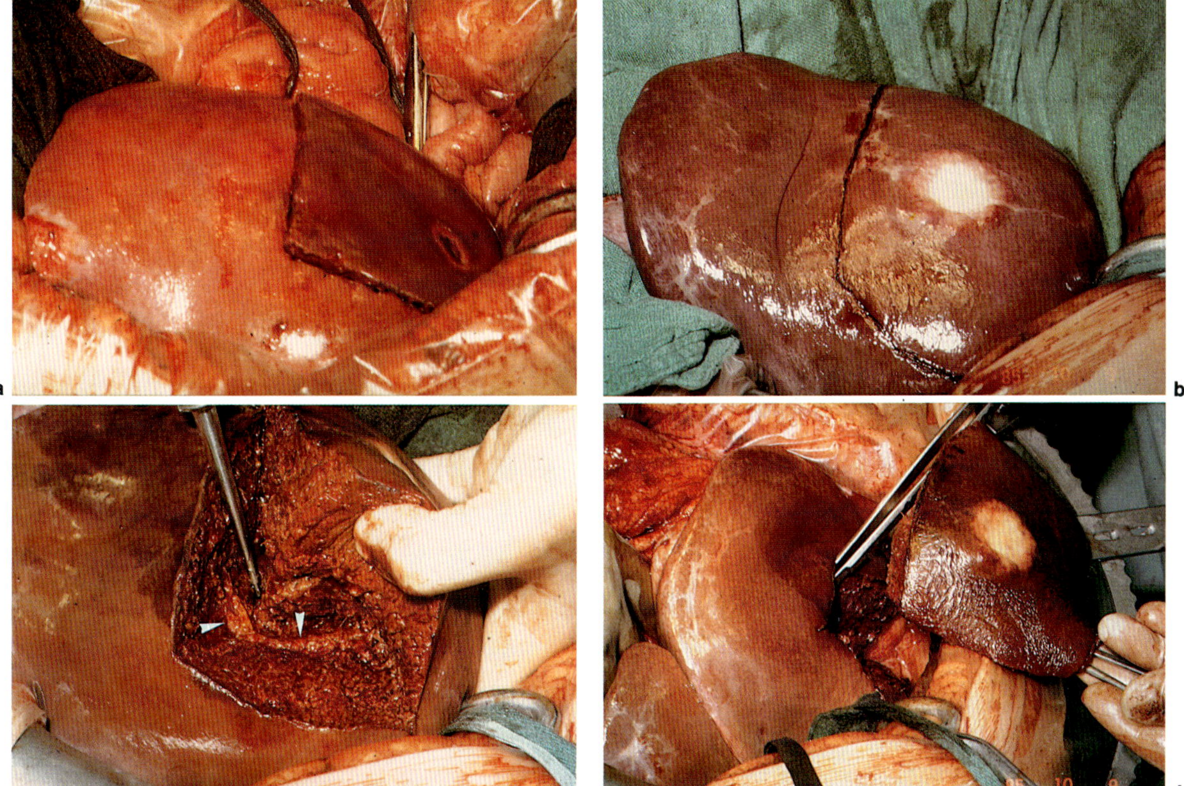

Fig. 6.5.30   Segmentectomy and perisegmentectomy of segment VII
a   True segmentectomy with preliminary ultrasound-guided biopsy after division of the portal pedicle VII. This segment
shows typical color change, while the liver remnant retains optimal blood supply
b   Perisegmentectomy encroaching on segments V, VI, and VIII
c   Portal pedicles to segment V and VIII are preserved (arrows) while the pedicle VII is exposed for ligation using the
CUSA-dissector
d   Specimen and liver remnant with slight impairment of blood supply to superficial parts of segment V

Fig. 6.5.27   Advanced cancer of the gallbladder resected by a polysegmentectomy (IVb−VI) and partial gastrectomy
a   Marking of the transverse resection plane
b   Hepatic resection completed
c   Raw surface, dissected ligament and gastroduodenal anastomosis
d   Postoperative CT scan showing the parenchymal defect

Fig. 6.5.28   Resection of an adenoma in segment V
a   Tumor at the lower side of segment V at a considerable distance from the main fissure and the clearly visible boundary
V/VI (arrows)
b   Parenchymal defect after only a partial resection of segment V covered with fibrinogen adhesive in spray technique

Fig. 6.5.29   Bisegmentectomy (V + VI) with complementary cholecystectomy for a symptomatic focal nodular hyperplasia of segment V
a   Situs after marking of the transection planes
b   Specimen with the tumor pushing the V/VI boundary (arrows) considerably to the right

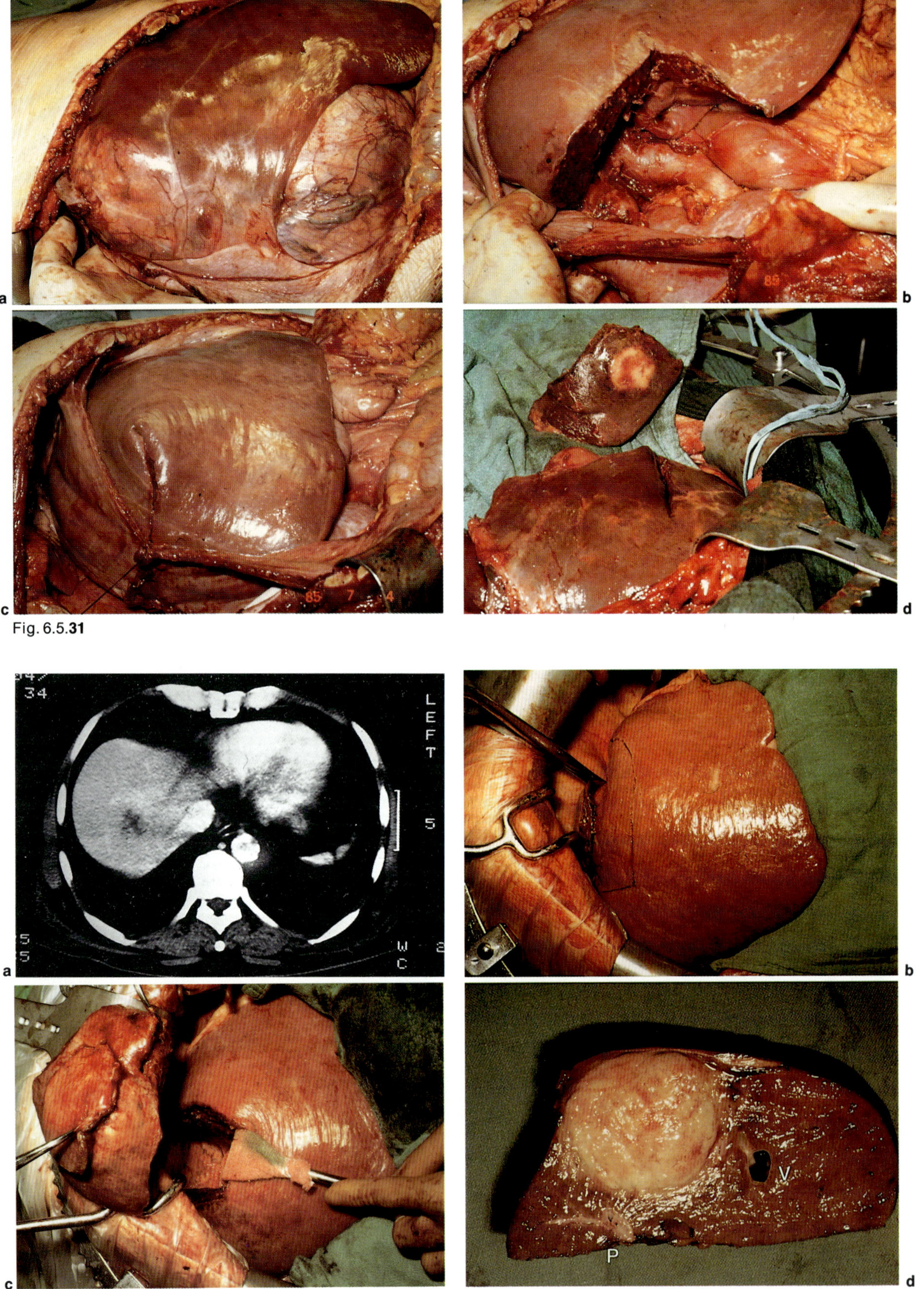

Fig. 6.5.**31**

Fig. 6.5.**32**

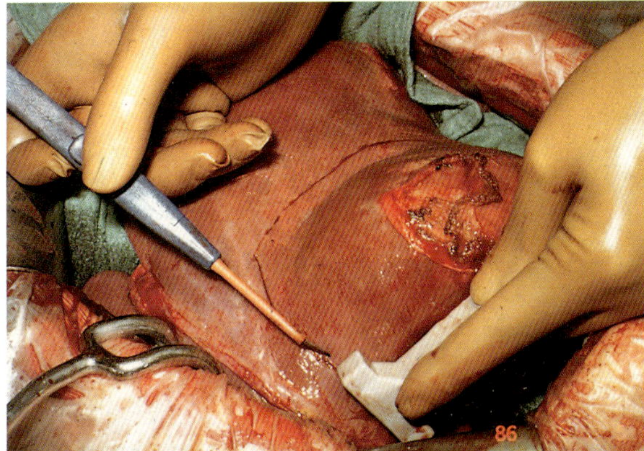

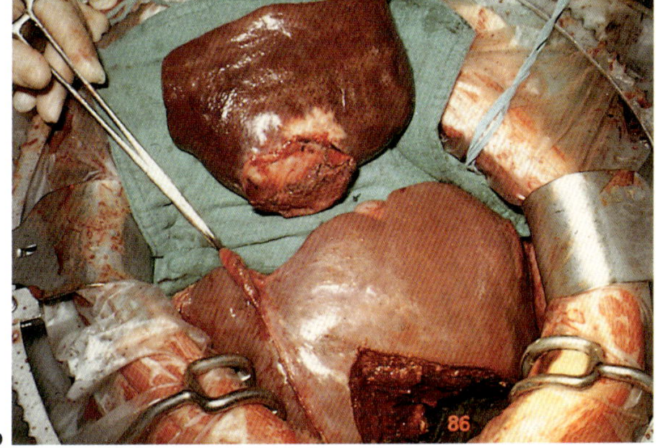

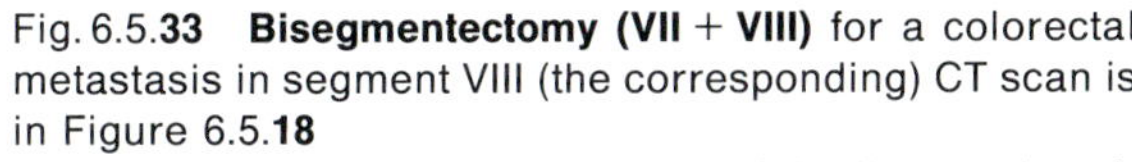

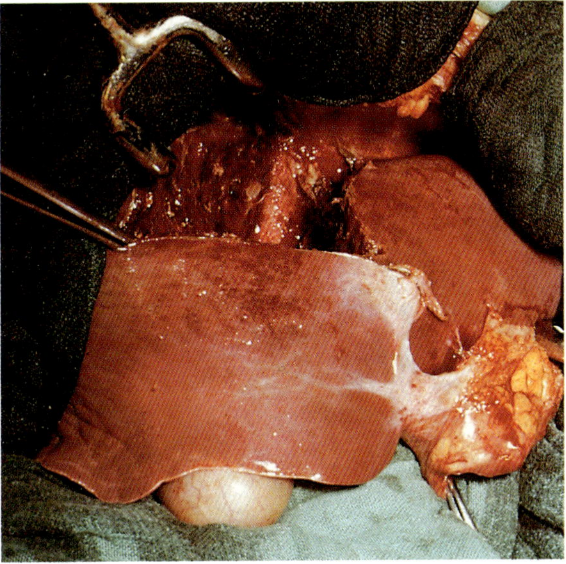

Fig. 6.5.**34**   **Bisegmentectomy (IV a + VIII)** with ligation of the middle hepatic vein and partial excision from the left hepatic vein for a solitary metastasis at the venous confluence. The venous drainage of both segments IV b and V is not compromised

Fig. 6.5.**33**   **Bisegmentectomy (VII + VIII)** for a colorectal metastasis in segment VIII (the corresponding) CT scan is in Figure 6.5.**18**

a   Following complete mobilization of the liver and excision of the adherent diaphragm, the transection planes are marked using ultrasound

b   Intact post-resectional venous drainage of segments V and VI despite ligation of the right hepatic vein

Fig. 6.5.**31**   **Closure of the parenchymal defect following peripheral segmentectomies**

a   Huge adrenal cancer invading the diaphragm and the neighboring liver

b   Defect after en bloc resection including a segmentectomy VII

c   Closure of the hepatic defect and repair of the widely excised diaphragm

d   Specimen and liver remnant after a comparable monosegmentectomy VI

Fig. 6.5.**32**   **Monosegmentectomy VIII** for a small hepatocellular carcinoma with mild cirrhosis present

a   CT scan with the subdiaphragmatic lesion

b   After excision of the adherent diaphragm, the resection planes are marked on the liver capsule

c   Liver remnant with normal blood supply and venous drainage

d   Specimen with portal pedicle (P) and branch of the right hepatic vein (V)

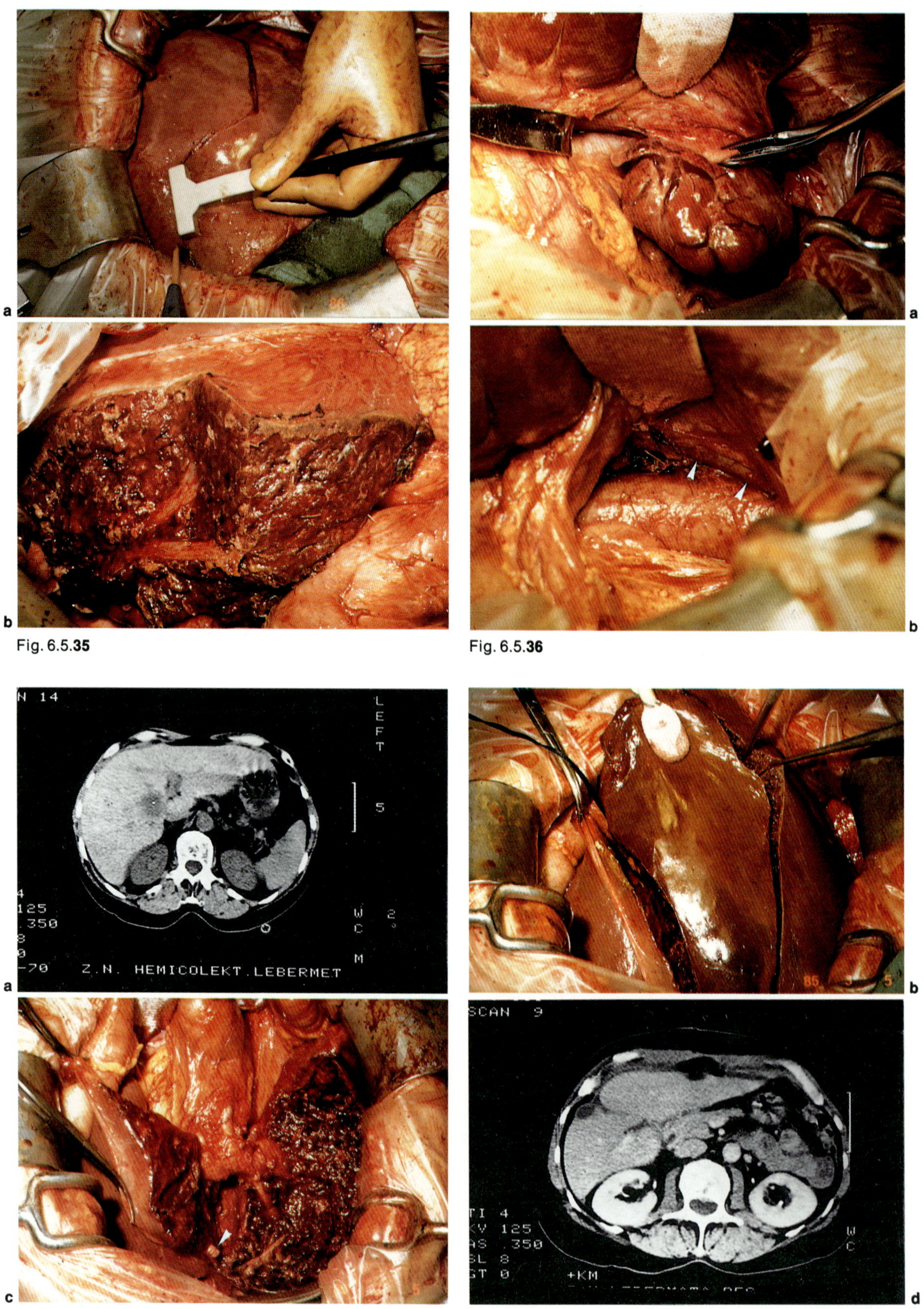

Fig. 6.5.**35**

Fig. 6.5.**36**

Fig. 6.5.**37**

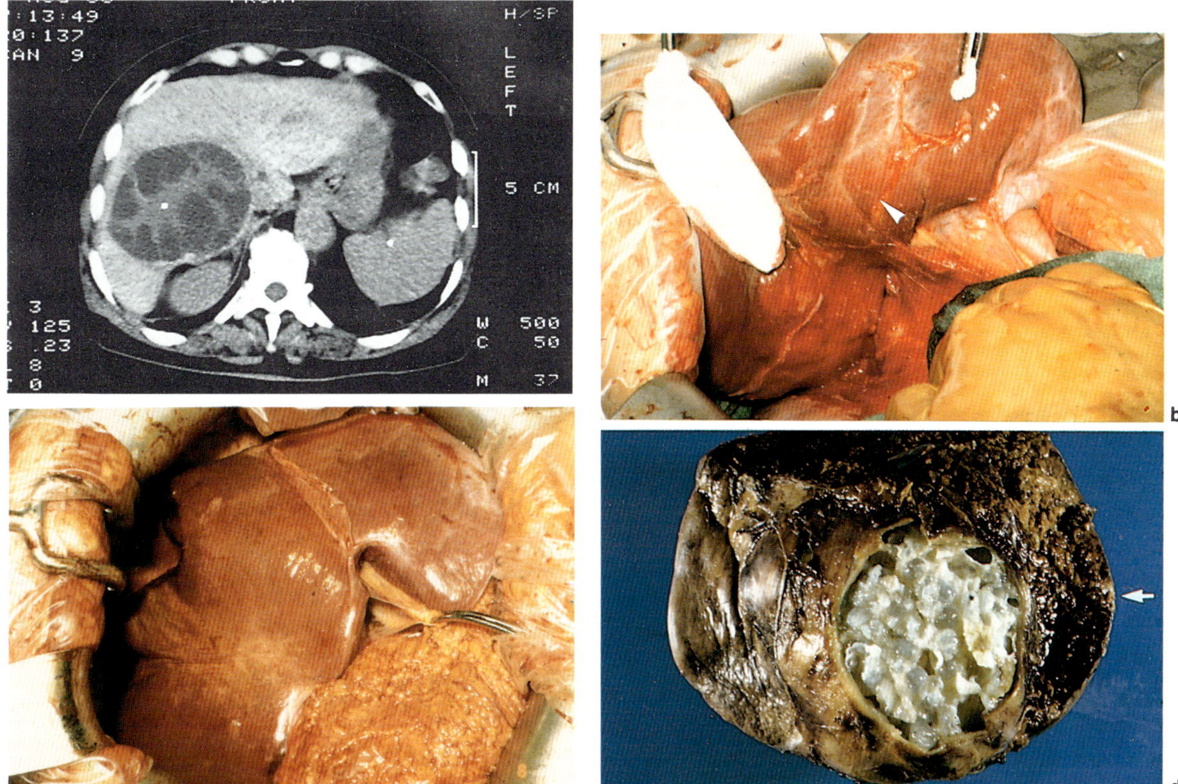

Fig. 6.5.**38** **Plurisegmentectomy** (I + VII + VIII) for an extensive hydatid cyst located in the caudate process
a Preoperative CT scan
b After mobilization of the right lobe, the hydatid cyst and a retrohepatic vein (arrow) become visible
c Hepatic defect with intact venous drainage after resection with ligation of the right hepatic vein
d Specimen in a posterior view with the hydatid cyst opened (arrow: longitudinal resection plane)

Fig. 6.5.**35** **SOR modifications of common anatomical resections of the right lobe**
a Marking of the stepped resection plane for a segmentectomy (VI–VIII) in a case of a large solitary metastasis in segment VII
b SOR [IVa + (V–VIII)] with both the middle and umbilical veins exposed

Fig. 6.5.**36** **Monosegmentectomy I** for a focal nodular hyperplasia
a Step-by-step mobilization of the tumor from the vena cava
b Following resection, the trunk of the middle hepatic vein (arrow) is visible anteriorly at the raw surface

Fig. 6.5.**37** **Bisegmentectomy (I + IV)** for a small colorectal metastasis in the caudate process
a Preoperative CT scan
b Simultaneous preparation of two resection planes along the main fissure and falciform ligament
c After completion of the resection, the hilar branching, the right and left hepatic veins and the anterior surface of the vena cava are exposed (arrow: stump of the middle hepatic vein)
d Postoperative CT scan with the two parts of liver remnant close together

of the middle hepatic vein is exposed at the end (Fig. 6.5.**36**).

Access to lesions lying in front of the vena cava in the caudate process is more difficult. These lesions can attain considerable size, regardless of whether they are benign or malignant. They require various operative procedures depending on their size and on the involvement of the left caudate portion. Smaller lesions, limited to the pre-vena caval area, can be tackled with a (IV + I) bisegmentectomy (Fig. 6.5.**37**). In the case of pronounced extension to the right, a cranially-directed poly-segmentectomy should be considered to avoid the right hepatectomy including segment I otherwise required. Depending on the venous drainage of segment VI, the SOR (I + VII + VIII) or stepped extension with additional removal of an otherwise congested segment VI come under consideration (Fig. 6.5.**38**). A tumor affecting both the caudate lobe and pre-vena caval process may usually require a right-sided, sometimes a slightly modified left-sided hepatectomy because of the close relationship with the left portal pedicles. In view of the proximity to the anterior main portal trunk cranially to the right, segment VIII needs to be at least partially included (Fig. 6.5.**39**).

Recent Clinical Experience

Segmentectomy was introduced together with the intraoperative ultrasound equipment at our institution in October 1984. During the 39 months up to

Table 6.5.**1**   **Liver resections performed**, 1 October 1984 – 1 January 1988

	Malignant tumor	Benign tumor	Other indications	Total
Standard resection	86	9	8	103
Segment-orientated resectomy	84	14	17	115
Non-anatomical procedures	46	20	32	98
Total	216	43	57	316

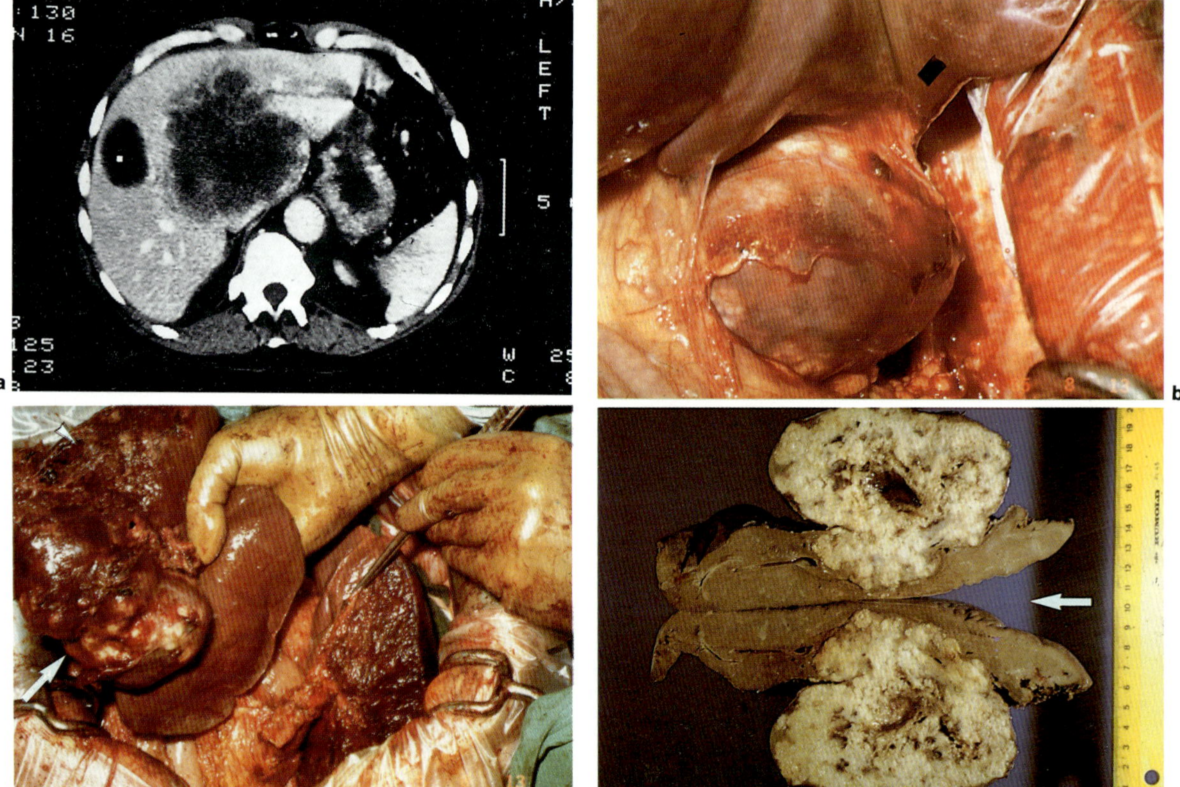

Fig. 6.5.**39**   **Resection of segments I–IV encroaching on segment VIII** for a large solitary colorectal metastasis involving the entire caudate lobe and process
a   Preoperative CT scan demonstrating additionally a benign cyst of segment VIII
b   Tumor in the caudate lobe with close contact to the left hilar structures
c   Resection completed. Small arrow: parts of the cyst wall; large arrow: sulcus of the vena cava
d   Transverse section of the specimen. Arrow: resection site

Table 6.5.2   Relative risk of postoperative hepatic failure and consequent mortality in anatomical forms of hepatic resection of the right lobe

| | Standard resection required | | | | | |
| | Right lobectomy | | | Right hepatectomy | | |
Operation performed	n	Hepatic failure	Death	n	Hepatic failure	Death
Standard resection	17**	6**	2**	40**	7**	2*
SOR preserving one additional segment	9	2	–	11**	2*	1*
SOR preserving more than 2 segments	21	–	–	31*	–	–

SOR: segment-orientated resection. Each asterisk represents one cirrhotic patient

January 1988, a total of 316 liver resections have been performed, of which 297 were elective operations. There was an even distribution between the three resectional approaches, with the anatomical procedures being performed predominantly for malignant disease. Non-anatomical excisions represent the largest proportion for other indications (Table 6.5.1).

Two basic issues arising from traditional resections were mentioned initially in this chapter: post-resectional functional capacity of the liver remnant and radicality as define by histological examination.

Post-operative liver failure was most pronounced in cirrhotic patients, resulting in an unacceptably high mortality rate (Table 6.5.2). In the non-cirrhotic group the probability of hepatic failure largely depended on the amount of functional intact parenchyma removed, with a significant increase in the respective risk following a greater than 50% reduction (Table 6.5.3). Calculated on the basis of the number of segments removed, the risk was increased considerably where four segments or more were removed, as in right hepatectomy, whereas all the related segmental modifications preserving one or two additional segments resulted in a complete prevention of this functional sequela in all but one of the patients. Following right lobectomy, hepatic failure occurred in 35% and resulted in two deaths. In this context the segment-orientated modifications of the right lobectomy have to be divided into two subgroups. Removal of less than 4 segments (e.g. [IV a + VII + VIII] resection) excluded hepatic insufficiency completely. The [IV a + (V – VIII)] modification showed a comparable risk to a right hepatectomy. However, although one severe course required intensive care for 10 days, all 9 patients who underwent this type of surgery survived.

With regard to the aim of achieving a clear margin, SOR procedures proved superior to both standard and non-anatomical resections (Table 6.5.4). The reason for some unforced errors in

Table 6.5.3   Influence of the proportion of liver volume removed and of preexisting cirrhosis on hepatic failure following anatomical resection on the right hepatic lobe

Liver volume removed	> 50%	< 50%
Cirrhotics		
Patients	4	3
Postoperative hepatic failure	4	1
Consequent death	3	1
Non-cirrhotics		
Patients	62	60
Postoperative hepatic failure	11	1
Consequent death	1	–

common hepatectomies and lobectomies may be a certain lack of flexibility. More important, however, is the continuing high proportion of positive margins in non-anatomical procedures, despite all the surgeons involved in liver resection during the period presented having been fully aware of this problem.

The all-important preservation of negative margins is, in my own opinion, greatly aided by the routine application of intraoperative ultrasound. In the 165 operations where it was performed, this investigation modified the initial operative intent in 25 cases (15%). The planned resection had to be extended because of additional nodules in five, and due to an unexpectedly close tumor–anatomical relation in six patients. Conversely, in four patients the extent of the procedure could be reduced in view of a surprisingly wide margin, and in another four because non-palpable lesions could be localized exactly (Fig. 6.5.15). In the remaining case the CT scan clearly indicated a lesion located deep in the right lobe which could not be confirmed by palpation. In this equivocal situation thorough intraoperative re-imaging excluded the presence of a tumor and made an objective decision to avoid further surgery possible.

Table 6.5.4   Risk of histologically proved non-radical tumor removal. Only those patients for whom complete tumor removal was both intended and theoretically possible are included

	Malignant tumor		Benign tumor		Total	
	n	Non-radical	n	Non-radical	n	Non-radical
Standard resection	79	5	8	1	87	6 = 6.9%
Segment-orientated resection	78	2	14	–	92	2 = 2.2%
Non-anatomical procedures	43	9	18	2	61	11 = 18%
Total	200	16 = 8%	40	3 = 7.5%		

From the technical point of view, the ultrasonic dissector is a great step forward. Surprisingly, the median blood loss for various extents of resection was not diminished, though unforeseen severe bleeding could be almost completely ruled out.

Conclusion

At the moment, complete surgical resection represents the only treatment for malignant tumors of the liver which offers the chance of long-term tumor-free survival. The SOR approach appears to be a fundamental improvement in preventing incomplete tumor removal as well as wastage of non-involved hepatic tissue. It guarantees an optimum of local radicality with a maximum of parenchymal preservation. The use of modern diagnostic and surgical aids such as intraoperative ultrasound, liver transection using the ultrasonic aspirator and control of bleeding using infrared coagulation or fibrin tissue adhesive, expedites these technically sophisticated types of liver resection and permits their safe and low-risk implementation.

References

Adson MA. Resection of liver metastases: when is it worthwhile. World J Surg 1987; 11: 511–520.

Adson MA. Primary hepatocellular cancers: western experience. In: Blumgart LM, ed. Surgery of the liver and biliary tract; vol 2. Edinburgh: Churchill Livingstone, 1988.

Andrus CH, Kaminsky DL. Segmental hepatic resection utilizing the ultrasonic dissector. Arch Surg 1986; 121: 515–520.

Bismuth H. Surgical anatomy and anatomical surgery of the liver. World J Surg 1982; 6: 3–9.

Bismuth H, Moussin D, Castaing D. Major and minor segmentectomies "réglées" in liver surgery. World J Surg 1982; 6: 10–24.

Bismuth H, Castaing D. Operative ultrasound of the liver and biliary ducts. Berlin: Springer, 1987a.

Bismuth H, Castaing D, Garden OJ. The use of operative ultrasound in surgery of primary liver tumors. World J Surg 1987b; 11: 610–614.

Blumgart LM. Liver resection: liver and biliary tumors. In: Blumgart LM, ed. Surgery of the liver and biliary tract; vol 2. Edinburgh: Churchill Livingstone, 1988: 1251–1280.

Blumgart LM, Leach KG, Karran SJ. Observations on liver regeneration after right hepatic lobectomy. Gut 1971; 12: 922–928.

Brown DA, Pommier RF, Woltering EA, Fletcher WS. Nonanatomic hepatic resection for secondary hepatic tumors with special reference to hemostatic technique. Arch Surg 1988; 123: 1063–1066.

Cantlie J. On a new arrangement of the right and left lobes of the liver. Proc Anat Soc Great Britain/Ireland 1988; 32: 4.

Couinaud C. Le foie: Études anatomiques et chirurgicales. Paris: Masson, 1957.

Ekberg H, Tranberg K-G, Andersson R, Lundstedt C, Hagerstrand J, Ranstram J, Bengmark S. Determinants of survival in liver resection for colorectal secondaries. Br J Surg 1987; 74.

Elias H, Petty D. Gross anatomy of the blood vessels and ducts in the human liver. Am J Anat. 1952; 90: 59–111.

Fortner JG, Papachristou DN. Surgery of liver tumors. Int Adv Surg Oncol 1979; 2: 251–275.

Franco D, Bonnet P, Smadja C, Grange D. Surgical resection of segment VIII (anterosuperior subsegment of the right lobe) in patients with liver cirrhosis and hepatocellular carcinoma. Surgery 1985; 98: 949–954.

Gall FP, Scheele J. Die operative Therapie von Lebermetastasen. In: Schildberg FW, Chirurgische Behandlung von Tumormetastasen. Melsungen: Bibliomed, 1987: 223–240.

Goldsmith NA, Woodburne RT. The surgical anatomy pertaining to liver resection. Surg Gynecol Obstet 1957; 195: 310–318.

Guthy E. Die Infrarotkontaktkoagulation. In: Reifferscheid M, ed. Neue Techniken in der operativen Medizin. Berlin: Springer, 1986.

Healey JE Jr, Schroy PC. Anatomy of the biliary ducts within the human liver: analysis of the prevailing pattern of branchings and the major variations of the biliary ducts. Arch Surg 1953; 66: 599–616.

Hjortsjö C-H. The topography of the intrahepatic duct systems. Acta Anat 1951; 11: 599–615.

Hobsley M. Intrahepatic anatomy: a surgical evaluation. Brit J Surg 1958; 45: 635–644.

Hodgson WJB, DelGuercio LRM. Preliminary experience in liver surgery using the ultrasonic scalpel. Surgery 1984; 95: 230–234.

Hodgson WJB, Kemmney M, Scheele J, Tranberg KG. Does the ultrasonic dissector improve the quality of HPB surgery? In: Bengmark S, ed. Progress in surgery of the liver, pancreas and biliary system. Dordrecht: Nijhoff, 1988: 205–219.

Hughes K, Scheele J, Sugarbaker PH. Surgery for metastatic colorectal cancer to the liver: optimizing the results of treatment. Surg Clin North Am 1989; 69: 339–360.

Hugnet CJ, Moniel J, eds. Les tumeurs primitives du foie chez l'adult. Paris: Masson, 1983.

Köckerling F, Scheele J, Gall FP. Die chirurgische Therapie des Gallenblasencarcinoms. Chirurg 1988; 59: 236–243.

Lee CS, Chao CC, Lin TY. Partial hepatectomy on cirrhotic liver with a right lateral tumor. Surgery 1985; 98: 942–948.

Lin TY, Lee LS, Chen CC, Lian KY, Lin WSJ. Regeneration of

human liver after hepatic lobectomy studied by repeated liver scanning and repeated needle biopsy. Ann Surg 1979, 190: 48–53.

Makuuchi M, Hasegawa H, Yamanzaki S. Ultrasonically guided subsegmentectomy. Surg Gynecol Obstet 1985; 161: 346–350.

Makuuchi M, Hasegawa H, Yamazaki S, Takayasu K, Moriyama N. The use of operative ultrasound as an aid to liver resection in patients with hepatocellular carcinoma. World J Surg 1987; 11: 615–621.

Masselot R, Leborgne J. Anatomical study of the hepatic veins. Anat Clin 1978; 1: 109–125.

Mizumoto R, Suzuki H. Surgical anatomy of the hepatic hilum with special reference to the caudate lobe. World J Surg 1988; 12: 2–10.

Mukai JK, Stack CM, Turner DA, Gould RJ, Petasnick JP, Matalon TAS, Doolas AM. Imaging of surgically relevant hepatic vascular and segmental anatomy, part 1: normal anatomy. AJR 1987a; 149: 287–292.

Mukai JK, Stack CM, Turner DA, Gould RJ, Petasnick JP, Matalon TAS, Doolas AM, Nurakami M. Imaging of surgically relevant hepatic vascular and segmental anatomy, part 2: extent and resectability of hepatic neoplasms. AJR 1987b; 149: 293–297.

Nakashima T, Kojiro M, eds. Hepatocellular carcinoma: an atlas of its pathology. Berlin: Springer, 1987.

Neuhaus P. Vereinfachte Technik der transhepatischen Gallengangs-Drainage bei zentralen Gallengangscarcinomen. Chirurg 1984; 55: 413.

Okuda K, Obata H, Nakajima Y, Ohtsuki T, Okazaki N, Ohnishi K. Prognosis of primary hepatocellular carcinoma. Hepatology 1984; 4: 35–65.

Ottow RT, Barbiere SA, Sugarbaker PH, Wesley RA. Liver transsection: a controlled study of four different techniques in pigs. Surgery 1985; 97: 596–601.

Priesching A. Leberresektionen: chirurgische Anatomie, Indikationen, Technik. München: Urban and Schwarzenberg, 1986.

Rex H. Beiträge zur Morphologie der Säugerleber. Morphol Jahrb 1888; 14: 517.

Sales JP, Hannoun L, Sichez JP, Hiniger J, Levey E. Surgical anatomy of segment IV. Anat Clin 1984; 6: 295–304.

Scheele J. Indikation, Technik und Ergebnis der Fibrinklebung nach Leberresektionen. In: Scheele J, ed. Fibrinklebung. Berlin: Springer, 1982.

Scheele J. Neue Möglichkeiten in der Behandlung von Metastasen – aus der Sicht des Chirurgen. In: Bundesärztekammer. Fortschritt und Fortbildung in der Medizin. Köln: Deutscher Ärzte-Verlag, 1988: vol 12, 205–219.

Scheele J. Die segmentorientierte Leberresektion: Grundlagen, Technik, Stellenwert. Chirurg 1989a; 60: 251–265.

Scheele J. Gefäßorientierte Segmentresektion der Leber. Langenbecks Arch Chir 1989b (in press).

Starzl TE, Bell RH, Beart RW, Putnam CW. Hepatic trisegmentectomy and other liver resections. Surg Gynecol Obstet 1975; 141: 429–437.

Thompson HH, Tompkins RK, Longmire WP Jr. Major hepatic resection: a 25-year experience. Ann Surg 1983; 197: 375–388.

Ton That Tung. Résections majeures et mineures du foie. Paris: Masson, 1979.

6.6 Liver Transplantation for Hepatic Malignancy

D. A. Rouch, J. C. Emond, J. R. Thistlethwaite, and C. E. Broelsch

Liver transplantation has been used liberally by some centers in the past for the treatment of primary hepatic malignancy. Long-term observation following liver transplantation in this population has demonstrated poor survival mainly due to a high rate of tumor recurrence. Even if resection involves considerable risk, as in patients with concomitant liver disease (i.e. liver cirrhosis or hepatitis) it may warrant the attempt because of the ultimate incurability of malignant hepatic disease.

At the present time, liver transplantation should be used highly selectively in patients with primary hepatic malignancy. The first approach in all patients with hepatic malignancy should be liver resection, even at a price of considerable risk. If hepatic involvement by tumor is too great to be cured by surgical resection, and no extrahepatic metastasis can be identified, the patient can be considered for total hepatectomy and orthotopic liver transplantation (OLTx). Each case is individualized with respect to tumor histology, general health of the patient and availability of donors. Follow-up should be in conjunction with an oncologist, and adjuvant therapy should be recommended, especially to patients with multicentric intrahepatic disease. Although results of long-term survival are disappointing, ocassional cures are encountered. In some patients, palliation with probable life extension is achieved with OLTx even though the patients may eventually succumb to metastatic disease. The need to understand the natural course of transplanted livers in tumor patients better and the need to develop better adjuvant therapy justifies continued attempts at liver transplantation in selected patients with liver tumors.

Pretransplant Assessment

The preoperative work-up is the same as one would do to assess a patient for liver resection (Hockerstedt 1986, Soriede et al. 1985, Calne 1982, Broelsch et al. 1985). Abdominal computed tomography (CT) is done to evaluate the extent of tumor involvement in the liver and surrounding viscera. A chest X-ray and chest CT scan are done to rule out pulmonary metastasis. Angiography of the celiac trunk and SMA is done to evaluate the anatomical confines of the tumor in the liver and possible involvement of the hepatic artery. The venous phase of the mesenteric arteriogram is used to assess patency of the portal vein and possible involvement of the portal vein with the tumor.

Upper and lower endoscopy or barium studies should be done to rule out primary gastrointestinal tumors that may have spread to the liver. As experience is gained with magnetic resonance imaging (MRI), this may be utilized in the future to evaluate liver tumors and the extent of disease. If it is determined that extrahepatic disease is present, the patient may still benefit from a limited resection (as in the case of obstructing tumors).

If it is determined that the tumor is confined to the liver, a laparotomy is performed with the intention of performing a curative resection. If at the time of laparotomy the tumor is found to be too far beyond the anatomical confines of the segmental anatomy of the liver to permit a curative resection, the patient can be staged for a liver transplant. A careful exploration of the abdominal cavity is done to rule out evidence of extrahepatic tumor spread. Any lymph node that is suspicious in addition to random lymph node biopsies in the portal and celiac regions is examined. The diaphragm is inspected, and any non-contiguous spread to the diaphragm or peritoneal surface is a contra-indication to transplantation. If any evidence exists for extrahepatic tumor spread, the patient is not a candidate for a liver transplant.

If at the time of the laparotomy the patient has a multicentric hepatic malignancy negating the chances of cure by partial resection, even if the disease appears to be confined to the liver, we do not routinely recommend liver transplantation. In these instances the patient is informed of the morbidity and possible mortality following OLTx, the morbidity of long-term immunosuppression, including possible hastening of tumor growth, and the small chance of cure even with OLTx. Chemotherapy is recommended to follow OLTx, which also adds to the morbidity. If, after such counseling, the patient and family request OLTx, and no extrahepatic disease can be demonstrated, the patient is placed on the transplant list. OLTx is performed as quickly as possible, but if a patient with end-stage liver disease is in need of the organ, the tumor patient must wait for the next available organ. The patient is allowed to go home when sufficiently recovered from the laparotomy, and is called in from home at the time of transplantation.

An alternative approach has been chosen by the Pittsburgh group in an attempt to save the tumor patient a laparotomy prior to transplantation (personal communication). Based upon non-invasive diagnostic tests, including angiography and/or laparoscopy that indicate no extrahepatic involvement by tumor, laparotomy is performed with a donor organ readily available. If the tumor turns out to be resectable or if extrahepatic disease is found, the patient is either treated by partial hepatectomy or the abdomen is closed and the donor organ is used in another patient who has been alerted for such an eventuality (usually a cirrhotic patient). The alternatives are discussed with the patient preoperatively without knowing the details of the tumor status, which are incomplete prior to laparotomy. This places a considerable psychological burden on the patient. The patient must be mentally prepared not only to accept a liver transplant, but also to accept no surgery at all (as in the case of extrahepatic disease found during laparotomy). In addition, the need to wait for a donor and suitable back-up recipient to schedule the laparotomy is too inconvenient to apply this practice widely except in a center, such as Pittsburgh, performing daily liver transplants as a routine.

Post-Transplant Assessment

Post-operative management includes assessment for adequate liver function (detection of rejection, biliary complication, etc.) as well as detection of chemotherapy toxicity and tumor recurrence. The progress of the transplant patient is monitored weekly for the first two months, biweekly for the next two months, and then every three months for the next year. Liver function tests, glucose, complete blood count (CBC), blood urea nitrogen (BUN), creatinine and cyclosporine A levels are monitored at each visit. The patient is evaluated with respect to energy level, appetite, muscle weight gain and strength. Each patient is examined for evidence of peripheral edema, high blood pressure or cyclosporine A toxicity (tremulousness, hirsutism, gingival hyperplasia, renal dysfunction). Once the patient has sufficiently recovered from the transplant, with stable liver function tests, chemotherapy is initiated. This is usually one month after the transplant.

Tumor markers, if elevated preoperatively, should be measured prior to discharge as a baseline. Thereafter, the tumor markers can be monitored every two to three months for the first two years. Repeat CT scan of the liver and abdomen, chest X-ray, bone scan and serum chemistries should be performed at three, six, nine, twelve and eighteen months to evaluate for tumor recurrence. MRI may also prove helpful in postoperative monitoring. The significance of all these tests is certainly disputable, because following transplantation there is no measurable disease left to be treated directly. Success of the therapy can therefore only be judged by the absence or delayed onset of metastatic disease. However upon recognition of the recurrence by any marker or direct visualization, the likelihood of cure by further measures is very small and efforts should be focused on palliation and control of the recurrent disease.

Results

The early experience with liver transplantation included many liver tumor patients, including those with metastatic disease to the liver (Williams et al. 1973, Starzl et al. 1976). Patients with metastatic liver disease were left with limited options with regard to alternative therapies. The long-term survival rate following total hepatectomy and liver transplantation was unknown, and patient selection for liver transplantation was less restrictive. It soon became apparent that patients with metastatic liver disease had poor survival rates following transplantation. Following OLTx the patients were found to develop early recurrence, possibly hastened by the immunosuppression on which they were maintained to prevent rejection. Patients with metastatic cancer to the liver should no longer be considered for liver transplantation.

Patients with primary liver cancer can be considered for OLTx selectively. OLTx should be limited to patients who cannot be cured by partial resection and in whom there is no evidence of extrahepatic disease. The patient should be made aware of the risks of the procedure and the disappointing experience so far with long-term results following OLTx for hepatic malignancy.

The liver transplant procedure is technically easier to perform in patients with hepatic malignancy than in cirrhotics (Table 6.6.1). Even if the patient has had a previous laparotomy to evaluate the extent of the tumor, the lack of portal hypertension, general good nutrition and normal coagulation in the tumor patient makes the operation easier. As a result of the shorter operative time,

Table 6.6.**1** **Perioperative and postoperative courses following orthotopic liver transplantation:** tumor patients compared with cirrhotic patients

	Tumor patients	Cirrhotic patients
Operative time	7 ± 3 h	11 ± 5 h
Blood loss	0.8 ± 1.0 vol	3.5 ± 4.0 vol
Period in intensive care	3 ± 2 days	7 ± 9 days
Days on the ventilator	2 ± 1 days	5 ± 7 days
Hospital stay	15 ± 6 days	35 ± 20 days
One-month survival	95 %	90 %
One-year survival	26 %	72 %

Table 6.6.2   Histology and survival data for 111 patients with orthotropic liver transplantations for primary hepatic malignancy. Data published through January 1987 from Hanover, Cambridge, MA, Pittsburgh and the University of Chicago (Calne 1982, 1985, Pichlmayr et al. 1983, 1984, Iwatsuki et al. 1982)

Histology	n	%	One year survival	Long-term survival	
HCC	73	65.7	19	8	3 incidental 1 with recurrence
Cholangiocarcinoma	21	18.9	3	0	
Klatskin	8	6.3	2	0	
Hepatoblastoma	4	3.6	3	3	2 incidental tumors 1 alive with recurrence
Hemangioendothelial sarcoma	3	2.7	1	1	alive with recurrence
Other sarcomas	2	1.8	1	1	
Overall	111		29 (26.1%)	13 (11.7%)	5 incidental tumors 3 alive with recurrence

lower blood loss and good condition of the patient, the recovery time is shorter and smoother than for the typical cirrhotic. The incidence of reoperation for bleeding is smaller, and overall morbidity (renal insufficiency, fluid overload, length of ventilatory support and intubation, numbers of transfusions, length of bed rest, length of urinary catheterization) is also smaller in comparison with the cirrhotic who requires a liver transplant.

At the present time, it is unclear whether the tumor patient has an altered immunologic response to the liver graft. The incidence of rejection is probably similar to other patients who require a liver transplant. The early results of the liver transplant can be expected to be good in tumor patients, but late results will be disappointing due to recurrence.

Recurrence

Recurrence of tumor in the graft, or distant metastasis, usually occurs in the first year and gives rise to disappointing long-term results (Table 6.6.2). Adjuvant chemotherapy may prove to be beneficial for tumor patients following liver transplantation in the hope of improving cure rates or prolonging disease-free survival. A multidisciplinary approach should be taken toward these patients, with input from the hepatologist, oncologist and radiation therapist. When used, chemotherapy is instituted after sufficient recovery, with stabilization of liver function tests, has taken place. This is usually one month following the transplant. Once recurrence of the disease takes place, the approach should be that of controlling the disease rather than further attempts at cure. Further adjuvant treatment depends on the histology, site of recurrence, adjuvant therapy already received, and the general condition of the patient. Tumor histology plays a significant

role in prognosis following liver transplant, and experience with survival rates for different liver tumors varies.

Prognosis and Tumor Histology

Hepatocellular Carcinoma (HCC)

The most common primary hepatic malignancy is hepatocellular carcinoma (HCC). This represents approximately two-thirds of all primary hepatic malignancies. It commonly occurs in the setting of liver cirrhosis (Liver Cancer Study Group of Japan 1984, Shikata 1976), especially cirrhosis caused by chronic active hepatitis B (Arthur et al. 1984, World Health Organization 1983, Chisari 1984, Kew 1984, Vyas et al. 1984). Since chronic active hepatitis with cirrhosis is the most common indication for liver replacement, incidental HCC is occasionally identified only after total hepatectomy and liver transplant. Survival statistics are excellent for patients undergoing OLTx for cirrhosis in whom an incidental HCC is identified, and therefore should be considered in a different light than in patients presenting with HCC. The incidental nature of the malignancy and good survival statistics should also be taken into account when a report includes these patients in the survival statistics for patients with hepatic malignancy. Ocassionally the first indication that a patient has HCC is a rising serum level of alphafetoprotein (AFP). For that reason every patient with chronic active hepatitis B and cirrhosis should have periodic AFP levels monitored. A rising AFP may herald the occurrence of an otherwise occult HCC, hastening the decision in favor of OLTx while the tumor is still occult. The chances of cure at this stage while the HCC is not identifiable by CT scan or other radiologic measures remain good.

Another form of HCC that carries a favorable prognosis after surgical removal is fibrolamellar carcinoma. This tumor tends to occur in a younger age group, in an otherwise normal liver. Long-term cures are approximately 70% following total removal of the disease (either by resection or OLTx) (Starzl et al. 1986). In patients with recurrence, the tumor has slow progression.

When a patient presents with the diagnosis of clinically evident HCC as the indication for OLTx, the prognosis following transplantation is poor. Experience so far shows a one-year survival of 15–25% (Calne 1982, 1985, Pichlmayr et al. 1983, 1984, Iwatsuki et al. 1982).

A patient with solitary HCC should undergo an attempt at resection, and if total removal of the tumor cannot be accomplished by partial resection, an OLTx can be considered. Or, if the patient presents with a solid unilocular HCC of less than 10 cm diameter in a cirrhotic liver with no evidence of extrahepatic spread, major resection may not be tolerated and OLTx can be considered. Full consideration should be given to resection in any event prior to OLTx.

When a patient presents with multicentric HCC, even if it seems confined to the liver, the disease has at this point become a systemic one. With microscopic systemic disease, OLTx only debulks the tumor, and OLTx should not be routinely recommended. We counsel the patient that the chances of cure are small even if apparent total removal of disease is accomplished with OLTx. We educate the patient about the risks of the procedure and the possible tumor proliferation as an effect of immunosuppression. If the patient still has interest in accepting the morbidity of the operation and subsequent chemotherapy with a small chance of cure, we proceed with OLTx and recommend adjuvant chemotherapy as part of the follow-up. A small percentage of patients will be cured by this plan of management.

The longest-surviving patient with clinically evident HCC treated by OLTx has now survived for 13 years. Her tumor was a primary solitary lesion that presented itself with a very slow progression prior to the decision that transplantation should be performed. This tumor was not graded specifically as a fibrolamellar carcinoma but was a primary HCC in a noncirrhotic liver. This patient subsequently presented with a solitary pulmonary metastasis that was removed 10 years ago. She continues to remain free of disease. Another patient with a multilocular giant HCC (low-grade malignancy), possibly derived from an adenoma of the liver, underwent a hepatic trisegmentectomy first and subsequently experienced recurrence of the disease in the remaining left lateral segment. The tumor developed into a 6 kg hepatic mass and

presented itself as an adenoma on CT and Tc-HIDA scans. Resection was attempted but not completed due to involvement of the only remaining hepatic venous outflow. When alphafetoprotein markers started to increase, OLTx was successfully performed. The patient is alive and well three years from the initial resection and 28 months after the OLTx with no evidence of recurrence. Both tumors, the solitary tumor and the multilocular tumor, had in common a very slow natural progression that is described for some types of HCC.

Cholangiocarcinoma and Klatskin Tumor

OLTx has been used to treat patients with cholangiocarcinoma (cholangiocellular carcinoma of the intrahepatic bile ducts) and Klatskin tumor (bile duct cancer at the confluence) with little success. The rate of cure following apparent curative resection of these diseases is very poor with five-year survival rates less than 5%. Initially it was hoped that total hepatectomy and liver transplantation would be applicable for these patients. However, their survival statistics following OLTx have been extremely disappointing, even in highly selected patients such as those with Klatskin tumor. Out of 29 patients transplanted for either cholangiocarcinoma or Klatskin tumor, there was 17% one-year survival and no long-term survivors (Table 6.6.2). Early recurrence was common, often in the new graft itself. Many centers consider the diagnosis of cholangiocarcinoma or Klatskin tumor an absolute contra-indication to OLTx.

Other Forms of Primary Hepatic Malignancy

Less common primary liver tumors include hepatoblastoma, various well-differentiated sarcomas (such as hemangio-endothelial sarcoma) and poorly-differentiated sarcomas. Except for instances where the tumor is an incidental finding, these tumors also have a poor prognosis following transplantation. In cases of hepatoblastoma or sarcoma of the liver, as in cases of HCC or Klatskin tumor, resection should be tried first. If a curative resection cannot be performed by partial removal of the liver, a liver transplant can be recommended, with the understanding that the likelihood of recurrence following OLTx is high.

A three-year-old male presented with a recurrent hepatoblastoma. He had had a right hepatectomy and chemotherapy 10 months earlier for hepatoblastoma. Non-invasive studies and laparotomy showed that he had disease that was confined to the remaining portion of liver. He underwent removal of the remainder of his liver and was transplanted in what was felt to be a curative resection. After an initial good recovery, he presented two months later with extensive replacement of his liver graft by recurrent tumor. He died one month later due to pulmonary failure.

A thirty-four-year-old female presented with RUQ pain, and preoperative studies suggested – that she had a benign hemangioma of the right lobe of the liver. At laparotomy she was found to have hemangioendothelial sarcoma. The primary site was the right lobe of the liver, but in addition she had miliary spread throughout the entire liver. There was no evidence of intraperitoneal spread, and random lymph node biopsies were performed in the portal and celiac regions, which were free of disease. No resection was performed. She was closed up, and further investigative studies were performed which included a normal chest CT scan and a bone scan that showed no evidence of metastatic disease. The operative risks were explained to the patient and her husband, and they opted for an aggressive approach, even though the chance of cure was stated to be less than 20%. She underwent total hepatectomy and liver transplantation, followed by a full course of doxorubicin. She tolerated the transplant and subsequent chemotherapy well. Nine months after transplant, she was asymptomatic, but a bone scan and CT scan demonstrated a lytic lesion in her T4 vertebral body. She has now reached 12 months after the transplant and is still asymptomatic, but with recurrent disease. She has had good palliation of the disease, but her final outcome is uncertain.

Comments

Soriede (1985) described 13 patients with primary hepatic malignancy who underwent liver resection, most having an extended liver resection. 12 of them had what was felt to be a curative resection. The hospital survival was 100%, and one-year survival was 92%. Long-term cure was accomplished in 9 patients, or 69%. The experience in Hanover and in the University of Chicago has been similar. Hospital survival has been 90% in non-cirrhotic patients undergoing liver resection for primary hepatic malignancy. Long-term cure has been achieved in 6 out of 9 patients requiring major resection. The better results following resection have in part been due to patient selection, but other factors also favor patients undergoing resection rather than OLTx. Patients undergoing liver resection have less perioperative mortality compared to OLTx due to the difference in magnitude of the two operations. Also, such patients are not exposed to the postoperative risks of immunosuppression or rejection. Ultimate survival is dependent on curing the malignant disease. Unfortunately, the patient undergoing OLTx does not experience any significant advantage compared to the resection patient, because of the high rate of recurrence following OLTx. The patient with OLTx therefore has the added risks of morbidity and mortality from the transplant procedure without significant benefit compared to the patient treated with resection. The immunosuppression necessary to prevent rejection may even hasten the growth of occult metastatic disease. Major liver resection performed at centers experienced in liver surgery should carry low hospital mortality, especially in non-cirrhotic patients.

Cirrhotic patients do not tolerate major liver resection well, and the motivation to perform total removal and liver replacement will be higher in order to accomplish the removal of malignant disease and prevent liver failure. Some patients require total hepatectomy as their only chance for cure. OLTx has application in a select group of informed patients with hepatic malignancy in whom partial liver resection offers no chance of cure.

Patients with solitary tumors that require total hepatectomy and transplantation for cure have a better chance of survival than patients with multicentric tumors. Tumors that are multicentric, yet confined to the liver, may arise in three different ways. First, the tumors may represent simultaneous yet separate primary sites of malignancy as a result of genetic predetermination. This is unlikely. Another possibility is that the tumor invades a vascular structure and grows retrograde within a branch of the hepatic artery or portal vein, with metastatic deposits breaking off at points of bifurcation, spreading tumor deposits throughout the liver. It is possible that this occurs, at least on occasion. Another more likely explanation of miliary spread within the liver is that some primary hepatic malignancies are systemic diseases at the time of discovery, but that the systemic deposits only grow to noticeable size in the fertile environment of the liver. This would explain the poor long-term outcome for patients with apparent curative removal of disease by OLTx who then develop early recurrence, often in the transplanted graft itself. After counselling the patient with multicentric disease on the small chance of cure if the decision is made to undergo a transplant, chemotherapy should be administered postoperatively. With this practice it may occasionally be possible to eradicate microscopic disease or at least prolong disease-free survival following transplantation. More experience needs to be gained in this area.

Summary

The survival results of patients with primary hepatic malignancy treated with curative liver resection are better than when treated with transplantation. In both cases, long-term survival is disappointing. The first approach in all patients with primary hepatic malignancy should be resection. If the tumor cannot be totally removed with partial liver resection, and there is no evidence of extrahepatic spread, the patient can be considered for total hepatectomy and liver transplantation. This is especially true of patients with solitary liver tumors. Following transplantation there are some long-term cures, and most patients will have good palliation even if they eventually succumb to recurrent disease. Patients must be informed of the potential morbidity and mortality from the transplant procedure, with the small chance of long-term cure. Patients with multicentric disease should be considered to have systemic disease, and are not routinely considered transplant candidates. In the event that the decision is made to perform OLTx in patients with multicentric primary hepatic malignancy, adjuvant chemotherapy should be used as part of the postoperative management. Patients with secondary metastatic liver disease should not be considered for liver transplantation.

References

Arthur MJP, Hall AJ, Wright R. Hepatitis B, hepatocellular carcinoma, and strategies for prevention. Lancet 1984; i: 607–610.

Broelsch CE, Neuhaus P, Wonigeit K, Pichlmayr R. Liver transplantation for hepatic tumors. Gips CH, Krom RAF, eds. Progress in liver transplantation. 1985: 189–195.

Calne RY. Liver transplantation for liver cancer. World J Surg 1982; 76–80.

Calne RY, ed. Liver and biliary disease. 2nd ed. London: Baillière Tindall, 1985: 1422.

Chisari FV, ed. Advances in hepatitis research. New York: Masson, 1984.

Hockerstedt K. Liver transplantation in liver cancer. Ann Chir Gynaecol 1986; 75 (suppl 200): 65–68.

Iwatsuki S, Klintmalm GB, Starzl TE. Total hepatectomy and liver replacement (orthotopic liver transplantation) for primary hepatic malignancy. World J Surg 1982; 6: 81–85.

Kew MC. Hepatic tumors. Semin Liver Dis 1984; 4: 2.

Lee NW, Wong J, Ong GB. The surgical management of primary carcinoma of the liver. World J Surg 1982; 6: 66–75.

Liver Cancer Study Group of Japan. Primary liver cancer in Japan. Cancer 1984; 54: 1747–1755.

Pichlmayr R, Broelsch CE, Neuhaus P, Lauchart W, Grosse H, Creutzig H, Schnaidt U, Vonnahme F, Schmidt E, Burdelski M, Wonigeit K. Report on 68 human orthotopic liver transplantations with special reference to rejection phenomena. Transplant Proc 1983; 15: no 1.

Pichlmayr R, Broelsch CE, Wonigeit K, Neuhaus P, Siegismund S, Schmidt FW, Burdelski M. Experiences with liver transplantation in Hannover. Hepatology 1984; 4 (1): 56–60.

Shikata T. Primary liver carcinoma and cirrhosis. In: Okuda K, Peters RL, eds. Hepatocellular carcinoma. London: Wiley, 1976: 53–72.

Soriede O, Czerniak A, Blumgart LH. Large hepatocellular cancers: hepatic resection or liver transplantation? Br Med J 1985; 291: 853–857.

Starzl TE, Porter KA, Putnam CW, Schroter GPJ, Halgrimson CG, Weil R III, Hoelscher M, Reid HAS. Orthotopic liver transplantation in ninety-three patients. SGO 1976; 142: 487–505.

Starzl TE, Shaw BW, Nolesnik MA, Forhi DC, van Thiel DH. Treatment of fibrolamellar hepatoma with partial or total hepatectomy and transplantation of the liver. SGO 1986; 162: 145–148.

Vyas GN, Dienstag JL, Hoofnagle JH, eds. Viral hepatitis and liver disease. New York: Grune and Stratton, 1984.

Williams R, Smith M, Shilkin KB, Herbertson B, Path MC, Joysey V, Calne RY. Liver transplantation in man: the frequency of rejection, biliary tract complications, and recurrence of malignancy based on an analysis of 26 cases. Gastroenterology 1973; 64: 1026–1048.

Willis RA, ed. Pathology of tumours. 45th ed. New York: Appleton-Century-Crofts, 1967: 181–182.

World Health Organisation. Prevention of liver cancer. WHO Tech Rep Ser 1983; no 691.

6.7   Complications of Liver Surgery and their Management

P. Neuhaus

Foster and Berman (1977), in their standard monograph on solid liver tumors, stated, "the distressingly high rates of morbidity and mortality reported after liver resection can be reduced significantly by a skilled surgical team." Now, ten years later, this is still true, and an increasing number of general surgeons are becoming interested in liver surgery. The surgical techniques have been described, but it must be stressed again that intraoperative prevention of complications by adequate resection techniques and careful hemostasis is more important even than ideal treatment of complications.

Complications after liver resection can be divided into general complications as the result of major abdominal surgery, specific complications related to surgical techniques, and complications related to surgical decisions and to the underlying liver disease.

The group of patients with liver tumors represents all age groups, benign as well as malignant conditions, and extremely ill as well as otherwise healthy subjects. Although postoperative complications like pneumonia, superficial wound infection, deep vein thrombosis, pulmonary embolism and gastrointestinal bleeding are rare after uncomplicated liver resections, efforts towards their prevention are important and follow exactly the same routes as in any other form of major abdominal surgery (Ekberg et al. 1986). These include the use of perioperative prophylactic antibiotic treatment, low-dose heparin, H_2-receptor antagonists and adequate physiotherapy.

The most disappointing complication for the surgeon is intraoperative death from exsanguinating hemorrhage. Right lobectomies always carried the highest risk of such intraoperative and of postoperative life-threatening complications often due to technical problems (Table 6.7.1) (Ekberg et al. 1986, Foster and Berman 1977, Thompson et al. 1983).

Table 6.7.1   Operative mortality after resection of solid liver tumors (Foster and Berman 1977)

Type of resection	n	Total	%
Right lobectomy	44	173	25.4
Extended right lobectomy	10	40	25.0
Left lobectomy	5	57	8.7
Extended left lobectomy	5	69	7.2
Wedge resection	18	282	6.3
Total	82	621	13.2

Table 6.7.2   Causes of operative deaths in 76 patients after resection of solid liver tumors (Foster and Berman 1977)

Cause	n
Intraoperative death	18
Postoperative hemorrhage	11
Liver failure for technical reasons	13
Error of judgement	5
Sepsis	4
Total	51 = 67.1%
Liver failure in cirrhotic patients	12
Liver failure, cause unknown	3
Cardiopulmonary, gastrointestinal bleeding	8
Recurrent cancer	2
Total	25 = 32.9%

In Foster and Berman's survey, there were 18 intraoperative deaths in 621 liver resections, 15 due to a failure to control hemorrhage, and probably 3 due to air embolization (Table 6.7.2). Although this will occasionally also happen in the future, surgical techniques nowadays should make it a rare event. One last resort can sometimes be packing of the liver wound and relaparotomy for definitive hemostasis after stabilization of vital functions and correction or restoration of coagulation factors and thrombocytes. Nevertheless, failure to achieve complete hemostasis at the resected liver surface is still the main reason for complications after liver surgery. Postoperative hemorrhage, biliary leakage and biliary fistula, subphrenic abscess formation and right pleural effusion, sepsis and liver failure are often directly related to incomplete hemostasis and inadequate surgical technique (Joishij 1980, Lee 1982, Lin 1979).

Rare complications also directly related to surgery are hematobilia, intrahepatic abscess formation, sepsis and liver failure when parenchymal necrosis results from devascularization by deep sutures (Neuhaus and Pichlmayr 1986). Other technical complications after major resection include vascular and biliary problems either due to accidental lesion or to unnoticed malposition of the liver remnant, especially after right hepatectomy.

Some complications are clearly related to the underlying liver disease. Above all, the possibility of liver failure after any sort of liver surgery in cirrhotic patients must be mentioned here. Also, extended resections in normal livers sometimes carry the risk of liver failure. But often "borderline surgery" of this sort is the only chance of a cure for patients with liver tumors (Mizumoto et al. 1979, Nagao et al. 1987, Nagasue et al. 1986, Okamoto et al. 1984).

Postoperative Investigations after Liver Resection

As postoperative routine investigations, red and white blood count, blood sugar, electrolytes, prothrombin time, thrombocytes and blood gases are checked twice daily or more during the first three days after operation. Daily bilirubin, AST, ALT, GLDH, AP and y-GT, albumin and creatinine testing, together with a clotting profile give a picture of hepatic parenchymal damage as well as of the remaining liver function. These values lose their prognostic significance, of course, when massive substitution of blood products becomes necessary due to severe intra- and postoperative hemorrhage. A rise in bilirubin may then be caused by degradation of erythrocytes. On the other hand, liver enzymes, albumin and clotting factors are influenced by dilution and substitution and can only with difficulty be used for functional assessment of the remaining liver.

The most valuable non-invasive tool for postoperative investigation is ultrasound examination, which can detect swelling of the parenchyma, dilation of blood vessels and bile ducts, fluid collections, necrotic areas and even vascular thrombosis. The same information can be obtained by axial computed tomography. Hepatobiliary sequential scintigraphy can show signs of poor excretion and small biliary leakages. Routine postoperative chest X-rays detect right pleural effusions often due to subphrenic hematoma, bile and pus collection. But atelectasis, pneumonia and signs of hyperhydration or pulmonary capillary damage after prolonged hypotension or massive transfusions can also be diagnosed in this way.

Operative Complications

Surgical complications are mostly related to unexpected operative problems, either brought about by problematic decisions, e. g. to undertake extended resection, or by technical difficulties.

Intraoperative Hemorrhage

Failure to control hemorrhage is always mentioned as the primary complication in liver surgery. In Foster and Berman's series of 621 liver resections, 18 out of 82 operative deaths occurred in the operating room, and the high quantities of blood transfusion often needed intra- and postoperatively point to the same problem (Table 6.7.2).

Interestingly, most of the intraoperative deaths from hemorrhage (11 out of 15) occurred when the major hepatic veins were dissected. Surgical exposure of this area was possibly sometimes inadequate (Foster and Berman 1977). To avoid bleeding from the liver wound, dissection should no longer be done with crude finger fracture or "crush technique." Either the ultrasonic knife or fine dissection with the back of Metzenbaum scissors should be used, so that multiple small vessels can be identified and ligated. Definite hemostasis may then be achieved with infrared sapphire coagulation and fibrin glue, or both. Both methods can be regarded as important advances in hepatic surgery (Guthy et al. 1979, 1984, Scheele 1984).

Using these modern technical tools during the last two years in 62 major liver resections, there were no intraoperative deaths or surgical complications related to excessive intraoperative hemorrhage. Only one biliary fistula occurred after left trisegmentectomy, and this closed spontaneously 4 weeks after the operation. Subphrenic abscesses or sepsis were not encountered. One patient in this series died of liver failure after right trisegmentectomy, possibly due to vascular thrombosis, at the end of the first postoperative week (Table 6.7.3).

If intraoperative bleeding seems to be uncontrollable, one should realize that there is a hepatic vein problem and be prepared to correct it surgically. But if the bleeding is diffuse from the liver surface – especially after massive transfusion and a prolonged operating time, it can be wise to postpone definitive hemostasis, pack the wound with towels, and take the patient to intensive care until organ function, coagulation profile, body temperature and other metabolic processes are corrected (Neuhaus and Pichlmayr 1986). Hemostasis can then often be achieved easily 24 hours later, when packing is removed and the wound can finally be drained and closed. But these events can only be a rare exception nowadays. In the author's

Table 6.7.3 Complications and perioperative mortality in 62 patients after liver resection. Neuhaus, 1986–1987

	Complications	Deaths
Intraoperative deaths	–	–
Hemorrhage	–	–
Subphrenic abscess	–	–
Biliary fistula*	1	–
Wound infection	1	–
Liver failure**	1	1
Sepsis	–	–

* Left trisegmentectomy
** Right trisegmentectomy

personal experience, neither massive blood-transfusion nor packing has ever been necessary, and almost one-third of the anatomical hemi-hepatectomies has been performed without any transfusion.

Postoperative Intra-abdominal Hemorrhage

In discussing postoperative intra-abdominal hemorrhage, one has to distinguish between continuous postoperative bleeding from the liver wound and subphrenic hematoma or intra-abdominal blood collections without active further blood loss.

If blood loss via wound drains, measured by the requirement for transfusion, is not more than 2 units of blood during the first 12 hours postoperatively, with a tendency to improve, the time should be taken to correct metabolic disturbances and replace blood cells, clotting factors and albumin as needed. In many cases, bleeding from the cut liver surface is significantly reduced after 12 to 24 hours, and if ultrasound examination does not show subphrenic hematoma of more than 200–300 ml in volume, because the blood loss has been quantitatively drained to the outside, no operative intervention is needed.

Continuous bleeding on the first morning after the operation usually makes relaparotomy advisable, especially after major hepatic resection, where the early postoperative course is often of vital importance in view of secondary problems like impaired renal function, ventilation and gas exchange, catabolism and infection. Often only 2 or 3 sutures are needed to stop bleeding completely, and the following postoperative period will be better than after a prolonged period of incomplete hemostasis and blood replacement.

If measurable intra-abdominal or subphrenic hematoma is found postoperatively by ultrasound examination or suspected clinically, without further active bleeding, relaparotomy and removal of the old blood is advisable. Large hematomas and also the absorption of larger quantities of blood can cause severe problems after hepatectomy, whereas the trauma of a short second operation is usually well tolerated. In all cases of relaparotomy when complete hemostasis cannot be achieved, when poorly perfused portions of parenchyma are visible, or when there is dead space which is not readily occupied by the remaining liver lobe, it can be useful to fill it with a piece of omentum majus placed against the resected liver surface. A soft drain (in our case an "easyflow" or "Jackson Pratt" drainage system) is placed between the omentum and the liver to prevent further blood accumulation and eventually form a track for the discharge of necrotic material, bile and pus if necessary.

Table 6.7.4 Postoperative complications in 55 patients after major liver resections (Thompson et al. 1983)

Type of complication	n	%
Postoperative intra-abdominal hemorrhage	7	12.7
Biliary fistula	8	14.5
Intra-abdominal infection, abscess	18	32.7
Fever over more than 1 week after operation	29	52.7
Postoperative mortality	8	14.5

Subphrenic Abscess and Intra-abdominal Infection

Intra-abdominal infection and subphrenic abscesses occurred in 18 out of 55 patients after major liver resections reported by Thompson and coworkers in 1983 (Table 6.7.4). The mortality rate in patients with abscesses is considerable, because sepsis and liver failure can result, especially with inadequate therapy (Bengmark and Hasselgren 1987, Foster and Berman 1977, Thompson et al. 1983, Yanaga et al. 1986). Hemorrhage and incompletely evacuated hematomas, biliary leaks from the resected liver surface, and devascularized necrotic tissue left behind are the main causative factors in abscess formation (Figs. 6.7.1, 6.7.2) (Bengmark and Hasselgren 1987, Eng et al. 1981). Early diagnosis with ultrasound examination or CT scan is most important if any disturbance of the postoperative course is suspected.

Intra-abdominal infections and subphrenic abscesses should be treated aggressively either by surgical drainage or, especially when more than two weeks have passed since the operation, by ultrasound-guided percutaneous drainage. This method has been developed in recent years mainly for intrahepatic abscesses, but is has been shown to be of great value for all sorts of well-localized intra-abdominal pus collections as well (Gamstätter et al. 1983).

Parenchymal Necrosis

Necrotic areas after standard liver resection are usually the result of technical errors. If possible, such sources of severe complication should be resected primarily. But if, after extended right or left resection with little parenchyma remaining, a small edge looks bluish, the decision whether or not to resect this can be difficult. Here careful drainage and coverage of the surface with viable omentum can be better than resection, especially when the functional reserve of the liver seems to be marginal.

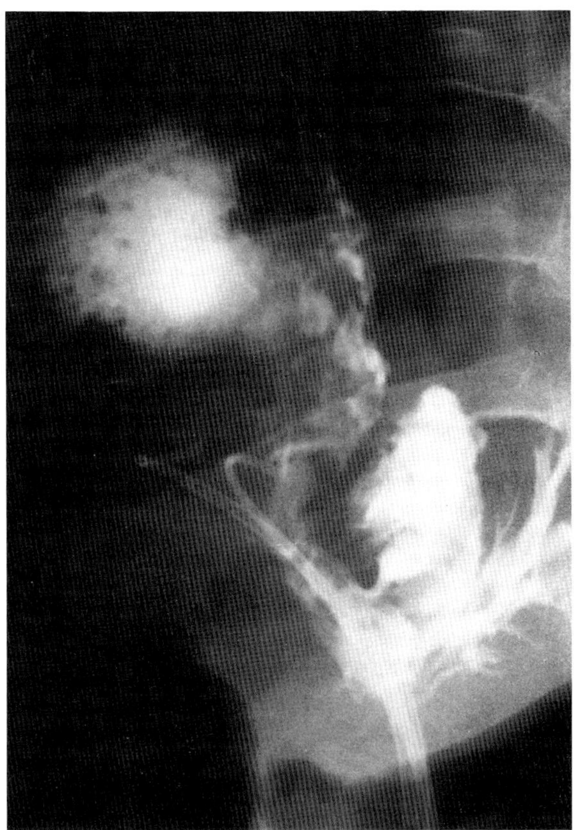

Fig. 6.7.**1 Biliary leakage and abscess formation** after right hemihepatectomy. Repair by direct suture and viable omentum

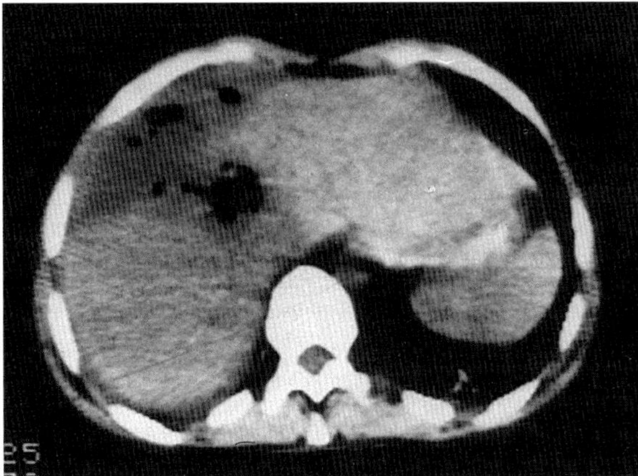

Fig. 6.7.**2 Hematoma, biliary leakage and abscess formation** after central wedge resection (segment 4) for liver metastasis. Uneventful course after surgical drainage

There is still the chance that the poorly-perfused segment may yet survive, or that drainage and omentum may help to localize the demarcation process. In any case, the postoperative course of a patient of this sort must be closely observed so that the correct point for any surgical reintervention which may be necessary is not missed. This is certainly the case when signs of pulmonary involvement, renal impairment and incipient sepsis follow.

Parenchymal necrosis after liver resection must have been common with earlier "crush" and "fracture" techniques, with deep "compression sutures" or with the still-popular adaptation of the liver wound edges. There is no place for any of these in modern liver surgery. They account for the majority of postoperative complications, whether life-threatening complications or simply the prolonged postoperative fever seen in 50% of the patients reported by Thompson (1983).

Biliary Fistula

The two main factors in the development of external biliary fistulas are surgical mistakes and anatomical problems when extended resections are necessary. Ultrasound dissection and (equally effective) dissection with fine scissors, especially in an almost bloodless field when inflow occlusion is used, have reduced the danger of biliary leaks from open bile ducts considerably. (Delva et al. 1984, Huguet et al. 1976). Small ducts will always still be open, even when 30 or 40 ligatures are used in a hemihepatectomy. But these either close spontaneously, or with infrared coagulation or fibrin glue, when the main bile ducts are patent.

Routine T-tube drainage of the common bile duct cannot be advised. It does not lower the incidence of biliary leaks and is potentially harmful, especially in small ducts (Bengmark and Hasselgren 1987). In right hemihepatectomies, the danger of biliary leaks from the resection surface is not very high with standard techniques, but the positioning of the remaining left liver is important. If the falciform ligament and left triangular ligament are divided, complete rotation of the hilus can cause vascular problems and biliary outflow obstruction. Deep sutures may also impair bile ducts and blood vessels near the surface and then lead, directly or via necrosis and abscess formation, to biliary fistula. The same is also true of "adaptation" of the liver wound edges.

In left hemihepatectomies it has to be kept in mind that in some cases bile ducts for the medial and posterior segments of the right liver can drain into the left hepatic duct, and that the bile duct of the caudate lobe also drains into the left hepatic duct (Mizumoto and Suzuki 1988, Smadja and

Blumgart 1988). Biliary fistulas are thus more frequent after left than after right hemihepatectomy.

In any case of visible bile leakage, the source should be identified and repaired. This can either be by means of simple suture ligation or, if larger bile ducts are involved, repair with T-tube placement. Preferably, one side of the T-tube is placed above the lesion. If direct repair is not possible, Roux-en-Y bilioenteric anastomosis with a transhepatic stent, as used after resection of Klatskin tumors, must be performed. Usually one or two drains are placed near the leak and carefully covered with viable omentum, so that the leak is localized. If the main ducts are intact and a leak does not close after a few days, it is likely that the bile duct for a small segment of the liver has been cut or ligated. In this case one should wait for three to six weeks, by which time the fistula usually closes and the parenchymal segment becomes atrophic. In rare cases, the fistula track must later be drained into a jejunal loop. Careful monitoring for signs of cholangitis and abscess formation must be performed.

If a mechanical biliary outflow problem is presumed, endoscopic retrograde cholangiography can be of value in localizing the side of the obstruction or kinking. But a negative cholangiogram can never exclude biliary leaks (see above)! Here a hepatobiliary sequential scintigraphy (HBSS) can sometimes be of value.

Hematobilia and Bilhemia

These are extremely rare cases which can occur as a result of deep sutures through the bile duct and portal veins, or after intrahepatic abscess formation. Sandblom (1948) first described hematobilia after trauma, and since then many cases have been reported, although none after elective liver surgery. Late symptoms following liver resection such as upper abdominal pain, hematemesis and melena, and possibly icterus and hemorrhagic shock, can point to hematobilia. About 50% of affected patients die, so aggressive, active treatment is necessary (Sandblom et al. 1984, Wittrin et al. 1978).

Localization of the fistula or of atypical arterial findings by angiography are also sometimes possible without active bleeding. Preferably, surgical treatment should be attempted either by resection or if possible by suture ligation. Alternatively, embolization, and occasionally also careful conservative treatment, have been successful (Curet et al. 1984).

Liver Failure

Temporary liver insufficiency must not be confused with liver failure. Especially after right trisegmentectomy, a period of rising serum bilirubin and other signs of impaired liver function is normal. Substitution of coagulation factors and albumin as necessary, bowel cleaning with magnesium sulfate, lactulose and neomycin, and the infusion of glucose and branched-chain amino acids are usually recommended. Whether prophylactic parenteral antibiotics are helpful is an open question. Metronidazole is recommended against gram-negative anerobic bacteria from the gut. The prevention of hypoxemia, hypovolemia and electrolyte or metabolic imbalances is most important. Respirator treatment should be avoided if possible, since it causes harmful hemodynamic changes in the liver (Neuhaus et al. 1983).

Normally this temporary liver insufficiency shows signs of improvement through regeneration of the liver cells after 5–8 days. If postoperative liver insufficiency proceeds to liver failure with secondary organ failure there is, as yet, almost nothing that can be done (Brölsch 1985). But before the diagnosis of irreversible liver failure is accepted, a careful search should be made for surgical problems like thrombosis of the hepatic artery or portal vein, hepatic venous outflow and biliary obstruction. Usually these complications can no longer be treated when hepatic failure has developed, but vascular problems diagnosed early by a rise in glutamate dehydrogenase (GLDH) and by Doppler sonography and angiography may be successfully corrected at reoperation. Artificial liver support has not yet been developed to the point of practical usefulness. Liver transplantation, if available, may occasionally be successful, for example after resection of benign liver processes, but is probably not of value for patients with malignant tumors (Brunner 1978, Brunner and Schmidt 1981).

References

Bengmark S, Hasselgren PO. Septische Probleme in der Leberchirurgie. Chir Gastroenterol 1987; 3: 105–114.

Brölsch CE, Neuhaus P, Ringe B, Sturm J, Pichlmayr R. Postoperative Leberinsuffizienz nach leberchirurgischen Eingriffen. In: Encke A et al., eds. Chirurgische Intensivmedizin. München: Urban and Schwarzenberg, 1985: 237–244.

Brunner G. Approaches to an "artifical liver". Acta Hepatogastroenterol 1978; 25: 77–86.

Brunner G, Schmidt FW. Artificial liver support. Berlin: Springer, 1981.

Curet P, Baumer R, Roche A, Grellet J, Mercadier M. Hepatic hemobilia of traumatic or iatrogenic origin: recent advances in diagnosis and therapy, review of the literature from 1976 to 1981. World J Surg 1984; 8: 2–8.

Delva E, Barberousse HP, Nordlinger B, Ollivier JM, Vacher B, Guilmet C, Huguet C. Hemodynamic and biochemical monitoring during major liver resection with use of hepatic vascular occlusion. Surgery 1984; 95: 309–318.

Ekberg H, Tranberg K-G, Andersson R, Jeppsson B, Bengmark S. Major liver resection: perioperative course and management. Surgery 1986; 100: 1–8.

Eng RHK, Tecson-Tumang F, Corrado ML. Blunt trauma and liver abscess. Am J Gastroenterol 1981; 76: 252–255.

Foster JH, Berman MM. Solid liver tumors. In: Major problems in clinical surgery; vol 13. Philadelphia: Saunders 1977: 255–266.

Gamstätter G, Rothmund M, Braun B, Dähnert W, Günther R. Perkutane oder offene chirurgische Drainage beim Leberabszeß. In: Häring R, ed. Chirurgie der Leber. Weinheim: Edition Medizin, 1983: 439–444.

Guthy E, Kiefhaber P, Nath G, Kreitmair A. Infrarot-Kontakt-Koagulation: klinische Anwendung an Leber und Milz. Langenbecks Arch Chir 1979; 348: 105–108.

Guthy E, Brölsch C, Neuhaus P, Pichlmayr R. Infrarot-Kontakt-Koagulation an der Leber: Technik, Taktik, Ergebnisse. Langenbecks Arch Chir 1984; 363: 129–138.

Huguet C, Nordlinger B, Galoppin JJ. Normothermic hepatic vascular exclusion for extensive hepatectomy. Surg Gynecol Obstet 1976; 147: 689–693.

Joishij SK, Balasegaram M. Hepatic resection for malignant tumors of the liver. Am J Surg 1980; 139: 360–369.

Lee NW, Wong J, Ong G-B. The surgical management of primary carcinoma of the liver. World J Surg 1982; 6: 66–75.

Lin T-Y. Resectional therapy for primary malignant hepatic tumors. Int Adv Surg Oncol 1979; 2: 25–54.

Mizumoto R, Suzuki H. Surgical anatomy of the hepatic hilium with special reference to the caudate lobe. World J Surg 1988; 12: 2–10.

Mizumoto R, Kawarada Y, Noguchi T. Preoperative estimation of operative risk in liver surgery, with special reference to functional reserve of the remnant liver following major hepatic resection. Jpn J Surg 1979; 9: 343–349.

Nagao T, Inoue S, Goto S, Mizuta T, Omori Y, Kawano N, Morioka Y. Hepatic resection for hepatocellular carcinoma: clinical features and long-term prognosis. Ann Surg 1987; 205: 33–40.

Nagasue N, Yukaya H, Ogawa Y, Sasaki Y, Chang Y-C, Niimi K. Clinical experience with 118 hepatic resections for hepatocellular carcinoma. Surgery 1986; 99: 694–702.

Neuhaus P, Pichlmayr R. Postoperative Komplikationen nach Versorgung von Leberrupturen. In: Siewert JR, Pichlmayr R, eds. Das traumatisierte Abdomen. Berlin: Springer 1986: 95–101.

Neuhaus P, Neuhaus R, Vonnahme F, Pichlmayr R. Verbesserte Möglichkeiten des temporären Leberersatzes durch ein neues Konzept der extracorporalen Leberperfusion. Langenbecks Arch Chir 1983; supl: 223–228.

Okamoto E, Kyo A, Yamanaka N, Tanaka N, Kuwata K. Prediction of the safe limits of hepatectomy by combined volumetric and functional measurements in patients with impaired hepatic function. Surgery 1984; 95: 586–592.

Sandblom PH, Saegesser F, Mirkovitvh V. Hepatic hemobilia: hemorrhage from the intrahepatic biliary tract: a review. World J Surg 1984; 8: 41–50.

Scheele J. Indikation, Technik und Ergebnisse der Fibrinklebung nach Leberresektionen. In: Scheele J, ed. Fibrinklebung. Berlin: Springer, 1984: 86–94.

Smadja C, Blumgart LH. The biliary tract and the anatomy of biliary exposure. In: Blumgart LH, ed. Surgery of the liver and biliary tract. Edinburgh: Churchill Livingstone, 1988: 11–22.

Thompson HH, et al. Major hepatic resection: a 25-year experience. Ann Surg 1983; 197: 375–387.

Wittrin G, Clemens M, Safrany L, Schönleben K. Hämobilie und Bilhämie-Komplikationen beim Lebertrauma. Zentralbl. Chir 1978; 103: 1463–1470.

Yanaga K, Kanematsu T, et al. Intraperitoneal septic complications after hepatectomy. Ann Surg 1986; 203: 148–152.

7 Surgical Management of Pancreatic Malignancies

7.1 Subtotal Duodenopancreatectomy for the Management of Pancreatic Duct, Distal Common Bile Duct and Ampullary Carcinoma

N.J. Lygidakis and M.N. van der Heyde

Introduction

For a proportion of patients with pancreatic head carcinoma resectional surgery can nowadays be considered to be an optimal form of treatment. Overall, the results after resection are more satisfactory than after any form of palliative medical or surgical management (Chapter 7.6) (Brooks and Culebras 1976). Subtotal pancreatectomy (Fig. 7.1.1) is generally considered to be the optimal form of resection. It is, however, regarded by some with reservation and scepticism. Their attitude is supported by a number of arguments in favor of total pancreatectomy (Brooks and Culebras 1976, Ihse et al. 1977).

Subtotal resection is considered to be less radical, particularly since, in view of the incidence of multifocal localization of the process, the pancreatic remnant could contain residual pathology. Furthermore, total pancreatectomy obviates complications of anastomotic dehiscence of the pancreaticojejunostomy (Brooks and Culebras 1976, Ihse et al. 1977). Nevertheless, the advocates of subtotal duodenopancreatectomy are growing in number (Braasch and Gray 1977, Crist et al. 1987, Grace et al. 1986, Mannell et al. 1986, Sato et al. 1977, Tsuchiya et al. 1986, Trede 1987, Van Heerden et al. 1981). The factors which have contributed to this change in attitude are the impressive decrease in the early mortality rate, which is at present below 5 %

(Crist et al. 1987, Trede 1987), the satisfactory long-term survival rate even in pancreatic duct carcinoma (Crist et al. 1987), and the adequate quality of post-operative life, which is of great importance (Braasch and Gray 1977, Braasch et al. 1986, Cooperman et al. 1982, Crist et al. 1987, Grace et al. 1986, Lerut et al. 1984, Sato et al. 1977, Trede 1987).

Subtotal duodenopancreatectomy is our policy in Amsterdam and, based on the results, we consider it to be the treatment of choice for the majority of patients with resectable pancreatic head carcinoma. In essence, subtotal duodenopancreatectomy is carried out in every patient with pancreatic head carcinoma which is considered resectable on the basis of preoperative and peroperative evaluation studies. Biopsies from the margins of the pancreatic remnant and the rim of the pancreatic duct are routinely taken. Should there be residual pathology in these sections, we continue with total pancreatectomy. The presence of a very narrow pancreatic duct (less than 1 mm) and the presence of diabetes or steatorrhea constitute further indications for total pancreatectomy. In the first 100 patients who underwent resectional pancreatic surgery following the criteria mentioned above, 78 underwent subtotal pancreatectomy and 22 total pancreatectomy.

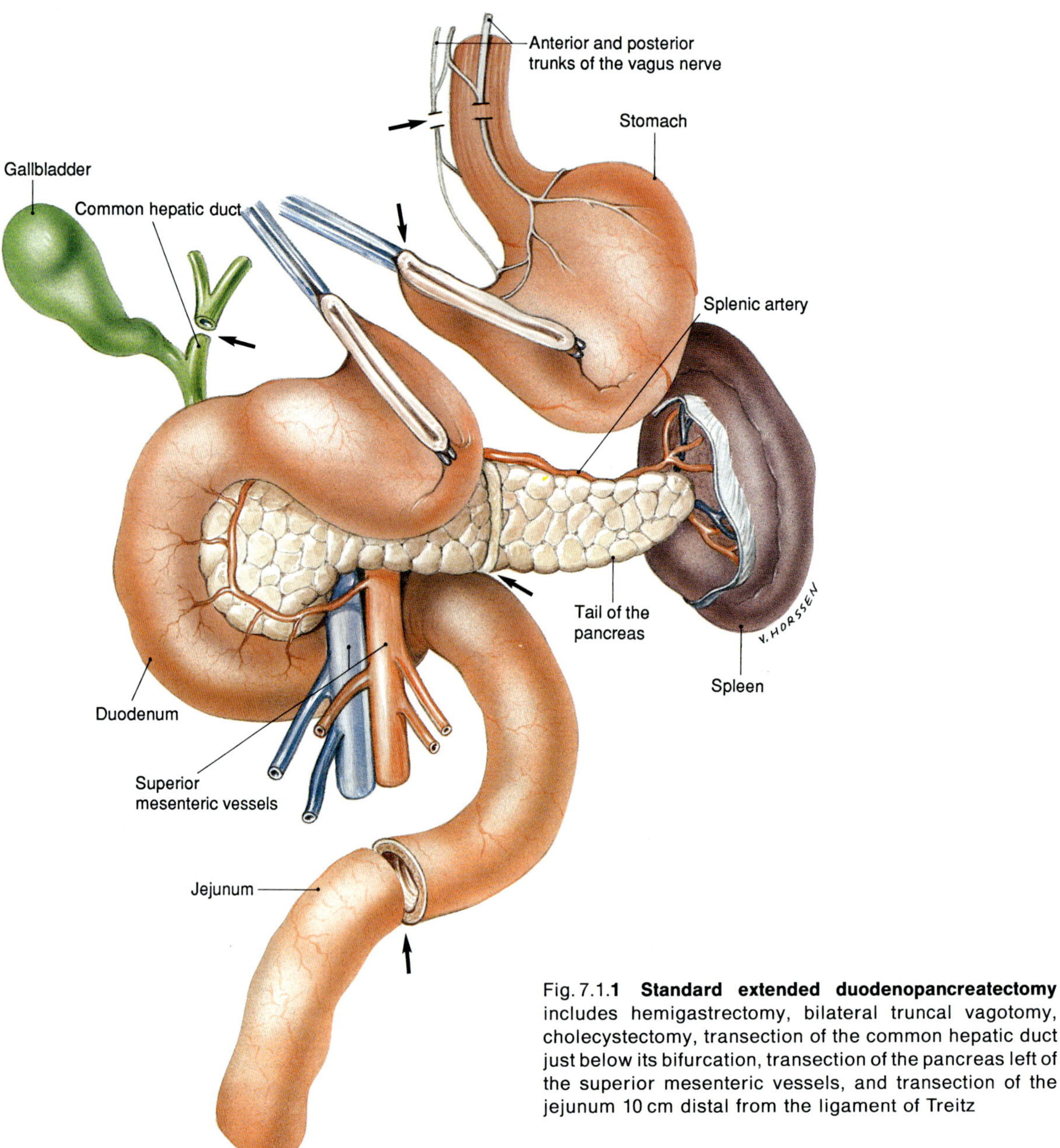

Fig. 7.1.**1   Standard extended duodenopancreatectomy** includes hemigastrectomy, bilateral truncal vagotomy, cholecystectomy, transection of the common hepatic duct just below its bifurcation, transection of the pancreas left of the superior mesenteric vessels, and transection of the jejunum 10 cm distal from the ligament of Treitz

Technique

The topography of the surgical site is depicted in Figure 7.1.**2**. All operations which involve pancreatic and biliary malignant disease start with a bilateral subcostal incision in order to obtain good access to the upper abdomen (Fig. 7.1.**3**). The liver, hepatoduodenal ligament, lesser omentum and gastrocolic ligament are carefully evaluated (Fig. 7.1.**4**). We start with the mobilization of the head of the pancreas and duodenum by opening the posterior peritoneum 2 cm to the right of the right margin of the caval vein. With a sharp dissection, the retroperitoneal duodenum, pancreatic head,

lymph nodes and retroperitoneal fat are completely freed all along the vena cava and aorta. In this way, both the inferior vena cava and the aorta are cleared from their lymphatics (Fig. 7.1.**5**). We continue with bimanual palpation of the head of the pancreas and with evaluation of the existing anatomical situation with regard to the extent and spread of the tumor, and most particularly whether the tumor is stuck in the aorta and in the region of origin of the superior mesenteric artery (Fig. 7.1.**6a, b**). The base of the mesentery is similarly carefully inspected (Fig. 7.1.**7a, b**), and the stomach is separated from the colon by transection of the gastrocolic ligament (for the transection line, see Fig. 7.1.**4**), allowing

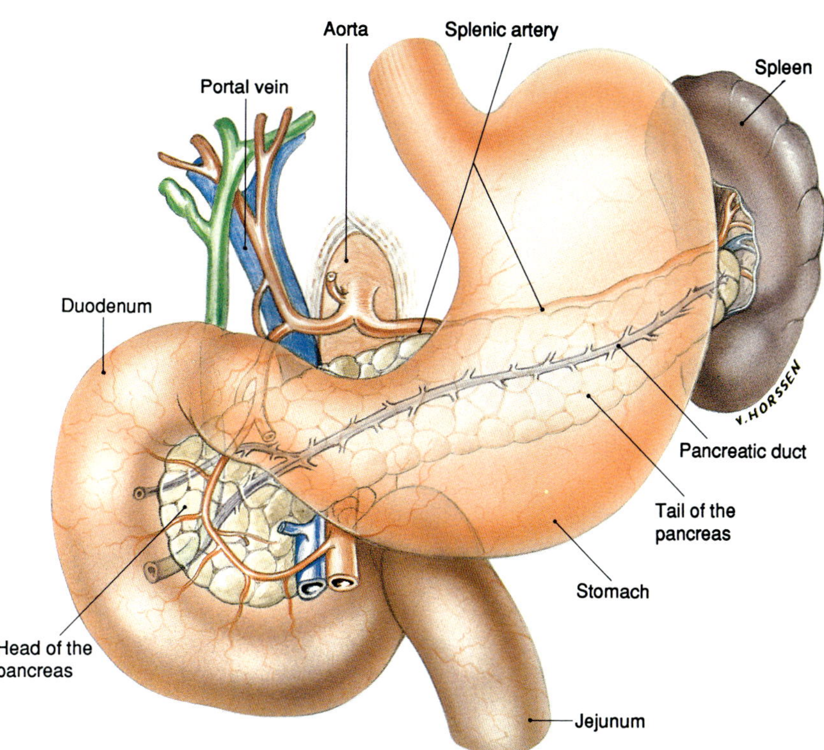

Fig. 7.1.**2** **Overview of the anatomic relationship** between the pancreas and the surrounding organs

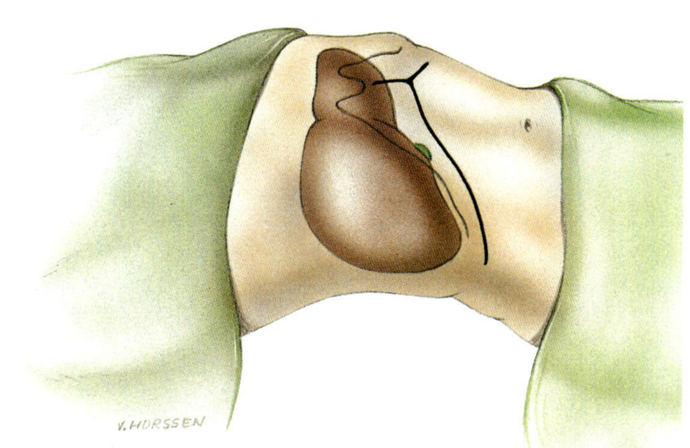

Fig. 7.1.**3** **Routine bilateral subcostal incision** for major pancreatic and biliary surgery

access to the anterior surface of the pancreas (Figs. 7.1.**4** and 7.1.**8**). The inspection includes the transverse mesocolon, the ligament of Treitz, the abdominal aorta and the regional peritoneum.

At this stage, provided the lesion is resectable, we continue with dissection of the hepatoduodenal ligament. The following must be identified, skeletonized (freed from lymphatics) and isolated via vessel loops: the common bile duct, common hepatic duct, cystic duct, portal vein, and hepatic artery (Fig. 7.1.**9**).

The common hepatic duct is transected just below its bifurcation, and cholecystectomy (see Chapter 8.3) is carried out. Both transected segments of the bile duct are closed after biopsies from the proximal segment are taken (Fig. 7.1.**10**).

The distal segment of the transected common hepatic duct is dissected down its right side, offering access to the underlying portal vein. The common hepatic artery and its junction with the gastroduodenal artery are dissected, while a number of small branches to the posterior pancreatic arcade are identified, ligated and transected.

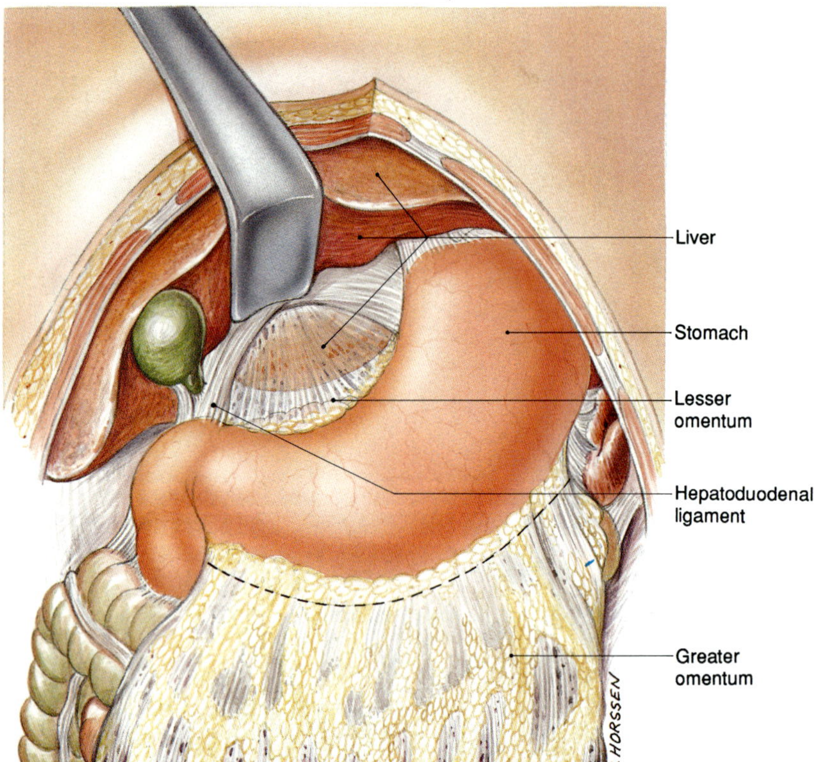

Fig. 7.1.4   Assessment of the liver, stomach, lesser omentum, hepatoduodenal ligament and greater omentum. The dotted line indicates the subsequent line of transection of the gastrocolic ligament

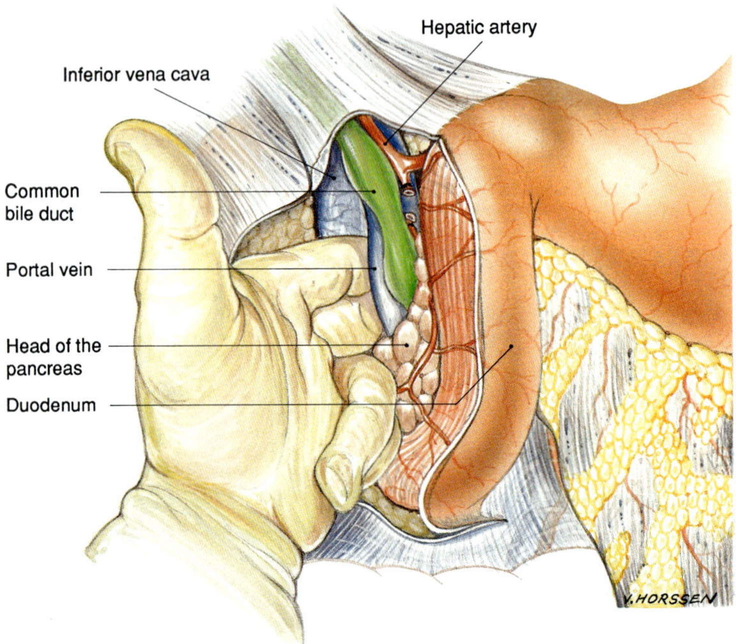

Fig. 7.1.5   Mobilization of the duodenum and head of the pancreas. By sharp dissection all along the inferior vena cava and aorta, the retroperitoneal duodenum, pancreatic head, surrounding lymphatics and retroperitoneal fat are dissected and completely freed from the underlying aorta and inferior vena cava

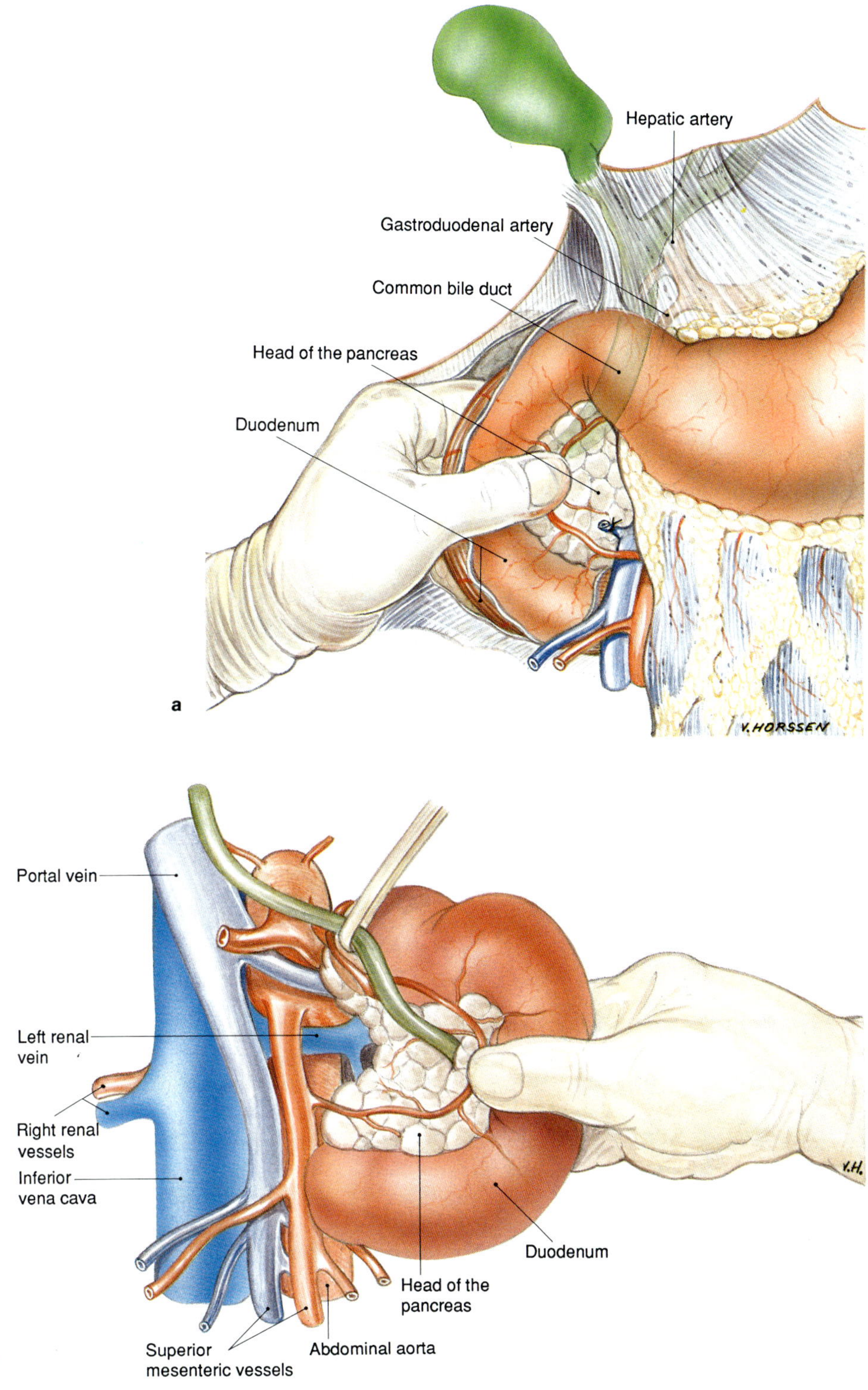

Fig. 7.1.6 Bimanual assessment of the mobilized duodenum and head of the pancreas.
a Anterior view.
b Posterior view: note the extent of mobilization of the duodenum, pancreas and surrounding lymph nodes and retroperitoneal fat, and the extent of clearance of the underlying inferior vena cava and aorta. The course of the superior mesenteric vein and portal vein is indicated for clarity

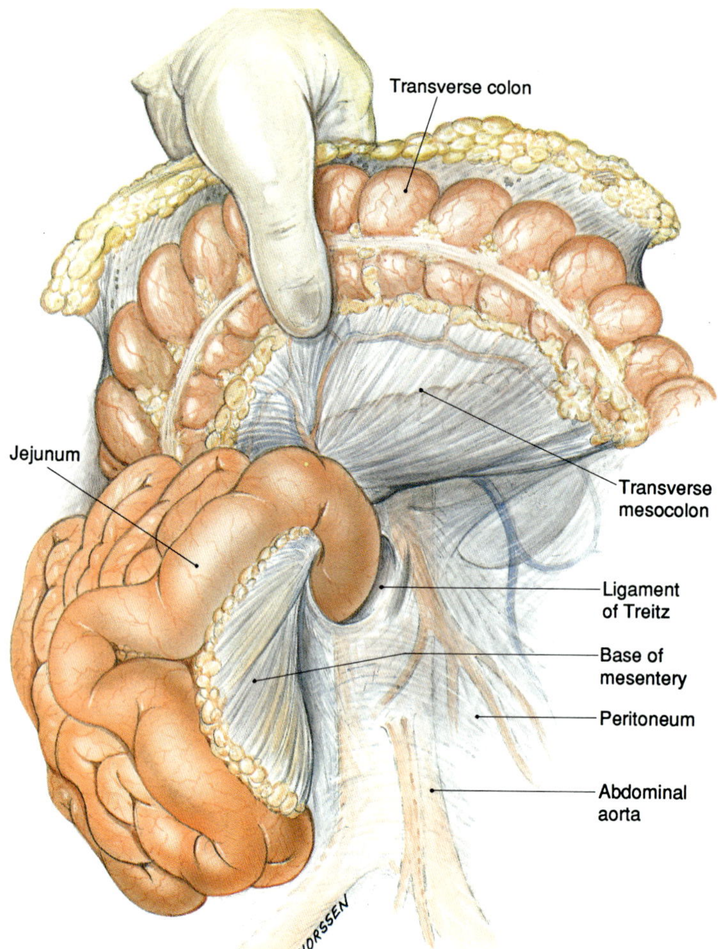

Fig. 7.1.**7 a**

Fig. 7.1.**7 a**, **b**   **Careful evaluation of the base of the mesentery and ligament of Treitz** for possible spread of the disease

The gastroduodenal artery is doubly ligated and then transected (Fig. 7.1.**10**). The portal vein now becomes more clearly visible. It is now possible to determine whether the portal vein is free of the posterior surface of the pancreas. To achieve this, we continue with dissection of the right gastrocolic ligament. By further downward dissection, we reach the anterior surface of the pancreas, the base of the superior mesenteric vessels and the retroperitoneal part of the duodenum up to its junction with the proximal jejunum (Fig. 7.1.**11**).

Inspection is now possible to determine whether or not there is any vascular involvement and whether invasion or compression of the portal vein is present (Fig. 7.1.**11**). One should follow the portal vein all the way along its anterior surface with the left index finger, and all the way along the base of the mesenteric and superior mesenteric vessels, and try to assess whether or not it is free from the posterior surface of the pancreas (Fig. 7.1.**11**). Care is taken to avoid creating tension during this maneuver. When the two fingers touch, we confirm that the portal vein is free. (For patients with compromised mesenteric vessels secondary to tumor invasion, see Chapter 7.3). At this point we continue with hemigastrectomy and bilateral truneal vagotomy. Having performed this, the ligament of Treitz is dissected, and the jejunum is transected 10 to 15 cm distally. The proximal segment is transferred to the right abdomen. The pancreas is now transected to the left of the mesenteric vessels (Figs. 7.1.**12**, 7.1.**13**, 7.1.**14**).

The body of the pancreas is now further freed from the underlying splenic artery and splenic veins for subsequent anastomosis with the jejunum (Fig. 7.1.**13**). The head of the pancreas is reflected to the right and freed from the portal vein by means of a meticulous step-by-step dissection (Figs. 7.1.**12**–7.1.**14**). The splenic vein, splenic artery, hepatic artery, and superior mesenteric vein and artery are clearly visible. The proximal jejunal loop is freed from its mesentery (Fig. 7.1.**14**). The com-

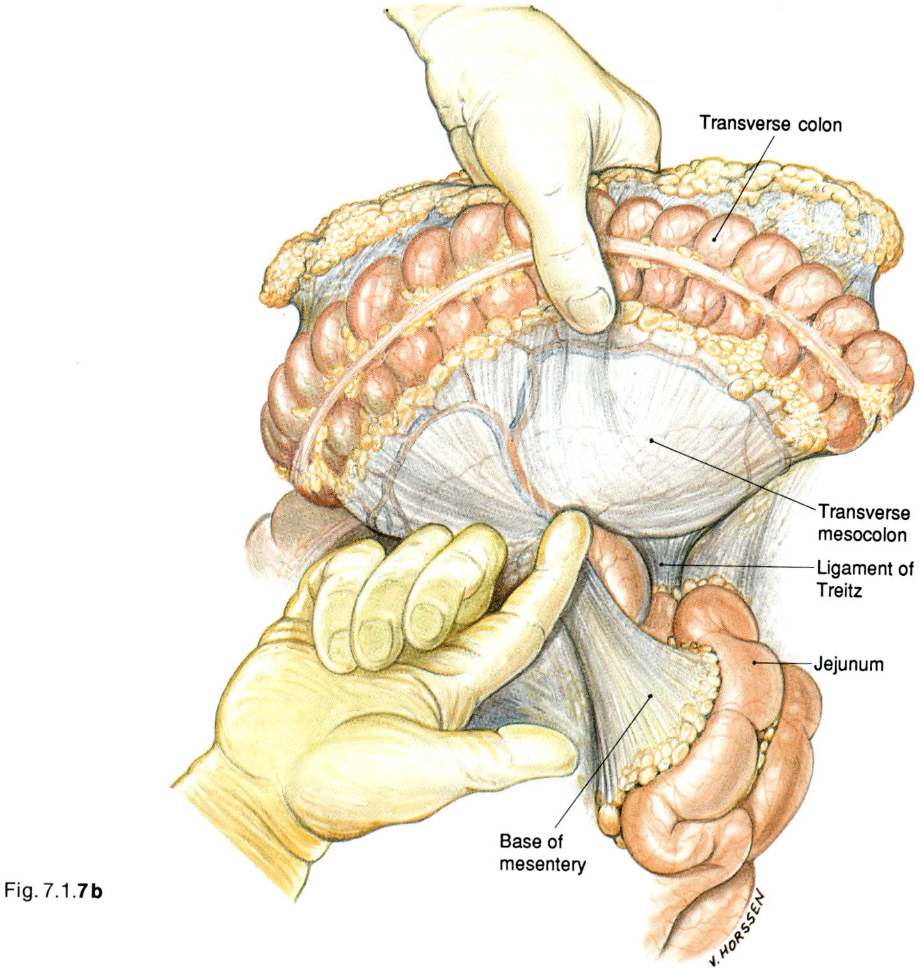

Fig. 7.1.**7 b**

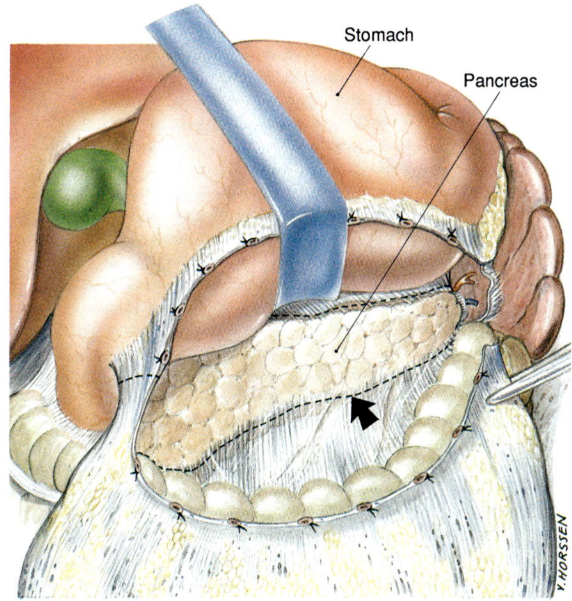

Fig. 7.1.**8 Transection of the gastrocolic ligament.** The stomach is mobilized and lifted up by means of a retractor in order to obtain an ample view of the anterior surface of the pancreas. The dotted lines demonstrate the margins of the subsequent resection along the superior and inferior borders of the pancreas. The other dotted line indicates the later resection of the right gastrocolic ligament and downward dissection of the right colic flexure

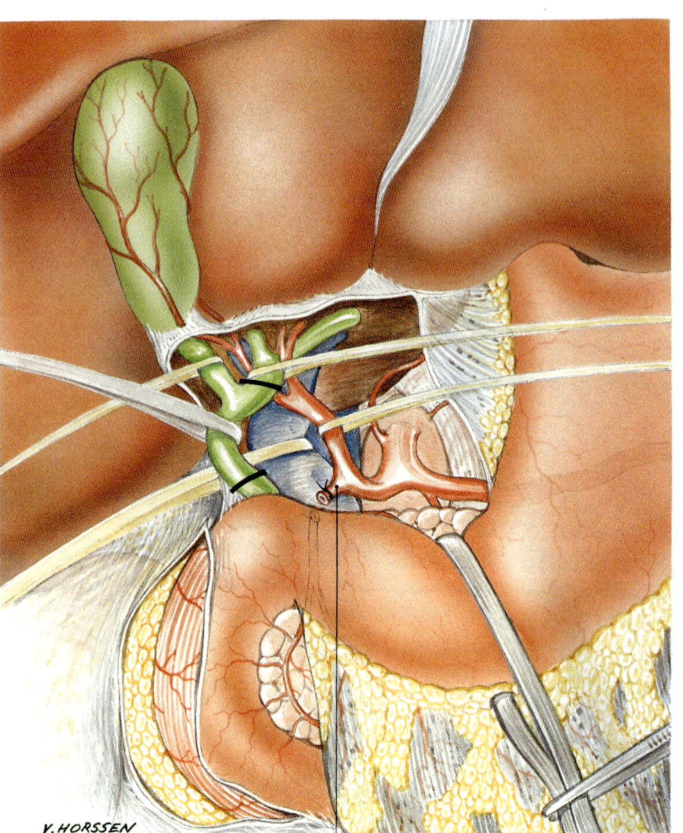

Fig. 7.1.**9 Dissection of the hepatoduodenal ligament** and identification and isolation of the common bile duct, portal vein and hepatic artery. The lines indicate the transections of the common hepatic duct and common bile duct in preparation for cholecystectomy. The gastroduodenal artery is transected

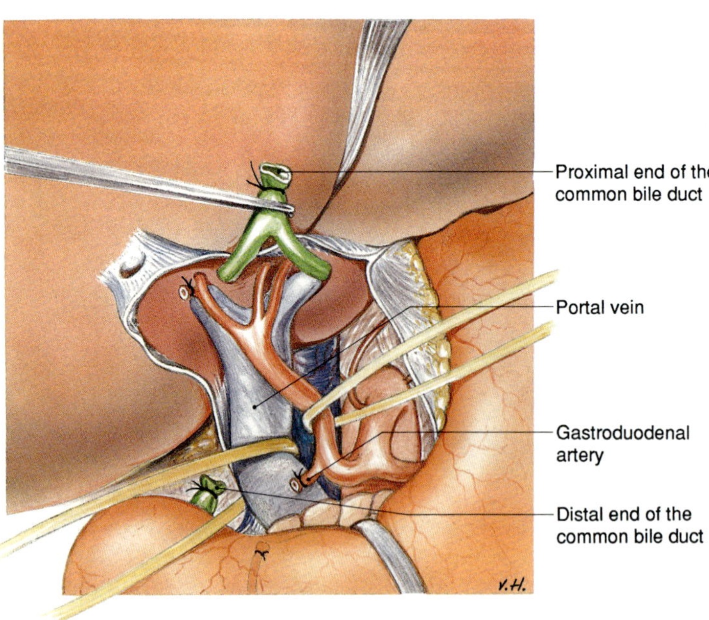

Fig. 7.1.**10 The retropancreatic segment of the portal vein is visualized** after ligation of the gastroduodenal artery. Cholecystectomy has been carried out, and the common bile duct is transected. Its proximal end is reflected cephalad and is closed to avoid spillage of bile in the operative field. Its distal end is ligated

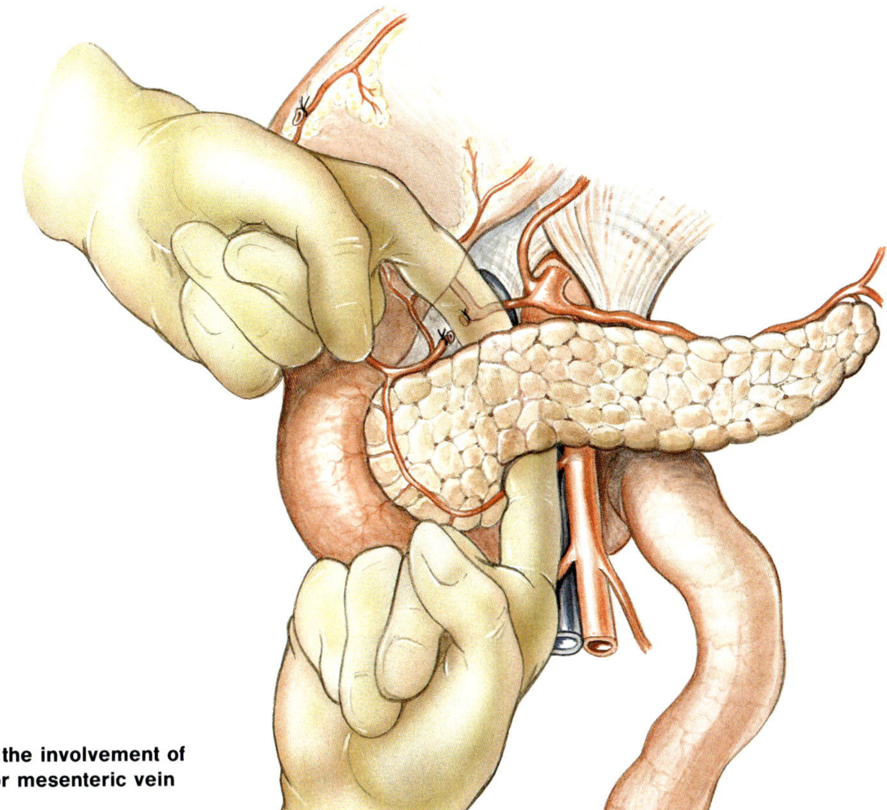

Fig. 7.1.**11** **Assessment of the involvement of the portal vein and superior mesenteric vein** in the tumor process

pletely mobilized portal vein is lifted up by means of a vessel loop (Fig. 7.1.**15**). This offers access to a number of venous branches which originate from its posterior surface. These branches are also isolated, ligated and transected (Fig. 7.1.**14**). By further dissecting the portal vein on its right side, we reach the superior mesenteric artery, which is carefully dissected and isolated by means of vessel loops (Fig. 7.1.**16**). The superior mesenteric artery is skeletonized from its lymphatics and completely freed. During this dissection, we isolate, ligate and transect a number of arterial branches which originate from the superior mesenteric artery in order to secure good hemostasis and complete clearance all along the aforementioned space (Fig. 7.1.**17**). The superior mesenteric artery is the limit of the resectional plane. When dissecting the superior mesenteric artery, it must be remembered that the right hepatic artery may originate from it in a number of patients.

At this point, the head of the pancreas and the uncinate process, with the distal stomach, duodenum and the 10 cm of jejunum attached, together with the gallbladder, the surrounding lymphatics, the retroperitoneal fat, and the distal end of the common hepatic duct are completely resected and taken out. The operative site is shown in Figures 7.1.**17** and 7.1.**18**.

We now prepare to reconstruct gastrointestinal continuity, according to our policy, by preparing two jejunal loops. Figure 7.1.**18** illustrates the isolated proximal jejunal segment which is to be used to construct pancreatic and biliary anastomoses. Reconstruction of gastrointestinal continuity is carried out using a standard technique outlined in Chapter 7.4.

Comments

Of our first 100 patients with pancreatic head carcinoma who were deemed feasible for pancreatic resection, 78 patients were treated with subtotal duodenopancreatectomy. In recent years, the number of patients who could be treated with this kind of pancreatic resection has increased due to growing expertise in fashioning the pancreatic anastomosis. This is possible even in the presence of a narrow pancreatic duct and of a friable pancreas.

The argument against subtotal duodenopancreatectomy are not justified (Braasch and Gray 1977, Cooperman et al. 1982, Crist et al. 1987, Grace et al. 1986, Trede 1987, Van Heerden et al. 1981). With the surgical technique outlined in Chapter 7.4, it appears possible to minimize the risk and the consequences of dehiscence of the pancre-

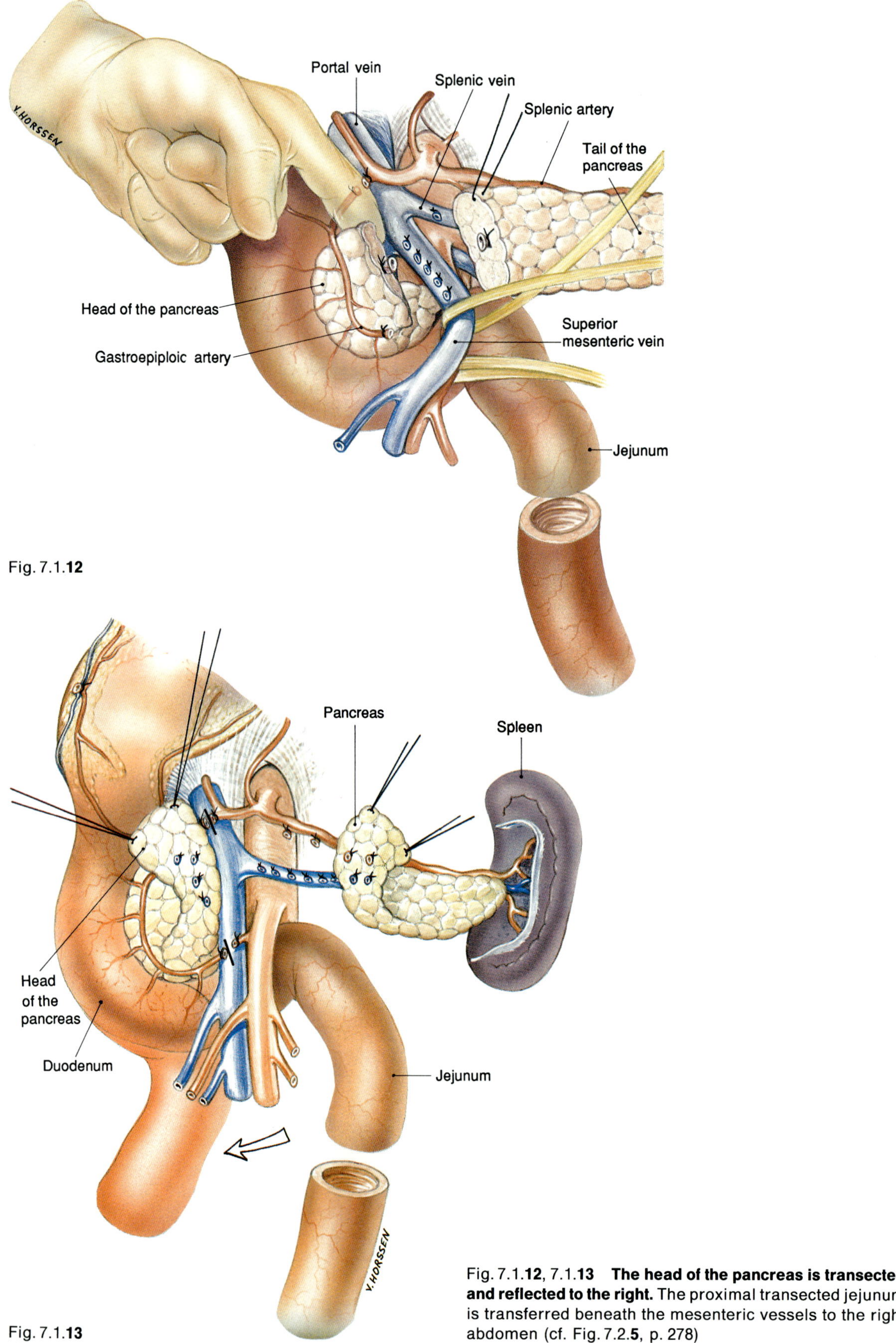

Fig. 7.1.**12**

Fig. 7.1.**13**

Fig. 7.1.**12**, 7.1.**13**   **The head of the pancreas is transected and reflected to the right.** The proximal transected jejunum is transferred beneath the mesenteric vessels to the right abdomen (cf. Fig. 7.2.**5**, p. 278)

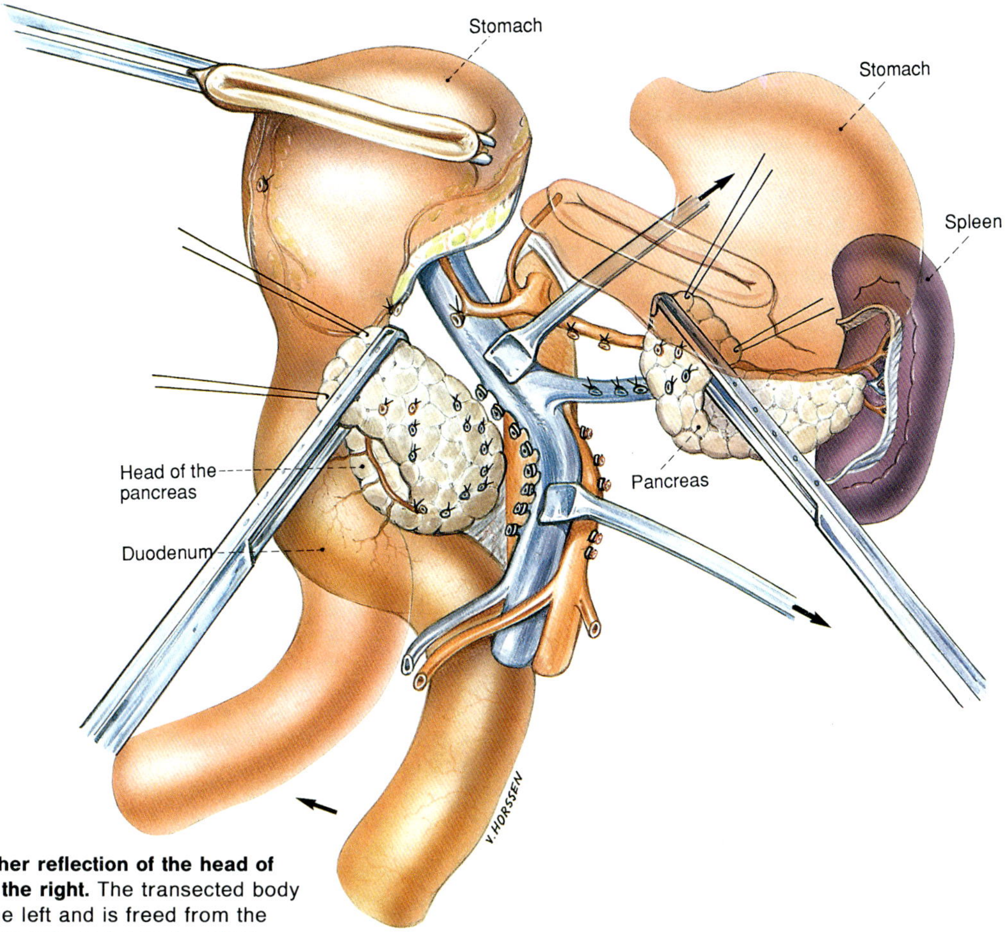

Fig. 7.1.**14   Further reflection of the head of the pancreas to the right.** The transected body is reflected to the left and is freed from the underlying splenic vein and splenic artery after careful isolation, ligation and transection of a number of venous and arterial branches. The head of the pancreas is freed from the superior mesenteric vessels (artery and vein) all along its attachments to the base of the mesentery

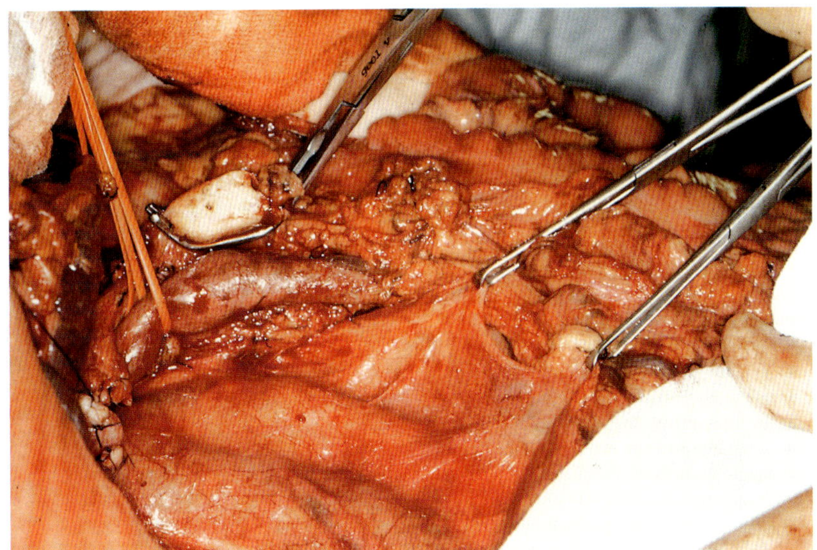

Fig. 7.1.**15   The portal vein is mobilized and lifted up with a vessel loop.** This allows isolation, ligation and transection of a number of venous branches originating from its posterior surface

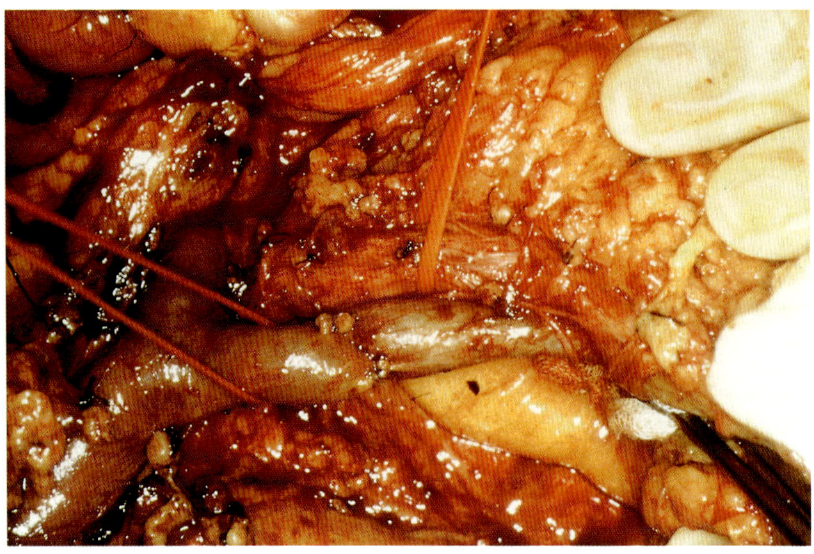

Fig. 7.1.**16   The superior mesenteric artery is dissected free from lymphatics** and isolated with vessel loops

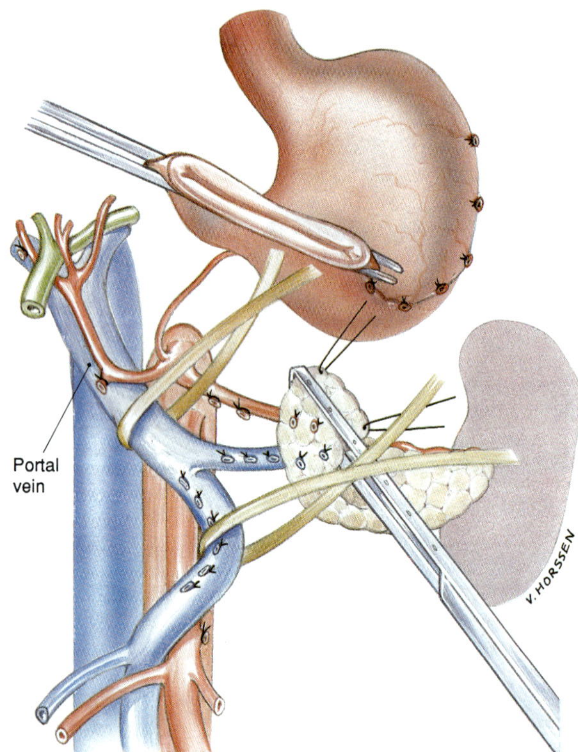

Fig. 7.1.**17   After resection of the uncinate process,** the entire specimen is removed

aticojejunal anastomosis, and thus to perform the whole procedure with an acceptable early mortality.

We feel that subtotal duodenopancreatectomy is associated with a better quality of life than total pancreatectomy, and that is justified when we consider the method of choice for the management of patients with pancreatic duct, ampullary and distal bile duct carcinoma (Trede 1987).

References

Ashton SJ, Longmire WP Jr. Pancreaticoduodenal resection: twenty years experience. Arch Surg 1981; 106: 813.

Braasch JW, Gray BN. Considerations that lower pancreatoduodenectomy mortality. Am J Surg 1977; 133: 480–484.

Braasch JW, Deziel DJ, Rossi RL, et al. Pyloric and gastric preserving pancreatic resection: experience with 87 patients. Ann Surg 1986; 204: 411–418.

Brooks JR, Culebras JM. Cancer of the pancreas: palliative operation, Whipple procedure or total pancreatectomy. Am J Surg 1976; 131: 516–523.

Cooperman AM, et al. Pancreatoduodenal resection and total pancreatectomy: an institutional review. Surgery 1982; 90: 703–707.

Crist DW, Sitzmann JV, Cameron JL. Improved hospital morbidity, mortality and survival after the Whipple procedure. Ann Surg 1987; 206: 358–365.

Edis AJ, Kierman PD, Taylor WF. Attempted curative resection of ductal carcinoma of pancreas: review of Mayo Clinic experience. Mayo Clin Proc 1980; 55: 531–539.

Grace PA, Pitt HA, Tompkins R, den Besten L, Longmire WP Jr. Decreased morbidity and mortality after pancreaticoduodenectomy. Am J Surg 1986; 151: 141.

Hertner FP, Cooperman AM, et al. Surgical experience with pancreatic and periampullary cancer. Ann Surg 1982; 195: 274–281.

Ihse I, Lilja P, Arnesjö B, Bengmark S. Total pancreatectomy for cancer: an appraisal of 65 cases. Ann Surg 1977; 186: 675–703.

Lerut JP, Gianello PR, Otte JB, Kestens PJ. Pancreaticoduodenal resection: surgical experience and evaluation of risk factors in 103 patients. Ann Surg 1984; 199: 432–437.

Longmire WP, Traverso LW. The Whipple procedure and other standard operative procedures to pancreatic cancer. Cancer 1981; 47: 1706–1711.

Mannell A, van Heerden J, Weiland LH, Ilstrup DM. Factors influencing survival after resection for ductal adenocarcinoma of the pancreas. Ann Surg 1986; 203: 403–407.

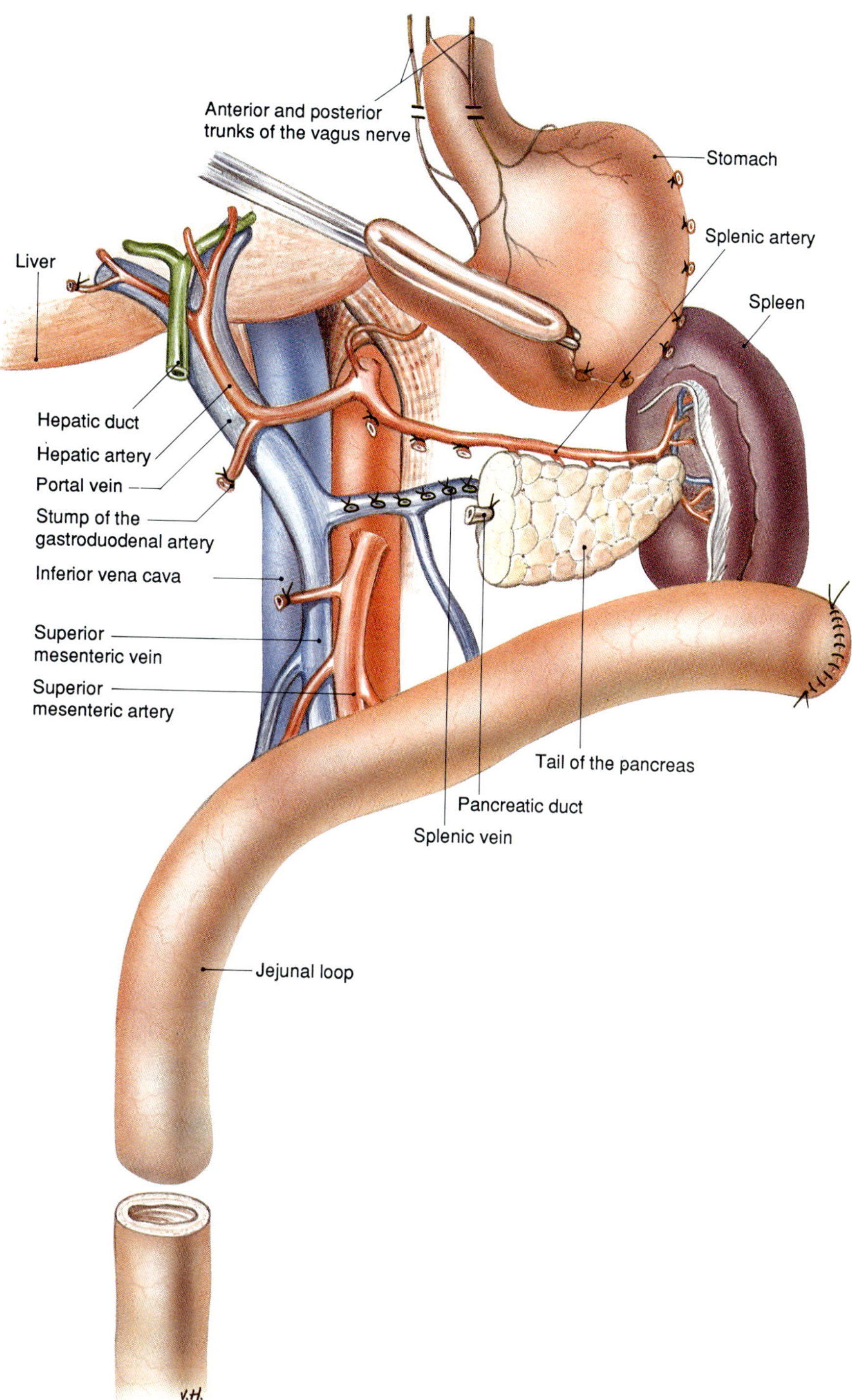

Fig. 7.1.**18**   **Preparation for the reconstruction of gastrointestinal continuity** with isolation of a proximal jejunal segment

Sato T, Saitoh Y, Moto N, Matsuno S. Follow-up studies of radical resection for pancreaticoduodenal cancer. Ann Surg 1977; 186: 581–587.

Scott WH, Dean RH, Parker T, Anant G. The role of vagotomy in pancreaticoduodenectomy. Ann Surg 1980; 192: 688–696.

Tsuchiya R, Tomioka T, Izawa K, et al. Collective review of small carcinomas of the pancreas. Ann Surg 1986; 203: 77–81.

Trede M. The surgical treatment of pancreatic carcinoma: the surgeon's dilemma. Br J Surg 1987; 74: 79–80.

Van Heerden JA, McIlrath DC, Dozois RR, et al. Radical pancreatoduodenectomy: a procedure to be abandoned. Mayo Clin Proc 1981; 56: 601–700.

7.2   Total Pancreatectomy

N.J. Lygidakis and M.N. van der Heyde

Introduction

Currently, total pancreatectomy is regarded with scepticism concerning its value as a procedure of choice for the management of pancreatic duct, distal common bile duct and ampullary carcinoma. The arguments in favor of total pancreatectomy, associating it with lower mortality, a higher rate of radical resection, and longer survival than subtotal duodenopancreatectomy, no longer find support (Trede 1987). Mortality, early morbidity and long-term survival are not directly related to the extent of pancreatic resection. Moreover, total pancreatectomy is associated with significant side-effects and postoperative sequelae that mar the quality of postoperative life (Braasch et al. 1986, Crist et al. 1987, Grace et al. 1986, Hertner et al. 1982, Jones et al. 1985, Mannell et al. 1986, Pram and McLine 1975, Trede 1985, 1987, Tsuchiya et al. 1986, Van Heerden et al. 1981).

Total pancreatectomy is carried out in our department in patients with 1) carcinoma located in the body or tail of the pancreas; 2) positive histological results from frozen biopsies taken from the margins of the resected pancreas during sub-total duodenopancreatectomy; and 3) occasionally in patients with a small pancreatic duct of less than 1 millimeter in transverse diameter and very friable pancreatic tissue.

Technique

Standard total pancreatectomy involves resection of the entire pancreas with the duodenum, gallbladder, the distal portion of the common bile duct, the distal half of the stomach, the spleen and 10–15 cm of the proximal jejunum (Fig. 7.2.**1**). We start with a bilateral subcostal incision (Fig. 7.1.**3**, p. 263), which gives access to both the right and left portions of the gland. We continue by mobilizing the duodenum and the head of the pancreas from the inferior vena cava and aorta in order to obtain maximum mobility of the pancreatic gland for a precise assessment of the existing pathological situation (Figs. 7.1.**5**, 7.1.**6**, p. 264, 265).

The gastrocolic ligament is severed after previous step-by-step dissection and ligation of the gastrocolic vessels (Fig. 7.1.**8**, p. 267). The stomach is reflected cephalad, and the anterior surface of the pancreas is now completely free for further exploration (Fig. 7.2.**2**). The hepatoduodenal ligament is

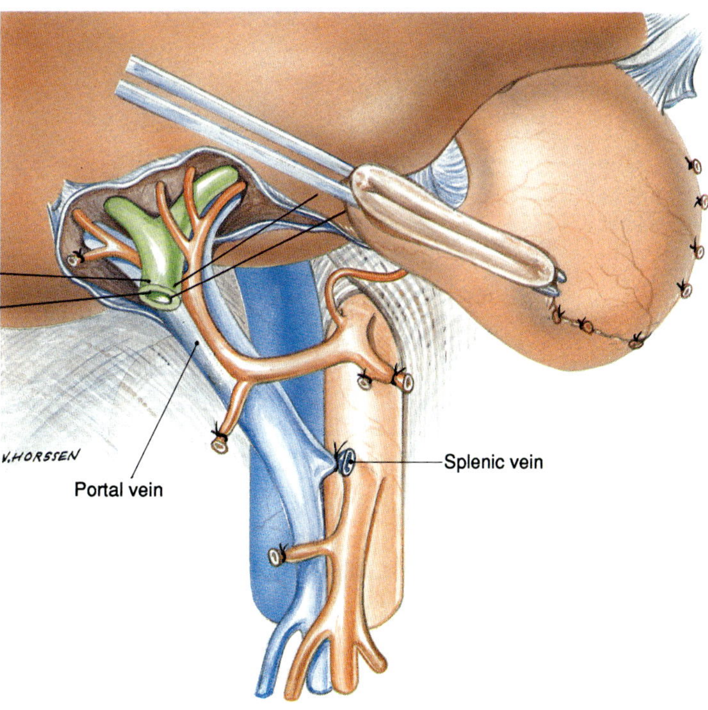

Fig. 7.2.**1** **Operative site** following total pancreatectomy

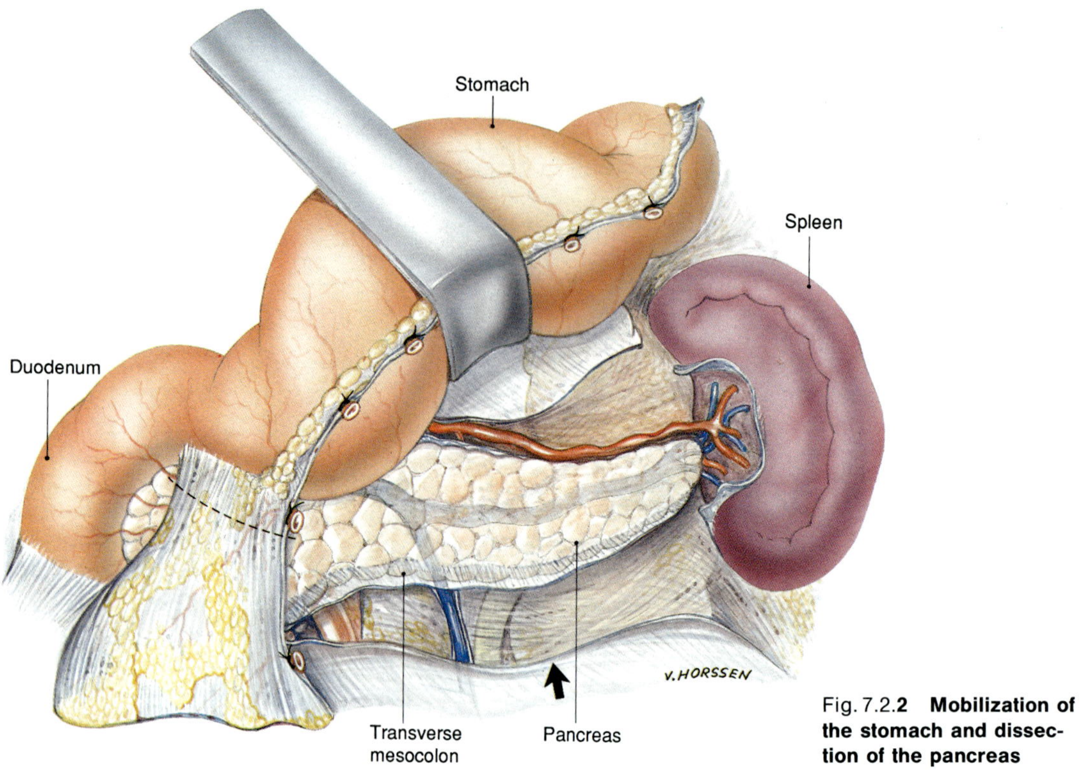

Fig. 7.2.**2 Mobilization of the stomach and dissection of the pancreas**

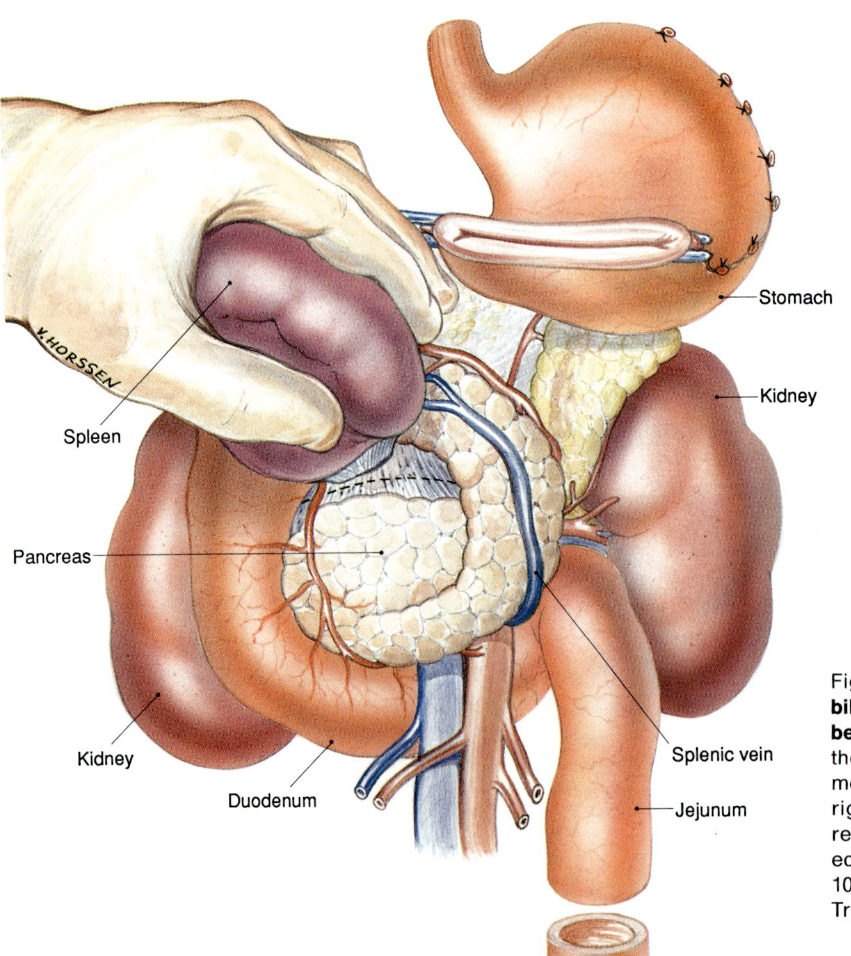

Fig. 7.2.**3 Hemigastrectomy and bilateral truncal vagotomy have been carried out.** The spleen and the tail of the pancreas are mobilized and reflected to the right. The splenic artery has already been ligated and transected. The jejunum is transected 10 cm distal from the ligament of Treitz

dissected and the gallbladder is removed after transection of the common hepatic duct just below its bifurcation (Figs. 7.1.**9**, 7.1.**10**, p. 268).

Frozen biopsies are taken from the proximal margin of the transected common hepatic duct, and its distal end is further dissected all along its right side, just lateral from the hepatic artery and just above the portal vein, which is visible in the depths of the plane of dissection. During the dissection, the left index finger is interposed between the anterior surface of the portal vein and the posterior surface of the common bile duct in order to have full control of the portal vein.

The portal vein and hepatic artery are isolated via vessel loops and completely skeletonized from the surrounding lymphatics. Via a further dissection all along the hepatic artery, we reach its junction with the gastroduodenal artery, which is doubly ligated and transected. The hepatic artery is further dissected up to its origin at the celiac axis. This gives access to the origin of the splenic artery, which is also dissected, skeletonized, ligated and

transected. At this point, hemigastrectomy with bilateral truncal vagotomy is routinely carried out.

The spleen is then freed from its attachments to the splenic flexure, diaphragm and stomach. It is dissected together with the tail of the pancreas from the underlying left kidney and left adrenal gland (Fig. 7.2.**3**) and reflected to the right. The proximal jejunum is transected 10–15 cm from the ligament of Treitz.

The pancreas is carefully dissected along its superior and inferior border and freed from the underlying structures. This gives access to the aorta and superior mesenteric artery. The latter is now dissected and skeletonized from its surrounding lymphatics (Fig. 7.1.**16**, p. 272). By means of further reflection to the right, the splenomesenteric junction is reached, and we proceed with double ligation and transection of the splenic vein (Fig. 7.2.**4**). After double ligation of the venous branches from the superior mesenteric vein and the portal vein, the pancreas is prepared for resection. The superior mesenteric vein and artery are now dissected and

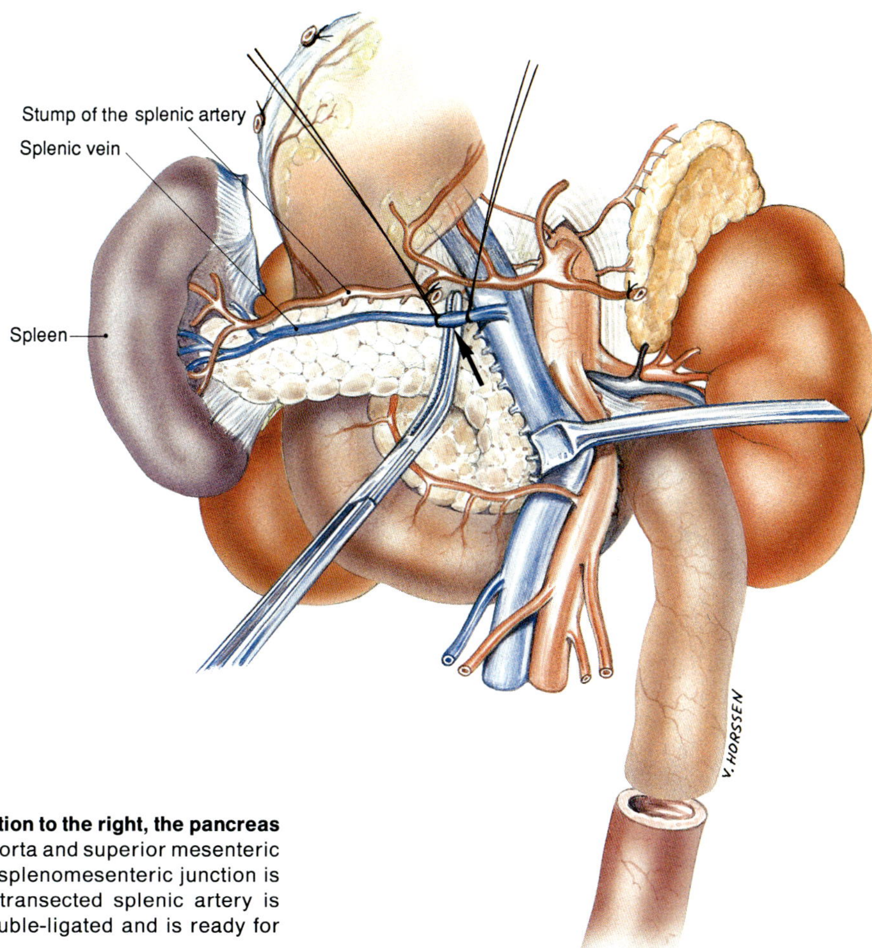

Fig. 7.2.**4   With further reflection to the right, the pancreas is freed** from the underlying aorta and superior mesenteric artery until the region of the splenomesenteric junction is reached. The stump of the transected splenic artery is seen. The splenic vein is double-ligated and is ready for transection

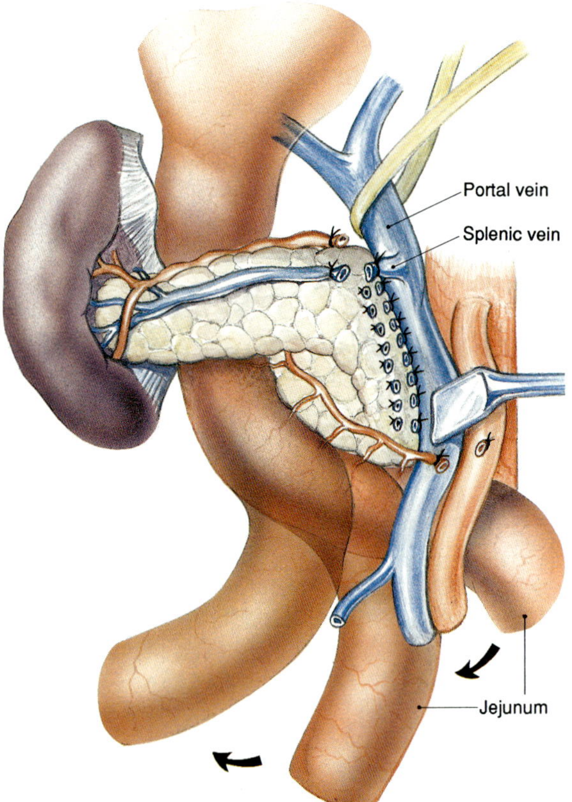

Fig. 7.2.5 The splenic vein is transected. The various branches arising from the posterior surface of the portal vein are one by one isolated, ligated and transected, and the transected jejunum is transferred step-by-step under the mesenteric vessels to the right abdomen

their posterior branches to the pancreas are individually isolated, ligated and transected. We are now ready to complete the resection of the pancreas up to the border of the superior mesenteric artery, which is isolated.

Dissection of the gastrocolic ligament is now completed. The right gastroepiploic artery is ligated and transected. The ligament is further dissected up to the anterior surface of the pancreatic head, and the retroperitoneal part of the duodenum up to the duodenojejunal junction. This junction is completely freed from the ligament of Treitz by means of meticulous dissection. The jejunum is now transected 10–15 cm from the ligament of Treitz. The dissection of the jejunum is continued and its proximal segment is transferred beneath the mesenteric vessels into the right abdomen (Figs. 7.1.**12**, 7.1.**13**, p. 270, Fig. 7.2.**5**). Using the technique described in Chapter 7.1, the entire pancreas with the uncinate process is transected from the base of the mesentery and taken out with the specimen, consisting of the spleen, the distal part of the stomach,

the duodenum, 10 centimeters of the proximal jejunum, the gallbladder and the distal common bile duct (Fig. 7.2.**1**). Alimentary continuity is restored by a side-to-side gastrojejunostomy and an end-to-side hepaticojejunostomy (Fig. 7.2.**6**).

Another variant of total pancreatectomy is necessary when, during subtotal pancreatectomy, the results of the frozen biopsy indicate that there is residual disease in the pancreatic remnant. Under these circumstances one may proceed with further dissection and transection after double ligation of the splenic artery and splenic vein. Dissection is continued all the way along the superior and inferior borders of the pancreas, which is freed from the underlying structures in the retroperitoneal space and taken out with the spleen after mobilization from its attachments.

Discussion

Total pancreatectomy is not to be considered as an operation of choice but as a necessity in extensive pancreatic malignancy involving the body and tail, and in a number of patients suffering from pancreatic head carcinoma (Braasch et al. 1986, Crist et al. 1987, Grace et al. 1986, Hertner et al. 1982, Jones et al. 1985, Mannell et al. 1986, Pram and McLine 1975, Trede 1985, 1987, Tsuchiya et al. 1986, van Heerden et al. 1981).

Of our first 100 pancreatic resections for pancreatic head carcinoma, 78 patients underwent subtotal duodenopancreatectomy and 22 patients total pancreatectomy. The proportion of patients with free resectional margins after total pancreatectomy was not significantly different from that after subtotal pancreatectomy (see Chapter 7.7).

Comments

Theoretically, total pancreatectomy should improve the results of surgical treatment of pancreatic carcinoma. The tumor may be well-disseminated and may spread during pancreatic duct transection, the process may be multifocal, and the spread and extent of the tumor may be difficult to assess during the operation, even when frozen biopsies are taken from the margins of the transected pancreas. Apart from these considerations, leakage at the pancreaticojejunostomy contributes to increased mortality and morbidity. Leaving behind the spleen and the tail of the pancreas removes the possibility of optimal lymphadenectomy. In dealing with an aggressive disease like pancreatic cancer, therefore, an aggressive rather than a defeating approach might be thought

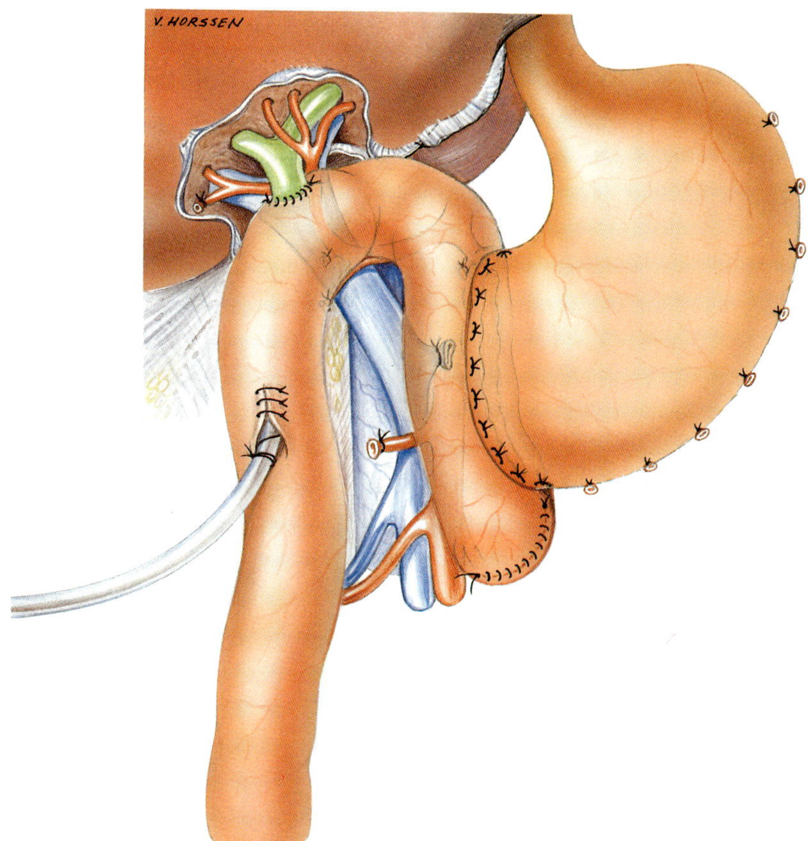

Fig. 7.2.**6   Reconstruction of alimentary continuity after total pancreatectomy** via a side-to-side gastrojejunostomy and end-to-side hepaticojejunostomy

to deserve consideration (Levine et al. 1978, Moossa et al. 1979, Tryka and Brookes 1979). In practice, however, reported results do not support this view (see the references cited at the beginning of this section). Today, with improvements in surgical technique, subtotal duodenopancreatectomy should be considered as the operation of choice for the majority of patients, and can be recommended as such.

References

Braasch JW, Deziel DJ, Rossi RL, et al. Pyloric and gastric preserving pancreatic resection: experience with 87 patients. Ann Surg 1986; 204: 411–418.

Crist DW, Sitzmann JV, Cameron JL. Improved hospital morbidity, mortality and survival after the Whipple procedure. Ann Surg 1987; 206: 358–365.

Grace PA, Pitt HA, Tompkins RK, et al. Decreased morbidity and mortality after pancreatoduodenotomy. Am J Surg 1986; 152: 141–149.

Hertner F, Cooperman A, Ahlborn T, Antinou C. Surgical experience with pancreatic and periampullary cancer. Ann Surg 1982; 195: 274–281.

Jones BA, Langer B, Tailor B, Giroti M. Periampullary tumors: which ones should be resected. Am J Surg 1985; 149: 47–52.

Levine B, Remine WH, Herman RF, et al. Cancer of the pancreas. Am J Surg 1978; 135: 185–191.

Mannell A, van Heerden JA, Weiland LH, Ilstrup DM. Factors influencing survival after resection from ductal adenocarcinoma of the pancreas. Ann Surg 1986; 203: 403–407.

Moossa AR, Lewis JH, Malkie CR. Surgical treatment of pancreatic cancer. Mayo Clin Proc 1979; 54: 468–472.

Pram MB, McLine WH. Further evaluation of total pancreatectomy. Arch Surg 1975; 110: 506–512.

Trede M. The surgical treatment of pancreatic carcinoma. Surgery 1985; 97: 28–35.

Trede M. Treatment of pancreatic carcinoma: the surgeon's dilemma. Br J Surg 1987; 74: 79–80.

Tsuchiya R, Noda T, Harada N, et al. Collective review of small carcinomas of the pancreas. Ann Surg 1986; 203: 77–81.

Tryka AF, Brookes JR. Histopathology in the evaluation of total pancreatectomy for ductal carcinoma. Ann Surg 1979; 190: 373–381.

Van Heerden JC, McIlrath DC, Dozois RR, et al. Radical pancreatoduodenectomy: a procedure to be abandoned. Mayo Clin Proc 1981; 56: 601–700.

7.3   The Contribution of Vascular Surgery to the Surgical Management of Pancreatic Head Carcinoma

N.J. Lygidakis and M.N. van der Heyde

Introduction

Pancreatic head carcinoma, i.e. pancreatic duct, distal common bile duct and ampullary carcinoma, offers a number of options for management. The lesions may be bypassed without resection, as suggested by some authors (particularly in patients with suspected pancreatic duct carcinoma) in order to reduce the mortality and morbidity of resection when cure or long-term palliation cannot realistically be expected (Cotton 1984, Crile 1970, Leduska et al. 1977, Shapiro 1975). This policy requires an exact preoperative differentiation between ampullary, pancreatic and distal common bile duct carcinoma, in order to avoid bypassing potentially curable ampullary, distal bile duct and duodenal tumors. This may be difficult and unreliable (see Chapter 7.8). From the practical point of view, resection remains the only chance of cure.

There is no doubt that the results after various kinds of palliative medical or surgical management are associated with short-term survival (Braasch et al. 1986, Crile 1970, Leduska et al. 1977, Shapiro 1975). Should pancreatic resection therefore be carried out whenever feasible, even in the form of en bloc resection of the pancreas combined with lymph node clearance and if necessary with resection of the superior mesenteric artery, middle colic artery, celiac axis and portal vein? (Fortner 1985) From the literature available, it seems likely that this approach is not justified (Cotton 1984, Crist et al. 1987, Grace et al. 1986, Jones et al. 1985, Lygidakis et al. 1986, Mannell et al. 1986, Trede 1985). There is evidence that carcinoma which extends outside the confines of the pancreas and peripancreatic tissues is not amenable to treatment with resectional surgery (Jones et al. 1985).

Occasionally, however, the surgeon has to anticipate a situation in which the tumor invades regional vascular structures without further extension. In these cases, vascular resectional techniques may be indicated.

In this chapter, the surgical techniques used with our first 100 patients who underwent vascular resection are outlined.

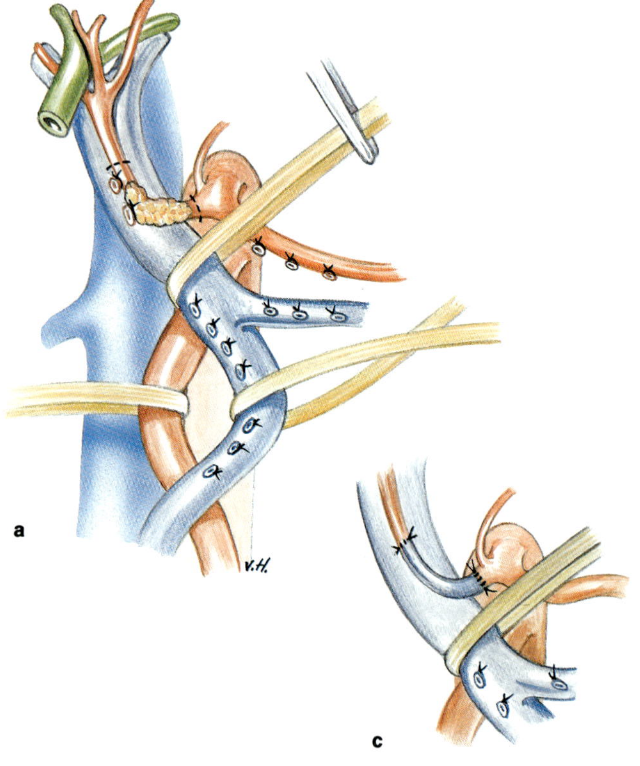

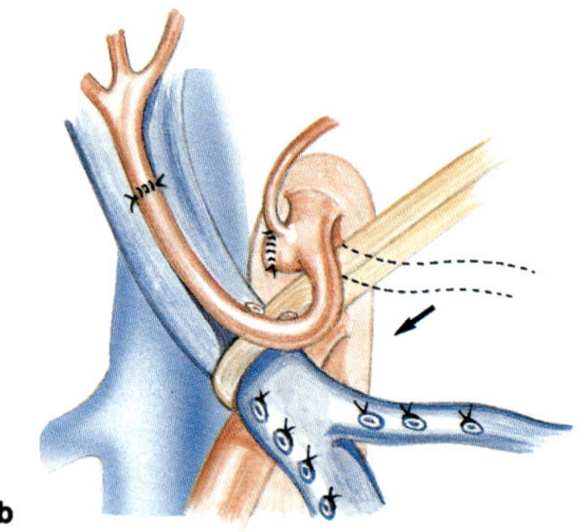

Fig. 7.3.1 **Resection and reconstruction of the common hepatic artery** after invasion by cancer
a End-to-end anastomosis after resection
b Reconstruction via an end-to-end anastomosis between the transected proximal margin of the hepatic artery and the splenic artery
c Reconstruction by means of a venous graft

Technique

Vascular resection during pancreatic resection for pancreatic duct, distal common bile duct or ampullary carcinoma is feasible in both total and subtotal pancreatectomy (Fortner 1985).

The technical options in resection of the hepatic artery are shown in Figures 7.3.**1a**, **b** and **c**. Reconstruction after resection is carried out by an end-to-end anastomosis, by interposing a venous graft, or by using the splenic artery, which can be anastomosed end-to-end with the transected proximal margin of the common hepatic artery. In the latter case, splenectomy is always carried out as a supplementary procedure, whether the pancreatic resection was total or subtotal.

The technical options for the portal vein are illustrated in Figures 7.3.**2a**, **b** and **c**. Portal resection is carried out after prior isolation of the portal vein above and below its invaded segment. In the case of en bloc total pancreatectomy, the tail of the pancreas and the mobilized spleen are reflected to the right, and the splenic vein and splenic artery are ligated and transected (Fig. 7.2.**3**, p. 276). The portal vein is isolated above and below its invaded segment using vascular clamps, and transected (Fig. 7.3.**3a**, **b**). Through a further reflection of the entire pancreas to the right and the transected segment of the portal vein, we reach the border of

the superior mesenteric artery. The uncinate process is resected after previous isolation, ligation and transection of a number of small arterial branches originating from the posterior surface of the superior mesenteric artery. Reconstruction of the transected portal vein takes place either by means of a venous graft or by end-to-end anastomosis, depending on the length of the transected segments (Figs. 7.3.**2b**, **c**, 7.3.**3b**).

In subtotal pancreatectomy, we mobilize the superior and inferior border of the pancreas and free its posterior surface from the underlying splenic vein and splenic artery by ligating and transecting a number of venous and arterial branches (Fig. 7.3.**4**). The pancreas is transected to the left of the splenomesenteric junction, while its proximal and distal margins are further dissected and freed from the underlying splenic vein and splenic artery (Fig. 7.3.**5**).

The pancreatic head and duodenum are reflected to the right, as in en bloc total pancreatectomy (Fig. 7.3.**6**). The portal vein is transected after isolation of the splenomesenteric junction, and of the proximal and distal margins of its invaded segment, by vascular clamps. Reconstruction takes place either with an end-to-end anastomosis, or with a venous transplant, with or without inclusion of the splenic vein (Fig. 7.3.**6**, inset).

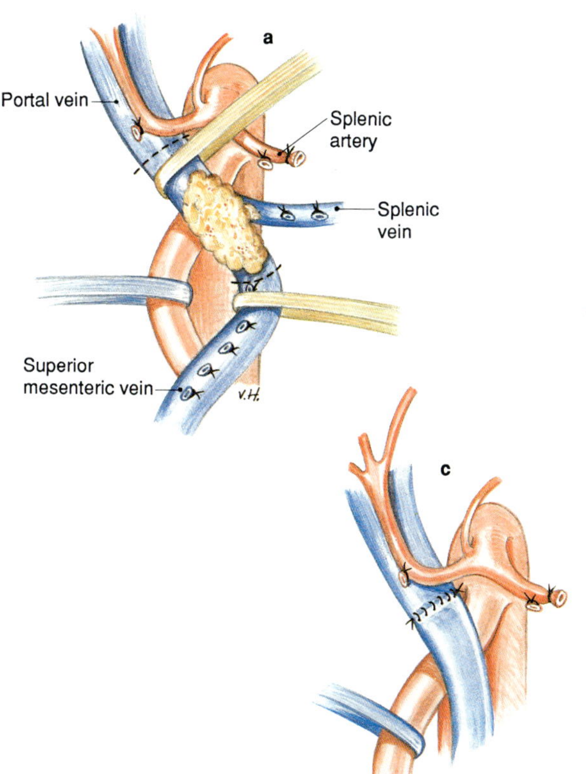

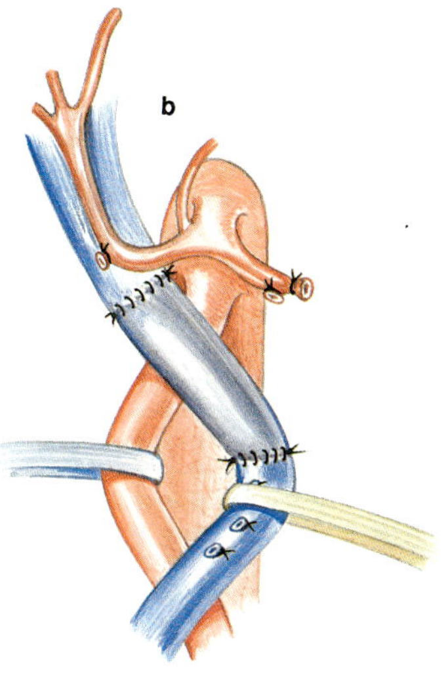

Fig. 7.3.2 Resection and reconstruction of the portal vein after invasion in the region of the splenomesenteric junction
a Extent of invasion
b Reconstruction using a venous graft
c Reconstruction by direct end-to-end anastomosis

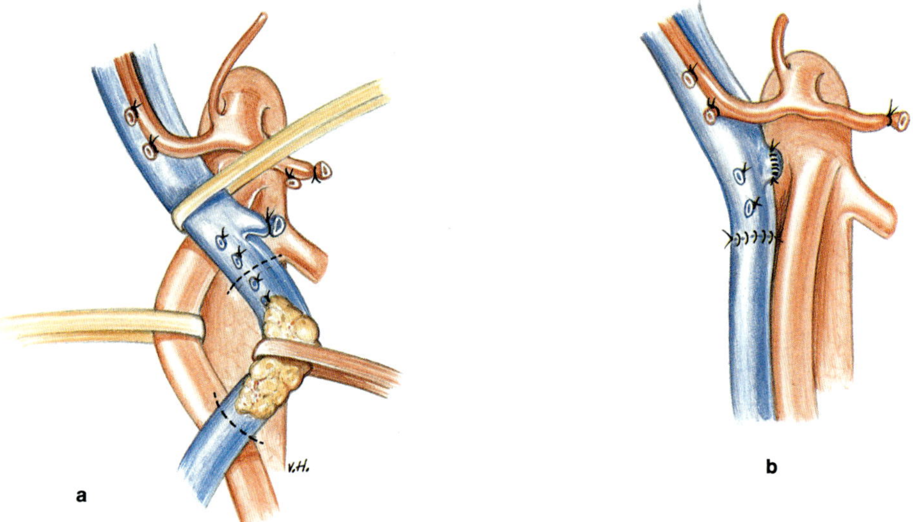

Fig. 7.3.**3a**   **Invasion of the portal vein below the splenomesenteric junction**
b   Resection and reconstruction via an end-to-end anastomosis

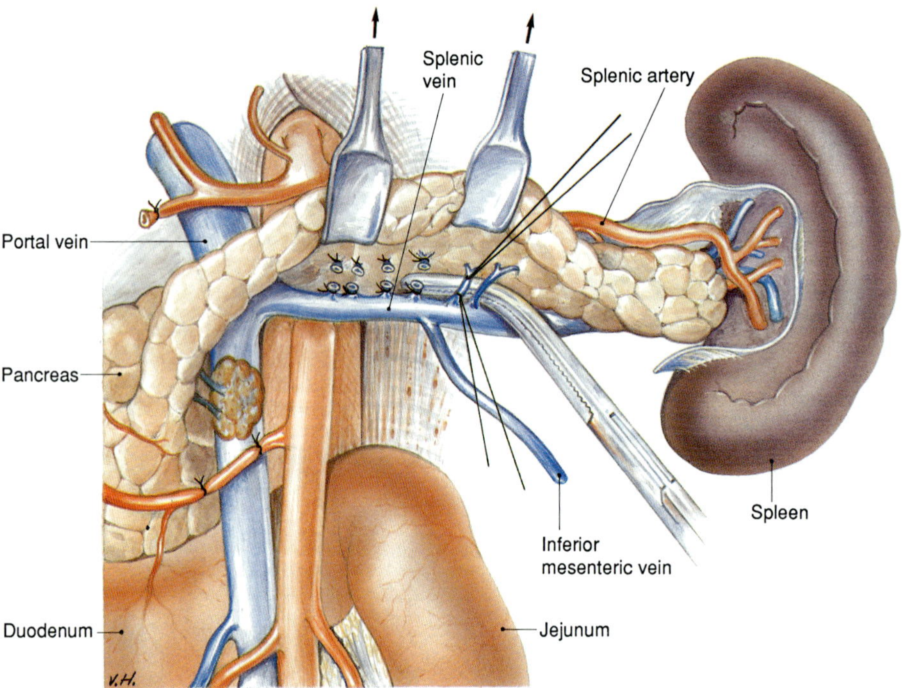

Fig. 7.3.**4**   **Dissection of the superior and inferior borders of the pancreas** and dissection of its posterior surface from the underlying splenic vein

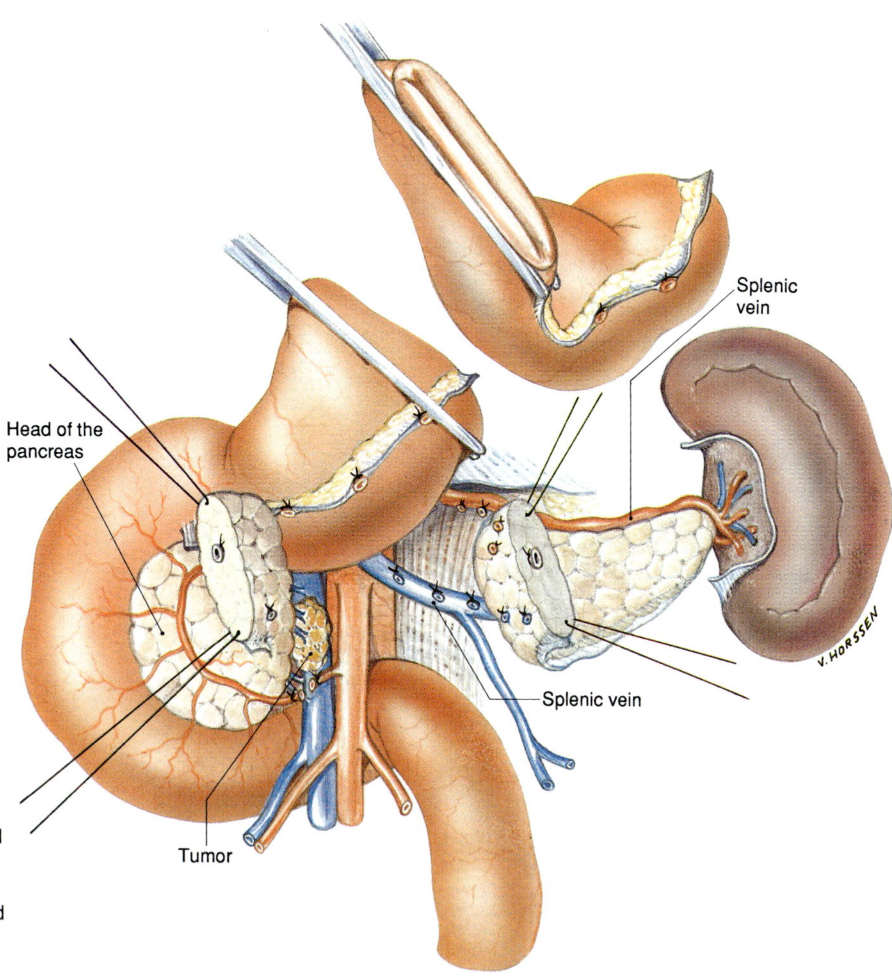

Fig. 7.3.**5   Transection of
the pancreas.** The splenic
artery and splenic vein
are isolated, and the head
of the pancreas is reflected to the right. The portal
vein is well visualized and
its invaded segment can
be easily traced

The various forms of invasion of the superior mesenteric artery and the surgical options for correction are shown in Figures 7.3.**7 a**, **b** and **c**. It is important to mobilize the body and tail of the pancreas sufficiently, reflecting them to the right (Fig. 7.3.**8**), in order to obtain adequate access to the aorta. This allows the isolation, after step-by-step dissection, of the superior mesenteric artery from its origin. The invaded segment is resected and reconstructed with an end-to-end anastomosis, or with a venous graft interposed between the transected margins of the superior mesenteric artery, or by means of the splenic artery, which is anastomosed end-to-end with the transected distal segment of the superior mesenteric artery (Figs. 7.3.**7**, 7.3.**9**).

Finally, in the case of invasion of the inferior vena cava, the involved segment is isolated and the inferior vena cava is transected above and below the invaded segment and then reconstructed with an end-to-end anastomosis (Fig. 7.3.**10**) or with a venous graft.

Discussion

Vascular resection and reconstruction is considered as a procedure of necessity during pancreatic resection when we face local vascular invasion which has not been assessed before surgery. During the period under study, a total of 100 patients underwent pancreatic resection. Thirteen of these patients underwent resection and reconstruction of the vessels. Eleven survived the operation and remained alive for various intervals. We believe that eventually the presented technical options may well be used in order to enable the surgeon to overcome difficult situations of unexpected vascular invasion during pancreatic resection for carcinoma. We did not consider these procedures as curative, but they are a useful alternative which enables us to overcome unexpected situations.

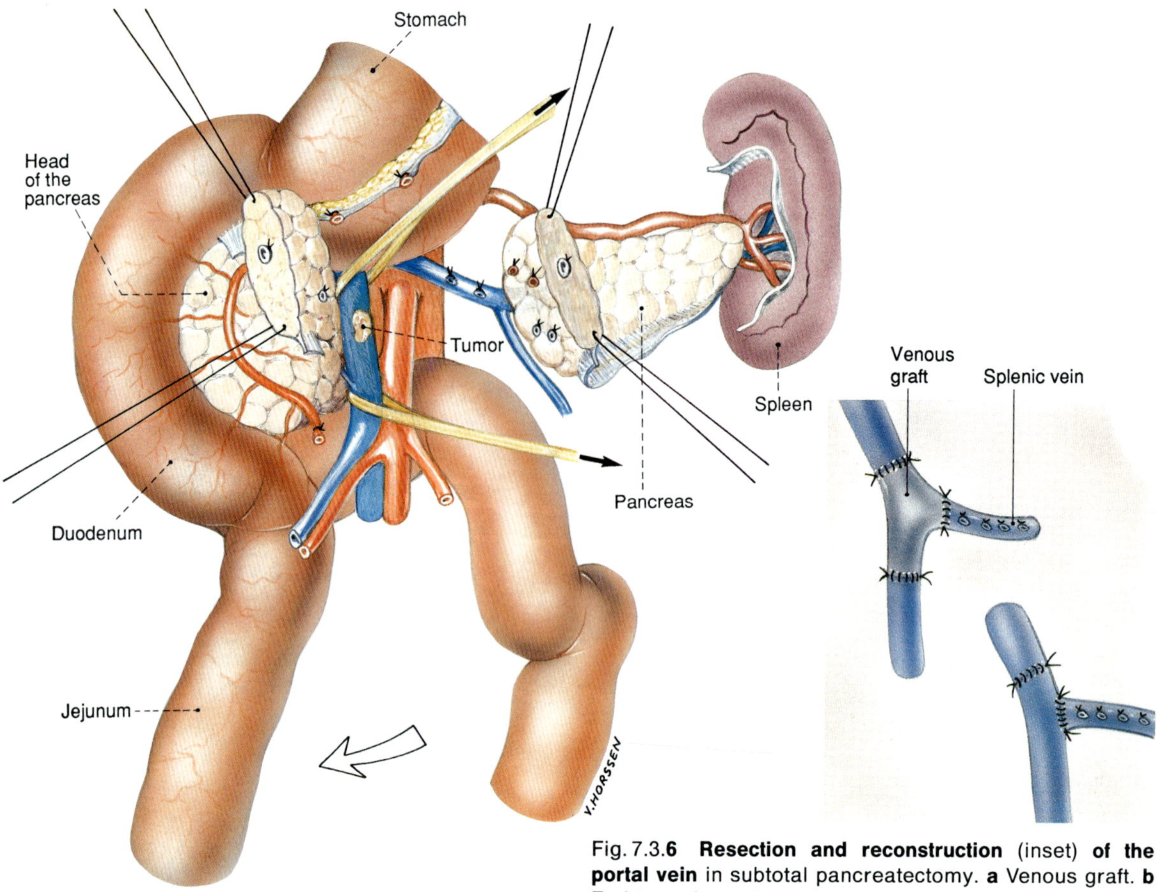

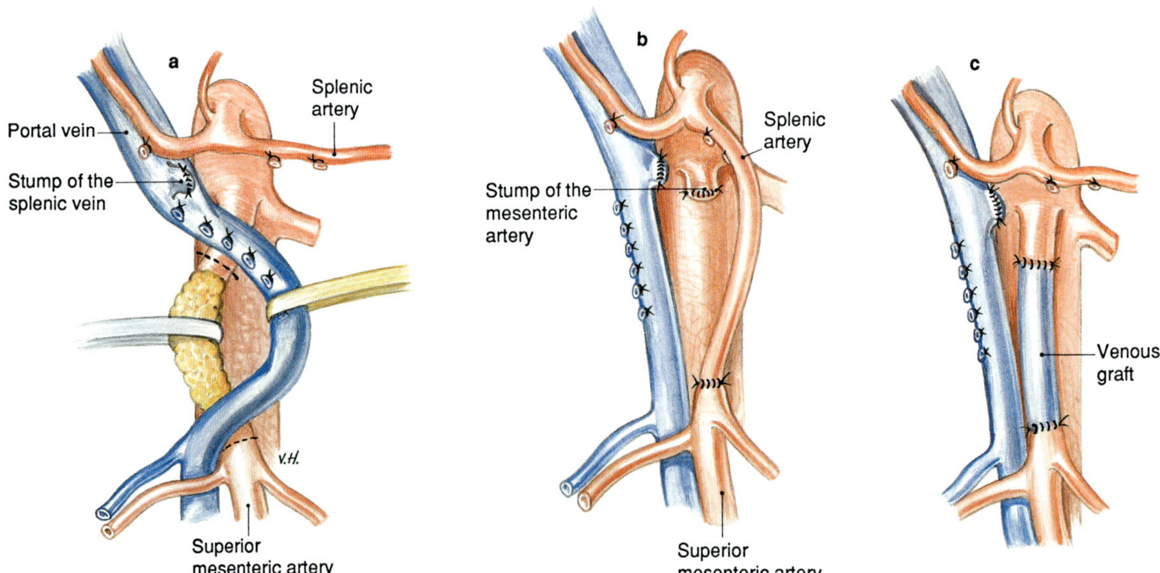

Fig. 7.3.**6** **Resection and reconstruction** (inset) **of the portal vein** in subtotal pancreatectomy. **a** Venous graft. **b** End-to-end anastomosis

Fig. 7.3.**7** **Invasion of the superior mesenteric artery**
a Resection of the superior mesenteric artery from its origin at the aorta
b Reconstruction with an end-to-end anastomosis using the splenic artery
c Reconstruction with a venous graft interposed between the transected segments of the superior mesenteric artery

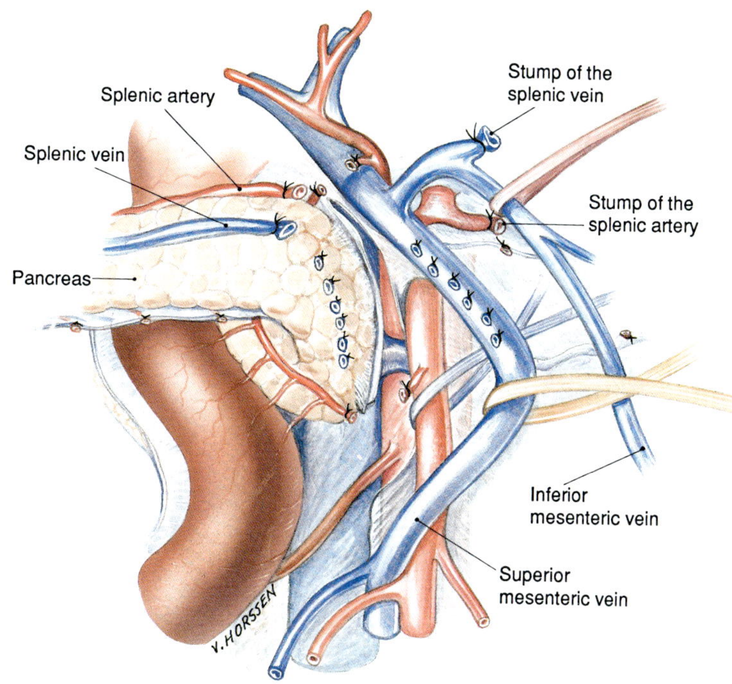

Fig. 7.3.**8**   **Mobilization of the pancreas**

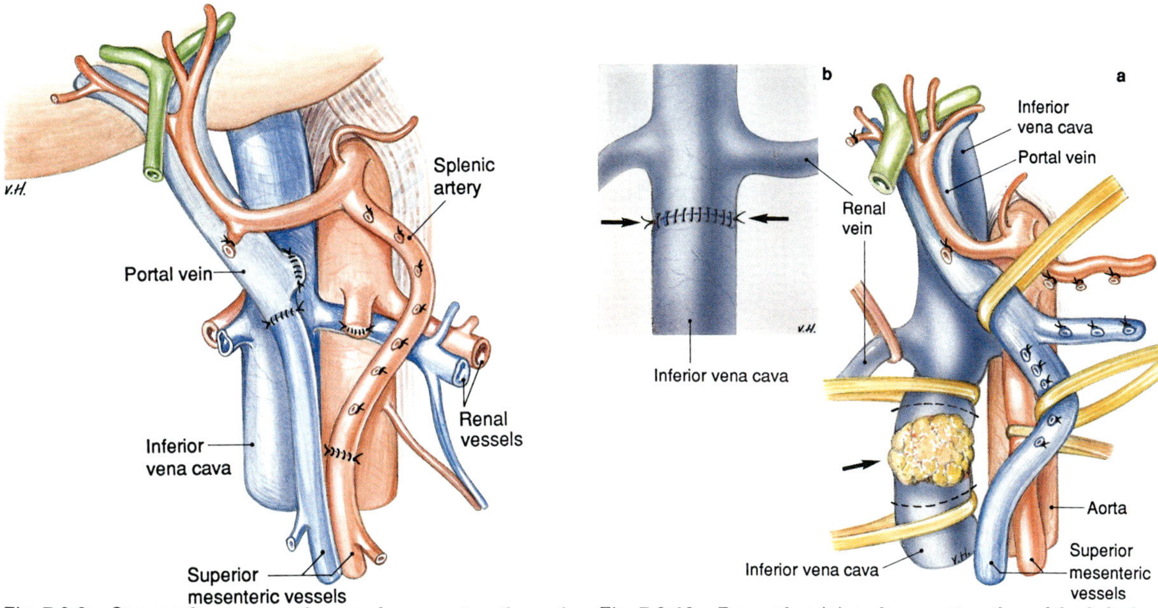

Fig. 7.3.**9**   **Concomitant resection and reconstruction of both the portal vein and the superior mesenteric artery**

Fig. 7.3.**10**   **Resection (a) and reconstruction of the inferior vena cava** by end-to-end anastomosis (**b**). Transection lines: – – –

References

Braasch S, Rossi R, Watkins E, et al. Pyloric and gastric preserving pancreatic resection. Ann Surg 1986; 204: 411–418.

Cotton PB. Endoscopic methods for relief of malignant obstructive jaundice. World J Surg 1984; 8: 542–562.

Crile G Jr. Advantages of bypass operations over radical pancreaticoduodenectomy in treatment of pancreatic carcinoma. Surg Gynecol Obstet 1970; 130: 1049.

Crist DW, Sitzmann JV, Cameron JL. Improved hospital morbidity, mortality and survival after the Whipple procedure. Ann Surg 1987; 206: 358–365.

Fortner JG. Technique of regional subtotal and total pancreatectomy. Am J Surg 1985; 150: 539.

Grace PA, Pitt HA, Tompkins R, den Besten L, Longmire WP. Decreased morbidity and mortality after pancreaticoduodenectomy. Am J Surg 1986; 151: 141.

Jones BA, Langer B, Taylor B, Giroti M. Periampullary tumors: which ones should be resected. Am J Surg 1985; 149: 46–52.

Leduska NJ, Dent TH, Lindemander SM. Results of palliative operation for carcinoma of the pancreas. Arch Surg 1977; 103: 330–334.

Lygidakis NJ, Brummelkamp WH, Tytgat GNJ. Periampullary and pancreatic head carcinoma: facts and factors influencing mortality, survival and quality of postoperative life. Am J Gastroenterol 1986; 82: 968.

Mannell H, van Heerden J, Weiland LH. Factors influencing survival after resection for ductal adenocarcinoma of pancreas. Ann Surg 1986; 203: 403–407.

Shapiro TM. Adenocarcinoma of the pancreas: a statistical analysis of bypass vs Whipple resection in good-risk patients. Ann Surg 1975; 182: 15–21.

Trede M. Surgical treatment of pancreatic carcinomas. Surgery 1985; 97: 28–35.

7.4 Reconstruction of Alimentary Continuity After Subtotal Duodenopancreatectomy

N.J. Lygidakis and M.N. van der Heyde

Introduction

One of the main problems the surgeon faces after subtotal duodenopancreatectomy concerns the kind of reconstruction of alimentary continuity. This is reflected in the various technical approaches suggested by surgeons from all over the world (Ashton and Longmire 1981, Braasch et al. 1986, Cattell and Warren 1953, Kapur 1986, Lygidakis and Brummelkamp 1985, Ruilova and Hershey 1976, Sato et al. 1977, Shin 1982, Traverso and Longmire 1978). All of these approaches are specifically directed to overcoming the problems of anastomotic dehiscence (Pliam and Remine 1975), in particular the high risk of pancreaticojejunostomy leakage (Papachristou and Fortner 1981, Traverso and Longmire 1978), and the problems of long-term functional results with regard to steatorrhea, reflux gastropathy, peptic ulceration, dumping, etc. It is beyond question that the unpopularity of subtotal duodenopancreatectomy can be ascribed to the threat of leakage from the pancreatic anastomosis, which is associated with high morbidity and mortality (Gilsdorf and Spanos 1973, Pliam and Remine 1975). The incidence of anastomotic leakage has in the past been high (Cattell and Warren 1953, Gillsdorf and Spanos 1973, Pliam and Remine 1975, Shin 1982).

In September 1983, we developed a new technique for the reconstruction of alimentary continuity, the main objective of which was to anticipate and avoid these potential problems (Fig. 7.4.1) (Lygidakis and Brummelkamp 1985). When we designed this technique, we postulated that we

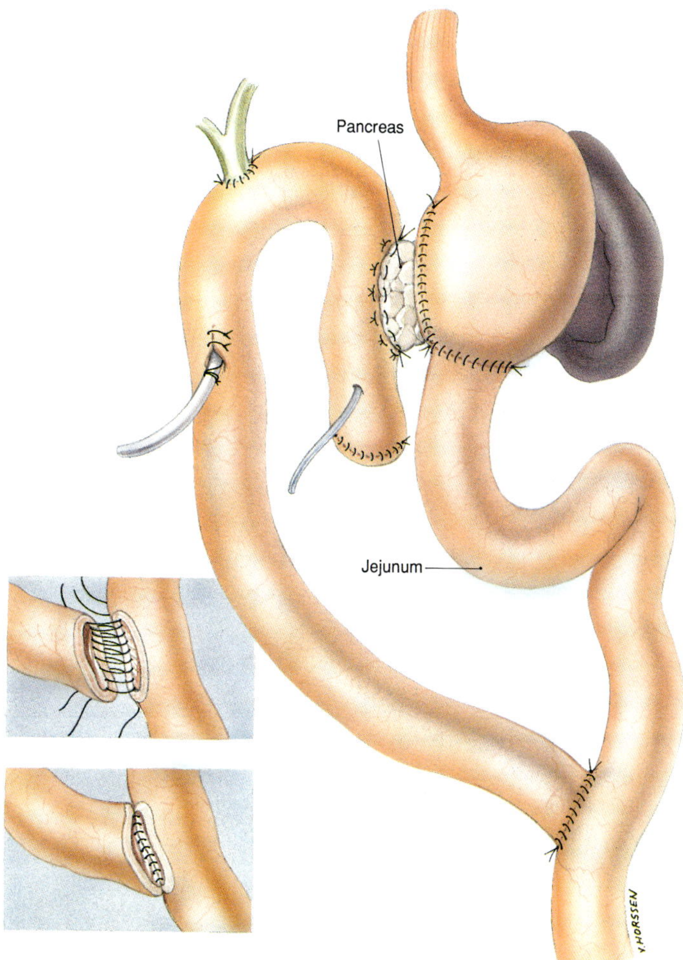

Fig. 7.4.1 **Reconstruction of alimentary continuity after subtotal duodenopancreatectomy** using two separate jejunal loops in a Roux-en-Y fashion, according to the technique developed at the Amsterdam clinic. Insets: creation of the end-to-side jejunojejunostomy

could possibly overcome or fulfill the following points. Firstly, any kind of overload of the jejunal loop used for fashioning the gastric, pancreatic and biliary anastomosis. We achieve this by using two separate jejunal loops, which are completely independent of each other, in a Roux-en-Y fashion. One is a 20–30 cm long isolated anisoperistaltic loop for the pancreatic and biliary anastomosis. The other forms the gastric anastomosis. In this way, oral feeding is possible early in the postoperative period, resulting in the patient being in a better nutritional condition.

Secondly, optimal conditions must be provided for the anastomotic healing process, particularly with regard to the pancreatic anastomosis, since this anastomosis remains the crucial point in the whole procedure (Papachristou and Fortner 1981). To achieve these optimal conditions, advantage is taken of the excellent healing potential of the jejunal mucosa. Jejunal mucosa is applied all along the rough surface of the pancreatic remnant, promoting a satisfactory healing process in the pancreaticojejunostomy.

Thirdly, the isolated anisoperistaltic jejunal loop used for the pancreatic and biliary anastomosis is designed to serve as a substitute for the patient's alimentary tract, and to imitate, or at least resemble, normal anatomic conditions. The purpose of joining this loop with the other loop in an end-to-side fashion, 60 cm distal from the gastrojejunostomy, is to achieve a function resembling that of the duodenum and ampulla of Vater.

From September 1983, 78 patients underwent consecutive subtotal duodenopancreatectomy and alimentary reconstruction for pancreatic head carcinoma using the aforementioned technique (cf. Chapter 7.1).

Technique

After the duodenopancreatectomy is completed, the proximal jejunal loop is transected 20–30 cm distal from its proximal end (Fig. 7.1.**18**, p. 273). The so-called proximal jejunal segment is now transferred, via an opening which is made in the transverse mesocolon, to the upper abdomen, where it is used to create the pancreatic and biliary anastomosis (Fig. 7.4.**2**). The remaining distal jejunal segment is eventually used to create the gastric anastomosis.

A 3–4 cm long seromyotomy is carried out 5 cm proximal from the proximal end of the proximal jejunal loop. The posterior surface of the residual pancreas is freed from the underlying portal vein and splenic vein, making it possible to

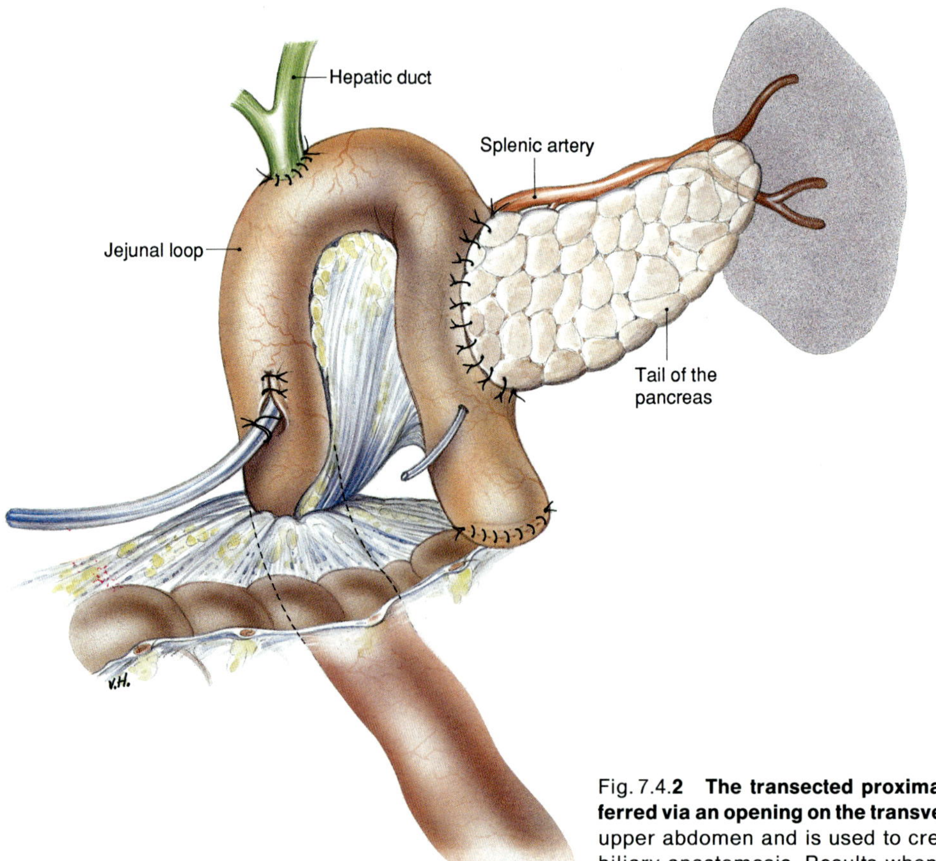

Fig. 7.4.**2 The transected proximal jejunal loop is transferred via an opening on the transverse mesocolon** into the upper abdomen and is used to create the pancreatic and biliary anastomosis. Results when completed

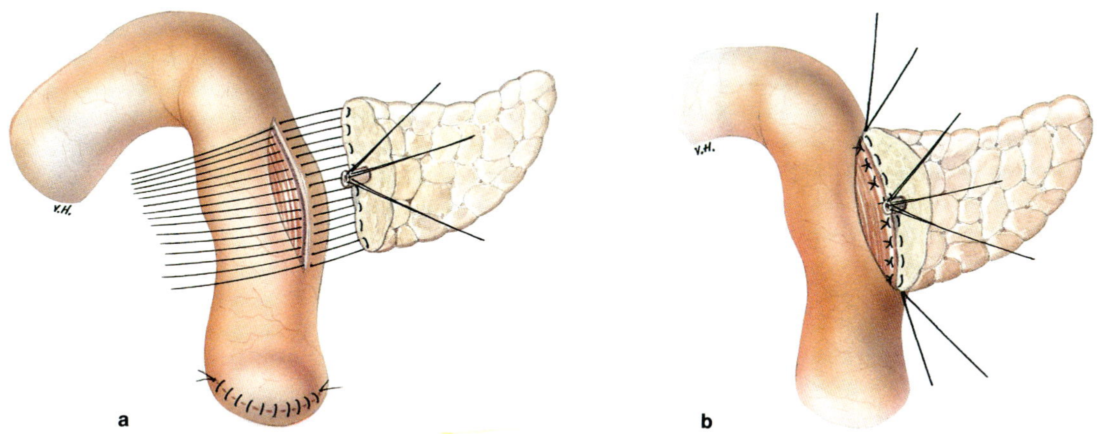

Fig. 7.4.**3a**   **Seromyotomy is carried out.** Interrupted 6-0 Vicryl sutures are inserted in the anterior leaf of the pancreatic duct
b   **The posterior layer of the pancreaticojejunostomy is completed.** The jejunal mucosa lies opposite the rough surface of the pancreas

create the posterior layer of the pancreaticojejunostomy using 4 or 5 interrupted 4-0 Vicryl® sutures, which are inserted between the seromuscular layer of the posterior border of the jejunal seromyotomy and the posterior surface of the pancreas (Fig. 7.4.**3a**). The sutures are tied one by one, completing the posterior layer of the pancreaticojejunostomy (Fig. 7.4.**3b**). The jejunal loop is now anchored to the pancreatic remnant, with the pancreatic duct lying opposite to the protruding jejunal mucosa. Using 6-0 interrupted Vicryl sutures, which are inserted all along the anterior aspect of the pancreatic duct, we are able to keep the stoma of the pancreatic duct open and delineate its posterior aspect.

An opening is made in the jejunal mucosa opposite to the stoma of the pancreatic duct (Fig. 7.4.**4a**). The mucosal opening has the same diameter as the pancreatic duct. Using interrupted Vicryl sutures between the posterior surface of the jejunal mucosa opening and the posterior aspect of the pancreatic duct, we create the posterior layer of the anastomosis of the pancreatic duct and jejunal mucosa opening (Fig. 7.4.**4b**). The pancreatic duct is stented with a no. 8 rubber silicone tube, which is anchored to the posterior aspect of the pancreatic duct with a catgut suture. Through a separate opening, 2 to 3 centimeters distal from the seromyotomy of the jejunum, a clamp is introduced and guided out of the jejunum via the posterior layer of the anastomosis between the pancreatic duct and the jejunal mucosa opening (Fig. 7.4.**4c**). The free end of the transanastomotic tube is grasped with the open tip of the clamp and brought out via a Witzel jejunostomy (Fig. 7.4.**4d**). We complete the anastomosis between the anterior aspect of the pancreatic duct and the anterior surface of the jejunal mucosa by using the already inserted sutures on the anterior aspect of the pancreatic duct (Fig. 7.4.**4e**, **f**). These sutures are tied after being inserted as full-thickness sutures on the jejunal mucosa, and the anterior layer of the anastomosis between the pancreatic duct and the jejunal mucosa opening is then completed (Fig. 7.4.**4f**). Finally, 4-0 Vicryl full-thickness interrupted sutures between the anterior border of the jejunal seromyotomy and the anterior surface of the pancreas complete the pancreaticojejunostomy (Fig. 7.4.**5a**, **b**).

The biliary anastomosis is carried out in an end-to-side fashion 8–10 cm to the right of the pancreatic anastomosis. Interrupted 4-0 Vicryl sutures are inserted in the anterior aspect of the common hepatic duct (Fig. 7.4.**6a–c**). The posterior layer of the hepaticojejunostomy is carried out with interrupted 4-0 full thickness Vicryl sutures interposed between the posterior border of the jejunum and the posterior aspect of the common hepatic duct (Fig. 7.4.**6d**, **e**). These sutures are tied. The transanastomotic tube is introduced into the common hepatic duct (Fig. 7.4.**6e**). The stent is anchored on the posterior aspect of the anastomosis and is brought out with a Witzel jejunostomy (Fig. 7.4.**6f**, **g**). The anterior layer of the hepaticojejunostomy is fashioned with the sutures which already were inserted on the anterior aspect of the common hepatic duct. These sutures are inserted as full-thickness interrupted sutures on the anterior surface of the jejunal opening and are then tied (Fig. 7.4.**6h**, **i**).

The gastrojejunostomy is created using the distal jejunal segment. The alimentary reconstruction is completed by creating an end-to-side jejunostomy 50-60 cm distal from the gastrojejunos-

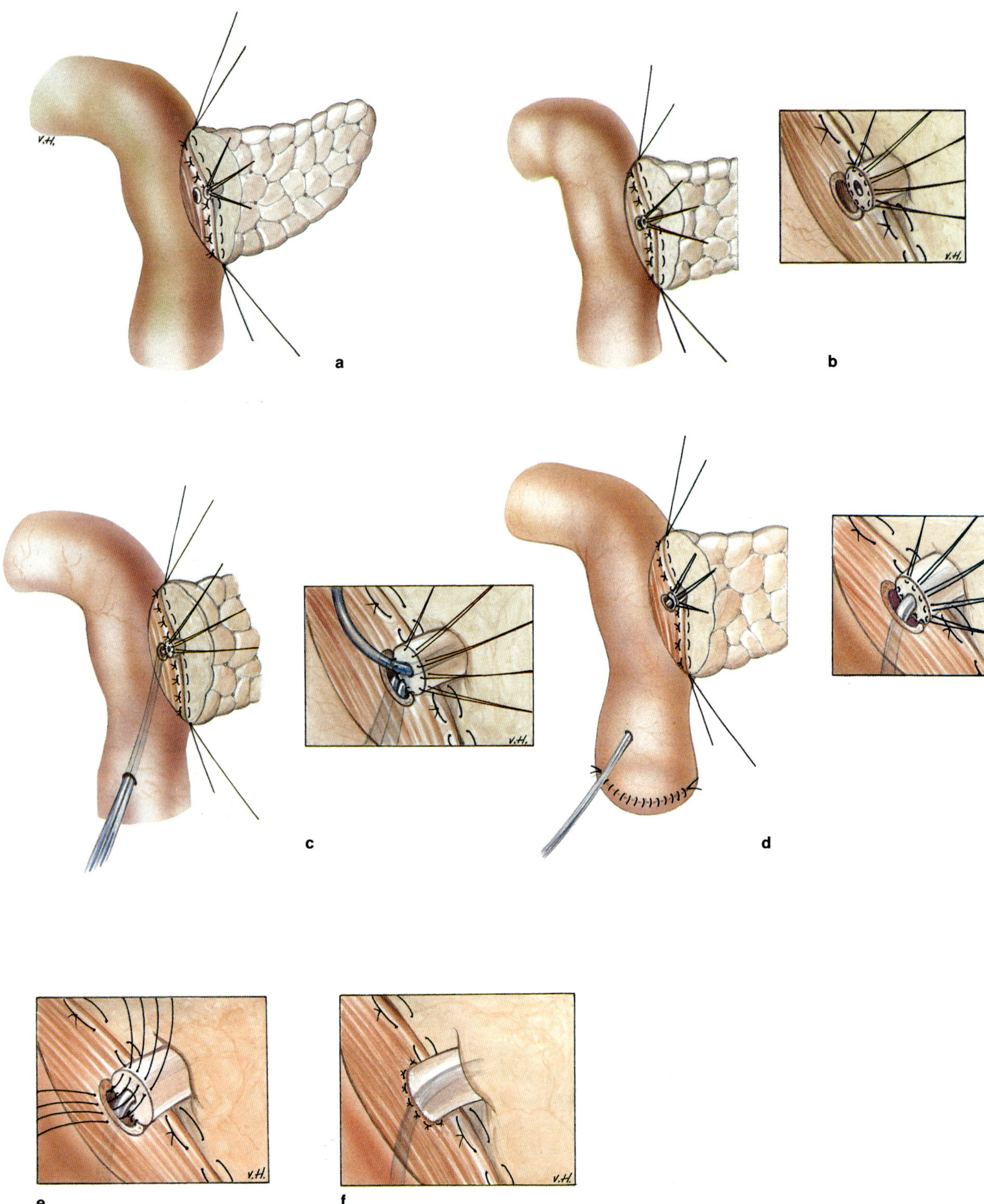

Fig. 7.4.4 a   An opening is made on the jejunal mucosa precisely opposite the opening of the pancreatic duct. Care is taken to ensure that both openings have the same diameter
b   The posterior layer of the anastomosis between the pancreatic duct and the jejunal mucosa opening is created
c   The anastomosis between the pancreatic duct and the jejunal mucosa opening is stented
d   The transanastomotic tube is brought out via a Witzel jejunostomy
e   The anterior layer of the anastomosis between the anterior leaf of the pancreatic duct and the anterior surface of the jejunal mucosa opening is created using the holding sutures one by one
f   The anterior layer of the anastomosis between the pancreatic duct and the jejunal mucosa opening is completed

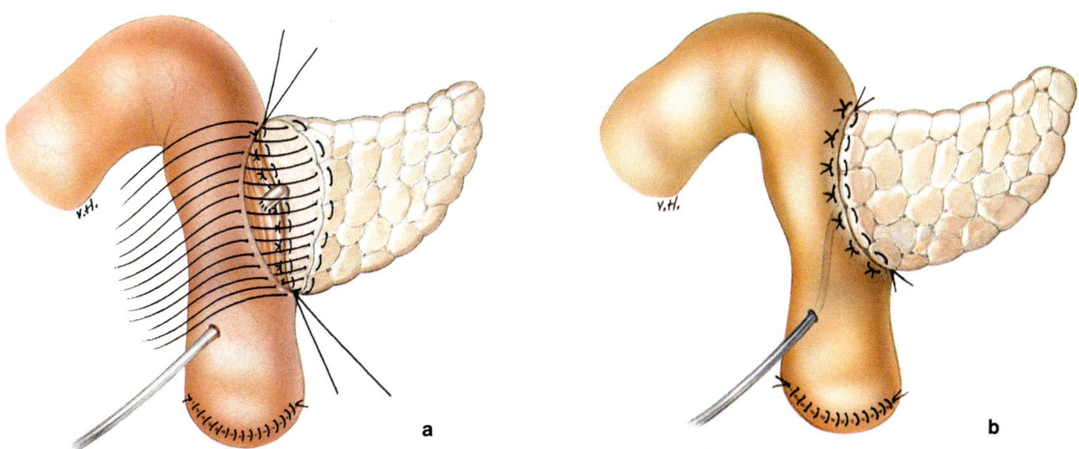

Fig. 7.4.**5a, b   The anterior layer of the pancreaticojejunostomy is created.** The jejunum mucosa is attached to the rough surface of the pancreas

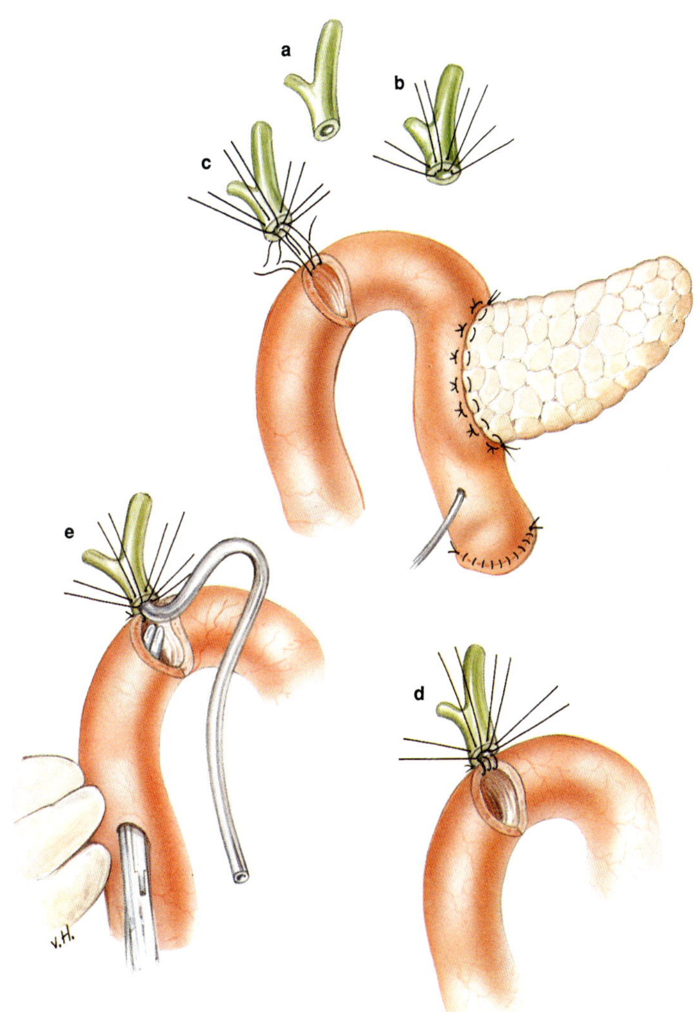

Fig. 7.4.**6a**   The transected common hepatic duct and the jejunal opening
b   Interrupted sutures are inserted in the anterior leaf of the common hepatic duct
c, d, e Creation of the posterior layer of the hepaticojejunostomy
f, g The transanastomotic tube is brought out via a Witzel jejunostomy
h, i The anterior layer of the hepaticojejunostomy is created and completed

tomy. This anastomosis is made between the distal end of the proximal jejunal segment and the distal jejunal loop (Fig. 7.2.**6**, p. 279).

Discussion

There are a number of advantages with this type of reconstruction. It is associated with a low early mortality rate and with satisfactory long-term results. Only one of the 78 patients who underwent this type of reconstruction died. Temporary gastric retention lasting 5–6 days occurred in most patients. The whole procedure is technically easy and promotes healing of the pancreatic anastomosis, taking advantage of the excellent healing properties of the jejunal mucosa which, after seromyotomy, comes into direct contact with the rough surface of the pancreas. Although the incidence of pancreatic anastomotic leakage was high, as routinely recorded by fistulography (Fig. 7.4.**7**, 7.4.**8**), the clinical course was asymptomatic in the majority of

patients. All but one patient responded well to conservative management. The absence of long-term complications such as reflux gastropathy (Chapter 7.6), marginal ulceration, and dumping resulted in a satisfactory quality of life.

The favorable results in our patients can be ascribed to the method of reconstructing alimentary continuity which was used (Lygidakis and Brummelkamp 1985). In our opinion, the use of two separate jejunal loops joined in a Roux-en-Y fashion anticipates dumping and reflux gastropathy in two ways. Firstly, it leads to slow propulsion of food through the jejunal loop. Secondly, it eliminates any reflux of bile and pancreatic juice in the gastric remnant (Fig. 7.4.**9**). Finally, supplementary vagotomy and hemigastrectomy reduce the incidence of marginal ulceration. None of our patients had marginal ulceration during the period of follow-up. The mucosa-to-mucosa anastomosis for the pancreatic duct promotes a good healing process with long-term patency, which is extremely

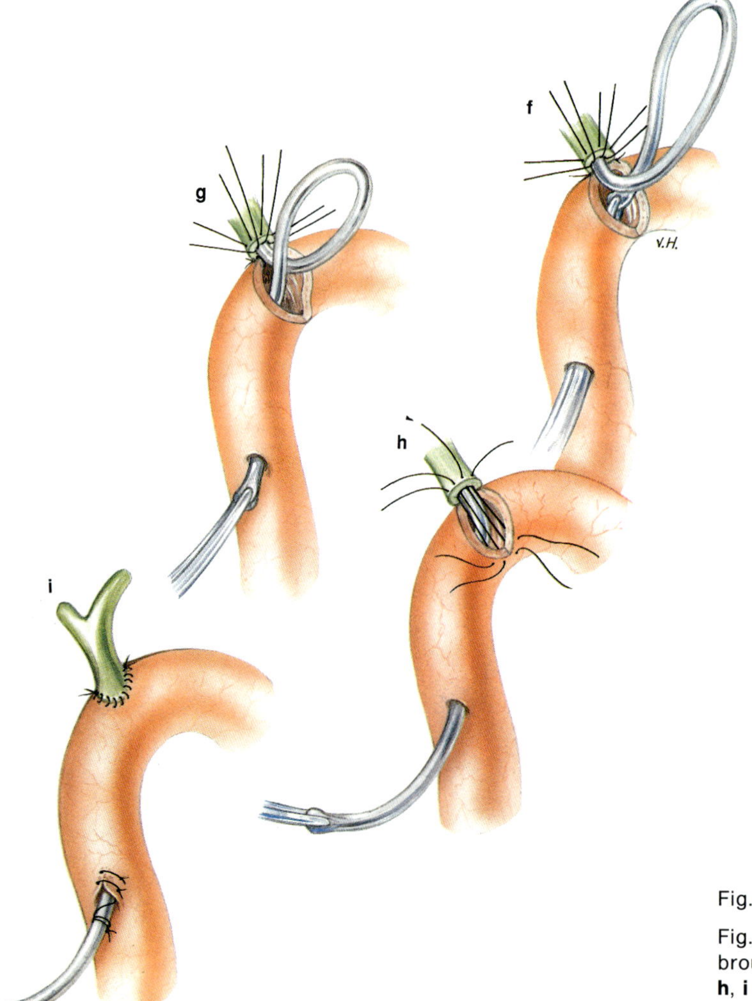

Fig. 7.4.**6 f–i**

Fig. 7.4.**6 f, g** The transanastomotic tube is brough out via a Witzel jejunostomy
h, i The anterior layer of the hepaticojejunostomy is created and completed

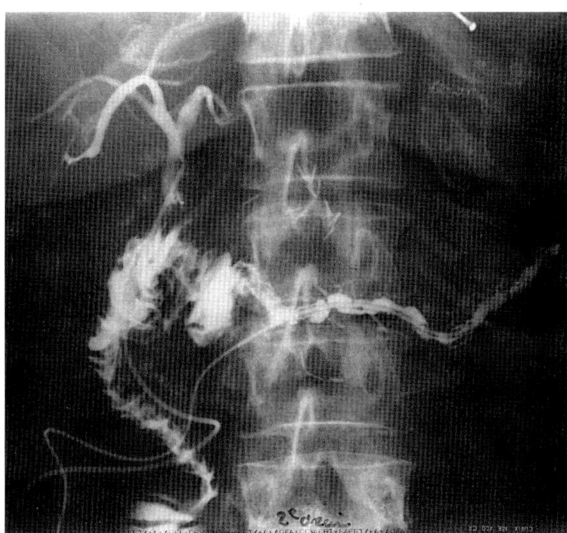

Fig. 7.4.**7 A fistulogram showing the pancreatic and biliary anastomoses,** which are completely isolated from the gastric anastomoses

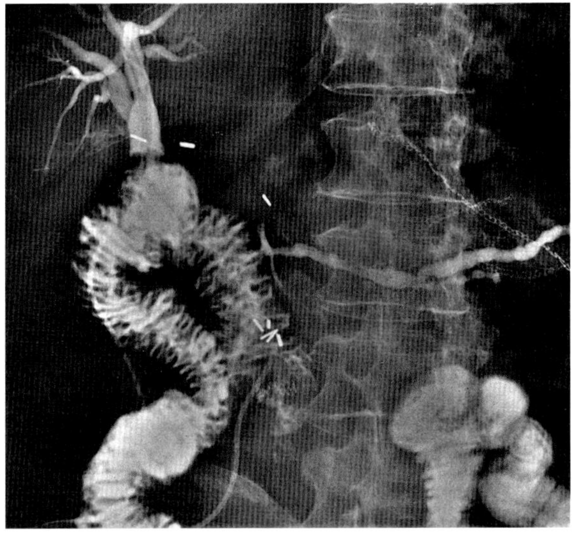

Fig. 7.4.**8 A fistulogram showing an anastomotic leak in the pancreaticojejunostomy.** This patient had no clinical symptoms

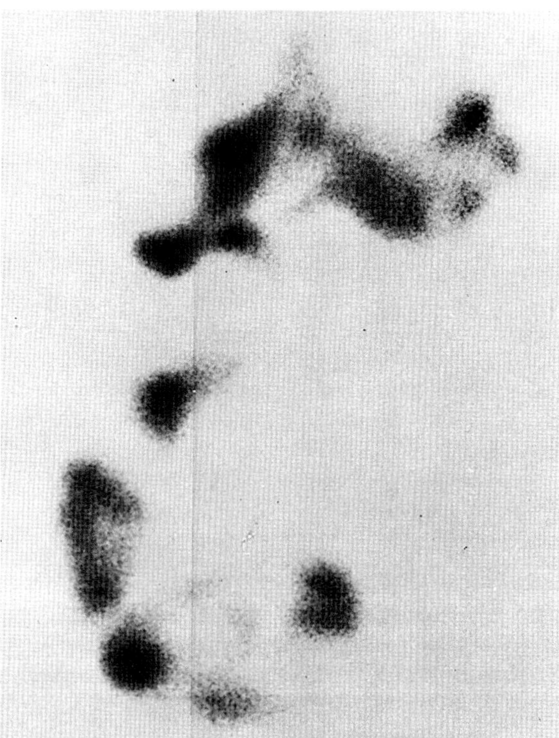

Fig. 7.4.**9 High-frequency ^{99m}Tc scintigraphy** demonstrates a delayed transit time all along the isolated jejunal loop which was used to create the pancreatic and biliary anastomoses. Note the lack of reflux in the gastric remnant

important for an adequate function of the pancreatic remnant (Figs. 7.4.**10**, 7.4.**11**). The low number of our patients who developed diabetes underlines the value of a patent pancreatic anastomosis for the adequate function of the pancreatic remnant (Braasch et al. 1986, Grace et al. 1986, Lygidakis et al. 1986, Lygidakis and Brummelkamp 1985). Occlusion of the pancreatic duct, whether it is primary, as some surgeons consider, or secondary, following stenosis of the pancreatic anastomosis, certainly initiates fibrosis of the pancreatic rem-

nant, causing further impairment of function and an increased incidence of steatorrhea.

Satisfactory results have also been reported after other methods of reconstructing alimentary continuity following subtotal duodenopancreatectomy (Ashton and Longmire 1981, Braasch et al. 1986, Cattell and Warren 1953, Kapur 1986, Mashado et al. 1976, Ruilova and Hershey 1976, Sato et al. 1977, Traverso and Longmire 1978). Particularly for pylorus-preserving technique (Traverso and Longmire 1978), it seems likely that there are some disadvantages in these methods, at least in patients with a malignant process of the periampullary and pancreatic region, because the procedures reported do not make radical resection of the tumor easy. In addition, there is a high incidence of gastric retention in the immediate postoperative period which poses a number of problems necessitating prolonged nasogastric suction, which is a further inconvenience to the patient (Braasch et al. 1986, Traverso and Longmire 1978). Finally, there is the risk of marginal ulceration to be considered when embarking on this kind of reconstruction (Braasch et al. 1986, Traverso and Longmire 1978). In our opinion, the technique we employ overcomes these liabilities and offers acceptable and satisfactory

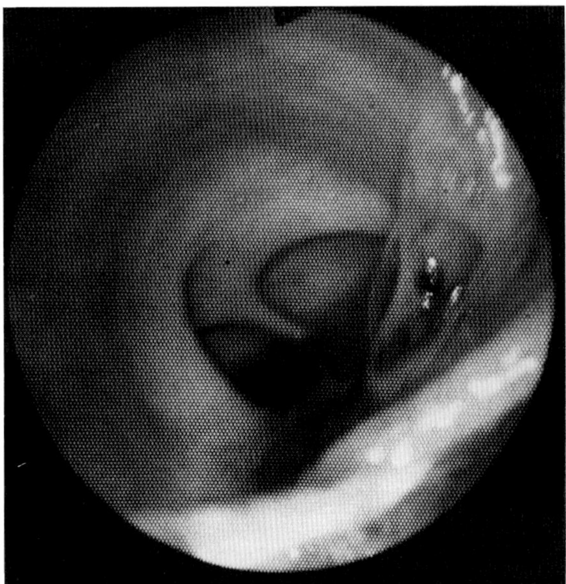

Fig. 7.4.**10   An endoscopic view of the hepaticojejunostomy,** 16 months after the initial surgery: It is large and well-functioning

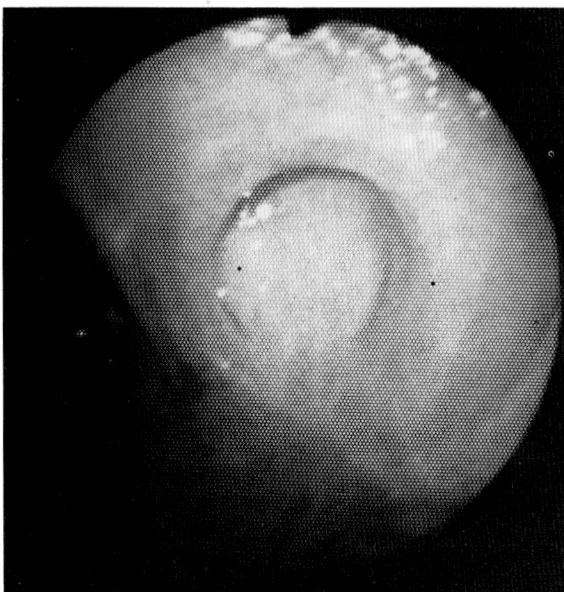

Fig. 7.4.**11   An endoscopic view of the pancreaticojejunostomy** in the same patient. Note the patency of the anastomosis between the pancreatic duct and the jejunal mucosa

early and late results. Based on our experience, we recommend this approach as a promising alternative in the reconstruction of alimentary continuity after subtotal duodenopancreatectomy. There is ongoing evidence that subtotal duodenopancreatectomy in general offers optimal results for the management of patients with pancreatic head carcinoma (Grace et al. 1986). A reconstructive procedure contributing to the success of the operation as a whole is therefore very important.

References

Ashton SJ, Longmire WP Jr. Pancreaticoduodenal resection: twenty years experience. Arch Surg 1981; 106: 813–818.

Braasch JW, Rossi R, Watkins E, Deziel D, Winter P. Pyloric and gastric preserving pancreatic resection: experience with 87 patients. Ann Surg 1986; 204: 411–418.

Cattell RB, Warren KW, eds. Surgery of the pancreas. Philadelphia: Saunders, 1953.

Grace PA, Pitt HA, Tompkins R, den Besten L, Longmire WP Jr. Decreased morbidity and mortality after pancreaticoduodenectomy. Am J Surg 1986; 151: 141.

Gilsdorf RB, Spanos P. Factors influencing morbidity and mortality in pancreaticoduodenotomy. Ann Surg 1973; 177: 332.

Kapur BML. Pancreaticogastrostomy in pancreaticoduodenal resection for ampullary carcinoma: experience in 31 cases. Surgery 1986; 100: 489–493.

Lygidakis NJ, Brummelkamp WH. A new approach for the reconstruction of continuity of the alimentary tract after pancreaticoduodenectomy. Surg Gynecol Obstet 1985; 160: 453–458.

Lygidakis NJ, Brummelkamp WH, Tytgat GNJ. Periampullary and pancreatic head carcinoma: facts and factors influencing mortality, survival and quality of postoperative life. Am J Gastroenterol 1986; 81: 968–973.

Mashado MCC, et al. A modified technique for the reconstruction of the alimentary tract after pancreaticoduodenectomy. Surg Gynecol Obstet 1976; 143: 271–279.

Papachristou DN, Fortner JG. Pancreatic fistula complicating pancreatectomy for malignant disease. Br J Surg 1981; 68: 238–241.

Pliam MB, Remine N. Further evaluation of total pancreatectomy. Arch Surg 1975; 110: 506–512.

Ruilova LA, Hershey CD. Experience with 21 pancreaticoduodenectomies. Arch Surg 1976; 111: 27–31.

Sato T, Saitoh Y, Moto N, Matsuno S. Follow-up studies of radical resection for pancreaticoduodenal cancer. Ann Surg 1977; 186: 581–587.

Shin MN. Resection of pancreas without production of fistula. Surg Gynecol Obstet 1982; 154: 497–501.

Traverso LW, Longmire WP Jr. Preservation of the pylorus in pancreaticoduodenectomy. Surg Gynecol Obstet 1978; 146: 950–963.

7.5   Pylorus-Preserving Pancreatoduodenectomy

R. L. Rossi and J. W. Braasch

Introduction

Pancreatoduodenectomy has become the operation of choice for the management of patients with resectable tumors of the periampullary area and the head of the pancreas and for some patients with chronic pancreatitis. In 1935, Whipple et al. described a two-stage procedure for the excision of periampullary tumors. The first stage consisted of cholecystogastrostomy to relieve obstructive jaundice and gastrojejunostomy. The second stage included transection of the duodenum beyond the pylorus and excision of the duodenum and head of the pancreas. Whipple et al. sutured and ligated the transected border of the pancreas. In 1945, he reported on a one-stage operation that was associated with a lower cumulative morbidity and mortality than the two-stage operation and avoided the difficulties of reoperation (Whipple 1945). When Whipple performed the one-stage operation, he used the common bile duct instead of the gallbladder to reestablish biliary flow, and he resected the distal stomach and duodenum.

Since then, modifications of the Whipple operation have been introduced (Hunt 1941, Cattell 1943, 1948, Mackie et al. 1975) that use different techniques of pancreaticojejunostomy and gastric resection, with or without truncal vagotomy. Currently, the standard pancreatoduodenectomy is a one-stage operation that includes hemigastrectomy and resection of the duodenum, distal common bile duct, head of the pancreas, and proximal jejunum. Pancreaticojejunostomy, hepaticojejunostomy, and gastrojejunostomy are required for reconstruction of the gastrointestinal tract.

Although the original technique did not include gastric resection, partial gastrectomy was thought to be a necessary step in the Whipple procedure until 1978 when Traverso and Longmire reported on two patients who underwent pancreatoduodenectomy with preservation of the entire stomach and a segment of duodenum and reconstruction of the gastrointestinal tract by end-to-side duodenojejunostomy. The goals of this modification were to maintain gastric capacity and gastric mixing ability and to decrease the side effects of gastrectomy, such as dumping, diarrhea, and fecal fat loss. We have used this modification to treat patients with chronic pancreatitis as well as patients with periampullary carcinoma, distal bile duct carcinoma, carcinoma of the head of the pancreas, and other nonductal neoplasms of the head of the pancreas (Fig. 7.5.1).

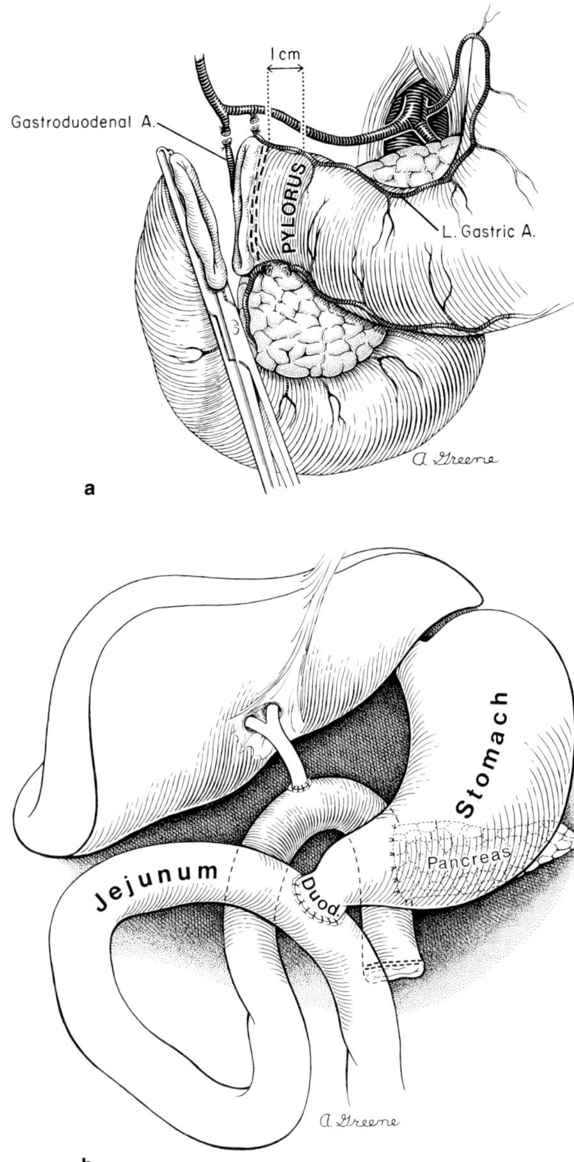

Fig. 7.5.1a, b   Pancreatoduodenectomy with pylorus preservation. (From Rossi and Braasch 1982, with permission)

Technique

The first step of the operation we perform includes abdominal exploration, diagnosis of the tumor, and assessment of resectability. Tissue samples can be obtained from a distant metastatic tumor, from nodes, or from the primary site using direct knife biopsy, transduodenal needle biopsy, or aspiration cytology. Lesions of the head of the pancreas are

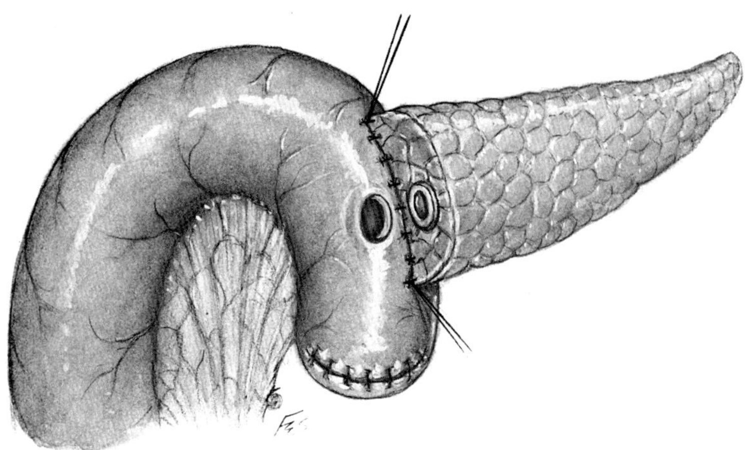

Fig. 7.5.**2   End-to-side mucosa-to-mucosa pancreaticojejunostomy.** A layer of interrupted 3-0 silk sutures is placed between the posterior border of the transected pancreas and the jejunum. (From Rossi and Braasch 1985, with permission)

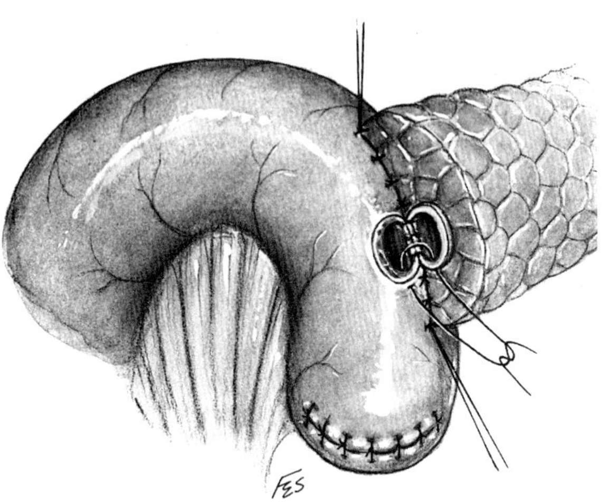

Fig. 7.5.**3   Enterostomy is performed in the jejunum, and 4-0 silk sutures are used to anastomose the pancreatic duct and jejunum.** (From Rossi and Braasch 1985, with permission)

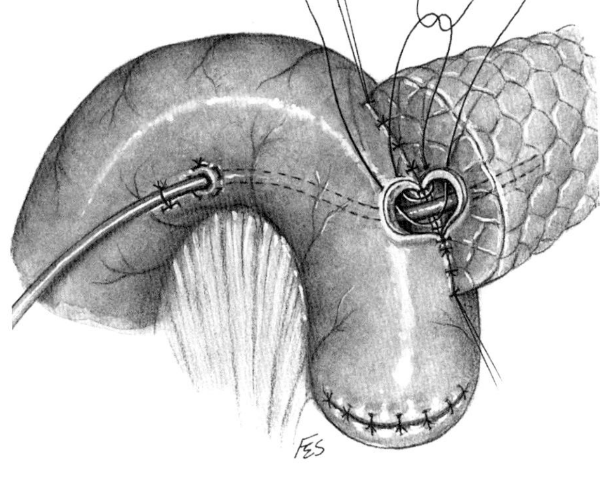

Fig. 7.5.**4   A stent is placed through a separate enterotomy and passed through the anastomosis** before the anterior anastomotic sutures are placed. A purse string suture of silk prevents leakage of the jejunum around the insertion site of the stent. The stent is secured with an absorbable suture. (From Rossi and Braasch 1985, with permission)

considered unresectable when they have metastasized or involve nodes or when they extend to the transverse mesocolon, superior mesenteric vessels, or retroperitoneum. For adequate assessment of the primary site, an extensive Kocher maneuver and opening the gastrocolic ligament are required. The gastrocolic ligament is opened outside the gastroepiploic arcade so as to preserve blood supply to the stomach as far distally as possible in the event that pylorus-preserving resection is needed. When the lesion is resectable, basic steps of the operation include identification and division of the gastroduodenal artery, dissection of the plane between the superior mesenteric vein and the neck of the pancreas, division of the common bile duct,

takedown of the angle of Treitz and transection of the proximal jejunum, transection of the duodenum approximately 1–2 cm beyond the pylorus, transection of the neck of the pancreas over the superior mesenteric vessels, dissection of the head of the pancreas and uncinate process from the superior mesenteric vessels, and gastrointestinal reconstruction.

Technical details of importance when performing this modification of pancreatoduodenectomy include preservation of the nerves of Latarjet and ligation of the gastroepiploic artery as far distally as possible to preserve the blood supply to the greater curvature of the stomach and antropyloric area. When possible, we try to preserve the supra-

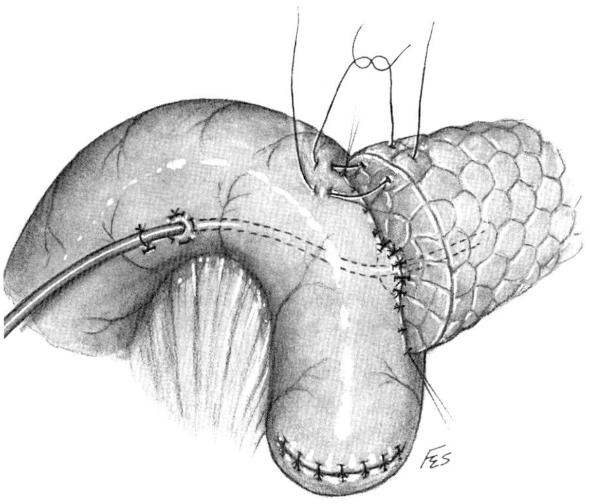

Fig. 7.5.**5 After completion of the anterior aspect of the ductal anastomosis, the anterior border of the pancreas is sutured to the jejunum.** (From Rossi and Braasch 1985, with permission)

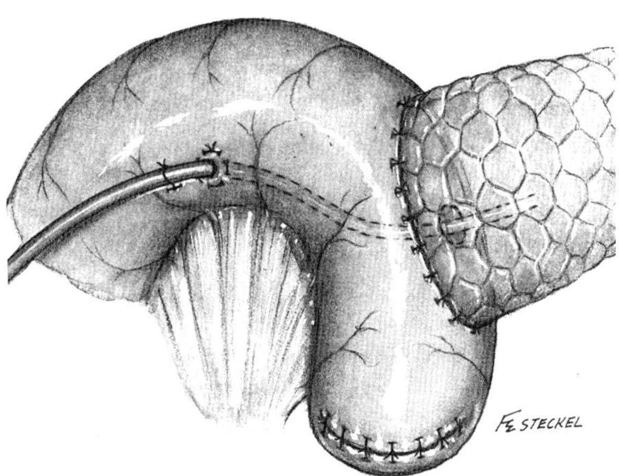

Fig. 7.5.**6 Completed end-to-side mucosa-to-mucosa pancreaticojejunostomy.** (From Rossi and Braasch 1985, with permission)

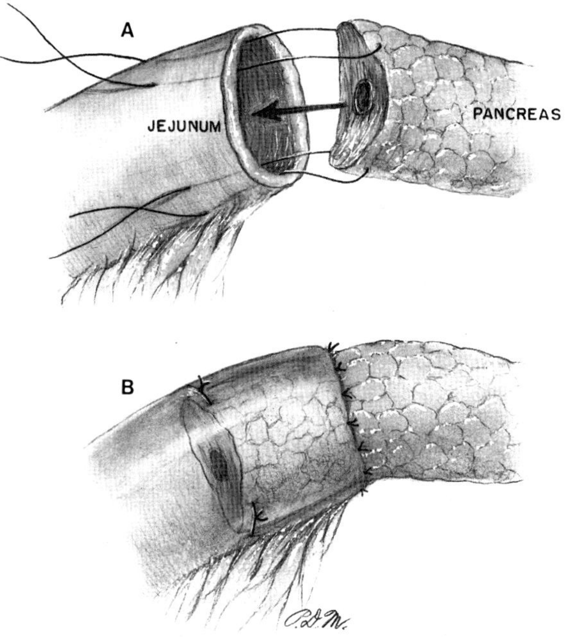

Fig. 7.5.**7a Dunking technique: one-layer anastomosis.** Two guide sutures are placed through the border of the pancreas and the jejunum at about 3 cm from the end of the intestine. Traction achieves dunking of the pancreas.
b A row of silk sutures is placed around the pancreas and jejunum, with care being taken to invert the jejunal mucosa. The stay sutures are tied individually. (From Braasch and Rossi 1985, with permission)

duodenal artery that arises from the hepatic artery and proceeds to the first portion of the duodenum and the pylorus. A safe pancreaticojejunostomy is mandatory for low morbidity and mortality.

Requirements for a safe pancreatoduodenectomy include appropriate patient selection, identification of such vascular abnormalities as a replaced hepatic artery, and performance of a safe pancreaticojejunostomy. At the Lahey Clinic from 1965 to 1975, Whipple operations were performed so that the pancreaticojejunostomy was an end-to-side mucosa-to-mucosa anastomosis. The operative mortality rate was 6%, and most of the deaths were related to intra-abdominal causes, such as bleeding and sepsis.

A multifactorial analysis showed that the increased morbidity and mortality were related to the size of the pancreatic duct and the consistency of the gland. Patients with small ducts and soft glands were more likely to have complications than those with large ducts and firm glands. The type of pancreaticojejunostomy we perform now is based on the condition of the pancreas. Patients with a soft gland and a small pancreatic duct are treated with a dunking pancreaticojejunostomy while those with a firm gland and a large duct are treated with an end-to-side mucosa-to-mucosa anastomosis of the duct and gland. Figures 7.5.**2** through 7.5.**10** illustrate the different types of pancreaticojejunostomy (Rossi and Braasch 1985).

In 120 pylorus-preserving pancreatoduodenectomy procedures performed since 1979, the operative mortality rate has been 4%. Patients now die of extra-abdominal causes, that is, associated illnesses, rather than of complications of the pancreaticojejunostomy. The incidence of pancreatic leakage is 6–7%, but its morbidity is low, perhaps as a result of the type of anastomosis performed, an

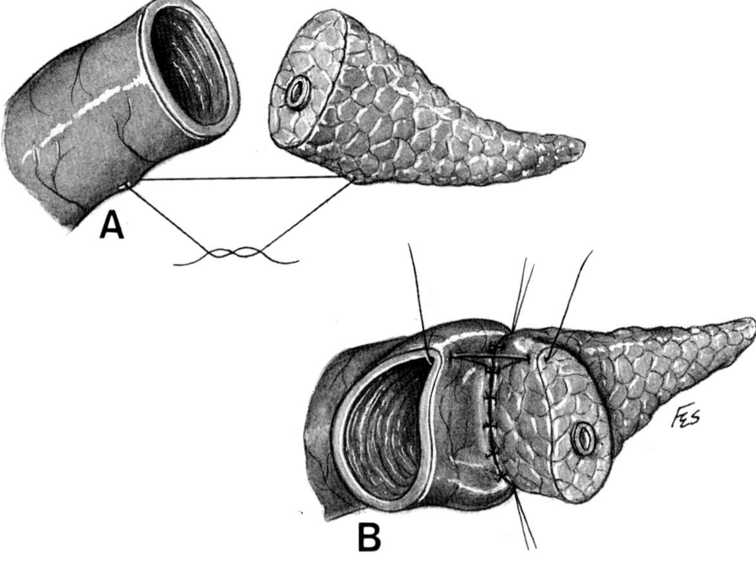

Fig. 7.5.**8**   **Two-layer dunking anastomosis**
a   Posterior layer of sutures placed at about 2 cm from the end of the jejunum and 2 cm from the border of the transected pancreas
b   Sutures placed between the posterior border of the transected pancreas and the border of the posterior wall of the jejunum. (From Rossi and Braasch 1985, with permission)

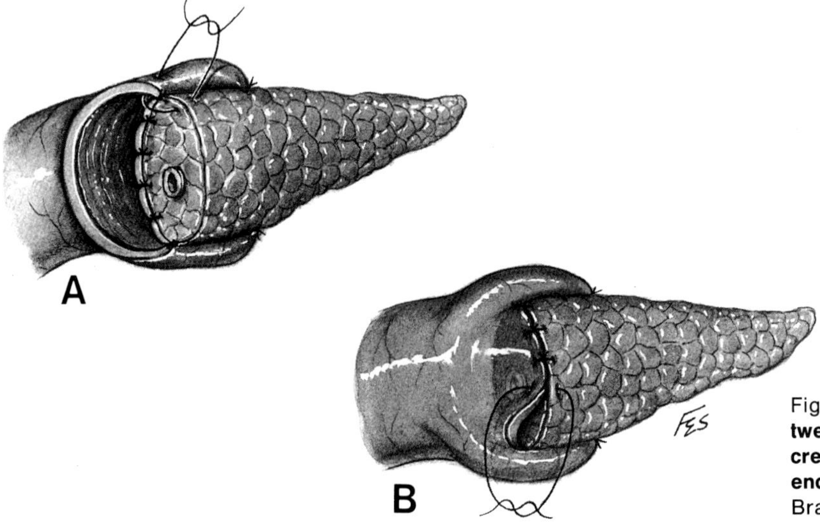

Fig. 7.5.**9a, b**   **Sutures placed between the anterior border of the pancreas and the anterior wall of the end of the jejunum.** (From Rossi and Braasch 1985, with permission)

improved drainage system, and enhanced medical support.

After the pancreaticojejunostomy has been completed, an end-to-side hepaticojejunostomy is performed using a single layer of absorbable interrupted monofilament sutures. The end-to-side duodenojejunostomy is constructed in two layers with absorbable interrupted sutures in the inner row and silk sutures in the outer seromuscular row. A fine pediatric feeding tube is left in place as a pancreatic stent in most patients. A T tube through the hepatic duct or tube gastrostomy and needle catheter jejunostomy is used selectively. Two or three closed-system drains are placed near the pancreaticojejunostomy and another drain in the area of the hepaticojejunostomy.

Results

We have compared this modification of the pancreatoduodenectomy with the standard procedure to determine whether it improves gastrointestinal function and to document its effect on cancer survival, postoperative morbidity and mortality, and the incidence of jejunal ulceration. From 1979 to 1987, 120 such procedures have been performed at the Lahey Clinic Medical Center. We have reported on the first 87 patients (Braasch et al. 1986), of whom 57 had cancer, 28 had chronic pancreatitis, and 2 had miscellaneous benign conditions. Seventy-one patients had hemipancreatectomy, 13 patients had total pancreatectomy, and 3 other patients had completion total pancreatectomy, since they had had a distal pancreatectomy.

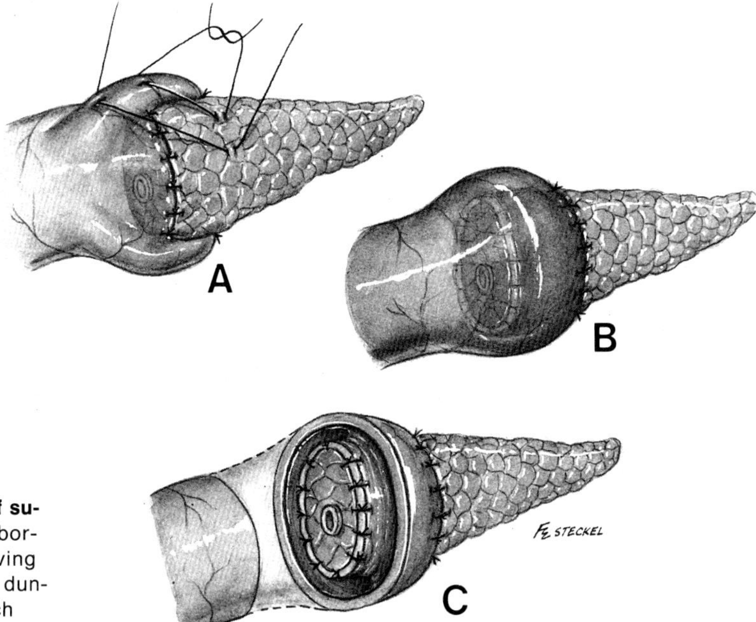

Fig. 7.5.**10a, b   Second anterior layer of sutures,** placed at about 2–3 cm from the border of the pancreas and jejunum, achieving intussusception. **c** Completed two-layer dunking technique. (From Rossi and Braasch 1985, with permission)

The commonest postoperative complication was transient gastric stasis that required gastric suctioning for more than seven days (median, 11 days) after operation in about half of the patients. The incidence of pancreatic fistula was 6 % and was similar for the dunking and end-to-side mucosa-to-mucosa types of pancreaticojejunostomy (Braasch et al. 1986). A diagnosis of marginal ulcer was suggested in five patients. Three patients were treated successfully medically, one patient underwent reoperation because of pain, and one patient had transthoracic vagotomy. However, no ulcer was found in either of the latter two patients. The incidence of presumed marginal ulceration is no higher than with the standard pancreatoduodenectomy. Warren and Williams (1988) reduced the incidence of jejunal ulceration after standard pancreatoduodenectomy from 17 % to 7 % by adding truncal vagotomy or by extending the gastric resection to subtotal gastrectomy. Pearlman et al. (1986) reported that the pylorus-preserving pancreatoduodenectomy did not result in hypergastrinemia or gastric hyperacidity.

Gastric resection has been associated with fast gastric emptying, loss of body weight, increased fecal loss of fat (Doty and Meyer 1987, Wollaeger et al. 1963), dumping, diarrhea, and bile gastritis, and it may adversely affect the accurate regulation of the blood sugar in the diabetic patient (Hongo et al. 1987). When indium-111 in water or technetium-99m sulfur colloid absorbed into the white of scrambled eggs was used in a study of gastric emptying after pylorus-preserving pancreatoduodenectomy, gastric emptying was normal compared

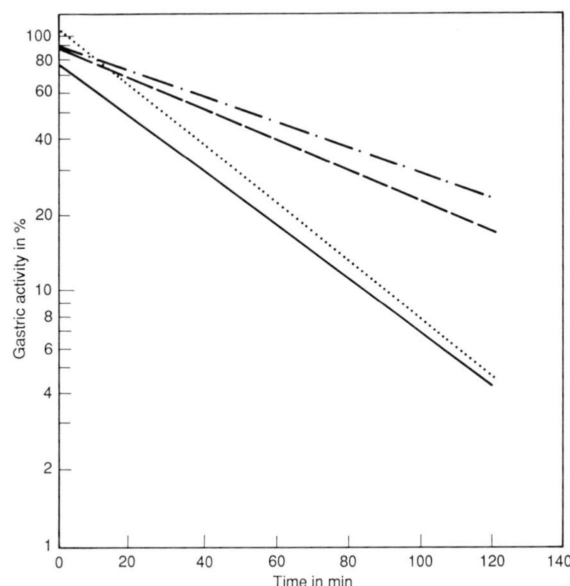

Fig. 7.5.**11   Gastric emptying for solids and liquids** in patients who underwent pylorus-preserving pancreatectomy and in normal subjects. (From Braasch et al. 1986, with permission). Pancreatectomy patients (liquids): –·–·–; normal subjects (liquids): – – – –; pancreatectomy patients (solids): ·········; normal subjects (solids): ———

with the control group (Fig. 7.5.**11**). Enterogastric reflux was studied with the use of technetium-99m bound to hepatobiliary iminodiacetic acid (HIDA) that is excreted in the bile. Patients treated with pylorus-preserving pancreatoduodenectomy had less reflux than patients who were treated by gastric

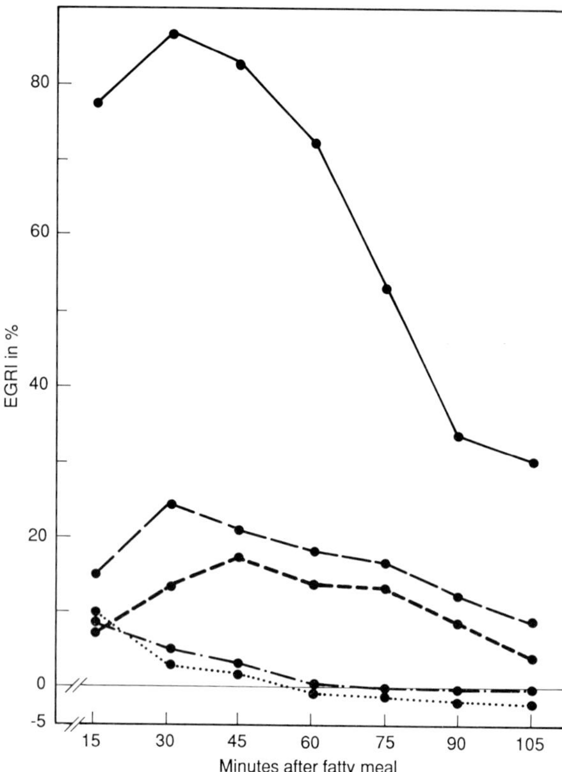

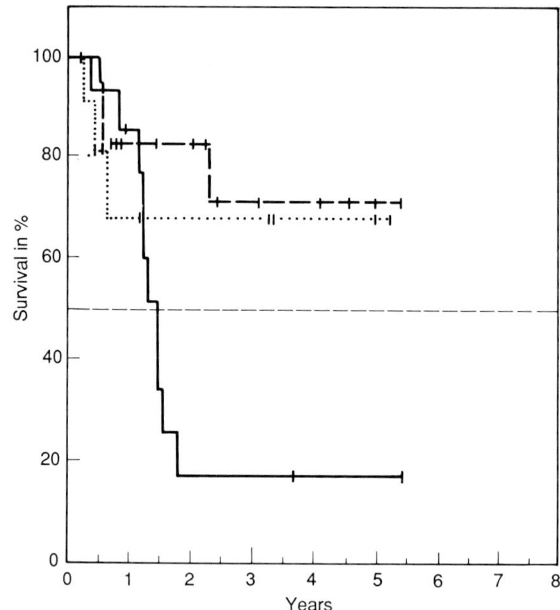

Fig. 7.5.**12 Enterogastric reflux** in patients who underwent gastrectomy and pylorus-preserving pancreatectomy and in normal subjects. (From Braasch et al. 1986, with permission). Billroth II (alkaline gastritis) (Tolin et al.): ———; Billroth II (asymptomatic) (Tolin et al.): –––––; normal subjects (Lahey Clinic): ·········; normal subjects (Tolin et al.): ———; pancreatectomy patients (Lahey Clinic): ––––. EGRI: enterogastric reflux indication

Fig. 7.5.**13 Adjusted actuarial survival after pylorus-preserving pancreatectomy** for periampullary carcinoma. (From Braasch et al. 1986, with permission). Ampullary adenocarcinoma (18 patients, median survival time + 65 months): –+–+–; bile duct adenocarcinoma (12 patients, median survival time + 63 months): ·········; pancreatic head adenocarcinoma (14 patients, median survival time 18 months): ———

resection and Billroth II anastomosis, with or without symptoms of bile reflux gastritis (Fig. 7.5.**12**).

Long-term gastrointestinal function and nutritional status were assessed in patients who were followed up for at least four months after operation and had no evidence of recurrent cancer (Braasch et al. 1986). These patients weighed more than 100 % of their preoperative weight and 95 % of their pre-illness weight (median values). Only one instance of mild dumping was noted.

Actuarial analysis of survival calculated by the Kaplan-Meier product-limit method revealed an adjusted actuarial five-year survival rate of 70.6 % ± 13.5 % for patients with periampullary carcinoma, 68.2 % ± 15.8 % for patients with bile duct adenocarcinoma, and 17 % ± 10.9 % for patients with adenocarcinoma of the pancreatic head (Fig. 7.5.**13**). Two patients with carcinoma of the pancreas were long-term survivors and were free of disease. Compared with historical controls, the differences between the long-term survival of pa-

tients with carcinoma of the periampullary area and the head of pancreas treated with a pylorus-preserving pancreatoduodenectomy and patients treated with a standard Whipple operation do not appear to be appreciable. It is our view that the biologic behavior of periampullary and pancreatic tumors is such that widespread metastasis is likely to occur if the tumor involves the wall of the stomach, proximal duodenum, or lymph nodes about the lesser or greater curvature of the stomach, and that adding gastrectomy as is included in the standard pancreatoduodenectomy would therefore be unlikely to influence survival. Results reported to date have not demonstrated a benefit of total pancreatectomy over pancreatoduodenectomy in the management of patients with carcinoma of the periampullary area, and the resultant insulin-dependent diabetes can be difficult to manage. The biologic importance of multicentricity is unclear because higher survivals have not been obtained with total pancreatectomy, and the potential benefits of avoiding pancreaticojejunostomy and decreasing the operative mortality and morbidity have not been documented. Therefore, we perform total pancreatectomy selectively, for instance, when the transected margin of the pancreas contains tumor on frozen section, when we are unsatisfied with pancreaticojejunostomy and believe the chance of leakage from the anastomosis is high, or when the patient is insulin-dependent before the operation and the prevention of diabetes is not a concern. On occasion, for patients with large tumors, such as cystadenocarcinomas or islet cell tumors that are attached to the antrum and proximal duodenum, and in some unusual types of pancreatitis, the standard pancreatoduodenectomy with gastric resection will be performed rather than a pylorus-preserving technique.

Conclusions

After reviewing our experience with approximately 120 pylorus-preserving pancreatoduodenectomy procedures, we believe this technique represents an advance over standard pancreatoduodenectomy because it shortens operative time, benefits the patient by permitting normal gastric capacity and gastric emptying, diminishes bile reflux, and avoids the dumping syndrome. It may also decrease the amount of fecal fat loss, and in diabetic patients, may facilitate control of diabetes through more steady gastric emptying compared with the fast emptying that occurs after gastric resection. Observations that would justify the concern that this operation could be ulcerogenic have not been noted by us. As a cancer procedure, pylorus-preserving pancreatoduodenectomy appears to be associated with survival rates that are similar to those with the standard pancreatoduodenectomy.

References

Braasch JW, Rossi RL. Pyloric preservation with the Whipple procedure. Surg Clin North Am 1985; 65: 270.

Braasch JW, Deziel DJ, Rossi RL, Watkins E Jr, Winter PF. Pyloric and gastric preserving pancreatic resection: experience with 87 patients. Ann Surg 1986; 204: 411–418.

Cattell RB. Resection of pancreas: discussion of special problems. Surg Clin North Am 1943; 23: 753–766.

Cattell RB. Technic for pancreatoduodenal resection. Surg Clin North Am 1948; 28: 761–775.

Doty JE, Meyer JH. Vagotomy and antrectomy impairs absorption of fat from solid, but not liquid dietary sources (abstract). Gastroenterology 1987; 92 (suppl 2): 1374.

Hongo M, Satake K, Sanoyama K, Lin YF, Ujiie H, Toyota T, Goto Y. Regulation of insulin demand by gastric emptying in diabetics (abstract). Gastroenterology 1987; 92 (suppl 2): 1440.

Hunt VC. Surgical management of carcinoma of ampulla of Vater and of periampullary portion of the duodenum. Ann Surg 1941; 114: 570–602.

Mackie JA, Rhoads JE, Park CD. Pancreaticogastrostomy: further evaluation. Ann Surg 1975; 181: 541–545.

Pearlman NW, Stiegmann GV, Ahnen DJ, Schultz AL, Fink LM. Acid and gastrin levels following pyloric-preserving pancreaticoduodenectomy. Arch Surg 1986; 121: 661–664.

Rossi RL, Braasch JW. Biliary cancer surgery: When to do what. Contemp Surg 1982; 20: 21.

Rossi RL, Braasch JW. Techniques of pancreaticojejunostomy in pancreatoduodenectomy. Probl Gen Surg 1985; 2: 506–513.

Tolin RD, Malmud LS, Stelzer F, Menin R, Makler PT Jr, Applegate G, Fisher RS. Enterogastric reflux in normal subjects and patients with Bilroth II gastroenterostomy: measurement of enterogastric reflux. Gastroenterology 1979; 77: 1027–1033.

Traverso LW, Longmire WP Jr. Preservation of the pylorus in pancreaticoduodenectomy. Surg Gynecol Obstet 1978; 146: 959–962.

Warren KW, Williams C. Reoperative pancreatic surgery. In: Tompkins R, ed. Reoperations on the gastrointestinal tract. Philadelphia: Lippincott, 1988 (in press).

Whipple AO. Pancreaticoduodenectomy for islet carcinoma: five-year follow-up. Ann Surg 1945; 121: 847–852.

Whipple AO, Parsons WB, Mullins CR. Treatment of carcinoma of ampulla of Vater. Ann Surg 1935; 102: 763–779.

Wollaeger EE, Waugh JM, Power MH. Fat-assimilating capacity of the gastrointestinal tract after partial gastrectomy with gastroduodenostomy (Billroth I anastomosis). Gastroenterology 1963; 44: 25–32.

7.6 Surgical Palliation of Cancer of the Pancreas

B. Launois

Introduction

Cancer of the pancreas, once a rare disease, has increased during the past 35 years all over the world. In the United States it is the fifth most common cause of cancer death. The prognosis of the disease remains poor, despite recent advances in diagnostic and operative techniques (Czernchow et al. 1985).

In a review of 15000 patients with pancreatic cancer, the absolute 5-year survival rate was 0.4 per cent (Gudjonsson et al. 1978). It is of interest that in another study, the average length of survival of all patients diagnosed as having cancer of the pancreas was 3–4 months, with over 90% of patients dying in under a year (Cancer Incidence 1978). These figures reflect the fact that at the time of diagnosis the disease is already very advanced, so that the majority of patients are considered as not being eligible for pancreatic resection. For such patients, the remaining possibilities are surgical palliative bypass (Brooks and Culebras 1976, Crile Jr. 1970), endoscopic palliative bypass (Huibregtse et al. 1986), and transcutaneous transhepatic bypass (Cotton 1986). The choice between these alternatives must be an individual one, as the results obtained remain more or less similar (cf. Chapter 7.8).

Generally, excision was considered the treatment of choice. Palliative surgery is only indicated when the tumor appears to be unremovable (DuVal 1954, Fortner et al. 1977, Grossetti and Launois 1980, Ihse et al. 1977, Launois 1983, Lawrence and Gosh 1977, Lewis et al. 1987, Matsui et al. 1979, Moossa 1979, Moossa et al. 1984, Pliam 1975).

Technique

For the great majority of patients, we recommend gastrojejunostomy combined with biliary drainage procedures. We prefer choledochojejunostomy rather than cholecystojejunostomy, since in our experience the former offers better results (Lewis et al. 1987). We consider that the combination of gastric and biliary bypass surgery is necessary to eliminate the need for further surgery, which may be indicated in patients in whom biliary bypass alone is performed (Grossetti and Launois 1980, Sarr and Cameron 1984). Biliary enteric anastomosis is usually carried out in an end-to-side fashion using one-layer interrupted 5-0 Vicryl sutures.

We prefer a Roux-en-Y jejunal loop, to avoid the incidence of bile reflux into the stomach which can be very troublesome for most of these patients. We do not favor cholecystojejunostomy because of a high incidence of cystic duct occlusion, which renders the anastomosis useless. Whenever feasible and possible, we proceed with choledochojejunostomy.

We are against other recommended procedures, such as cholecystogastrostomy or choledochoduodenostomy, because they are associated with poor palliation and a poor quality of postoperative life (Grossetti and Launois 1980).

Results

The operative mortality for palliative surgical bypass remains high (19.3%). However, the mortality is related to patient age, at 5% for patients younger than 65, and 30% for those older than 65 (Grossetti and Launois 1980). The mortality in a series of 10814 patients who had palliative surgical bypass for pancreatic head carcinoma was 18% (Sarr and Cameron 1984). In the same collective study, the median survival was 5.5 months after palliative surgical bypass for pancreatic head carcinoma (Sarr and Cameron 1984).

Comments

These results are inferior to those after medical palliative management, where the mortality is about 10% and the survival 5–6 months (Huibregtse et al. 1986). However, it seems difficult to compare the results of surgical drainage with endoscopic or percutaneous drainage with regard to mortality, morbidity, survival and quality of palliation. Surgery is obligatory in patients presenting with jaundice caused by periampullary cancer, unless there are contra-indications of a general nature. Cytological or histological proof, and particularly histological typing, of the cancer is imperative. The diagnosis of cancer should not be made on the sole basis of ultrasound or CT-scan images. If cancer is confirmed, excision should be attempted, especially when the common bile duct is affected. Should resection prove impossible, a double biliary digestive and gastrojejunal bypass is performed of necessity. Choledochojejunal anastomosis is advocated in young patients. Choledochoduodenal anastomosis is quicker to perform in elderly patients. If the patient is over 70, an elective palliative double bypass is only considered, due to age.

In making the decision as to which kind of palliative measure to employ, the choice should be based on each patient's anatomical and mechanical peculiarities and on the patient's general condition with regard to age, presence of associated disease and stage of the disease. In patients with short life expectancy, endoscopic or percutaneous drainage should be preferred. For patients who are in good general condition and who have less advanced disease and better life expectancy, surgical drainage is a valid palliative approach.

References

Brooks JR, Culebras JM. Cancer of the pancreas: palliative operation, Whipple procedure or total pancreatectomy. Am J Surg 1976; 131: 16–20.

Cancer Incidence and Mortality in the USA: SEER 1973–1976; NIH publication, no 78. Bethesda: US Department of Health, Education and Welfare, 1978: 1837.

Cotton PB. Endoscopic biliary stents: trick or treatment. Gastrointest Endosc 1986; 32: 364–365.

Crile G Jr. Advantages of bypass operations over radical pancreaticoduodenectomy in treatment of pancreatic carcinoma. Surg Gynecol Obstet 1970; 130: 1049.

Czernchow P, Lerebeurs B, Hecketsweiler P, Colin R. Epidémiologie temperospatiale du cancer du pancréas: Etude de mortalité internationale et française. Gastroenterol Clin Biol 1985; 9: 767–775.

DuVal MK. Caudal pancreatic jejunostomy for chronic relapsing pancreatitis. Ann Surg 1954; 140: 775–785.

Fortner JG, Kim DK, Cubilla A, et al. Regional pancreatectomy: en bloc pancreatic portal vein and lymph-node resection. Ann Surg 1977; 186: 42–50.

Grossetti D, Launois B. Le traitement palliatif du cancer du pancréas. Rennes: 2èmes Journées de Chirurgie Digestive, 1980.

Gudjonsson B, Livstone EM, Spiro HM. Cancer of the pancreas diagnostic accuracy and survival statistics. Cancer 1978; 42: 2492.

Huibregtse K, Katon RM, Coene PO, Tytgat GNJ. Endoscopic palliative treatment in pancreatic cancer. Gastrointest Endosc 1986; 32: 334–338.

Ihse I, Lilja P, Arnesjö B, Bengmark S. Total pancreatectomy for cancer: an appraisal of 65 cases. Ann Surg 1977; 186: 675–680.

Launois B. La chirurgie du pancréas pour cancer. Bordeaux Med 1983; 17: 115–118.

Lawrence AG, Gosh BC. Total pancreatectomy for carcinoma of the pancreas. Am J Surg 1977; 77: 244–246.

Lewis WD, Cady B, Rohrer RJ, Jenkins RL, Benotti PN, Dermott WV. Avoidance of transhepatic drainage prior to hepaticojejunostomy for obstruction of the biliary tract. Surg Gynecol Obstet 1987; 165: 381–386.

Matsui Y, Aoki Y, Ishikawa O, et al. Ductal carcinoma of the pancreas: rationales for total pancreatectomy. Arch Surg 1979; 114: 722–726.

Moossa AR. Reoperation for pancreatic cancer. Arch Surg 1979; 114: 502–504.

Moossa AR, Scott MM, Lavell-Jones M. The place of total and extended total pancreatectomy in pancreatic cancer. World J Surg 1984; 8: 895–899.

Pliam MB, Remine WH. Further evaluation of total pancreatectomy. Arch Surg 1975; 110: 506–512.

Sarr MG, Cameron JL. Survival palliation of unresectable carcinoma of the pancreas. World J Surg 1984; 8: 906–918.

Wilson SM, Block GE. Periampullary carcinomas. Arch Surg 1974; 108: 539–544.

7.7   Early Complications After Pancreatic Resection for Pancreatic Head Carcinoma

N.J. Lygidakis and M.N. van der Heyde

Introduction

Pancreatic resection as a modality for the management of pancreatic head carcinoma (Fig. 7.7.**1**) remains a major surgical procedure associated with a range of early and late complications (Bergstrand et al. 1978, Björk et al. 1981, Edis et al. 1980, Forrest and Longmire 1979, Langer et al. 1979, Longmire 1984, Nakase et al. 1977, Papachristou and Fortner 1981, Piorkowski et al. 1982, Van Heerden et al. 1981, Walsh 1982). Progress in diagnostic technique and accumulated experience in a number of highly specialized surgical centers, however, have contributed to a dramatic decline in early mortality and thus initiated renewed interest in the clinical application of pancreatic resection (Braasch et al. 1986, Crist et al. 1987, Mannell et al. 1986, Moossa et al. 1984, Trede 1985). A number of recent publications confirm the hypothesis that resectional surgery remains the only chance of cure for the patient with pancreatic duct, distal bile duct and ampullary carcinoma (Crist et al. 1987, Trede 1985).

In this chapter, the various problems and challenges which we faced in a consecutive series of 100 pancreatic resections carried out in patients with pancreatic head carcinoma are presented.

Technique

The series included 62 men and 38 women with a mean age of 60 years (range 23–74 years). After extensive screening and staging (Table 7.7.**1**), the patients had been judged eligible for pancreatic resection. Exception was made in cases of (a) presence of distant metastases, (b) presence of non-compensated respiratory and cardiovascular disease, and (c) presence of invasion of the celiac axis or of the superior mesenteric artery. At the time of admission, the clinical presentation varied. Before surgery, patients were routinely prepared for the operation (Table 7.7.**2**). A number of patients had biliary drainage by means of an endoprosthesis inserted after papillotomy during the initial endoscopic retrograde cholangiopancreatography (ERCP).

Initial surgical management included extended subtotal duodenopancreatectomy in 78 patients (group A) and total pancreatectomy in 22 patients

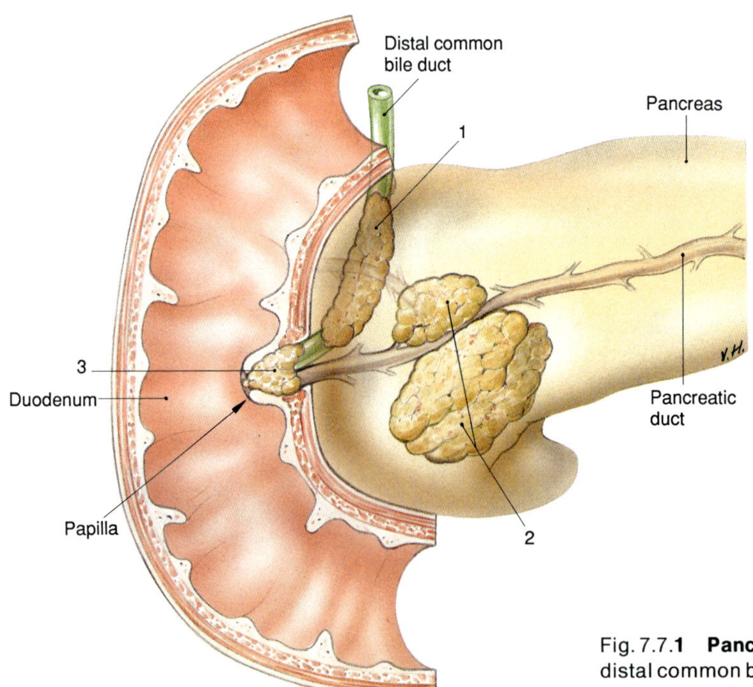

Fig. 7.7.**1**   **Pancreatic head carcinoma** 1 Carcinoma of the distal common bile duct; 2 carcinoma of the pancreatic duct and pancreatic head; 3 ampullary carcinoma

Table 7.7.1   Techniques in the preoperative diagnosis of pancreatic head carcinoma

Endoscopic retrograde cholangiopancreatography (ERCP)
Histopathology of biopsies taken during ERCP
Percutaneous transhepatic cholangiography
Computed tomography
Ultrasonography
Echo-endoscopy
Angiography of hepatic and superior mesenteric arteries
Late-phase splenography
Liver tests (SGOT, SGPT, alkaline phosphatase, total bilirubin, γ-GT)
Pancreas tests (serum amylase, serum glucose)
Coagulation profile (bleeding and clotting time, PTT, thrombocytes)

SGOT: serum glutamic-oxaloacetic transaminase; SGPT: serum glutamic-pyruvic transaminase; γ-GT: gamma-glutamyl transpeptidase; PTT: partial thromboplastin time

Table 7.7.2   Preoperative preparation in patients with pancreatic head carcinoma

Total parenteral nutrition*
Whole-gut irrigation**
Correction of coagulopathy*
Preoperative biliary drainage*
(range: 1–24 weeks, mean: 5 weeks)

* In a proportion of patients
** In all patients

Table 7.7.3   Histological diagnosis of 100 resected specimens of total or subtotal pancreatectomy

	Pancreatectomy	
	Total (n = 22)	Subtotal (n = 78)
Ampullary carcinoma (n = 33)	3	30
Distal bile duct carcinoma (n = 32)	6	26
Pancreatic duct carcinoma (n = 31)	13	22

(group B). Pancreatic resections were carried out following the techniques described in Chapters 7.1, 7.2, and 7.3, and reconstruction of alimentary continuity as outlined in Chapter 7.4. Bile samples for anaerobe and aerobe cultures were taken routinely during initial surgery. Resected specimens were assessed in the department of pathology (Table 7.7.3).

Postoperative care was completed, and after an overnight stay in the recovery room, most patients were transferred to the specialized HPB ward. During the first 2–3 years, patients were routinely admitted to the intensive care unit. On the 14th postoperative day, a fistulography was made via the transanastomotic tube to assess healing of the anastomosis in the majority of patients. Extensive diagnostic procedures were carried out at the slightest clinical suspicion or sign of postoperative complication. These included chest X-rays, ultrasound and computed tomography (CT) studies of the abdominal cavity, leukocyte scans and, in case of gastrointestinal bleeding, selective angiography of the celiac trunk or superior mesenteric artery, or both, and erythrocyte scan in a number of patients.

Operative mortality was defined as the number of deaths that occurred during the first 30 postoperative days. Complications were characterized as "major" if surgical re-intervention was indicated, and as "minor" if they could be treated conservatively. The decision on whether to reoperate or not was based on clinical grounds, i.e. persistent hyperthermia, tachycardia, signs of peritoneal irritation, signs of gastrointestinal or abdominal bleeding, or signs of ileus, and on the results of the examinations mentioned above.

Surgical management during re-exploration included a wide exposure of the abdominal cavity by entering the former incision. Management was aggressive, in an attempt to eradicate any residual area of sepsis. In many patients in whom it was considered that sepsis remained, we preferred to leave the abdominal cavity open by just closing the edges of the wound with an interposed Vicryl mesh. Patients were kept under complete respiratory control, and were intubated as long as this was considered necessary. By doing this we could follow a program of 'planned relaparotomy' and re-explore the patient every two or three days if this was necessary, based on his or her general condition. The number of re-interventions ranged per patient from one to 6 interventions, with a mean of 2. A total of 30 re-interventions were performed in 18 patients.

Minor complications were treated conservatively by means of percutaneous CT-guided drainage or selective embolization. The choice depended on the kind of complication (abscess or bleeding) and from its location and extent.

Results

Three patients died during the first 30 days after operation, two after total pancreatectomy and one after subtotal pancreatectomy. Causes of death were bleeding, sepsis and thrombosis of the superior mesenteric vein anastomosis. Two of these patients had re-interventions.

Sepsis and septic complications. Sepsis was the main cause of postoperative complications, and occurred in 35 patients (35 %). Sepsis included the

Table 7.7.4   Localization of abscess in patients who underwent pancreatic resection for pancreatic head carcinoma (n = 100).
In parentheses, the number of patients with more than one intervention

	Group A (n = 78)	Group B (n = 22)
Generalized peritonitis		1
Subphrenic or subhepatic abscess	6 (4)	1
Intrahepatic abscess		2 (1)
Retroperitoneal abscess secondary to infected hematoma	2	2 (1)

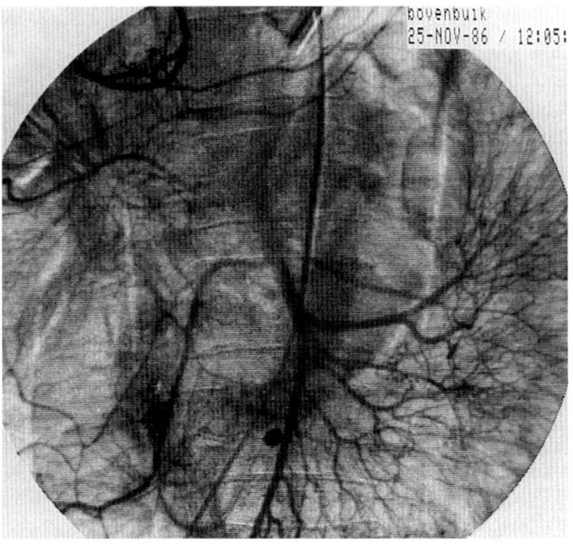

Fig. 7.7.**2   Selective superior mesenteric angiography** shows the site of origin of bleeding in the area of the jejunojejunal anastomosis in a patient with Roux-en-Y reconstruction after subtotal duodenopancreatectomy

formation of an intra-abdominal abscess (14 patients) or abdominal wall infiltration (9 patients), known to be associated with persistent hyperpyrexia and was characterized by absence of intraperitoneal fluid collection. Intra-abdominal abscesses required re-intervention in 14 patients, and were present in several locations (Tables 7.7.**4**). Nine of the 14 patients with intra-abdominal abscesses had positive bile cultures. Eight of the 9 patients with abdominal wall infiltration had positive bile cultures, as did 8 of the 12 patients with wound infection. The micro-organisms isolated from the abscess exudates were identical with those isolated from the bile cultures.

Bleeding. Bleeding in the gastrointestinal tract occurred in 7 patients, 3 of them requiring early re-intervention. Another 4 patients developed intra-abdominal bleeding with early re-intervention in 3 patients. Selective angiography of the celiac trunk or superior mesenteric artery, or both, proved to be of great benefit in defining the site of bleeding precisely (Figs. 7.7.**2** and 7.7.**3**) and in assessing its severity. Selective angiography also proved its value in the control of bleeding. Four of the 7 patients with gastrointestinal bleeding were successfully treated either by infusion of somatostatin or vasopressin, or with embolization of the bleeding vessels. Bleeding was not related to the age of the patients, nor was there any relationship to serum bilirubin levels, or to the installation of preoperative biliary drainage, or to the presence of positive bile cultures.

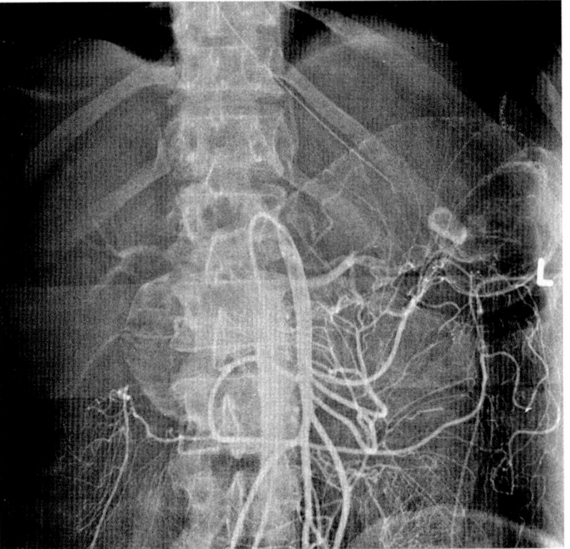

Fig. 7.7.**3   Selective angiography** via the superior mesenteric artery shows the origin of bleeding from a jejunal vessel all along the gastrojejunostomy

Table 7.7.5   Relation between the histological diagnosis and the incidence of major complications after pancreatic resection (n = 100)

	Sepsis (n = 14)	Pancreatic or biliary anastomotic leakage (n = 3)	Intra-abdominal and gastrointestinal tract bleeding (n = 6)
Pancreatic duct carcinoma (n = 35)	6		3
Distal common bile duct carcinoma (n = 32)	4	1	1
Ampullary carcinoma (n = 33)	4	2	2

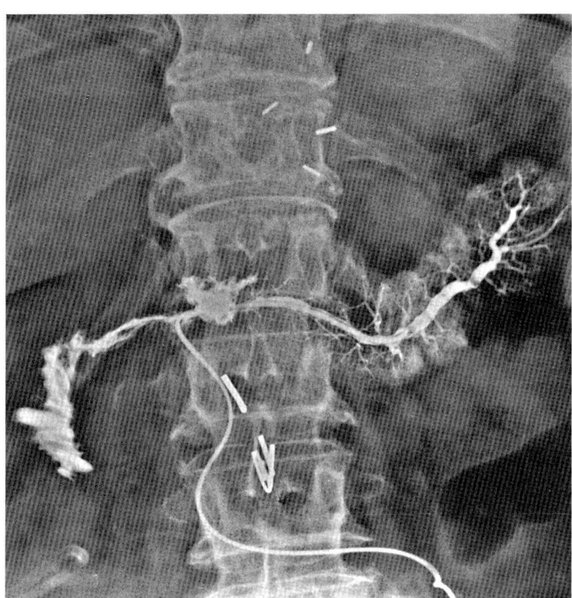

Fig. 7.7.**4** **Fistulogram** shows leakage of the pancreaticojejunal anastomosis

Anastomotic leakage. Another aspect concerns the incidence of anastomotic leakage, and more specifically the incidence of pancreatic anastomotic leakage. Although 11 patients were seen to have pancreaticojejunostomy leakage on fistulograms (Fig. 7.7.**4**) only 1 patient required early re-intervention. In all 10 patients, the leakages healed spontaneously under conservative management. Conservative treatment consisted of antibiotics, adequate drainage via the already in situ abdominal drains, and total parenteral nutrition. Only one of the 10 patients required percutaneous drainage of a subphrenic abscess.

Fistulography in another 5 patients showed biliary anastomotic leakage. Only 2 patients required reoperation. The remaining 3 responded well to the same type of conservative management.

The relationship between the histological diagnosis of the disease and the incidence of the various complications is presented in Table 7.7.**5**.

Discussion

Despite encouraging results, pancreatic resection is still associated with major operative risks and a considerable incidence of serious postoperative complications. Close monitoring and recording of the postoperative status of each patient, and the use of modern diagnostic techniques for early and precise detection of the various complications, make early and precise identification of complications possible and prevent any delay in the decision for early re-intervention. In our opinion, early re-intervention is the main factor contributing to

the overall results of the present series. We believe that the timing of the re-exploration is of the utmost importance, since exploration should be done at an early stage, before the various adverse reactions of sepsis or bleeding become irreversible. With a well-planned policy of early re-intervention and the pre-planned relaparotomies mentioned above, together with optimal use of modern diagnostic techniques, we were able to treat a number of patients successfully. Among these techniques, angiography was of value for the precise localization of bleeding (Fig. 7.7.**5**) and in estimating its severity. Additionally, computed tomography and ultrasound contributed to the diagnosis of abdominal symptoms, and were an aid in differentiating between intra-abdominal abscess and abdominal wall infiltrations (Fig. 7.7.**6**). Fistulography showed the presence and extent of anastomotic leakage, and this, in combination with the clinical presentation of the patient and the outcome of the abdominal CT scan and ultrasound studies, enabled the decision to be made on whether treatment should be surgical or medical.

Although the incidence of leakage of both pancreatic and biliary anastomoses remains high, it is certainly lower than reported in other series (11–22 %) (Langer et al. 1979, Longmire 1984, Piorkowski et al. 1982, Walsh 1982). The majority of the patients had no clinical evidence of leakage. Moreover, the anastomotic leakage healed spontaneously with conservative management (Fig. 7.7.**7**). We believe that a number of factors contribute to the ultimately favorable outcome, such as the

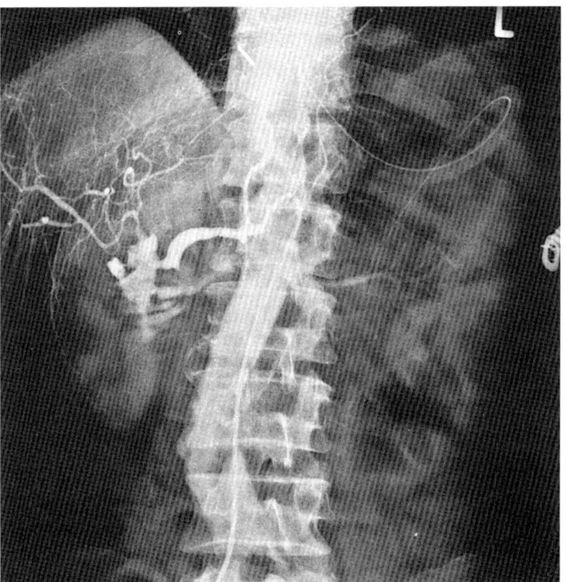

Fig. 7.7.**5** **Selective hepatic artery angiography** shows the origin of bleeding from a traumatic aneurysm of the right hepatic artery 45 days after extensive (regional) subtotal duodenopancreatectomy

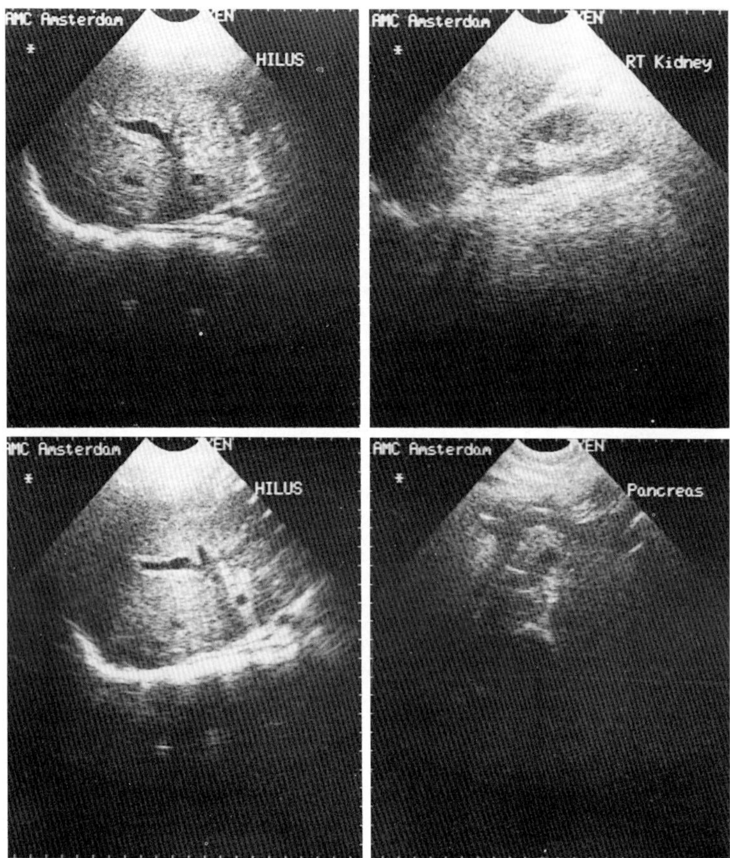

Fig. 7.7.**6** **Ultrasound findings** in a patient with right subphrenic and subhepatic fluid collections

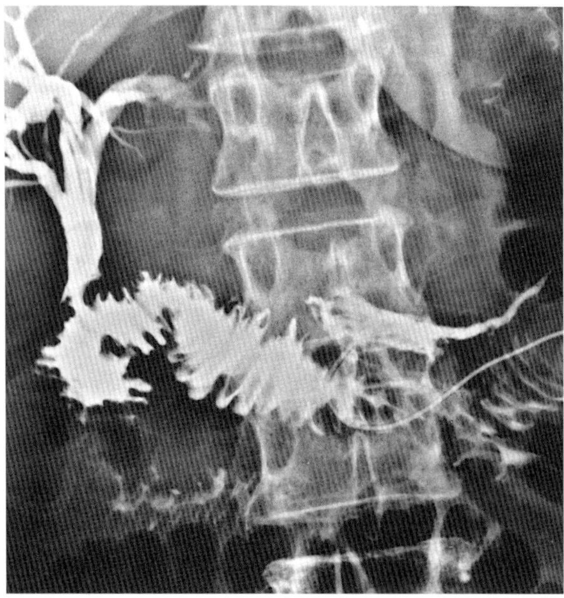

Fig. 7.7.**7** **Leakage of the pancreatic anastomosis** in a patient in whom the leakage healed without surgical intervention

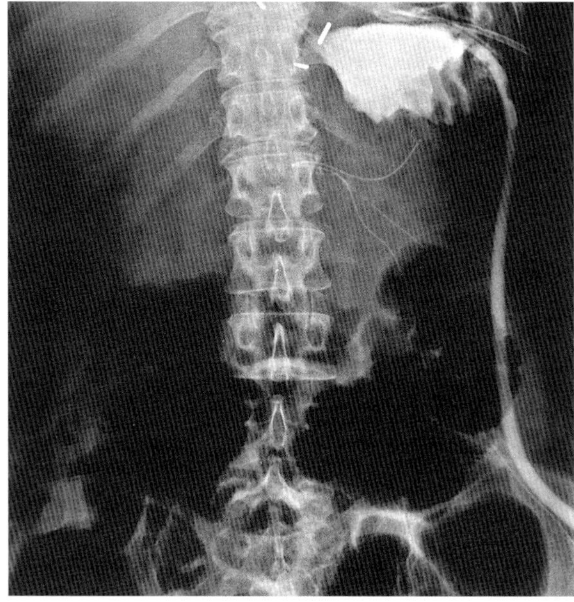

Fig. 7.7.**8** **Laceration of the gastric wall** after total pancreatectomy and splenectomy, seen in an X-ray control via the left subphrenic tube

method of reconstruction, in which healing is promoted by means of a separate jejunal loop for the pancreatic and biliary anastomoses. With a reconstruction of this sort, overloading of the anastomotic line with gastric content is avoided, while at the same time early oral feeding is feasible, even in the case of anastomotic leakage along the loop of the pancreatic and biliary anastomoses. Another contributing factor is the use of transluminal drains by means of which a so-called blow-out of the anastomosis is avoided, since postoperative edema may temporarily obstruct the flow of pancreatic secretion and bile. This difference after anastomotic leakage is, in our opinion, an interesting and important factor with regard to the outcome for the patient. If the various factors responsible for postoperative complications are evaluated, the incidence of septic complications associated with infected bile after the introduction of endoprostheses is certainly a major enabling factor. However, the majority of these septic complications occurred or were linked to incidents secondary to technical faults, such as thrombosis of the right hepatic artery after regional subtotal pancreatectomy, laceration of the gastric wall after total pancreatectomy, splenectomy with subsequent damage to the vascular supply of the gastric remnant (Fig. 7.7.**8**), and finally, in the region of the uncinate process all along the right retroperitoneal space, large hematomas caused by persistent diffuse bleeding secondary to inadequate hemostasis during pancreatic resection. The presence of large hematoma and infected bile may certainly provoke the onset of an abscess. Refined surgical technique, meticulous hemostasis, and avoidance of necrosis and spilling of bile during pancreatic resection, are of paramount importance. Also, careful monitoring of the patient during the early postoperative period is vital.

References

Bergstrand O, et al. A retrospective study of carcinoma of the pancreas with special reference to the results of surgical treatment. Acta Chir Scand 1978; 26 (suppl 482).

Björk S, Svenson JO, et al. Cancer of the head of the pancreas and choledochoduodenal junction: a clinical study of 88 Whipple resections. Acta Chir Scand 1981; 147: 353–361.

Braasch JW, Deziel DJ, Rossi RL, et al. Pyloric and gastric preserving pancreatic resection: experience with 87 patients. Ann Surg 1986; 204: 411–418.

Crist DW, Sitzmann JV, Cameron JL. Improved hospital morbidity, mortality and survival after the Whipple procedure. Ann Surg 1987; 206: 358–365.

Edis AJ, Kierman PD, Taylor WF. Attempted curative resection of ductal carcinoma of the pancreas: review of Mayo Clinic experience. Mayo Clin Proc 1980; 55: 531.

Forrest JF, Longmire WP Jr. Carcinoma of the pancreas and periampullary region: a study of 279 patients. Ann Surg 1979; 189: 129–135.

Grace PA, Pitt HA, Tompkins RK, et al. Decreased morbidity and mortality after pancreatoduodenectomy. Am J Surg 1986; 152: 141–149.

Langer B, et al. Periampullary tumors: advances in diagnosis and surgical treatment. Can J Surg 1979; 22: 34.

Longmire WP Jr. Cancer of the pancreas: palliative operation, Whipple procedure or total pancreatectomy. World J Surg 1984; 8: 872–879.

Mannell A, van Heerden JA, Weiland LH, Ilstrup DM. Factors influencing survival after resection for ductal adenocarcinoma of the pancreas. Ann Surg 1986; 203: 403–407.

Moossa AR, Scott MM, Lavell-Jones M. The place of total and extended total pancreatectomy in pancreatic cancer. World J Surg 1984; 8: 895–899.

Nakase A, Matsumoto Y, et al. Surgical treatment of cancer of the pancreas and periampullary region: cumulative results in 57 institutions in Japan. Ann Surg 1977; 177: 185–193.

Papachristou DN, Fortner JG. Pancreatic fistula complicating pancreatectomy for malignant disease. Br J Surg 1981; 68: 238–242.

Piorkowski RJ, Blievernicht SW, Lawrence W Jr, et al. Pancreatic and periampullary carcinoma: experience with 200 patients over a 12 year period. Am J Surg 1982; 143: 189–193.

Trede M. The surgical treatment of pancreatic carcinoma. Surgery 1985; 97: 28–35.

Van Heerden JA, McIlrath DC, Dozois RR, et al. Radical pancreatoduodenectomy: a procedure to be abandoned. Mayo Clin Proc 1981; 56: 601–700.

Walsh DB. Adenocarcinoma of the ampulla of Vater: diagnosis and treatment. Ann Surg 1982; 195: 152.

7.8   Resectional Surgery for Pancreatic Head Carcinoma: Can the Prognosis Be Predicted?

N.J. Lygidakis and H.J. Houthoff

Introduction

Carcinoma of the pancreatic head (pancreatic duct, distal bile duct and ampullary carcinoma) remains a subject of controversy with regard to its management and prognosis. The incidence of carcinoma of the pancreatic head is increasing, and an estimated 25000 new cases of primary pancreatic carcinoma are diagnosed annually in the United States. This number corresponds to the estimated number of patients who die of this disease each year in the USA (Moossa and Dawson 1981). Recently, pancreatic resection has gained ground and it can at present be considered as the only possibility of cure (Braasch et al. 1986, Carter 1987, Crist et al. 1987, Grace et al. 1986, Lygidakis et al. 1986, Mannell et al. 1986, Trede 1985, Tsuchiya et al. 1986). Unfortunately, the number of patients amenable to resectional surgery is low at the time of diagnosis, and is limited even in the best series to 22.1 % of patients with cancer of the head of the gland and to only 7 % of those with cancer of the body and tail of the pancreas (Matsumo and Sato 1986). Although the tumor may be locally invasive, this does not mean that there is diffuse spread, and that in itself does not mean that surgical resection is excluded (Carter 1987).

The acceptance of pancreatic resection as the procedure of choice for the management of pancreatic head carcinoma is the result of an impressive decline in mortality after pancreatectomy (Braasch et al. 1986, Crist et al. 1987, Grace et al. 1986, Mannell et al. 1986, Tsuchiya et al. 1986). Mortality after subtotal pancreatectomy can be as low as 2 %, and may be associated with low late morbidity as well as with promising long-term survival (Chapters 7.1, 7.2) (Braasch et al. 1986, Crist et al. 1987, Grace et al. 1986, Mannell et al. 1986, Tsuchiya et al. 1986). To appreciate this change, the figures previously obtained for morbidity and mortality have to be recalled. The average mortality rate amongst 4622 patients treated for malignant tumors of the pancreas recorded over the past 20 years was 17.7 % (Warren et al. 1975). Another series of 3610 patients showed mortality rates of 25.3 % after duodenopancreatectomy and 37.5 % after total pancreatectomy (Nakase et al. 1977). In general, the mortality varied from 10–30 % and was associated with a high morbidity rate and short survival (Bergstrand et al. 1978, Hines and Bruens 1976, Webster et al. 1975).

Palliative biliodigestive bypass surgery is associated with dismal results with regard to morbidity and mortality, which are higher than after pancreatic resection. Mortality after palliative surgical procedures for pancreatic head carcinoma ranges from 11–30 %, with a mean of 22 % (Braasch et al. 1986, Crile 1979, Hertner et al. 1982, Longmire 1984, Shapiro 1975, Van Heerden et al. 1980, Zollinger et al. 1982). The reported figures with regard to survival are also disappointing. Survival in all reported series is limited, with a poor quality of life (Crile 1979, Hertner et al. 1982, Leduska et al. 1977, Longmire 1984). Endoscopic palliation, usually carried out in end-stage patients who are unfit for surgical therapy, is associated with significant mortality and with survival rates which are more or less similar to those reported after surgical palliative procedures (Huibregtse et al. 1986).

With all this information in mind, it is clear that pancreatic resection has much to offer, and may lead to more satisfactory short- and long-term results in surgically-fit patients. However, predictive criteria, based on preoperative findings, which would assist in deciding which patients with pancreatic head carcinoma will benefit more, do not as yet exist. In an attempt to define the relation of a number of morphological findings to the prognosis and outcome in each individual patient, we retrospectively assessed a number of histological findings from each resected specimen, using a standard morphological protocol. The present study reports our results.

Methods

Specimens from our first 100 pancreatic resections for ampullary, bile duct and pancreatic duct carcinoma were evaluated retrospectively.

Morphological evaluation. All resected specimens were evaluated in the department of pathology. To set a standard protocol for staging, a number of parameters were used. These are presented in Table 7.8.1. The specimens were processed according to the same protocol, defining the macroscopic and microscopic procedures. After inspection and orientation, the specimens were sectioned in an anteroposterior direction. The slices of the whole ampullary region, including the head of the pancreas, were routinely embedded in paraffin. The surgical resection margins, e. g. in the small intestine, stomach, head or tail of the pancreas, common bile duct and mesenteric soft tissues around the superior mesenteric artery and vein, were all examined. The soft tissues around the head of the pancreas, present in all surgical specimens and representing the cleavage margins, were marked with ink and subsequently embedded to evaluate the radicality of tumor resection in these regions. The local lymph nodes located around the portal vein and common bile duct, the portal area of the liver and the region of the stomach, were separately enclosed for staging of lymph node involvement.

Classification and grading of the tumors were carried out on the basis of their site of origin and microscopic characteristics. Tumors superficial to the muscularis propria of the duodenum which originated from the mucous membrane of the common or ampullary part of the ductal system and ampullary region were classified as ampullary carcinoma (Fig. 7.7.1, p. 304). Tumors which clearly originated from the epithelial lining of the pancreatic ducts were defined as pancreatic duct tumors, and tumors which originated from the distal part of the common bile duct were diagnosed as bile duct tumors.

Follow-up included detailed clinical history and meticulous physical examination to assess the symptoms and sequelae related to the operation or the disease.

Statistical analysis. The results were analyzed using a number of statistical techniques, the Mantel-Haenzel test, the log-rank test and the proportional hazards model.

Results

Pathological evaluation showed ampullary carcinoma in 33 patients, distal common bile duct carcinomas in 32 patients, and pancreatic duct tumors in 35. Adenocarcinomas were well, moderately or poorly differentiated and classified according to the commonly accepted cytonuclear and histological criteria. Perineural invasion, e. g. inva-

Table 7.8.1   Parameters for histological staging

		Staging
Tumor size less than 2 cm	* T	T1
Tumor size 2–4 cm		T2
Tumor size 4–6 cm		T3
Tumor size more than 6 cm	*	T4
No pancreactic capsule involvement	S	S0
pancreatic capsule involvement		S1
No retroperitoneal extension of disease	Rp	Rp0
retroperitoneal extension		Rp1
No vascular involvement	V	V0
vascular involvement		V1
No lymph node involvement	N	N0
Lymph node involvement		N1
Local lymph node involvement		N1a
Regional lymph node involvement (portal/mesenteric)		N1b
Distant lymph node involvement (para-aortic)		N1c

* The tumor diameter is not used as a staging parameter

Table 7.8.2   Histopathological diagnosis in 100 patients with pancreatic head carcinoma in relation to size, differentiation and spread of tumor and residual pathology in the surgical margins

	n	Bile duct	Pancreatic duct	Ampullary
Total	100	32	35	33
Differentiation				
High	20	5	7	8
Moderate	40	13	16	11
Poor	40	14	12	14
mean diameter, cm		1.7	2.8	2.4
(range, cm)		(0.4–4.5)	(1–6)	(0.5–7)
Invasive growth				
soft tissue	60	18	24	18
blood vessels	56	19	22	15
perineural	51	16	18	17
Lymphnode involvement				
Local	49	15	18	16
Regional	3	0	2	1
Distant	0			
Surgical margins				
Cleavage margins	31	8	17	6
Blood vessels	16	5	10	1
Pancreatic ducts	1	0	2	0

Table 7.8.3 Correlation between 2 cm tumor diameter and the stage of the tumor according to the histopathological findings in the resected specimen, demonstrating the lack of direct relation between the two parameters

	n	Diameter > 2 cm (n = 60)			Diameter < 2 cm (n = 40)		
		Stage I	II	III	Stage I	II	III
Ampullary carcinoma	33	3	5	7	4	6	8
Distal common bile duct carcinoma	32	3	6	8	2	5	8
Pancreatic duct carcinoma	35	1	13	14	2	3	2
Total	100	7	24	29	8	14	18

Table 7.8.4 Staging systems for pancreatic head carcinoma adopted according to the results of the present study. (Stage IV patients were not eligible for resection)

	Stage I	Stage II	Stage III	Stage IV
Diameter of the tumor (T)*	1–3	1–3	1–3	1–4
Pancreatic capsule involvement (S)	0	1	1/0	1
Retroperitoneal extension of disease (Rp)	0	1	1/0	1
Vascular involvement (V)	0	1	1/0	1
Lymph node involvement (N)	0	0	1a, 1b	1c

* The tumor diameter is not used as a staging parameter

sion of tumor cells in and around the peripheral nerves, was present in the majority of the malignant specimens, as was vasoinvasive growth in the small lymphatic or blood vessels. Even in small tumors, this invasive growth could be extensive (Table 7.8.1, 7.8.2). The presence of free margins of resection was often more dependent on invasive growth than on the size of the tumor. Resections were defined as having free margins when the distance between the surgical margins and the infiltrative growth was 1.5 mm or more. Specimens which were considered not to have free margins were those with a clear tumor mass around the ducts, vessels or nerves, or in the connective tissue of the surgical margins. Further histological assessment in each patient showed a not significant relation between the diameter of the tumor and its stage (Table 7.8.3) (Mantel-Haenzel test stratified by cancer type. These figures were the same irrespective of whether ampullary, pancreatic duct or distal bile duct carcinoma was involved. Indeed, the invasive and metastatic potential of large tumors (diameter more than 2 cm) equalled that of small tumors (less than 2 cm). This prompted us to adopt an adapted staging system (Table 7.8.4).

Staging of the malignant tumors and, more particularly the extension of invasive growth as assessed by the histological parameters in the resected specimen, were not related to the type or site of origin of the tumors (Tables 7.8.5, 7.8.6). In fact, only 10–15% of malignant tumors – irrespec-

tive of the site of the tumor – were in stage I of the disease. Therefore, so-called early cancer (malignant mass confined to the region of origin with only local infiltrative growth and without metastasis) was only encountered in a small number of patients. With the Mantel-Haenzel test stratified by cancer type, it was possible to confirm that there was no association between the tumor stage and its site of origin (p > 0.20). Staging of the tumor, however, was related to the grading, i.e. differentiation, of the malignant tumor. The differentiation of the tumor was not related to the site of origin of the neoplasm (Table 7.8.2).

Evaluation of the invasive growth of the tumors showed that 18 of the 33 patients with periampullary carcinoma had retroperitoneal and perineural spread of the tumor. Sixteen of these 18 patients had lymph node involvement. Eighteen of the 32 patients with distal common bile duct carcinoma also had retroperitoneal and perineural spread, with lymph node involvement in 15 of these in addition. Similarly, 24 of the 35 patients with pancreatic duct carcinoma showed spread in 18 associated with lymph node involvement.

Pathological evaluation of the resected specimens showed that 52 of the 100 patients had free resectional margins, while 48 had involved resectional margins. The presence of free resectional margins was not influenced by the extent of the pancreatic resection. The presence of free resectional margins was not related to the size of the

Table 7.8.5 Correlation between tumor classification, stage of the disease and the presence of free resectional margins (bracketed figures). Mantel-Haenzel test

	n	Stage I	Stage II	Stage III
Ampullary adenocarcinoma	33 (26)	6 (6)	15 (10)	12 (10)
Distal common bile duct carcinoma	32 (19)	4 (4)	12 (8)	16 (7)
Pancreatic duct carcinoma	35 (7)	3 (3)	15 (2)	17 (2)
Total	100 (52)	13 (13)	42 (20)	45 (19)

Table 7.8.6 Correlation between 2 cm tumor diameter and the presence of free resectional margins (bracketed figures). No direct relation between the two parameters is evident.

	n	Diameter > 2 cm	Diameter < 2 cm
Ampullary carcinoma	33	15 (11)	18 (15)
Distal common bile duct carcinoma	32	17 (9)	15 (10)
Pancreatic duct carcinoma	35	28 (4)	7 (3)
Total	100	60 (24)	40 (28)

Table 7.8.7 Comparison of the survival rate with the tumor classification and radicality of resection.

	n	Alive	Free from disease
Ampullary carcinoma	33	26	22
Distal common bile duct carcinoma	32	19	12
Pancreatic duct carcinoma	35	20	6
Total	100	65	40

lesion. Large and small-sized tumors had equal potential for radical resection (Table 7.8.6). Local or regional lymph node involvement did not preclude radical resection. This was mainly seen in patients with ampullary carcinoma. Twenty-one out of 49 patients with positive lymph nodes had free resectional margins. Irrespective of the site of origin of the tumor, patients with stage I tumors had equally good potential for free resectional margins. Free resectional margins in stage II and stage III tumors were related to the type of neoplasm, and showed a higher incidence in patients with ampullary and distal common bile duct carcinoma than in those with pancreatic duct carcinoma (Table 7.8.5).

Operative results. Three patients died during the first 30 postoperative days as a consequence of the operation (sepsis in 2 patients, bleeding in one patient).

Sixty-five patients are alive at the time of writing (October 1988) (Table 7.8.7). Survival has ranged from 3–50 months and is related to the presence of free resectional margins: 40 of the 52 patients with free resectional margins are alive with a satisfactory quality of life. In contrast, only 25 of the 48 patients with involved resectional margins are alive. Any factor which influences the presence of resectional margins also influences the survival.

Survival was not related to the size of the tumor or to lymph node involvement. Of the total of 40 patients with small tumors (less than 2 cm), 29 are alive compared with 36 of the 60 patients with large tumors (more than 2 cm). The mean survival for the group with small tumors was 28 months, compared with 30 months for those with large tumors (p > 0.15). Lymph node involvement did not preclude long-term survival, and 27 of the 49 patients with lymph node involvement are alive. By

Table 7.8.**8**   **Results of proportional hazards regression analysis** on survival time

Covariate	Regression coefficient	Estimated standard error	Z-statistic
Presence of free resectional margins	1.56	0.69	2.26 significant
Stage I	1.32	0.67	2.17 significant
Diameter	− 0.59	0.55	− 2.09 not significant
Differentiation	1.29	0.68	2.09 significant
Site of origin of ampullary, pancreatic duct and distal bile duct in stage I and II	1.23	0.66	2.19 significant

contrast, the survival was related to the site of origin of the tumor (Table 7.8.**7**, 7.8.**8**).

In conclusion, the survival is significantly influenced by the presence of free resectional margins, differentiation of the tumor, early stage-I tumors irrespective of their origin, and as far as stage-II and stage-III tumors are concerned, the nature of the tumor. Ampullary and distal bile duct tumors have a far better prognosis than pancreatic duct tumors.

Discussion

The present study shows that resectional pancreatic surgery offers satisfactory prospects for patients with ampullary, pancreatic duct and distal bile duct carcinomas. Although at the time of surgery the proportion of patients with a malignant process which is confined to the region of origin (stage I) remains low, the results with respect to the survival are acceptable and are by no means related to the site of origin. As far as the other patients are concerned (stages I and II), those with ampullary lesions are more effectively treated. However, the results so far in the case of pancreatic duct carcinoma offer some encouragement.

Thus, the overall numbers of patients who are alive after resectional surgery for ampullary, distal bile duct and pancreatic duct carcinoma are 26 out of 33, 19 out of 32, and 20 out of 35 patients, respectively.

In our opinion, the results of the present series of patients confirm the conclusion of other studies that pancreatic resection remains the optimal type of management for patients who are considered eligible for this treatment (Braasch et al. 1986, Crist et al. 1987, Grace et al. 1986, Mannell et al. 1986, Trede 1985). Our policy is that a patient is considered eligible for pancreatic resection if the following factors apply: 1) there are no distant metastases (liver); 2) there is no associated non-compensated disease (cardiopulmonary); 3) the patient is younger than 75; 4) the patient is found by CT or US to have a tumor mass of less than 6 cm; 5) there

is no vascular involvement of the celiac axis (common hepatic artery) or superior mesenteric artery; and 6) no invasion of the base of the mesentery and no peritoneal spread are found in the peroperative assessment. Lymph node involvement or limited involvement of the portal vein are not considered to be contra-indications for resection.

There are several considerations in favor of this policy. In the first place, resectional surgery can be carried out with an acceptably low mortality (3 %) (1.4 % after subtotal pancreatectomy and 8 % after total pancreatectomy), with an encouraging long-term survival and with a satisfactory quality of life for the patient following the operation. These figures are in agreement with those of other studies (Braasch et al. 1986, Crist et al. 1987, Grace et al. 1986, Mannell et al. 1986, Trede 1985, Tsuchiya et al. 1986). The results are superior to those following surgical or medical palliative management (Brooks and Culebras 1979, Cotton 1984, Crile 1979, Huibregtse et al. 1986, Leduska et al. 1977, Longmire 1984, Shapiro 1975, Zollinger et al. 1982). Secondly, it became clear from the results of the histological evaluation of each resected specimen that it was not possible to predict the prognosis and outcome of the disease in a substantial number of patients by means of preoperative or peroperative diagnostic investigations. Indeed, we demonstrated that the survival was only related to the degree of differentiation of the tumor, to the presence of free resectional margins and, as far as stage-II and stage-III tumors were concerned, with the site of origin.

None of the aforementioned parameters could be precisely defined before or during the operation, at least not for every individual patient. Only resection can offer eventual cure for the patient with ampullary, pancreatic duct or distal bile duct carcinoma.

Pre- and peroperative screening should be evaluated with care and caution, and the decision on whether a patient is a good or poor candidate for resection should be taken after consideration of the fact that neither the tumor size nor its site of origin can predict the prognosis and outcome. The fact that only pancreatic resection offers a number of patients the possibility of cure means that every effort should be made to assess whether or not every patient under consideration is fit for this kind of management (Crist et al. 1987, Ihse et al. 1977). Finally, even after resection with involved resectional margins, the overall results regarding mortality, morbidity and survival are reasonable (Cotton 1984, Huibregtse et al. 1986, Shapiro 1975). They can certainly not be compared with the results obtained after palliative medical or surgical management, where patients are already at an advanced stage of the disease and are therefore not considered eligible for resectional surgery. However, the fact that the quality of life after palliative resection is acceptable supports our policy of favoring resectional surgery, even in patients in whom it is likely that resection may be non-radical.

References

Akwari OI, van Heerden JA, Adson MA. Radical pancreaticoduodenectomy for cancer of the papilla of Vater. Arch Surg 1977; 112: 451–459.

Braasch JW, Gray NJ. Considerations that lower mortality after pancreatoduodenectomy. Am J Surg 1977; 133: 480–484.

Braasch JW, Deziel DS, Rossi RL, Martinus E, Winter P. Pyloric and gastric preserving pancreatic resection: experience with 87 patients. Ann Surg 1986; 204: 411–418.

Bergstrand O, et al. A retrospective study of pancreas cancer with special reference to the results of surgical treatment. Acta Chir Scand 1978; 26 (suppl 482).

Brooks JR, Culebras JM. Cancer of the pancreas: palliative operation, Whipple procedure or total pancreatectomy. Am J Surg 1979; 131: 516–523.

Carter DC. Carcinoma of the pancreas. Current Opin Gastroenterol 1987; 3: 736–743.

Cotton PB. Endoscopic methods for relief of malignant obstructive jaundice. World J Surg 1984; 8: 854–862.

Crile G Jr. Advantages of bypass operations over radical pancreaticoduodenectomy in treatment of pancreatic carcinoma. Surg Gynecol Obstet 1979; 130: 1049–1053.

Crist DW, Sitzman JN, Cameron JL. Improved hospital morbidity, mortality and survival after Whipple procedure. Ann Surg 1987; 206: 358–365.

Fortner JG. Technique of regional subtotal and total regional pancreatectomy. Am J Surg 1985; 150: 539–545.

Fortner JG. Surgical principles for pancreatic cancer: regional total and subtotal pancreatectomy. Cancer 1981; 47: 1712–1718.

Grace PA, Pitt HA, Tompkins RK, et al. Decreased morbidity and mortality after pancreatoduodenectomy. Am J Surg 1986; 151: 141–143.

Hertner F, Coopermann A, Ahlborn T, Antinou C. Surgical experience with pancreatic and periampullary cancer. Ann Surg 1982; 195: 274–281.

Hines LH, Bruens RP. 10 years experience treating pancreatic and periampullary cancer. Am Surg 1976; 42: 441.

Huibregtse K, Katon RM, Coene PP, Tytgat GNJ. Endoscopic palliative treatment in pancreatic cancer. Gastrointest Endosc 1986; 32: 334–338.

Ihse I, Lilja PM, Arnesjö B, Bengmark S. Total pancreatectomy for cancer by appraisal of 65 cases. Ann Surg 1977; 186: 675–681.

Leduska NJ, et al. Results of palliative operations for carcinoma of the pancreas. Arch Surg 1977; 103: 330–334.

Longmire WP Jr. Cancer of the pancreas: palliative operation, Whipple procedure or total pancreatectomy. World J Surg 1984; 8: 872–879.

Lygidakis NJ, Brummelkamp WH. A new approach for the reconstruction of continuity of the alimentary tract after pancreaticoduodenectomy. Surg Gynecol Obstet 1985; 160: 453–458.

Lygidakis NJ, Brummelkamp WH, Tytgat GNJ, et al. Periampullary and pancreatic head carcinoma: facts and factors influencing mortality, survival and quality of post-operative life. Am J Gastroenterol 1986; 82: 968–974.

Mannell A, van Heerden J, Weiland LH, et al. Factors influencing survival after resection for ductal adenocarcinoma of the pancreas. Ann Surg 1986; 203: 403–407.

Matsumo S, Sato T. Surgical treatment for carcinoma of the pancreas: experience in 272 patients. Am J Surg 1986; 152: 499–503.

Moossa AR, Dawson PJ. The diagnosis of pancreatic cancer. Pathobiol Annu 1981; 11: 299.

Moossa AR, Scott MH, Jones ML. The place of total and extended total pancreatectomy in pancreatic cancer. World J Surg 1979; 3: 516.

Nakase A, Matsumoto Y, Vichiada K, et al. Surgical treatment of cancer of the pancreas and periampullary region: cumulative results in 57 institutions in Japan. Ann Surg 1977; 185: 52–57.

Nagai H, Kuroda A, Morioka Y. Lymphatic and local spread of T1 and T2 pancreatic cancer. Ann Surg 1986; 204: 65–71.

Shapiro TH. Adenocarcinoma of the pancreas and statistical analysis of bypass vs Whipple resection in good-risk patients. Ann Surg 1975; 182: 715–721.

Trede M. The surgical treatment of pancreatic carcinoma. Surgery 1985; 97: 28–35.

Tsuchiya R, Tomioka T, Izawa K. Collective review of small carcinomas of the pancreas. Ann Surg 1986; 203: 77–84.

Van Heerden JA, Heath PM, Alden GR. Biliary bypass for ductal adenocarcinoma of the pancreas: Mayo Clinic experience 1970–1975. Mayo Clin Proc 1980; 55: 537–542.

Van Heerden JA, McIlrath DC, Dozois RR, Adson MA. Radical pancreatoduodenectomy: a procedure to be abandoned? Mayo Clin Proc 1981; 56: 601.

Warren KW, Choe DS, Plaza J, Relihan M. Results of radical resection for periampullary cancer. Ann Surg 1975; 181: 534–542.

Webster DJT. Carcinoma of the pancreas and periampullary region: a clinical study in a district general hospital. Br J Surg 1975; 62: 130.

World Health Organization: Geneva, WHO Offset Publication no 6–8, p 7.

Zollinger RM, Tremolade C, Baccaglini C, et al. Cancer of the pancreas: the surgeon's dilemma. Am J Surg 1982; 43: 279–286.

7.9   Gastrinoma of the Pancreas

T. J. Howard and Edward Passaro, Jr.

Introduction

In 1955, Zollinger and Ellison first described the syndrome of fulminant peptic ulceration, gastric hypersecretion and non-beta islet cell tumors of the pancreas. These tumors were found to secrete an ulcerogenic factor which was later identified as the gastrointestinal hormone gastrin (Gregory et al. 1960). Early therapeutic options were limited, as patients were identified late in the course of their disease. Approximately half of the patients had metastatic disease at the time of the initial diagnosis (McCarthy 1980), and 80 % had had at least one previous ulcer operation (Ellison et al. 1987). As a result of these limitations, successful resection of gastrinomas was felt to be possible in only 5 % of cases (Jensen et al. 1983, Thompson et al. 1975, McCarthy 1980).

Recent advances in radioimmunoassay techniques, anti-secretory medications, and radiographic imaging studies have provided an effective means of early diagnosis and localization (Wolfe and Jensen 1987). Improved understanding of the biological characteristics of these tumors has allowed for better patient selection (Zollinger 1985). As a result of these advances, a third of all patients with gastrinomas may currently be cured by surgical resection (Ellison et al. 1987). Our intent in this chapter is to discuss important developments in the understanding of gastrinomas and the influence of these developments on our ability to resect this tumor successfully for cure.

Historical Background

As early as 1946 (Seiler and Zinninger 1946, Brown et al. 1950, Forty and Barrett 1952), surgeons recognized the presence of a non-insulin-producing islet-cell tumor associated with marked gastric acid secretion and severe peptic ulcer disease. It was not until 1955 that Zollinger and Ellison first postulated an "ulcerogenic humoral factor" secreted by the islet cell tumor as being responsible for the clinical manifestations of this disease. The theory of an ulcerogenic factor of pancreatic origin was not new, having been proposed by Poth et al. (1948) nearly seven years earlier. However, the ability to study this hypothesis in a patient group selected from a large number of patients with peptic ulcer disease was new. Intense interest in this syndrome followed, as clinicians believed that this ulcerogenic factor, if present, might be the key to understanding peptic ulcer disease.

In 1960, Gregory reported on finding gastrin-like activity present in tumor extracts from patients with the Zollinger–Ellison syndrome. Other investigators (Code et al. 1962, Friesen et al. 1962, Grossman et al. 1961) soon corroborated this finding, and the islet-cell tumor elaborating this peptide became known as a gastrinoma. A tumor registry was established by Ellison and Wilson (1964). Its purpose was the collection, centralization and analysis of the available data on a large group of patients with gastrinoma with the intention of developing an optimal standardized treatment regimen.

The development of a rapid, sensitive and reproducible radioimmunoassay for serum gastrin (McGuigan and Grieder 1968, Yalow and Berson 1970) was a major advance in the diagnosis and study of gastrinomas. Serum gastrin radioimmunoassay soon became routine in the evaluation of patients suspected of having a gastrinoma (Jaffee et al. 1972). Although helpful, an elevated serum gastrin level was not diagnostic. Difficulty arose in distinguishing between patients with peptic ulcer disease (Walsh et al. 1975, Stage and Stadil 1979) and gastrinoma patients with mildly elevated serum gastrin levels. To assist in this differentiation, provocative tests were developed measuring the effect of secretin (Isenberg et al. 1972), calcium (Passaro et al. 1972), and bombesin (Basso et al. 1981) on the serum gastrin level. The secretin stimulation test has become the provocative test of choice in making the diagnosis of gastrinoma (McGuigan and Wolfe 1980).

Before effective medical control of the hypersecretory state was developed, total gastrectomy was the best treatment for patients with the Zollinger–Ellison syndrome (Thompson et al. 1982). All other therapeutic endeavors were uniformly unsuccessful (Ellison and Wilson 1967). In 1977, H_2 receptor antagonists became available, and medical control of the hypersecretory state and fulminant ulcer disease became possible (Richardson and Walsh 1976). Cimetidine (McCarthy 1978) controlled the diarrhea common to this group of patients and promoted ulcer healing. Not all patients, however, could be satisfactorily maintained on cimetidine (Stabile et al. 1983, Bonfils et al. 1979). Newer anti-secretory agents are being developed and tested with the hope of developing a more complete medical control of this disease (Lamers et al. 1980). Despite these limitations, the use of anti-secretory agents has now made the need for total gastrectomy rare.

These advances have allowed clinicians to

focus on the long-term consequences of tumor growth and metastasis (Norton et al. 1986a). It is believed that 60% of these tumors are malignant (Zollinger et al. 1976). From a surgical standpoint, it is now possible to have a planned operation with aggressive resection of the primary tumor at an earlier clinical stage. The ideal would therefore be to perform an early, aggressive resection safely to prevent late mortality from metastatic disease.

Embryology

The endocrine pancreas is a complex structural and functional unit which includes the islets of Langerhans plus a number of ill-defined intrapancreatic extra-islet endocrine cells (Deconinck 1971, Larsson and Sunder 1976). The presence of gastrin in islet-cell tumors of the pancreas has been convincingly established (Gregory et al. 1967). Identification of the specific cell type responsible for the production of gastrin in the adult human pancreas has not been established. Although some studies (Erlandsen and Hegre 1976, Polak 1975) show that gastrin is produced in the D cells of the pancreatic islet along with somatostatin, others (Creutzfield 1975, Lofstra 1974, Alumets and Hakanson 1983) have been unable to substantiate these findings. If gastrin-producing cells are not a normal constituent of the islets of Langerhans in man, the ontogeny of gastrinomas becomes important in understanding the biology and location of these tumors.

The precise embryological origin of endocrine cells of the digestive tract, especially the cells composing the islet of Langerhans, remains controversial. Both classic work (Robb 1961) and recent studies (Pusyrev 1979) propose that islet cells similar to pancreatic exocrine cells are derived from the same layer, namely the endodermal cells lining the buds of the primitive gut. Feyrter (1969) disagreed, and felt that the islets of Langerhans are part of a diffuse endocrine system composed of cells dispersed throughout the body. In support of this concept, Pearse (1966, Pearse et al. 1973) demonstrated that cells producing peptide hormones as diverse as the cells of the islets of Langerhans, corticomedullary cells of the adrenal gland, and glomus cells of the carotid body, have a number of common cytochemical and ultrastructural features. The acronym APUD (Pearse 1968) (*amine precursor uptake and decarboxylation*) was coined and applied to these cells to describe their ability to take up material such as dopa or 5-hydroxytryptophan and decarboxylate them to produce biogenic amines. The embryological assumption was made that cells displaying similar structural and biochemical features should have a common origin. All APUD cells were therefore considered to be derived from neuroectodermal (neural crest) precursors (Pearse 1969).

The embryological evidence to support this hypothesis was forthcoming. A neuroectodermal origin of ultimobrachial C-cells of the thyroid, type I cells of the carotid body and corticomedullary cells of the adrenal gland has been completely validated using an allograph marker technique in quail-chick embryos (Le Douarin 1973). Tapia (1981) and Teitelman provided enzymatic evidence of a neural crest origin of pancreatic endocrine cells. Circumstantial evidence for this theory was offered by the clinical syndromes of multiple endocrine neoplasia (MEN), types I and II. These syndromes, associated with cells of the APUD system, involve the familial inheritance of pluriglandular and polyhormonal abnormalities, suggesting a primary genetic defect in the totipotential cells of a common precursor (Friesen et al. 1972). Despite these observations, however, the ontogeny of endocrine cells in the pancreas remains controversial (Andrews 1976, Orci et al. 1970).

In summary, there is no definitive evidence for the presence of a gastrin-secreting cell type in the adult human pancreas. There is also uncertainty with regard to the ontogeny of gastrin-secreting islet-cell tumors of the pancreas. In addition, although the APUD concept is a useful model for understanding the MEN syndromes, experimental evidence has been unable to support its validity. The inability to resolve these fundamental questions has limited our understanding of these tumors. Specific questions concerning tumor location, i.e. pancreatic/duodenal/extrapancreatic/ extraintestinal, and concerning the benign clinical course of resected tumor from lymph nodes, might well be elucidated by an understanding of the ontogeny of gastrinomas.

Pathology

Gastrinomas are usually small tumors, with the majority being less than two centimeters in diameter at most (Norton et al. 1986a). Multiple tumors are found in 10–33% of patients with the sporadic form of the disease (Norton et al. 1986a, Ellison et al. 1987). Multiple tumors are present in all patients with familial gastrinoma associated with the MEN I syndrome. Unfortunately, depending on the experience of the operating surgeon, in 7–30% of patients with biochemical evidence for gastrinoma, no tumor will be found at exploration (Friesen 1982, Deveney et al. 1978, Stabile et al. 1984). The reason for this is as yet unknown. On gross examination, the tumors appear ovoid to round, with a smooth tan appearance (Fig. 7.9.1). The

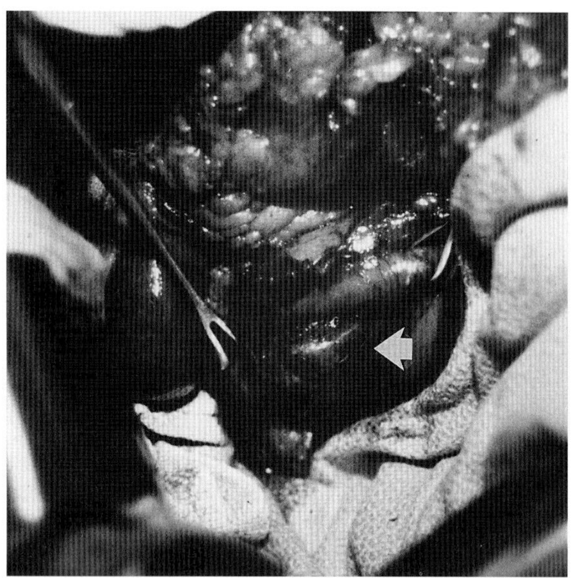

Fig. 7.9.**1**   **After a Kocher maneuver has been performed, Babcock clamps lift the duodenum superiorly and the tumor is found** on the inferior surface of the pancreatic head (arrow)

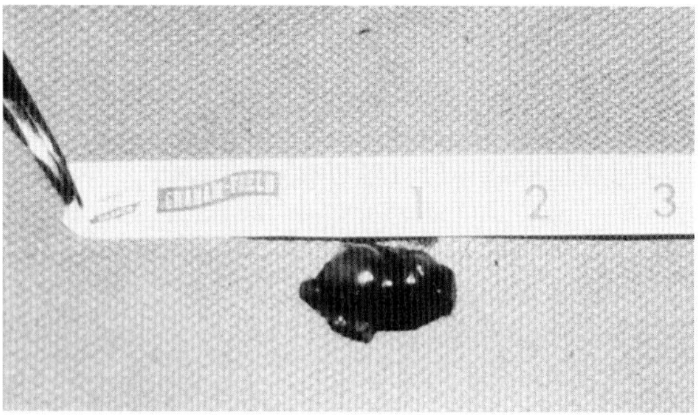

Fig. 7.9.**2**   **Surgical specimen of gastrinoma** excised from the inferior pancreatic head

consistency is firm on palpation. On cut section, a thin fibrous capsule surrounds a brownish, red core of tumor (Fig. 7.9.**2**). Histologically, the tumor closely resembles a carcinoid (Fig. 7.9.**3**). The cells are notably uniform, with eosinophilic cytoplasm and fine granular stippling. The nuclei are oval, with clumps of chromatin and one or more nucleoli. The morphologic pattern is variable. Commonly the tumor cells are in solid sheets or nests of tumor cells with associated trabeculae (Wilson 1973). Follicular or rosette patterns are sometimes seen. Ultrastructurally, the tumor cells have been shown to contain two types of secretory granules (Rosai 1974). One type is round, 150–200 µm in size, resembling the secretory granules of the gastrin-secreting cells in the gastric antrum. The other is pleomorphic and larger, 150–350 µm in size, resembling the secretory granules in the delta cells of the pancreatic islet.

Although it is generally mentioned that 60 % of gastrinomas are malignant (Wolfe et al. 1982, Zollinger et al. 1976), there is confusion as to how malignancy should be defined. Histologic and ultrastructural characteristics are of little value in deciding the malignant potential of a gastrinoma. Based on clinical experience, the presence of tumor in the liver is the sole criterion for malignant disease (Stabile and Passaro 1985). This is important, as a number of surgical series have reported cures from resection of gastrinoma in peripancreatic lymph nodes (Norton et al. 1986a, Stabile and Passaro 1985, Friesen 1982, Malagelada et al. 1983) and ovaries (Norton et al. 1986a) without identification of the primary tumor. The histologic finding of gastrinoma in lymph nodes does not therefore seem to have the same clinical or biological significance as it does for most other tumors.

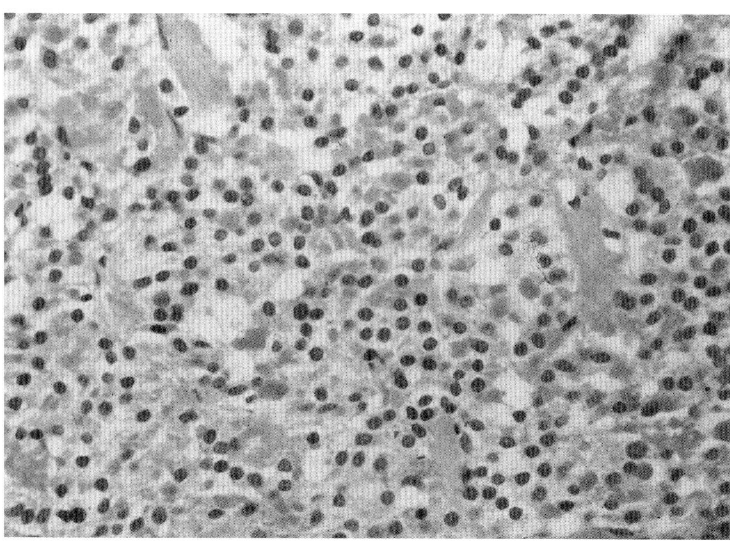

Fig. 7.9.**3**   **Histologic section of a gastrinoma**

Pathophysiology

The pathophysiology of gastrinoma can be explained entirely by accentuation of the known biological effects of gastrin (Isenberg et al. 1973). Gastrin is a potent stimulant of acid secretion and, to a lesser extent, pepsin secretion by the gastric mucosa (Grossman 1960). In addition, gastrin has a direct trophic effect on the gastric mucosa, causing hyperplasia and an increased parietal cell mass (Polacek and Ellison 1963).

The two clinical manifestations of this altered physiology are fulminant peptic ulcer disease and severe diarrhea (Wolfe and Jensen 1987). The peptic ulcers are the result of gastric acid hypersecretion from the direct stimulation by gastrin of the parietal cell mass. The cause of the diarrhea in patients with a gastrinoma is multifactorial (Isenberg et al. 1973). The delivery of large volumes of acid to the duodenum and a decrease in small bowel absorption due to the direct action of gastrin have been suggested as possible mechanisms (Isenberg et al. 1973). It is unlikely that the diarrhea in patients with a gastrinoma is due solely to the direct effect of gastrin on intestinal absorption, as the symptoms are relieved after total gastrectomy (Soergel 1969). Other mechanisms contributing to the diarrhea include mucosal damage from the acid load leading to direct malabsorption, inactivation of pancreatic enzymes by the low intraduodenal pH, and an increased gastro-intestinal motility (Grossman 1960). Clinical observation has shown that patients undergoing gastric juice aspiration for secretory studies uniformly report a decrease in diarrhea and ulcer symptoms.

Clinical Features

The incidence of gastrinoma in the general population has been estimated at up to 0.1 % of all patients with duodenal ulcer disease (Wolfe and Jensen 1987). From the available data there appears to be no significant racial or geographic distribution. The peak onset for symptoms is between the 3rd and 5th decade, although tumors have been reported in the very old (Ellison and Wilson 1967) and very young (Wilson 1982). Most series show a preponderance in males, who form approximately 65 % of the patients studied (Norton et al. 1986a, Thompson et al. 1982).

The most common presenting symptom of patients with gastrinoma is abdominal pain, which occurs in 70–95 % of patients (Ellison and Wilson 1964, Way et al. 1968). The pain is typically mid-epigastric in location, burning in nature, and associated with peptic ulceration. In approximately 20 % of patients, diarrhea will be the presenting symptom (Ellison and Wilson 1964). The duration of ulcer symptoms prior to diagnosis averages 4 years (Ellison et al. 1987). The clinical spectrum of patients with gastrinomas has changed since the introduction of the gastrin radioimmunoassay in 1970 and histamine H_2 antagonists in 1977. To emphasize this point, Ellison et al. (1987) have shown that prior to 1970, 80 % of patients had serious complications from peptic ulcer disease including bleeding, perforation, or obstruction. In contrast, only 20 % of patients after 1970 had these complications. Currently, patients are presenting with more chronic, indolent symptoms. It is not unusual to see patients who have suffered from intermittent abdominal pain for years on cimetidine and antacids prior to their presention to the surgeon.

Patients with gastrinoma typically have no abnormal findings on physical examination. Mild weight loss or gain, tenderness in the mid-epigastrium or a guaiac-positive stool are sometimes found. Unlike other pancreatic islet-cell tumors, patients with gastrinomas have no characteristic cutaneous stigmata (Wilkinson 1973).

Radiology

The roentgenographic appearance of the upper gastrointestinal tract in patients with the Zollinger–Ellison syndrome is quite characteristic (Cope and Warwick 1974, Zboralske and Amberg 1968). The pathologic changes reflect the underlying pathophysiologic state. Despite the overnight fast, the hypersecretory state produces increased intraluminal fluid, detected on the initial flow of barium into the stomach. Large gastric rugal folds, particularly in the body and fundus, reflect the parietal cell hyperplasia which occurs in the presence of persistent hypergastrinemia. Dilation of the duodenum and jejunum is associated with edematous mucosal folds (Weber et al. 1959) (Fig. 7.9.**4**). A floccular, granular appearance of the barium is noted. Motility of the bowel is variable, with the stomach and duodenum being described as large and atonic, but with the small bowel having rapid transit. Ulcers in the distal part of the duodenum or jejunum are highly suggestive of a gastrinoma, but are rare.

Abdominal ultrasound has been reported to detect pancreatic tumors in 28 % of patients with the Zollinger–Ellison syndrome (Hancke 1979). Other studies substantiate this low sensitivity when used preoperatively (Norton et al. 1986a). Ultrasound's utility may be more fully realized intraoperatively as an adjunct to manual palpation in the localization of small intrapancreatic tumors (Klotter et al. 1987, Cromack et al. 1987).

Computed tomography (CT) was initially re-

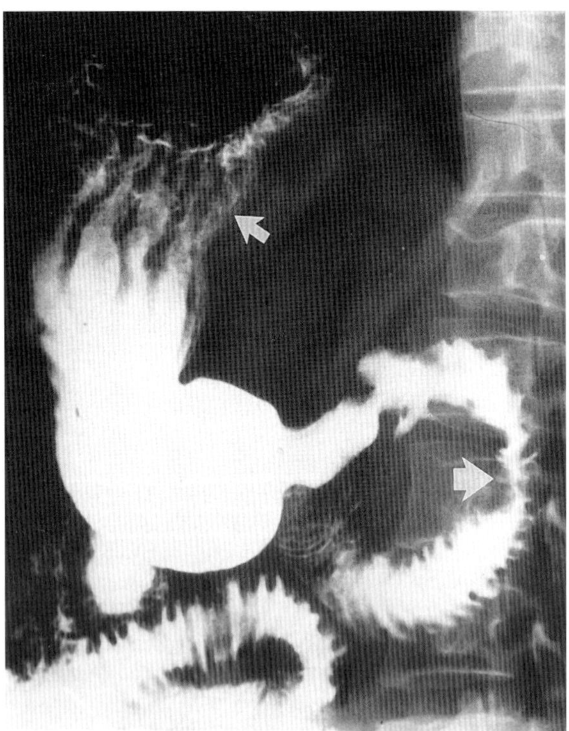

Fig. 7.9.**4 Upper gastrointestinal series** of a patient with the Zollinger–Ellison syndrome. Note the large rugal folds (small arrow) and the edematous mucosal folds (large arrow)

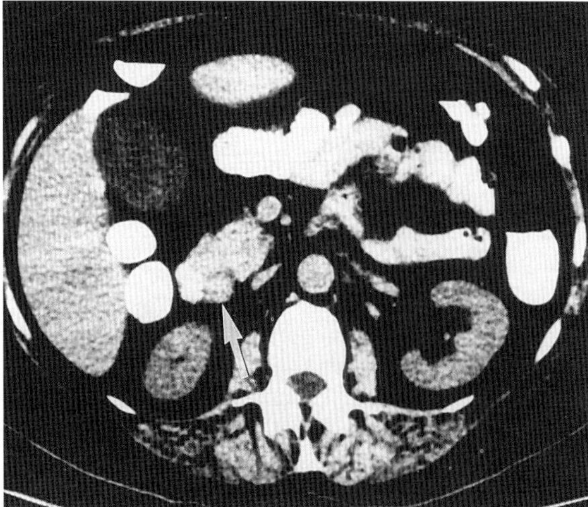

Fig. 7.9.**5 Computed tomography revealing a well-circumscribed mass on the inferior surface of the pancreatic head**, just medial to the second portion of the duodenum (arrow)

ported to be unreliable in the localization of gastrinomas preoperatively (Dunnick et al. 1980, Dangaard-Peterson and Stage 1979). Newer-generation CT scanners with improved spatial resolution, and the development of bolus intravenous contrast techniques, have improved the sensitivity markedly (Stark et al. 1984) (Fig. 7.9.**5**). Currently, 40–59% of gastrinomas can be localized preoperatively with the CT scan (Gunther et al. 1983, Wank et al. 1987). The CT scan has proved particularly useful in preoperative screening for metastatic disease. For gastrinoma metastatic to the liver, the CT scan has a sensitivity of 72% and a specificity of 98% (Wank et al. 1987).

Selective angiography of the pancreas is useful in demonstrating the presence of gastrinomas. Initial small series and individual case reports indicated success with this technique (Moritz et al. 1969, Clemett and Park 1967). Other series have reported a lack of success (Mills et al. 1979, Thompson et al. 1982). In the largest, most well-controlled study to date, Maton (1987) reports a sensitivity of 68% and a specificity of 94% for extrahepatic gastrinomas and a sensitivity of 86% and specificity of 100% for hepatic gastrinomas.

Percutaneous transhepatic portal venous sampling (PVS) was developed in Sweden in an attempt to localize pancreatic secretory tumors better (Reichardt and Ingemansson 1980). The technique used in performing this procedure is critical in obtaining valid, reproducible results. Some of the important technical points were summarized by Roche (1982): a) tumor localization is inaccurate with large trunk blood samplings; b) hyperselective PVS is necessary to localize abnormal secretions; c) calcium and secretin do not improve tumor localization; d) levels of several different components in the same blood sample determine the significance of the unique elevated component; and e) blood sample contamination with contrast material should be kept to a minimum. Despite this attempt at standardizing the technique, vastly different results with the use of PVS have been reported in the literature (Thompson et al. 1982, Ingemansson et al. 1977, Cherner et al. 1986). Those groups with good results recommend its use routinely in the preoperative localization of gastrinomas. Others (Thompson et al. 1982, Norton et al. 1986a) believe that selective venous sampling offers no advantage over detailed imaging studies and a careful exploration by the operating surgeon during laparotomy. In addition, this technique is invasive, technically demanding, and the results are difficult to interpret.

In summary, ultrasound and CT remain the initial screening tests in the search for primary tumor and for hepatic metastasis in patients with gastrinomas. Both tests have excellent specificity, adequate sensitivity, and a high degree of patient

Table 7.9.**1**   **Sensitivity and specificity of radiographic procedures**

	Hepatic Metastasis			Primary Gastrinoma		
	Sens	Spec	PPV	Sens	Spec	PPV
Ultrasound (Norton et al. 1986a)	21%	92%	80%	28%	93%	85%
Computed tomography (Wank et al. 1987)	72%	98%	93%	59%	95%	96%
Angiography (Maton et al. 1987)	86%	100%	100%	68%	94%	97%
Portal venous sampling (Cherner et al. 1986)				73%	33%	55%

acceptance (Table 7.9.**1**). Angiography is particularly useful as an adjunct, to delineate hepatic metastasis in cases where the CT scan is equivocal. Percutaneous transhepatic portal venous sampling should be reserved for specialized centers with expertise in this technique. Until better standardization becomes available, it should not be used routinely in the preoperative evaluation of patients with gastrinomas.

Diagnosis

Historically, the principal method of making the diagnosis of gastrinoma was by documenting the presence of marked gastric acid hypersecretion. The two most useful parameters of acid secretion used were the rate of basal acid secretion (Aoyagi and Summerskill 1966) and the ratio of basal to maximal acid secretion (Isenberg et al. 1973). A basal acid output that exceeded 15 mEq/h in patients without, or 5 mEq/h in patients with a previous acid-reducing operation or a basal acid output : maximal acid output ratio of 0.6, was considered highly suggestive of the presence of a gastrinoma (Jensen et al. 1983). Both of these tests lacked sensitivity and specificity in discriminating between those patients with gastrinomas, those with duodenal ulcers, and those with ordinary peptic ulcer disease (Kaye et al. 1970, Regan and Malagelada 1978, Thompson et al. 1975).

The development of the gastrin radioimmunoassay (McGuigan and Grieder 1968) made the direct measurement of the hormone possible. The assumption was that all patients with gastrinoma would have hypergastrinemia that could be detected by the gastrin radioimmunoassay. Soon, however, it became apparent that not only do serum gastrin values fluctuate from day to day in the same patient, but hypergastrinemia is not limited to patients with gastrinoma, and some patients with documented gastrinomas do not have hypergastrinemia (Table 7.9.**2**) (Walsh et al. 1975).

Table 7.9.**2**   **Disease states with hypergastrinemia that mimic gastrinomas**

Retained excluded gastric antrum syndrome (REAS)
Gastric outlet obstruction
Chronic Gastritis
Pernicious anemia
Antral G-cell hyperfunction
Antral G-cell hyperplasia
Renal failure

Provocative tests, as discussed above, were developed to assist in making this distinction (Isenberg et al. 1972, Passaro et al. 1972, Basso et al. 1981). The secretin stimulation test is the provocative test of choice in establishing the diagnosis of the Zollinger–Ellison syndrome (Lamer and Van Tongeren 1977). To perform the test, current recommendations are the intravenous bolus injection of 2 U/kg body weight of Secretin-Kabi and measuring the serum gastrin levels 10 min and 1 min before, and 2, 5, 10, 20, and 30 min after administration (Jensen et al. 1983). The response is usually maximal at 2 to 5 min. An absolute increase of 200 pg/ml in serum gastrin level is generally regarded as diagnostic (McGuigan and Wolfe 1980).

In the differential diagnosis of patients with hypergastrinemia and hyperchlorhydria, two entities are of particular importance, retained gastric antrum and primary G-cell hyperplasia. The retained gastric antrum syndrome is a rare condition. It occurs in patients who have undergone a partial gastrectomy and Billroth II reconstruction in which part of the antrum is left attached to the excluded proximal duodenal stump (Van Heerden 1971). Because the antrum is excluded from the acid stream, the normal inhibitory mechanism of gastric acid on gastrin release by the antral G-cells is lost, resulting in hypersecretion and hypergastrinemia (Jensen et al. 1983). The clinical presentation of these patients is very similar to that of patients with gastrinoma. These patients are distinguished from patients with gastrinomas by the secretin stimulation test (Korman et al. 1972). Patients with retained gastric antrum show a fall in serum gastrin in response to secretin challenge, whereas patients with gastrinomas show a marked increase.

The syndrome of primary antral G-cell hyperplasia has been referred to as the pseudo-Zollinger–Ellison syndrome (Friesen and Tomita 1981). Gastric hypersecretion and basal hypergastrinemia is caused by antral G-cell hyperplasia, and no tumor is found. This syndrome can also be distinguished from gastrinomas by the secretin stimulation test (McGuigan and Wolfe 1980). With secretin stimulation, these patients show either a decrease in serum gastrin or a slight increase, in contrast to the marked increase in patients with gastrinomas (Lamers et al. 1968). In addition, these patients have a rise in serum gastrin concentration following a meal, whereas patients with a gastrinoma do not (Jensen et al. 1983).

Multiple Endocrine Neoplasia I

Patients with gastrinomas and the Zollinger–Ellison syndrome are found to have associated non-pancreatic endocrine tumors in 20–30% of cases (Deveney et al. 1983, Friesen 1982). This association is now commonly referred to as the multiple endocrine neoplasia type I syndrome (MEN I). MEN I is a familial syndrome inherited in an autosomal-dominant fashion with variable expressivity. The tumors are parathyroid hyperplasia, pituitary adenomas, and islet-cell tumors of the pancreas. Hyperplasia of the parathyroid glands is usually of the chief cell variety, while the pituitary tumors may be chromophil, eosinophil, or basophil in type (Modlin 1979). In patients with gastrinomas who belong to the MEN I syndrome, 73–88% have parathyroid involvement, 16–65% have pituitary involvement, and 9–19% have adrenal cortical involvement (Table 7.9.3). As with most dominantly inherited disorders, there is considerable variation in expressivity of the syndrome between family members. This leads to patients and family members with subtle

clinical findings who are asymptomatic. Expression of multiglandular dysfunction in patients with MEN I increases with follow-up; from 0% in the first year of life to 50% by the 5th decade (Friesen et al. 1972). The incidence of MEN I therefore appears to be a function of both the thoroughness of the screening measures applied and of the length of time a particular family is followed up.

The initial evaluation includes a thorough history from the patient, with special reference to kidney stones, visual changes or other tumors which have been removed. A detailed family history should also be obtained, emphasizing other family members with ulcer disease or previous gastric operations, as well as the presence of kidney stones, visual changes or other endocrine tumors. Routine screening tests for hyperparathyroidism or a serum prolactin level should be performed.

The clinical importance of identifying patients with gastrinomas who belong to the MEN I syndrome cannot be overemphasized. The tumors present are biologically distinct from those patients with gastrinomas without the familial component (Friesen 1972). Thompson et al. (1984) have shown that these patients all have multiple small islet-cell tumors. Due to their multiplicity and size, the prospects of resection for cure are extremely poor (Van Heerden et al. 1986). It is generally agreed that these patients should initially be managed medically (Deveney et al. 1983, Stabile and Passaro 1985, Van Heerden et al. 1986, Ellison et al. 1987). Correction of hyperparathyroidism via parathyroidectomy can facilitate control of gastric hypersecretion and increase patients' responsiveness to antisecretory medications (Norton, in press). Although some series report an improved survival over patients with sporadic non-familial gastrinoma (Zollinger 1985), others (Stabile et al. 1984) have found no evidence of improved survival. What is clear is that a significant percentage of patients with MEN without the possibility of tumor excision will die from metastatic disease. For this reason, Norton et al. (1986a) advocate exploration in these patients, with tumor resection when imaging studies localize a specific tumor mass. This resection is performed solely on the basis of malignant potential, without expectation of cure.

Table 7.9.**3** **Incidence of associated endocrinopathies in MEN I patients** with the Zollinger–Ellison syndrome

	No. of patients	Parathyroid	Pituitary	Adrenocortical
van Heerden et al. (1986)	25	22 (88%)	4 (16%)	0
Ellison and Wilson (1967)	16	14 (88%)	3 (19%)	3 (19%)
Thompson et al. (1984)	11	8 (73%)	3 (27%)	1 (9%)
Ballard et al. (1964)	85	75 (88%)	55 (65%)	16 (19%)

Treatment

The optimal treatment for gastrinomas has been the subject of recurrent debate since its original description in 1955. Much of the discussion has centered on the issue of whether a primarily medical (McCarthy 1980) or surgical (Zollinger et al. 1980) approach should be taken. Historically, as mentioned above, the treatment of choice for patients with gastrinoma was total gastrectomy (Fox et al. 1974). This procedure was directed solely toward controlling the fulminant peptic ulceration and its complications. A direct, effective method of treatment was needed, since there was a 28 % mortality rate in these patients, attributed to the complications of peptic ulcer disease (Deveney et al. 1978). In the pre-cimetidine era it was found that attempts at tumor resection, or lesser gastric resections such as subtotal gastrectomy or vagotomy and drainage procedure, carried a 50–100 % mortality rate (Ellison and Wilson 1967). It was noted that these patients developed severe, often fatal complications within days of acid-reducing operations involving less than total gastrectomy (Isenberg et al. 1973). Also, most attempts at tumor resection were limited, as 50 % of these patients had hepatic metastases at the time of diagnosis (Ellison and Wilson 1964).

The H2 blockers have facilitated the perioperative control of these patients and allowed for safer exploration (Thompson et al. 1982) as well as more aggressive attempts at tumor removal (Norton et al. 1986b). Combined with the improved ability to diagnose gastrinomas (McGuigan and Wolfe 1980), better tumor localization (Norton et al. 1986a), and improved patient selection, operations are now being performed earlier, more safely, and with minimal morbidity and mortality.

It is now apparent that the natural history of malignant gastrinoma has become the most important prognostic factor in the long-term survival of these patients (Norton et al. 1986b). Initial series reported a 42 % 5-year survival rate (Zollinger et al. 1980) and a 36 % 10-year survival rate (Zollinger 1985) for patients with hepatic metastases. Other studies (Norton et al. 1986) suggest a poorer prognosis, with the actuarial 5-year survival rate for metastatic disease being only 20 %.

The current focus of surgical management is on resection of gastrinoma for cure. Surgical cure is defined as resection of all gastrinoma tumor such that the patient is rendered eugastrinemic, requires no antisecretory medications, has a negative secretin stimulation test, and no evidence of recurrent disease on long-term follow-up. Oberhelman (1961) was the first surgeon to recognize that effective excision of gastrinomas was possible. His experience (Oberhelman 1977) with duodenal tumors showed 9 out of 11 patients remaining disease-free 2–11 years after tumor resection, which was often by a Whipple procedure. In addition, only one patient in this series required a total gastrectomy. Others (Jaffee et al. 1972, Bonfils et al. 1981) substantiated this finding. Despite these reports, many authors (Stage and Stadil 1979, Jensen et al. 1983, McCarthy 1980) continued to cite cure rates of 2–5 % overall for patients with gastrinomas. One reason for the continuingly low cure rate was the inclusion of patients with MEN I in these series. The duodenal wall tumors which occur in 13 % of patients with gastrinomas were felt to be a special subset of patients, with a higher cure rate (Wolfe and Jensen 1987, Hoffman et al. 1973). As experience with these tumors grew, reports of surgical cures in extrapancreatic, extraintestinal sites (Wolfe et al. 1982) and lymph nodes (Norton et al. 1986a, Stabile and Passaro 1985, Friesen 1982, Malagelada et al. 1983) were published. Soon the aggressive localization and resection of tumors was advocated to prevent death from metastatic disease and tumor progression (Norton et al. 1986b, Wolfe and Jensen 1987, Zollinger et al. 1980). It has recently been shown, in a compilation of several large series (Ellison et al. 1987), that the cure rate for resection of gastrinomas is approximately 30 %. In the large surgical series of Norton (1986a) Ellison (1987) and Friesen (1982), the surgical cure rates are 30 %, 40 %, and 43 %, respectively. In our own series, we now have 69 patients, and have operated on fifty-six. There are 9 patients who have been cured, based on postoperative gastrin radioimmunoassay and a negative secretin stimulation test. These patients have been followed from 1–124 months. Excluding those patients with MEN, the surgical cure rate is 24 % (9 out of 38).

All patients with gastrinomas who do not show MEN I syndrome, and who have no preoperative evidence of hepatic metastases, should undergo surgical exploration with resection for potential cure (Wolfe and Jensen 1987). The procedure used has been well described (Zollinger et al. 1976). An upper midline or bilateral subcostal incision is made, and inspection and palpation of the viscera is carried out. If hepatic metastasis is present, a biopsy is taken for histologic confirmation, and a decision is made on whether or not to perform a total gastrectomy. Patients who are noncompliant with the prescribed medical regimen, or have failed medical therapy, undergo total gastrectomy. Patients well-controlled on their medical regimens are simply closed.

In patients without evidence of hepatic metastasis, a diligent and systematic search for primary and regional metastatic tumor is undertaken. It has been shown that 89 % of tumors will be found within the anatomic confines of the gastrinoma triangle (Stabile et al. 1984) (Fig. 7.9.**6**). This

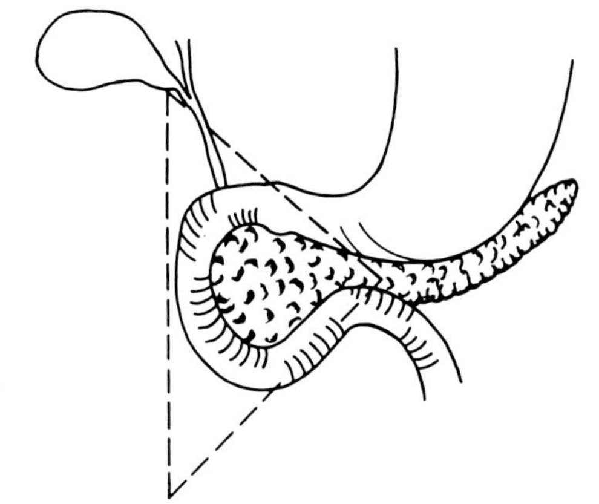

Fig. 7.9.**6   The gastrinoma triangle.** From: Am J Surg 1984; 147: 25–31

triangle is defined as the junction of the cystic duct and common bile duct superiorly, the junction of the second and third portions of the duodenum inferiorly, and the junction of the neck and body of the pancreas medially. It is in this area that the surgeon must concentrate his visual and tactile senses when looking for the tumor. 85–90 % of pancreatic tumors will be found in a superficial location amenable to enucleation or local excision. Beginning at the superior aspect of the gastrinoma triangle, the confluence of the cystic and common bile duct is visualized and the porta hepatis examined. The lesser omental sac is widely opened by detaching the gastrocolic omentum from the transverse colon. The head of the pancreas is completely mobilized using a generous Kocher maneuver. The body and the tail of the gland are mobilized by incising the retroperitoneum along its inferior margin.

Using direct visualization and bimanual palpation, the entire pancreas and duodenum are carefully examined, and all palpable masses are meticulously excised and submitted as frozen sections for histologic examination. Intraoperative ultrasound may provide assistance in the evaluation of nodules within the pancreatic substance (Cromack et al. 1987). All regional lymph nodes found within the anatomic triangle are excised and submitted for frozen section. The greater and lesser omenta are systematically searched. The splenic hilum, celiac axis and the root of the mesentery are explored for metastatic tumor. The duodenum down to the ligament of Treitz and proximal jejunum is palpated for small adenomas through the serosal surface. If at this point no tumor is found, a longitudinal pyloroduodenotomy is performed, and the duodenal wall is examined by palpation between the index finger intraluminally and the thumb extraluminally. If a lesion is discovered, it is excised

with a full-thickness margin of grossly normal duodenum. In most instances, the longitudinal pyloroduodenotomy is reconstructed anatomically, unless total gastrectomy is also carried out.

Tumors in the pancreas are enucleated or excised locally. Distal pancreatectomy may be necessary in some instances in which a lesion which is otherwise curable is unable to be enucleated or locally excised. Rarely, in patients with an otherwise curable tumor in the pancreatic head or duodenum which cannot be excised locally and who are good surgical candidates, a pancreaticoduodenectomy of the Whipple type is performed. The morbidity and mortality of this procedure must be balanced against the benefits of possible curative resection. Tumors so large or locally invasive that a primary resection cannot be performed are only biopsied.

Despite extensive preoperative localization and a thorough intra-abdominal exploration, approximately 7–30 % of patients will have no identifiable tumor (Friesen 1982, Deveney et al. 1978, Stabile et al. 1984). The reason for this wide variation in intraoperative localization is that the ability to find these tumors is a function of the experience and familiarity of the operating surgeon with gastrinomas. Those patients controlled preoperatively with antisecretory medications are closed and restarted on their medical regimens. Patients who are refractory to H_2-receptor antagonists (Stabile et al. 1983) or non-compliant with the medication, undergo a total gastrectomy. Our current management includes the option of participating in the clinical trials using omeprazole (McArthur et al. 1985) postoperatively rather than total gastrectomy in those patients who are refractory to standard H_2-receptor blockers. For those patients who decline to participate in the study, and for treatment failures on omeprazole (Lloyd-Davis et al. 1986), we would continue to recommend a total gastrectomy.

Treatment regimens for patients with metastatic gastrinoma have been disappointing. Chemotherapy using streptozotocin and fluorouracil, with or without doxorubicin, has been reported to be effective in 50–70 % of patients with metastatic disease (Howard et al. 1984, Moertel et al. 1980). Unfortunately, these studies are small, lack consistent protocols, and suffer from insufficient follow-up (Wolfe and Jensen 1987). Other studies using hepatic artery embolization (Carrasco et al. 1983), hormonal therapy (Shepard and Senator 1986), and treatment with interferon (Grikson et al. 1986), are much less clear. A recent protocol by Norton et al. (1986 b) utilizing aggressive surgical resection of all metastatic gastrinoma in 3 out of 20 patients resulted in 2 patients being eugastrinemic postoperatively. Further clinical evaluation is needed before the usefulness of these various modalities for metastatic gastrinoma is truly known.

Prognosis

It is difficult to predict a given patient clinical course on the basis of the available literature. The reasons for this are the diversity of clinical presentations, non-standardization of treatment protocols, and the relatively short follow-up available. Despite these limitations, some general statements concerning these tumors may be made. Their slow growth allows one to express mortality in terms of 10-year survival rates. A broad stratification can be made in terms of favorable vs. unfavorable prognosis (Zollinger 1985). There is a 70% 10-year survival rate in patients with duodenal wall tumors, tumors which could not be located at laparotomy, and patients with gastrinoma showing the MEN I syndrome. In contrast, patients with unresectable tumors, hepatic metastasis, and gastrinoma *not* associated with the MEN I syndrome, comprise the unfavorable group, and have an approximately 30% 10-year survival.

References

Alumets J, Hakanson R. Ontogeny of endocrine cells in porcine gut and pancreas. Gastroenterology 1983; 85: 1359–1372.

Andrews A. An experimental investigation into the possible neural crest origin of pancreatic APUD (islet) cells. J Embryol Exp Morphol 1976; 35(3): 577–593.

Aoyagi T, Summerskill WHJ. Gastric secretion with ulcerogenic islet cell tumor: importance of basal acid out-put. Arch Intern Med 1966; 117: 667–672.

Ballard HS, Frame B, Harstock RJ. Familial multiple endocrine adenomapeptic ulcer complex. Medicine (Baltimore) 1964; 43: 481.

Basso N, Lezoche E, Materia A, Passaro E Jr, Speranza V. Studies with bombesin in the Zollinger–Ellison syndrome. Br J Surg 1981; 68: 97–100.

Bonfils SM, Bernades P. Zollinger–Ellison syndrome: natural history and diagnosis. Clin Gastroenterol 1974; 3: 359.

Bonfils S, Mignon M, Gratton J. Cimetidine treatment of acute and chronic Zollinger–Ellison syndrome. World J Surg 1979; 3: 597–604.

Bonfils S, Landor JH, Mignon M, Hervoir P. Results of surgical management in 92 consecutive patients with Zollinger–Ellison syndrome. Ann Surg 1981; 194: 693–697.

Brown CH, Neville WE, Hazard JB. Islet cell adenoma without hypoglycemia causing duodenal obstruction. Surgery 1950; 27: 616.

Carrasco UT, Chuang VS, Wallace S. APUDoma metastatic to the liver: treatment of hepatic artery embolization. Radiology 1983; 149: 79–83.

Cherner JA, Doppman JL, Norton JA, Miller DL, et al. Selective venous sampling for gastrin to localize gastrinoma. Ann Intern Med 1986; 105: 841–847.

Clemett AR, Park WM. Arteriographic demonstration of pancreatic tumor in the Zollinger–Ellison syndrome. Radiology 1967; 88: 32–34.

Code CF, Hollenbeck GA, Summerskill WHJ. Extraction of a gastric secretogogue from primary and metastatic islet cell tumors in two cases of the Zollinger–Ellison syndrome. J Surg Res 1962; 2: 136.

Cope V, Warwick F. The role of radiology in the detection of endocrine tumors of the gastrointestinal tract. Clin Gastroenterol 1974; 3: 621.

Creutzfield N. Pancreatic endocrine tumors: the riddle of their origin and hormone secretion. Isr J Med Sci 1975; 11: 762.

Cromack DT, Norton JA, et al. The use of high resolution intraoperative ultrasound to localize gastrinomas: an initial report of a prospective study. World J Surg 1987; 11: 648–653.

Dangaard-Pedersen K, Stage JG. CT scanning in patients with the Zollinger–Ellison syndrome and carcinoid syndrome. Scand J Gastroenterol 1979; 14: 117–122.

Deconinck JF. The ultrastructure of the human pancreatic islet. Diabetologia 1971; 7: 266–282.

Deveney CW, Deveney CS, Way LW. The Zollinger–Ellison syndrome: 23 years later. Ann Surg 1978; 188: 384–393.

Deveney CW, Deveney KE, Stark D. Resection of gastrinomas. Amer Surg 1983; 198: 446–533.

Dunnick NR, Doppman JL, Mills SR, McCarthy DM. Computed tomographic detection of nonbeta pancreatic islet cell tumors. Radiology 1980; 135: 117–120.

Ellison EC, Carey LC, Sparks J, et al. Early surgical treatment of gastrinoma. Am J Med 1987; 82(5B): 17.

Ellison EH, Wilson SD. The Zollinger–Ellison syndrome: reappraisal and evaluation of 260 registered cases. Ann Surg 1964; 160: 512–530.

Ellison EH, Wilson SD. Ulcerogenic tumor of the pancreas. Proc Clin Cancer 1967; 3: 225–244.

Erlandsen SL, Hegre OD. Pancreatic islet cell hormone distribution of cell types in the islet and evidence for the presence of somatostatin and gastrin within the D cells. J Histochem Cytochem 1976; 24: 883–897.

Feyrter F. Die peripheren endokrinen (parakrinen) Drüsen. In: Kaufmann E, Staemler M, eds. Lehrbuch der speziellen pathologischen Anatomie; vol 11, 12. Berlin: De Gruyter, 1969.

Forty R, Barrett GM. Peptic ulceration of third part of duodenum associated with islet cell tumors. Br J Surg 1952; 40: 60.

Fox PS, Hoffman JW, Decosse JJ, Wilson SD. The influence of total gastrectomy to survival in malignant Zollinger–Ellison tumors. Ann Surg 1974; 180: 558–566.

Friesen SR. Treatment of the Zollinger–Ellison syndrome: a 25 year assessment. Am J Surg 1982; 143: 331–338.

Friesen SR, Tomita J. Pseudo-Zollinger–Ellison syndrome: hypergastrinemia, hyperchlorhydria without tumor. Ann Surg 1981; 194: 481–493.

Friesen SR, Tracy HJ, Gregory RA. Mechanism of gastric hypersecretion in the Zollinger–Ellison syndrome: successful extraction of gastrin-like activity from metastases and primary pancreatico-duodenal islet cell carcinoma. Ann Surg 1962; 155–167.

Friesen SR, Schinke RN, Pearse AGE. Genetic aspects of the Zollinger–Ellison syndrome: prospective studies in two kindred; antral gastrin cell hyperplasia. Ann Surg 1972; 176: 370–383.

Gregory RA, Tracy HJ, French JM, Sircus N. Extraction of a gastrin-like substance from a pancreatic tumor in a case of Zollinger–Ellison syndrome. Lancet 1960; i: 1045.

Gregory RA, Grossman MI, Tracey HJ, Bentley PH. Nature of the gastric secretogogue in the Zollinger–Ellison tumors. Lancet 1967; ii: 543.

Grikson B, Oberg K, Alm G, et al. Treatment of malignant endocrine pancreatic tumors with human leukocyte interferon. Lancet 1986; ii: 1307–1309.

Grossman MI. Gastrin and its activities. Nature 1960; 228: 1147–1150.

Grossman MI, Tracy HJ, Gregory RA. Zollinger–Ellison syndrome in a Bantu woman with isolation of gastrin-like substance from primary and secondary tumors, II: extraction of gastrin-like activity from tumors. Gastroenterology 1961; 41: 87–91.

Gunther RW, Klose KJ, Ruckert K, Kuhn FP, et al. Islet-cell tumors: detection of small lesions with computer tomography and ultrasound. Radiology 1983; 148: 485–488.

Hancke S. Localization of hormone-producing gastrointestinal tumor by ultrasonic scanning. Scand J Gastroenterol 1979; 14 (suppl 53): 115–116.

Hoffman JW, Fox PS, Nelson SD. Duodenal wall tumors and the Zollinger–Ellison sndrome: surgical management. Arch Surg 1973; 107: 334–339.

Howard JM, Collen MJ, Raufmans JP, et al. Comparison of the effect of chemotherapy on tumor size, serum gastrin, and gastric acid secretion in patients with Zollinger–Ellison syndrome (ZES). Gastroenterology 1984; 84: 1192 (abstract).

Ingemansson S, Larsson LI, Lunderquist A, Stadil F. Pancreatic vein catheterization with gastrin assay in normal patients and in patient with Zollinger–Ellison syndrome. Am J Surg 1977; 134: 558–563.

Isenberg JI, Walsh JH, Passaro E Jr, et al. Unusual effect of secretin on serum gastrin, serum calcium and gastric acid secretion in a patient with suspected Zollinger–Ellison syndrome. Gastroenterology 1972; 62: 626.

Isenberg JI, Walsh JH, Grossman MI. Zollinger–Ellison syndrome. Gastroenterology 1973; 65: 140–165.

Ippoliti AF. Zollinger–Ellison syndrome: provocative diagnostic tests. Ann Intern Med 1977; 87: 787–788.

Jaffee BM, Peskin G, Kaplan EL. Diagnosis of occult Zollinger–Ellison tumors by gastrin radioimmunoassay. Cancer 1972; 3: 694–700.

Jensen RT, Gardener JD, Raufman JP, Pandol SJ, et al. Zollinger–Ellison syndrome: current concepts and management. Ann Intern Med 1983; 98: 59–75.

Kaye MD, Rhodes J, Beck P. Gastric secretion in duodenal ulcers with particular reference to the diagnosis of Zollinger–Ellison syndrome. Gastroenterology 1970; 58: 476–481.

Klotter HJ, Ruckert K, Kummerle F, Rothmund M. The use of intraoperative sonography for endocrine tumors of the pancreas. World J Surg 1987; 11: 635–641.

Korman MG, Scott DF, Hansky J, Wilson H. Hypergastrinemia due to excluded gastric antrum: a proposed method for differentiation from the Zollinger–Ellison syndrome. Aust NZ J Med 1972; 3: 266–271.

Lamers CBH, Van Tongeren JHM. Comparative study of the value of the calcium, secretin, and meal stimulated increase in serum gastrin to the diagnosis of the Zollinger–Ellison syndrome. Gut 1977; 18: 128–134.

Lamers CBH, Ruland CM, Joosten HJM, Verkooyen HCM, et al. Hypergastrinemia of antral origin in duodenal ulcer. Dig Dis Sci 1968; 23: 988–1002.

Lamers CBHW, Lind T, Moberg S, Jansen JBMJ, Olbe L. Omeprazole in Zollinger–Ellison syndrome. N Engl J Med 1984; 310: 758–761.

Larsson LI, Sunder F. Pancreatic polypeptide: a postulated new hormone. Diabetologia 1976; 12: 211–226.

Le Douarin NA. A biological cell-labelling technique and its use in experimental embryology. Dev Biol 1973; 30: 217.

Lloyd-Davis KA, Rutgersson K, Solvell L. Omeprazole in Zollinger–Ellison syndrome: four year international study. Gastroenterology 1986; 90: 1523 (abstract).

Lofstra F. Are gastrin cells present in mammalian pancreatic islets? Diabetologia 1974; 10: 291.

Malagelada JR, Edis AJ, Adson MA, et al. Medical and surgical options in the management of patients with gastrinomas. Gastroenterology 1983; 84: 1524–1532.

Maton PN, Miller DL, Doppman JL, Collen MJ, et al. Role of selective angiography in the management of patients with Zollinger–Ellison syndrome. Gastroenterology 1987; 92: 913–918.

McArthur KE, Collen MJ, Maton PN, Cherner JA, et al. Omeprazole: effective, convenient therapy for Zollinger–Ellison syndrome. Gastroenterology 1985; 88: 939–944.

McCarthy DM. Report on the United States experience with cimetidine in Zollinger–Ellison syndrome and other hypersecretory state. Gastroenterology 1978; 74: 453–458.

McCarthy DM. The place of surgery in the Zollinger–Ellison syndrome. N Engl J Med 1980; 302: 1344–1347.

McGuigan JE, Grieder MH. Immunochemical measurement of elevated levels of gastrin in the serum of patients with pancreatic tumors of the Zollinger–Ellison variety. N Engl J Med 1968; 278: 1308–1313.

McGuigan JE, Wolfe MM. Secretin injection test in the diagnosis of gastrinoma. Gastroenterology 1980; 79: 1324–1331.

Mills SR, Doppman JL, Dunnick NR, McCarthy DM. Evaluation of angiography in Zollinger–Ellison syndrome. Radiology 1979; 131: 317–320.

Modlin IM. Endocrine tumors of the pancreas. Surg Gynecol Obstet 1979; 149: 751–769.

Moertel CG, Hanley JA, Johnson LA. Streptozotocin alone compared with streptozotocin plus fluorouracil in the treatment of advanced islet cell carcinoma. N Engl J Med 1980; 303: 1188–1194.

Moritz M, Kahn PC, Callow AD, et al. Unusual clinical manifestations and angiographic findings in a patient with the Zollinger–Ellison syndrome. Ann Intern Med 1969; 71: 1133–1140.

Norton JA, Doppman JL, Collen MJ, Harmon JW, et al. Prospective study of gastrinoma localization and resection in patients with Zollinger–Ellison syndrome. Ann Surg 1986a; 204(4): 468–479.

Norton JA, Sugarbaker PH, Doppman JD, Wesley RA, et al. Aggressive resection of metastatic disease in selected patients with malignant gastrinoma. Ann Surg 1986b; 203: 352–359.

Norton JA, Cornelius MJ, Doppman JL, Maton PN, et al. Effect of parathyroidectomy in patients with hyperparathyroidism and Zollinger–Ellison syndrome and MEN type I: a prospective study. Surgery (in press).

Oberhelman HA Jr. Excisional therapy for ulcerogenic tumors of the duodenum. Arch Surg 1977; 104: 447–453.

Oberhelman HA Jr, Nelson TS, Johnson AN Jr, et al. Ulcerogenic tumors of the duodenum. Ann Surg 1961; 153: 214–227.

Orci L, Rufener G, Pictet R. Present state and evidence for mixed endocrine and exocrine pancreatic cells in spray mice. In: Falkner S, Hellman B, Täljedal IB, eds. The structure and metabolism of pancreatic islet. Oxford: Pergamon, 1970: 37–52.

Passaro E Jr, Basso N, Walsh JH. Calcium challenge in the Zollinger–Ellison syndrome. Surgery 1972; 72: 1.

Pearse AGE. Common cytochemical properties of cells producing polypeptide hormones with particular reference to calcitonin and thyroid C cells. Vet Rec 1966; 79: 587–590.

Pearse AGE. Common cytochemical and ultrastructural characteristics of cells producing polypeptide hormones (the APUD series) and their relevance to thyroid and ultimobrachial C cells and calcitonin. Proc R Soc Lond 1968; 170: 71–80.

Pearse AGE. The cytochemical and ultrastructure of polypeptide-hormone producing cells of the APUD series and the embryologic, physiologic, and pathologic implications of the concept. J Histochem Cytochem 1969; 17: 303–312.

Pearse AGE, Polak JM, Heath CM. Development, differentiation, and derivation of endocrine polypeptide cells of the mouse pancreas: immunofluorescence, cytochemical, and ultrastructural studies. Diabetologia 1973; 9: 120–129.

Polacek MA, Ellison EH. A comparative study of parietal cell mass and distribution in normal stomachs, in stomachs with duodenal ulcer, and in stomach of patient with pancreatic adenoma. Surg Forum 1963; 14: 313–315.

Polak JM. A growth-hormone release-inhibiting hormone in gastrointestinal and pancreatic D cells. Lancet 1975; i: 1220.

Poth E, Manhoff LJ, Deloach AW. The relation of pancreatic secretion to peptic ulcer formation. Surgery 1948; 24: 62.

Pusyrev AA. The formation of endocrine cells in the human pancreas from epithelium of acini and ducts. Arkh Anat Gistol Embriol 1979; 1: 20–25.

Regan PT, Malagelada JR. A reappraisal of clinical, roentgenologic, and endoscopic features of the Zollinger–Ellison syndrome. Mayo Clin Proc 1978; 53: 19–23.

Reichardt W, Ingemansson S. Selective vein catheterization for hormone assay in endocrine tumors of the pancreas: technique and results. Acta Radiol 1980; 21: 177–187.

Richardson CT, Walsh JH. The value of a histamine H_2-receptor antagonist in the management of patients with Zollinger–Ellison syndrome. N Engl J Med 1976; 294: 133.

Robb P. The development of the islet of Langerhans in the human fetus. Q J Exp Physiol 1961; 46: 335–343.

Roche A, Raisonnier A, Gillon-Savoniet MC. Pancreatic venous sampling and arteriography in localizing insulinomas and gastrinomas: procedure and results in 55 cases. Radiology 1982; 145: 621–627.

Rosai J, Greider MH, McGuigan JE. Morphologic, histochemical, ultrastructural and biochemical observation in 21 human ulcerogenic and diarrheagenic islet cell tumors. Am J Pathol 1974; 41: 312–315.

Seiler S, Zinninger MM. Massive islet cell tumor of the pancreas without hypoglycemia. Surg Gynecol Obstet 1946; 82: 301.

Shepard JJ, Senator GB. Resection of liver metastasis in patients with gastrin secreting tumor treated with SMS 201–995. Lancet 1986; iii: 574.

Soergel KH. Mechanism of diarrhea in the Zollinger–Ellison syndrome, non-insulin-producing tumors of the pancreas. In: Demling L, Ottenjann R, eds. Non-Insulin-producing tumors of the pancreas. Modern aspects on Zollinger–Ellison syndrome and Gastrin. International Symposium at Erlangen, July 16th and 17th, 1968. Stuttgart: Thieme, 1969: 152–164.

Stabile BE, Passaro E Jr. Benign and malignant gastrinomas. Am J Surg 1985; 149: 144–150.

Stabile BE, Ippoliti AF, Walsh JH, Passaro E Jr. Failure of histamine H_2-receptor antagonist therapy in Zollinger–Ellison syndrome. Am J Surg 1983; 145: 17–23.

Stabile BE, Morrow DJ, Passaro E Jr. The gastrinoma triangle: operative implications. Am J Surg 1984; 147: 25–31.

Stage JG, Stadil F. The clinical diagnosis of the Zollinger–Ellison syndrome. Scand J Gastroenterol 1979; 14 (suppl 53): 79–91.

Stark DD, Moss AA, Goldberg HI, Deveney CW. CT of pancreatic islet cell tumors. Radiology 1984; 150: 491–494.

Tapia FJ, Polak M, Barbosa MJ. Neuron specific enolase is produced by neuro-endocrine tumors. Lancet 1981; i: 808–811.

Teitelman G, et al. Transformation of catecholaminergic precursors into glucagon cells in mouse embryonic pancreas. Proc Natl Acad Sci USA 78: 5225–5229.

Thompson JC, Reeder DD, Villar HV, Fender HR. Natural history and experience with diagnosis and treatment of the Zollinger–Ellison syndrome. Surg Gynecol Obstet 1975; 140: 721–739.

Thompson JC, Lewis BG, Weiner I, Townsend CM. The role of surgery in the Zollinger–Ellison syndrome. Ann Surg 1982; 197: 594–607.

Thompson NV, Lloyd RV, Nishiyama RH, et al. MEN I pancreas: a histological and immunochemical study. World J Surg 1984; 8: 561–574.

Van Heerden JA, Bernatz PE, Rovelstad RA. The retained antrum: clinical considerations. Mayo Clin Proc 1971; 46: 25–27.

Van Heerden JA, Smith JL, Miller LJ. Management of the Zollinger–Ellison syndrome in patients with multiple endocrine neoplasia type I. Surgery 1986; 100: 971–976.

Walsh JH, Grossman MI. Gastrin. N Engl J Med 1975; 292: 1324–1334, 1377–1384.

Wank SA, Doppman JL, Miller DL, Collen MJ, et al. Prospective study of the ability of computed axial tomography to localize gastrinoma in patients with Zollinger–Ellison syndrome. Gastroenterology 1987; 92: 905–912.

Way L, Goldman L, Dunphy JE. Zollinger–Ellison syndrome: an analysis of 25 cases. Am J Surg 1968; 116: 293–303.

Weber JM, Lewis S, Heasley KH. Observation on small bowel pattern associated with Zollinger–Ellison syndrome. AJR 1959; 82: 973–977.

Wilkinson DS. Necrolytic migratory erythema with carcinoma of the pancreas. Trans St Johns Hosp Dermatol Soc 1973; 59: 244–250.

Wilson SD. Ulcerogenic tumors of the pancreas: the Zollinger–Ellison syndrome. In: Carey LC, ed. The Pancreas. St. Louis: Mosby, 1973: 295–318.

Wilson SD. The role of surgery in children with the Zollinger–Ellison syndrome. Surgery 1982; 92(4): 682–692.

Wolfe MM, Jensen RT. Zollinger–Ellison syndrome. N Engl J Med 1987; 317: 1200–1209.

Wolfe MM, Alexander RV, McGuigan JE. Extrapancreatic extraintestinal gastrinoma effective treatment by surgery. N Engl J Med 1982; 306: 1533–1536.

Yalow RS, Berson S. Radioimmunoassay of gastrin. Gastroenterology 1970; 58: 1.

Zboralske FW, Amberg JR. Detection of the Zollinger–Ellison syndrome: the radiologist's responsibility. AJR 1968; 104: 529–543.

Zollinger RM. Gastrinomas: factors influencing prognosis. Surgery 1985; 97: 49–54.

Zollinger RM, Ellison EH. Primary peptic ulcerations of the jejunum associated with islet cell tumors of the pancreas. Ann Surg 1955; 142: 709–728.

Zollinger RM, Martin EW, Carey LC, et al. Observations on the postoperative tumor growth of certain islet cell tumor. Ann Surg 1976; 184: 525–530.

Zollinger RM, Ellison EC, Fabri PJ, Johnson JJ, et al. Primary peptic ulcerations of the jejunum associated with islet cell tumors: twenty-five year appraisal. Ann Surg 1980; 192: 422–430.

7.10 Endocrine Tumors of the Pancreas

H.G. Beger and M. Büchler

Classification

Endocrine tumors of the pancreas are classified as benign or malignant tumors derived from the diffuse neuroendocrine system of the pancreas. Neuroendocrine cells are characterized by the biosynthesis and secretion of either biogenic amines or peptide hormones such as insulin, gastrin, glucagon, vasoactive intestinal polypeptide (VIP), pancreatic polypeptide (PP), or neurotensin (Friesen and Tomita 1987, Klöppel and Seifert 1988). According to the well-characterized clinical signs and symptoms caused by the uncontrolled release of large amounts of peptides and hormones from these tumors, we have learned to describe and classify these tumors as insulinomas, gastrinomas, glucagonomas, VIPomas, PPomas, or neurotensinomas. In contrast to the World Health Organization classification, which differentiates between islet-cell tumors, carcinoids of the pancreas and poorly-differentiated endocrine carcinomas, the functional classification of endocrine pancreatic tumors seems to be the most reliable for clinical practice. In addition, we can now demonstrate by immunohistochemistry the hormone or peptide causing the clinical syndrome in most cases. The functional classification of endocrine tumors of the pancreas, with morphological support from the immunohistochemical identification of the hormone responsible, has therefore led to the acceptance of a classification system for endocrine tumors which is used throughout the world (Table 7.10.1).

Most endocrine tumors of the pancreas are benign. The only criterion for malignancy is evidence of lymph node involvement, distant metastases, or direct infiltration of other organs by the tumor (Klöppel 1983). No other pathomorphologic criteria for malignancy are of any value in endocrine tumors of the pancreas. Table 7.10.1 shows the rates of malignancy in different types of endocrine pancreatic tumors.

Endocrine pancreatic tumor is a very rare disease, occurring at a rate of less than one in 100000 people (Schein et al. 1973). In West Germany, the frequency of operations for endocrine pancreatic tumors is between 20 and 30 a year (Kümmerle and Rückert 1978). Our own experience (Department of General Surgery, University of Ulm, 1982–1987) comprises 19 endocrine pancreatic tumors over a 6-year period (Table 7.10.2).

This chapter describes the surgical approach to endocrine tumors of the pancreas, excluding gastrinomas, which are described in Chapter 7.9.

Insulinoma

About 70–80% of all endocrine pancreatic tumors are insulinomas. Less than 10% of these B-cell tumors of the pancreas are malignant, and almost

Table 7.10.1 **Classification of endocrine tumors of the pancreas**

Type	Incidence	Rate of malignancy	Hormone	Cellular origin	Extrapancreatic localization
Insulinoma	75%	< 10%	Insulin	B-cell	1%
Gastrinoma	15–20%	> 50%	Gastrin	G-cell	20–40%
VIPoma	1–2%	> 50%	vasoactive intestinal polypeptide	D_1-cell	5–20%
Glucagonoma	1–2%	> 70%	Glucagon	A-cell	rare
Somatostatinoma	< 1%	> 50%	Somatostatin	D-cell	frequent
PPoma	< 1%	?	pancreatic polypeptid	PP-cell	?
Carcinoid	?	?	Serotonin	EC-cell	?
Corticotropinoma	< 1%	> 99%	Corticotropin, melanocyte-stimulating hormone	?	?
Parathyrinoma	< 1%	> 99%	?	?	?
Neurotensinoma	?	?	Neurotensin	?	?
Calcitoninoma	?	?	Calcitonin	?	?
Non-peptide tumors	< 5%	?	–	?	?

According to Stefanini et al. 1974, Klöppel 1983, Creutzfeld 1985, Friesen and Tomita 1987, Reber 1987

Table 7.10.2 Endocrine tumors of the pancreas. Department of General Surgery, University of Ulm, 1982–1987

Type	Number	Localization
Insulinoma (benign)	14	13 Pancreas (1 extrapancreatic?)
Insulinoma (malignant)	1	Pancreas (+ lymph node metastasis)
Nesidioblastosis	2	Pancreas
Gastrinoma	1	Pancreas
Carcinoid	1	Pancreas
Total:	19	

Table 7.10.3 Insulinoma: Pathological findings in 951 completely documented cases

	No. of patients	%
Localization		
Head	305	32
Body	285	30
Tail	323	34
Uncinate	29	3
Ectopic	9	1
Size		
< 0.5 cm	47	5
0.5–1.0 cm	323	34
1.0–5.0 cm	504	53
> 5.0 cm	77	8
Number		
Single	789	83
Multiple	123	13
Multiple endocrine adenopathy	39	4
Parathyroid	16	1.7
Pituitary	10	1.0
Adrenal cortex	10	1.0
Thyroid	3	0.3
Type		
Benign	798	84
Malignant	153	16
metastases	47	5

According to Stefanini et al. 1974

Table 7.10.4 Insulinoma: Incidence of symptoms

Symptom	% of patients
Neurological	
Temporary, non-focal or transient (apathy, dizziness, clouded sensorium, behavioral disturbance, coma, seizures)	92
Temporary focal neurologic deficit (paralysis/paresis, sensory loss, diplopia)	5
Permanent neurological deficit (stroke)	7
Cardiovascular	
Episodic palpitation, pallor, precordial pain	17
Gastrointestinal	
Hunger, nausea, vomiting	9

According to Stefanini et al. 1974

The clinical picture of the insulinoma syndrome is usually characterized by neurological signs and symptoms (Table 7.10.4) caused by hyperinsulinemic hypoglycemia. Cardiovascular or gastrointestinal symptoms of insulin-producing pancreatic tumors only appear in 22% of patients. The diagnosis of insulinoma is mainly based on high serum insulin along with hypoglycemia, demonstrating autonomous insulin secretion. A fasting test proves the insulinoma diagnosis in 95% of patients (Friesen and Tomita 1987). In insulinoma patients, the plasma glucose level falls, but the circulating insulin level remains elevated because of the tumor's autonomous secretion. The ability to analyze the C-peptide in the plasma has greatly assisted in the diagnosis of insulinoma syndrom (Rubenstein et al. 1977). A wide range of differential diagnoses must be taken into account to confirm the diagnosis of an insulin-producing pancreatic tumor. In particular, endocrine or hepatic diseases and congenital enzyme defects may cause hypoglycemia similar to the insulinoma syndrome (Friesen and Tomita 1987).

Imaging and Localization

After establishing the diagnosis of insulinoma, every insulin-producing tumor of the pancreas should be localized preoperatively. The surgical approach and the operative strategy are greatly facilitated by adequate localizing investigations. For practical reasons, the localizing approach should start with ultrasonography (US) of the pancreas. With modern US machines and highly-developed, experienced centres for pancreatic surgery, many endocrine tumors of the pancreas can be demonstrated by this technique. The second step in imaging an endocrine pancreatic tumor is computed tomography (CT) (Günther 1983). This

all insulinomas are localized in the pancreas. According to Stefanini and co-workers (1974), who reviewed a large series of 1067 insulin-producing pancreatic tumors, insulinomas are localized in one-third of patients in the head of the pancreas, in one-third in the body, and in one-third in the tail of the pancreas (Table 7.10.3). 80% of insulinomas are single tumors, with an average size of 1–5 cm. In our own patient population, we had 13 out of 15 with single insulinomas, 1 patient with 2 tumors and 1 with 4 tumors. The median size was 2 cm, and 9 out of 13 single insulinomas were localized in the tail, 3 within the pancreatic body, and in only 1 patient in the pancreatic head.

technique entails similar problems to those of ultrasonography, because both are able to localize endocrine tumors above 2 cm in diameter, while diagnostic sensitivity in tumors smaller than this seems to be low. A real advantage is demonstrated by i. v. contrast enhancement during the CT investigation, because endocrine tumors of the pancreas normally enhance very quickly (Günther 1983). Angiography has been shown to be the best of the tests commonly used in preoperative localization of insulinomas, with a sensitivity of up to 88 % (Edis et al. 1976, Fulton et al. 1976). Selective or superselective arteriography of pancreatic vessels is therefore obligatory for all patients with insulinoma if ultrasonography or computed tomography have not been able to localize the tumor lesion. There is a further localization approach, using selective pancreatic vein catheterization in combination with a hormone assay (Ingemansson et al. 1978, Lunderquist et al. 1978). This is a difficult and very invasive method, because the catheterization of small pancreatic veins via the transhepatic route is intended. In our opinion, this technique should be restricted to patients in whom the extensive diagnostic measurements mentioned above have not been conclusive. It should be taken into account that, in most cases, the surgeon's hand during laparotomy is more sensitive than preoperative CT, ultrasonography, or angiography. We therefore use the technique of selective pancreatic vein catherization only after an inadequate primary operation and before starting surgical re-intervention.

Indication for Surgery

The only possible and curative therapy for insulinoma is surgical removal of the pancreatic tumor. The indication for surgery should be considered as early as possible to avoid late and irreversible consequences of the insulinoma syndrome such as persistent neurologic damage. Even in malignant insulinoma, the indication for surgery should be considered, since most patients benefit from the partial or total removal of tumor mass through an improvement in the clinical symptoms of hypoglycemia.

Preoperative and Intraoperative Management

When the diagnosis of insulinoma has been established, patients should be protected from the risk of hypoglycemia until the operation is performed. This may be done either by feeding or intravenous glucose infusion.

During the operation, we use an artificial beta-cell, which determines and records the serum glucose values at various intervals (Schwartz et al. 1979). By means of this machine the patient is protected from hypoglycemia, and after removal of the insulin-producing tumor the rise in blood glucose can be detected very early.

Surgical Approach

The authors use either a bilateral subcostal or a median abdominal incision, depending on the weight and physique of the patients. In overweight patients, a frequent finding in insulinoma disease, we favour a transverse incision. The operating surgeon should have a clear strategy in localizing and removing the endocrine pancreatic tumor. The most important task is adequate mobilization of the pancreas. The second step is macroscopic inspection, followed by extensive bidigital palpation of the pancreatic gland. A step-by-step guide to the intraoperative approach is given in Table 7.10.5.

We start the exploration by performing an extensive Kocher maneuver. The duodenum and the pancreatic head should be fully explored and mobilized to the aorta. To approach the pancreatic body and tail, the gastrocolic ligament is dissected together with the ligamentary adhesions between the pancreas and the stomach, pancreas and spleen, and between the pancreas and the splenic flexure of the colon. In some instances, the spleen should be fully mobilized to explore the pancreatic tail. In addition, it is necessary to dissect the tissue around the lower border of the pancreatic body and tail. After this, a palpatory approach to the posterior wall of the pancreatic body and tail is possible. The second step entails full macroscopic inspection of the pancreatic gland. In most cases, and especially if there has been a positive preoperative localization, the insulinoma is visible due to its distinct color, normally darker than the pancreatic parenchyma. If there is no tumor visible, we commence bidigital palpation of the whole pancreatic organ. By this means the insulinoma becomes detectable from its consistency, which, in all cases, is more solid than that of the normal pancreatic parenchyma. It should always be remembered that in up to 10 % of patients with insulinoma syndrome, there are multiple tumor lesions. After identifying one tumor lesion, the bidigital palpation of the gland should therefore be continued to ensure that further insulinomas are not missed. Most insulin-producing

Table 7.10.5 **Step-by-step intraoperative approach**

1	Extensive mobilization of the pancreas
2	Macroscopic inspection
3	Bidigital palpation
4	Fine-needle puncture, biopsy
5	Intraoperative ultrasonography
6	In vivo staining (toluidine blue)
7	Intraoperative selective catheterization of the pancreatic veins

tumors will be identified after mobilization, inspection, and extensive bidigital palpation of the pancreas.

If the insulinoma can still not be identified, there are four other techniques to carry out (Table 7.10.5). Suspicious parenchyma lesions should either be subjected to fine-needle puncture, or biopsies should be taken and the samples should be sent for frozen-section diagnostic evaluation. Recently, intraoperative ultrasonography of the pancreas has been introduced to localize undetected pancreatic tumors. Experience is as yet limited, but this seems to be a suitable method of detecting small insulinomas in otherwise unaltered pancreatic parenchyma (Sigel et al. 1981). Another way of identifying the insulinoma is in vivo staining with toluidine blue (Hurvitz et al. 1967, Spelsberg et al. 1976). This technique is either performed by peripheral intravenous injection or by intra-arterial injection (splenic artery, gastroduodenal artery). Some authors have been able to demonstrate selective in vivo tumor staining after toluidine blue injection. The final but obviously good method of detecting the insulinoma is intraoperative selective catherization of the pancreatic veins, with determination of insulin via the splenic vein or superior mesenteric vein (Turner et al. 1978, Teichmann et al. 1981).

Surgical Treatment

The surgical therapy of choice is enucleation of the insulinoma, because only the pathological lesion should be removed, with healthy pancreatic parenchyma being preserved. Enucleation begins after anterior or posterior incision of the pancreatic capsule. Afterwards, the tumor should carefully be mobilized and totally removed. Careful hemostasis of the pancreas with 5-0 prolene transfixion sutures is essential. After enucleation, the pancreatic capsule is resutured by 5-0 prolene sutures and a drainage is placed. If the insulinoma is localized in the pancreatic tail or body, a pancreatic tail or a 50% left resection represent an alternative operative procedure to enucleation. The authors prefer enucleation of the tumor, whenever possible, to preserve healthy pancreatic tissue. If a pancreatic tail or left resection is performed, it is possible in most cases to preserve the spleen by careful preparation. Insulinomas of the pancreatic head should always be treated by enucleation. Care must be taken to avoid a lesion of the main pancreatic duct or the common bile duct in the pancreatic head. In the case of an obvious lesion of the common bile duct, the intrapancreatic choledochus should be resutured and a T-tube should be inserted.

In the case of preoperatively and intraoperatively undetectable insulinoma, we do not assume an indication or a need for a so-called "blind" left or right pancreatectomy. Instead, we finish the operation as an exploratory laparotomy. It is better to exhaust all of the available diagnostic tools mentioned above and to prepare for a second laparotomy after the initial operation. Only in very rare cases is there an indication for subtotal left resection (Child) or total pancreatectomy at the secondary operation if the insulinoma still cannot be detected. In our own patient population we were able to identify 14 out of 15 insulinomas at the first operative exploration. Seven were treated by enucleation and seven by pancreatic tail or left resection. The remaining one was treated by a subtotal left resection during the second surgical approach.

Malignant insulinoma should be treated in the same manner as pancreatic ductal adenocarcinoma, i.e. by partial duodenopancreatectomy if the tumor is localized in the pancreatic head, or by left or subtotal left resection if the malignant lesion is demonstrated in the pancreatic body or tail. A lymph node dissection seems useful in malignant insulinoma. We had one patient with malignant insulinoma of the pancreatic body, treated by subtotal left resection and lymph node dissection, who was obviously cured one year after therapy.

Results of Surgery and Complications

The most frequent complication is pancreatic fistula after enucleation or left resection. In the large series of Stefanini and co-workers (1974), 12% of patients suffered from pancreatic fistula after enucleation therapy for insulinoma, whereas only 4.5% had this type of complication after left resection (Table 7.10.6). In our patients, we had two fistulas after seven enucleation procedures. One was cured by conservative management and the other one by relaparotomy and fistuloduodenostomy. Other complications arising after insulinoma surgery are pseudocysts (6.5%) and acute pancreatitis (Table 7.10.6). We had 2 abscesses (Table 7.10.7) after 8 distal resections. One was cured by relaparotomy, and the other by an ultrasonography-guided drainage procedure.

Hospital mortality after enucleation therapy has been shown to be 5.7% in the literature (Stefanini et al. 1974, Moss and Kaplan 1987) and 5.5% after distal resection, respectively. There was no mortality in our own group. 9.2% of 1012 cases in the review by Stefanini had persistent hypoglycemia due to endocrine tumors missed during operation. Obviously, these operative failures will be less frequent in the future when new diagnostic techniques and methods of preoperative and intraoperative localization gain widespread acceptance. In general, the long-term prognosis for benign insulinoma is excellent after surgery.

Table 7.10.**6** **Postoperative complications** after surgery for insulinoma

	No. of patients	Fistulas No.	%	Pseudocysts No.	%	Acute pancreatitis No.	%	Other complications No.	%
Enucleation	428	51	12	28	6.5	5	1.2	34	8
Distal resection	335	16	4.5	1	–	11	3.4	20	6
Pancreaticoduodenectomy	61	–	–	–	–	7	12	5	8
Other types of operation	58	–	–	–	–	–	–	9	15

According to Stefanini et al. 1974

Table 7.10.**7** **Results after surgical treatment** for benign insulinoma (n = 14). Department of General Surgery, University of Ulm, 1982–1987. Mortality: 0

	Type of operation	No.	Complications	Follow-up
Primary operation	Enucleation	7	2 fistulas	All cured
	Tail resection	5	1 abscess	All cured
	Left resection	2	–	All cured
Second operation	Subtotal left resection	1	1 abscess	?

Nesidioblastosis

Nesidioblastosis is clinically characterized by persistent hyperinsulinemic hypoglycemia in the neonatal period. The morphological equivalent of nesidioblastosis is either generalized or multifocal B-cell hyperplasia, or a focal adenomatosis of the endocrine pancreas (Heitz et al. 1977, Klöppel 1983). All infants suffer from recurrent hypoglycemia in the first six months, with symptoms of pallor, sweat, apathy and convulsions. The diagnosis is made on the basis of an inappropriately elevated circulating insulin level with hypoglycemia, an absence of ketone bodies, a positive glucagon test, and increased glucose utilization (Aynsley-Green 1981).

Surgical treatment. If medical treatment such as somatostatin infusion or diazoxide administration fails to normalize the glucose levels, surgical intervention is indicated. The surgical therapy of choice is a subtotal left resection preserving the spleen, removing about 85% of the pancreas, and leaving only a small amount of pancreatic tissue in the area of the common bile duct and duodenum. Although most of these infants will become diabetic after this type of surgery, subtotal left resection is the only chance of avoiding the consequences of recurrent hypoglycemia, such as severe neurological problems. Our own experience consists of two neonates with nesidioblastosis. They were cured by spleen-preserving subtotal left resection of the pancreas.

Glucagonoma

The glucagonoma syndrome is characterized by an islet-cell tumor with hypersecretion of glucagon. The most important clinical signs and symptoms are diabetes mellitus, a specific skin rash, weight loss, anemia, glossitis, cheilosis and venous thrombosis (Mallison et al. 1974, Prinz et al. 1987) (Table 7.10.**8**). The diagnosis is made by an elevated level of fasting serum immunoreactive glucagon together with the characteristic clinical picture.

Glucagonoma is usually localized in the pancreatic body and tail, and only rarely in the pancreatic head (Prinz et al. 1987). Most glucagonomas are greater than 3 cm in diameter when recognized. In contrast to small insulinomas, therefore, there is generally no problem in localizing glucagonomas. Ultrasonography, computed tomography and especially arteriography are suitable for localizing glucagonomas in the pancreas. About 70% of glucagon-producing endocrine pancreatic tumors have been shown to be malignant (Prinz et al. 1987). The most frequent sites for metastasis are the liver and peripancreatic lymph nodes.

Surgical treatment. When the tumor appears to be benign, complete surgical removal by means of enucleation or distal resection can completely reverse all of the clinical manifestations of the glucagonoma syndrome. However, in most cases, only palliative surgery is possible because of malignant glucagonoma with metastatic disease. Glucagon-producing endocrine tumors of the pan-

Table 7.10.8 Clinical signs and symptoms in glucagonoma syndrome (n = 70)

Sex (70)	Female: Male, 40 : 30 or 1.3 : 1
Age range	
Females (37)	19–71 yrs, mean 50
Males (30)	32–84 yrs, mean 58
Diabetes, or abnormal glucose tolerance test (67)	94 %
Marked hyperglucagonemia	100 %
Skin rash (65)	80 %
Glossitis (46)	80 %
Anemia, normocytic/normochromic (54)	90 %
Weigth loss > 4.5 kg (54)	91 %
Pathology	
Benign (20)	29 %
Malignant (50)	71 %
Less common findings:	No. of individuals manifesting this finding
Hypoaminoacidemia	22
Thrombosis	17
Diarrhea	13
Mental changes	10
Neurologic changes	4
Scotomata	?
Part of the MEA type I syndrome	?
Hypocholesterolemia	?

Numbers in brackets represent the number of individuals for whom information concerning this parameter was available..
According to Prinz et al. 1987

creas are usually slowly growing neoplasms. The reduction of the glucagon-secreting tumor mass may thus lead to significant palliation by reducing signs and symptoms. It therefore seems reasonable to resect as much tumor mass as possible if a radical removal of the tumor cannot be attained (Prinz et al. 1987).

There are some other options after palliative surgery, such as chemotherapy or somatostatin treatment, to reduce the symptoms of glucagonoma and provide an acceptable quality of life for these patients.

VIPoma

To date, about 200 patients have been described as having the Verner–Morrison syndrome, which is caused by a VIP-producing endocrine pancreatic tumor (Verner and Morrison 1958, Smale and Reber 1987). The clinical picture is characterized by a watery diarrhea, hypokalemia, achlorhydria and flushing in about 15 % of the patients (Smale and Reber 1987). 10–20 % of VIPomas are localized outside of the pancreas, especially in the retroperitoneal sympathetic chain and the adrenal medulla (Long et al. 1981). 40–60 % of vipomas have been demonstrated to be malignant.

The specific diagnosis of a VIP-producing tumor requires the demonstration of an elevated fasting concentration of plasma VIP by radioimmunoassay, together with the characteristic clinical picture. Localization of VIP-producing pancreatic tumors should be carried out by ultrasonography, computed tomography, and selective arteriography, as in the other endocrine pancreatic tumors mentioned above.

Surgical treatment. Patients with VIPoma syndrome and proved diagnosis by VIP radioimmunoassay should undergo surgery. The surgical treatment of choice is the same as for glucagonoma syndrome. If possible, there should always be radical pancreatic surgery to remove all tumor lesions. If palliative surgery has to be performed, a debulking of the primary tumor and metastases should be carried out to decrease VIPoma symptoms and allow more effective medical management (Nagorney et al. 1983). Postoperatively, a serial determination of VIP in the plasma allows follow-up of any recurrence of the original disease. Again, there are various medical treatment protocols, including chemotherapy and hormonal therapy with somatostatin, to give patients symptomatic relief.

Patients with benign VIPomas can be cured by surgical excision. The average survival for those with malignant VIPoma syndrome has been shown to be about one year (Smale and Reber 1987).

Other Endocrine Pancreatic Tumors

MEA-1 Syndrome

Multiple endocrine adenopathy is characterized by multiple tumors in two or more of the endocrine glands (Wilson 1978, Friesen 1982). In MEA-1 syndrome, in most of the cases there is an endocrine adenoma of the pancreas together with hyperparathyroidism caused by parathyroid adenoma. In some cases, the pancreatic endocrine tumor is accompanied by tumors of the pituitary gland, the adrenal medulla, or the thyroid gland. Most of the endocrine pancreatic tumors in multiple endocrine adenopathy are non-B-cell tumors, for example gastrinomas. If an insulinoma syndrome is evident in MEA-1, there are often multiple pancreatic adenomas or even an adenomatosis of the pancreatic gland.

The surgical strategy in MEA-1 is dependent on the preponderant clinical picture. First of all, hyperparathyroidism should be treated by removal of the parathyroid adenoma. Secondly, the pancreatic endocrine tumor should be treated surgically like all other endocrine pancreatic tumors mentioned above, i.e. either by enucleation or by pancreatic tail or left resection. If insulinoma syndrome is caused by adenomatosis, a subtotal left resection is sometimes necessary.

Somatostatinoma

Up to now, about 20 patients with somatostatin-producing tumors of the pancreas have been mentioned in the literature (Schusdziarra et al. 1983, Reber 1987). Somatostatin is a pancreatic hormone found in D-cells of the pancreatic islets. Somatostatin causes a release inhibition of all gastrointestinal hormones that are known. In addition, the emptying of the gallbladder, gut motility and gastric emptying are inhibited or delayed. Patients with somatostatinoma syndrome exhibit diabetes mellitus, cholelithiasis, diarrhea, steatorrhea and gastric hypochlorhydria. The tumor seems to show a high potential for malignancy (50%). Most somatostatinomas described in the literature were located within the pancreatic head.

Surgical treatment is mandatory in somatostatinoma, as in other endocrine pancreatic tumors. The aim is to remove the whole tumor mass by the surgical techniques described above or to achieve at least palliation by reducing the tumor burden.

PPoma

To date, less than 20 patients with PPoma have been described (Reber 1987). In contrast to the other endocrine syndroms, the PPoma picture has no characteristic signs or symptoms. Morphologically, it is characterized by single or multiple pancreatic endocrine tumors producing pancreatic polypeptide. The malignant potential of these tumors seems to range between 20 and 40%.

Surgical treatment should be performed in the same manner as described for the glucagonoma or VIPoma syndrom.

Very Rare Endocrine Pancreatic Tumors

There are some patients described with neurotensinomas, corticotropinomas, parathyrinomas, calcitoninomas, and carcinoid syndrome of the pancreas. To date, all of them are case reports, and general rules for treatment should relate to the number and quality of pancreatic tumors: i.e. the decision as to what kind of surgery should be performed depends, above all, on the questions of whether the tumor is malignant and whether multiple lesions are present or not.

References

Aynsley-Green A. Nesidioblastosis of the pancreas in infancy. Dev Med Child Neurol 1981; 23: 372.

Bloom SR, Polak JM, Wellborn RB. Pancreatic APUDomas. World J Surg 1979; 3: 587.

Creutzfeld W. Endocrine tumors of the pancreas. In: Arquilla E, Volk BW, eds. The diabetic pancreas. 2nd ed. New York: Plenum, 1985.

Edis AJ, et al. Insulinoma: current diagnosis and surgical management. Curr Probl Surg 1976; 13: 1.

Friesen SR. Tumors of the endocrine pancreas. N Engl J Med 1982; 306: 580.

Friesen SR, Tomita T. The APUD concept of the pathology of islet cell tumors. In: Howard JM, Jordan GL, Reber HA, eds. Surgical diseases of the pancreas. Philadelphia: Lea and Febiger, 1987: 803–813.

Fulton RE, et al. Preoperative localization of insulin-producing tumors of the pancreas. AJR 1975; 123: 367.

Günther R. Lokalisation von endokrinen Pankreastumoren. In: Kümmerle F, Rückert K, eds. Chirurgie des endokrinen Pankreas. Stuttgart: Thieme, 1983: 80–95.

Heitz PU, Klöppel G, Häcki WH, Polak JM, Pearse AGE. Nesidioblastosis: the pathologic basis of persistent hyperinsulinemic hypoglycemia in infants: morphologic and quantitative analysis of seven cases based on specific immunostaining and electron microscopy. Diabetes 1977; 26: 632–642.

Hurvitz RJ, Perzik SL, Morgenstern L. In vivo staining of the parathyroid glands and pancreas. Arch Surg 1967; 95: 274–277.

Ingemannson E, et al. Localization of insulinomas and islet cell hyperplasia by pancreatic vein catherization and insulin assay. Surg Gynecol Obstet 1978; 146: 725.

Klöppel G. Pathologie der endokrinen Tumoren des Pankreas. In: Kümmerle F, Rückert K, eds. Chirurgie des endokrinen Pankreas. Stuttgart: Thieme, 1983: 1–43.

Klöppel G, Seifert G. Pathologische Anatomie des Pankreas. In: Hollender LF, Peiper HJ, eds. Pankreaschirurgie. Berlin: Springer 1988: 37–82.

Kümmerle F, Rückert K. Chirurgie des endokrinen Pankreas in der Bundesrepublik. Dtsch Med Wochenschr 1978; 103: 729–732.

Long RG, et al. Clinicopathologic study of pancreatic and ganglioneuroblastoma tumors secreting vasoactive intestinal polypeptide (VIPomas). Br Med J 1981; 282: 1767.

Lunderquist A, et al. Selective pancreatic vein catheterization for hormone assay in endocrine tumors of the pancreas. Cardiovasc Intervent Radiol 1978; 1: 117.

Mallison CN, et al. A glucagonoma syndrome. Lancet 1974; ii: 1.

Moss NH, Kaplan EL. Insulinoma and Nesidioblastosis. In: Howard JM, Jordan GL, Reber HA, eds. Surgical diseases of the pancreas. Philadelphia: Lea and Febiger, 1987: 814–828.

Nagorney DM, et al. Resolution of recurrent Verner–Morrison syndrome by resection of metastatic VIPoma. Surgery 1983; 93: 348.

Prinz RA, Sugimoto J, Lorincz AL, Kaplan EL. Glucagonoma. In: Howard JM, Jordan GL, Reber HA, eds. Surgical diseases of the pancreas. Philadelphia: Lea and Febiger, 1987: 848–859.

Reber HA. Rare islet cell tumors of the pancreas. In: Howard JM, Jordan GL, Reber HA, eds. Surgical diseases of the pancreas. Philadelphia: Lea and Febiger, 1987: 865–872.

Rubenstein AH, Kuzuya H, Horwitz DL. Clinical significance of circulating C-peptide in diabetes mellitus and hypoglycemic disorders. Arch Intern Med 1977; 137: 625.

Schein PS, De Lellis RA, Kahn CR, Gordon P, Kraft AR. Islet cell tumors: current concepts and management. Ann Intern Med 1973; 79: 239.

Schusdziarra V, et al. Somatostatinoma syndrome: clinical, morphological and metabolic features and therapeutic aspects. Klin Wochenschr 1983; 61: 681.

Schwartz SS, et al. Continuous monitoring and control of plasma glucose during operation for removal of insulinomas. Surgery 1979; 85: 702.

Sigel J, Coelho JLU, Nyhus LM, Donahue PE, Velasco JM, Spignos DG. The role of ultrasound scanning during biliary and pancreatic surgery. Lecture on the 29th congress of the Societé Internationale de Chirurgie, September 13–19, 1981, Montreux.

Smale BF, Reber HA. Vasoactive intestinal peptide (VIP) producing tumors. In: Howard JM, Jordan GL, Reber HA, eds. Surgical diseases of the pancreas. Philadelphia: Lea and Febiger, 1987: 860–864.

Spelsberg F, Kemkes BM, Landgraf R. Intraoperative Vitalfärbung von Insulinomen mit Toluidinblau. Chirurg 1976; 47: 50–51.

Stefanini P, Carboni M, Patrassi N. Surgical treatment and prognosis of insulinoma. Clin Gastroenterol 1974; 3: 697.

Teichmann RK, Spelsberg F, Heberer G. Intraoperative biochemische Lokalisation von Insulinomen. Fortschr Med 1981; 99: 535–536.

Turner RC, Morris PJ, Lee ECG, Harris EA. Localization of insulinomas. Lancet 1978; i: 515–518.

Verner JV, Morrison AB. Islet cell tumor and a syndrome of refractory watery diarrhea and hypokalemia. Am J Med 1958; 25: 374.

Wilson SD. Wermer's syndrome: multiple endocrine adenopathy, type I. In: Friesen SR, ed. Surgical endocrinology: clinical syndromes. Philadelphia: Lippincott, 1978.

7.11 Intraoperative Radiotherapy of Pancreatic Carcinoma

S. Swanson, J. E. Tepper, W. U. Shipley, C. Willett, and A. L. Warshaw

Forty percent of patients with adenocarcinoma of ductal origin of the pancreas who are selected for exploratory laparotomy have localized, unresectable disease (Shipley et al. 1984a). Treatment with surgical bypass of the biliary tract and postoperative chemotherapy and external beam radiation therapy (EBRT) produces a median survival time of 6–12 months (Cancer of the Pancreas Task Force 1981). To improve local tumor control, palliation, and possibly survival time, investigators added intraoperative electron beam radiation therapy (IORT) to this treatment.

The focus of this chapter will be on an evaluation of IORT in the treatment of localized, unresectable carcinoma of the pancreas; however, the one trial of IORT in the treatment of resectable carcinoma of the pancreas will be discussed as well.

IORT is a technique of radiation therapy that has gained renewed interest in recent years in both Japan and the United States. It involves the application of a large single dose of radiation to a defined area that has been surgically exposed. This area may be either an unresectable localized tumor or the tumor bed that remains after resection. The tumor bed may include areas of gross residual disease or areas that are at high risk for local recurrence after resection of a known disease.

Seven centers in Japan and over 20 in the U.S. use IORT primarily as a boost dose of radiation in conjunction with perioperative EBRT. Analysis of cell survival curves suggests that 20 Gy of IORT may be the equivalent of 40 to 60 Gy given as fractionated EBRT (Gunderson et al. 1983).

Patient Selection

At the Mayo Clinic and the Massachusetts General Hospital (MGH), IORT is performed in patients with localized, unresectable pancreatic carcinoma in whom: (1) there are no contra-indications to surgical exploration, (2) carcinoma is histologically proven, (3) the tumor is located such that the intraoperative approach permits direct irradiation of the lesion with a minimum of intervening radiosensitive normal tissue (this may require dividing a gastrojejunostomy for exposure), (4) the entire tumor or tumor bed can be localized and can be included in the high-dose intraoperative boost volume (less than 9 cm in diameter), and (5) no metastases are present.

To select such patients, preoperative evaluation has included history, physical examination, routine chest roentgenography, and standard laboratory tests. Preoperative ultrasound-guided percutaneous needle biopsy is done to obtain a histological diagnosis. Unresectability is suggested by occlusion or stenosis of the superior mesenteric vessels or the portal vein at angiography or by loss of the fat planes around these vessels on computed tomography (CT) scan.

The possibility of metastasis of pancreatic carcinoma is particularly difficult to evaluate preoperatively. Mayo Clinic researchers reported performing exploratory surgery in 40 patients with pancreatic carcinoma and finding that 12 were inappropriate for IORT because of metastases (liver, 6; peritoneal seeding, 4; peritoneal seeding and liver metastases, 2) (Gunderson et al. 1984).

In order to improve the detection rate of peritoneal or liver metastases in patients with pancreatic carcinoma, 40 patients with biopsy-proven pancreatic carcinoma underwent laparoscopy at the MGH after complete staging studies (including imaging studies and angiography) failed to detect metastatic disease (Warshaw et al. 1986). Fourteen patients had positive examinations. Six had single, small (1–2 mm) nodules in the liver, 7 had parietal peritoneal nodules, and 1 had omental nodules. All nodules were confirmed to be metastatic disease by histological examination. The size and location of the nodules suggested that some may have been overlooked at laparotomy, especially the three in the pelvis. The positive laparoscopic findings altered the treatment plan in all 14. All were excluded from receiving IORT. Nine patients were discharged immediately, as they had tumor in the body or tail of the pancreas and did not require either biliary or gastric bypass for obstructive symptoms. Two patients underwent endoscopic placement of biliary stents. Only 3 of the 14 patients required laparotomy for biliary and gastric bypass.

Of the 26 who had negative examinations, all underwent laparotomy, and no metastatic disease was found in 23. Three had metastatic disease in the liver that had been overlooked at laparoscopy. Two of these patients had had what were now considered incomplete examinations. The third patient had a metastatic nodule in the central liver that was detected by palpation at laparotomy; it was not visible.

At the MGH, laparoscopy is currently used as a final examination before exploratory laparotomy in patients who have not had abdominal surgery.

Technique

The technique of IORT of the pancreas, as practiced at the MGH, involves the following. Selected patients undergo exploratory laparotomy in a standard operating room. If possible, excision is performed and IORT is not. Those with localized, unresectable pancreatic carcinoma are evaluated for IORT intraoperatively by the surgeon and the radiotherapist. If no metastatic disease is present and if the tumor can be encompassed by a specially-designed lucite cylinder to allow delivery of electron beam irradiation, the IORT is considered possible. The patient's wound is closed with temporary nylon sutures and covered with multiple drapes. The patient is then placed in a Surgi-Lift (a flexible lifter) and transported to the radiotherapy suite where the linear accelerator room has been prepared as an operating room. Anesthesia during the transfer requires 100% oxygen (to maximize oxygenation during IORT), sodium pentothal, and appropriate narcotics. In the radiotherapy suite, the patient is re-draped, the wound is opened, the tumor is exposed, and the lucite cylinder is applied (Fig. 7.11.1). The lucite cylinder extends from the

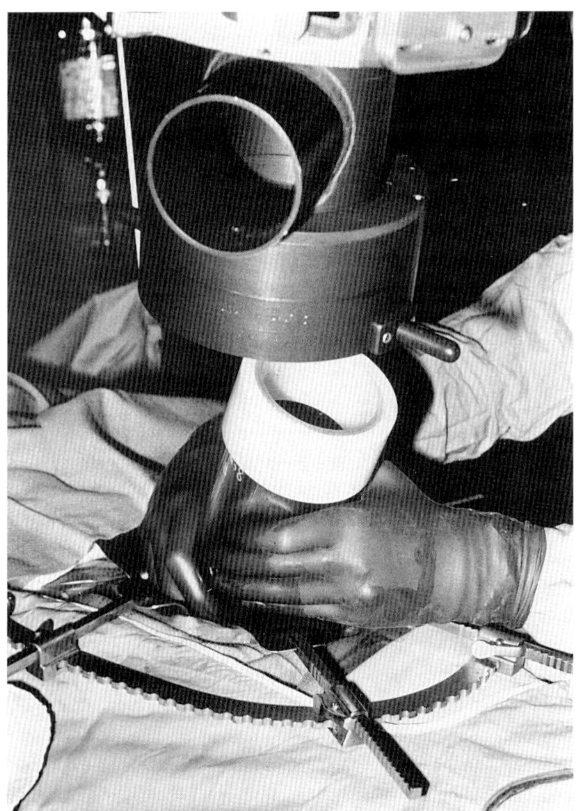

Fig. 7.11.**1 Lucite cone** (clear with white rim) held in position over a pancreatic carcinoma while the linear accelerator is maneuvered to dock with the cone

tumor to the linear accelerator. It collimates the electron beam, delineates the treatment volume, and retracts normal structures outside its circumference. Cylinders are 6–9 cm in diameter. All personnel move outside the linear accelerator suite, where closed-circuit television provides a constant view of the patient, the respirator, and measurements of blood pressure and ECG. Using a Clinac 35 linear accelerator, the patient is irradiated over three to five minutes with 15–20 Gy to the 90% isodose line. The patient is then returned to the operating room, if anastomoses are required; otherwise, the patient's wound is closed in the linear accelerator suite and the patient is taken to the recovery room.

The obvious disadvantage of the MGH technique is the transfer of the patient between the operating room and the radiotherapy suite. Although it has not caused morbidity, it is time-consuming for the surgeon, the radiotherapist, and the staffs of the operating room and radiotherapy department. At the MGH, one operating room and the linear accelerator suite are reserved for IORT one morning each week. During this time, 20 patients would normally receive out-patient radiation treatments. One solution to this problem is to place radiotherapy units in a standard operating room, obviating the need for travel between the operating room and radiotherapy suite. The MGH plans to install a linear accelerator in a standard operating room. This is a very expensive solution and should probably be done only by a limited number of centers at this stage.

Many patients are referred for IORT after recent laparotomies. The timing of the reoperation for IORT is important. Because of the development of inflammation and adhesions, it is best to reoperate less than 1 week or between 3 and 6 weeks after the initial laparotomy.

Localized, unresectable pancreatic carcinoma is treated with 15 to 20 Gy of IORT and perioperative EBRT. EBRT is given preoperatively in 1.8 to 2.0 Gy daily fractions up to a dose of 10 to 20 Gy to decrease the risk of tumor implantation at laparotomy. Postoperatively, EBRT is administered in 1.8 to 2.0 Gy daily fractions to a total perioperative EBRT dose of 50 Gy.

Unresectable Carcinoma of the Pancreas

IORT Results

In 1980, seven institutions in Japan began a clinical trial to evaluate surgery alone, surgery plus IORT, or surgery plus IORT and EBRT in the treatment of patients with pancreatic carcinoma that was localized, impossible to excise completely, and without evidence of metastases to the liver or peritoneum (Abe 1985). Each group included patients treated with biliary bypass (80–90%) or incomplete excision (10–20%). Median survival times were 5.5 months in the surgery group, 5.5 months in the surgery plus IORT group, and 12.0 months in the surgery plus IORT and EBRT group. The significantly increased median survival time in the surgery plus IORT and EBRT group is encouraging, but the groups were not identical and a surgery plus EBRT group was not evaluated. An extremely useful benefit of IORT was demonstrated by this study: over 70% of patients became pain-free one week after receiving a single dose of 20 Gy or more of IORT.

Complications in this Japanese pilot study were significant (Abe et al. 1987). In the study, some patients received 20–35 Gy of IORT. In patients who received more than 25 Gy, diarrhea and hematochezia occurred in 30%, and duodenal ulcers in 10%. One patient developed prepyloric obstruction that required laparotomy and gastrojejunostomy. One patient, who received 35 Gy to the stump of the resected pancreas, died 10 days after IORT. Acute pancreatic necrosis was considered the cause of death. Two patients bled from the prepyloric area 6 and 8 months after 25 Gy IORT and 45 Gy EBRT. These complications responded to medical therapy. From these results, and those from canine studies, most investigators now limit the IORT does to 20 Gy and defunctionalize irradiated loops of bowel.

Of the centers in the United States employing IORT, three have reported detailed results of the treatment of unresectable pancreatic cancer with IORT. The Mayo Clinic researchers compared two treatment regimens for locally advanced, unresectable pancreatic cancer (Roldan et al. 1986, Gunderson et al. 1987). Exploratory laparotomies were performed, and the majority of patients had biliary and gastric bypass. Further treatment was either IORT of 20 Gy and postoperative EBRT of 45–55 Gy in the "IORT" group (37 patients) or postoperative EBRT of 40–60 Gy without IORT in the "EBRT" group (145 patients). Many received chemotherapy. Median survival times showed no differences between the groups: EBRT; 12.7 months and IORT 12.4 months: Although tumor size, tumor grade, type of pancreatic biopsy, or size of EBRT field did not alter the survival rate, location of the tumor did; the survival rate was 18% at two years for patients with tumors in the head versus 4% for those with tumors located elsewhere. The most impressive finding of the study was that local control was significantly improved with IORT; two-year local control was 65% in the IORT group, but only 19% in the EBRT group. In the IORT group, only 7% failed within the IORT or EBRT fields; failure was predominantly caused by distant metastases or peritoneal seeding.

Complications in patients treated at the Mayo Clinic included gastric outlet obstruction in patients who did not undergo gastric bypass at the time of IORT. They also reported three postoperative infections in patients who underwent IORT one seven days after initial exploratory laparotomies.

Investigators at the National Cancer Institute (NCI) recently reported results of IORT in the treatment of patients with unresectable pancreatic carcinoma (Sindelar and Kinsella 1986 b). Thirty-two patients with unresectable stage III (locally advanced; positive nodes) or stage IV (visceral or peritoneal metastases) pancreatic carcinoma underwent biliary and gastric bypass and were randomized to receive either IORT of 25 Gy and postoperative EBRT of 50 Gy to the upper abdomen or postoperative EBRT of 60 Gy without IORT. Both groups were treated with postoperative fluorouracil (5-FU). Median survival times for patients with stage III and stage IV disease did not differ between the IORT and EBRT groups (8 months); however, for those with stage III disease, median survival time and time to disease progression were superior in the IORT group.

Complications in patients treated at the NCI included late duodenal hemorrhage in 3 out of 16 patients. There was one early death from respiratory failure in their IORT group.

The largest United States experience with the longest follow-up of treatment of pancreatic carcinoma with IORT comes from the MGH, where treatment began in 1978 and over 80 patients have been treated. A report published in 1984 detailed the results of treatment of the first 29 patients at the MGH (Shipley et al, 1984 b). Patients received 15 to 20 Gy IORT; during the study, the IORT dose was gradually increased as it became clear that normal tissue tolerance was reasonable and that local failures were occurring with the lower doses. Treatment included perioperative EBRT of 50 Gy and biliary and gastric bypass. Most patients received chemotherapy. Median survival time was 16.5 months for all patients, and 17 months for the 27 patients who completed the full course of EBRT. There was a trend toward increased survival time in patients who had smaller tumors. The actuarial probability of local control at 12 months was 64%. This study from the MGH is important, as it reports the best median survival time (16.5 months) for patients with unresectable pancreatic carcinoma. However, there are two concerns: (1) although other studies have notable differences, no other study has confirmed the MGH findings, and (2) as Gunderson and colleagues (1987) note, the MGH results may be due to selection, as 22 out of

29 patients underwent second operations for IORT six to 10 weeks after the initial surgery.

One significant finding of this study is that IORT is effective in pain relief. Of 16 patients with preoperative pain, 12 were totally relieved of pain with IORT and 4 noted significant improvement.

Complications in patients treated with IORT at the MGH were acceptable. No patient developed anesthetic complications or infection; thus, there was no morbidity that could be attributed to the transfer of the patient from the operating room to the radiotherapy department. In the 29 patients reported, 3 developed duodenal bleeding and one, who had not had a gastric bypass, developed duodenal obstruction that was corrected by a gastroenterostomy. Two patients developed non-malignant common bile duct obstruction that was corrected surgically. One patient developed upper small bowel necrosis at 36 months; autopsy revealed pancreatic fibrosis, generalized atherosclerosis, and superior mesenteric artery occlusion form intimal proliferation. Finally, one patient developed a pancreatic abscess with Candida that was treated with systemic antifungal therapy.

Recently, the MGH reported their results of the use of misonidazole as a hypoxic cell sensitizer in the treatment with IORT of unresectable localized pancreatic cancer (Tepper et al. 1987). Between 1982 and 1985, 41 patients were given intravenously 3.5 gm/m^2 of misonidazole 30 min before IORT. The results from this group were compared with those from patients treated with IORT between 1978 and 1982 who did not receive misonidazole. Median survival time was worse in the misonidazole group (12 months) than the other group (16.5 months). The reason for the different survival times may be due to patient selection (patients in the misonidazole group tended to have larger tumors); however, the investigators felt the results of this study were sufficient to argue against the use of misonidazole in this manner.

The MGH experience of treatment of pancreatic carcinoma with IORT and EBRT included 73 patients as of October 1986. Of these, 53 had evidence of disease progression, with only 24 having failure within the IORT field. Of the 73 patients, 57 had died as of October, 1986 (Fig. 7.11.2). While the results of the MGH are encouraging in terms of improved local control, the high mortality, primarily from disease progression outside the IORT field, underscores the need for effective systemic therapy for this disease.

IORT Alternatives

The treatment results, including median survival times of 12 to 16.5 months, and complications of IORT need to be compared with the results of alternative treatments of localized, unresectable carcinoma of the pancreas. Survival after biliary bypass alone is about 6 months (Cancer of the Pancreas Task Force 1981). Postoperative EBRT with 60–70 Gy coupled with chemotherapy can improve survival to 10 to 12 months (Dobelbower et al. 1980, Gunderson et al. 1987).

Several groups have used EBRT and interstitial irradiation with radioactive iodine as an alternative method of delivering an intraoperative boost. From 1975 to 1978, before the availability of electron-beam IORT, 12 patients with localized, unresectable pancreatic cancer were treated at the MGH with surgical bypass, radioactive iodine implantation of the tumor, and postoperative EBRT of 40 to 45 Gy (Shipley 1984a). The median survival time was 11 months, with the longest surviving patient living 31 months. The potential problems of significant bleeding, pancreatic fistula, pancreatitis, or tumor implantation did not occur in this small series. At Thomas Jefferson University (Philadelphia, PA), 54 patients were treated with this method (Mohiuddin et al. 1986). There were four deaths and significant morbidity in 28. Median survival time was 14.5 months. Although this median survival time is encouraging, the 7.4% mortality and 52% morbidity are unacceptably high for a palliative procedure. The EBRT dose used at Thomas Jefferson University was 60 Gy which may have added importantly to the morbidity.

Although more cumbersome, electron-beam IORT has four advantages over Iodine-125 implants: (1) larger tumors may be treated, (2) smaller tumors may be treated with 1–2 cm margins, (3) treatment is less traumatic, and (4) the possibility of seeding tumor from the needle placements is avoided.

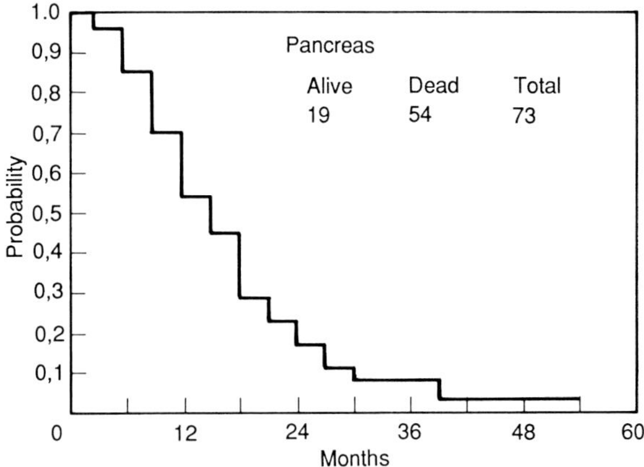

Fig. 7.11.2 **Actuarial survival as of October 1986** of all patients with unresectable pancreatic carcinoma treated with IORT at the Massachusetts General Hospital

Resectable Carcinoma of the Pancreas

NCI researchers studied adjuvant IORT (Sindelar and Kinsella 1986a). Thirty-two patients with locally advanced pancreatic cancer underwent resection and were randomly assigned to treatment with IORT of 20 Gy for stages I to III or the control regimen consisting of no adjuvant therapy for stage I (confined to the pancreas) and postoperative EBRT of 50 Gy for stages II (tumor outside of pancreas; nodes negative) and III (positive nodes). Operative mortality was unacceptably high (28%), but did not differ between the IORT and control groups. Similarly, complications occurred in 12 patients (sepsis, fistulae, and cardiopulmonary problems), yet were no different between the groups. Thus, IORT did not add morbidity or mortality in this small study. Overall median survival did not differ (12 months), yet it tended to be longer in those with stages II and III who were treated with IORT. Finally, local control was superior in the IORT group; the one-year local control rate was over 80% in the IORT group and nil in the control group. This study is important as it is the only randomized, controlled trial that specifically considers IORT as an adjunct in resected pancreatic cancers. It shows that local control can be improved. It suggests that survival time can be improved for those with locally advanced tumors.

Summary

The results of IORT use in pancreatic carcinoma thus far are encouraging, although the approach is still experimental. It relieves pain. It appears to improve local control. It may improve survival, especially in stage III disease (a common finding in the results from the Japanese, NCI, and MGH studies), but significant survival benefit is not anticipated until effective systemic therapy is developed.

References

Abe M, Intraoperative radiotherapy for carcinoma of the stomach and the pancreas. Proceedings XVI International Congress of Radiology, 1985: 207–210.

Abe M, Shibamoto Y, Takahashi M, Manabe T, Tobe T, Inamoto T. Intraoperative radiotherapy in carcinoma of the stomach and pancreas. World Surg 1987; 11: 459–464.

Cancer of the Pancreas Task Force. Staging of cancer of the pancreas. Cancer 1981; 47: 1631–1637.

Dobelbower RR, Borgelt BB, Strubler KA, Kutcher GJ, Suntharalingam N. Precision radiotherapy for cancer of the pancreas: technique and results. Int Radiat Oncol Biol Phys 1980; 6: 1127–1133.

Gunderson LL, Tepper JE, Biggs PJ, Goldson A, Martin JK, McCullough EC, Rich TA, Shipley WU, Sindelar WF, Wood WC. Intraoperative and/or external beam irradiation. Curr Probl Cancer 1983; 7: 1–93.

Gunderson LL, Martin JK, Earle JD, Byer DE, Voss M, Fieck JM, Kvols LK, Rorie DK, Martinez A, Nagorney DM, O'Connell MJ, Weber FC. Intraoperative and external beam irradiation with or without resection: Mayo pilot experience. Mayo Clin Proc 1984; 59: 691–699.

Gunderson LL, Martin JK, Kvols LK, Nagorney DM, Fieck JM, Wieand HS, Martinez A, O'Connell MJ, Earle JD, McIlrath, DC. Intraoperative and external beam irradiation +/− 5-FU for locally advanced pancreatic cancer. Int J Radiat Oncol Biol Phys 1987; 13: 319–329.

Mohiuddin M, Cantor RJ, Biermann WA, Weiss SM, Rosato FE. Combined modality treatment of localized unresectable adenocarcinoma of the pancreas. Int J Radiat Oncol Biol Phys 1986; 12 (suppl 1): 119–120.

Roldan GE, Gunderson LL, Nagorney DM, Martin JK, Illstrup DE, Holbrook MA, Kvols LK. External beam vs. intraoperative and external beam irradiation for locally advanced pancreatic cancer. Int Radiat Oncol Biol Phys 1986; 12 (suppl 1): 149.

Shipley WU, Tepper JE, Warshaw AL, Orlow EL. Intraoperative radiation therapy for patients with pancreatic carcinoma. World Surg 1984a; 8: 929–934.

Shipley WU, Wood WC, Tepper JE, Warshaw AL, Orlow EL, Kaufman SD, Battit GE, Nardi GL. Intraoperative electron beam irradiation for patients with unresectable pancreatic carcinoma. Ann Surg 1984b; 200: 289–296.

Sindelar WF, Kinsella TJ. Randomized trial of intraoperative radiotherapy in resected carcinoma of the pancreas. Int J Radiat Oncol Biol Phys 1986a; 12 (suppl 1): 148.

Sindelar WF, Kinsella TJ. Randomized trial of intraoperative radiotherapy in unresectable carcinoma of the pancreas. Int J Radiat Oncol Biol Phys 1986b; 12 (suppl 1): 148–149.

Tepper JE, Shipley WU, Warshaw AL, Nardi GN, Wood WC, Orlow EL. The role of misonidazole combined with intraoperative radiation therapy in the treatment of pancreatic carcinoma. J Clin Oncol 1987; 5: 579–584.

Warshaw AL, Tepper JE, Shipley WU. Laparoscopy in the staging and planning of therapy for pancreatic cancer. Am J Surg 1986; 151: 76–80.

8.1 Surgery for Primary Cholangiocarcinoma of the Porta Hepatis

N.J. Lygidakis and M.N. van der Heyde

Introduction

Although Courvoisier claimed that bile duct carcinoma was described for the first time in 1885, Fardal is to be credited with the first description of a patient in 1840 (Blumgart et al. 1984). The incidence of carcinoma of the confluence of the common hepatic duct varies in large patient series from 0.01–0.85% of autopsy studies (Alexander et al. 1984). In the United States alone, the estimate is 4,500 new patients per year (Ottow et al. 1985). It seems likely that there has been an increase, or that many cases which had been misdiagnosed in the past are now discovered more frequently. Early diagnosis based on clinical and cholangiographic findings is difficult, despite recent advances in direct cholangiography (Cameron et al. 1982). There are only a few definite signs for the differential diagnosis, and usually early infiltration of carcinoma into the portal vein, hepatic artery and surrounding tissues renders the management challenging and problematic, both for the surgeon and the patient (Alexander et al. 1984, Lai et al. 1987). Bile duct tumors, however, have little tendency to metastasize, and for that reason even palliative resection can offer long-term survival (Alexander et al. 1984, Cameron et al. 1982, Lai et al. 1987, Lygidakis et al. 1986).

Bile duct tumors can be classified in three types according to location. Type I represents tumors confined to the common hepatic duct (above the cystic duct-common bile duct junction, and below the bifurcation, Fig. 8.1.1a. Type II represents tumors of the bifurcation (Fig. 8.1.1b), and type III represents tumors of the bifurcation with extension to the left or right or both hepatic ducts (Fig. 8.1.1c). However, from the practical point of view the classification means nothing, as it does not predict the prognosis of the individual patient.

Management of primary cholangiocarcinoma of the porta hepatis remains controversial. Endoscopists (Cotton 1982, Dudley et al. 1979, Huibregtse and Tytgat 1984), radiologists (Dudley et al. 1979, Wiechel et al. 1982) and surgeons are advocates of their own therapeutic approaches. Results reported regarding survival are disappointing (Malt et al. 1980). Improvements in prognosis and outcome remain a desideratum, despite advances in preoperative diagnosis and management (Lai et al. 1987). Even surgeons are not yet in agreement on whether surgical management should attempt to be radical (Evander et al. 1980, Launois et al. 1979, Mizumoto et al. 1986, Sakaguchi and Nakamura 1986) or whether treatment should be limited to an attempt at pure palliation (Alexander et al. 1984, Cameron et al. 1982, Lai et al. 1987, Malt et al. 1980, Wiechel 1982). Radical resection is seldom achieved by simple resection of the tumor (Lai et al. 1987). However, even with combined tumor and major liver resection the radicality rate remains low (Lai et al. 1987, Lygidakis et al. 1988), while the mortality increases dramatically (Lai et al. 1987). On the other hand, there is ample evidence that if patients with cholangiocarcinoma are left untreated, their life expectancy will range from only 2–5 months (Ottow et al. 1985).

Palliation via endoscopic, percutaneous or surgical transtumoral or anastomotic drainage is associated with significant mortality, morbidity and limited overall survival (Cotton 1982, Dudley

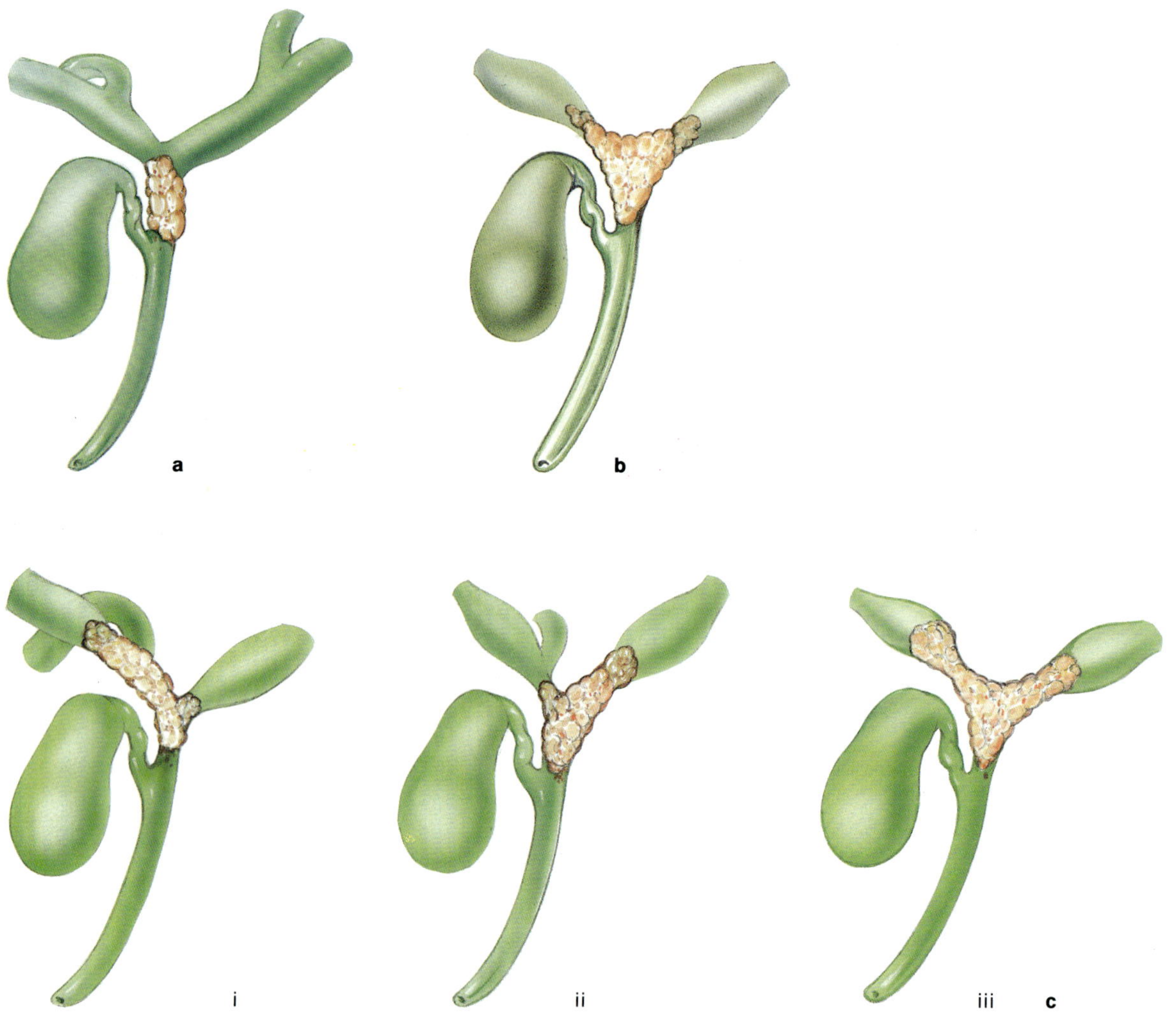

Fig. 8.1.**1 a**   **Type I cholangiocarcinoma:** confined to the common hepatic duct
b   **Type II cholangiocarcinoma:** confined to the bifurcation of the common hepatic duct
c   **Type III cholangiocarcinoma:** affecting the bifurcation of the common hepatic duct with spread of the disease to i) the right, ii) the left or iii) both hepatic ducts

1979, Huibregtse and Tytgat 1984, Malt et al. 1980, Terblanche et al. 1972, Wiechel 1982). The quality of postoperative life remains poor, and patients suffer from frequent attacks of cholangitis and problems with anastomotic drainage tubes. They become cripples of their illness, with frequent readmission to hospital due to sepsis, and they usually do not die from their tumor, but from failure to control septic complications (Lai et al. 1987).

Simple resection of the tumor, although it is seldom radical, offers satisfactory results and long-term palliation secondary to adequate drainage of the intrahepatic biliary tree (Cameron et al. 1982). Our personal experience with simple tumor resection and drainage of the biliary tree via intrahepatic cholangiojejunostomies between segmental hepatic ducts and a Roux-en-Y jejunal loop, is promising (Lygidakis et al. 1986). Thus, the dilemma of how to approach these patients still remains today. Even liver transplantation has failed to control the disease and has given disappointing results (Blumgart et al. 1984).

Surgical Treatment

Today, patients with cholangiocarcinoma who are eligible for surgical treatment have the following options:

1. Simple, complete macroscopic or partial resection of the tumor and drainage of the intrahepatic biliary tree via intrahepatic cholangiojejunostomies between segmental hepatic ducts and a Roux-en-Y jejunal loop (Lygidakis et al. 1986).
2. Combined tumor and liver resection, with or without resection of the regional vascular structures, based on the well-known principles of liver segmentation (Lygidakis et al. 1988, Mizumoto et al. 1986, Sakaguchi and Nakamura 1986).
3. Surgical drainage procedures, such as anastomotic or transtumoral drainage, without further resection (Lai et al. 1987, Wiechel 1982).

Simple Resection of the Tumor

The division of the liver into segments (Fig. 6.4.1, p. 195) forms the basis for the present technique, which was first described by Cameron et al. (1982) and subsequently modified by us (Lygidakis et al. 1986).

The operation is carried out with a bilateral incision (Fig. 7.1.3, p. 263). After entering the abdominal cavity, the porta hepatis is assessed (Chapter 7.1), followed by dissection of the common bile duct, of the portal vein and of the hepatic artery. All of these structures are isolated with vessel loops and completely dissected and skeletonized from their lymphatics (Fig. 8.1.2). We continue with a cholecystectomy and transection of the common bile duct. The common bile duct is transected as distal towards the duodenum as possible. The distal end is closed with transfixion sutures and the proximal end is reflected cephalad towards the porta hepatis (Fig. 8.1.3).

Via upward reflection and downward traction, the common hepatic duct is dissected more proximally up to its confluence and the underlying confluence of the portal vein and hepatic artery. The portal trunk, right and left portal veins, common hepatic artery, and right and left hepatic arteries are dissected and isolated with vessel loops. Following the intrahepatic course of the right and left branches of the portal vein, the intrahepatic course of the right and left hepatic ducts becomes clear (Fig. 8.1.4).

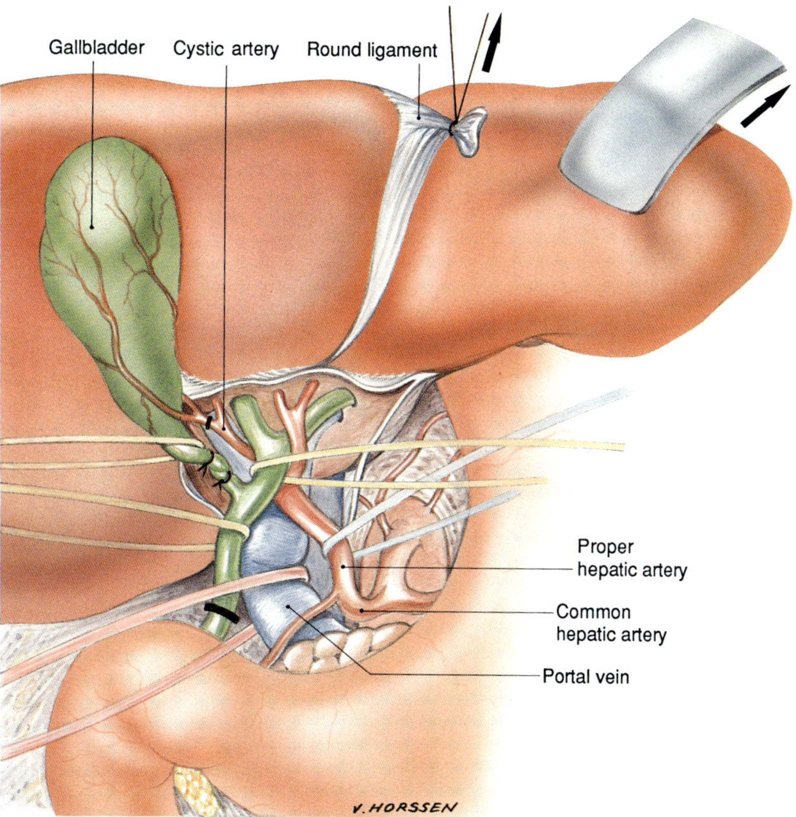

Fig. 8.1.2 Dissection of the hepatoduodenal ligament, identification and isolation of the portal vein, hepatic artery, cystic duct and common bile duct. The cystic duct has been doubly ligated. The cystic artery is ligated next, and cholecystectomy can be performed

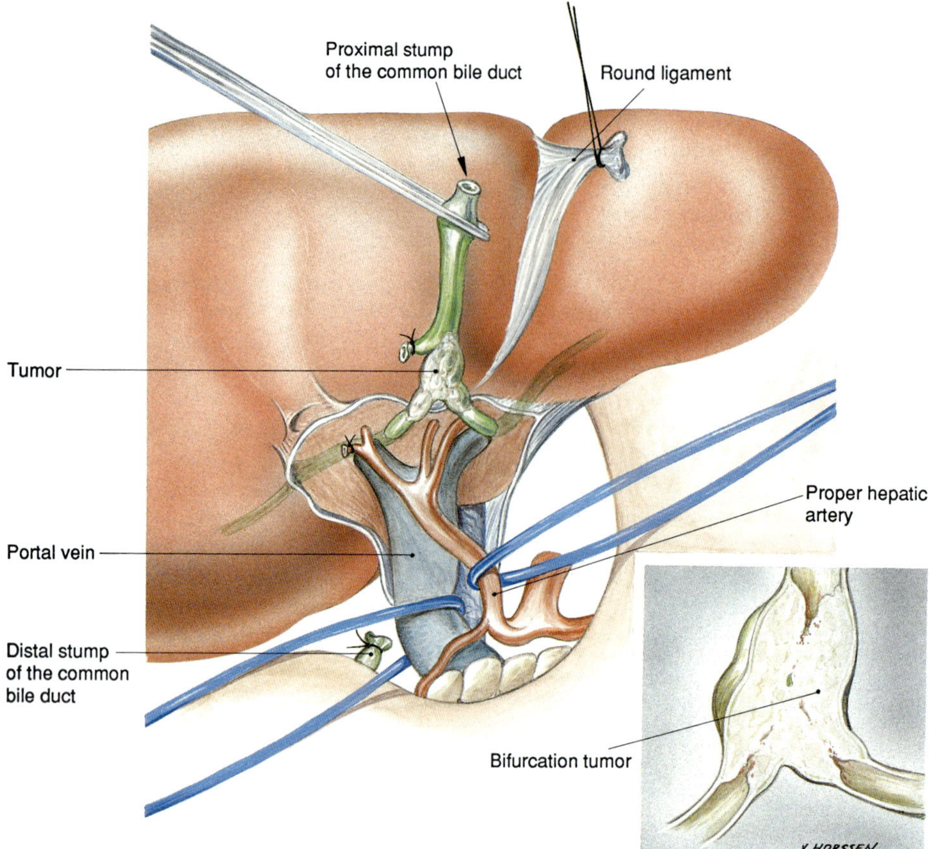

Fig 8.1.3 **After cholecystectomy, the common bile duct is transected.** Its distal end is closed, and its proximal end is reflected cephalad towards the porta hepatis

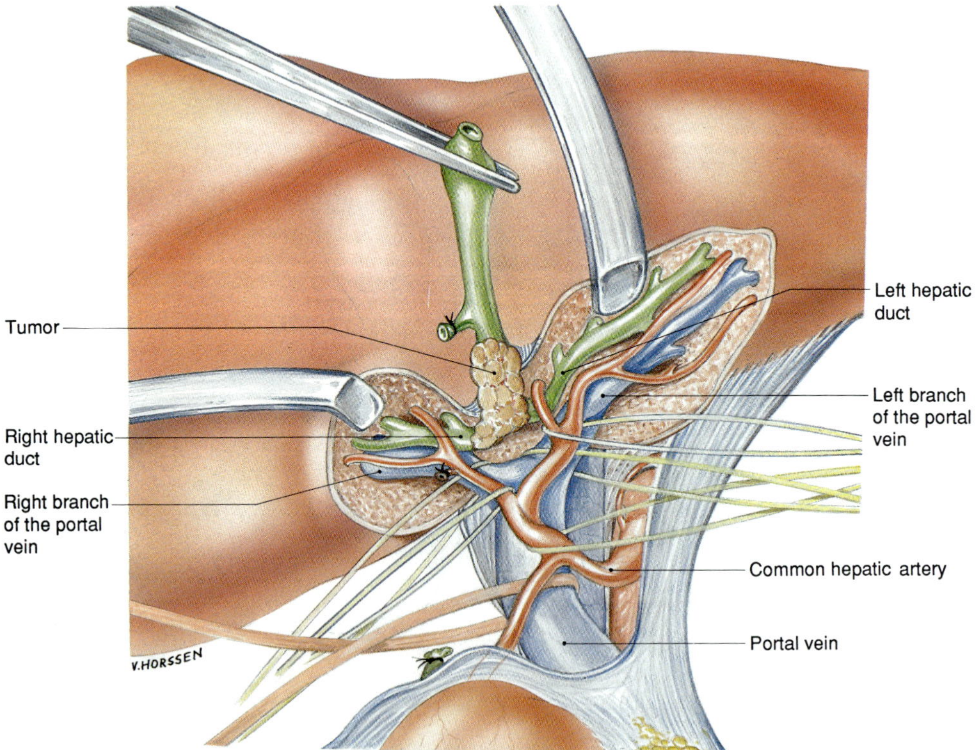

Fig. 8.1.4 **Following the intrahepatic course of the right and left branches of the portal vein** we get access to the intrahepatic course of the right and left hepatic ducts, till the level of their subsequent segmental bifurcation

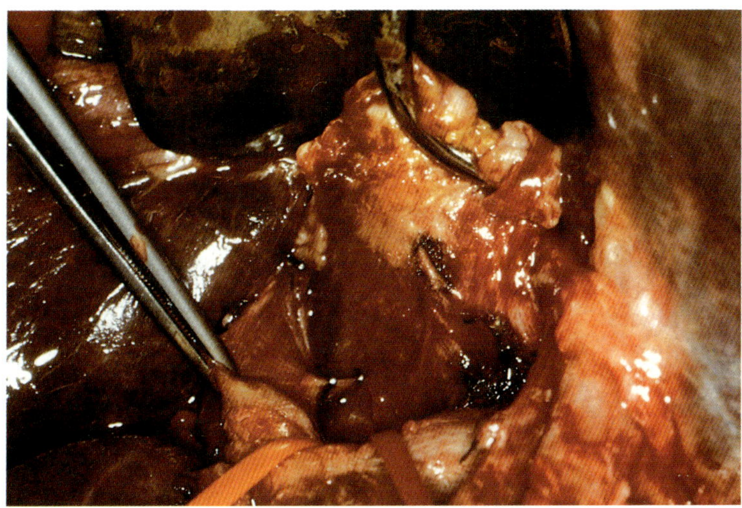

Fig. 8.1.**5** **Small side branches all along the intrahepatic course of the right and left branches of the portal vein are isolated, ligated and transected**, preferably using clips. This offers access to an avascular plane along which we can follow the intrahepatic course of the main hepatic ducts

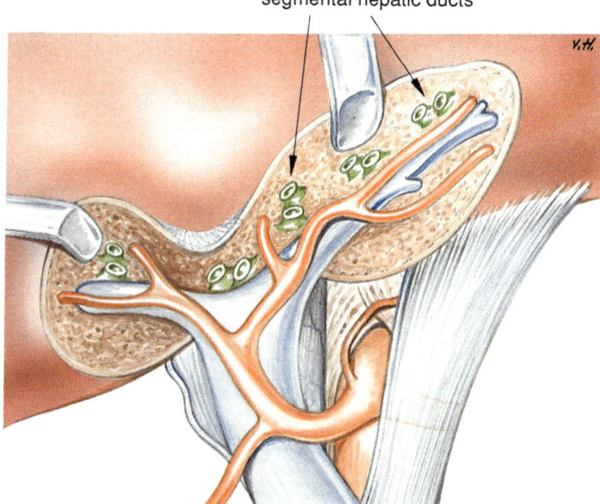

Fig. 8.1.**6** **Segmental hepatic ducts that appear after the transection of the main right and left hepatic ducts.** They vary in number depending on the level of transection of the main hepatic ducts

During dissection, the minor segmental branches of both the portal vein and the hepatic artery are isolated, ligated and transected, preferably using clips. In this way we gain access to an avascular plane via which we split the liver and gain better access to the intrahepatic course of the main right and left hepatic ducts up to the level of their segmental bifurcations (Fig. 8.1.**5**). The ducts are transected here proximal to the confluence of the common hepatic duct and proximal to the tumor.

The tumor, together with the right and left hepatic ducts, the confluence and the common hepatic duct are resected. In the space left, there is a variable number of segmental hepatic ducts, de-pending on the level of transection of the main hepatic ducts (Fig. 8.1.**6**). By side-to-side anastomosis between adjunct segmental hepatic ducts, common segmental hepatic duct stomata are fashioned where feasible (Fig. 8.1.**7**). Drainage of the biliary tree is carried out by means of separate one-layer mucosa-to-mucosa anastomoses between common or single segmental hepatic duct stomata and an isolated Roux-en-Y jejunal loop (Fig. 8.1.**8a, b**).

The steps involved in creating the anastomosis with single hepatic duct stomata are outlined in Figure 8.1.**9**. Figure 8.1.**10** demonstrates the creation of intrahepatic cholangiojejunostomies between common segmental hepatic duct stomata and the Roux-en-Y jejunal loop. In both cases, interrupted full-thickness 6-0 Vicryl (polyglycolic acid) sutures are used for the anastomoses. A row of full-thickness sutures is inserted on the anterior aspect of the hepatic duct stomata (Fig. 8.1.**9a**). Lifting these sutures up causes the lumen of the segmental hepatic duct stomata to remain open, facilitating the creation of the posterior layer of the cholangiojejunostomy. This layer is created with full-thickness interrupted sutures inserted between the posterior aspect of the common segmental hepatic duct stomata and the lower edge of the jejunostomy (Lygidakis 1987). In general, we use 5 or 6 sutures which are inserted and then tied.

Now that the posterior wall of the cholangiojejunostomy has been created (Fig. 8.1.**10a**), the transanastomotic tube can be secured with a separate suture on the posterior wall of this anastomosis, if used. It is brought out via a Witzel jejunostomy (Fig. 8.1.**10b**). The next step is the creation of the anterior layer of the cholangiojejunostomy by using the sutures already inserted on the anterior aspect of the segmental hepatic duct stomata (Fig. 8.1.**9c, d**). These sutures are inserted

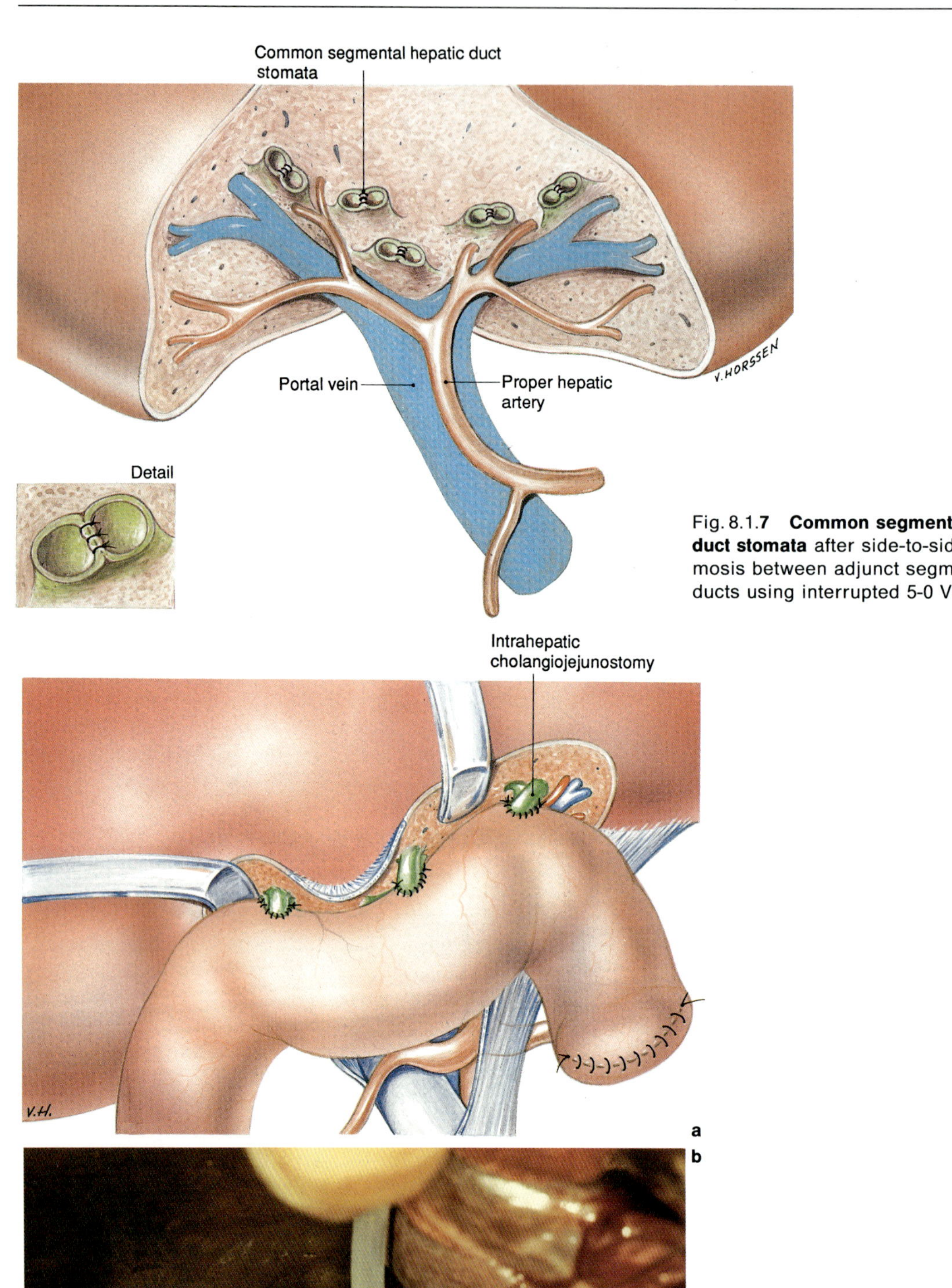

Fig. 8.1.**7   Common segmental hepatic
duct stomata** after side-to-side anastomosis between adjunct segmental hepatic
ducts using interrupted 5-0 Vicryl sutures

Fig. 8.1.**8 a   Intrahepatic cholangiojejunostomy** between common segmental
hepatic duct stomata and a Roux-en-Y
jejunal loop.
b   A segmented hepatic duct stoma is
shown

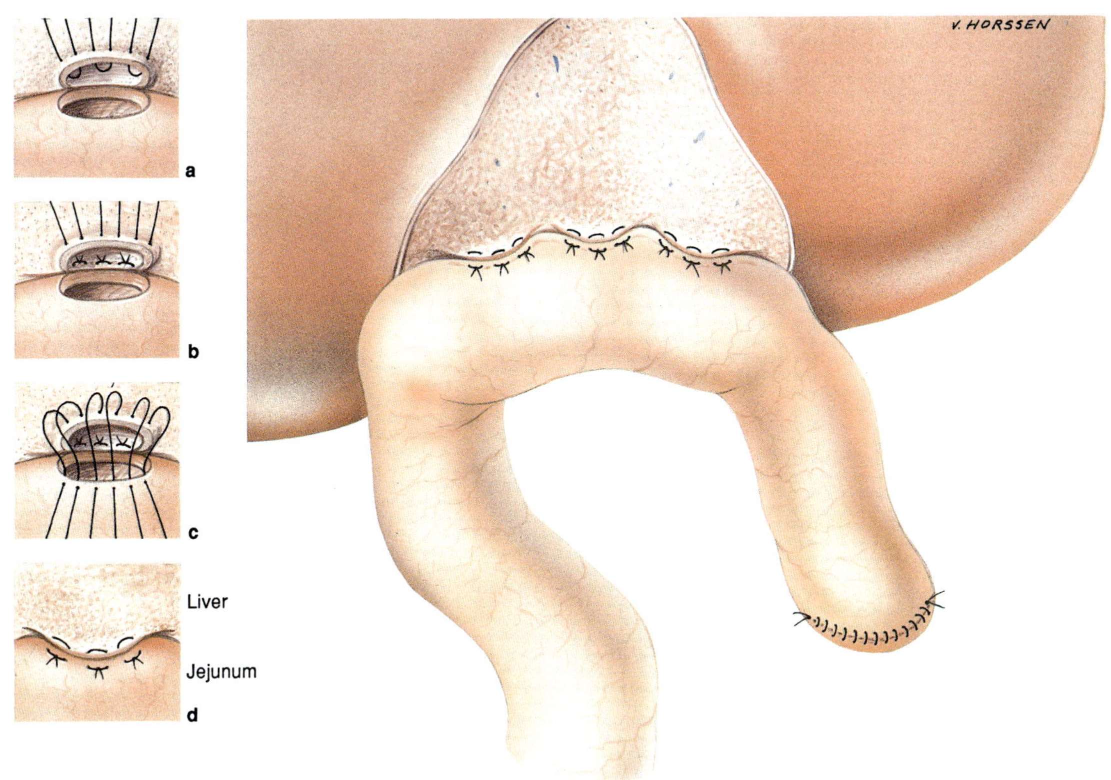

Fig. 8.1.9 Various steps in the technique of intrahepatic cholangiojejunostomy. a Sutures are inserted on the anterior aspect of the single segmental duct stoma. **b** The posterior layer of the anastomosis is fashioned using full-thickness sutures. The anastomosis is completed with steps **c** and **d**

one by one on the upper edge of the jejunostomy and then tied (Fig. 8.1.**10b**). The intrahepatic cholangiojejunostomy is now completed.

In general, 2 or 3 separate intrahepatic cholangiojejunostomies are used to drain the intrahepatic biliary tree. The anastomosis described above can also be created without transanastomotic tubes. Indeed since 2 years we obviate the use of transanastomotic tubes without any impact on the outcome of our patients. The wound is closed and transanastomotic and transabdominal tubes are then secured separately (Fig. 8.1.**11**).

Results

Figure 8.1.**12** shows two separate intrahepatic cholangiojejunostomies in a patient operated on for primary cholangiocarcinoma of the confluence of the common hepatic duct. Cholangiography was performed two weeks after the operation, and the transanastomotic tubes were removed at the same time. The patient was able to be discharged without tubes and without any jaundice. In similar findings (Figs. 8.1.**13** and 8.1.**14**), separate intrahepatic cholangiojejunostomies with segmental hepatic ducts can be seen. From September 1983 to January 1988, 30 patients underwent simple resection of the

tumor and drainage of the intrahepatic biliary tree according to the principle of intrahepatic cholangiojejunostomies. Three patients died during the first 30 postoperative days. Two patients had radical resection, and in 28 resection was not radical. Quality of life was satisfactory. Survival ranged from 4–43 months (mean 26 healthy).

We attribute these results to the efficacy of biliary drainage using the principle of intrahepatic cholangiojejunostomies. Adequate biliary drainage is an essential prerequisite for the elimination of biliary stasis and for prevention of cholangitis (Cameron et al. 1982). Use of anastomotic tubes is limited to the first 15 postoperative days, and this is certainly an advantage of the present technique (Lygidakis et al. 1986). We consider the present results better than after any other kind of surgical or medical palliative management (Alexander et al. 1984, Blumgart et al. 1984, Cotton 1982, Dudley 1979, Huibregtse and Tytgat 1984, Lai et al. 1987, Malt et al. 1980, Ottow et al. 1985, Terblanche et al. 1972, Wiechel 1982). We agree with others (Cameron et al. 1982) that because of the peculiarities of primary cholangiocarcinoma of the porta hepatis, the main cause of death in such patients is sepsis secondary to cholangitis (Cameron et al. 1982). There remains no question that the greater

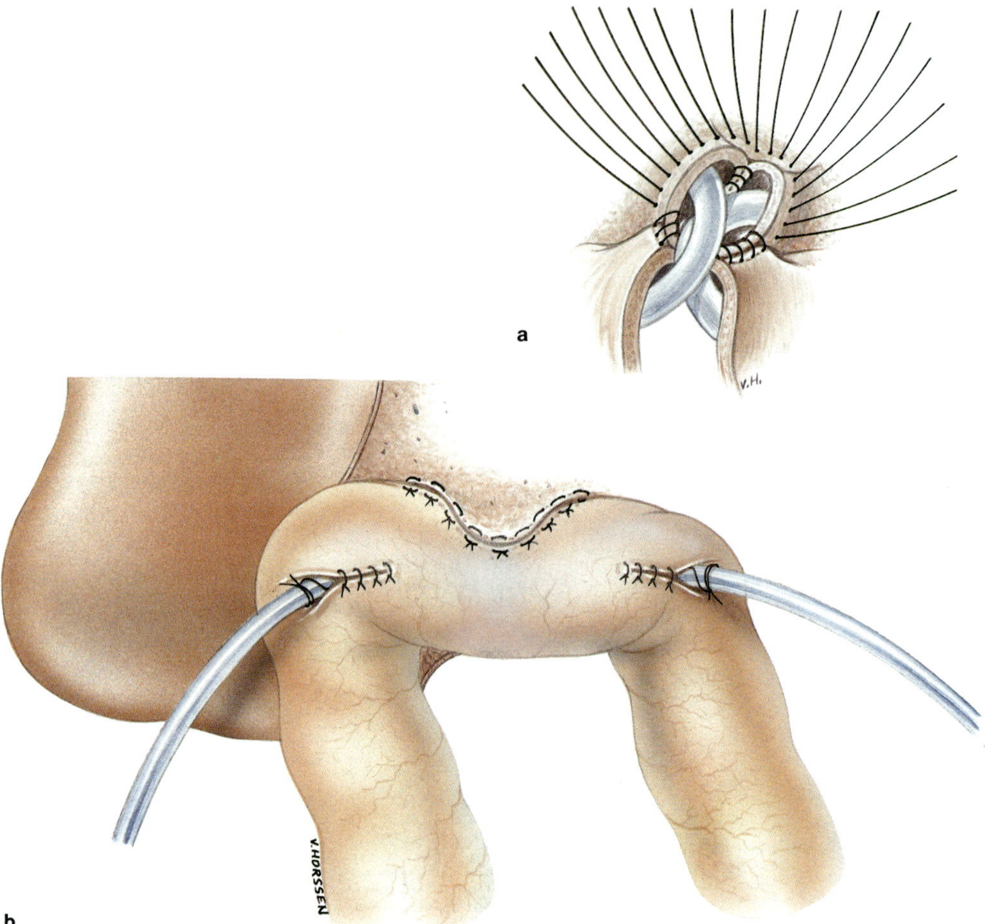

Fig. 8.1.**10 a** **Creating a cholangiojejunostomy** between the common segmental hepatic duct stomata and Roux-en-Y jejunal loop
b **Transanastomotic tubes** are brought out through Witzel jejunostomies

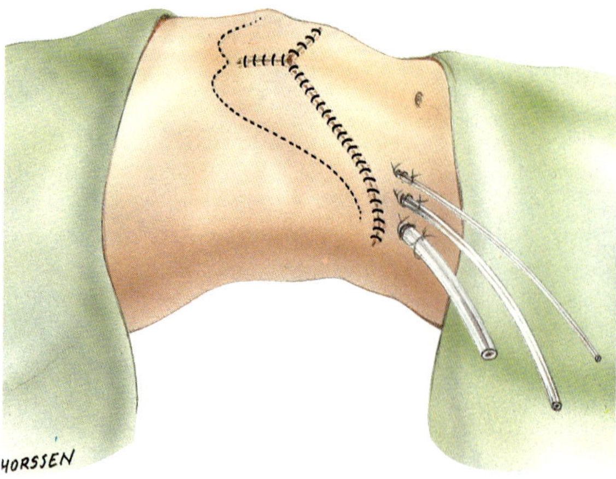

Fig. 8.1.**11**   **The abdominal wall is closed**, and the tubes are brought out through separate wounds

proportion of these tumors grow slowly and metastasize slowly, and that even partial resection is thus associated with long-term palliation.

Cholangitis is adequately prevented by the technique described, and overall survival, even after partial resection of the tumor, is therefore noticeably prolonged (Lygidakis et al. 1986). Presently, we supplement our patients routinely with postoperative radiotherapy using iridium wires for intraluminal irradiation combined with external beam irradiation.

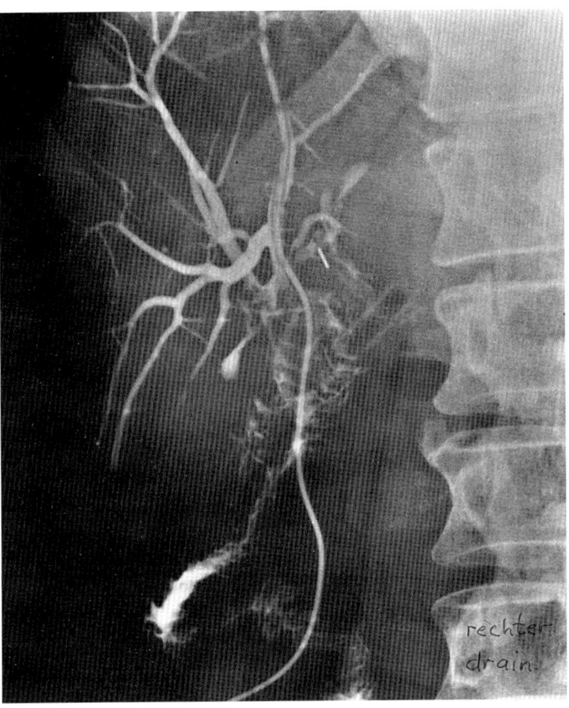

Fig. 8.1.**12   Intrahepatic cholangiojejunostomies** between the segmental hepatic ducts and a Roux-en-Y jejunal loop after left hemihepatectomy

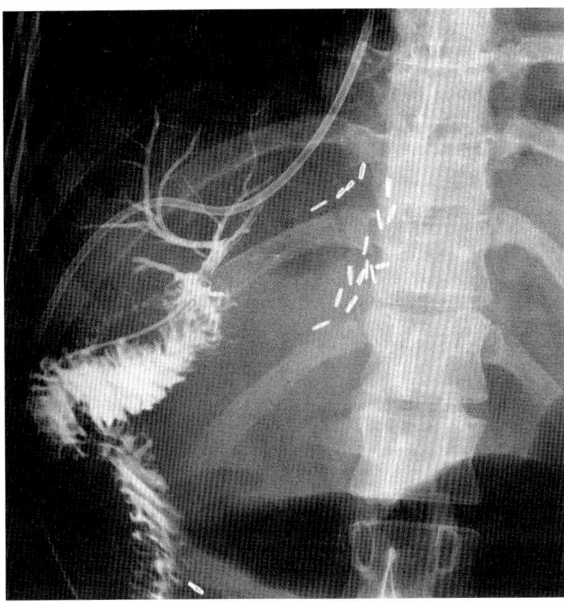

Fig. 8.1.**14   Extensive left hemihepatectomy:** anastomosis between the segmental hepatic ducts and a Roux-en-Y jejunal loop

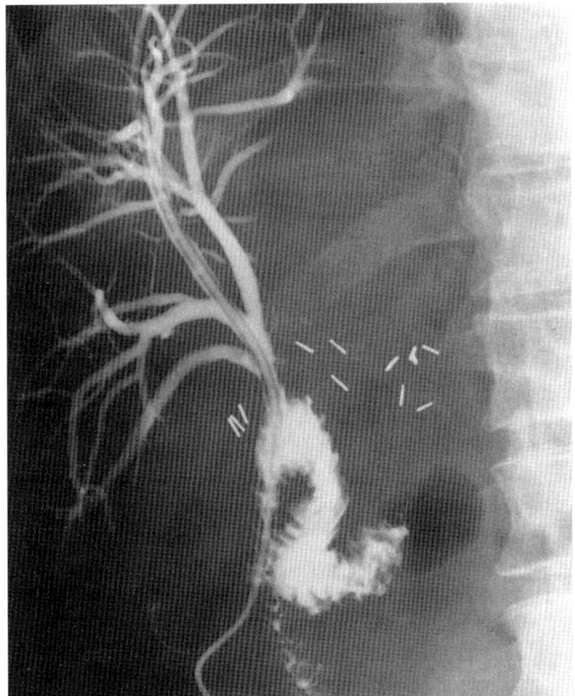

Fig. 8.1.**13   Biliary drainage after extensive left hemihepatectomy.** Note the common segmental hepatic duct stoma for segments VI and VIII

Combined Liver and Tumor Resection with or without Regional Vascular Resection

Indications and Contra-Indications

Combined tumor and liver resection is an appealing alternative in the surgical management of primary cholangiocarcinoma at the hepatic hilus in a proportion of patients. The main object is still to increase the number of patients amenable to resectional surgery and possibly to achieve an increased rate of radical resection, on the assumption that this will lead to longer survival and a more satisfactory quality of postoperative life. This approach, however, is associated with significant mortality, and for this reason is generally regarded with scepticism (Cameron et al. 1982, Lai et al. 1987, Malt et al. 1980, Ottow et al. 1985, Terblanche et al. 1972). On the other hand, there is recent evidence that this policy is indicated in patients who would otherwise be considered not eligible for surgical resectional management (Lygidakis et al. 1988, Mizumoto et al. 1986, Sakaguchi and Nakamura 1986). There is support for the view that the cost of a higher mortality is counterbalanced by an expected longer overall survival secondary to an increase of the number of patients amenable to resectional surgery. However, the criteria of selection must be firm and objective. Patients older than 65 years, those with an advanced stage of the disease in whose life expectancy is already limited, and those in poor

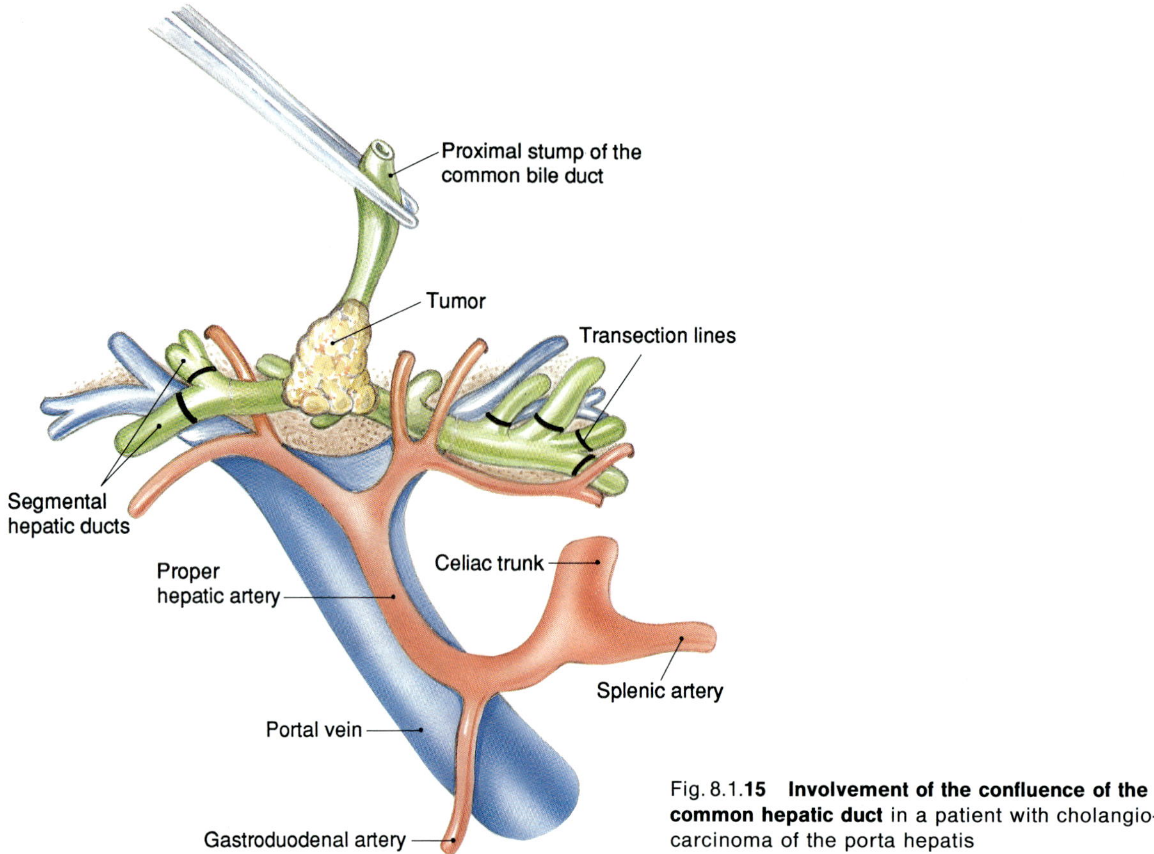

Fig. 8.1.**15** **Involvement of the confluence of the common hepatic duct** in a patient with cholangio-carcinoma of the porta hepatis

general condition, must certainly be excluded. The main risk factors remain sepsis, coagulopathy, and impaired renal and liver function. The value of preoperative biliary drainage, which has been studied by different groups in an attempt to reduce these risk factors, remains undefined. Attempts are being undertaken to improve the general condition of the average patient before surgery for extra-hepatic biliary obstruction by correcting immune deficiencies, malnutrition, coagulopathy and sepsis. It is hoped that we may succeed in achieving a lower mortality and thus a broadening of the indications for this kind of surgical management.

Surgical Technique

The same steps are followed as described above for simple resection of the tumor, up to the point of dissection of the confluence of the common hepatic duct and of the underlying bifurcation of the portal vein and hepatic artery (Fig. 8.1.**4**). At this stage, the presence of tumor growth towards the liver parenchyma and towards the regional vascular structures is carefully evaluated. It is important to assess precisely the extension of the tumor growth

in order to plan the extent of the liver and possibly vascular resection required. However, this is very difficult, and for the majority of patients there is microscopic spread of the disease via perineural lymph clefts, periductal lymphatic network and periductal venules and arterioles. The disease can be diffuse by submucosal infiltration, and may infiltrate the bile duct wall over a wide distance.

Figure 8.1.**15** shows involvement of bifurcation of the common hepatic duct with potential spread in the liver of a patient with cholangiocarcinoma of the hepatic hilus. Whether tumor resection should be supplemented by right or left liver resection, depends on the extension of the tumor towards the left or right hepatic ducts and on the extent of its spread in the liver (Figs. 8.1.**16a, b**; 8.1.**17a, b**).

Liver resection following oncological principles is carried out, firstly by transecting the main right or left hepatic duct intrahepatically proximal from the tumor and from the confluence of the common hepatic duct (Fig. 8.1.**18a**). Then, if a right hemihepatectomy or right trisegmentectomy are planned (example in Fig. 8.1.**18a, b** without vascular involvement) the left main hepatic duct is dissected

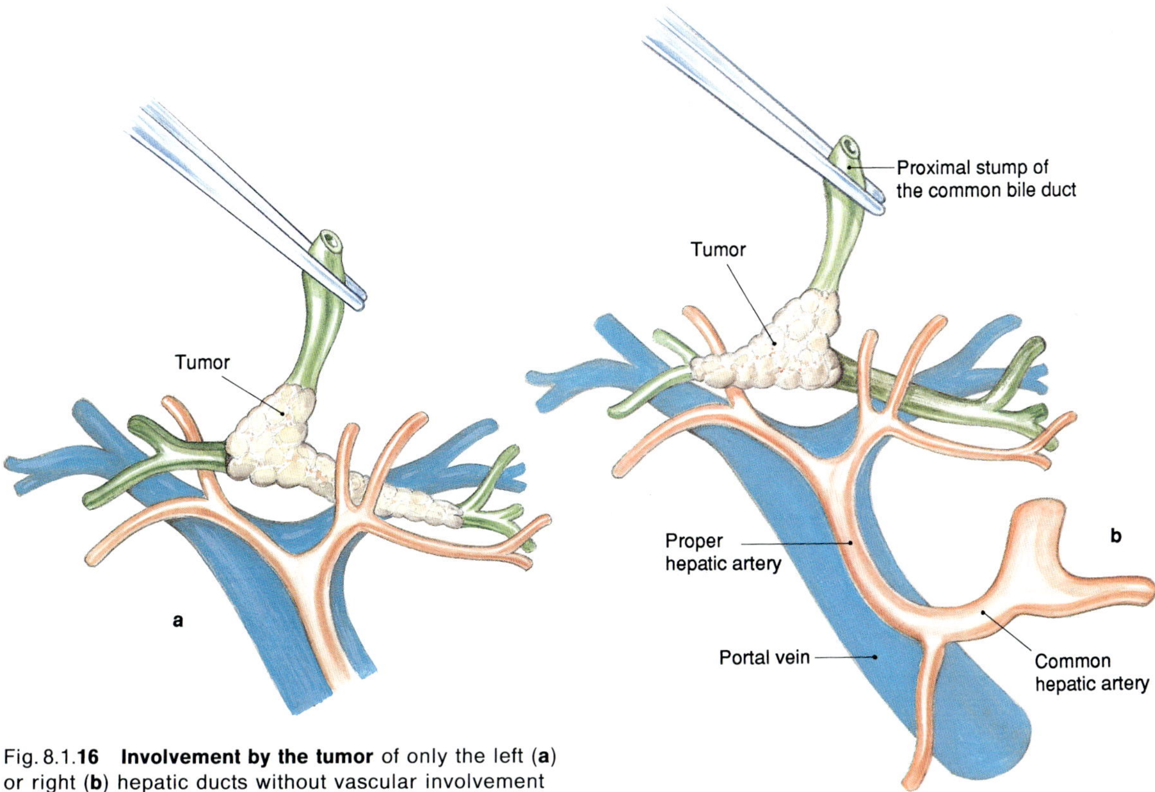

Fig. 8.1.**16 Involvement by the tumor** of only the left (**a**)
or right (**b**) hepatic ducts without vascular involvement

all along its intrahepatic course and then transected
at the level of its segmental bifurcation. Similarly if
a left hemihepatectomy or left trisegmentectomy is
planned (example in Fig. 8.1.**18c**) with vascular
involvement), the right main hepatic duct is dissected proximal from the confluence of the common hepatic duct and at the level of its segmental
bifurcation combined then transected with resection of the invaded segments of the hepatic
artery and portal vein of the residual liver
(Fig. 8.1.**18c–e**).

In both cases, the main hepatic ducts are
transected all along their intrahepatic course. The
proximal segment is kept open, and the distal
segment of the transected right or left hepatic duct
is pulled toward the contralateral region of the
porta hepatis. This offers access to the afferent
vessels of the porta hepatis, to their confluence and
their intrahepatic branches (Fig. 8.1.**18a–e**). Following the intrahepatic course of those vessels we
can, if necessary, isolate, ligate and transect the
segmental branches of the hepatic artery and portal
vein corresponding to additional liver segments
that are considered for resection. (For the technical
steps involved in liver resection, see Chapters
6.3–6.5.)

Liver resection can be supplemented by resection of both the portal vein and the hepatic artery of

the part of the liver that is going to be preserved
(Figs. 8.1.**19**, 8.1.**20**). Vascular reconstruction can
be accomplished either with an end-to-end anastomosis or by using venous grafts. The residual
liver is always drained via intrahepatic cholangiojejunostomies between the segmental hepatic
ducts and an isolated Roux-en-Y jejunal loop
(Figs. 8.1.**21**, 8.1.**22**).

Figure 8.1.**23** shows the cholangiographic findings in a patient after left trisegmentectomy and
intrahepatic cholangiojejunostomies between the
segmental hepatic ducts of segments VI and VII and
a Roux-en-Y jejunal loop.

**Option and Technique of Vascular Resection and
Reconstruction**

When there is vascular involvement (Fig. 8.1.**24**),
resection of the tumor and liver can be supplemented by regional vascular resection. If the infiltration
only affects the regional vascular structures, the
operation can be limited to tumor and vascular
resection.

Figure 8.1.**24** shows a patient with bilateral
involvement of both the portal vein and the hepatic
artery. In these patients we start with liver resection
and then continue with resection of the invaded

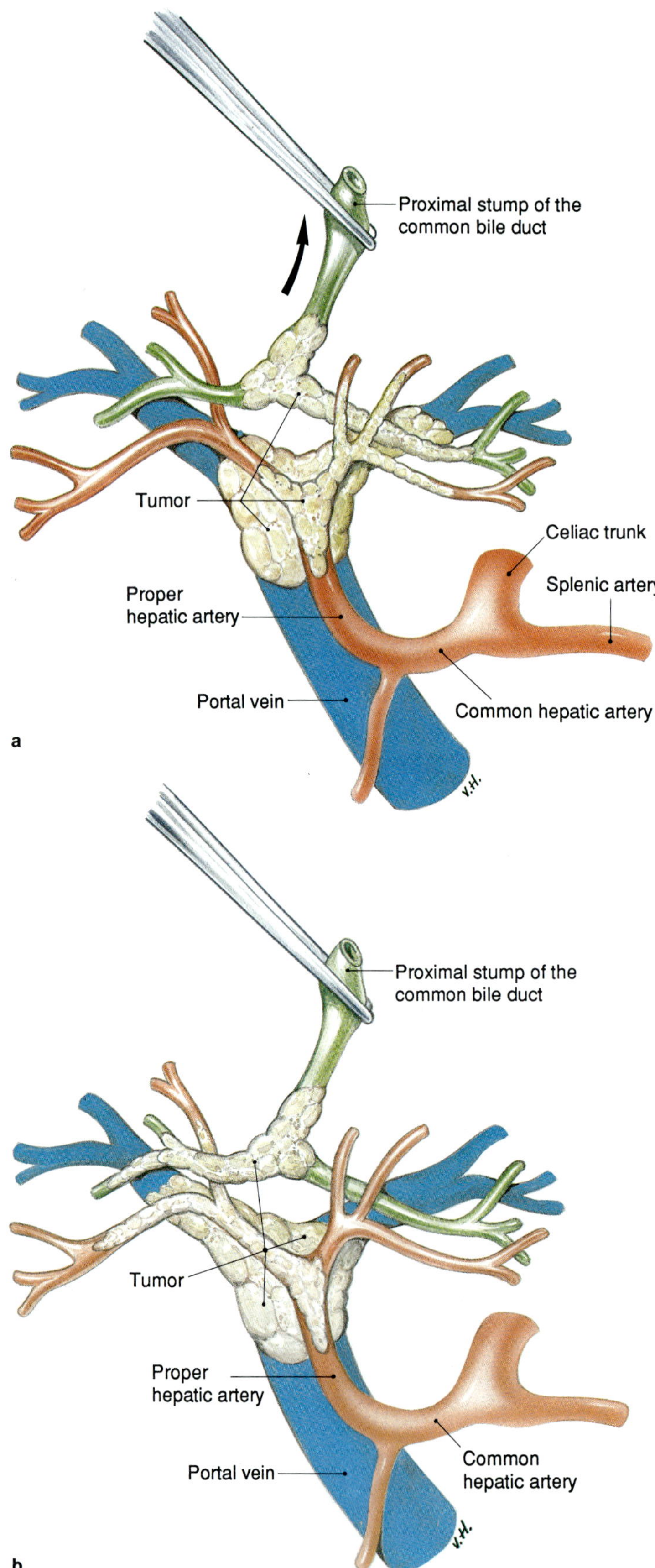

Fig. 8.1.**17 a   Extension of the tumor to the left hepatic duct, portal vein and hepatic artery**, with concomitant invasion of their confluence. Extensive left hemi-hepatectomy with resection and reconstruction of the right branch of the portal vein and right hepatic artery is indicated

b   Extension of the tumor to the right hepatic duct, portal vein and hepatic artery, with invasion of their confluence. Extensive right hemihepatectomy with resection and reconstruction of the left branch of the portal vein and hepatic artery is indicated

vascular segments of the portal vein and hepatic artery of the residual liver. This resection can be extended or limited, depending on the extent of neoplastic infiltration. Vascular reconstruction is carried out either via an end-to-end anastomosis or by using of venous grafts. Both the portal vein and the hepatic artery can be transected and reconstructed by use of venous grafts.

The technique described makes patients eligible for surgical resection who, according to adopted criteria of resectability, were considered unsuitable for resectional procedures because of bilateral biliary and vascular involvement (Alexander et al. 1984, Blumgart et al. 1984, Evander et al. 1980, Launois et al. 1979, Malt et al. 1980, Ottow et al. 1985, Tompkins et al. 1981, Terblanche et al. 1972, Wiechel 1982). Figure 8.1.**25** shows the anatomical distribution of arteries and veins to the liver. Figure 8.1.**26** illustrates the various techniques for resection and reconstruction of the hepatic artery and the arterial supply of the liver, showing methods of resecting the invaded vascular segment and reconstructing it using either an end-to-end anastomosis or (Fig. 8.1.**26b**) an interposed venous graft (Fig. 8.1.**26c**). The steps to be taken in the case of extensive tumor involvement with infiltration of the gastroduodenal artery (Fig. 8.1.**26d**) are shown in Figure 8.1.**26e, f**. The use of a venous graft here is mandatory. Another option in resecting and reconstructing the hepatic artery by use of the splenic artery is illustrated by Figure 8.1.**26h**. Here, the splenic artery is anastomosed end-to-end with the transected proximal margin of the common hepatic artery. Then the gastroduodenal artery is anastomosed end-to-side with the splenic artery.

The various steps to be taken to manage involvement of the portal vein are presented in Figure 8.1.**27**. Figure 8.1.**27a–e** shows minor vascular involvement which can be repaired by means of local incision and simple end-to-end anastomosis or filling of the defect with a venous patch graft. More extensive invasion of the portal vein is managed by means of reconstruction with a venous graft using end-to-end anastomoses (Figure 8.1.**27f–h**). It is this kind of combined liver and vascular resection, and this kind of intrahepatic biliary drainage, that represent a step forward in surgical techniques for the management of primary cholangiocarcinoma of the porta hepatis.

Indeed, extensive liver resection, extensive vascular resection with the feasibility of vascular reconstruction even at the level of segmental bifurcations of both hepatic artery and portal vein, combined with the possibility of adequate drainage of the intrahepatic biliary tree, viz. segmental hepatic ducts, open new horizons and new perspectives for a number of patients who, until recently,

were considered not eligible for resectional surgery (Blumgart et al. 1984, Lai et al. 1987).

Selective hepatic artery arteriography 90 days after resection and reconstruction of the right hepatic artery in a patient who had left hemihepatectomy with resection and reconstruction of the contralateral vascular structures is shown in Figure 8.1.**28**. Late-phase portography shows a patent and well-functioning vascular prosthesis, interposed between the trunk of the portal vein and the transected proximal margin of the right portal vein in the same patient (Fig. 8.1.**29**).

A hepatobiliary iminodiacetic acid (HIDA) scan in another patient (Fig. 8.1.**30**) shows a well-functioning intrahepatic cholangiojejunostomy of the residual liver in a patient who underwent left trisegmentectomy. Reconstruction of the intrahepatic biliary tree was carried out with intrahepatic cholangiojejunostomies between the segmental hepatic ducts and a Roux-en-Y jejunal loop.

Figure 8.1.**31** shows a cholangiogram of a patient who underwent extensive liver resection and the same type of biliary reconstruction. The segmental hepatic ducts of segments VI and VII were used.

Figure 8.1.**32** shows resection and reconstruction of both the portal vein and the hepatic artery with venous grafts, in a patient with bilateral vascular and biliary involvement. Vascular resection was combined with liver resection.

Figure 8.1.**33** shows resection and reconstruction of both the portal vein and the hepatic artery in a patient with bilateral vascular involvement. This patient had vascular resection without liver resection. The appearance of the segmental hepatic ducts after transection of the main right and left hepatic ducts at the level of their segmental bifurcation can be seen.

Another kind of combined tumor and central liver resection is illustrated in Figure 8.1.**34**. This resection is carried out by a step-by-step isolation, ligation and transection of the segmental branches of the right and left portal vein and hepatic artery, all along the intrahepatic course of the left hepatic artery and portal vein to begin with, and then all along the course of the right portal vein and hepatic artery. In this way we resect segments IV, V and VIII. The basis of this technique lies in anatomical knowledge of the segmental distribution of the portal vein, hepatic artery and hepatic veins.

Results

From September 1983 to January 1988, 20 patients underwent liver resection with or without reconstruction of regional vascular strucures. Five patients died.

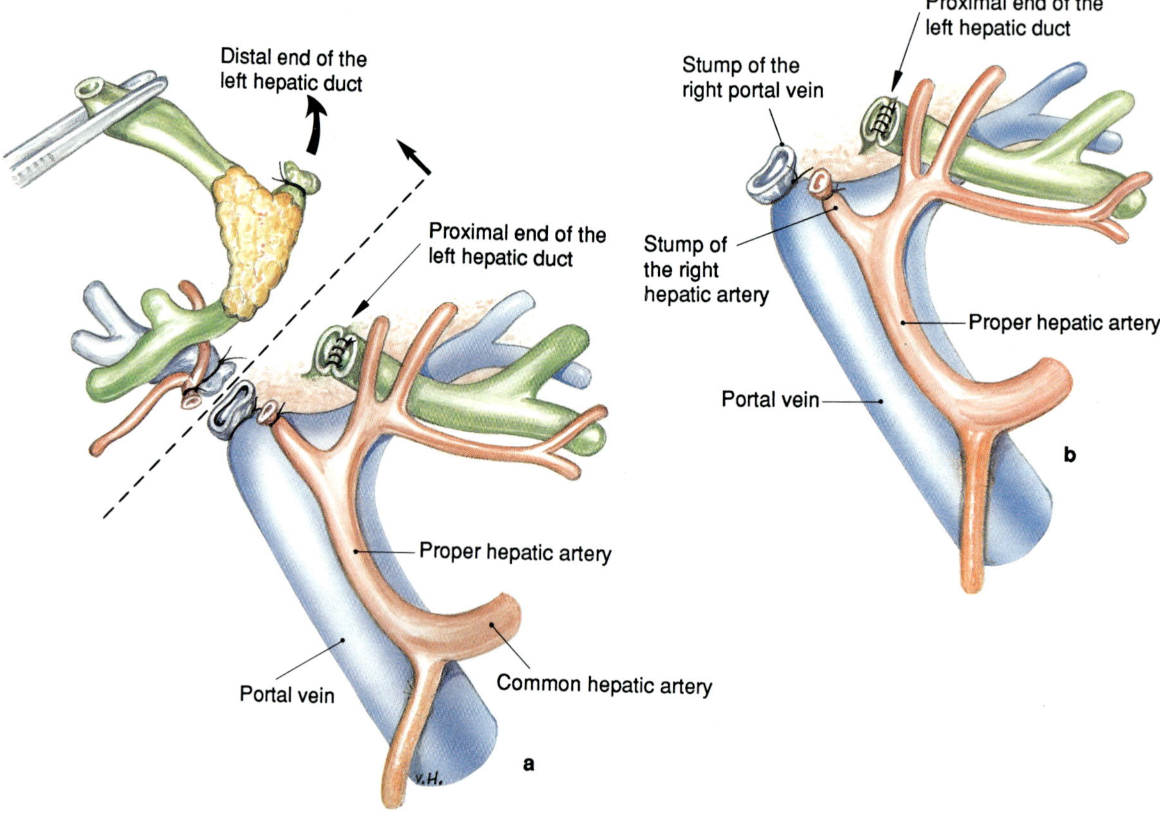

Fig. 8.1.**18a, b**

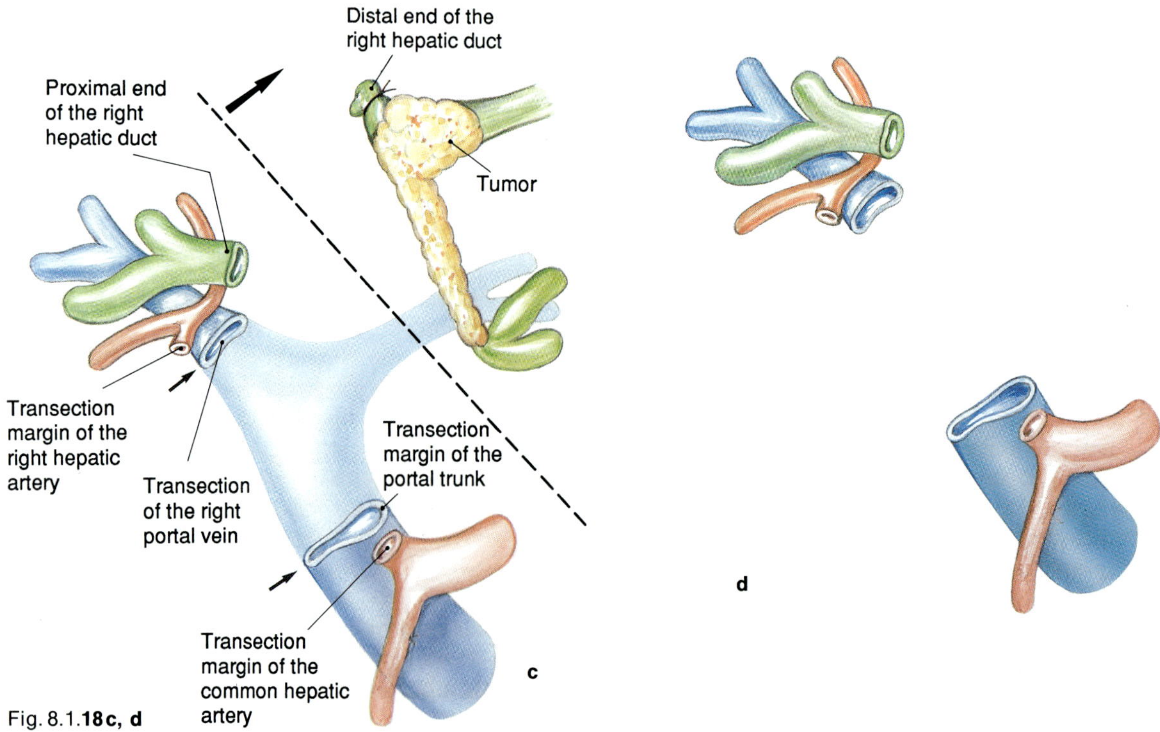

Fig. 8.1.**18c, d**

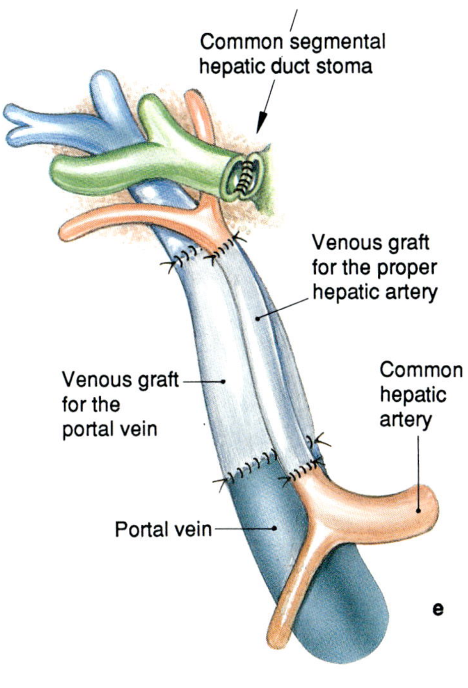

Fig. 8.1.**18e**

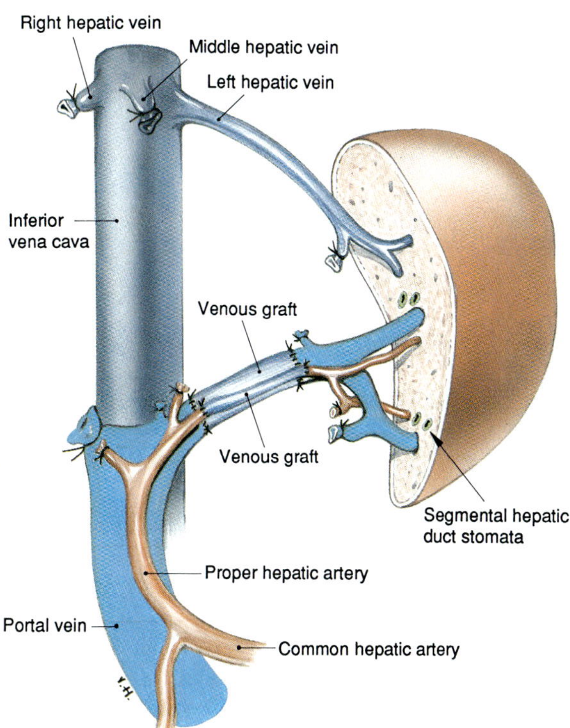

Fig. 8.1.**19 An extended right hemihepatectomy** combined with resection and reconstruction of the left hepatic artery and portal vein by means of venous grafts

The survival was satisfactory (Chapter 8.6). To appreciate these figures, it is necessary to realize that if these patients had been left untreated, their life expectancy would have been 4–5 months (Ottow et al. 1985). On the other hand, if these patients had not been treated in this way, tumor resection would have been abandoned according to the usual criteria for resectability (Alexander et al. 1984, Blumgart et al. 1984, Cameron et al. 1982, Evander et al. 1980, Iwasaki et al. 1986, Lai et al. 1987, Launois et al. 1979, Malt et al. 1980, Ottow et al. 1985, Tompkins et al. 1981, Terblanche et al. 1972, Wiechel 1982). In our opinion, the combination of tumor and liver resection with regional vascular resection, is an alternative for a number of patients with primary cholangiocarcinoma of the confluence of the common hepatic duct. This view is supported by recent publications (Lygidakis 1988, Mizumoto et al. 1986, Sakaguchi and Nakamura 1986).

Although the mortality is still high, we are convinced that with a precise selection of the patients and a better understanding of the various pathophysiological aspects of cholestasis, our results can be further improved. This will open some possibilities of cure for a number of patients who until recently were considered not to be eligible for resectional surgery and who were therefore condemned to a limited life-span and to a form of palliative management associated with a poor qual-

Fig. 8.1.**18a, b Extension of the tumor to the right of the liver without vascular involvement.** Dissection all along the intrahepatic course of the left hepatic duct. Note the subsequent transection lines for the duct and the lines for the transection of the right hepatic artery and the right branch of the portal vein which follow before right hemihepatectomy in this case

c, d Extension of the tumor towards the left part of the liver and involvement of vessels. Dissection of the right hepatic duct up to the level of its segmental bifurcation. Transection lines are indicated in black. In this case, extensive left hemihepatectomy combined with resection and reconstruction of the right branch of the portal vein and right hepatic artery is indicated

e Vascular reconstruction is carried out by means of two end-to-end anastomes with interposed venous grafts for both the portal vein and the hepatic artery

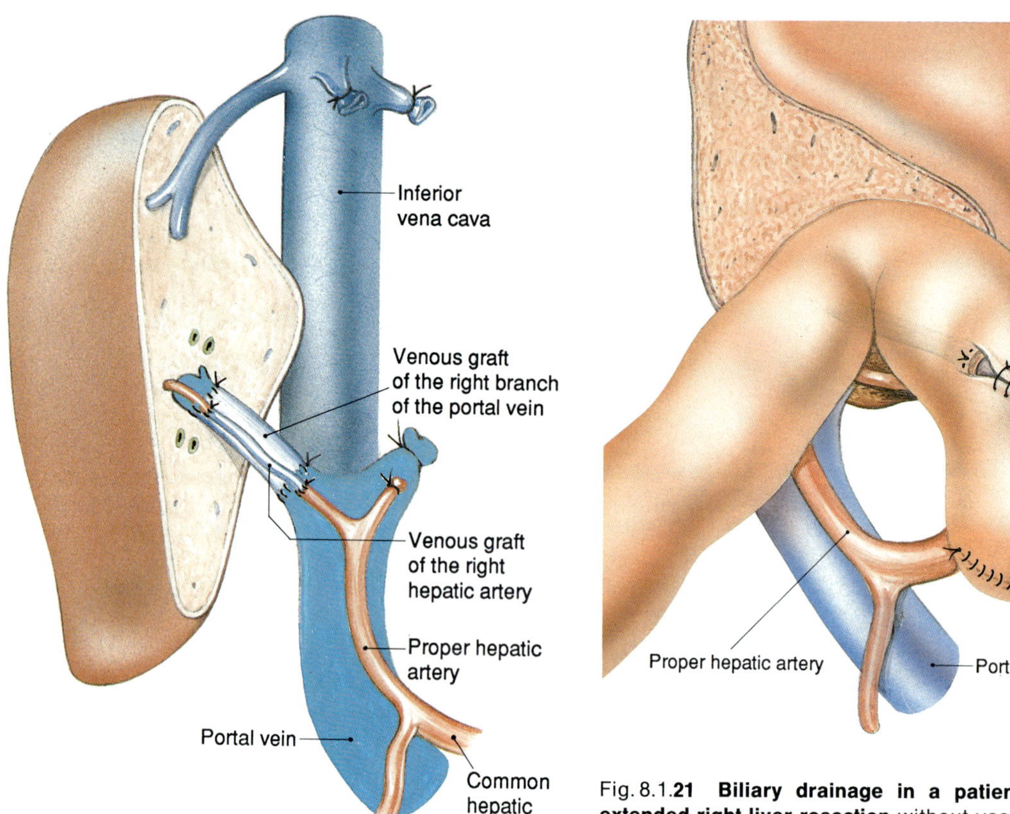

Fig. 8.1.**20**   **An extended left hemihepatectomy** combined with resection and reconstruction of the right portal vein and hepatic artery

Fig. 8.1.**21**   **Biliary drainage in a patient who had an extended right liver resection** without vascular resection. Intrahepatic cholangiojejunostomies between the segmental hepatic ducts of the residual liver and a Roux-en-Y jejunal loop

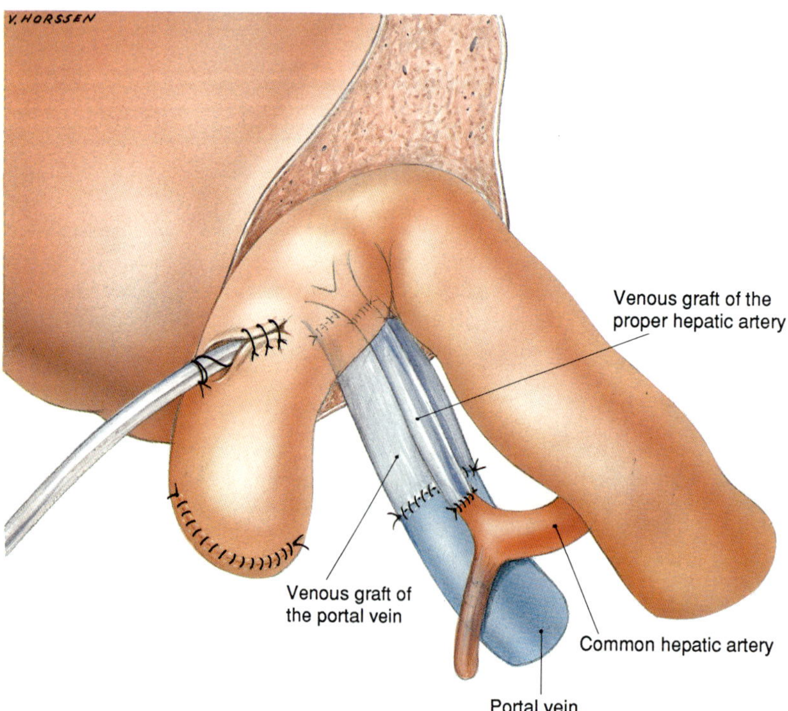

Fig. 8.1.**22**   **Biliary drainage of the residual liver via intrahepatic cholangiojejunostomies** between the segmental hepatic ducts and a Roux-en-Y jejunal loop, in a patient who had a combined extended left liver and vascular resection

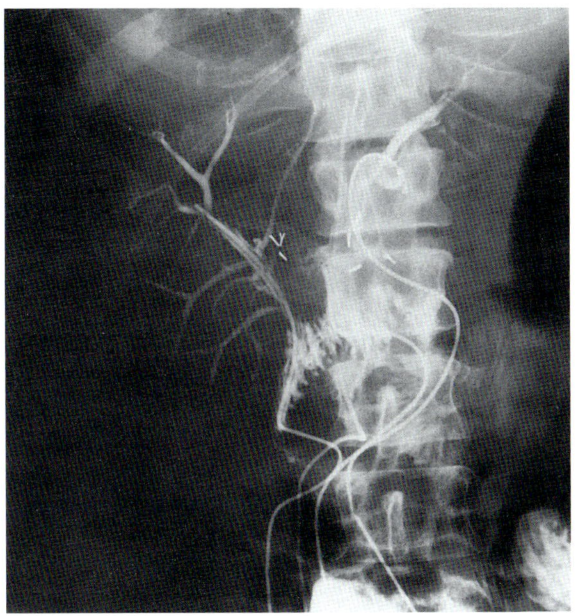

Fig. 8.1.**23 Cholangiography after extended left hemihepatectomy.** Intrahepatic cholangiojejunostomies with segmental hepatic ducts and a Roux-en-Y jejunal loop

ity of life (Alexander et al. 1984, Blumgart et al. 1984, Evander et al. 1980, Lai et al. 1987, Malt et al. 1980, Ottow et al. 1985, Tompkins et al. 1981, Terblanche et al. 1972, Wiechel 1982).

Conclusions

In our opinion, attempted radical surgery has to be regarded as the first choice whenever it is feasible. Despite the increased mortality, it increases the number of patients amenable to resection, and although it fails to increase the rate of radical resection significantly, it achieves better biliary drainage. This is achieved by eliminating biliary stasis by resection of the part of the liver that is more difficult to drain and by optimal biliary drainage of the residual liver through the segmental hepatic ducts. This is considered essential for the management of a disease which does not metastasize frequently, but has a tendency toward early infiltrative growth and is therefore rarely eradicated, even after more extensive resection.

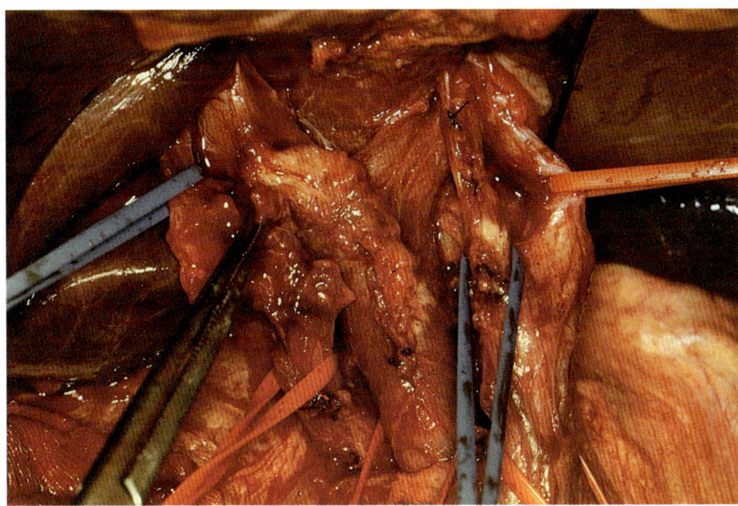

Fig. 8.1.**24 Bilateral involvement** of both the portal vein and the hepatic artery

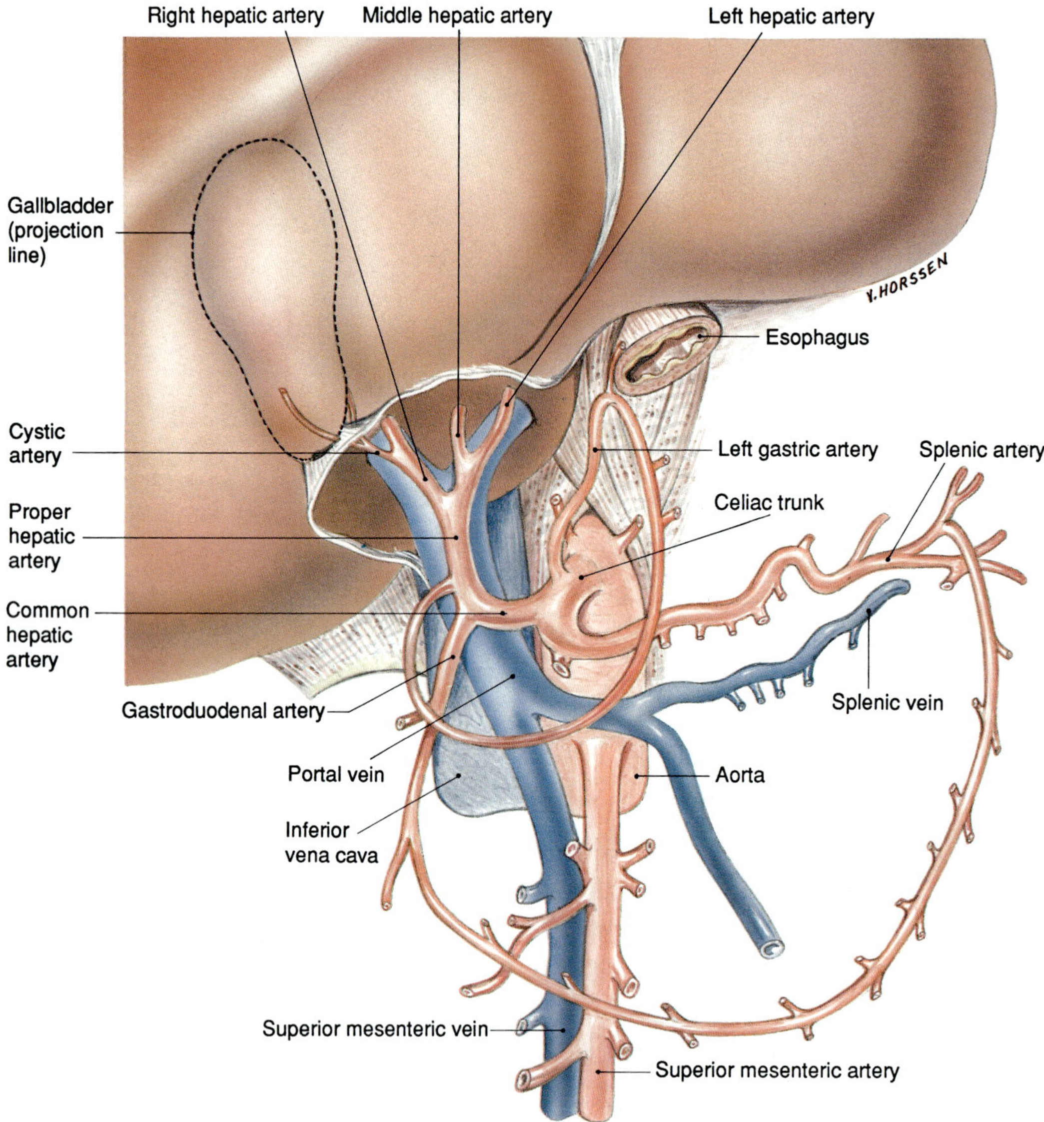

Fig. 8.1.**25** **Vascular supply of the liver** with normal anatomical distribution

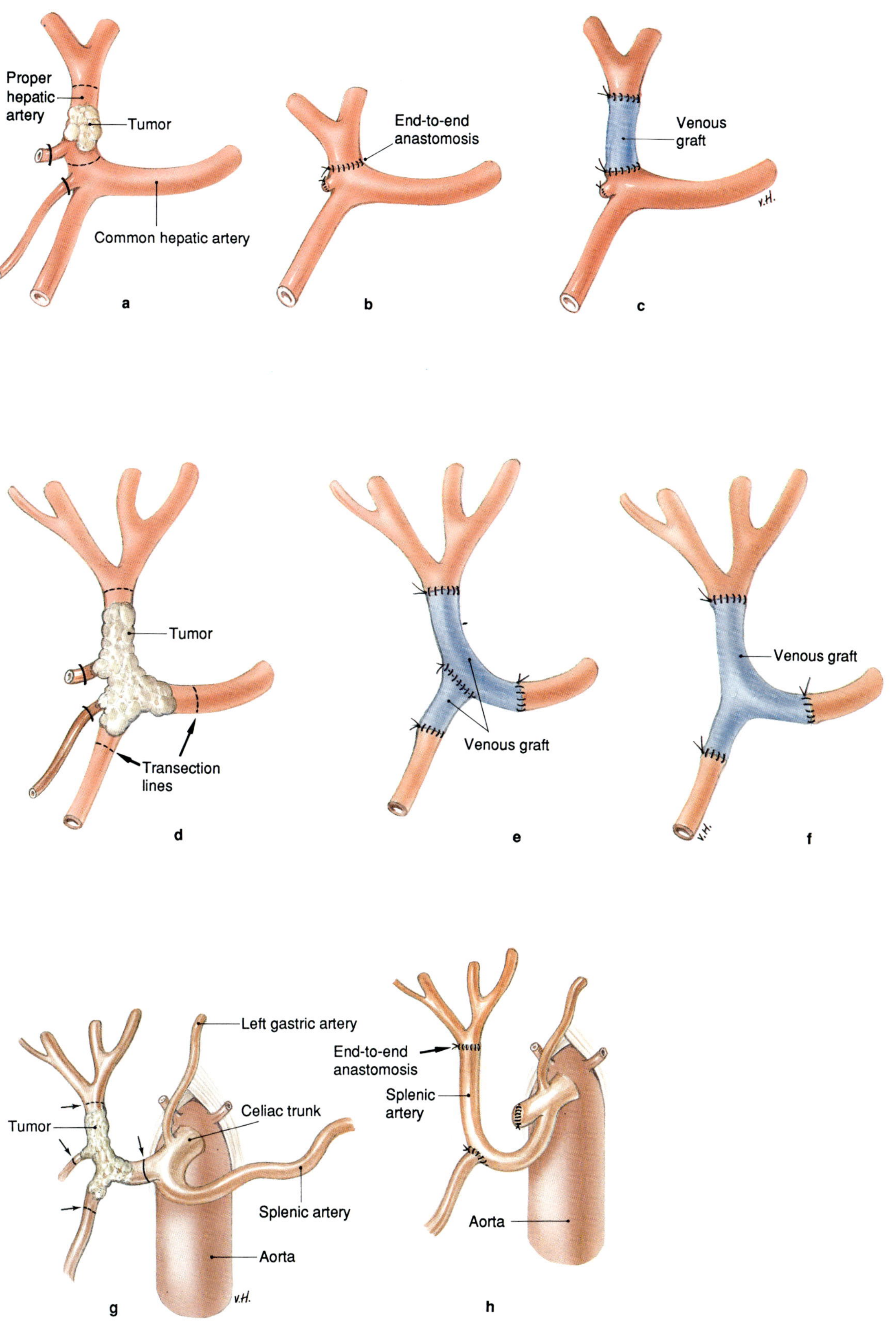

Fig. 8.1.26 a–h   Various steps in the resection and reconstruction of the hepatic artery in cases of tumor spread

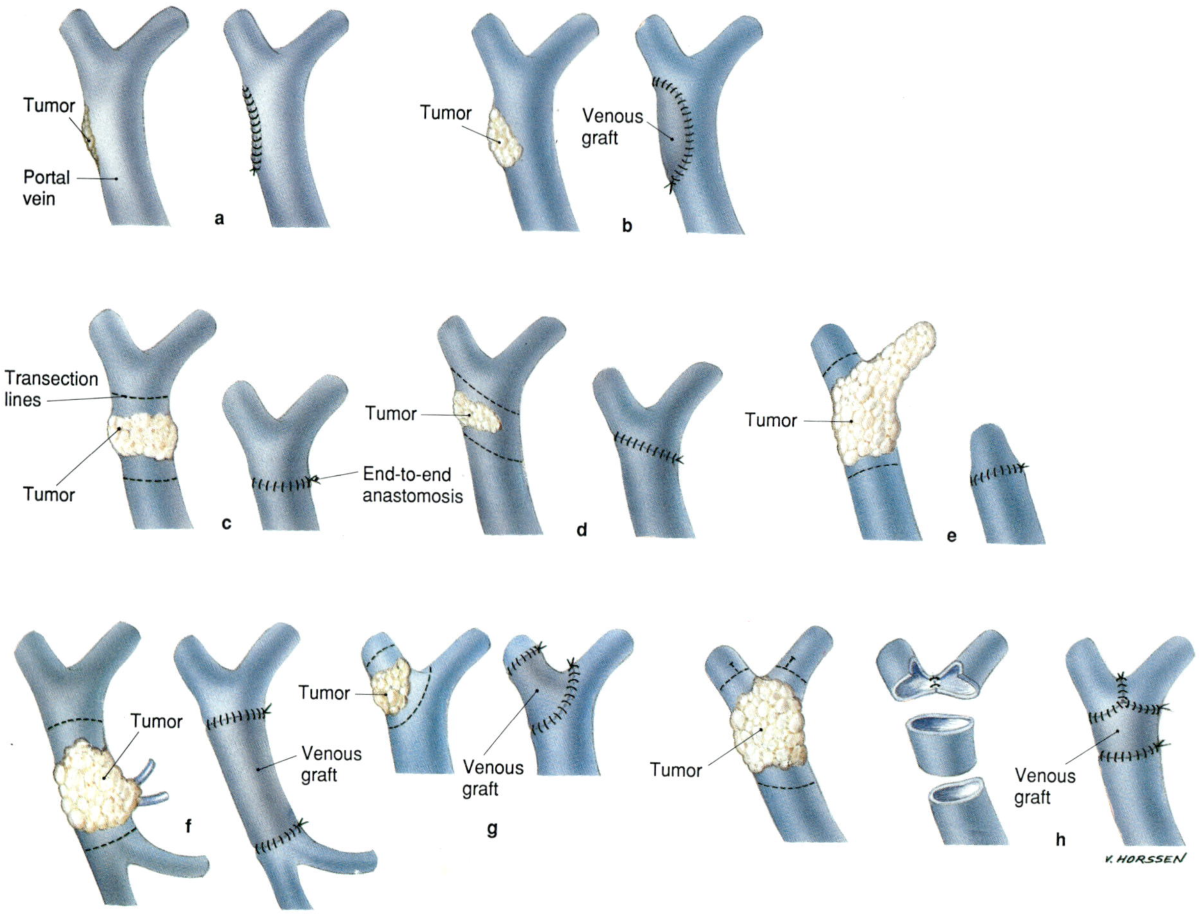

Fig. 8.1.**27 a–h**   **Various steps in the resection and reconstruction of the portal vein**

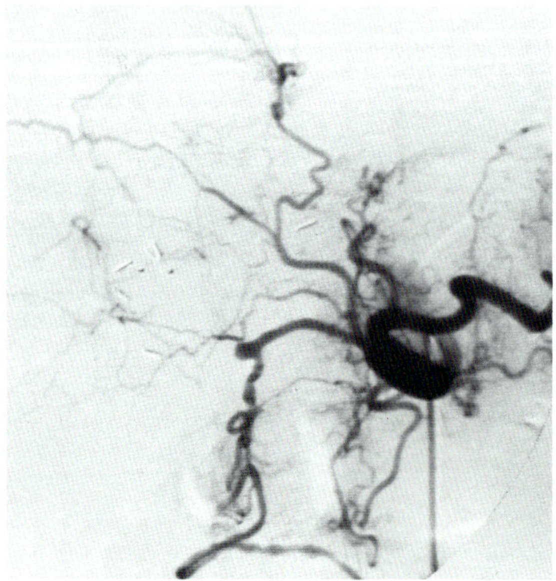

Fig. 8.1.**28 Selective hepatic artery angiography** after resection and reconstruction of the common hepatic artery using a venous graft. Patent and well-functioning vascular prosthesis

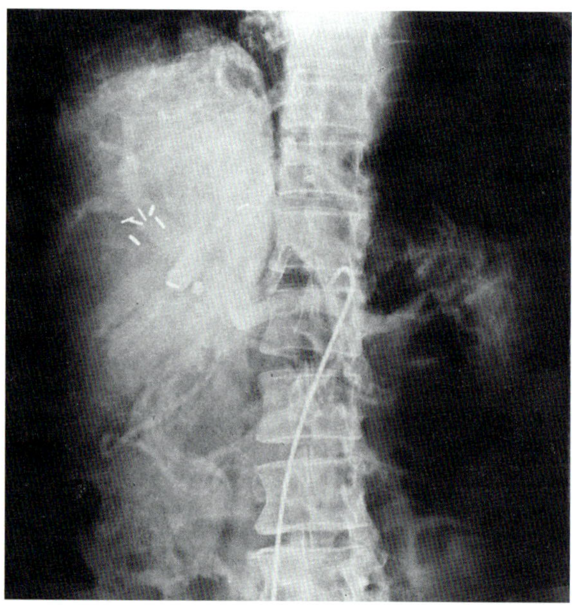

Fig. 8.1.**29 Late-phase portogram** after resection and reconstruction using a venous graft of the portal vein

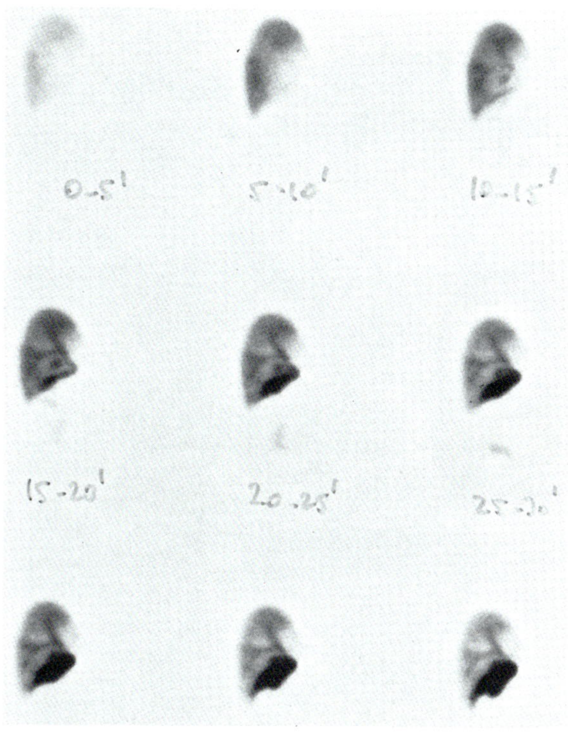

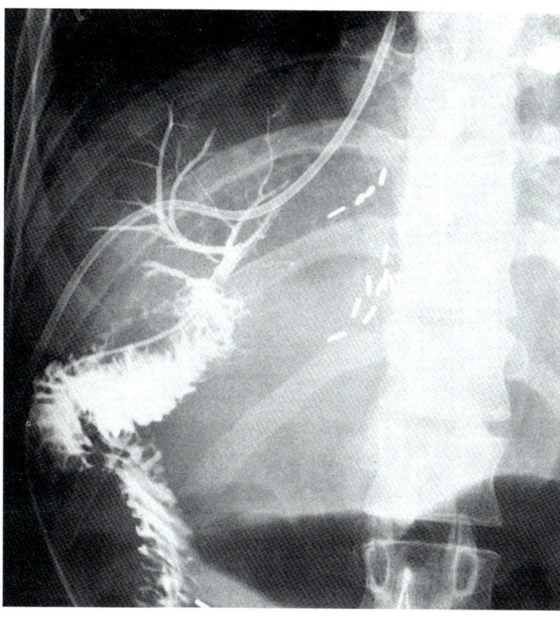

Fig. 8.1.**31** **Cholangiography after extended left hepatectomy**. Cholangiojejunostomies with the segmental hepatic ducts of the residual liver

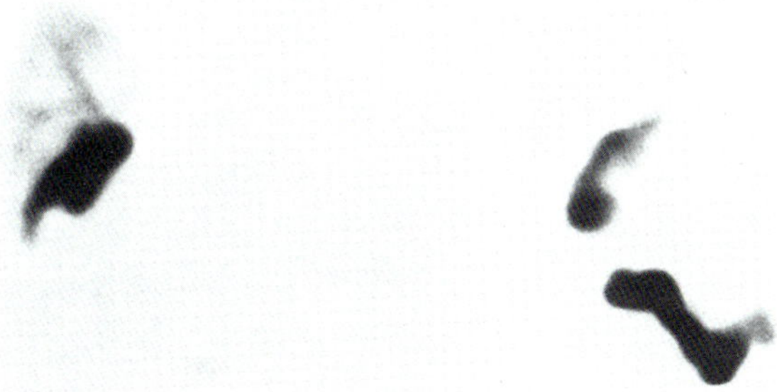

Fig. 8.1.**30a, b** **Hepatobiliary iminodiacetic acid (HIDA) scan** after extended left hemihepatectomy. Well-functioning cholangiojejunostomies of the residual liver

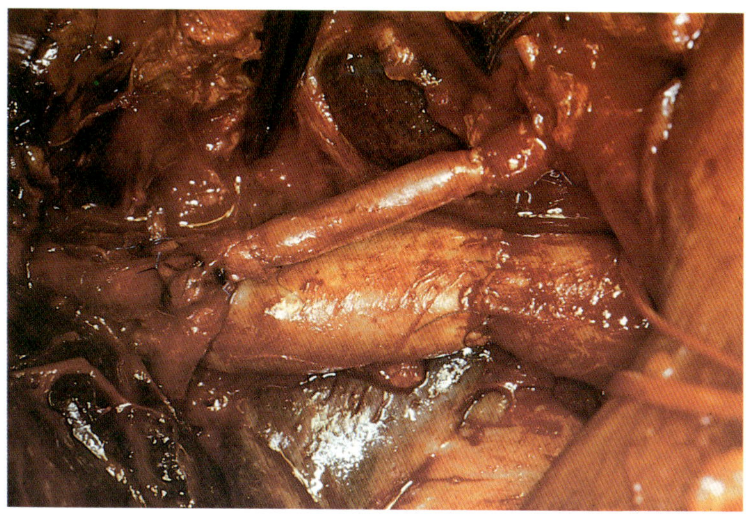

Fig. 8.1.**32** After an extended right hemihepatectomy, this patient underwent resection and reconstruction of the portal vein and hepatic artery using venous grafts

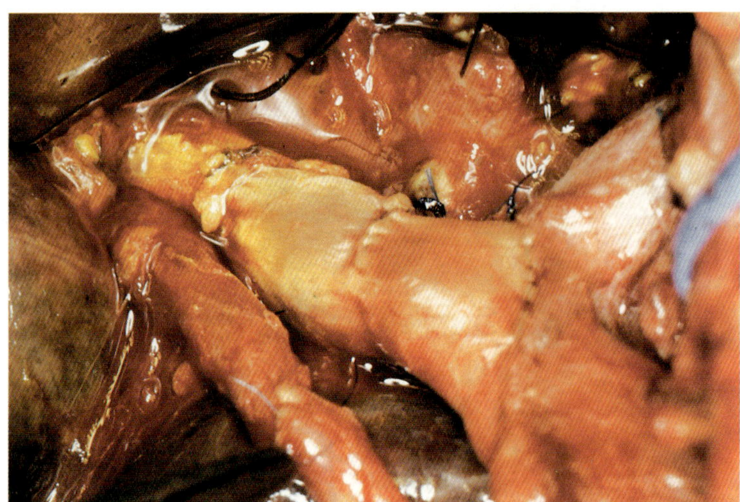

Fig. 8.1.**33** **Resection and reconstruction of the portal vein and hepatic artery** using venous grafts without liver resection

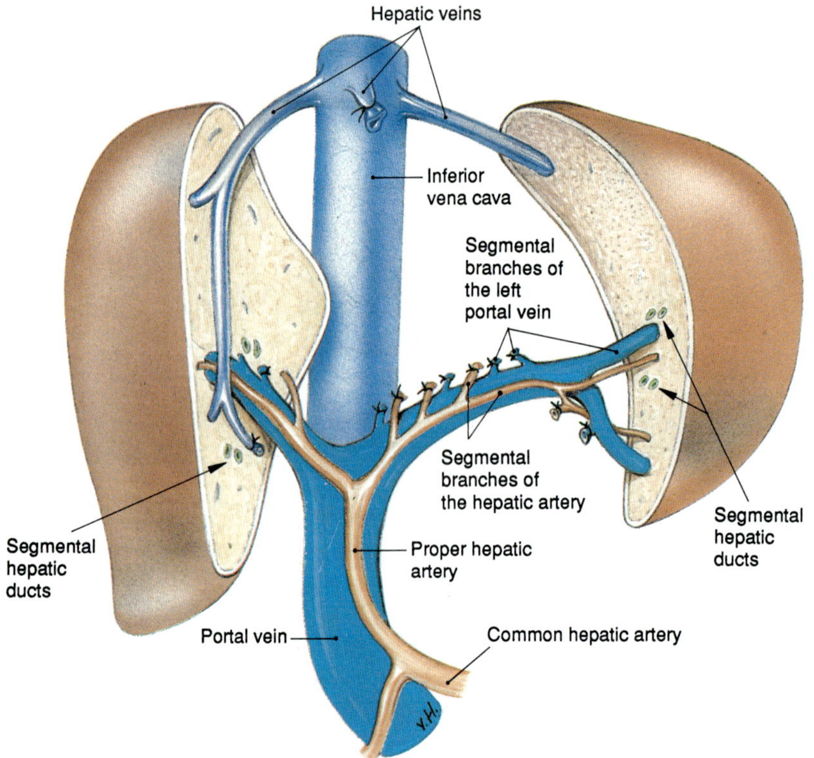

Fig. 8.1.**34** **Central liver resection of segments I, IV, V and VIII,** showing the residual liver from segments II, III, VI and VII, with their afferent and efferent vessels and segmental hepatic ducts

References

Alexander F, Rossi RL, O'Bryan M, Khettry U, Braasch J, Watkins E. Biliary carcinoma: a review of 109 cases. Am J Surg 1984; 147: 503.

Blumgart LH, Benjamin R, Hadjis NJ, Beazley R. Surgical approaches to cholangiocarcinoma at confluence of the hepatic ducts. Lancet 1984; i: 66.

Cameron JL, Broe P, Zuidema PGD. Proximal bile duct tumors: surgical management with silastic transhepatic biliary stents. Ann Surg 1982; 196: 412.

Cotton PB. Duodenoscopic placement of biliary prosthesis to relieve malignant obstructive jaundice. Br J Surg 1982; 69: 501.

Dudley SE, Ely J, Adson MA. Biliary decompression in hilar obstruction. Arch Surg 1979; 144: 519.

Evander A, Fredlund P, Hoevels J, Ihse J, Bengmark S. Evaluation of aggressive surgery for carcinoma of the extrahepatic bile ducts. Ann Surg 1980; 191: 23.

Huibregtse K, Tytgat GNJ. Endoscopic placement of biliary prostheses. In: Salmon P, ed. Advances in gastrointestinal endoscopy; vol 1. London: Chapman and Hall, 1984: 219–231.

Iwasaki Y, Okamura T, Okazi A, Todorote T, Takase Y. Surgical treatment of carcinoma of the confluence of the major hepatic ducts. Surg Gynecol Obstet. 1986; 162: 457.

Lai ECS, Tompkins RK, Roslyn JJ, Mann LL. Proximal bile duct cancer: quality of survival. Ann Surg 1987; 205: 111.

Launois G, Campion JP, Brisset P, Gosselin P. Carcinoma of the hepatic hilus: surgical treatment and the case of resection. Ann Surg 1979; 190: 151.

Lygidakis NJ. Kombinierte Rekonstruktion der Gallengänge und der Lebergefäße bei Carcinomen der Hapaticusgabel. Chirurg 1987; 58: 282.

Lygidakis NJ, Brummelkamp WH, Lubbers MJ, Huibregtse K, Tytgat GNJ, Schenk KE, van Gulik TM. A new surgical approach for the management of carcinoma of the junction of the main hepatic ducts. Surg Annu 1986; 18: 297.

Lygidakis NJ, van der Heyde MN, Van Dongen RJAM, Kromhout JG, Tytgat GNJ, Huibregtse K. Surgical approaches for unresectable primary carcinoma of the hepatic hilus. Surg Gynecol Obstet 1988; 166: 107–114.

Malt RA, Warshaw AL, Jamieson CG, Hawk JC III. Left intrahepatic cholangiojejunostomy for proximal obstruction of the biliary tract. Surg Gynecol Obstet 1980; 150: 193.

Mizumoto R, Kawarada Y, Suzuki H. Surgical treatment of hilar carcinoma of the bile duct. Surg Gynecol Obstet 1986; 162: 153.

Ottow RT, August DA, Sugarbaker PH. Treatment of proximal biliary tract carcinoma: an overview of techniques and results. Surgery 1985; 97: 251.

Sakaguchi S, Nakamura S. Surgery of the portal vein in the resection of cancer of the hepatic hilus. Surgery 1986; 99: 344.

Tompkins RK, Thomas D, While A, Longmire W Jr. Prognostic features in bile duct carcinoma. Arch Surg 1981; 194: 447.

Terblanche J, Saunders SJ, Louw SJ. Prolonged palliation in carcinoma of the main hepatic duct junction. Surgery 1972; 71: 720.

Wiechel KL. Diagnosis and treatment of primary extrahepatic bile duct tumors. Am J Surg 1982; 193: 99.

8.2   Palliative Surgical Drainage for Primary Cholangiocarcinoma of the Porta Hepatis

E. Moreno González, R. Gómez Sanz, I. Garcia Garcia, A. Calle Santiuste and J. Arias Diaz

Introduction

A large proportion of patients with primary malignant biliary tumors are not eligible for resection at the time of admission. For these patients, biliary decompression (medical or surgical), either in the form of bilioenteric anastomosis or in the form of transtumoral drainage, is the only remaining possibility. Thus, biliary drainage is the goal for patients who have unresectable tumors and cannot be treated by partial resection of the bifurcation and carrying out intrahepatic cholangiojejunostomies with the segmental hepatic ducts (Chapter 8.1). However, drainage procedures are associated with a high incidence of cholangitis. The relief of jaundice is transient and not universal, the overall survival is limited, and the quality of life is poor.

The various anastomotic techniques used for biliary drainage relate to the anatomical features of the intrahepatic biliary tree, which make a number of biliary diversion procedures feasible (Bismuth et al. 1978, Blumgart and Kelly 1984, Longmire and Sandford 1949, Rossi et al. 1973). Apart from surgical drainage, alternative endoscopic and percutaneous transhepatic drainage procedures are available (Chapters 10.4, 10.5) (Dooley et al. 1979, Ferrucci et al. 1981, Mark et al. 1985, Mueller et al. 1987). These procedures are also indicated for a proportion of patients considered not eligible for resection.

Technique

The main surgical biliary drainage procedures are outlined here.

Drainage with the Left Hepatic Duct

This procedure is indicated mainly when the right and left hepatic ducts communicate in the case of lesions restricted to the area below the hepatic duct confluence. In the case of lesions restricted to the area at or above the confluence, only the left liver is able to drain, and this is associated with an increased incidence of septic complications connected with the undrained, cholestatic right liver.

We start by dividing the round ligament. A clamp or suture is placed on the divided lower segment of the ligament so that it can be used as a retractor to elevate the undersurface of the liver and thus gain access to the hilar plate (Fig. 8.2.**1a**).

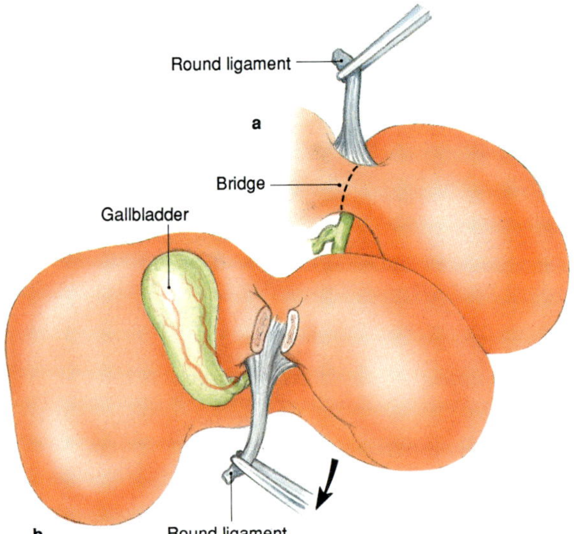

Fig. 8.2.**1a**   **The round ligament is transected** and then lifted up and used as retractor. Transection line: ----
b   After the bridge has been transected, the round ligament may be used to pull the liver downwards

The bridge of liver tissue connecting the left lobe of the liver to segment IV is divided using a thermic knife (Fig. 8.2.**1b**). We continue with a step-by-step dissection of the hilar plate, which is the space between the capsule of Glisson and the peritoneal reflection embracing the left portal triad (Fig. 8.2.**2a**). By means of this dissection, we identify the left portal vein and the left hepatic duct near it (Fig. 8.2.**2**). The duct is dissected, isolated and incised along its entire course (Fig. 8.2.**2b**). A row of 4-0 Vicryl sutures is inserted on the upper aspect of the left hepatic duct (Fig. 8.2.**2c**), a Roux-en-Y jejunal loop is transferred into the upper abdomen, and it is opened and sutured, using interrupted 4-0 Vicryl sutures, to the lower aspect of the left hepatic duct in a side-to-side fashion (Fig. 8.2.**2c**). The sutures already inserted on the upper aspect are now used as full-thickness sutures on the upper surface of the jejunal opening, completing the anastomosis (Fig. 8.2.**2c**).

Drainage with Segment III Hepatic Duct

In patients with advanced malignant tumors, the left hepatic duct may well be involved, thus being unsuitable for use in creating a bilioenteric anas-

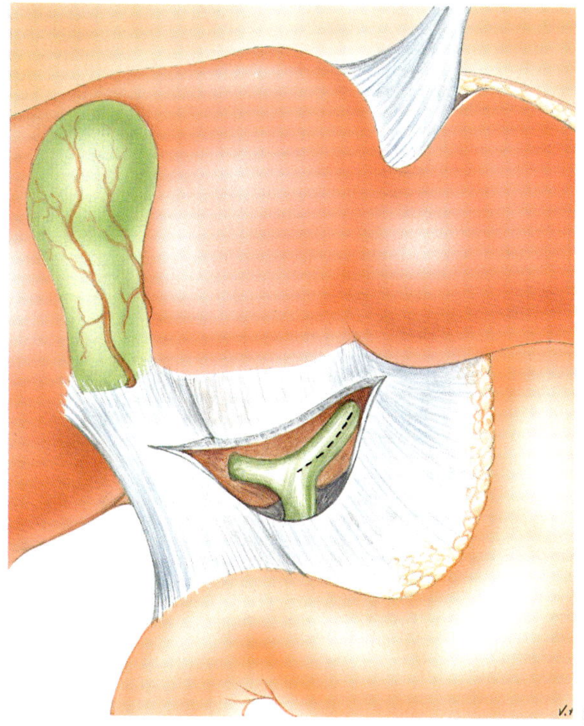

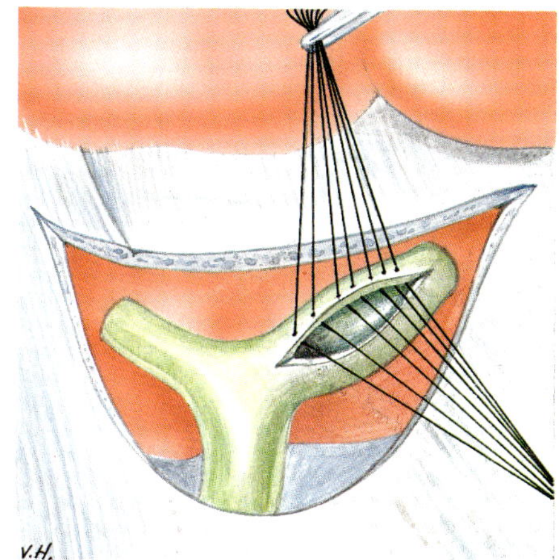

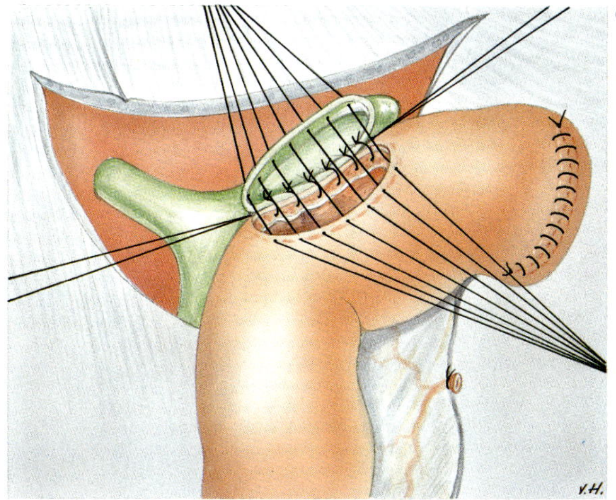

Fig. 8.2.**2a** **After dissection of the hilar plate**, the left hepatic duct can be seen

b **The left hepatic duct is opened all along its course.** Several sutures are inserted on its upper aspect

c **Creation of a side-to-side hepaticojejunostomy** between a Roux-en-Y jejunal loop and the left hepatic duct

tomosis. In such cases, the hepatic duct to segment III may be used (Fig. 8.2.**3**). We start in the same way as for left hepatic duct anastomosis, by transecting the round ligament. The liver is then pulled upwards, while the transected round ligament is pulled downwards. Dissection now has to take place on the left upper surface of the liver, at the base of the round ligament.

First we encounter the branch of the portal vein to segment IV and immediately after that, we gain access to the hepatic duct of segment III, which lies above and behind the portal vein. The portal branch to segment IV is carefully dissected, and its side branches are identified, isolated, ligated and transected. This provides access to the segment III hepatic duct and space to fashion the side-to-side anastomosis between the Roux-en-Y jejunal loop and the segment III hepatic duct, following the same principles as described for left hepatic duct anastomosis.

Longmire Procedure

Longmire and Sandford (1949) described a surgical technique for using the segment II hepatic duct in

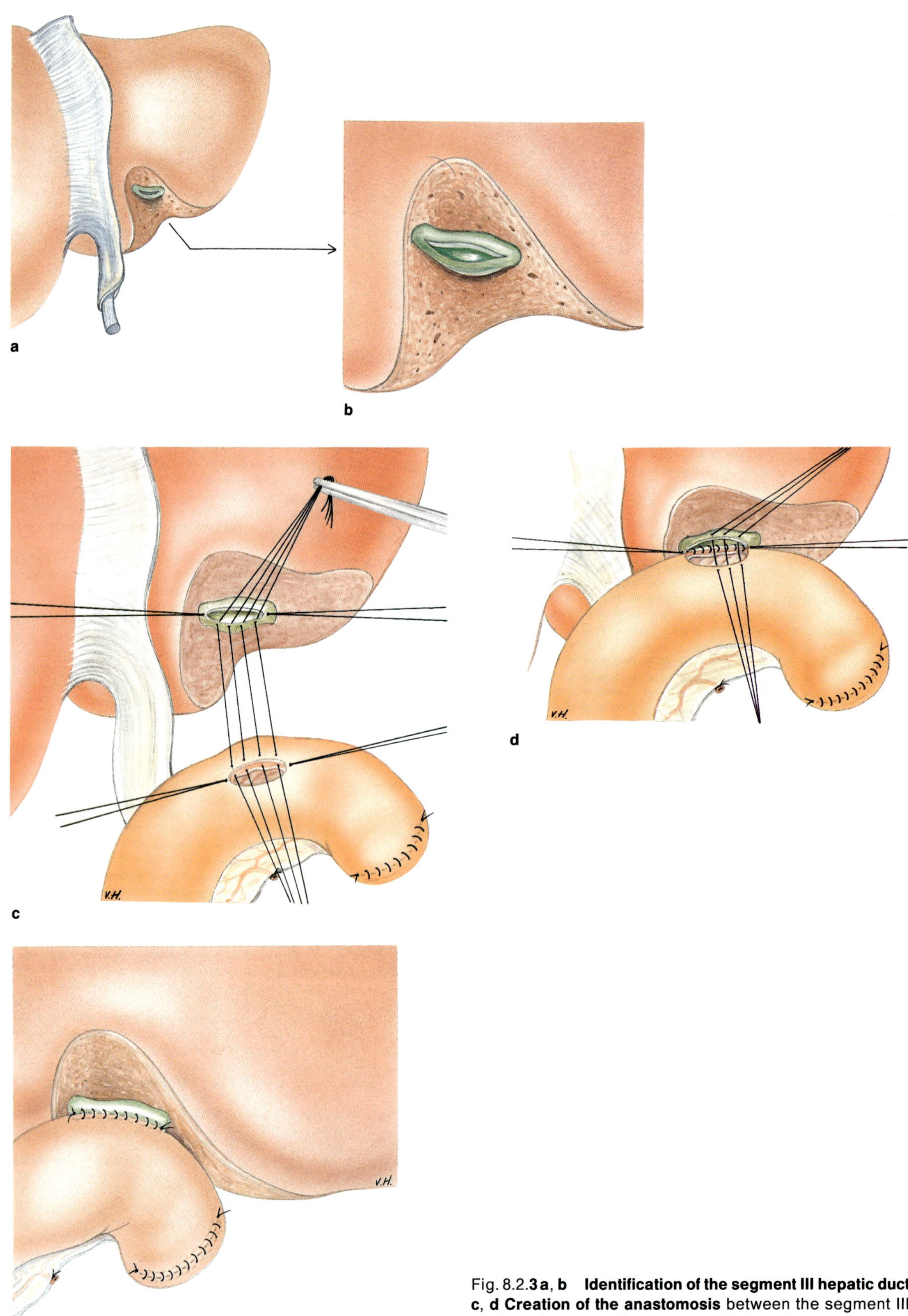

Fig. 8.2.**3 a, b   Identification of the segment III hepatic duct**
c, d Creation of the anastomosis between the segment III
    hepatic duct and a Roux-en-Y jejunal loop
e   The hepaticojejunostomy is completed

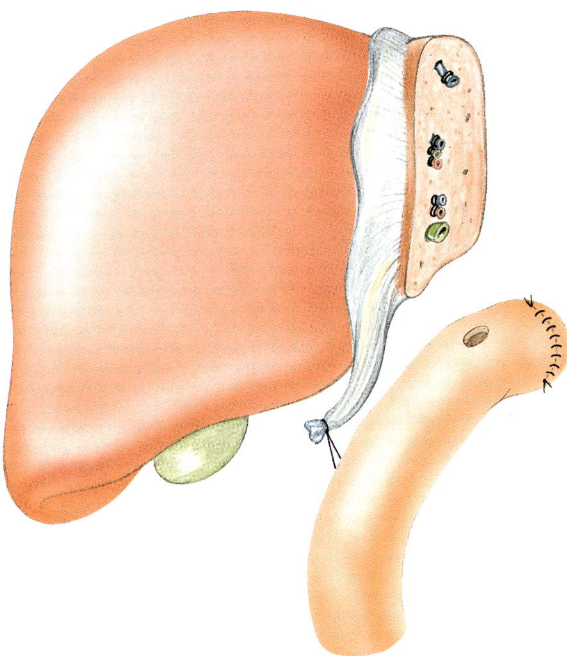

Fig. 8.2.**4**   **Longmire's approach**

cases with advanced obstruction of the bifurcation. This approach is reserved as a last resort when all the other surgical drainage approaches described are considered unfeasible (Fig. 8.2.**4**).

The Longmire procedure entails removal of part of the left lobe of the liver so as to get access to the dilated intrahepatic duct of segment II. The lateral segment of the left lobe is mobilized, a clamp is placed, and a wedge resection of the liver is carried out. By gradually releasing the pressure on the clamp, we identify and ligate the various vessels. A Roux-en-Y jejunal loop is prepared and sutured after being opened to the Glisson capsule. Single mattress sutures are used, inserted as full-thickness sutures through the jejunal wall and rough surface of the transected liver towards the Glisson capsule.

Right-Sided Hepaticojejunostomies

Occasionally, the right hepatic duct system can be reached by following a dissection of the hilar plate on the right side. This approach offers access to the right hepatic duct, similar to the technique described above for the left hepatic duct. The seg-

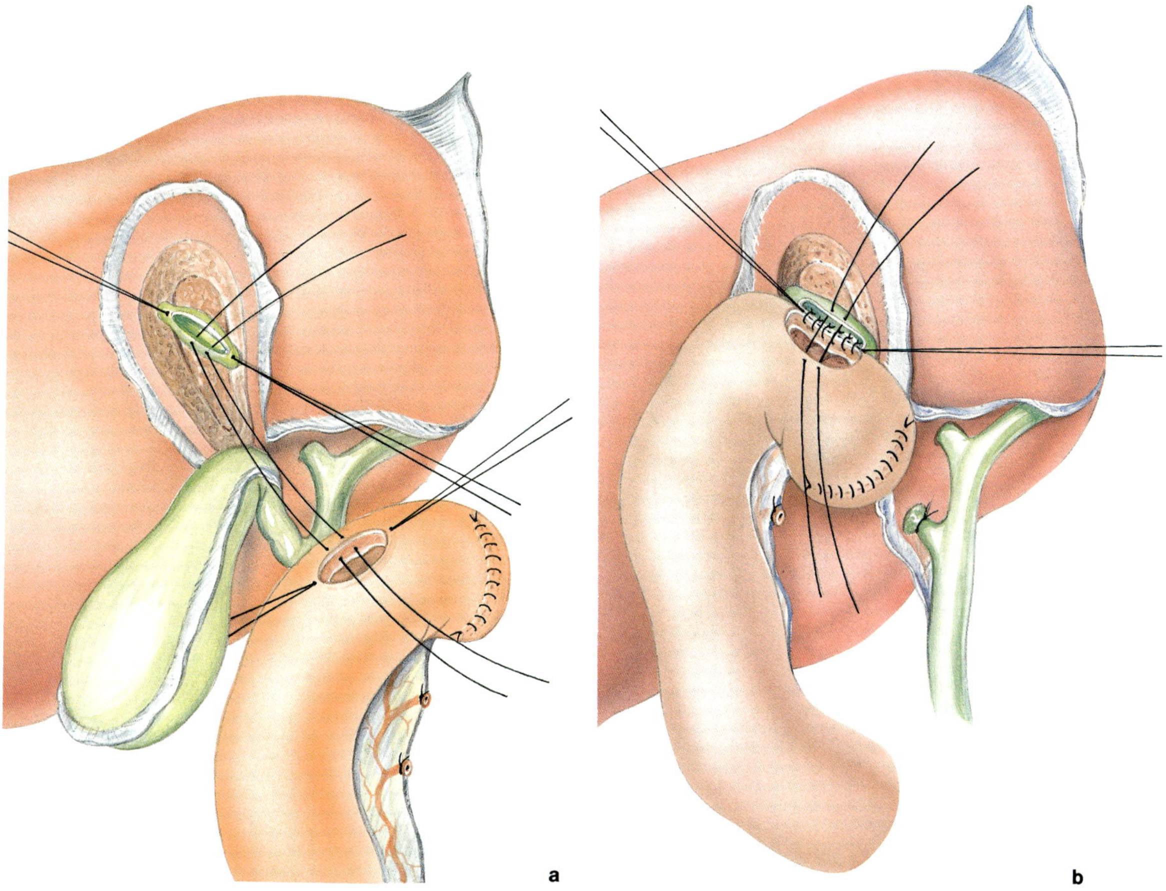

Fig. 8.2.**5a**, **b**   **Technique for use of right hepatic duct to segment V** via the gallbladder fossa

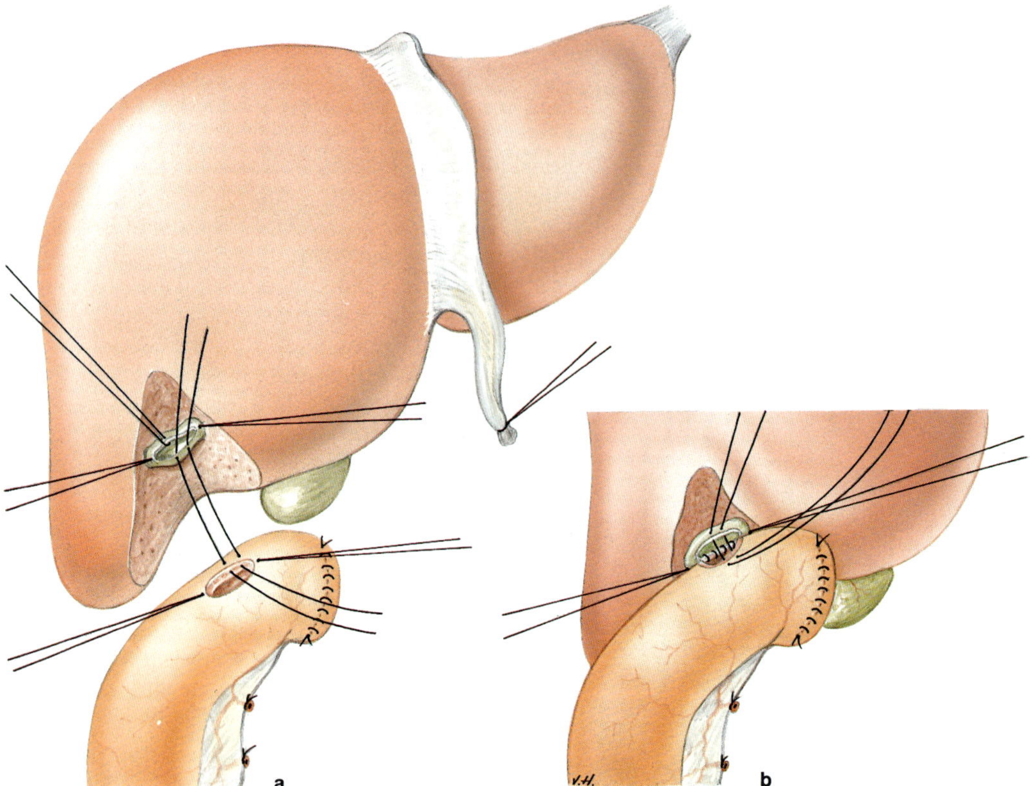

Fig. 8.2.**6a, b   Operative steps to create the hepaticojejunostomy** with the hepatic duct to segment VI

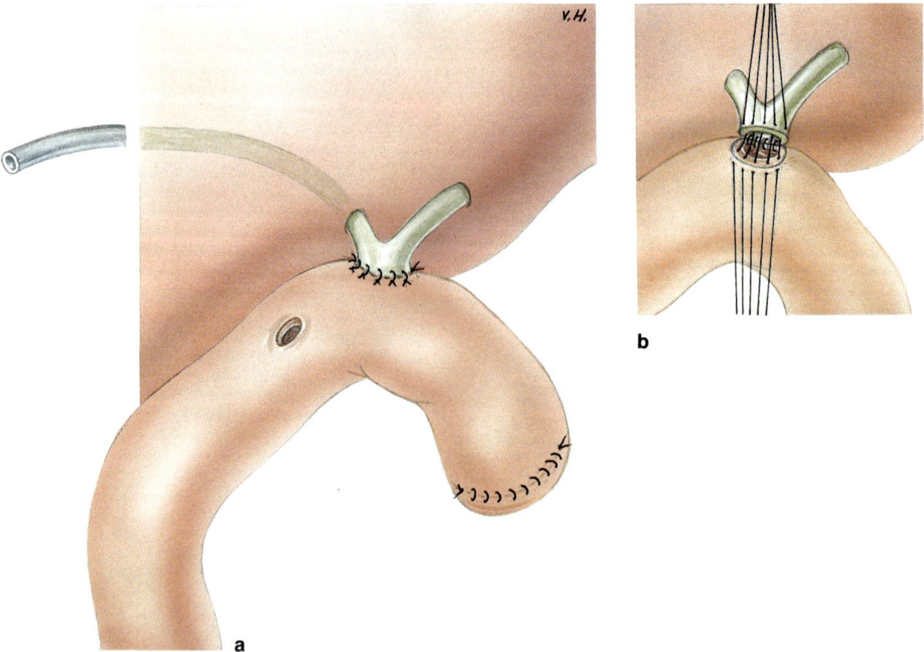

Fig. 8.2.**7a, b   Creating the hepaticojejunostomy.** Both hepatic ducts can be stented for transtumoral drainage

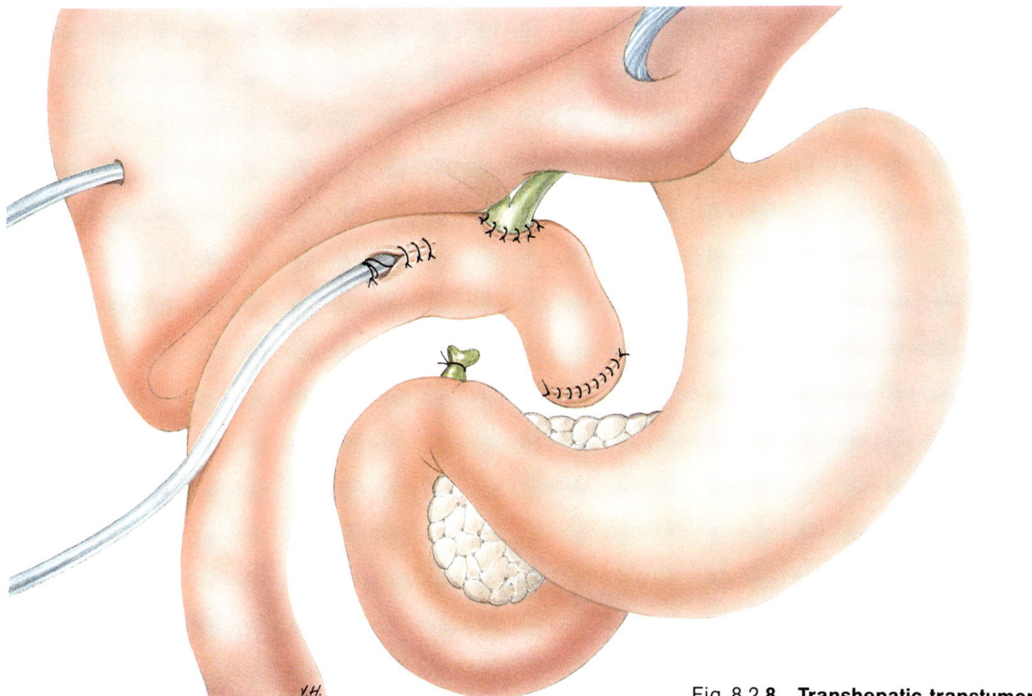

Fig. 8.2.**8**   **Transhepatic transtumoral drainage**

ment V hepatic duct can also be used and is approached after cholecystectomy by making an incision in the gallbladder fossa (Fig. 8.2.**5a, b**).

Alternatively, the segment IV duct can be used, following the techniques illustrated in Figure 8.2.**6a, b**).

Operative Intubational Techniques in Malignant Biliary Obstruction

Goetz and Praderi used transhepatic stents for biliary reconstruction. Today, stents are employed in dealing with advanced malignant process confined to, or located above, the bifurcation when we are unable to resect the tumor or the bifurcation of the common hepatic duct.

We start with dissection of the hepatoduodenal ligament, followed by identification and transection of the common bile duct. The distal end of the common bile duct is closed and its proximal end is reflected cephalad (Chapter 8.1). By further proximal dissection, we reach the bifurcation of the common hepatic duct and the underlying bifurcation of the portal vein. At this stage, we use Baker dilators in an attempt to overcome the obstruction caused by the tumor. We do this for both the right and the left hepatic ducts (Fig. 8.2.**7a, b**). The Baker dilators are gently pushed through the tumor and the liver parenchyma to the anterior surface of the liver. One or two tubes (for one or both hepatic ducts) are now attached to the tip of the dilator with double ligatures. By retracting the dilator, one end

of the tubes is pulled back through the liver, stenting the tumor. The hepaticojejunostomy is carried out between the transected proximal margin of the common hepatic duct and the jejunal loop. Both ends of the tube are subsequently brought out of the abdominal cavity using two separate wounds, and they are sutured to the abdominal wall (Fig. 8.2.**8**). The end of the tube stenting the anastomosis is brought out via the jejunal loop, forming a Witzel jejunostomy. This is referred to as a U-tube.

Comments

Transtumoral drainage gives palliation, but is also associated with increased mortality, morbidity and limited survival (Mark et al. 1985). It is not always easy to place a U-tube, and a false passage can be created during the attempt to dilate the tumor. However, there is no question that transtumoral transhepatic drainage has a place in the surgical management of proximal malignant biliary tumors.

References

Bismuth H, Franco D, Corlette M, Hepp J. Long-term results of hepaticojejunostomy Roux-en-Y. Surg Gynecol Obstet 1978; 146: 161–167.

Blumgart LH, Kelly CJ. Hepaticojejunostomy in benign and malignant high bile duct strictures: approaches to the left hepatic ducts. Br J Surg 1984; 71: 257–261.

Dooley JS, et al. Nonsurgical treatment of biliary obstruction. Lancet 1979; ii: 1040–1044.

Ferrucci JT, Mueller PR, Harbin WP. Percutaneous transhepatic biliary drainage: techniques, results and applications. Radiology 1981; 135: 1–3.

Longmire WP, Sandford MD. Intrahepatic cholangiojejunostomy with partial resection of the liver. Surgery 1949; 128: 330–347.

Mark A, Malangoni MA, et al. Effective palliation of malignant biliary duct obstruction. Ann Surg 1985; 201: 554–559.

Mueller PR, et al. Percutaneous biliary drainage: technical and catheter-related problems in 200 procedures. AJR 1987; 138: 17–23.

Rossi AP, Braasch JW, Warren KW. Carcinoma of the proximal bile ducts. Surg Gynecol Obstet 1973; 136: 923.

8.3 Surgery for Gallbladder Carcinoma

E. Moreno González, J. Arias Diaz, P. Rico Selas, J. Seoane González and M. Hidalgo Pascual

Introduction

Primary gallbladder carcinoma is a lethal disease resistant, the majority of patients to any form of treatment (Nevin 1976, Piehler 1978, Wanebolt et al. 1982). One explanation is that the diagnosis takes place too late and that the patients are already at an advanced stage of their disease when detected (Piehler 1978).

The disease is seen in 1–2% of cholecystectomy specimens, and was the cause of death in 2000 men and 3500 women in the UK between the years 1966 and 1970 (Diehl 1980). There is an increased incidence with age, particularly in female patients. Over 90% of patients are above 50 years of age, and the peak age incidence is 70–75 years, with a male to female ratio of 1 : 3 (Bergdahl 1980, Nevin 1976, Piehler 1978).

There is an established association between carcinoma of the gallbladder and cholelithiasis, although the precise causative role of gallstones in the formation of carcinoma is not yet clear (Broden and Bengston 1980). The estimated risk of developing cancer in patients with lithiasis of the gallbladder is 1–3% (Piehler 1978).

Clinical Presentation and Differential Diagnosis

The most common symptoms of gallbladder carcinoma are pain, weight loss and jaundice, with a 76%, 39% and 38% incidence respectively (Piehler 1978). A proportion of patients present a clinical picture of acute cholecystitis manifested by fever, leukocytosis, localized pain and tenderness. These patients are seen at an early stage, and have a better prognosis. Some patients present with a clinical picture of empyema, and others show more advanced signs of the disease, with a variety of symptoms such as anorexia, weight loss, vomiting and jaundice.

Serum alkaline phosphatase and bilirubin levels are the laboratory values most often elevated in patients with gallbladder carcinoma, but they do not assist the differential diagnosis between benign and malignant disease. Oral cholecystography in 90% of cases does not opacify the gallbladder, and intravenous cholangiography is unsuccessful in 93% of patients. Endoscopic retrograde cholangiopancreatography (ERCP) may be diagnostic (Ogoshi and Nima 1977). Angiography is not helpful in detecting early lesions, but it may help to demonstrate the extent of the disease. Ultrasound and computed tomography (CT) are not of value, and in general, preoperative diagnosis can only be made in 5 to 18% of patients (Abrams et al. 1970, Blumgart 1984, Collier et al. 1984, Fakim et al. 1962, Nevin 1976).

Surgical Management

The indications for the various operative procedures for gallbladder carcinoma depend on the general condition of the patient and the stage of the disease. At the time of diagnosis, the disease has already spread locally (regional lymph nodes and liver) in the majority of patients (Fakim et al. 1962). Poor-risk patients, and those with advanced disease (metastases, or histological invasion of all 3 layers of the gallbladder wall plus the cystic lymph node and the liver) are, in our opinion, not eligible for surgery, even for palliative procedures, unless severe duodenal obstruction exists. However, if the disease is not advanced, or if the diagnosis is made incidentally during or after cholecystectomy, the following surgical options are open.

In patients with limited spread of the disease (invasion of only 1–2 layers of gallbladder wall) extended cholecystectomy is indicated. This consists of cholecystectomy, regional lymphadenectomy and a wedged liver resection of the gallbladder fossa (Adson et al. 1982, Bismuth and Malt 1979, Bismuth et al. 1982, Blumgart 1984, Collier et al. 1984, Ische 1979, Koo et al. 1981, Wanebolt et al. 1982).

Alternatively, we prefer to proceed with formal anatomical right hemihepatectomy, as described in Chapter 6.3 (Abrams et al. 1970).

Technique

Extended Cholecystectomy

This procedure consists of resection of the gallbladder with a wedge resection of the liver parenchyma all along the gallbladder fossa of the lymphatic tissue of the Calot triangle, and of the lymphatics of the hepatoduodenal ligament.

Incision: although a medial supraumbilical laparotomy can be used, a right subcostal incision is generally preferable.

Dissection of the hepatoduodenal ligament: we proceed with a step-by-step dissection by means of which we isolate the portal vein, hepatic artery and common bile duct below and above the common hepatic duct–cystic duct junction, as in the initial steps for surgery of tumors of the porta hepatis (Fig. 8.1.2, p. 343). These structures are completely freed from their lymphatics all along their course. The hepatic artery is dissected free from the celiac axis up to and above its bifurcation, and the portal vein and common bile duct from the supraduodenal region up to and above the bifurcation.

The liver parenchyma is resected about 20 mm from the hepatovesicular implantation, leaving a tongue of liver parenchyma about 20 mm thick on the surface of the gallbladder when it is resected. Meticulous hemostasis is performed, and an external drainage is left in the area.

Disadvantages of extended cholecystectomy: the indication for this technique is a matter of debate, because although theoretically appealing, it has not been associated with satisfactory results in practice (Wanebolt et al. 1982, Warren et al. 1969). This approach is only recommended in the case of a small tumor confined to the gallbladder.

Cholecystectomy with Extended Right Hemihepatectomy

Tumors clearly infiltrating the gallbladder fossa are treated with this procedure by a number of surgeons (Adson et al. 1982, Ische 1979, Moossa et al. 1975, Wanebolt et al. 1982, Warren et al. 1969). However, the results show high morbidity and mortality, with limited overall survival (Koo et al. 1981). For the surgical technique, see Chapter 8.1.

Disadvantages of cholecystectomy with right extended hemihepatectomy: at present, it is under discussion whether extended liver resection embracing the entire right lobe and one segment of the left lobe is indicated for gallbladder carcinoma (Koo et al. 1981). However, it can certainly be considered for tumors of the fundus and body of the gallbladder, with extensive growth infiltrating segments V and VI but without infiltration of the hepatoduodenal ligament and without lymphatic metastases at the level of the porta hepatis.

Conclusions

It is our view that, although radical surgery is an attractive alternative for a small proportion of patients with gallbladder carcinoma, the majority of them present at an advanced stage of the disease which precludes such an approach (Blumgart et al. 1984, Collier et al. 1984, Koo et al. 1981, Wanebolt et al. 1982). Furthermore, even after radical surgery results remain poor and disappointing (Koo et al. 1981). Any consideration of further surgical treatment should be individualized and well assessed, taking into account all of the factors mentioned above regarding age, general condition, and stage of the disease.

References

Abrams RM, Meng CH, et al. Angiographic demonstration of carcinoma of gallbladder. Radiology 1970; 94: 277–282.

Adson MA, et al. Hepatobiliary cancer: surgical considerations. Mayo Clin Proc 1982; 56: 686–699.

Bergdahl L. Gallbladder carcinoma first diagnosed at microscopic examination of gallbladders removed for presumed benign diseases. Ann Surg 1980; 191: 19–22.

Bismuth H, Malt R. Carcinoma of the biliary tract. N Engl J Med 1979; 302: 704–706.

Bismuth H, Houssin D, Castaign D. Major and minor segmentectomies "regles" in liver surgery. World J Surg 1982; 6: 10–24.

Blumgart LH. Tumors of the gallbladder and bile ducts. In: Elis, Schwartz SI, eds. Maingot's abdominal operations. 8th ed. New York: Appleton-Century Crofts, 1984.

Broden G, Bengston L. Carcinoma of the gallbladder in relation to cholelithiasis and to concept of prophylactic cholecystectomy. Acta Chir Scand 1980; 500 (suppl): 15–18.

Collier NA, Carr D, Hemingway A, Blumgart LH. Preoperative diagnosis and its effect on the treatment of carcinoma of the gallbladder. Surg Gynecol Obstet 1984; 159: 465–470.

Diehl AK. Epidemiology of gallbladder cancer: a synthesis of recent data. J Nat Cancer Inst 1980; 65: 1209–1214.

Fakim RB, et al. Carcinoma of the gallbladder: a study of its mode of spread. Ann Surg 1962; 156: 114–124.

Ische I. Evaluation of intended radical surgery in carcinoma of gallbladder. Br J Surg 1979; 68: 158–160.

Koo J, Wong J, Cheng FCY, Ong GB. Carcinoma of the gallbladder. Br J Surg 1981; 68: 161–165.

Moossa AR, et al. The continuing challenge of gallbladder cancer: survey of thirty years experience at the University of Chicago. Am J Surg 1975; 130: 57–62.

Nevin JE. Carcinoma of the gallbladder. Cancer 1976; 37: 141–148.

Ogoshi K, Nima M. The diagnostic evaluation of ERCP in pancreatitis and biliary carcinoma. Gastroenterol Jpn 1977; 12: 218–223.

Piehler JM. Primary carcinoma of the gallbladder. Surg Gynecol Obstet 1978; 147: 929–942.

Wanebolt J, et al. Carcinoma of the gallbladder a curable lesion? Ann Surg 1982; 195: 624–631.

Warren K, et al. Primary neoplasia of the gallbladder. Surg Gynecol Obstet 1969; 126: 1036–1040.

8.4   Surgery for Cholangiocarcinoma of the Middle and Distal Common Bile Duct

N.J. Lygidakis and M.N. van der Heyde

Introduction

Primary cholangiocarcinomas at the middle and distal common bile duct are more amenable to surgical management and can be more easily diagnosed (Braasch 1983, Tompkins et al. 1981) (Figs. 8.4.1 and 8.4.2). In making the diagnosis, special attention has to be given to differentiate these malignancies from sclerosing cholangitis, benign iatrogenic structures and from structures secondary to chronic pancreatitis (Braasch et al. 1967). In many instances, these often multifocal cholangiocarcinomas spread diffusely under the biliary mucosa (Braasch et al. 1967). Care is required to obtain free margins during surgical resection. An extensive resection such as duodeno-pancreatectomy is indicated for distal bile duct lesions, while for those of the middle bile duct in

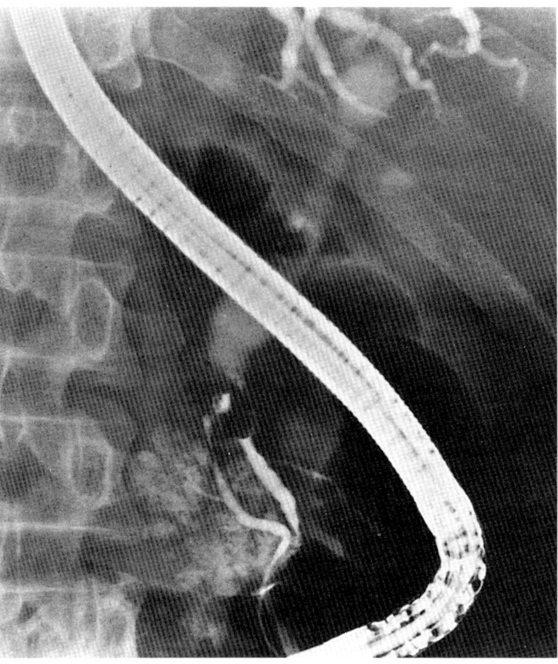

Fig. 8.4.**2**   Cholangiogram of a patient with cholangiocarcinoma confined to the distal end of the common bile duct

most cases a resection of the common hepatic duct confluence combined with duodenopancreatectomy is indicated.

These cholangiocarcinomas may occur concomitantly with inflammatory bowel disease, inflammatory polyposis and choledochal cysts (Braasch et al. 1967, Lees and Herman 1981). Nowadays, surgical management is promising, and with the advances in surgical techniques, the prognosis and prospects for this kind of lesion have markedly improved. The operation-related mortality after duodeno-pancreatectomy has dropped to 2 % (Grace et al. 1986, Mannell et al. 1986, Trede 1985, Tsuchiya et al. 1986). These results have therefore favorably influenced the indications for resectional management of these lesions.

Management

The operation begins with a bilateral subcostal incision (Fig. 7.1.3, p. 263). After opening the abdomen, the hepatoduodenal ligament is dissected and the common bile duct is identified in order to assess the precise location and extent of the tumor. The

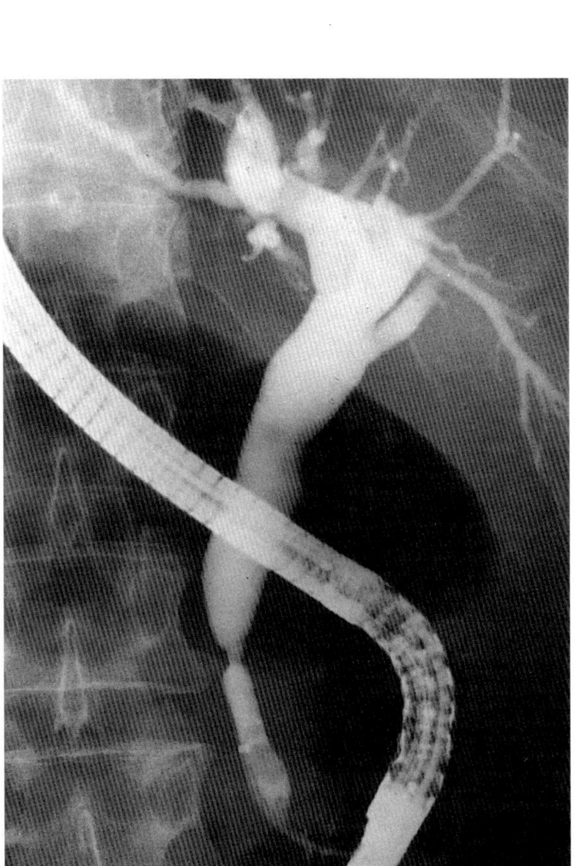

Fig. 8.4.**1**   **Cholangiogram** of a patient with cholangiocarcinoma confined to the middle third of the common bile duct

portal vein and hepatic artery are dissected, cleared from their lymphatics and isolated by means of vessel loops. The common bile duct is transected proximal to the tumor, and a frozen biopsy is taken from the proximal margins of transection (Fig. 8.1.**2**, p. 343). The transected proximal stump of the common bile duct is reflected cephalad, and its distal end is closed and further dissected from the portal vein and hepatic artery (Fig. 8.1.**3**, p. 344).

Subtotal duodenopancreatectomy is combined with hemigastrectomy, bilateral truncal vagotomy and with complete lymphatic clearance along the aorta, inferior vena cava, portal vein, hepatic and superior mesenteric artery (Fig. 7.1.**1**, p. 262) (Chapter 7.1). In patients with normal histology in the frozen biopsy from the proximal margin of the common bile duct and with a pancreatic duct with a diameter of more than 1 mm, reconstruction of alimentary continuity is carried out as described in Chapter 7.4.

In patients with a narrow pancreatic duct (less than 1 mm in transverse diameter) and a friable pancreas, we proceed to total pancreatectomy, thus anticipating the risk of dehiscence of the pancreatic anastomosis. Reconstruction of alimentary continuity in these patients, is carried out with an end-to-side hepaticojejunostomy and a side-to-side gastrojejunostomy (Fig. 7.2.**6**, p. 279). The end-to-side hepaticojejunostomy is carried out as a one-layer anastomosis with interrupted 4-0 or 5-0 Vicryl full-thickness sutures between an opening in the jejunal loop and the common hepatic duct (Fig. 7.4.**6h, i**, p. 291).

In patients in whom the malignant process extends at or above the bifurcation of the common hepatic duct, we proceed with a further proximal dissection of the cephalad-reflected proximal stump of the common hepatic duct up to the level of its bifurcation. We continue with dissection of the main left and right hepatic ducts along their intrahepatic course till the level of their segmental bifurcation (Fig. 8.1.**4**, p. 344).

Depending on the results of the frozen biopsies, the right and left hepatic ducts are transected proximal to the bifurcation of the common hepatic duct. The intrahepatic biliary tree is drained with a double anastomosis between the right and left hepatic ducts and a Roux-en-Y jejunal loop (Fig. 8.4.**3**) or with intrahepatic cholangiojejunostomies between the segmental hepatic ducts and a Roux-en-Y jejunal loop depending on the level of transection of the main hepatic ducts (Fig. 8.4.**4**). The anastomoses are carried out in one layer with 5-0 Vicryl full-thickness interrupted sutures.

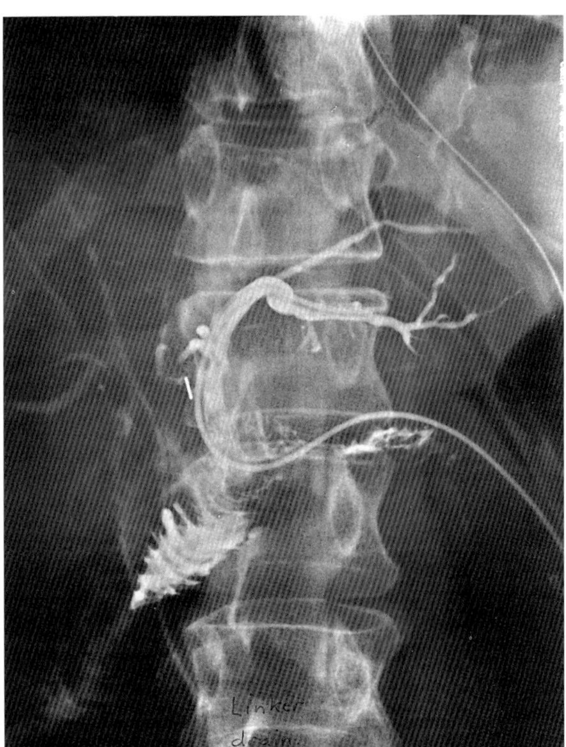
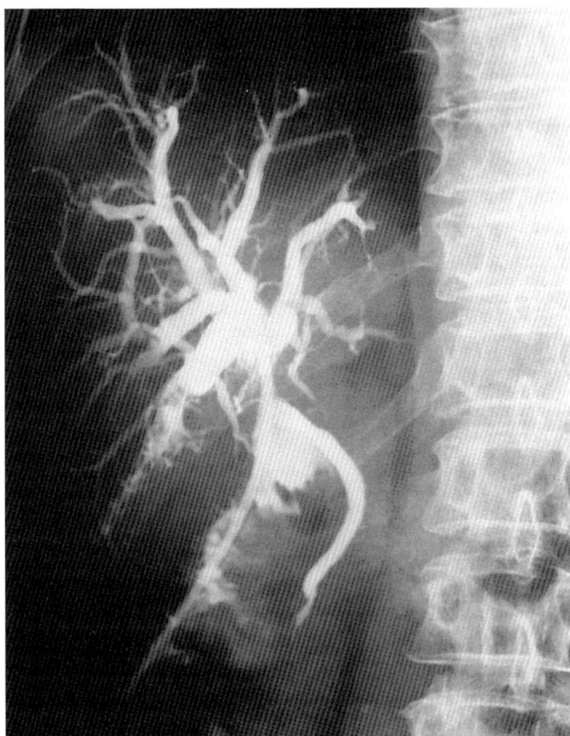

Fig. 8.4.**3a, b** **Cholangiogram** of a patient with hepaticojejunostomies between the right and left hepatic ducts and a Roux-en-Y jejunal loop

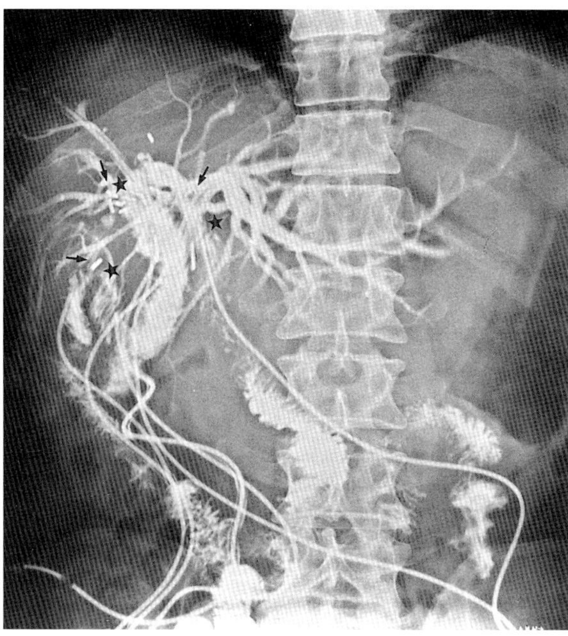

Fig. 8.4.**4 Three separate cholangiojejunostomies** (arrows) between the segmental hepatic ducts and a Roux-en-Y jejunal loop in a patient with a diffuse form of cholangiocarcinoma which affected a large part of the intrahepatic biliary tree

Results

From September 1983 to Januar 1988, 37 patients with cholangiocarcinoma underwent resectional surgery. In 5 patients, the tumor was confined to the middle common bile duct, and in 32 patients the distal common bile duct was involved. One patient died in the immediate postoperative period, and two patients needed early reoperation because of severe and life-threatening complications.

Comments

The results with regard to early mortality after subtotal duodenopancreatectomy in the present series of patients correspond to those in other series (Braasch et al. 1986, Grace at al. 1986, Mannell et al. 1986, Trede 1985, Tsuchiya et al. 1986), and offer a promising outlook for patients whose prospects, a few years ago, were limited to one year survival after the diagnosis (Braasch 1983, Lees et al. 1980, Walsh et al. 1983). At that time, the operative results were dismal and disappointing, with an operative mortality of 20 % after palliative bypass, 70 % after

Whipple resection, and 100 % after local tumor resection (Anderson et al. 1985). Also disappointing were the results of others who reported a 25 and 30 % mortality after resection in patients with middle and distal bile duct cholangiocarcinoma (Tompkins et al. 1981). Less disappointing results were also reported, but these were still far from satisfactory (Gibby et al. 1985).

Fortunately, the mortality decreased and the prospects with regard to the prognosis are improving. It is promising that near-identical figures are reported in connection with the mortality and survival after subtotal pancreatectomy (Braasch et al. 1986, Grace et al. 1986, Mannell et al. 1986, Trede 1985, Tsuchiya et al. 1986) (Chapter 7.1). Contributing towards these favorable prospects are the many factors related to improvement of diagnostic techniques, making early and more accurate diagnosis feasible, improvements in surgical techniques and enhanced surgical expertise in highly specialized centers, and finally a better understanding of the various problems secondary to cholestasis.

References

Anderson JB, Cooper MJ, Williamson RCV. Adenocarcinoma of the extrahepatic biliary tree. Ann R Coll Surg Engl 1985; 67: 139–143.

Braasch, JW. Malignant disease of the distal bile duct. In: Moody FF, ed. Advances in diagnosis and surgical treatment of biliary tract disease. New York: Masson 1983: 109–118.

Braasch JW, Warren KW, Kunen GA. Malignant neoplasms of the bile ducts. Surg Clin N Am 1967; 47: 627.

Braasch JW, Rossi R, Watkins E, Deziel D, Winter P. Pyloric and gastric preserving pancreatic resection: experience with 87 patients. Ann Surg 1986; 204: 411–418.

Gibby DG, Hanks J, Wanebo H, Kaiser D, et al. Bile duct carcinoma. Ann Surg 1985; 202: 139–144.

Grace PA, Pitt HA, Tompkins RM, den Besten L, Longmire WP Jr. Decreased morbidity and mortality after pancreatoduodenectomy. Am J Surg 1986; 151: 141.

Lees CD, Herman RE. Familial polyposis coli associated with bile duct cancer. Am J Surg 1981; 141: 378.

Lees CD, Zapolanski A, Cooperman AM. Carcinoma of the bile ducts. Surg Gynecol Obstet 1980; 151: 192–198.

Mannell A, van Heerden J, Weiland LH, Ilstrup DM. Factors influencing survival after resection for ductal adenocarcinoma of the pancreas. Ann Surg 1986; 203: 403.

Takasan H, Kim C, et al. Clinicopathologic study of seventy patients with carcinoma of the biliary tract. Surg Gynecol Obstet 1980; 150: 721–726.

Tompkins RK, Tomas D, Wile A. Prognostic factors in bile duct carcinoma: analysis of 96 cases. Ann Surg 1981; 194: 447–457.

Trede M. The surgical treatment of pancreatic carcinoma. Surgery 1985; 97: 28–35.

Tsuchiya R, Tomioka T, Izawa K. Collective review of small carcinomas of the pancreas. Ann Surg 1986; 203: 77–81.

Walsh DD, Eckhauer FE, Cronenwett JL. Adenocarcinoma of the ampulla of Vater. Ann Surg 1983; 195: 152–157.

8.5 Diagnosis and Treatment of Early Complications after Surgery for Primary Cholangiocarcinomas of the Porta Hepatis

N.J.Lygidakis and M.N. van der Heyde

Introduction

Surgery for cholangiocarcinoma of the porta hepatis is still associated with significant morbidity and mortality (Beazley et al. 1984, Lai et al. 1987, Pain et al. 1985, Pitt et al. 1981, Thompson et al. 1983). Despite advances in diagnostic and surgical techniques, complications such as sepsis, bleeding and impaired liver function, when superimposed on the postoperative course of a jaundiced patient, are life-threatening. This is reflected by the high morbidity (53.8%) and mortality (69.2%) reported in a recent series of 57 patients with proximal bile duct tumors (Lai et al. 1987). High morbidity and mortality have also been encountered in other series (Alexander et al. 1984, Anderson et al. 1985, Beazley et al. 1984, Pitt et al. 1981, Terblanche and Louw 1973). It is impressive, that the mortality after liver resection combined with tumor resection was 19% in a series of 61 patients while the mortality after bypass surgery (hepaticojejunostomy) was 26% (Beazley et al. 1984). The main cause of the mortality and morbidity in these patients was sepsis.

The incidence of septic complications varies from 12–32% (Iwatsuki et al. 1983, Thompson et al. 1983). The major focus for the development of sepsis is still bile spillage which is either due to leakage of the hepaticojejunostomy or to the rough surface of the liver after combined liver and tumor resection (Alexander et al. 1984, Beazley et al. 1984). The incidence of biliary fistulas is high, ranging from 25–56% (Alexander et al. 1984). Other foci for the development of sepsis are hematomas and necrotic tissue in the rough surface of the liver after resections which have not been carried out at the anatomical lines of liver segmentation. Furthermore, patients with jaundice are prone to develop sepsis for a variety of reasons, with a high incidence of endotoxemia (Fletcher et al. 1982, Hunt et al. 1982, Pain et al. 1985, Pitt et al. 1981), a high incidence of biliary infection and intrabiliary hypertension, with subsequent bacteremia (Lygidakis and Brummelkamp 1985), and a high incidence of immune deficiency secondary to impaired liver function (Drivas et al. 1976). Sepsis is a serious complication, with a mortality of up to 80%. In a series of 15 patients with a bypass for proximal bile duct tumors, 6 developed sepsis and 4 of them died. Sepsis in one of these 4 patients was concomitant with bleeding (Beazley et al. 1984).

Bleeding due to a number of factors, such as impaired liver function and thrombocytopenia secondary to sepsis, is another serious complication (Hunt et al. 1982, Pain et al. 1985, Pitt et al. 1981). Furthermore, there is decreased fibrinolysis which is associated with reactionary hyperfibrinogenemia (Hunt et al. 1982, Pain et al. 1985). In cholestasis, decreased fibrinolysis is secondary to increased serum lipids (Hunt et al. 1982).

In this chapter, an attempt will be made to share with the reader the various problems and challenges which we faced in a series of patients who underwent resectional surgery for primary cholangiocarcinoma of the porta hepatis.

Patients and Methods

From September 1983 to January 1988, 50 patients with primary cholangiocarcinoma of the porta hepatis underwent resectional surgery in our department. Eight of these 50 patients died during the first 30 days after the operation. They were part of a group of 16 patients who underwent early reoperation because of severe and life-threatening complications (Table 8.5.1). Eight other patients developed hepatic encephalopathy after extensive right or left hemihepatectomy (80% liver resection). All 8 were successfully treated by monitoring, parenteral nutrition, and controlled respiration in the intensive care unit.

Minor complications such as wound infections and minor anastomotic leaks were treated conservatively and are not discussed here.

Diagnosis of the complications was based on the clinical presentation as such, tachycardia, hypotension, oliguria, respiratory distress, mental confusion and disorientation, and on the outcome of the blood screening tests for hemoglobin, white blood cell count, thrombocytes, hematocrit, urea, glycose, serum glutamic-oxaloacetic transaminase (SGOT), serum glutamic-pyruvic transaminase (SGPT), alkaline phosphatase, serum ammonia, Electroencephalogram (EEG) tests, upper-abdominal ultrasound (US) and computed tomography (CT). Selective angiography of the celiac axis and superior mesenteric artery were also carried out in a small proportion of patients to define the source of bleeding or for embolization purposes. In all patients, records of coagulation profile, central venous pressure, arterial pressure and wedge pulmonary pressure were kept during the immediate and

Table 8.5.**1 Causes of morbidity and mortality** in 50 patients who underwent surgery for primary cholangiocarcinoma of the porta hepatis

Cause of complications	Treatment	No. of patients	Dead	Alive
Diffuse bleeding during liver resection and diffuse bleeding from overtransfusion	Packing Planned relaparotomy	4 (4/20)	3	1
Bleeding from the jejunojejunal anastomosis	Suture			
	Control focus	1 (1/30)	0	1
Bleeding cholangiojejunostomy caused by anastomotic disruption during withdrawal of anastomotic tubes	Suture Control focus			
	Re-anastomosis	1 (1/30)	0	1
Subphrenic abscess	Surgical drainage	(2/30)	2	0
		6 (4/20)	1	3
Intra-abdominal abscess	Surgical drainage	(1/30)	1	0
		4 (3/20)	1	2
Hepatic encephalopathy	Conservative management	8 (8/20)	0	8

early postoperative period after the re-intervention in the intensive care unit.

The decision on whether to reoperate or not was made after careful evaluation of the general condition of the individual patient, and particular care was taken to perform re-intervention as early as possible.

Surgical Techniques and Treatment Policy

Management of Bleeding

Angiography offered valuable information regarding the site of origin of the bleeding and also guided us in differentiating between bleeding secondary to coagulopathy and bleeding of traumatic origin (Fig. 8.5.1). Angiography was only carried out when the general condition of the patient allowed, and when the bleeding could be controlled. The latter could easily be anticipated after transfusion of blood at a rate of 300 cm^3 per hour and with an arterial pressure of 80–100 mmHg. In the case of diffuse bleeding, with bleeding from the abdominal cavity via the transabdominal tubes, the patient was immediately transferred to the operating theater where every effort was made to correct the coagulopathy (administration of fresh blood, transfusion of fresh frozen plasma and thrombocytes) in order to create the optimal conditions for operation. The same policy was followed in patients who showed diffuse bleeding, even without excess bleeding from the tubes, but with increased abdominal distension and with persistent tachycardia (more than 130 pulses/min and hemoglobin less than 6 g/l) and difficulty in maintaining a stable arterial pressure of 80–100 mmHg even after blood transfusion at a rate of 300 cm^3 per hour. Furthermore, we re-explore any patient who had a major episode of bleeding irrespective of whether the bleeding per-

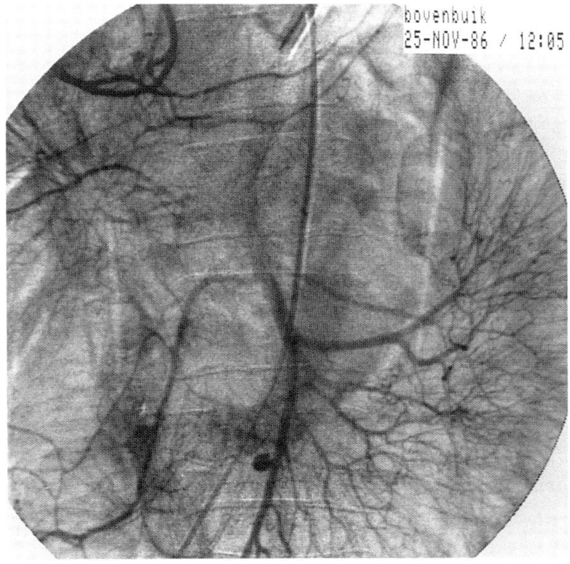

Fig. 8.5.**1 Bleeding jejunojejunostomy** demonstrated by angiography

sisted or had stopped, in order to evacuate the hematoma from the abdominal cavity and to prevent a life-threatening sepsis.

During surgery, the kind of management depends on the operative findings. Of prime importance is the identification of the site of origin of the bleeding and its immediate control. In this respect, correction of an eventual coagulopathy is also important and must always be considered.

In patients with diffuse and persistent bleeding, it may be wise to consider packing the bleeding area, closing the abdominal wall with Vicryl or collagen mesh, and reopening the abdomen 3 or 4 days later, depending on the progress of the bleeding and the patient's general condition. If the bleeding originates from specific points, the best approach is suturing and complete control of the bleeding area. Our experience with packing is satisfactory, and combined with planned relaparotomy the situation has good chances to be controlled.

Mangement of Septic Complications

In patients with subphrenic or intra-abdominal abscess, signs of sepsis such as persistent hyperpyrexia ($> 38.5°C$), tachycardia ($> 120/min$), metabolic acidosis (< 7.2), thrombocytopenia (< 100000 thrombocytes), oliguria ($< 500\ ml/24\ h$) and hypotension ($< 100\ mmHg$ central arterial pressure) were carefully evaluated in combination with upper-abdominal ultrasound and CT scans. Both US and CT were of great value in establishing the location and extent of the complication (Figs. 8.5.**2**, 8.5.**3**), and enabled us to choose between surgical and medical management by CT-guided percutaneous drainage (Fig. 8.5.**4**).

Unfortunately, despite the policy described, retrospective assessment of the septic complications in these patients showed that, particularly for patients with diffuse intra-abdominal abscesses, the decision to reoperate was taken too late. In our opinion, 3 of these patients should have been operated on at an earlier stage.

Apart from the 10 patients who underwent reoperation for manifest sepsis (Table 8.5.**1**), another 7 with subphrenic abscess were successfully treated by percutaneous drainage under CT control. During operation for subphrenic and subhepatic abscesses, the exposure was always wide, and care was taken to eradicate any form of sepsis by meticulous debridement of the region of the abscess.

Management of Encephalopathy

Our experience with the treatment of hepatic encephalopathy is limited to 8 patients who developed severe hepatic encephalopathy secondary to residual liver dysfunction after 80 % liver resection. All 8 patients had characteristic electroencephalo-

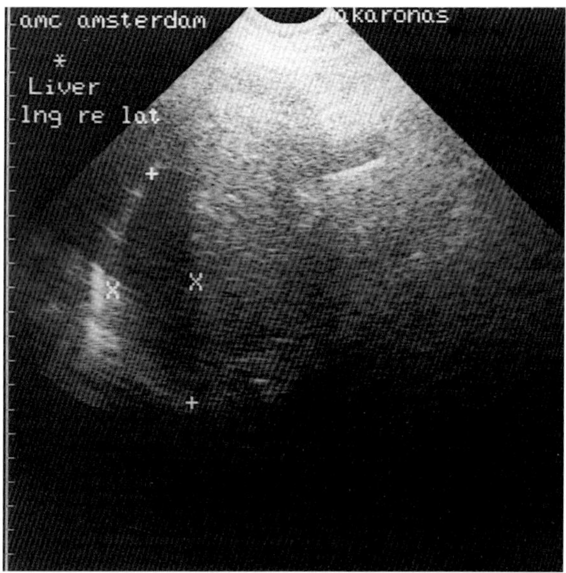

Fig. 8.5.**2** **Ultrasound scan** in a patient with subphrenic and subhepatic abscess

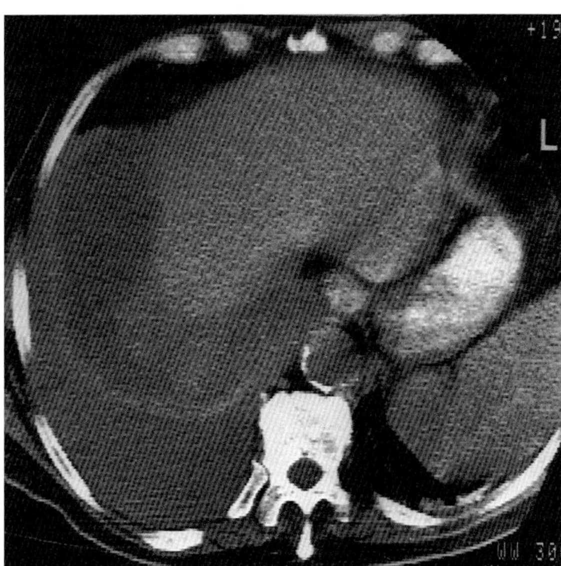

Fig. 8.5.**3** **Computed tomography** in a patient with subphrenic and subhepatic abscess

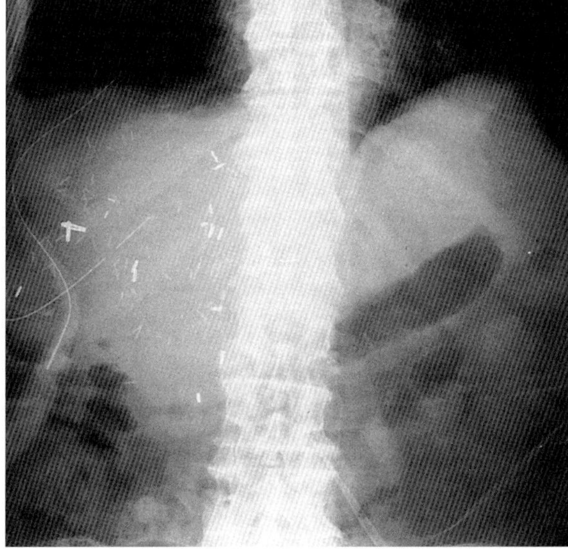

Fig. 8.5.**4** **Percutaneous drainage** of a subphrenic and subhepatic abscess under CT control

grams and increased serum-ammonia levels. Treatment consisted of nutritional support with total parenteral nutrition, respiratory support by artificial ventilation, antibiotics, and general surveillance of each patient.

In dealing with this type of complication, we had the impression, and found evidence, that the impaired liver function of the residual liver after extensive liver resection is significantly aggravated by large hematomas secondary to bleeding and by the presence of septic foci. Thus, 4 patients had a late-phase hepatic encephalopathy which had, surprisingly enough, developed on the 9th and 10th postoperative day, after an uneventful and smooth early postoperative phase during which they were fully conscious and alert. The development of encephalopathy coincided with hematomas in 2 patients and with a subphrenic abscess in 2 other patients. It seems likely that the residual liver, already handicapped by the magnitude of the major operation, fails to cope with the extra workload required to deal with huge hematomas or with localized or generalized abscesses.

Results

The mortality in 16 patients who underwent early reoperation because of severe postoperative complications is presented in Table 8.5.1. The overall mortality was 50%, caused predominantly by sepsis. Ten of the 17 patients with septic complications required urgent reoperation (59%). The mortality in these patients was very high (50%), and equalled that after reoperation for bleeding, where 3 of the 6 patients died. The fact that the remaining 7 patients with localized abscess who had conservative treatment by CT-guided puncture had an uneventful recovery is noteworthy, and should be considered.

Comments

We searched for factors which could have contributed to the morbidity and mortality, but we could not find any specific relationships, e. g. with regard to serumbilirubin levels and the incidence of postoperative bleeding and septic complications. We did find a close relationship between encephalopathy and the extent of the liver resection. All patients with hepatic encephalopathy had had 80% liver resection, and the majority had cholestasis. The age of the patients did not significantly influence the incidence of postoperative complications. The magnitude of the operation, however, influenced both the morbidity and mortality. Therefore, the incidence of postoperative complica-

tions after combined liver and tumor resection was higher than that in patients who had only tumor resection. Similarly, the overall mortality was higher for patients with combined liver and tumor resection compared to those with tumor resection alone (cf. Chapter 8.1).

The data presented in this chapter confirm again that surgery for primary cholangiocarcinoma of the porta hepatis continues to be a challenging task associated with significant morbidity and mortality (Alexander et al. 1984, Anderson et al. 1985, Beazley et al. 1984, Lai et al. 1987). There are, however a number of points which deserve closer consideration.

The overall mortality rate in the present series of 50 patients who had tumor resection (30 out of 50) or combined tumor and liver resection, with or without resection of vascular structures (20 out of 50) was 16% (8 out of 50). This can be considered as satisfactory when compared to the results in other series (Alexander et al. 1984, Anderson et al. 1985, Beazley et al. 1984, Lai et al. 1987). It is promising that the mortality after partial or complete tumor resection remained low (3 out of 30, 10%). This, in combination with the fact that the survival and the quality of life after the operation was good (Chapter 8.1), leads to the conclusion that the surgical approach described should be considered as a promising alternative for the average patient with primary cholangiocarcinoma of the porta hepatis. The mortality of 10% after such an approach contrasts sharply with the mortality of 26% which has been reported after bypass operations in the same category of patients (Anderson et al. 1985, Beazley et al. 1984). Certainly, our mortality rate (5 out of 20, 25%) in patients with combined tumor and liver resection with or without resection of regional vascular structures is high, but it is nervertheless lower than the mortality which has been reported after tumor and liver resection (Lai et al. 1987). All of the patients who had bilateral vascular involvement had an advanced stage of disease, and should have been considered as not eligible for surgical resection if the criteria of resectability (Chapter 8.1.) had been followed.

As far as the incidence of septic complications and their underlying causes are concerned, it is of interest that the incidence of biliary fistulas remained low and did not lead to abscess formation, and that the patients did not need to be reoperated.

The two patients with minor anastomotic leakage responded well to conservative management by percutaneous drainage of the small bile collections. The low incidence of anastomotic leakage in our series compares favorably with the results of other series, where a high incidence of hepaticojejunostomy leakage was observed (Beazley et al. 1984).

In our opinion, the difference between our results and those reported in the literature derives from our method of creating intrahepatic cholangiojejunostomies (Chapter 8.1). In conclusions, the low overall morbidity and mortality in patients who had tumor resection alone can be attributed to the following factors:

1. We were able to eliminate, or at least reduce, biliary stasis and to drain the entire biliary tree adequately by creating separate intrahepatic cholangiojejunostomies. Adequate biliary drainage is the best protection against sepsis and cholangitis.

2. By taking this surgical approach, we had a very low incidence of anastomotic leakage. In contrast, patients with combined tumor and liver resection have a higher mortality and morbidity which could be considered to result from a combination of many parameters responsible for cholestasis (Allisson et al. 1979, Drivas et al. 1976, Fletcher et al. 1982, Hunt et al. 1982, Pain et al. 1985, Pitt et al. 1981). In particular, carrying out liver resection and specifically extended liver resection in cholestatic patients diminishes the reserve of liver function to a remarkable extent. The liver remnant can therefore hardly cope with the metabolic and functional demands being put on it, handicapped as it is, firstly by the presence of cholestasis, secondly by damage during the operation and anesthesia, and thirdly by the decrease in its functional mass secondary to liver resection. Our results regarding the incidence of bleeding, sepsis, and encephalopathy for the second group of patients (n = 20), clearly support this hypothesis (Table 8.5.1).

Another aspect of interest is the way in which we treated the complications, and the fact that we reoperated on all patients with major complications. In case of bleeding, suturing of the bleeding focus remains the optimal form of treatment, and can clearly be recommended whenever feasible. In patients with diffuse uncontrolled bleeding of mixed etiology (coagulopathy plus sepsis), the decision is crucial and sometimes dramatic. However, the surgeon must realize that he has to stop somewhere and that there is no point in merely replacing blood losses without any prospect of control. The policy of packing the bleeding surface and attempting to correct the coagulopathy is warranted and must be recommended. This policy of 'wait and see' and of planned relaparotomy is sometimes life-saving, and has to be considered.

For the majority of patients with sepsis, surgery is the optimal form of treatment, and has to be carried out as soon as the diagnosis of this severe complication is confirmed. Well-planned medical management by percutaneous CT-guided puncture is also a possibility for a selected group of patients, and should be considered after evaluation of the patient's individual clinical condition.

Finally, we wish to emphasize that surgery for proximal bile duct tumors is very demanding. Awareness of the possible complications, and the alertness and ability to manage them appropriately, are necessary prerequisites for this kind of surgery.

References

Alexander F, Rossi R, Bryan M, et al. Biliary carcinoma. Am J Surg 1984; 147: 303–309.

Allisson M, Prentic CRM, Kenneth AC, Blumgart LH. Renal function and other factors in obstructive jaundice. Br J Surg 1979; 66: 392–397.

Anderson JB, Cooper MJ, Williamson RC. Adenocarcinoma of the extrahepatic biliary tree. Ann R Coll Surg Engl 1985; 67: 139–143.

Beazley R, Hadjis N, Benjamin I, Blumgart LH. Clinicopathological aspects of high bile duct cancer. Ann Surg 1984; 199: 623–636.

Drivas G, James O, Wardle N. Study of reticuloendothelial phagocytic capacity in patients with cholestasis. Br Med J 1976; i: 1558.

Fletcher MS, Westwick J, Kakkar VV. Endotoxins, prostaglandins and renal fibrin deposition in obstructive jaundice. Br J Surg 1982; 69: 625.

Hunt DR, Allison M, Prentice CRM. Blumgart LH. Endotoxemia disturbance of coagulation, and obstructive jaundice. Am J Surg 1982; 144: 325.

Iwatsuki S, Shaw BW, Starzl TE. Experience with 150 liver resections. Ann Surg 1983; 197: 247–253.

Lai ECS, Tompkins RK, Roslyn JL, Mann LL. Proximal bile duct cancer: quality of survival. Ann Surg 1987; 205: 111–118.

Lygidakis NJ, Brummelkamp WH. The significance of intrabiliary pressure in acute cholangitis. Surg Gynecol Obstet 1985; 161: 453–458.

Lygidakis NJ, Brummelkamp WH. Surgery for cholangiocarcinoma of the junction of the common hepatic duct: a new approach for a better quality of life. J. Exp Clin Cancer Res 1986; 5: 197–202.

Pain A, Cahill CJ, Bailey ME. Perioperative complications in obstructive jaundice: therapeutic considerations. Br J Surg 1985; 72: 942.

Pitt HA, Cameron JL, Postier RG, Gadacz TR. Factors influencing mortality in biliary tract surgery. Am J Surg 1981; 141: 66.

Terblanche J, Louw JH. U tube drainage in palliative therapy of carcinoma of the main hepatic duct junction. Surg Clin North Am 1973; 53: 1245–1256.

Thompson HH, Tompkins R, Longmire WP. Major hepatic resection: a 25-year experience. Ann Surg 1983; 1977: 375–388.

8.6 Carcinoma of the Biliary Tree: Prospects for the Patient

N.J. Lygidakis and M.N. van der Heyde

The prognosis for cholangiocarcinoma of the biliary tree is poor, especially for tumors located at or above the bifurcation of the common hepatic duct. The management of these tumors with regard to the outcome and the prognosis remain controversial. The life expectancy for this category of patients, if they are not treated, is limited to 2–3 months (Wheeler et al. 1981). It is clear from a review of the literature, that tumor resection is the only approach that offers a possibility of cure (Ottow et al. 1985). Resection can be limited to local removal of part, or of the entire tumor, this can be combined with liver resection or with liver and regional vascular resection (Alexander et al. 1984, Anderson et al. 1986, Blumgart et al. 1984, Cotton 1982, Dooley et al. 1979, Evander et al. 1980, Fortner et al. 1976, Huguet et al. 1981, Huibregtse and Tytgat 1984, Lai et al. 1987, Launois et al. 1979, Lees et al. 1980, Lygidakis 1987, Malt et al. 1980, Nakayama et al. 1978, Ottow et al. 1985, Sakaguchi and Nakamura 1986).

The operative mortality in a collective series of 75 cases of local resection of hilar cholangiocarcinoma was 11 % (Boerma 1983). The mean survival of these 75 patients was 19 months, without any survival after 5 years, the usual cause of death being recurrence and cholangitis. Cameron et al. (1982) described an elegant technique for the resection of the bifurcation of the common hepatic duct, associated with satisfactory results with regard to the overall mortality and survival after resection of the hepatic confluence. Indeed, they had no mortality and achieved a satisfactory long-term survival for the majority of patients.

Encouraged by these results, we started with a similar policy in September 1983 (Lygidakis et al. 1986). In our first 30 patients who had partial or macroscopically complete tumor resection, anastomotic stents were used in a proportion of them and always no longer than 15 days, after surgery. The mean survival was 26 months, with patients alive as long as 3 and 4 years. Three patients died during the first 30 postoperative days. The quality of postoperative life was satisfactory, free from serious postoperative sequelae and side effects. For the majority of patients, simple resection of the tumor is palliative, and only exceptionally may resection be radical. Only 2 of our patients who had simple tumor resection had a radical resection.

Simple resection of the tumor with the bifurcation of the common hepatic duct and drainage of the intrahepatic biliary tree via separate intrahepatic cholangiojejunostomies appears, at present, to be the best available surgical alternative in the management of primary proximal bile duct cholangiocarcinoma (Ottow et al. 1985). Indeed, after percutaneous, endoscopic or transtumoral drainage or even after surgical anastomotic bypass, there is a high 30-day mortality (20–30 %), a limited survival (5–9 months), and, most strikingly, a poor quality of life (Cotton 1982, Dooley et al. 1979, Huguet et al. 1981, Huibregtse and Tytgat 1984, Lai et al. 1987, Launois et al. 1979, Malt et al. 1980, Nakayama et al. 1978, Wheeler et al. 1981). The patients have frequent episodes of septic cholangitis, and require multiple hospital readmissions, and most of them die from sepsis. More extensive resections, including combined tumor and liver resections, are associated with increased mortality (27–60 %) without significant difference in the overall survival (Alexander et al. 1984, Anderson et al. 1986, Evander et al. 1980, Fortner et al. 1976, Launois et al. 1979, Lees et al. 1980, Lygidakis et al. 1986). Why we fail to gain a significant increase in the rate of radical removal of tumor even after extensive liver resection is not yet well understood. Bile ducts have thin walls, and bile duct tumors are apt to involve the bile duct walls and spread very easily to invade surrounding tissues. Bile duct tumors readily invade the periductal lymphatic network, perineural lymph clefts, and periductal venules and arterioles. For these reasons, the tumor cells often remain after macroscopic radical resection. Even if the resection is extended, eradication of the disease is extremely difficult, leaving a very small proportion of patients with genuinely radical resection.

Should radical resection be considered as an optimal goal of surgical management? The answer is not yet clear (Cameron et al. 1982), and at the moment, it is difficult to make any definite statement. Of our 20 patients with combined liver and tumor resection, only 7 had a radical resection, and 5 patients died during the first 30 postoperative days. The mean overall survival was 31 months, with a range of 6–45 months.

In general, we believe that with a few exceptions, bile duct tumors are slow-growing and small-sized scirrhous and annular adenocarcinomas. Because of their slow growth and lack of metastases, even non-radical resection can be associated with a satisfactory survival, provided that there is adequate biliary drainage and thus elimination of biliary stasis and cholangitis. Based on our results and the results of Cameron et al. (1982), it appears that the principle of intrahepatic cholangiojejunostomies between the segmental hepatic ducts and a Roux-en-Y jejunal loop, makes it possible to obtain optimal biliary drainage. This type of anastomosis offers a satisfactory quality of postoperative life and a reasonable survival, even in patients with partial tumor resection. The choice between tumor resection alone, and tumor resection supplemented with liver resection with or without regional vascular resection, remains difficult. Both alternatives have their pros and cons, and in our opinion the choice between the two should be based on the clinical and operative peculiarities of each individual patient. A decision must only be based on a careful and objective evaluation of the actual situation. We accept the increased mortality and morbidity of combined tumor and liver resection in the hope that we may obtain a longer survival. As far as the extent of liver resection is concerned, it seems that the majority of patients need an extended hemihepatectomy (Evander et al. 1980, Fortner et al. 1976, Lees et al. 1980, Mizumoto et al. 1986, Sakaguchi and Nakamura 1986).

Drainage of all parts of the liver is essential, and remains important in order to avoid septic complications and liver abscesses. We are inclined to embark on liver resection even in patients in whom, in our opinion, it is impossible to drain the intrahepatic biliary tree efficiently because of the spread of tumor. In carrying out liver resection, we are able to drain the residual liver adequately, and thus to reduce or eliminate the incidence of cholangitis and septic complications.

This view of the value of adequate drainage as a factor promoting survival and improving the quality of postoperative life is shared by others (Bismuth and Corlette 1975, Cameron et al. 1982, Evander et al. 1980).

Tumors arising at the middle and lower third of the common bile duct have a better prognosis, since the resectability rate is higher than that of hilar tumors. In addition, resectional surgery for such tumors is associated with a lower mortality and morbidity rate and with longer survival. The majority of patients will require subtotal duodenopancreatectomy, which can be carried out with a very low mortality (2–5%) and offers promising long-term survival (Chapter 7.1).

In conclusion, we believe that most patients with cholangiocarcinoma currently have reasonable prospects using up-to-date management. There is no question that the improvement in diagnostic techniques, the better understanding of the various individual problems of the jaundiced patient, have contributed to a dramatic change in recent years with regard to the prognosis and outcome for the patient with cholangiocarcinoma of the biliary tree. Today, surgery is a valid alternative and can provide satisfactory overall results in the management of a disease which, 10 years ago, was considered untreatable.

References

Alexander F, Rossi RL, O'Bryan M, Khettry U, Braasch J, Watkins E. Biliary carcinoma: review of 109 cases. Am J Surg 1984; 147: 503.

Anderson JB, Cooper MJ, Williamson RCN. Adenocarcinoma of the extrahepatic biliary tree. Ann R Coll Surg Engl 1986; 67: 139.

Bismuth H, Corlette MB. Intrahepatic cholangioenteric anastomosis of the hilus of the liver. Surg Gynecol Obstet 1975; 140: 170.

Blumgart LH, Benjamin IS, Hadjis NS, Beazley R. Surgical approaches to cholangiocarcinoma at confluence of the hepatic ducts. Lancet 1984; i: 66.

Boerma EJ. The surgical treatment of cancer of the hepatic duct confluence: a clinical anatomical and experimental study and literature survey (Dissertation). University of Amsterdam, 1983.

Cameron LJ, Broe P, Zuidema GD. Proximal bile duct tumors: surgical management with silastic transhepatic biliary stents. Ann Surg 1982; 196: 412.

Cotton PB. Duodenoscopic placement of biliary prostheses to relieve malignant obstructive jaundice. Br J Surg 1982; 69: 501.

Dooley JS, Olney J, Dick R, Sherlock S. Non-surgical treatment of biliary obstruction. Lancet 1979; ii: 1040.

Evander A, Fredlund P, Hoevels J, Ihse J, Bengmark S. Evaluation of aggressive surgery for carcinoma of the extrahepatic bile ducts. Ann Surg 1980; 191: 23.

Fortner JG, Kallum BO, Kim DK. Surgical management of carcinoma of the main hepatic ducts. Ann Surg 1976; 184: 68.

Huguet C, Hakami F, Bloch P. L'intubation transmurale des obstructions néoplastiques du hile du foie: a propos de trente-six observations. Ann Chir 1981; 35: 341.

Huibregtse K, Tytgat GNJ. Endoscopic placement of biliary prosthesis. In: Salmon P, ed. Advances in gastrointestinal endoscopy; vol 1. London: Chapman and Hall, 1984: 219–231.

Lai ECS, Tompkins RK, Roslyn JJ, Mann LL. Proximal bile duct cancer: quality of survival. Ann Surg 1987; 205: 111.

Launois B, Campion JB, Brissot P, Gosselin M. Carcinoma of the hepatic hilus: surgical treatment and the case of resection. Ann Surg 1979; 190: 151.

Lees CD, Zapolanski A, Cooperman AM, Herman RE. Carcinoma of the bile ducts. Surg Gynecol Obstet 1980; 151: 193.

Lygidakis NJ. Kombinierte Rekonstruktion der Gallengänge und Lebergefäße bei Carcinomen der Hepaticusgabel. Chirurg 1987; 58: 282.

Lygidakis NJ, Brummelkamp WH, Lubbers ME, Huibregtse K, Tytgat GN, Schenk KE, van Gulik TM. New surgical approach for the management of carcinoma of the junction of the main hepatic ducts. Surg Annu 1986; 18: 297.

Lygidakis NJ, van der Heyde MN, Tytgat GNJ. The unresectable primary cholangiocarcinoma of the porta hepatis: surgical approaches. Surg Gynecol Obstet (in press).

Malt RA, Warshaw AL, Jamieson CG, Hawks JC III. Left intrahepatic cholangiojejunostomy for proximal obstruction of the biliary tract. Surg Gynecol Obstet 1980; 150: 193.

Mizumoto R, Kawarada Y, Suzuki H. Surgical treatment of hilar carcinoma of the bile duct. Surg Gynecol Obstet 1986; 162: 153.

Nakayama T, Ikeda A, Okuda K. Percutaneous transhepatic drainage of the biliary tract: techniques and results in 104 cases. Gastroenterology 1978; 74: 544.

Ottow RT, Augst DA, Sugarbaker PH. Treatment of proximal biliary tract carcinoma: an overview of techniques and results. Surgery 1985; 97: 251.

Sakaguchi S, Nakamura S. Surgery of the portal vein in resection of cancer of the hepatic hilus. Surgery 1986; 99: 344.

Wheeler PG, Dawson JL, Nunnerley H, Brinkley D, Laws J, Williams R. Newer techniques in the diagnosis and treatment of proximal bile duct carcinoma: an analysis of 41 consecutive patients. Q J Med 1981; 50: 247.

9 Clinical Applications of the SLT Contact Nd:YAG Laser in Hepatobiliary and Pancreatic Malignancy

S. N. Joffe

Introduction

Despite well-standardized techniques for liver and pancreatic resection, operative mortality rates ranging from 5–40% are reported. Postoperative complications include bleeding, infection and sepsis. These complications are frequently related to intraoperative bleeding, the extent of necrotic tissue, and bile or pancreatic fluid leakage. Resection technique is an important factor in preventing these complications.

Liver. The CO_2 laser was first used in liver surgery in 1975 (Fidler et al. 1975). Subsequently, an experimental study used a combined CO_2 and neodymium:yttrium-aluminum-garnet (Nd:YAG) laser in performing a partial liver resection (Meyer and Haverkampf 1982). This was followed by a clinical report on 15 patients (Sultan et al. 1986). The CO_2 laser provided good cutting but inadequate hemostasis. The Nd:YAG laser provided good coagulation, but the necrotic zone of liver damage was 5 to 6 mm, which decreased to a mean of 1.7 mm when combined with the CO_2 laser.

A study comparing the ultrasonic dissector (CUSA) and the non-contact Nd:YAG laser with a conventional blunt dissection technique showed the CUSA was superior to the "finger fracture" technique in that it caused less postoperative tissue damage and reduced bleeding (Tranberg et al. 1985). The non-contact Nd:YAG laser had poor cutting properties and, although it produced hemostasis, the depth of tissue damage was considerable.

The Surgical Laser Technologies, Inc. (SLT) contact Nd:YAG laser scalpel, which uses a synthetic sapphire, has been developed (Daikuzono and Joffe 1985). This device has proved to be effective and safe in both endoscopic and open general surgery (Joffe 1986) along with the stable medium-powered SLT contact laser.

In a liver resection study, the contact Nd:YAG laser technique was shown to be more effective than the non-contact method (Joffe et al. 1986). SLT contact laser surgery required low power ranges (5 to 25 W) for a rapid hepatic lobe resection which was associated with reduced bleeding and smoke. Non-contact resection at low power (10 to 20 W) caused uncontrollable bleeding leading to death in experimental animals. Light microscopy showed laser tissue damage of 0.5 to 1.0 mm with the contact method, with evidence of healing, fibrosis and minimal necrotic material at 15 days. In the non-contact group, thermal damage was 2 to 4 mm in depth with accumulated necrotic material encapsulated by fibrous tissue at 15 days.

Pancreas. The trend in recent years in the treatment of pancreatic carcinoma and occasionally in the treatment of pancreatitis has been towards total pancreatectomy. The pancreas is also harvested for transplantation. Clinical experience with living related pancreatic transplantation (Ross et al. 1983) and the necessity for refining the technique of total pancreatectomy with duodenal preservation in chronic pancreatitis, has led to the development of contact laser surgery. This technique reduces operating time, blood loss and associated morbidity and mortality (Munda et al. 1983).

Pancreatic resection using the non-contact Nd:YAG laser in dogs (Berlatzky et al. 1985) was compared to the conventional multiple ligation technique. In both groups the blood loss was minimal, but the operative time was significantly shorter in the laser group. All animals survived and there were no differences in complications.

In a further study, the SLT contact Nd:YAG laser technique was compared to the older non-contact laser and conventional electrocautery method of performing proximal pancreatectomy in dogs with preservation of the duodenum (Schroder et al. 1987). Both electrocautery and the contact Nd:YAG laser were technically superior to the non-contact Nd:YAG laser. The latter was slower and caused more bleeding and smoke than the other two methods. Thermal injury to the pancreas by the contact Nd:YAG laser group was less than in the non-contact Nd:YAG laser group. When the pancreas was dissected using the contact laser, hemostasis was immediately achieved.

This Chapter presents some of the abdominal applications for the SLT contact laser system. The discussion focuses on the clinical applications and technical aspects of the various types of operative procedures in liver and pancreatic surgery.

Clinical Experience

Our clinical experience with the contact Nd:YAG laser consists of 55 abdominal operations (Table 9.1). These have involved liver resections, including a liver split, anatomical lobectomy, non-anatomical resections and tumor enucleation in 15 patients for both primary and metastatic tumors. Pancreatic resections, including distal, total, near-total and pancreatoduodenectomy, transduodenal sphincteroplasties and Puestow operations have been carried out in 10 patients for either chronic pancreatitis or tumors.

The SLT contact synthetic sapphires were used with a sterile, disposable SLT surgical handpiece for the abdominal operations. The Nd:YAG laser power ranges were 8 to 20 W, with a mean of 16 W for all procedures. Coaxial filtered air was used as the coolant for the fiber–probe interphase.

There were no direct complications related to using the Nd:YAG laser. A subtotal left and right hepatic lobectomy with minimal intraoperative bleeding was performed on each patient with metastatic carcinoma. The liver split for a high bile duct stricture was easily accomplished with mini-

mum blood loss in the whole operative procedure, which included the formation of a hepaticojejunostomy to both left and right ducts. Patients were discharged home on the 5th, 7th and 10th postoperative days respectively.

Pancreatic resections for chronic pancreatitis were performed easily, without excessive blood loss. In one patient undergoing a distal pancreatectomy, it was possible to isolate the pancreas from the splenic vein and artery up to the portal vein and thus to preserve the spleen. During one total pancreatectomy, the head of the pancreas and uncinate process were dissected free from the duodenal loop. The patient had undergone a previous choledochoduodenostomy and, as the duodenum was viable, it was not removed. All patients except one were discharged before the 10th postoperative day without evidence of sepsis. Among the total pancreatectomies, diabetes was well-controlled with insulin (30–40 units per day). At follow-up (6, 9, 10, and 18 months), all patients were asymptomatic. An insulinoma was excised without complications and the patient concerned is euglycemic.

The contact method of performing abdominal surgery with the Nd:YAG laser thus introduces a new era in laser surgery. Conventional non-contact air delivery Nd:YAG laser surgery is time-consuming, requires high laser energy (70–90 W), cannot be performed with sterile delivery systems, and is associated with excessive smoke production. Furthermore, the major problem, that the tips of the fibers melt and burn off when in contact with blood or tissue, has been totally eliminated using the contact synthetic sapphire probes. Coaxial water rather than gas is most useful. Previous experimental work with liver resection has indicated that the non-contact method of Nd:YAG laser surgery results in tissue necrosis at a depth of 3 to 5 mm, both vertical as well as lateral to the area being resected. The contact laser scalpel is associated with limited tissue damage of 0.5 to (rarely) 1 mm in depth. The SLT contact laser scalpel and cutting probes combine the coagulating properties of the Nd:YAG laser with cutting capabilities previously seen only with the CO_2 laser and electrocautery.

In what follows, potential applications of contact laser surgery in hepatic and pancreatic resection are discussed.

Table 9.1 **Abdominal operations in 55 patients** using the contact Nd:YAG laser system

Type of Operation	Pathology	No. of patients
Cholecystectomy	Gallstones	17
Liver resection	Tumors	15
Pancreatectomy	Pancreatitis, tumors	10
Adrenalectomy	Tumors	1
Gastric bypass	Obesity	9
Total colectomy	Ulcerative colitis	1
Exploratory laparotomy	Tumors, adhesions	2

Liver Resection

Indications

Hepatic resection is indicated for benign and malignant hepatic tumors, gallbladder or bowel carcinomas in continuity, cysts, abscess, or traumatic rupture of liver parenchyma. Metastases within the liver as solitary or multiple lesions are technically easy to resect provided the primary carcinoma (e. g. in the colon) has been removed. Possible hemorrhage associated with giant hemangiomas and the probability of malignant degeneration in adenomas are the main reasons for their excision. Resection for massive traumatic rupture confined to one anatomic lobe is usually preferred if multiple mattress sutures are inadequate in controlling blood loss.

Incision and Technique

Several incisions can be performed with the contact laser scalpel, but a bilateral subcostal (rooftop) or transverse supraumbilical incision is preferred. This can be extended into the chest through the seventh or eighth ribs on the right side. The diaphragm is incised and the phrenic nerve preserved to prevent diaphragmatic paralysis. A midline abdominal incision extended up as a median sternotomy also provides good exposure.

The SLT contact laser scalpel with a 0.2 to 0.4 mm diameter SLT frosted probe is used for the incision of subcutaneous tissue, muscle, fascia and peritoneum. Skin is incised either with a steel scalpel or with the laser scalpel. Power settings are 12 to 20 W with the laser set in the continuous wave (CW) and controlled by the foot switch. Coaxial air or CO_2 is used to cool the interphase between the quartz fiber and the synthetic sapphire probe. Water is never used.

The *principles* involved in the use of the SLT contact laser system are as follows. Laser power is *on* as the scalpel probe comes into contact with the tissue, and the laser is *off* as the probe comes off the tissue. If the probe sticks, it means that the power via the foot pedal was disengaged prior to the probe coming off the tissue. One must not pull the probe, but rather re-engage the laser: this will free the probe. Furthermore, the laser must not be on while the probe is not in direct contact with tissue. This may cause irreversible damage to the crystalline structure of the probe. If the probe begins to glow at its distal tip, the laser must be disengaged immediately or the tip will melt into a globular shape and the laser effect will be significantly diminished. The globular shape can be both seen and felt with the fingers, and the probe must be discarded.

Tissue adherent to the probe can easily be wiped off with a gauze swab. However, this is not necessary, as adherent tissue does not cause much impairment to the laser function. The tissue will become carbonized and burn off. Immediately after use, the probe is hot and should be allowed to cool for 20 to 30 seconds before being wiped with a wet sponge dipped in sterile water, saline or hydrogen peroxide. Alcohol should not be used, nor should the probe be cleaned with any abrasive material during the procedure.

The laser scalpel is not a mechanical cutting instrument. A "light touch" technique with gentle pressure is all that is required to obtain a cutting and coagulating effect. The laser energy must be allowed to do the incising. The more mechanical pressure used, the less effective the instrument is. The probe is therefore moved slowly and gently over the tissue in a continuous motion.

Traction and countertraction must be maintained at right angles to the incision at all times, either by manual pressure or by using retracting instruments. The laser power is controlled by the laser foot pedal in the continuous wave (CW) mode. This requires the surgeon to use eye–hand–foot coordination.

The laser power is set initially at 13 or 15 W, and the power is increased or decreased at 2 W increments until the desired tissue effect is obtained. The frosted laser probe with a tip diameter of 1.0 to 1.2 mm is used for liver resections, and may require higher laser power.

Major blood vessels are ligated or clipped. The technique for coagulating vessels 1 to 3 mm in size is to move the probe initially parallel to and on either side of the vessel to allow shrinkage and coagulation before transection. If bleeding occurs, it can be stopped using the lateral side of the frosted probe by "painting", or the vessel can be caught in a hemostat and the side of the probe applied directly to the transected vessel surface.

Initially the cutting process will appear slower than it is with a steel knife, but the major advantage is a hemostatic incision that does not need electrocautery or sutures. Increasing the speed of cutting can be achieved by increasing the power. The technique is rapidly learned, and experience is obtained by using the equipment frequently.

Anatomical Liver Resection Procedures

Resection of the liver with the SLT contact laser system can either be anatomical or nonanatomical (Table 9.2). Anatomical procedures are considered here first.

Right hepatic lobectomy. The line of liver resection extends from the gallbladder bed to the inferior vena cava (Fig. 9.1). Dissection is begun in the hilar region. The gallbladder is removed after division of the cystic artery and duct using the laser scalpel. The branches of the hepatic artery, portal vein, and bile ducts are carefully identified. The right hepatic duct and artery are ligated. If in doubt, a temporary occlusion is performed. If both the arterial and venous supplies to the right lobe are occluded, a line of color demarcation correspond-

Table 9.2   Operative procedures in the liver with the SLT contact Nd:YAG laser system

Disorder	Morbidity and Mortality	Treatment
Hepatic adenoma	Secondary intra-abdominal hemorrhage	Resection
Hemobilia	20 % mortality	Resection of hepatic segment with fistula
Hemangioma	Usually incidental, if large	Resection, if large, will rupture
Hepatocellular carcinoma (hepatoma)	High mortality	Resection
Metastatic nodules	Depends on primary malignancy and time interval	Enucleation, if single and no other sites of metastases; resection if multiple and technically possible

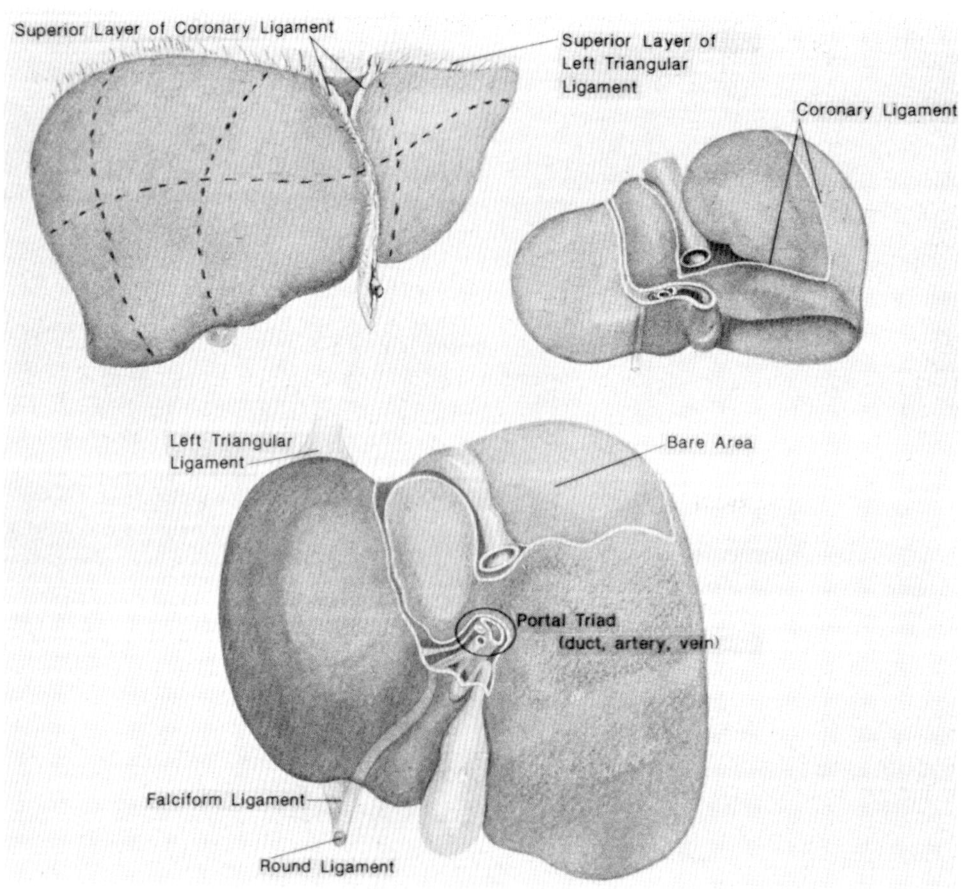

Fig. 9.1   **Normal anatomy of the liver** showing the ligaments, portal triad and sites of incision for hepatic lobectomies with the laser scalpel

ing to the anatomical division between the right and left lobes extending from the midpoint of the gallbladder fossa to the inferior vena cava is seen.

The right branch of the portal vein is doubly ligated and divided. The liver is rotated down and to the left to expose the inferior vena cava and the right hepatic veins. The right hepatic vein is ligated and divided carefully, as it is extremely short and easily torn. The line of liver resection is now marked out using the laser scalpel, leaving a margin of avascular liver for later identification of the middle hepatic vein. Dissection with the activated laser scalpel is begun just to the right of the center of the gallbladder fossa. The dissection is continued at a slight angle towards the left, following the trunk of the middle hepatic vein in the interlobar fissure.

Contact laser dissection is continued further into the liver substance, controlling the tributaries of the hepatic veins as they pass into the right lobe. This dissection is then carried down to the vena cava. This technique leaves a small amount of devitalized liver tissue along the margin, with preservation of the middle hepatic vein in the interlobar fissure. After the vena cava is reached, the right lobe is freed of its remaining attachments and removed. The new surface of the liver, if oozing, is "painted" over with the side of the laser scalpel. Large bleeding vessels are suture-ligated, and decompression of the biliary tree with a T-tube is not necessary. Catheter-type sump drains are placed in the wound and the incision is closed in layers.

Left hepatic lobectomy. The middle hepatic vein is the guideline for resection within the hepatic parenchyma, and should be preserved. Mobilization of the ductal structures proceeds in the same order as for right lobectomy. It is convenient to remove the gallbladder early on. The left triangular ligament is divided to mobilize the superior surface of the left lobe. By medial and downward traction on the liver, the hepatic veins are exposed. The left hepatic vein is carefully dissected into the liver substance. This locates the entrance of the middle hepatic vein. The left hepatic vein is carefully ligated and divided. Contact laser dissection is used to divide the liver substance, beginning just to the left of the gallbladder fossa and proceeding to the vena cava, leaving behind a border of the left lobe. The left lobe is freed of its remaining attachments and removed.

Left lateral segmental resection. The same abdominal incision as that described above is used. The left branches of the portal triad must not be ligated or divided, as this results in devitalization of the medial segment of the left lobe. The line of laser dissection should be approximately 1 cm to the left of the falciform ligament, to avoid damaging the structures of the medial segment of the left lobe and the left branch of the portal vein. In this resection the laser scalpel obviates the need for blunt dissection or multiple sutures through the liver. Individual large vessels are ligated. The falciform ligament can provide a peritoneal surface to cover the raw area of the liver. If oozing persists, the cut surface of the liver can be gently "painted" over using the side of the frosted laser scalpel.

Mesohepatectomy. Median hepatectomy is a method of resecting hilar cholangiocarcinomas, obtaining access to the bile ducts for anastomosis, or treating carcinoma of the gallbladder. The contact laser scalpel facilitates this anatomical procedure.

Non-Anatomical Liver Resection Procedures

Non-parasitic cysts. Small cysts discovered incidentally in surgical exploration or on CT scans require no treatment. Large cysts causing symptoms can be treated by surgical excision. If the cyst contains clear fluid and is difficult to excise because of its proximity to vascular or ductal structures, the cyst may be unroofed with the laser scalpel. Cystadenomas, cystadenocarcinomas and cysts associated with other neoplasms are excised with the laser scalpel.

Hepatocellular carcinoma. Tumors less than 3 cm in diameter should be resected non-anatomically with a good margin of normal liver (Fig. 9.2). The results of local wedge resection are similar to those of lobectomy. For larger, symptomatic tumors, the goal is to excise the tumor if possible. A standard laser hepatic lobectomy or extended hepatic resection is performed. However, in the case of extrahepatic spread, or where resection is not advisable, patients are treated with chemotherapy or radiation therapy, or both. The prognosis in this group is not good.

Metastatic tumors. The commonest origin of metastatic tumors in the liver is the colon. Five-year

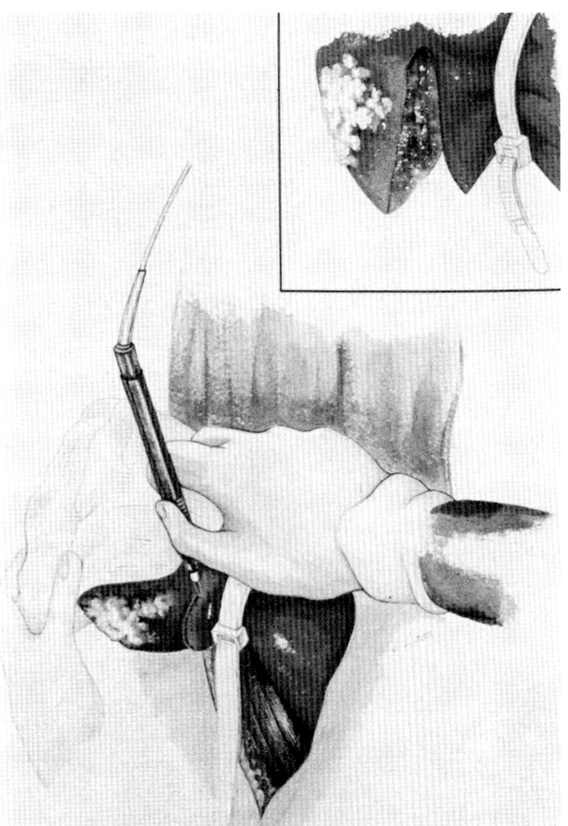

Fig. 9.**2** **Non-anatomical hepatic resection** using the SLT contact laser scalpel with a proximal liver strapper

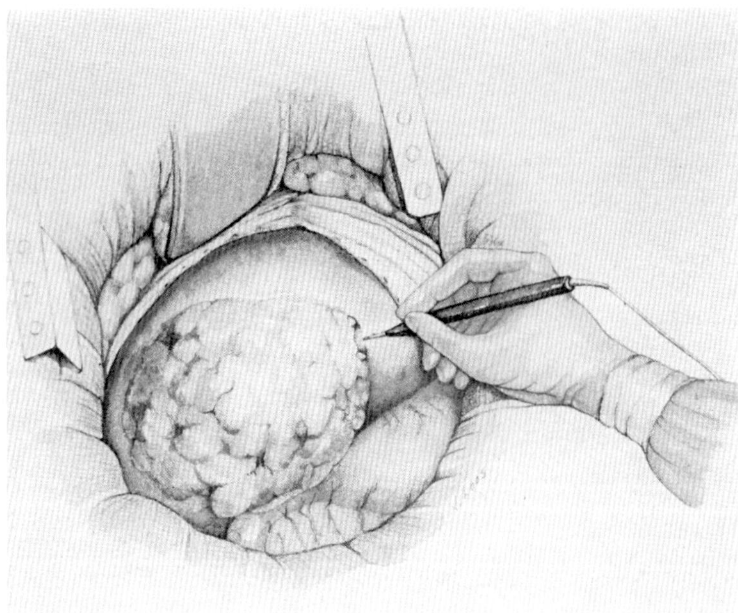

Fig. 9.**3** **Local excision of liver metastasis** using the SLT contact laser scalpel

survival in patients with resectable hepatic metastases is reported as high as 22 % after concomitant hepatic resection. Surgical treatment improves survival when the hepatic lesion is the only metastatic lesion. Complete curative resection of the primary lesion and resection of the metastases are therefore recommended. When hepatic metastases involve both lobes of the liver or when extrahepatic spread exists, surgical resection is not always indicated. Tumor debulking and excision of multiple liver metastases has been carried out using the laser scalpel with minimum blood loss (Fig. 9.3).

Complications with the Laser in Liver Surgery

One problem with the contact Nd:YAG laser in major liver surgery is the potential difficulty of identifying the largest central hepatic veins before partial perforation without adequate hemostasis. The SLT contact laser system is able to coagulate 80–85 % of the blood vessels. The remaining large vessels must be suture-ligated. This has led to the development of a modified technique for performing contact laser liver resection using a disposable plastic "strapper" as a proximal tourniquet to control the larger hepatic vessels (Schroder et al. 1986). The proximal resection surface is compressed by the "strapper", and the liver parenchyma distal to the tourniquet is resected with the laser scalpel (Fig. 9.2). This gives completely hemostatic resection without any bleeding, and liver resection can be completed rapidly. Thereafter all large vessels can be visualized and ligated during gradual release of the "strapper". Histological

studies have shown that this method did not cause any additional damage to the resected liver surface.

Liver resections are usually technically difficult, and are associated with problems in the control of bleeding. Laser techniques are not yet optimal, and all new techniques need to be evaluated critically. Use of the "strapper" with the SLT contact Nd:YAG laser system appears to be particularly promising. Larger clinical studies are needed to evaluate its application to human liver surgery.

Pancreatic Surgery

Indications

Major pancreatic surgery with the contact laser system is usually undertaken for tumors, trauma, pancreatitis, complications of pancreatitis, and congenital malformations (Table 9.3).

Incision

Transverse, bilateral subcostal or midline abdominal incisions are used. Occasionally, a left thoracoabdominal incision may be required. The SLT contact laser scalpel is used for this procedure.

Resection Procedures

Pancreatoduodenectomy. Using the SLT contact laser scalpel, the peritoneum lateral to the second part of the duodenum is divided to expose the inferior vena cava. The common bile duct is

Table 9.3 Types of pancreatic procedure using the SLT contact laser scalpel

Operation	Indications
Pancreatoduodenectomy	Carcinoma of the head of the pancreas, distal common bile duct, ampulla of Vater or duodenum
Total pancreatectomy	Carcinoma of the head or body of the pancreas Chronic pancreatitis
Distal pancreatectomy	Carcinoma of the tail of the pancreas Chronic pancreatitis Islet cell tumor
Pancreaticojejunostomy	Chronic pancreatitis
Cystogastrostomy or cystojejunostomy	Pseudocyst
Enucleation of a tumor	Insulinoma or pancreatic cystadenoma
Annuloplasty	Annular pancreas
Sphincteroplasty	Stenosis of the ampulla of Vater

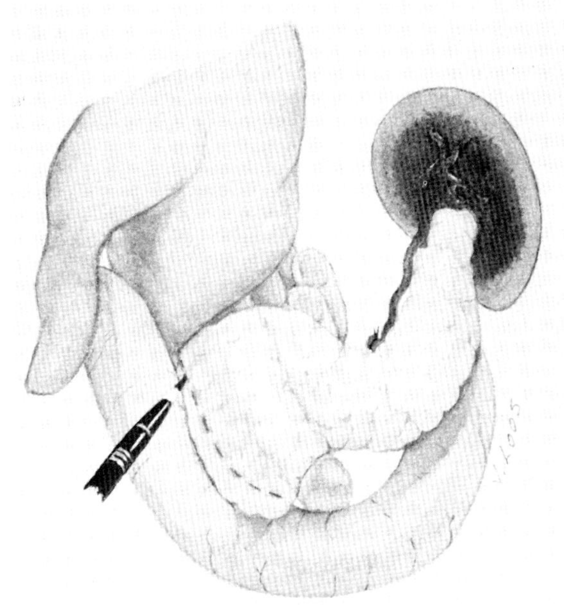

Fig. 9.4 Near-total pancreatectomy with preservation of the duodenum

retracted to the right. The right gastric artery is divided between ligatures, and the gastroduodenal artery is identified and ligated. A finger is inserted between the pancreas and the portal vein to ensure resectability. The stomach is divided between clamps with the laser scalpel, and the common bile duct transected at a selected point. The body of the pancreas to the left of the portal and superior mesenteric vessels is mobilized using the laser scalpel. A Kocher dissector is placed behind the pancreas at the selected site of division, and four stay sutures are placed in the pancreatic substance. The pancreas is then divided with the frosted 1.0 or 1.2 mm laser scalpel.

The whole of the duodenum and the upper few cm of the jejunum are removed using the laser scalpel, with ligation of the larger vessels. The pancreas to be removed is now detached from the superior mesenteric vessels, dividing the small vessels between the duodenum and the uncinate process. The inferior pancreatoduodenal artery is secured and divided. Using the laser scalpel, a thin slice of the uncinate process is left behind to protect the superior mesenteric vein. The tumor is now removed and a standard reconstruction is performed.

Total pancreatectomy. The operative technique is identical to that described above for pancreatoduodenectomy, except that instead of dividing the pancreas, the whole of the distal pancreas is mobilized so that the entire organ may be removed. Occasionally, for chronic pancreatitis, a near-total pancreatectomy is performed, with preservation of the duodenum. The laser scalpel is used to divide the pancreas and preserve the duodenum (Fig. 9.4).

Distal pancreatectomy. The body of the pancreas is exposed by dividing the gastrocolic omentum and widely opening the lesser sac. Using the laser scalpel, the spleen is mobilized from the posterior abdominal wall by dividing the lienorenal ligament. The gastrosplenic ligaments are then divided and the larger vessels ligated. With the stomach freed from the spleen, the peritoneum above and below the body and tail of the pancreas are incised with the laser scalpel. The distal pancreas and spleen are lifted forward. The body and tail of the pancreas and spleen are turned over to the right, exposing their posterior surfaces. The splenic vein is dissected to its proximal end and ligated and divided. At a slightly higher level the splenic artery is found, ligated and divided. The neck of pancreas is then mobilized from the portal vein using gentle dissection with the laser scalpel. Two stay sutures are inserted and the neck of the pancreas is divided with the laser scalpel. If indicated, the tail and part of the body of the pancreas are excised, with preservation of the spleen and splenic vessels. A small unobstructed pancreatic duct is ligated and divided, and the pancreatic neck is oversewn. If the pancreatic duct is dilated, an anastomosis of the duct to a loop of jejunum is undertaken using a standard technique.

Enucleation of a pancreatic cystadenoma or insulinoma. Removal of these tumors by enucleation is safe if they are encapsulated, with a well-defined plane of cleavage. Otherwise, partial pancreatectomy should be performed. The compressed pancreatic tissue overlying the cystadenoma is palpated and incised down to the capsule using the laser scalpel. Enucleation is performed using the finger or the laser scalpel between the pancreatic substance and the capsule of the mass. An insulinoma is similarly excised by obtaining a cleavage between the tumor and the normal pancreas. In the head, this is performed carefully to avoid a pancreatic fistula. If the cavity is small the incision is closed, but larger cavities are left open.

Conclusion

The SLT contact Nd:YAG laser system offers a new method of obtaining a hemostatic incision through the anterior abdominal wall, and is a surgical tool capable of performing various intra-abdominal resectional procedures, including liver and pancreatic surgery. Its advantages include a reduction in intraoperative bleeding, reduced tissue damage and tactile sensation with a reduction in laser power requirements. Sterile disposable laser scalpels and fibers, reusable synthetic sapphire probes and a user-friendly laser system offer a new dimension in liver and pancreatic surgery.

Potentially, all general surgical procedures could use the SLT contact laser, which may, in the future, replace conventional electrocautery and the surgical steel scalpel. Cost containment, physician education and an improvement in the quality of patient care will probably be the driving force for its acceptance.

Acknowledgment

"SLT contact Nd:YAG laser system" and "SLT contact laser scalpel" are registered trademarks of Surgical Laser Technologies, Inc., Malvern, PA, USA.

References

Berlatzky Y, Muggia-Sullam M, Munda R, Joffe SN. Use of Nd:YAG laser in pancreatic resections with duodenal preservation in the dog. Lasers Surg Med 1985; 5: 107–514.

Daikuzono N, Joffe SN. An artificial sapphire probe for contact photocoagulation and tissue vaporization. Med Instrum 1985; 19: 173–178.

Fidler JP, Hoeter RW, Polyani TG. Laser surgery in exsanguinating liver injury. Ann Surg 1975; 181: 74–80.

Joffe SN. Contact neodymium:YAG laser surgery in gastroenterology: a preliminary report. Lasers Surg Med 1986; 6: 155–157.

Joffe SN, Brackett KA, Sankar MY, Daikuzono N. Resection of the liver with the Nd:YAG laser. Surg Gynecol Obstet 1986; 163: 437–442.

Meyer H-J, Haverkampf K. Experimental study of partial liver resection with a combined CO_2 and Nd:YAG laser. Lasers Surg Med 1982; 2: 149–154.

Munda R, Berlatzky Y, Jonung M, Murphy RF, Brackett K, Joffe SN, Alexander JW. Studies of segmental pancreatic autotransplants in dogs. Arch Surg 1983; 118: 1310–1315.

Ross RL, Breasch JW, O'Bryan EM, Watkins E Jr. Segmental pancreatic autotransplantation for chronic pancreatitis. Gastroenterology 1983; 84: 621–626.

Schroder T, Joffe SN, Sankar MY, Brackett KM. Major liver resection in the pig using contact Nd:YAG laser: a new technique. Tokyo: International Nd:YAG Laser Symposium, 1986.

Schroder T, Brackett KA, Joffe SN. Proximal pancreatectomy: a comparison of electrocautery with the contact and noncontact Nd:YAG laser techniques in the dog. Am J Surg 1987; 5: 493–498.

Sultan RA, Fallouh H, Lefebvre-Vilardebo M, Ladouch-Badre A. Separate and combined use of Nd:YAG and carbon dioxide lasers in liver resections: a preliminary report. Lasers Med Sci 1986; 1: 101–105.

Tranberg KG, Rigotti P, Brackett KA, Bjornson HP, Fischer JE, Joffe SN. Liver resection: a comparison using the Nd:YAG laser, ultrasonic aspirator, or blunt dissection. Am J Surg 1985; 151: 368–372.

10 Postoperative and Palliative Management

10.1 Postoperative Evaluation: Complications, Risk Factors and Etiology

P.L.M. Jansen

Jaundice is often the presenting sign in hepatobiliary or pancreatic malignancy. The yellow discoloration of sclerae, skin, mucous membranes and urine is caused by retention of conjugated bilirubin as a result of impairment of complete blockage of bile flow by a tumor mass in the biliary tree or pancreas head. The dark urine and light stools show that, in these patients, renal excretion is the major pathway for elimination of bilirubin. Bile pigments in the serum of patients with extrahepatic obstruction consist of various forms of bilirubin: bilirubin diglucuronide and monoglucuronide, unconjugated bilirubin and bilirubin-albumin (Lauff et al. 1982). Bilirubin-albumin represents conjugated bilirubin which is covalently bound to albumin. Bilirubin is conjugated to albumin because the glucuronic acid moiety of bilirubin monoglucuronide or diglucuronide is replaced by a free amino acid group of albumin at the bilirubin binding site (Yoshida et al. 1987). In contrast, unconjugated bilirubin is non-covalently bound to albumin. The presence of bilirubin-albumin is a sign of chronic biliary obstruction. It becomes the predominant form of serum bilirubin in the early period after desobstruction of the bile duct. Unless there is sepsis, liver fibrosis or cirrhosis, the liver then rapidly resumes its excretory activities, and bilirubin glucuronides are cleared from the blood. However, bilirubin-albumin is retained, because this large molecular weight pigment cannot be excreted either via the bile or via the urine. Its disappearance only takes place with the biological degradation of albumin, which takes about twelve days. This is about the time that is required for a jaundiced patient's color to return to normal. (Weiss et al. 1983).

Pathophysiology of Jaundice

Toxicity of Bilirubin and Bile Salts

Extrahepatic biliary obstruction not only causes jaundice but also retention of bile salts, cholesterol, phospholipids, leukotrienes, and the enzymes alkaline phosphatase and γ-glutamyl transferase. Bilirubin and bile salts have toxic effects on various organ systems. Bilirubin inhibits the cellular immune response and spontaneous motility, chemotaxis and phagocytic activity of granulocytes (Rola-Pleszcynski et al. 1975, Rubaltelli et al. 1982). Patients with cholestasis have impaired phagocytic Kupffer cell function (Drivas et al. 1976). Bilirubin is a potent antioxidant, depresses cellular oxidation, and uncouples oxidative phosphorylation (Zetterstrom et al. 1956, Cowger et al. 1965). This may play a role in the brain damage caused by unconjugated bilirubin in kernicterus. It is an old dogma that after the neonatal period the „blood-brain barrier" becomes impermeable for bilirubin, but studies in rats have not shown any difference of blood-brain permeability in neonates and adults (Cornford et al. 1982). Hypoxia, acidosis and perhaps other factors may allow the penetration of bilirubin into the brain of neonates. Recently, it has been observed that also in adolescents with Crigler-Najjar disease (a genetic deficiency of bilirubin glucuronidation), high bilirubin levels can cause neurological damage (Blaschke et al. 1974). Other toxic effects of bilirubin include the *in vitro* depression of fibroblast function, inhibition of prolyl hydroxylase activity, and collagen synthesis (Taube et al. 1981, Than 1976; Greaney 1979). These various toxic effects of bilirubin may explain the impaired wound healing in jaundiced patients, although malnutrition and the presence of malignancy may be more important. Delayed wound healing in a group of jaundiced patients was restricted to patients with malignant disease and while patients with benign causes of jaundice had normal wound healing (Irvin et al. 1978). Factors like tumor necrosis factor (cachectin) may play a role under these circumstances (Beutler and Cerami 1987). Bilirubin, cholesterol and bile salts may affect biological membranes, in particular those of erythrocytes (Kawai et al. 1981, Sato et al. 1987, Lowe et al. 1981). However, clinically important hemolysis is not a feature of obstructive jaundice *per se*, except when complicated by endotoxemia or sepsis (Powell et al. 1968).

Leukotrienes

The metabolism of leukotrienes and endotoxins is highly relevant to an understanding of the complications that can occur in the postoperative period after biliary tract or pancreatic surgery. Although jaundice and pruritus are important clinical signs in patients with bile duct obstruction, the concomitant impairment of leukotriene disposition during bile duct obstruction may have a more profoundly adverse influence on vital organs. Leukotrienes are mediators of inflammatory action, causing such diverse effects as leucocyte accumulation, proliferation to T-lymphocytes, stimulation of natural cytotoxic cells (LTB-4), and smooth muscle contraction with effects on airways, coronary circulation, renal circulation and microvascular permeability (LTC-4, LTD-4 and LTE-4) (Lewis et al. 1984, Keppler et al. 1985). With regard to the latter activity, leukotrienes are about 5000 times more potent than histamine.

In the liver, major hepatobiliary excretion pathways are the bile salt transport system and the bilirubin transport pathway. Leukotrienes are predominantly cleared via the bile (Hagmann et al. 1984), and leukotriene excretion has been shown to occur via the bilirubin pathway (Huber et al. 1987). In extrahepatic biliary obstruction, both the bile salt and bilirubin transport pathways are blocked, causing retention of leukotrienes. Prolonged retention of these agents may cause

hypotension, reduction of cardiac output, impairment of renal blood flow and extensive extravasation of plasma, with contraction of circulatory volume and eventually shock (Lewis et al. 1984, Keppler et al. 1985). Intravascular biological inactivation by conjugation with glutathione represents an alternative to dispose of leukotrienes (Keppler et al. 1985 and 1987). Interestingly, γ-glutamyl transferase helps in the inactivation of leukotrienes. The other „enzyme of cholestasis‟, alkaline phosphatase, activates lipocortin by dephosphorylation. Activated lipocortin inhibits phospholipase, and thus diminishes arachidonate liberation from membrane phospholipids. Arachidonic acid is an important precursor of leukotrienes. Thus γ-glutamyl transferase and alkaline phosphatase may not only be markers of cholestasis, but may also play a role in inhibiting leukotriene activity (Keppler et al. 1985). Alkaline phosphatase synthesis in bile duct epithelium and hepatocytes is induced in early cholestasis, and is released from the membranes of the hepatocytes through the action of bile salts. Arachidonic acid, however, is a precursor not only of leukotrienes but also of other eicosanoids, such as the prostaglandins. Whether release of alkaline phosphatase into the circulation also causes inhibition of prostaglandin synthesis remains to be established.

Endotoxins

Leukotrienes are produced by macrophages, monocytes, neutrophils, eosinophils, mast cells and Kupffer cells. The various triggers for their synthesis include surgical trauma, bacterial endotoxins, platelet-activating and tumor necrosis factor (van Deventer et al. 1988). Bacterial endotoxins impair the hepatic elimination of bilirubin and not only stimulate the production of leukotrienes but also strongly inhibit their hepatic elimination (Hagmann et al. 1984). The gut is a rich source of bacterial endotoxins, where they are produced by gram-negative bacteria. Endotoxins reach the ciruclation via lymph and the thoracic duct, and via the portal vein (van Deventer et al. 1988). Endotoxemia probably plays a central and still underestimated role in many of the postoperative complications of biliary tract and pancreatic surgery (Bailey 1976). Problems with measuring endotoxin in the blood with the limulus test have recently been resolved and this test should be used to demonstrate endotoxemia in the postoperative period (Cooperstock and Riegle 1985).

Jaundiced patients have a high incidence of portal and systemic endotoxemia (Bailey 1976). Bile salts in the gut reduce the intestinal absorption of endotoxins (Kocsar et al. 1969). Absence of bile salts in the intestine of jaundiced patients, and surgical manipultion of the gut, may cause endotoxemia. Slight endotoxemia may occur commonly after abdominal operations, but the hepatic Kupffer cells and macrophage system can deal with this. However, overwhelming endotoxemia due to the absence of bile salts in the intestine of a jaundiced patient with a depressed Kupffer cell and macrophage system may cause problems. Endotoxins stimulate leukotriene synthesis. This may cause fever, thrombocytopenia, disseminated intravascular coagulation, drowsiness, renal failure, impairment of hepatic function, and occasionally shock (Lewis and Austen 1984, Kepler et al. 1985, van Deventer et al. 1988). Prevention of endotoxemia may be achieved by preoperative mechanical cleaning of the gut, oral administration of bile salts, or internal drainage procedures of the obstructed bile duct (Evans et al. 1982, Gouma et al. 1986). Antibiotics do not significantly reduce the amount of endotoxins in the gut, with the exception of polymyxin. Preoperative bowel preparation with antibiotics did not have any clinical benefit (van Deventer et al. 1988). In addition, preoperative external drainage of bile in jaundiced patients did not affect postoperative morbidity and mortality (Hatfield et al. 1982, McPherson et al. 1984, Pitt et al. 1985). Possible benefits of preoperative biliary decompression were offset by complications of the drainage procedures. This leaves open the question of whether newer endoscopic drainage procedures will have a beneficial effect on postoperative morbidity and mortality. Whatever procedure is attempted, the introduction of resistant hospital-acquired bacteria into the biliary tract should be avoided. Therefore, at present only patients with cholangitis or sepsis should be drained preoperatively. Unnecessary manipulation of the biliary tree should be avoided in jaundiced non-septic patients.

Postoperative Complications

Major postoperative complications are: 1 strictly surgical problems, such as dehiscence of anastomoses, leakage of bile and other fluids into the abdominal cavity causing fluid collections which may infect or cause ileus, hemorrhage, bile duct injury; 2 renal failure; 3 bacteremia and disseminated intravascular coagulation; 4 respiratory and cardiac failure; 5 liver failure when extensive hepatic resections are done; and 6 pancreatitis.

Risk Factors for Development of Postoperative Complications

Risk factors for the development of postoperative complications are jaundice, pre-existent medical disease, as diabetes mellitus, chronic pulmonary disease, cardiac arrhythmias, cholangitis, duration of operation and blood loss (Armstrong et al. 1984, Pitt et al. 1981, Stimpson et al. 1987, Blamey et al. 1983, Pellegrini et al. 1987). Liver cirrhosis is known to have a major adverse influence on postoperative morbidity and mortality of liver resections (Ong and Lee 1975, Nagao et al. 1985). Pitt et al. (1981) studied the factors affecting mortality in biliary tract surgery. Malignancy, jaundice, raised alkaline phosphatase, infection, renal failure, age above 60 years, anemia and hypoalbuminemia were the eight risk factors. When a combination of factors was present, mortality increased: with 5 risk factors present, mortality was 50%; 6 factors, 75%; and 7–8 factors, 100%. Patients underwent a wide variety of bile duct operations, with the exception of simple cholecystectomy. The overall mortality was 7.7%. The highest mortality was associated with hepatojejunostomy (19%). No hepatectomies were performed in this study. Blamey et al. (1983) reported that postoperative hemorrhage was more common in patients with preoperative bilirubin levels above 100 µmol/l, in the presence of malignancy and after surgical resections. Sepsis was more common after resections. Renal failure occurred more often in patients with preoperative serum creatinine levels above 130 µmol/l, serum bilirubin above 100 µmol/l, albumin below 30 g/l, and in the presence of malignancy and diabetes. Allison et al (1979) mention that a raised fibrin degradation product level preoperatively is associated with a poor postoperative outcome. Pellegrini et al. (1987) point out that morbidity and mortality after biliary surgery is not related to bilirubin levels *per se* but to concomitant diseases commonly found in patients with increased bilirubin levels, such as malignancy, cholangitis, cardiovascular, pulmonary, hepatic, renal and metabolic disease.

Renal Failure

Abdominal surgery in jaundiced patients is associated with a relatively high incidence of acute renal failure. About 6–18% seem to be affected postoperatively, and improvement of perioperative care and anesthesia has not influenced this figure (Armstrong et al. 1984, Pitt et al. 1981, Blamey et al. 1983). It is associated with a high mortality. Allison (1988) reported renal failure in 17% of jaundiced patients after hepatobiliary surgery and in 1% of non-jaundiced patients. Renal failure was associated with 100% mortality in this series. Potentially reversible prerenal oliguria often precedes irreversible renal failure. This is seen in patients with hypotension, hypovolemia and infection. Rapid correction of these conditions is mandatory to prevent further deterioration of renal function.

Why jaundiced patients are more prone to develop renal failure is not well understood. Obstructive jaundice by itself is associated with impaired renal function in 30% of patients (MCPherson et al. 1982). Impairment of urinary concentrating ability is seen in obstructive jaundice, and patients with obstructive jaundice are more prone to salt and water depletion (Allison et al. 1979). Cirrhotic patients are inclined to salt retention. Failure of the heart to elaborate enough auriculin or atrial natriuretic factor to overcome renal sodium retention may play an important role in the disturbance of sodium homeostasis in patients with liver cirrhosis (Laragh 1985). In addition, the renal vasculature in the jaundiced patient is more sensitive to the vasoconstrictive action of catecholamines (Bomzon and Kew 1983). Biliary constituents may have a cardiodepressor effect, a condition known as „the jaundiced heart". This „jaundiced heart" is not necessarily a depressed heart. Often the cardiac output is increased, and peripheral resistance and arterial pressure is decreased. This may be due to the presence of vasodilator substances. This explains the observation that relatively small volume losses tend to cause prolonged hypotension in jaundiced patients (Williams et al. 1960). Because of these pre-existent disturbances of renal and cardiac function, and diminished responsiveness of the cardiovascular system, meticulous fluid replacement should be carried out during operation of jaundiced patients. If renal failure occurs after operation, volume deficits and hypotension should be corrected without delay, and infections should be treated forthwith. Mannitol infusions are particularly helpful to induce diuresis and natriuresis (Allison et al. 1979, Dawson 1964). Wardle (1975) reported endotoxemia in 73% of patients with acute renal failure, and this author attributes renal failure to endotoxemia in a great number of cases. As we have seen above, the jaundiced patient is particularly prone to develop clinically important endotoxemia during or after abdominal surgery.

Renal prostaglandins are important for the maintenance of renal plasma flow, natriuresis, and glomerular filtration (Epstein 1986). Non-steroidal anti-inflammatory drugs are cyclo-oxygenase inhibitors which inhibit renal prostaglandin synthesis. Drugs like indomethacin, ibuprofen, naproxen, aspirin and probably also sulindac should be avoided, because they may precipitate or aggravate frank renal failure in jaundiced hypovolemic patients (Epstein 1986, Boyer et al. 1979, Zipser et al. 1979, Brater et al. 1985).

Hepatorenal Syndrome

The term hepatorenal syndrome should be reserved for „unexplained progressive renal failure occurring in patients with liver disease in the absence of clinical, laboratory or anatomic evidence of other known causes of renal failure" (Epstein 1988). Urine of patients with hepatorenal syndrome is practically sodium-free. Bleeding, hypovolemia, diuretics, aminoglycosides and non-steroidal anti-inflammatory drugs can precipitate hepatorenal syndrome in patients with liver disease. However, in contrast to prerenal failure, renal function in hepatorenal syndrome does not respond to blood volume replacement. Cortical vasoconstriction in the kidney is typically seen in hepatorenal syndrome. Hypovolemia may be the precipitating factor, but the factors that are responsible for the sustained supression of renal cortical flow have not been characterized yet.

Hepatic Failure

Surgical removal of cholangiocarcinoma located at the bifurcation of the right and left hepatic bile ducts usually involves partial hepatectomy. Partial hepatectomies are also carried out for primary liver cell carcinoma and metastatic liver disease. For these patients, preoperative evaluation of liver function is mandatory. The prognosis of partial hepatic resection in liver cirrhosis is poor (Ong and Lee 1975, Nagao et al. 1985). When this type of operation is planned, it is particularly important to avoid preoperative instrumental contamination of the biliary tract, because infectious complications after partial hepatectomy have a dismal prognosis.

Hepatic failure after extensive hepatectomies may be accompanied by hepatic encephalopathy, hemorrhagic diathesis, hypoglycemia, hepatorenal syndrome, and acute respiratory distress syndrome requiring mechanical ventilation. If hepatic encephalopathy occurs in the immediate postoperative period, an underlying cause is usually present, such as sepsis, endotoxemia, bleeding, dehydration or electrolyte imbalance. The liver has a considerable functional reserve capacity. Hepatic resections with removal of more than 70% of the liver in a patient with a good liver function can be done without running into severe hepatic failure. The liver is the principial organ for synthesis of clotting factors and albumin. After partial hepatectomy clotting factors and serum albumin decrease temporarily, but not to the degree expected on the basis of the liver volume removed. Furthermore, the synthesis of these factors is restored long before the liver has regenerated. The same applies for other liver functions (Zoli et al. 1986). In rats, a 70% hepatectomy caused only a 20% reduction of galactose elimination capacity (Yildirim and Poulsen 1981). Aminopyrene demethylation activity more closely follows the reduction of liver volume (Sendama et al. 1985). This is a cytochrome P-450-dependent activity.

Thus, drugs that are metabolized in the liver should be administered cautiously after partial hepatectomy, and the dose should be adjusted. In a study from Bologna, it was shown that removal of 50% of total liver volume in man was associated with about 25% reduction of albumin, 20% reduction of galactose elimination capacity, and only 10% reduction of prothrombin activity. Serum cholinesterase activity closely followed liver volume. Prothrombin activity returned to normal two weeks after operation (Zoli et al. 1986). In cirrhotics, no restoration of liver function occurred after partial hepatectomy in 3 out of 7 patients in a study from Taiwan (Lin and Chen 1965). In our hospital, a study was performed on liver function and liver regeneration in patients undergoing partial hepatectomy for Klatskin tumors and liver metastases. Liver volume was monitored scintigraphically (single photon emission computer tomography). The data in Table 10.1.1 show that caffeine clearance correlated with resected liver volume, whereas galactose elimination decreased to a relatively smaller degree.

Table 10.1.1 Liver function and liver volume after partial hepatectomy

	Before resection	After resection
Liver volume (ml)	2100 ± 300	980 ± 320
Caffeine clearance		
ml/min/kg body weight	1.5 ± 0.9	0.6 ± 0.3
l/min/ml liver	52 ± 27	54 ± 27
Galactose elimination		
mol/min/kg body weight	36 ± 7	23 ± 5
mol/min/ml liver	1.2 ± 0.5	1.5 ± 0.2

In the normal liver, hepatocytes divide approximately once a year. However, these cells have not lost their capacity to divide more rapidly. This capacity is used in acute viral or toxic hepatitis to replace dead cells by normally functioning hepatocytes. This latent potential for cell division is a fortunate quality of hepatocytes, since otherwise substantial liver resections would not be possible. The data from our study confirm this potential for liver regeneration. After removal of 50% of liver volume, the liver regenerated to about 80% of its original volume in 20 weeks.

The factors that trigger liver regeneration are not known precisely. After partial hepatectomy, three phases of cellular metabolism can be distinguished. First, there is a prereplicative phase of cellular hypertrophy. This coincides with a period of metabolic overload with increased electrolyte fluxes, increased Na/K ATPase activity, and increased ATP consumption. Protooncogenes are expressed in this period. This may be instrumental

for production of liver-derived hepatotrophic factors or receptor proteins. The next steps are those of DNA replication, followed by cell division. Several extrahepatic hepatotrophic factors such as insulin, glucagon, noradrenalin, and epithelial growth factor may play a role in liver regeneration. "Cytosolic hepatic stimulatory substance", purified from the cytosol of regenerating rat liver (LaBrecque and Pesch 1975), and "hepatopoietin", purified from rat serum after partial hepatectomy (Michalopoulos et al. 1984), cause DNA replication in cell culture, and increase the survival of rats after galactosamine-induced hepatitis. Serum of patients who underwent partial hepatectomy contains factors that increase DNA synthesis in cultured rat hepatocytes (Kubo et al. 1987). These investigations may lead to agents that can actively influence liver regeneration.

Recommendations for Postoperative Care after Liver or Biliary Tract Surgery

Attention Points

After liver or biliary tract surgery, several points of particular interest should be kept in mind. They are summarized in Table 10.1.2. Drug metabolism may be impaired after partial hepatectomy. Decreased serum albumin causes an increased volume of distribution for albumin-bound drugs and an increased free unbound fraction. Patients with latent encephalophathy have increased central sensitivity for benzodiazepines. In addition, hepatic drug metabolism is decreased, and dosage intervals must be increased to avoid drug accumulation. All anesthetics cause a decrease of liver blood flow and the blood flow-oxygen consumption ratio of the liver (Libonati et al. 1973, Strunin 1977.) Surgical manipulation of the intestines, relative hypoxia and hypercarbia, and increased sympathic tone decrease splanchnic blood flow and therefore tend to cause a relative ischemia of the liver during major

Table 10.1.2 Postoperative care of jaundiced patients: attention points

1 Meticulous water and electrolyte balance
2 Remove non-producing drains
3 Treat infections without delay
4 Supply clotting factors with fresh frozen plasma
5 In case of hepatic encephalopathy, look for precipitating factors such as electrolyte imbalance, hypoglycemia, gastrointestinal bleeding, inadvertent administration of benzodiazepines
6 Treat hepatic encephalopathy with lactulose or lactitol and protein restriction
7 In case of hepatic resection, adjust drug doses
8 Treat prerenal failure forthwith. Avoid non-steroidal anti-inflammatory drugs. Adjust aminoglycoside doses

abdominal operations. Increased serum transaminase activities after extensive liver or biliary tract operations can often be attributed to liver ischemia during the operation. This of course should be differentiated from halothane hepatitis, cytomegaly infection and non-A-non-B hepatitis. The interval between in increase of transaminases and the operation usually lead the way to the correct diagnosis.

Postoperative clotting abnormalities can be corrected by administration of fresh froozen plasma (10–20 ml/kg) and vitamin K (10 mg b.i.d.). Increased fibrinolysis can be counteracted by tranexamic acid. Bleeding from the upper gastrointestinal tract can be treated locally, depending on the cause, with injection sclerotherapy (bleeding ulcers or varices), laser coagulation or bicap thermal cauterization. For massively bleeding varices, balloon tamponade should be used. Intravenous administration of vasopressin or somatostatin is sometimes effective to stop bleeding from esophageal varices or other upper gastrointestinal lesions.

Electrolytes should be corrected, and a meticulous balance of fluids should be maintained. Electrolyte disturbances can be cofactors in the precipitation of hepatic encephalopathy. If hepatic encephalopathy occurs, protein intake should be restricted to 40 g daily, and lactulose or lactitol should be prescribed (Morgan and Hawley 1987). These laxatives inhibit ammonia production by gut bacteria, mainly by lowering the intestinal pH. If total parenteral nutrition is given, amino acid solutions can be replaced by branched-chain amino acids. Lipid solutions should not be given at all to patients with liver failure. To avoid hypoglycemia, concentrated 10% or 20% glucose solutions should be administered. Dehydration leads to prerenal failure, and may cause hepatorenal syndrome in patients with liver failure. Too much fluid, however, can cause ascites, with distension of the abdominal wall, impaired wound healing and, when extensive, dyspnoea.

Antibiotics

In this chapter, endotoxemia and sepsis have been stressed as important factors in the development of various postoperative complications. Judicious use of antibiotics either preoperatively or postoperatively is therefore very important. Preoperative administration of antibiotics should be started in a patient with a history of recent cholangitis, even if the fever has abated after endoscopic or percutaneous insertion of an endoprosthesis. The biliary ducts are probably still infected, and manipulation of the liver or bile ducts, intermittent cessation of bile flow during reconstruction procedures, and

spillage of bile into the peritoneal cavity, may reactivate a preexistent infection. The antibiotics administered should be bactericidal, aimed at gram-negative bacteria, and they should have good penetration in liver tissue, bile and stagnant bile present in obstructed liver segments. When a patient develops fever postoperatively, every effort should be made to obtain blood, urine, sputum or pus specimens for culture, since these are complicated patients who may be infected with multidrug-resistant bacteria. Often there is no time to await the results of cultures, and administration of antibiotics should be started on the basis of known resistance patterns in a particular hospital or a particular patient. Aminoglycosides are the drugs of choice for the treatment of gram-negative sepsis in combination with either a (synthetic) penicillin or a cephalosporin. Aminoglycoside serum levels should be monitored, and the dosage should be adjusted by prolonging the dose interval in patients with impaired renal function. Nomograms for dose adjustment in relation to the glomerular filtration rate are available (Bennet et al. 1977). In addition to the judicious use of antibiotics, measures should be taken to avoid contamination of the patient. Every day that a urinary catheter remains in situ increases the chances of a urinary tract infection by 5% (Wenzel 1985). Abdominal drains that do not drain should be repositioned or removed. Physical therapy to increase ventilation and assist the coughing up of sputum should be started as soon as possible. These simple measures shorten the hospital stay, reduce the costs of the operation, and prolong the life of the patient.

References

Allison MEM. The kidney and the liver: Pre- and postoperative factors. In: Blumgart LH, ed. Edinburgh; Churchill Livingstone, Surgery of the liver and biliary tract. 1988: 405–421.

Allison MEM, Prentice CRM, Kennedy AC, Blumgart LH. Renal function and other factors in obstructive jaundice. Br J Surg 1979; 66: 392–397.

Armstrong CP, Dixon JM, Taylor TV, Davies GC. Surgical experience of deeply jaundiced patients with bile duct obstruction. Br J Surg 1984; 71: 234–38.

Bailey ME. Endotoxin, bile salts and renal function in obstructive jaundice. Br J Surg 1976; 63: 774–778.

Bennet WM, Singer I, Golper T, et al. Guidelines for drug therapy in renal failure. Ann Intern Med 1977; 86: 754–783.

Beutler, B, Cerami A. Cachectin: more than a tumor necrosis factor. New Engl. J Med 1987; 316: 379–385.

Blamey SL, Fearon KCH, Gilmour WH, et al. Prediction of risk in biliary surgery. Br J Surg 1983; 70: 535–538.

Blaschke TF, Berk PD, Scharschmidt BF, et al. Crigler-Najjar syndrome: an unusual course with development of neurological damage at age eighteen. Pediatr Res 1974; 8: 573–590.

Bomzon L, Kew MC. Renal blood flow in experimental obstructive jaundice. In: Epstein M, ed. The kidney in liver disease. Amsterdam: Elsevier, 1983: 313–326.

Boyer TD, Zia P, Reynolds TB. Effect of indomethacin and prostaglandin A1 on renal function and plasma renin activity in alcoholic liver disease. Gastroenterology 1979; 77: 215–222.

Brater DC, Anderson S, Baird B, et al. Effects of ibuprofen, naproxen, and sulindac on prostaglandins in men. Kidney Int 1985; 27: 66–73.

Cooperstock M, Riegle L. Plasma Limulus gelation assay in infants and children: correlation with gram-negative bacterial infection and evidence for "intestinal endotoxemia". In: ten Cate JW, Buller HR, Sturk A, Levin J, eds. Bacterial endotoxins: structure, biomedical significance and detection with the Limulus amebocyte lysate test. New York: Liss, 1985: 307–314.

Conford EM, Braun LD, Oldendorp WH, Hill MA. Comparison of lipid-mediated blood-brain-barrier penetration in neonates and adults. Am J. Physiol 1982; 243: C161–C168.

Cowger ML, Igo RP, Labbe RF. The mechanism of bilirubin toxicity studied with purified respiratory enzyme and tissue culture. Biochemistry 1965; 4: 2763–2770.

Dawson JL. Jaundice and anoxic renal damage: protective effect of mannitol. Br Med J 1964; 1: 810–811.

Drivas G, James O, Wardle N. Study of reticuloendothelial phagocytic capacity in patients with cholestasis. Br Med J 1976; 1: 1568–1569.

Epstein M. Derangements of renal water handling in liver disease. Gastroenterology 1985; 89: 1415–1425.

Epstein M. Renal prostaglandins and the control of renal function in liver disease. Am J Med 1986; 80 (Suppl 1A): 46–55.

Evans HJR, Torrealba V, Hudd C, Knight M. The effect of preoperative bile salt administration on postoperative renal function in patients with obstructive jaundice. Br J Surg 1982; 69: 706–708.

Gouma DJ, Coelho JC, Fisher JD, et al. Endotoxemia after relief of biliary obstruction by internal and external drainage in rats. Am J Surg 1986; 151: 476–479.

Greaney MG, van Noort R, Symthe A, Irvin TT. Does obstructive jaundice adversely affect wound healing? Br J Surg 1979; 66: 478–481.

Hagmann W, Denzlinger C, Keppler D. Role of peptide leukotrienes and their hepatobiliary elimination in endotoxin action. Circ Shock 1984; 14: 223–235.

Hatfield ARW, Terblanche J, Fataar S, et al. Preoperative external biliary drainage in obstructive jaundice. Lancet 1982; ii: 896–899.

Huber M, Guhlmann A, Jansen PLM, Keppler D. Hereditary defect of hepatobiliary cysteinyl leukotriene elimination in mutant rats with defective hepatic anion excretion. Hepatology 1987; 7: 224–228.

Irvin TT, Vassilakis JS, Chattopadhyay DK, Greaney MG. Abdominal wound healing in jaundiced patients. Br J Surg 1978; 65: 521–522.

Kawai K, Cowger ML. Effect of bilirubin on ATPase activity of human erythrocyte membranes. Res Commun Chem Pathol Pharmacol 1981; 32: 123–135.

Keppler D, Hagmann W, Rapp S, et al. The relation of leukotrienes to liver injury. Hepatology 1985; 5: 883–891.

Keppler D, Huber M, Weckbecker G, et al. Leukotriene C4 metabolism by hepatoma cells and liver. Adv Enzyme Regul 1987; 26: 211–224.

Kocsar LT, Bertok, L, Varteresz V: Effect of bile acids on the intestinal absorption of endotoxin in rats. J Bacteriol 1969; 100: 220–223.

Kubo S, Matsui-Yuasa I, Otani S, et al: Liver regeneration factor detected in human serum after partial hepatectomy. Am J Gastroenterol 1987; 82: 1120–1126.

LaBrecque DR, Pesch LA. Preparation and partial characterization of hepatic regenerative stimulatory substance (SS) from rat liver. J Physiol 1975; 248: 273–284.

Laragh JH. Atrial natriuretic hormone, the renin-aldosteron axis and blood pressure-electrolyte homeostasis. N Engl J Med 1985; 313: 1330–1340.

Lauff JJ, Kasper ME, Wu TW, Ambrose RT. Isolation and preliminary characterization of a fraction of bilirubin in serum that is firmly bound to protein. Clin Chem 1982; 28: 69–637.

Lewis RA, Austen KF. The biologically active leukotrienes. J Clin Invest 1984; 73: 889–897.

Libonati M, Malsch E, Price HL, et al. Splanchnic circulation during methoxyflurane anesthesia. Anesthesiology 1973; 38: 466–472.

Lin TY, Chen CC. Metabolic function and regeneration of cirrhotic livers after hepatic lobectomy in man. Ann Surg 1965; 162: 959–972.

Lowe PJ, Coleman R. Membrane fluidity and bile salt damage. Biochim Biophys Acta 1981; 640: 55–65.

McPherson GAD, Benjamin IS, Habib NA, et al. Percutaneous transhepatic drainage in obstructive jaundice. Br J Surg 1982; 69: 61–264.

McPherson GAD, Benjamin IS, Hodgson HJF, et al. Preoperative percutaneous transhepatic biliary drainage. Br J Surg 1984; 71: 371–375.

Michalopoulos G, Houck KA, Dolan ML, Luetteke NC. Control of hepatocyte replication by two serum factors. Cancer Res 1984; 44: 4414–4419.

Morgan MY, Hawley KE: Lactitol vs lactulose in the treatment of acute hepatic encephalopathy in cirrhotic patients: a double-blind, randomized trial. Hepatology 1987; 7: 1278–1284.

Nagao T, Inoue S, Mizuta T, et al. One hundred hepatic resections. Ann Surg 1985; 202: 42–49.

Ong GB, Lee NW. Hepatic resection. Br J Surg 1975; 62: 421–430.

Perez-Ayuso RM, Arroyo V, Camps J, et al. Evidence that renal prostaglandins are involved in renal water metabolism in cirrhosis. Kidney Int 1984; 26: 72–80.

Pitt HA, Cameron JL, Postier RG, Gadacz TR. Factors affecting mortality in biliary tract surgery. Am J Surg 1981; 141: 66–72.

Pitt HA, Gomes AS, Lois JF, et al. Does preoperative percutaneous biliary drainage reduce operative risk or increase hospital cost? Ann Surg 1985; 201: 545–553.

Powell LW, Dunnicliff MA, Billing BH. Red cell survival in experimental cholestatic jaundice. Br J Haematol 1968; 15: 429–435.

Rola-Pleszczynski M, Hensen SA, Vincent MM, Bellanti JA. Inhibitory effects of bilirubin on cellular immune responses in man. J Pediatr 1975; 86: 690–696.

Rubaltelli FF, Granati B, Fortunato A, et al. Inhibitory effect of bilirubin and photobilirubin on neonatal and adult T lymphocytes and granulocytes. Biol. Neonate 1982; 42: 152–158.

Sato H, Aono S, Semba R, Kashiwamata S. Interaction of bilirubin with human erythrocyte membranes. bilirubin binding to neuraminidase- and phospholipase-treated membranes. Biochem J 1987; 248: 21–26.

Sendama I, de Hemptinne B, Lambotte L. Recovery of liver function in partially hepatectomized rats evaluated by aminopyrine demethylation capacity. Hepatology 1985; 5: 629–633.

Stimpso REJ, Pellegrini CA, Way LW. Factors affecting the morbidity of elective liver resection. Am J Surg 1987; 153: 189–196.

Strunin L. The liver and anesthesia. Philadelphia: WB Saunders, 1977.

Taube M, Elliot P, Ellis H. Jaundice and wound healing: a tissue culture study. Br J Exp Pathol 1981; 62: 227–231.

Than T. Skin prolyl hydroxylase and tensiometry in jaundice [Thesis]. University of Glasgow, 1976.

Van Deventer SJH, ten Cate JW, Tytgat GN. Intestinal endotoxemia: clinical significance. Gastroenterology 1988; 94: 825–831.

Wardle EN. Endotoxemia and the pathogenesis of acute renal failure. Quart J Med 1975; 44: 389–398.

Weiss JS, Gautam A, Lauff JJ, et al. The clinical importance of a protein-bound fraction of serum bilirubin in patients with hyperbilirubinemia. N Engl J Med 1983; 309: 147–150.

Wenzel RP. Prevention and treatment of hospital-acquired infections. In: Wijngaarden JB, Smith LH, eds. Cecil textbook of medicine. 18th Ed. Philadelphia: WB Saunders, 1988: 1541–1549.

Williams RD, Elliot DW, Zollinger RM. The effect of hypotension in obstructive jaundice. Arch Surg 1960; 81: 334–340.

Yared A, Kon V, Ichikawa I. Mechanism of preservation of glomerular perfusion and filtration during acute extracellular volume depletion. J Clin Invest 1985; 75: 1477–1487.

Yildirim SI, Poulsen HE. Quantitative liver functions after 70 % hepatectomy. Eur J Clin Invest 1981; 11: 469–472.

Yoshida H, Inagaki T, Hirano M, Sugimoto T. Analyses of azopigments obtained from the delta fraction of bilirubin from mammalian plasma (mammalian biliprotein). Biochem J 1987; 248: 79–84.

Zetterstrom R, Ernster L. Bilirubin, an uncoupler of oxidative phosphorylation in isolated mitochondria. Nature 1956; 178: 1335–1337.

Zipser RD, Hoefs JC, Speckart PF, et al. Prostaglandins: modulators of renal function and pressor resistance in chronic liver disease. J Clin Endocrinol Metab 1979; 48: 895–900.

Zoli M, Marchesini G, Melli A, et al. Evaluation of liver volume and liver function following hepatic resection in man. Liver 1986; 6: 286–291.

10.2 Postoperative Jaundice

P. L. M. Jansen

Liver function disturbances after operations are fairly common. Schemel (1976) reported unexplained and unexpected abnormalities of liver biochemistry in 1 out of 700 otherwise healthy patients admitted for elective surgery. About one third of this group was jaundiced. The causes of postoperative jaundice are summarized in Table 10.2.1. The clinical management of postoperative jaundice is often difficult, since the etiology may be obscured by the presence of more than one possible factor. For example, a somewhat increased bilirubin load in a patient with a mild postoperative liver function disturbance can lead to clinically manifest jaundice. These situations resolve spontaneously. On the other hand, jaundice may be a first sign of an abdominal abscess which calls for drainage. The immediate postoperative period for many patients is a critical phase, and a wrong clinical decision can have grave consequences.

Elevation of Mainly Unconjugated Bilirubin

Hemolysis

Postoperative hemolysis is common after transfusion of multiple units of blood. This type of jaundice is transient, only lasting a couple of days. Other causes of postoperative hemolysis include: mechanical injury to the red blood cells, for example after heart valve operations; mechanical injury to red blood cells due to fibrin strands in the case of disseminated intravascular coagulation, or due to microangiopathy in the case of thrombotic thrombocytopenic purpura; sickle-cell crisis; drug-induced hemolysis; sequestrational hemolysis associated with hypersplenism, for example due to splenic vein thrombosis. Congenital hemolytic anemias may become manifest after operations. For example, patients with glucose-6-phosphate dehydrogenase deficiency may start to hemolyse after operations.

Drugs that are implicated in drug-induced hemolytic anemia are: penicillin, sulfonamides, phenothiazines, quinine, methyldopa or levodopa, nitrofurantoin, and aspirin. In addition, amphotericin may cause hemolysis. A decreased plasma haptoglobin and an increased serum LDH activity and reticulocyte count are compatible with hemolysis. Resorption of hematomas can also cause a mild transient jaundice. In this case plasma haptoglobin is not decreased, since free hemoglobin does not enter the circulation but is converted via biliverdin to bilirubin within the hematoma.

Table 10.2.1   Postoperative Jaundice

Elevation of unconjugated bilirubin
   Hemolysis
   Resorption of hematomas
   Gilbert's syndrome

Elevation of conjugated bilirubin with
or without raised alkaline phosphatase
 i. Intrahepatic causes
   Endotoxin-induced
   Total parenteral nutrition
   Drug-induced
   Idiopathic postoperative jaundice
   Circulatory failure
   Pre-existing liver disease
   Viral hepatitis
   Stauffer's syndrome
   Hodgkin's disease
   Dubin-Johnson syndrome
   Rotor syndrome
ii. Extrahepatic obstruction
   Common duct stone or tumor
   Bile duct injury
   Pancreatitis

Gilbert's syndrome

Gilbert's syndrome is very common among the population: about 12% of men and 5% of women have this syndrome (Sieg et al. 1987). Its main characteristic is an elevated unconjugated serum bilirubin level, which rises upon fasting or during infectious diseases. It is almost invariably associated with a decreased activity of the enzyme that glucuronidates bilirubin in the liver. Due to this decreased enzyme activity, the liver has lost its reserve capacity to conjugate bilirubin and therefore the serum bilirubin concentration can rise dramatically in the postoperative period due to increased loads of bilirubin. Small loads of bilirubin that in normal people remain without clinical relevance, can cause prolonged jaundice in patients with Gilbert's syndrome. This can be a source of confusion in complicated postoperative situations.

Elevation of Conjugated Bilirubin with or without Raised Alkaline Phosphatase

Endotoxin-induced jaundice. Gram-negative bacteria within the bowel can be sources of endotoxins. Normal bowel mucosa is apparently an effective barrier for endotoxins, since portal blood from normal persons does not contain endotoxins, as determined with the limulus test (Van Deventer et al. 1988). Abdominal operations, however, can cause an increase in bowel mucosa permeability, thus allowing endotoxins to enter the portal blood. In the liver the blood is effectively cleared of endotoxins by the Kupffer cells. Endotoxins, however, can impair liver function and cause retention of tetrabromosulphthalein (BSP) and bilirubin (Utili et al. 1977). In mice that are first primed with dead bacteria so that the liver is filled with mononuclear cells, exposure to endotoxins causes fulminant hepatic failure (Mizoguchi et al 1987). Whether such a Shwartzman–Sanarelli phenomenon can also cause fulminant hepatic failure in the human liver is uncertain, but is theoretically not impossible.

Venous congestion of the bowel can damage the mucosal barrier to such an extent as to cause endotoxin shock in patients with, for example, impaired Kupffer cell function of the liver. It seems therefore advisable to clean the bowel, or prepare a patient with oral lactulose, before extensive bowel operations or shunt surgery are undertaken. Bile acids also bind endotoxins within the bowel lumen (Kocsar et al. 1969). Patients with biliary obstruction are at risk of developing endotoxin-mediated complications such as endotoxin shock, disseminated intravascular coagulation, and renal failure. This risk can be dealt with by preoperative internal drainage procedures, for example by an endoscopically-placed biliary stent.

Total parenteral nutrition (TPN). Prolonged intravenous administration of carbohydrate–amino acid mixtures with high calorie nitrogen ratios can lead to fatty liver. This does not usually cause overt jaundice, but can cause elevated alkaline phosphatase levels. Judicious use of lipid emulsions can prevent fatty liver during total parenteral nutrition. Jaundice during total parenteral nutrition is not rare and in particular is frequently seen in infants receiving TPN (Rodgers et al. 1976; Zarif et al. 1976). The cause is unknown. High loads of amino acids may cause impairment of hepatic transport processes. Amino acid uptake in the liver requires sodium ions. This sodium must be removed from the hepatocyte by the sodium pump, Na/K ATPase. This removal of sodium causes an electronegatively charged cell interior. This electronegative charge is probably the main driving force for the excretion of the bile acid anions from hepatocyte to bile. Excretion of bile acids into the bile attracts sodium and water, and this causes bile to flow (Erlinger 1988). If too many amino acids are taken up in the liver, the capacity of the liver to remove sodium effectively may be exceeded, sodium then accumulates in the hepatocyte, and this dissipates the electropotential. As a result, bile acids cannot be excreted, and bile flow is impaired. This can either produce cholestasis and jaundice, or

bile which is relatively poor in bile acids and supersaturated in cholesterol. This pathophysiological mechanism not only offers an explanation for the cholestasis frequently observed during TPN, but also for the biliary sludge which is often found in the biliary tree and gallbladder of patients on TPN. Experimental work along these lines may clarify this important phenomenon.

Drug-induced jaundice. Many drugs can impair liver function. Some drugs relevant for the postoperative period are mentioned in Table 10.2.2. Hepatic necrosis is a rare complication of halothane anesthesia. The incidence is 1 in 7000 exposures. However, the mortality rate from halothane-induced hepatic necrosis is 20 to 50 % (Touloukian and Kaplowitz 1981). Risk factors for halothane hepatitis include female sex, obesity, age over 40 years, previous exposure within 28 days, and previous unexplained postoperative fever.

Other drugs mentioned under the heading "hepatocellular damage" can all cause more or less severe hepatic necrosis, with high to very high serum transaminase activity and sometimes eosinophilia. In order to diagnose drug-induced hepatitis, other causes of postoperative liver function disturbances have to be excluded, notably circulatory failure during the operation, right-sided heart failure and viral hepatitis, and non-A non-B hepatitis in particular. Most helpful is a study of the relation between the occurrence of the liver function disturbances and the time of exposure. Sometimes the patient's history reveals previous adverse reactions. Liver histology can be helpful. Sometimes fairly characteristic patterns are seen: centrilobular necrosis in halothane or paracetamol hepatitis; diffuse spotty necrosis in isoniazid hepatitis; microvesicular steatosis after exposure to tetracycline or valproic acid; macro-vesicular steatosis with phospholipidosis after amiodarone; pure intrahepatic

Table 10.2.2 Drug-induced postoperative jaundice

Hepatocellular damage	Cholestasis
Halothane	Phenothiazines, Chlorpromazine
Nitrous oxide	Chlorothiazide
Thiopentone	Chlorthalidone
Paracetamol	Methyltestosterone
Isoniazide	Nitrofurantoin
Rifampicin	Erythromycin estolate
Pyrazinamide	
Para-aminosalicylic acid	
Sulfonamides	
Salicylates	
Penicillin	
Tetracycline	
Methyldopa	
Ketoconazole	
Phenytoin	

cholestasis after estrogens; and cholestasis with more or less periportal infiltrate after chlorpromazine (Zimmermann and Ishak 1987). Nitrofurantoin and methyldopa can cause chronic hepatitis. Certain drug reactions occur more often in patients on anti-epileptic therapy or in alcoholics. These patients have an induced cytochrome-P450 system and many drugs are converted to toxic intermediate metabolites by this enzyne system. One of the important cell-protecting compounds is glutathione. Glutathione is depleted in alcoholics or in patients who use drugs that are conjugated with glutathione. Glutathione can be rapidly repleted by administration of N-acetylcysteine. This compound provides the liver cell with cysteine, which is a precursor of glutathione. Administration of this sometimes life-saving drug in, for example, paracetamol intoxications, has to be done within the first 8 hours after ingestion of the intoxicating dose, since otherwise the toxic intermediates will already have damaged the hepatocytes irreversibly (Prescott and Critchley 1983).

Idiopathic postoperative jaundice. Patients who have undergone major surgery and received several units of blood, sometimes become jaundiced one to ten days after the operation. Conjugated bilirubin and alkaline phosphatase are increased, and the transaminases and the synthetic functions of the liver remain normal. Histologically the picture is purely cholestatic, and signs of hepatocellular damage or inflammatory infiltrate are absent. The etiology of this idiopathic postoperative jaundice is unknown (LaMont and Isselbacher 1979). Since this complex of symptoms suggests extrahepatic bile duct obstruction, it is sometimes necessary to rule out damage to the bile ducts by ultrasonography or endoscopic retrograde cholangiography. Sepsis, bile peritonitis and an intra-abdominal abscess can all present with very similar symptoms, and should be differentiated from idiopathic postoperative jaundice, which spontaneously resolves, usually in two to three weeks.

Circulatory failure. Many anesthetic agents cause splanchnic vasoconstriction and decreased portal flow (Strunin 1977). Normal livers can cope with this transient decreased oxygen supply, but in cirrhotics, with intra- and extrahepatic shunting of blood, anesthesia may cause hypoxic damage of the hepatocytes with postoperative liver failure as a result. Operative blood loss and hypotension should therefore be rapidly corrected in patients with liver cirrhosis. Surgical shock or prolonged hypotension can damage the liver function of patients without pre-existing liver disease. LaMont and Isselbacher (1979) describe two common presentations after circulatory failure. Most common is the presentation with cholestatic jaundice occurring on the second or third hospital day, with peak levels of bilirubin up to 500 μmol/l on the seventh to tenth day. The alkaline phosphatase is about normal, and the transaminases are mildly elevated. The pattern is indistinguishable from idiopathic postoperative jaundice. After prolonged shock, a more severe disease is seen which curiously, sometimes does not occur until the seventh or tenth day after the operation. Massive centrilobular necrosis with very high transaminase levels is seen, sometimes with a fatal outcome.

Pre-existing liver disease. Acute cholecystitis with or without choledocholithiasis may cause jaundice. In these situations, transaminases may be elevated but usually not more than two to three times. In the pre-endoscopic era, patients with acute viral hepatitis were occasionally operated on, on the assumption that they had acute cholecystitis. The higher transaminase level in these patients should have pointed the way to the correct diagnosis. However, these non-indicated operations have taught us the danger of anesthesia and surgery in acute hepatitis. This should be avoided, since these patients have an unacceptably high postoperative morbidity and mortality rate. Also, in patients with liver cirrhosis or chronic active hepatitis, surgery carries an increased risk of postoperative complications such as deterioration of liver function, ascites, renal failure, sepsis, variceal bleeding and hepatic encephalopathy. In many centers, sclerotherapy of esophageal varices is the treatment of choice after a first hemorrhage. Prophylactic sclerotherapy in patients who have not yet bled is at present of no proved benefit. However, it could be argued that prophylactic sclerotherapy in patients who need elective surgery may be indicated.

A raised alkaline phosphatase level in patients who have been operated on for inflammatory bowel disease may be the first manifestation of primary sclerosing cholangitis. This is a chronic disease which runs a course of exacerbations and remissions. The exacerbations are characterized by jaundice and cholangitis. The diagnosis is made by endoscopic retrograde cholangiography. Two types can be distinguished: i) involvement of the large extrahepatic bile ducts, with a beaded pattern of multiple stenoses and dilations; ii) involvement of the small intrahepatic bile ducts. Both types can be present *at once* (Wee and Ludwig 1985). This disease has to be differentiated from cholangiocarcinoma. The diagnosis of type ii can be made by liver biopsy. Histologically a characteristic picture is seen, with periductal fibrosis with a typical onion-skin pattern, bile duct proliferation and eventually vanishing bile ducts and cirrhosis (Ludwig et al. 1981). The latter stage is difficult to differentiate from primary biliary cirrhosis. Antimitochondrial antibody in primary sclerosing cholangitis is negative. There is a strong correlation with ulcerative colitis.

Viral hepatitis. Non-A non-B hepatitis is at present the major form of post-transfusion hepatitis. The incidence is 0.5–1.0% after transfusions of blood, plasma and clotting factors (Dienstag 1983). With a recently developed test for this form of hepatitis, also called hepatitis C, antibodies can be derected about 8 weeks after the acute onset. Transmission of hepatitis B by blood and blood products has become rare since blood donors have been routinely screened for hepatitis B surface antigen (HB_s – Ag). It is to be expected that screening of blood donors with the new test will also diminish the incidence of C hepatitis. The incubation time ranges from 2 to 20 weeks, with an average of 8 weeks. The acute phase resembles acute hepatitis B, and may present with acute massive liver cell necrosis or anicteric hepatitis. It may be difficult to differentiate fulminant viral hepatitis from halothane hepatitis. The incidence of chronic hepatitis after post-transfusion C hepatitis exceeds 25%, and about half of these cases eventually develop liver cirrhosis. Other forms of post-transfusion hepatitis include cytomegalovirus and Epstein–Barr virus hepatitis. Hepatitis A and delta hepatitis may also become manifest in the postoperative period. Pre-existing chronic hepatitis can become reactivated by an operation. Motivated by the appearance of AIDS as a post-transfusion problem, an increasing number of patients prefer transfusion of autologous blood during elective surgery.

Stauffer's syndrome is a rare cause of jaundice in patients with Grawitz carcinoma. The patient has conjugated hyperbilirubinemia and elevated alkaline phosphatase activity, whereas the liver is free of tumor. Surgical removal of the kidney tumor causes disappearance of the jaundice (Strickland and Schenker 1977).

Hodgkin's disease can also present with conjugated jaundice in the absence of hepatic or bile duct localization of the disease (Perera et al. 1974). Sometimes the jaundice disappears when Hodgkin's disease is brought to remission, but in our own experience this can take a year after curative treatment of the lymphoma.

Dubin–Johnson syndrome is characterized by conjugated hyperbilirubinemia, with bilirubin levels usually between 30 and 90 µmol/l, in the absence of any other liver function abnormality. The livers of these patients have a dark brown appearance due to a melanin-like intralysosomal pigment. The syndrome usually becomes manifest during puberty, and the jaundice deepens during pregnancy. The hepatobiliary excretion of conjugated bilirubin, the glutathione conjugate of BSP, and the oral X-ray contrast agent used for visualization of the gallbladder, iopanoic acid, is impaired. Bile acid excretion is normal. Dubin–Johnson syndrome can be differentiated from other hepatobiliary disorders such as Rotor syndrome by determining the urinary coproporphyrin isomer I. In Dubin–Johnson syndrome, total urinary coproporphyrin excretion is normal, but 80% is isomer I (Roy Chowdhury et al. 1988).

Rotor syndrome is a rare disorder manifested by predominantly conjugated hyperbilirubinemia, delayed plasma BSP disappearance, and normal liver histology. Total urinary coproporphyrin excretion is 2.5 to 5 times greater than in normal persons and in patients with Dubin–Johnson syndrome (Roy Chowdhury et al. 1988).

References

Dienstag JL. Non-A, non-B hepatitis I: recognition, epidemiology and clinical features. Gastroenterology 1983; 85: 439–462.

Erlinger S. Bile flow. In: Arias IM, Jakoby WB, Popper H, et al., eds. The liver: biology and pathobiology. New York: Raven, 1988.

Kocsar LT, Bertok L, Varteresz V. Effect of bile acids on the intestinal absorption of endotoxin in rats. J Bacteriol 1969; 100: 220–223.

Kuo G, Choo Q-L, Alter HJ, et al. An assay for circulating antibodies to a major etiologic virus of human non-A, non-B hepatitis. Science 1989; 244: 362–364.

LaMont JT, Isselbacher KJ. Postoperative jaundice. In: Wright R, Alberti KGMM, Karran S, Millward-Sadler GH, eds. Liver and biliary disease. London: Saunders, 1979.

Ludwig J, Barham SS, LaRusso NF, et al. Morphologic features of chronic hepatitis associated with primary sclerosing cholangitis and chronic ulcerative colitis. Hepatology 1981; 1: 632–640.

Mizoguchi Y, Tsutsui H, Miyajima K, et al. The protective effects of prostaglandin E_1, in an experimental massive hepatic cell necrosis model. Hepatology 1987; 7: 1184–1188.

Perera DR, Greene ML, Fenster LF. Cholestasis associated with extrabiliary Hodgkin's disease. Gastroenterology 1974; 67: 680–685.

Prescott LF, Critchley JAJH. The treatment of acetaminophen poisoning. Annu Rev Pharmacol Toxicol 1983; 23: 87–101.

Rodgers BM, Hollenbeck, JI, Donnelly WH, Talbert JL. Intrahepatic cholestasis and parenteral hyperalimentation. Am J Surg 1976; 131: 149–154.

Roy Chowdhury J, Wolkoff AW, Arias IM. Heme and bile pigment metabolism. In: Arias IM, Jakoby WB, Popper H, et al., eds. The liver: biology and pathobiology. New York: Raven, 1988.

Schemel WH: Unexpected hepatic dysfunction found by multiple laboratory screening. Anesth Analg 1976; 55: 810–881.

Sieg A, Arab L, Schlierf G, et al. Die Prävalenz des Gilbert-Syndroms in Deutschland. Dtsch Med Wochenschr 1987; 112: 1206–1208.

Strickland RC, Schenker, S. The nephrogenic hepatic dysfunction syndrome: a review. Dig Dis Sci 1977; 22: 49–55.

Strunin L. The liver and anaesthesia London: Saunders, 1977.

Touloukian J, Kaplowitz N. Halothane-induced hepatic disease. Semin Liver Dis 1981; 1: 134–142.

Utili R, Abernathy CO, Zimmerman HJ. Endotoxin effects on the liver. Life Sci 1977; 20: 553–568.

Van Deventer SJH, ten Cate JW, Tytgat GN. Intestinal endotoxemia: clinical significance. Gastroenterology 1988; 94: 825–831.

Wee A, Ludwig J. Pericholangitis in chronic ulcerative colitis: primary sclerosing cholangitis of the small bile ducts? Ann Intern Med 1985; 102: 581–587.

Zarif MA, Pildes RS, Szanto PB, Vidyasagar D. Cholestasis associated with administration of L-amino acids and dextrose solutions. Biol Neonate 1976; 29: 66–76.

Zimmermann HJ, Ishak KG. Hepatic injury due to drugs and toxins. In: MacSween RNM, Anthony PP, Scheuer PJ, eds. Pathology of the liver. Edinburgh: Churchill Livingstone, 1987.

10.3 Chemotherapy; Options and Possibilities

C.H.N. Veenhof

Pancreatic Cancer

Pancreatic cancer is often diagnosed at a late stage of the disease. Pain and weight loss are then the main signs and symptoms indicating the presence of locally advanced or metastatic disease. Surgery is considered the best option for management. However, only a small minority of patients present themselves as suitable candidates. Recent reviews indicate 5-year survivals of 3–18 % (average 7 %) (Longmire and Traverso 1981). These data do emphasize the need for some kind of effective postoperative treatment (radiotherapy with or without chemotherapy) and effective systemic treatment for palliation in patients with locally advanced and metastatic disease. This section will deal with the options for systemic therapy, with or without radiotherapy, for tumors of the exocrine pancreas.

Despite the overall impact of the increasing incidence of pancreatic cancer and the need of the majority of patients with this disease for an effective systemic treatment modality, no standard treatment is available at the moment. Efforts to identify effective cytostatic treatment are hampered by several factors. Both the intrinsic sensitivity or resistance of this particular tumor type, and the condition of the patient at the moment that systemic treatment is considered, play an important role. A poor performance status (weight loss, pain, anorexia, malabsorption) makes patients unsuitable for chemotherapy. Obstructive jaundice and hepatic dysfunction are other contra-indications for the use of specific cytotoxic agents. Moreover, objective parameters for response to treatment are often difficult to obtain with the available diagnostic tools.

All of these factors make it very difficult to perform well-designed trials and formulate a special problem when comparing literature data. Comparison is further hampered by lack of information on patient selection, lack of proper definitions of response criteria, and very often by the small number of patients evaluated. Some more recent studies do report better response rates. But it needs to be evaluated whether these improved response rates also lead to a prolongation of (disease-free) survival, meaning a contribution to a better quality of life, the most important option in palliation.

Chemotherapy

Single Agents

5-Fluorouracil (5-FU) is the drug most extensively studied in patients with pancreatic cancer. Most trials report responses of about 20 % (Carter and Comis 1975), although a wide range between 0 and 67 % can be found. The drug has been used in many dosages and schedules including 2-hour, 8-hour, 24-hour and 5-day continuous infusion, single large doses and weekly small doses, but none of these schedules has proved to be superior (Moertel 1977).

Mitomycin-C has been reported to have single-agent activity comparable to that of 5-FU (Crooke and Bradner 1976, Schein et al. 1978b, Smith and Schein 1979). Of the nitrosourea derivatives, streptozotocin showed response rates of 31 to 50 % in studies with a small number of patients (Du Priest et al. 1975). The other nitrosourea (BCNU, CCNU, methyl-CCNU) are considered as not active. In a series of phase 2 studies performed by the American Gastrointestinal Tumor Study Group (GITSG), no activity could be found for doxorubicin, methotrexate or actinomycin D (Schein et al. 1978a).

From these data, it is clear that treatment with single agents is of little benefit for patients with pancreatic cancer. Agents showing evidence of clinical benefit in 20 % or more of patients, where significant numbers of individuals have been treated, include only 5-FU, mitomycin-C and streptozotocin (Carter and Comis 1975, Crooke and Bradner 1976, DuPriest et al. 1975, Smith and Schein 1979). The newer drugs may deserve some more attention because of their activity as single agents. Epirubicin, an analogue of doxorubicin, demonstrated activity in 3 out of 10 patients (Hochster et al. 1984). The EORTC Gastrointestinal Cancer Cooperative Group confirmed this activity with responses in 8 out of 34 previously untreated patients, including 2 complete responses (Wils et al. 1985). Because of its low toxicity profile, this drug could be a candidate for incorporation in combination chemotherapy. Ifosfamide, a structural analogue of cyclophosphamide, was reported to be highly active, producing responses in 10 out of 13 patients (Brühl et al. 1976) and in 6 out of 10 patients (Gad-El-Mawla 1981). In contrast, a study from the United States reported only 6 responses out of 27 patients (22 %) (Loehrer et al. 1985). The role of this drug still remains to be established due to the response rate, probably comparable to that of other single agents, and because of the small number of patients being treated.

Combination Chemotherapy

Although chemotherapeutic agents have been used in various combinations, no drug regimen has produced uniformly high response or survival rates. Because some clinical benefit is derived from a few combination regimens, they will be discussed briefly.

Disturbing inconsistencies are found when comparing the data of combination chemotherapy with those of single agents. The underlying causes may again be the problems of patient selection and the lack of definition of response criteria. This emphazises the urgent need for well-designed, randomized prospective trials. Mallison et al. (1980) performed such a trial, comparing combination chemotherapy (21 patients) with no treatment (19 patients). In this study, a multi-drug regimen was used, including 5-FU, cyclophosphamide, methotrexate and vincristine as the initial course, followed by courses of 5-FU and mitomycin-C. Although no objective response rates were reported, there was a median survival advantage in favor of the treated group: 44 weeks versus 9 weeks. If this is a real difference it can only be attributed to the two known active drugs in this combination: 5-FU and mitomycin-C.

A comparison of fluorouracil versus fluorouracil plus doxorubicin versus fluorouracil plus doxorubicin plus mitomycin (F vs FA vs FAM) showed that all three regimens were equivalent with regard to disease progression, objective response rates and palliative effects (Cullinan et al. 1985). The toxicity and the costs were higher for the combination regimens, thus favoring treatment with 5-FU alone.

Among the studies reported as producing response rates of 40% are those with the combinations FAM and streptozotocin, mitomycin and fluorouracil (SMF) (Smith et al. 1980, Wiggans et al. 1978). The Cancer and Leukemia Group B (CALGB) compared these two regimens (Oster et al. 1982) and found disappointingly low response rates of 14% on FAM and 4% on SMF, not comparable to the response rates of around 40%

mentioned for both regimens. According to other studies, the lower response rates should be considered as more realistic than the higher ones. Addition of chlorozotocin (Smith et al. 1982) or hexamethylmelamine (Smith et al. 1983) to FAM produced low response rates of 13% and 17% in contrast to the higher response rate with FAM alone (37%) found by the same group of authors, and more in line with the 14% found by the CALGB study. In conclusion, these results cannot be considered superior to 5-FU alone.

Other studies using various combinations of cytostatic drugs proved not to be able to obtain survival benefit, in spite of sometimes "high" response rates (Table 10.3.1). This table shows remarkably clearly that no evident correlation exists in these studies between the wide range in response rates (4–48%) and the median survival times (with a range of only 10 weeks).

Combined Modality Therapy

The combination of radiotherapy with chemotherapy can only be considered for patients with locally unresectable disease in whom the anatomic distribution of the tumor also lends itself to radiotherapy. Earlier reports showed improvement in median survival in favor of 35–40 Gy of split course with 5-FU administered in daily doses on the first 3 days of the course of radiation, as compared to radiotherapy alone (Moertel et al. 1969). This difference appeared significant (p = 0.05), with a median survival of 10.4 months versus 6.3 months. The Gastrointestinal Tumor Study Group reported a gain in median survival in favor of a group of patients treated with radiotherapy plus 5-FU: 40 weeks, versus 23 weeks for radiotherapy alone (Moertel et al. 1981). Studies are now going on in an attempt to answer the question of whether combination chemotherapy (as, for instance, FAM) plus radiotherapy is superior to radiotherapy alone. Other studies question the value of the combination of chemotherapy and radiotherapy, and compare chemotherapy alone to chemotherapy plus radiotherapy. An important problem is that there is no

Table 10.3.**1**   **Response and survival rates** using various combinations of cytostatic drugs

Chemotherapy	No. of patients	Remission percentage	Median survival (weeks)	References
SMF	56	34	18	Bukowski et al. 1983
SMF	66	4	18	Oster et al. 1982
FAM	27	37	24	Smith et al. 1980
FAM	56	9	28	Oster et al. 1982
FAM-S	25	48	26	Bukowski et al. 1982
FAM-S	68	18	22	Bukowski et al. 1985

S = streptozotocin; M = mitomycin; F = 5-fluorouracil; A = doxorubicin

uniformly outstanding chemotherapeutic regimen that can be considered the optimal candidate to be included in a combined modality program.

In combining chemotherapy with radiotherapy, more attention should be paid to better timing and sequencing. As no single agent or combination of cytotoxic drugs appears superior to 5-FU, this latter drug should be considered the drug of choice to be used in combination with radiotherapy. Variations in administration procedures and in timing with regard to the radiotherapy are as worthwhile to investigate as to combine radiotherapy with all kind of other combinations of drugs. From in vitro data, it can be deduced that reductions in cell survival can be produced when exposure times to 5-FU are extended beyond the cell cycle time (Byfield et al. 1982, Calabro-Jones et al. 1982, Nakajiama et al. 1979).

Prolonged 5-FU concentrations can quantitatively enhance cell killing by X-rays. The data suggest that X-rays may sensitize the cells to 5-FU. The enhanced cell killing is maximized if the cells are continuously exposed to 5-FU for 48 h following X-ray exposure. Moreover, this post-radiation phenomenon is a direct function of 5-FU concentration. In vitro, the sensitization phenomenon becomes apparent with 5-FU levels in the range of $0.1-0.5\ \mu g/ml$. These levels can be achieved with continuous infusion of 5-FU in doses of 25 mg/kg/24 h. Moreover, these doses can be combined with radiotherapy, as can be deduced from studies using continuous infusion of 5-FU plus radiotherapy in the treatment of various tumor types (Barone et al. 1979, Byfield et al. 1980, 1983, 1984, Rotman et al. 1986, 1987).

Adjuvant Therapy

The 5-year survival after surgery for pancreatic cancer is limited. Many attempts are being made to improve this distressing figure with postoperative radiotherapy, chemotherapy, or a combination of these. However, no randomized trials have been reported showing definite benefit from these postoperative treatments. One study by the GITSG (Kalser et al. 1985) does not permit definitive statements, but does offer a suggestion on the prolongation of postresection survival time. Of the 49 patients in this study, 43 were evaluated. The adjuvant treatment consisted of radiotherapy plus 5-FU and this was compared with the effects following no adjuvant treatment. The median survival for the treated group was 20 months, as compared to 11 months for the control group. Because of the very slow accrual for this study and the likelihood of benefit in the treatment arm, the study was terminated and 30 additional patients were treated with the same combined treatment of radiotherapy plus 5-FU (Gastrointestinal Tumor Study Group 1987). The median survival time for this additional group of patients was 18 months. Ten patients were alive at 18.9 to 42.4 months (median 25.0). Both survival and the disease-free survival surpass those of the control group of the first study (Kalser and Ellenberg 1985). The question is whether these data are strong enough to consider this form of adjuvant treatment as the best option, with which other regimens should be compared in a prospective randomized way.

Cancer of the Gallbladder and Extrahepatic Bile Ducts

Carcinoma of the biliary system represents an uncommon malignancy. About two-thirds of biliary carcinomas arise in the gallbladder, the remainder are of ductal origin. Only in a small percentage of patients are the tumors resectable at the time of the initial diagnosis. The natural history suggests that cholangiocarcinoma is more indolent in its course than gallbladder carcinoma. Similarly, distal common bile duct carcinoma has a far better prognosis than cholangiocarcinoma arising at the middle and upper third of the biliary tree.

Surgery is the first option for these tumors. However, only a limited proportion of patients can be considered as candidates for this treatment modality because of the advanced stage of the disease at presentation. Moreover, local relapses or distant metastases (most frequently in the liver) occur, demanding other treatment procedures. The radiotherapeutic options are dealt with elsewhere. Relatively little information is available on chemotherapy for these tumors, either as single agents or in combination. The results are often difficult to interpret because of the limited number of patients treated per trial. Data collected from the literature present a wide range of response rates (9–25%) with single agents or combination chemotherapy.

Although no single agents have shown to have predictable activity in either gallbladder or bile duct cancer, combinations have been tried. The Eastern Cooperative Oncology Group (ECOG) compared oral 5-FU with oral 5-FU plus streptozotocin and with oral 5-FU plus methyl-CCNU (MeCCNU) in patients with inoperable gallbladder and bile duct cancer (Falkson et al. 1984). No difference was found between the three treatment groups with respect to response (ranging from 5–12%) and survival.

The largest series reported consisted of 17 patients with biliary cancer treated with FAM (5-fluorouracil–doxorubicin–mitomycin-C) (Harvey et al. 1984). This combination was chosen because of response rates of around 40 and 30% in gastric and pancreatic cancer found by the same group of investigators. They expanded their studies to the biliary tract, although no single-agent studies had proved activity for each of the drugs separately. Of the 17 patients studied, 14 had objectively measurable disease; four of these patients achieved a partial response (28 %). The median duration of the response was 8.5 months (range 5–18 months); the median survival 11.5 months. Another 7 patients experienced disease stabilization for three or more months. From this phase 2 study, it was concluded that further large, controlled trials should establish a more definitive estimate of the efficacy of the FAM regimen. The authors suggested a possible role for this combination with radiotherapy for less advanced stages of the disease.

Since biliary tract cancers are usually confined to the liver and/or surrounding area, some investigators thought the use of hepatic artery infusion (HAI) of cytostatic drugs a rational approach (Smith et al. 1984). Eleven patients with only hepatic or extrahepatic disease were treated with HAI of 5-FU and mitomycin-C. The results of this study with a small number of patients were remarkable: complete response in 1 patient (9 %) and partial responses in 6 patients (55 %). Both tumor types were equally represented amongst the responders. The median survival for all patients from the start of the first treatment was 12.5 + months; for the patients with gallbladder carcinoma it was 12.5 months, while not being reached for patients with cholangiocarcinoma. These data suggest an improvement, compared to the natural history of both tumor localizations, of 2.5 and 8.0 months respectively.

The intra-arterial route for the administration of drugs to the liver is controversial. Usually this method is used when the disease is limited to the liver. Even in that situation, the value of HAI has not yet been established, because of the lack of significant gain in survival (although high response rates may be achieved) and because of the development of extrahepatic disease manifestations. HAI as the only treatment appears to be insufficient and should be combined simultaneously with systemic treatment. The treatment with HAI of extrahepatic disease is more controversial. If systemic effects are also needed, the advantages of local treatment will loose their importance. But at the moment no systemic treatment for biliary cancer can be recommended as a standard therapy, based upon the results in the literature.

No reports of studies can be found in the literature concerning combined treatment with chemotherapy and radiotherapy. As no effective cytotoxic drugs are known for gallbladder or bile duct cancer, the only option for the combined modality could be the use of drugs as sensitizers for radiotherapy. As far as adjuvant chemotherapy is concerned, after radical resection at the moment the best advice seems to be to stick to the rule that adjuvant chemotherapy can only be considered if drugs are available which are effective in the advanced or metastatic state of the disease.

Hepatocellular Carcinoma

In hepatocellular carcinoma, surgery represents the best hope of cure. But only 10–20 % of primary hepatomas are amenable to operative resection; the expected 5-year survival ranges from 20 to 50 % (Adson and Weiland 1981, Hanks et al. 1980, Inouye and Whelan 1979, Starzl et al. 1980). The cytotoxic treatment of hepatocellular carcinoma has not been successful. A number of chemotherapy trials are reported, from which can be deduced that only treatment containing doxorubicin has been to any extent effective. However, the results of these studies do not in general confirm one other. In some trials, doxorubicin was found to be quite active (Olweny et al. 1975), whereas other authors reported low response rates (Ihde et al. 1977, Vogel et al. 1977). The response rate of single-agent doxorubicin in this disease is in the range of 10–20 %. Its analogue, epirubicin, produces the same minimal response rate (less than 20 %) (Shiu et al. 1986). Mitoxantrone, a synthetic anthracenedione, has been shown in some clinical studies to be as effective and less toxic than doxorubicin in a number of malignancies (Smith 1983). Several phase 2 studies have been reported on mitoxantrone in hepatocellular carcinoma (Dunk et al. 1985, Falkson and Coetzer 1985, Van Echo et al. 1984). In dosages of 10 to 14 mg/m^2 the response rate is in the range of 10–20 %, and thus comparable to that of doxorubicin. The advantage of mitoxantrone could be the lower toxicity also evident in patients with hepatocellular carcinoma, even in the case of hyperbilirubinemia (Dunk et al. 1985).

In phase 2 trials with cisplatin, a low response rate has been reported: a partial response in 1 out of 13 patients (Melia et al. 1981), in 1 out of 20 patients (Ravry et al. 1986) and in 2 out of 35 patients (Falkson et al. 1987). Combining doxorubicin with other cytotoxic agents did not improve the results, as appeared from the 12.5 % partial response with FAM (Al-Idrissi et al. 1985).

Intra-arterial administration of cytotoxic agents via the hepatic artery is also under study for this tumor. Although the reported response rates are higher than in systemic treatments with the same drugs, no significant effect on survival is seen (Al-Jurf et al. 1984, Shildt et al. 1984, Urist et al. 1984).

In the search for new drugs and new treatment modalities for insensitive tumors radioactive monoclonal antibodies are also in use. Radioactive monoclonal antibodies to ferritin have been studied in particular (Order et al. 1984, Order and Leibel 1984). Ferritin can be demonstrated immunohistochemically in most hepatocellular tumor tissue (Order et al. 1985). In 105 patients, treatment with ^{131}I-ferritin took place after an induction with external beam irradiation and chemotherapy with doxorubicin and 5-FU. In 66 evaluated patients, 4 complete and 24 partial responses were described. Problems of immune sensitization and immune complex formation were circumvented by the use of several animal species for the production of antibody and by the alternate use of these antibodies. The development of antibodies labeled with iodine 131 (Order et al. 1985) was recently followed by labeling with yttrium-90 (Order et al. 1986), which is an isotope emitting more powerful beta-radiation. In their most recent report (Sitzmann et al. 1987), the authors state that in 7 out of 11 patients this treatment converted non-resectable lesions to possible resectability. In one patient, the lesion could be partially resected, and 6 patients had complete resections. These new developments in the production of antibodies and labeling techniques promise advantages in higher response rates and improvement of survival.

Of the biological response modifiers, the interferons have been studied in connection with this tumor because of their known ability to modulate cell-mediated cytotoxicity. No clinical activity was seen, however (Forbes et al. 1985, Nair et al. 1985, Sachs et al. 1985).

Another interesting finding in the investigation of treatment options for hepatocellular carcinoma is the detection of hormone receptors in liver tissue, and in this tumor type in particular. High levels of androgen receptors have been found in tissue from hepatocellular carcinomas in comparison with surrounding non-tumor tissue and normal liver tissue (Iqbal et al. 1983, Nagasue et al. 1985, Ohnishi et al. 1986). In a number of patients estrogen receptors could also be detected in the tumor tissue (Nagasue et al. 1986). It is very challenging to investigate whether hormone therapy with antiandrogens or antiestrogens can be used in the treatment of hepatocellular carcinoma. In the few patients treated up till now, some partial responses have been reported (Demanes et al. 1982, Friedman et al. 1982). The Gastrointestinal Tract Cancer Cooperative Group of the European Organization for Research and Treatment of Cancer (EORTC) has recently initiated a double-blind clinical trial of an antiandrogen therapy versus placebo in unresectable hepatocellular carcinoma.

References

Adson MA, Weiland LH. Resection of primary solid hepatic tumors. Am J Surg 1981; 141: 18–21.

Al-Idrissi HY, Ibrahim FM, Abdel Satir A et al. Primary hepatocellular carcinoma in the eastern province of Saudi Arabia: treatment with combination chemotherapy using 5-fluorouracil, adriamycin and mitomycin-C. Hepatogastroenterol 1985; 32: 8–10.

Al-Jurf AS, Jochimsen PR, Shirazi SS, et al. Hepatic artery ligation and chemotherapeutic infusion in the treatment of hepatic malignancy. J Surg Oncol 1984; 27: 119–123.

Barone RM, Byfield JE, Frankel S. Combination infusional 5-fluorouracil and radiation therapy for the treatment of metastatic carcinoma of the colon to the liver. Dis Colon Rectum 1979; 22: 376–382.

Brühl P, Gunther V, Hoefer-Janker H, et al. Results obtained with fractionated ifosfamide massive dose treatment in generalized malignant tumors. Int J Clin Pharmacol Biopharm 1976; 14: 29–39.

Bukowski RM, Schacter LP, Groppe CW, et al. Phase II study of 5-fluorouracil, adriamycin, mitomycin-C and streptozotocin (FAM-S) in pancreatic carcinoma. Cancer 1982; 50: 197–200.

Bukowski RM, Balcerzak SP, O'Bryan RM, et al. Randomized trial of 5-fluorouracil and mitomycin-C with or without streptozotocin for advanced pancreatic cancer: a South West Oncology Group study. Cancer 1983; 52: 1577–1582.

Bukowski RM, Inamuasu M, Taylor S, et al. Randomized trials of combination chemotherapy vs a phase II drug in metastatic adenocarcinoma of the pancreas: South West Oncology Group study. Proc Am Soc Clin Oncol 1985; C-311 (abstract): 80.

Byfield JE, Barone R, Mendelsohn J, et al. Infusional 5-fluorouracil and X-ray therapy for non-resectable esophageal cancer. Cancer 1980; 45: 703–708.

Byfield JE, Calabro-Jones P, Klisak I, et al. Pharmacologic requirements for obtaining sensitization of human tumor cells in vitro to combined 5-fluorouracil or ftorafur and X rays. Int J Radiat Oncol Biol Phys 1982; 8: 1923–1933.

Byfield JE, Stanton W, Sharp TR, et al. Phase I–II Study of 120-hour infused 5-FU and split-course radiation therapy in localized non-small cell lung cancer. Cancer Treat Rep 1983; 67: 933–936.

Byfield JE, Sharp TR, Frankel SS, et al. Phase I and II trial of five-day infused 5-fluorouracil and radiation in advanced cancer of the head and neck. J Clin Oncol 1984; 2: 406–413.

Calabro-Jones PM, Byfield JE, Ward JF, et al. Time-dose relationships for 5-fluorouracil cytotoxicity against human epithelial cancer cells in vitro. Cancer Res 1982; 42: 4413–4420.

Carter SK, Comis RL. The integration of chemotherapy into a combined modality approach for cancer treatment, VI: pancreatic adenocarcinoma. Cancer Treat Rev 1975; 2: 193–214.

Crooke ST, Bradner WT. Mitomycin-C: a review. Cancer Treat Rev 1976; 3: 121–129.

Cullinan SA, Moertel CG, Fleming TR, et al. A comparison of three chemotherapeutic regimens in the treatment of advanced pancreatic and gastric carcinoma. JAMA 1985; 253: 2061–2067.

Demanes DJ, Friedman MA, McKerrow JH, et al. Hormone receptors in hepatoblastoma: a demonstration of both estrogen and progesterone receptors. Cancer 1982; 50: 1828–1832.

Dunk A, Scott S, Johnson P, et al. Mitoxantrone as single agent therapy in hepatocellular carcinoma. J Hepatol 1985; 1: 395–404.

DuPriest RW, Huntington MC, Massey WH, et al. Streptozotocin therapy in 22 cancer patients. Cancer 1975; 35: 358–367.

Falkson G, McIntyre JM, Moertel CG. Eastern Cooperative Oncology Group experience with chemotherapy for inoperable gallbladder and bile duct cancer. Cancer 1984; 54: 965–969.

Falkson G, Coetzer BJ. Phase II studies of mitoxantrone in patients with primary liver cancer. Invest New Drugs 1985; 3: 187–189.

Falkson G, Ryan LM, Johnson LA, et al. A random phase II study of mitoxantrone and cisplatin in patients with hepatocellular carcinoma. Cancer 1987; 60: 2141–2145.

Forbes A, Johnson PJ, Williams R. Recombinant human gamma-interferon in primary hepatocellular carcinoma. J R Soc Med 1985; 78: 826–829.

Friedman MA, Demanes DJ, Hoffman, PG Jr. Hepatomas: hormone receptors and therapy. Am J Med 1982; 73: 362–366.

Gad-El-Mawla N, Ziegler JL. Ifosfamide treatment of pancreatic cancer. Cancer Treat Rep 1981; 65: 357–358.

Gastrointestinal Tumor Study Group: Further evidence of effective adjuvant combined radiation and chemotherapy following curative resection of pancreatic cancer. Cancer 1987; 59: 2006–2010.

Hanks JB, Meyers WC, Filston HC, et al. Surgical resection for benign and malignant liver disease. Ann Surg 1980; 191: 584–592.

Harvey JH, Smith FP, Schein PS. 5-fluorouracil, mitomycin, and doxorubicin (FAM) in carcinoma of the biliary tract. J Clin Oncol 1984; 2: 1245–1248.

Hochster H, Green M, Speyer R, Blum R, Wernz J, Muggia F. Activity of 4′-epidoxorubicin (Epidx) in hepatoma (Hep) and pancreatic cancer (Panc). Proc. Am Soc Clin Oncol 1984; C-574 (abstract): 147.

Ihde DC, Kane RC, Cohen MH, et al. Adriamycin therapy in American patients with hepatocellular carcinoma. Cancer Treat Rep 1977; 61: 1385–1387.

Inouye AA, Whelan TJ. Primary liver cancer: a review of 205 cases in Hawaii. Am J Surg 1979; 138: 53–61.

Iqbal MJ, Wilkinson ML, Johnson PJ, et al. Sex steroid receptor proteins in foetal, adult and malignant human liver tissue. Br J Cancer 1983; 48: 791–796.

Kalser MH, Ellenberg SS. Pancreatic cancer: adjuvant combined radiation and chemotherapy following curative resection. Arch Surg 1985; 120: 899–903.

Loehrer PJ, Williams SD, Einhorn LH, Ansari R. Ifosfamide: an active drug in the treatment of adenocarcinoma of the pancreas. J Clin Oncol 1985; 3: 367–372.

Longmire WPJr, Traverso LW. The Whipple procedure and other standard operative approaches to pancreatic cancer. Cancer 1981; 47: 1706–1711.

Mallison CN, Rake MO, Cocking JB, et al. Chemotherapy in pancreatic cancer: results of a controlled prospective, randomised multicentre trial. Br Med J 1980; 281: 1589–1591.

Melia WM, Westaby D, Williams R. Diammino-dichloride platinum (cis-platinum) in the treatment of hepatocellular carcinoma. Clin Oncol 1981; 7: 275–280.

Moertel CG, Childs DS, Reitermeier RJ, et al. Combined 5-fluorouracil and supervoltage radiation therapy of locally unresectable gastrointestinal cancer. Lancet 1969; 2: 865–867.

Moertel CG. Chemotherapy of gastrointestinal cancer. In: Tagnon HJ, Staquet MJ, eds. Recent advances in cancer treatment. New York: Raven, 1977: 311–321.

Moertel CG, Frytak S, Hahn RG, et al. Therapy of locally unresectable pancreatic carcinoma: a randomized comparison of high dose (6000 rads) radiation alone, moderate dose radiation (4000 rads + 5-fluorouracil), and high dose radiation + 5-fluorouracil (The Gastrointestinal Tumor Study Group). Cancer 1981; 48: 1705–1710.

Nagasue N, Ito S, Yukaya H, et al. Androgen receptors in hepatocellular carcinoma and surrounding parenchyma. Gastroenterology 1985; 89: 643–647.

Nagasue N, Ito A, Yukaya H, et al. Estrogen receptors in hepatocellular carcinoma. Cancer 1986; 57: 87–91.

Nair PV, Tong MJ, Kempf R, et al. Clinical, serologic and immunologic effects of human leukocyte interferon in HBsAg-positive primary hepatocellular carcinoma. Cancer 1985; 56: 1018–1022.

Nakajiama Y, Miyamoto T, Tanabe M, et al. Enhancement of mammalian cell killing by 5-fluorouracil in combination with X-rays. Cancer Res 1979; 39: 3763–3767.

Ohnishi S, Murakami T, Moriyama T, et al. Androgen and estrogen receptors in hepatocellular carcinoma and in surrounding non-cancerous liver tissue. Hepatology 1986; 6: 440–443.

Olweny CLM, Toya T, Katongole-Mbidde E, et al. Treatment of hepatocellular carcinoma with adriamycin: preliminary communication. Cancer 1975; 36: 1250–1257.

Order SE, Leibel S. Radiolabeled antibodies in the treatment of primary liver cancer. Appl Radiol 1984; 13: 67.

Order SE, Klein J, Leichner P, et al. I–131 radiolabeled antibody (antiferritin) in the treatment of hepatoma: an update. Proc Am Soc Clin Oncol 1984; C-538 (abstract): 138.

Order SE, Stillwagon GB, Klein JL, et al. Iodine 131 antiferritin: a new treatment modality in hepatoma, a Radiation Therapy Oncology Group study. J Clin Oncol 1985; 3: 1573–1582.

Order SE, Klein JL, Leichner PK, et al. ^{90}Yttrium antiferritin: a new therapeutic radiolabeled antibody. Int J Radiat Oncol Biol Phys 1986; 12: 277–281.

Oster MW, Theologides A, Cooper MR, et al. Fluorouracil (F) + adriamycin (A) + mitomycin (M) FAM in advanced pancreatic cancer. Proc. Am Soc Clin Oncol 1982; C-350 (Abstract): 90.

Ravry MJR, Amura GA, Bartolucci AA, et al. Phase II evaluation of cisplatin in advanced hepatocellular carcinoma and cholangiocarcinoma: a Southeastern Cancer Study Group trial. Cancer Treat Rep. 1986; 70: 311–312.

Rotman M, Kuruvilla AM, Choi K, et al. Response of colo-rectal hepatic metastases to concomitant radiotherapy and intravenous infusion 5-fluorouracil. Int J Radiat Oncol Biol Phys 1986; 12: 2179–2187.

Rotman M, Macchia R, Silverstein M, et al. Treatment of advanced bladder carcinoma with irradiation and concomitant 5-fluorouracil infusion. Cancer 1987; 59: 710–714.

Sachs E, Di Bisceglie AM, Dusheiko GM, et al. Treatment of hepatocellular carcinoma with recombinant leucocyte interferon: a pilot study. Br J Cancer 1985; 52: 105–109.

Schein PS, Lavin PT, Moertel CG. Randomized phase II clinical trial of adriamycin in advanced measurable pancreatic carcinoma: a Gastrointestinal Tumor Study Group report. Cancer 1978 a; 42: 19–22.

Schein PS, McDonald JS, Hoth D, et al. Mitomycin-C: experience in the United States, with emphasis on gastric cancer. Cancer Chemother Pharmacol 1978 b; 1: 73–75.

Shildt R, Baker L, Stuckey W. Hepatic artery infusion (HAI) with 5FUDR (F), adriamycin (A) and streptozotocin (ST) in unresectable hepatoma: a South-West Oncology Group study. Proc Am Soc Clin Oncol 1984; C-587 (abstract): 150.

Shiu W, Mok SD, Tsao S, et al. Phase II trial of epirubicin in hepatoma. Cancer Treat Rep 1986; 70; 1035–1036.

Sitzmann JV, Order SE, Klein JL, et al. Conversion by new treatment modalities of nonresectable to resectable hepatocellular cancer. J Clin Oncol 1987; 5: 1566–1573.

Smith FP, Schein PS. Chemotherapy of pancreatic cancer. Semin Oncol 1979; 6: 368–377.

Smith FP, Hoth DF, Levin B, et al. 5-fluorouracil, adriamycin and mitomycin-C (FAM) chemotherapy for advanced carcinoma of the pancreas. Cancer 1980; 46: 2014–2018.

Smith F, Rustgi V, Schertz G, et al. Phase II study of 5-FU, doxorubicin and mitomycin (FAM) and chlorozotocin in advanced measurable pancreatic cancer. Cancer Treat Rep 1982; 66: 2095–2096.

Smith F, Brigo V, Lokey L, et al. Phase II evaluation of hexamethylmelamine plus FAM in advanced measurable pancreatic cancer. Proc Am Soc Clin Oncol 1983; C-493 (abstract): 126.

Smith GW, Bukowski RM, Hewlett JS, et al. Hepatic artery infusion of 5-fluorouracil and mitomycin C in cholangiocarcinoma and gallbladder carcinoma. Cancer 1984; 54: 1513–1516.

Smith IE. Mitoxantrone (novantrone): a review of experimental and early clinical studies. Cancer Treat Rev 1983; 10: 103–115.

Starzl TE, Koep LJ, Weil R, et al. Right trisegmentectomy for hepatic neoplasms. Surg Gynecol Obstet 1980; 150: 208–214.

Urist MM, Balch CM. Intra-arterial chemotherapy for hepatoma using adriamycin administered via an implantable constant infusion pump. Proc Am Soc Clin Oncol 1984; C-579 (abstract): 148.

Van Echo DA, Leone R, Davis B, et al. A phase II study of mitoxantrone (NSC 301 739) in patients with primary liver cancer (PLC). Proc Am Soc Clin Oncol 1984; C-558 (abstract): 143.

Vogel CL, Bayley AC, Brooker RJ, et al. A phase II study of

adriamycin (NSC 123 127) in patients with hepatocellular carcinoma from Zambia and the United States. Cancer 1977; 39: 1923–1929.

Wiggans R, Wooley P, McDonald J, et al. Phase II trial of streptozotocin, mitomycin C and 5-fluorouracil (SMF) in the treatment of advanced pancreatic cancer. Cancer 1978; 41: 387–391.

Wils J, Bleiberg H, Blijham G, Dalesio O, Duez N, Lacave Splinter T. Phase II study of epirubicin in advanced adenocarcinoma of the pancreas. Eur J Cancer Clin Oncol 1985; 21: 191–194.

10.4 Radiotherapy: Options and Possibilities

D. Gonzalez Gonzalez and C. Koedooder

Introduction

Adenocarcinomas of the extrahepatic bile duct and pancreatic adenocarcinomas are generally considered to be radioresistant tumors. It is important, however, to distinguish radioresistance from radiocurability. In fact, the intrinsic sensitivity of tumor cells to radiation is only one of the factors involved in the radiocurability of tumors. The radiation dose that can be administered within the tolerance of the normal tissues as well as the number of tumor cells and the extent of the tumor burden present at the time of treatment are equally important factors. Adenocarcinomas of the uterine body, for example, are radioresistant tumors, but it is possible to achieve about 50% tumor cure if a high radiation dose is administered by using intracavitary radioactive sources. Due to rapid fall-off of radiation, this high tumor dose does not compromise the tolerance of the normal tissues. If the number of tumor cells present in the treated area is not too large, so-called radioresistant tumors can also be radiocurable. This is the case in rectal adenocarcinomas and soft-tissue sarcomas, where microscopic remnants remaining after surgery can be sterilized using postoperative radiation.

In pancreatic adenocarcinomas, radiation has been administered in situations in which the tumor is locally unresectable. Data on the possible role of postoperative radiation, either as an adjuvant therapy or for the treatment of microscopic residual tumor, are scarce. The same is true of extrahepatic bile duct cancer. With the development of new diagnostic techniques, it will probably be possible within the next few years to diagnose hepatobiliary and pancreatic tumors at an earlier stage. In addition, radiation techniques are now available which allow radiation treatment to be administered with high precision.

We shall discuss here options and possibilities available in radiation therapy, and we shall compare data from the literature with our own experience.

Extrahepatic Bile Duct Tumors

In this section we shall consider tumors in the left and right hepatic ducts, at the confluence (Klatskin tumor) and in the middle portion of the bile duct. Carcinomas of the gallbladder are discussed separately, and carcinomas of the distal bile duct and periampullary region will be considered together with pancreatic cancer below.

The first option in the treatment of extrahepatic bile duct tumors is surgery. Radical resection achieves about 30% 2-year survival (Evander et al. 1980, Blumgart et al. 1984). However, radical resection can only be performed in a small proportion of patients. The main objective of surgery is to achieve adequate biliary drainage. In a review by Kopelson et al. (1977) of 94 patients reported in 16 series, the average survival with curative surgery was 16.9 months. Local recurrence after surgery is a common cause of failure, probably higher than 26%. In patients who only underwent a biliary drainage, the average survival is 2–9.5 months with a better prognosis when the drainage was done during surgery (Passariello et al. 1985, Gabrielsson et al. 1985, Qualman et al. 1984).

The role of radiation therapy in extrahepatic bile duct tumors has not yet been established. As noted above, these tumors have been considered radioresistant. However, this has never been proved. Table 10.4.1 gives a review of data from the literature. In patients who only have an external or internal biliary drainage, external beam irradiation achieved an average survival rate of between 9.5–27 months (Kopelson et al. 1977, Whelton et al. 1969, Green et al. 1973, Terblanche 1976, Mornex et al. 1984, Johnson et al. 1985, Fogel et al. 1984, Mittal et al. 1985). The series by Karani et al. (1985) deserves special consideration. In 30 patients receiving intraluminal irradiation with iridium-192 following biliary drainage, the mean survival was 16.8 months, which is similar to the survival reported in the so-called "curative" series with surgery. In patients with microscopic residual tumor in the surgical margin, the average survival was 15.7 months when postoperative irradiation was administered (Qualman et al. 1984).

Our own experience with irradiation in extrahepatic bile duct cancer is limited to 20 patients, 12 treated postoperatively for microscopic residual tumor and 8 after biliary drainage alone. This experience has been accumulated in the period 1981–1986. In the group of patients receiving postoperative irradiation, 6 were treated with external beam irradiation and 6 received combined external and intraluminal irradiation with iridium-192. Irradiation was given with a linear accelerator with a 10 megavolt (MV) photon beam. The target volume was defined with the use of all available pre- and postoperative information, i.e. computed tomography (CT) scan, surgical report, endoscopic retrograde cholangiopancreatography (ERCP), angiography and endosonography. The CT scan was performed in the treatment position to deline-

Table 10.4.1 Review of reported results in extrahepatic biliary duct cancer treated with radiation therapy

Author	No. of patients	Surgery	Dose (Gy)	Intraluminal iridium-192	Survival
Whelton et al. (1969)	5	Biliary drainage	50	–	Mean: 27 months
Green et al. (1973)	4	"	20–53	–	Mean: 11 months
Terblanche et al. (1976)	5	"	60	–	Range: 2.5–5 years
Qualman et al. (1984)	7	"	–	–	Mean: 9.5 months only 1XRT: 15 months
Qualman et al. (1984)	9	Resection positive margins	50	In 3 patients	Mean: 15.7 months
Karani, J. et al. (1985)	30	Biliary drainage	–	44.7 Gy (0.5 cm)	Mean: 16.8 months
Mornex et al. (1984)	7	Resection, drainage	20–50	30–57 Gy	Range: 1.5–23 months; 4 patients alive
Johnson et al. (1985)	7	External drainage	21–50	31–60 Gy	Mean: 15.4 months
Fogel et al. (1984)	34	Resection (8), drainage (25) (6 recurrences)	50	18–38 Gy (1.5 cm) in 3 patients	Mean: 11 months
Kopelson et al. (1977)	8	Drainage	38–72	–	Mean: 16.8 months
Mittal et al. (1985)	16	Resection, drainage	7.5–60	–	Mean: 8.7 months (drainage); 13 months (resection)

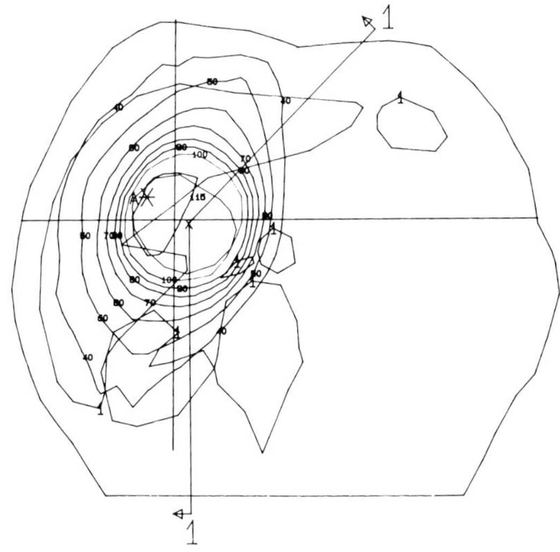

Fig. 10.4.1 **Computer planning dosimetry** derived from a computed tomography (CT) scan in treatment position. This patient had a right hemihepatectomy and cholangiojejunostomy. A rotation technique was used. Doses in regenerating liver, kidneys and spinal cord are within the tolerance of these organs

ate the target volume and plan dosimetry. In general, the liver hilum, the location of the hepaticojejunal anastomosis, and the distal part of the bile duct were included in the radiation fields. A multifield or rotational technique was used (Fig. 10.4.1). Two patients received conventional fractionation and the other 10 patients three fractions per day. The radiobiological arguments in favor of multiple fractions per day have already been reported (Schuster-Uitterhoeve et al. 1986). Apart from these arguments, the use of multiple fractions per day is more comfortable for the patient, as the overall treatment time is reduced to 19 days as compared to 42 days with conventional fractionation. The intraluminal irradiation was given with the microselectron afterloading system (Nucletron Engineering). In surgery, the extremity of the jejunal Roux-en-Y loop was not closed but instead brought to the abdominal wall, creating a jejunostomy. Through this loop it is easy to localize the anastomosis of the cholangiojejunostomy and to position the iridium wires (Fig. 10.4.2). When the intraluminal treatment is finished, the jejunostomy is surgically closed. The active length of the iridium wires was 5 cm, and one or more wires were used per application, depending on the technical possibility of crossing the jejunal loop. The dose distribution around the sources is presented in Figure 10.4.2.

The results, as well as some patient characteristics in the group treated with postoperative irradiation, are presented in Table 10.4.2. All the patients had a palliative tumor resection and a cholangiojejunostomy. In 4 cases, tumor resection was accompanied by resection of a part of the liver. Two patients died 7.5 and 9 months after surgery. In one of these two patients, the first sign of relapse was observed in the operation scar. Soon afterwards, this patient developed peritonitis carcinomatosa. The second patient also developed peritonitis carcinomatosa. The other patients are alive with survival periods of 8–34 months. The irradiation was well tolerated by all patients, and no significant acute reactions were observed. Two patients had late complications due to fibrosis of the jejunal loop, confirmed during reoperation. These two

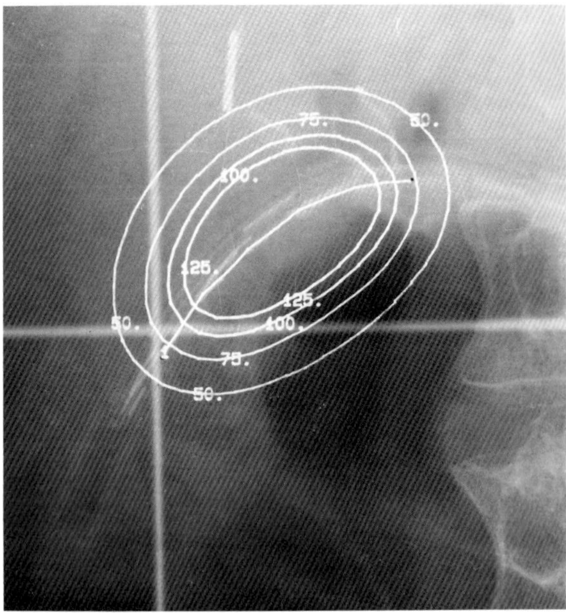

Fig. 10.4.**2 Control X-ray of the catheter** introduced through the Roux-en-Y loop. In this particular case, four iridium wires, each 5 cm in length, were positioned at the location of the cholangiojejunostomy. The dose distribution pattern (cGy/h) is also shown

patients have recovered well and are now alive without evidence of disease. Eight patients in the group as a whole have resumed their normal life.

The other group of patients was treated with radiation following external or internal biliary drainage. Only one patient received iridium-192 intraluminal irradiation through a nasobiliary probe. The results are presented in Table 10.4.**3**. Average survival was 10 months. All but one of the patients are now dead. This rate of survival seems to be superior to that reported for biliary drainage alone.

Gallbladder Cancer

Carcinoma of the gallbladder is often found by chance after simple cholecystectomy. In this favorable group, however, local relapse will occur in about 48% of patients (Kopelson et al. 1977). Reasons for local failure are the high incidence of local lymph node metastases, varying from 26–52% (Vaittinen 1970, Fahim 1962), and direct extension to the liver in 52–66% (Vaittinen 1970). Extension through the gallbladder wall increases the risk of microscopic residual disease and local

Table 10.4.**2 Patient characteristics, type of surgery, and radiation doses** in patients with extrahepatic bile duct cancer receiving postoperative irradiation

Age	Sex	Surgery	Differential grade	Lymph nodes	Perineural invasion	Dose/Fraction/Days (Gy)	Dose (Gy) of intraluminal iridium-192 (at 1 cm)	Last follow-up
31	M	Resection, cholangio-jejunostomy	G_1	−	+	44/41/19	−	34 months, alive
53	M	Resection, cholangio-jejunostomy	G_1	−	−	45/42/19	−	31 months, alive
58	M	Resection, cholangio-jejunostomy	G_2	−	+	45/42/19	−	36.5 months, alive
61	M	Resection, cholangio-jejunostomy	G_3	−	+	63/60/42	−	7.5 months, dead
57	M	Resection, cholangio-jejunostomy	G_2	−	+	45/41/19	−	12 months, alive
66	M	Resection, cholangio-jejunostomy	G_2	−	+	49/43/19	12	17 months, alive
57	M	Resection, cholangio-jejunostomy	G_1	+	+	45/41/21	10.5	9 months, dead
46	F	Resection, cholangio-jejunostomy	G_1	−	+	43/41/18	9.8	12 months, alive
58	M	Resection, cholangiojejunostomy hemihepatectomy	G_2	−	+	46/42/18 + 10/ 6/ 3	−	13 months, alive
59	M	Resection, cholangiojejunostomy hemihepatectomy	G_2	−	−	45/41/18	10	14 months, alive
31	M	Resection, cholangiojejunostomy hemihepatectomy	G_3	−	+	45/41/18	10.9	17 months, alive
63	F	Resection, cholangiojejunostomy hemihepatectomy	G_1	−	+	43/36/16	13.7	10 months, alive

Table 10.4.**3** **Results in inoperable extrahepatic bile duct cancer** after biliary drainage and radiation therapy

Age	Sex	Dose (Gy)/Fraction/Days	Last follow-up	Site of failure
72	F	64/32/44	3.5 months, dead	local + metastases
33	M	68/61/42	16 months, dead	local, ascites
36	M	60/30/41	20 months, dead	local
71	M	69/60/42	8.5 months, dead	local, ascites
62	F	69/60/42	4 months, dead	local, ascites
60	M	59/30/40	8 months, alive	–
64	F	45/41/21*	2 months, dead	local
48	F	64/32/42	18.6 months, dead	local

* (+ iridium-192, 20 Gy)

recurrence after surgery (Kopelson 1977). More radical surgical procedures do not seem to increase the chance of cure (Litwin 1967, Warren 1968). In the review by Kopelson et al. (1977), the 5-year survival rate in gallbladder cancer was 6–7%.

The role of radiation therapy in gallbladder cancer is not well established. In a series of 24 patients, postoperative irradiation following curative surgery achieved a median survival of 63 months as compared to 29 months with surgery alone (Vaittinen 1970). In patients treated palliatively or not treated, irradiation seemed to increase survival: the mean survival was 7 months as opposed to 4.6 months for the surgical palliation group (Kopelson 1977). In a series in which gross residual tumor was left after surgery, radiation doses of 12.5–59 Gy achieved a mean survival of 6.5 months (Mittal 1985).

Pancreatic Carcinoma

The best treatment option in pancreatic cancer is surgery. At the time of diagnosis, however, only 10–20% of patients are candidates for surgery (Bayler et al. 1973, Shapiro 1975, Brooks et al. 1976, Tepper et al. 1976). The mean survival after radical surgical procedures varied in older series between 8 and 17 months (Tepper et al. 1976, Najera et al. 1973, Gallitano et al. 1968, Feduska et al. 1971, Crile 1970). In more recent series, the mean survival has increased to 26–33 months (Moossa 1982). The role of postoperative irradiation in resected pancreatic carcinoma has not been investigated until recently. Rich (1985) reported on 10 patients treated with postoperative irradiation after complete surgical removal (Whipple procedure or total pancreatectomy). This group of patients had unfavorable features such as positive microscopic margins, gross unresected tumor, positive lymph nodes and perineural infiltration. Total radiation doses were 40–45 Gy, two patients with gross residual tumor receiving in addition an intraoperative boost of 12.5 Gy. The median survival was 10 months. It is noteworthy in this study that local failure was observed in only one patient. Nguyen et al. (1982) reported on 9 patients receiving 60 Gy after a Whipple procedure. Median survival was 13 months in carcinomas of the head of the pancreas and 17 months in carcinomas of the periampullary region. The Gastrointestinal Tumor Study Group (Kaiser et al. 1985) has conducted the only published randomized study with adjuvant combined radiation and chemotherapy following curative resection. Patients included in this study must have free margins of the surgical specimen. Positive lymph nodes were not a criterion for exclusion. Radiation therapy was given in two courses of 20 Gy each, separated by an interval of 2 weeks. A fluorouracil 500 mg/m^2 intravenous bolus was given once a week for two years or until recurrence. Twenty-two patients were randomized to the control group and 21 to the combined treatment. Median survival in the combined treatment group was 20 months, versus 11 months in the group treated with surgery alone. This difference in survival was statistically significant (p value 0.035). These data have recently been confirmed in 30 additional patients who received the same combined treatment (Gastrointestinal Tumor Study Group 1987). The two-year survival was 18% in the group treated with surgery alone versus 43% in the group with adjuvant therapy.

Our preliminary experience with postoperative irradiation after resection of pancreatic carcinoma is summarized in Table 10.4.4. All of the patients had microscopic residual tumor in the margins of the surgical specimen. Positive lymph nodes, perineural invasion and angioinvasion were also frequent features. Radiation fields encompassed the tumor area, as defined with clips during surgery, plus a margin of about 2 cm. Three isocentric fields were generally used, and when possible the target volume was reduced in the last week of irradiation. Four patients received 55.8–66 Gy total doses with conventional fractionation, 1.8–2 Gy per fraction over 6–7 weeks. The other 9 patients were treated

Table 10.4.4 Postoperative irradiation in resected pancreatic cancer

Age	Sex	Type of Surgery	Location	Pathology	Dose/Fraction/Days (Gy)	Last follow-up	Site of Failure
64	M	Total pancreatectomy	Distal common bile duct, head of the pancreas	G_2 microscopic residual in common bile duct; 1 positive lymph node; perineural invasion; angioinvasion	45/41/20	9 months, alive	–
70	F	Whipple	body and tail of the pancreas	G_1 microscopic residual, posterior margin	62/63/42	8.5 months, dead	Local
39	M	Whipple	Head of the pancreas	G_3 microscopic residual; posterior margin; negative lymph nodes; perineural invasion; angioinvasion	56/29/41	5 months, dead	Scar relapse, local ascites
62	F	Total pancreatectomy	Head of the pancreas, distal common bile duct	G_3 microscopic residual, lateral margin; negative lymph nodes	45/41/18	12 months, alive	–
69	M	Whipple	Head of the pancreas, distal common bile duct	G_3 microscopic residual, pancreatic margin; positive lymph nodes	52/25/35	8 months, alive	–
63	F	Whipple	Head of the pancreas, confluence of common bile duct and pancreatic duct	G_2 microscopic residual, pancreatic margin; positive lymph nodes; perineural invasion; angioinvasion	45/40/20	11 months, alive	–
65	F	Whipple	Ampulla of Vater	G_3 microscopic residual, posterior margin; negative lymph nodes; vasoinvasion	66/32/47	14 months, dead	Local
65	M	Whipple	Ampulla of Vater	G_1 microscopic residual, posterior margin; negative lymph nodes; perineural invasion; angioinvasion	60/30/44	7 months, alive	Local
62	F	Whipple	Head of the pancreas	G_2 microscopic residual, pancreatic margin; negative lymph nodes	66/60/42	4.5 months, alive	–
50	F	Total pancreatectomy	Head of the pancreas	G_3 microscopic residual tumor in all margins; positive lymph nodes; perineural invasion; vasoinvasion	23/20/ 9	10 months, dead	Local
63	M	Whipple	Ampulla of Vater	G_2 microscopic residual, posterior margin; negative lymph nodes; perineural invasion; vasoinvasion	45/41/21	10 months, alive	–
51	M	Whipple	Head of the pancreas, distal common bile duct	G_3 microscopic residual, posterior margin; positive lymph nodes	45/41/18	12 months, alive	–
61	F	Whipple	Head of the pancreas	G_3 microscopic residual, posterior margin; negative lymph nodes; perineural invasion; vasoinvasion	45/41/18	11.5 months, alive	–

Table 10.4.**5   Review of recently reported series on localized unresectable pancreatic carcinoma** treated with radiation therapy and chemotherapy

Authors	No. of patients	Dose (Gy)	Iodine implant	Chemotherapy	Survival (mean)	
Whittington et al. (1984)	36	63–70	–	–	7.3	months
Whittington et al. (1984)	19	63–70	–	+	12.4	months
Whittington et al. (1984)	13	55–60	+	–	5.5	months
Whittington et al. (1984)	20	55–60	+	+	11.3	months
Moertel et al. (1981)	25	60	–	–	5.5	months
randomized	83	40	–	5-FU	10	months
	86	60	–	5-FU	10.6	months
Gastrointestinal Tumor Study Group (1985)	73	60	–	5-FU	9.25	months
randomized	70	40	–	Doxorubicin	8.25	months
Klaassen et al. (1985)	44	–	–	5-FU	8.2	months
randomized	47	40	–	5-FU	8.3	months
Dobelbower et al. (1980)	12	60–70	–	+	15	months
Dobelbower et al. (1980)	28	60–70	–	–	12	months

5-FU: fluorouracil

with three fractions per day, either continuously over 3 weeks or in three courses of 20–22 Gy over 7 days with two weeks' interval. The rationale for this schedule has already been reported (Schuster-Uitterhoeve 1986). Four patients died 5–14 months from the date of surgery. The other 9 patients are alive without evidence of disease 4.5–12 months after surgery.

Radiation therapy alone, or in combination with chemotherapy, has been frequently used in the palliative treatment of localized unresectable pancreatic carcinoma. Recent reported data are summarized in Table 10.4.5 (Whittington et al. 1984, Moertel et al. 1981, Klaassen et al. 1985, Dobelbower et al. 1980). From these studies, the following conclusions can be drawn: it is possible to administer a high dose of radiation with modern techniques without compromising the tolerance of the normal tissues in neighboring organs (liver, kidneys, duodenum, spinal cord). The median survival is improved as compared with untreated patients. Chemotherapy in combination with radiation therapy is superior to radiation alone. Good palliation of symptoms can be obtained in about 70% of patients. The differences in survival between the series could be attributed to selection criteria as well as other factors, such as radiation and chemotherapy schedules.

Our own experience with radiation therapy in unresectable pancreatic carcinoma is limited (Schuster-Uitterhoeve et al. 1986). Twelve patients with locally unresectable carcinoma were treated with 3 fractions per day in 3 courses of 23 Gy over 7 days separated by 2-week intervals. The total dose was 63–69 Gy. The median survival was 6.3 months. These results compare quite well with those obtained with radiation alone by Moertel et

al. (1981) (5.5 months) and Whittington et al. (1984) (7.3 months), but are clearly inferior to those of Dobelbower et al. (1980) (12 months). There were no severe complications. Six patients died as consequence of local failure alone, and the other 6 of local failure combined with distant metastases.

Conclusions and Future Prospects

At present, the only therapy offering a chance of cure in extrahepatic biliary duct cancer, gallbladder cancer and pancreatic cancer is surgery. Unfortunately, only a relatively small proportion of patients with cancer in these sites are candidates for surgery at the time of diagnosis. The best hope for the future is that new diagnostic techniques might detect tumors at an earlier stage, so that surgical tumor resection can be performed in a larger number of patients.

Preliminary results seem to support the role of postoperative irradiation in extrahepatic biliary duct cancer. Our experience in this group of patients with postoperative external beam irradiation, whether combined with iridium-192 intraluminal implant or not, is encouraging and deserves further study. In unresectable extrahepatic biliary duct cancer, the results reported by Karani et al. (1985) with intraluminal application of iridium-192 wires are very promising. It remains to be established whether intraluminal treatment alone is better than external beam irradiation alone or a combination of both. Unfortunately, randomized studies in this relatively rare tumor are difficult to perform.

The role of postoperative irradiation in gallbladder cancer also deserves further investigation. In a small group of patients, postoperative radiation therapy improved survival by a factor of 2 as compared to surgery alone (Vaittinen 1970). Radiation therapy also seems to improve the prognosis in unresectable patients (Kopelson et al. 1977).

In a randomized study, postoperative radiation therapy combined with chemotherapy has been shown to improve the survival in "curative" resected pancreatic carcinoma as compared with surgery alone. This result needs further confirmation in future studies, but our own data support it. Optimum radiation doses and fractionation also need further investigation. There is now clear evidence that radiation therapy combined with chemotherapy prolongs survival and has a good palliative effect in unresectable pancreatic carcinoma. However, these treatments do not offer a relatively high chance of long-term survival.

Other avenues of investigation in extrahepatic bile duct, gallbladder and pancreatic cancer are:

1) *Intraoperative electron-beam radiotherapy*. This technique offers the possibility of administering a high tumor dose while at the same time avoiding damage to normal tissue. In unresectable extrahepatic bile duct cancer, Todoroky et al. (1980) have reported 10.9 months' overall survival, with a good palliative effect. Encouraging results have also been reported in unresectable pancreatic carcinoma by various authors, with a median survival of more than 15 months (Wood et al. 1982, Tepper et al. 1981, Gunderson et al. 1982).

2) *Interstitial radiotherapy* with iodine-125 or other radioactive sources should be a subject of further investigation. Implantation of iodine-125 in unresectable pancreatic carcinoma increased local control from 22 to 81 %, but did not increase survival (Whittington et al. 1984).

3) *Hyperthermia combined with radiation therapy* has proved to be effective in the treatment of various tumor sites. Hyperthermia has a radiosensitizing effect by inhibiting repair of sublethal damage, and further hypoxic cells are sensitive to heat. At present, however, it is difficult to reach high temperatures in deep-seated tumors.

References

Bayler SM, et al. Cross-classification and survival characteristics of 5000 cases of cancer of the pancreas. J Surg Oncol 1973; 5: 335–358.

Blumgart L, et al. Surgical approaches to cholangiocarcinoma at the confluence of hepatic ducts. Lancet 1984; 66–69.

Brooks JR, et al. Cancer of the pancreas: palliative operation, Whipple procedure or total pancreatectomy? Am J Surg 1976; 131: 516–520.

Crile G Jr. The advantages of bypass operations over radical pancreaticoduodenectomy in the treatment of pancreatic carcinoma. Surg Gynecol Obstet 1970; 130: 1049–1053.

Dobelbower RR, et al. Precision radiotherapy for cancer of the pancreas: technique and results. Int J Radiat Oncol Biol Phys 1980; 6: 1127–1133.

Evander A, et al. Evaluation of aggressive surgery for carcinoma of the extrahepatic bile ducts. Ann Surg 1980; 191: 23–29.

Fahim RB, et al. Carcinoma of the gallbladder: a study of its mode of spread. Ann Surg 1962; 156: 114–124.

Feduska NI, et al. Results of palliative operations for carcinoma of the pancreas. Arch Surg 1971; 103: 330–335.

Fogel TD, et al. The role of radiation therapy in carcinoma of the extrahepatic bile ducts. Int J Radiat Oncol Biol Phys 1984; 10: 2251–2258.

Gabrielsson N, et al. Endoscopically inserted endoprosthesis in inoperable biliary obstruction. Acta Radiol Diagn 1985; 26: 57–61.

Gallitano A, et al. Carcinoma of the pancreas, results of treatment. Cancer 1968; 22: 939–944.

Gastrointestinal Tumor Study Group. Radiation therapy combined with adriamycin or 5-fluorouracil for the treatment of locally unresectable carcinoma. Cancer 1985; 56: 2563–2568.

Gastrointestinal Tumor Study Group. Further evidence of effective adjuvant combined radiation and chemotherapy following curative resection of pancreatic cancer. Cancer 1987; 59: 2006–2010.

Green N, et al. Cancer of the common hepatic bile ducts. Palliative radiotherapy. Radiology 1973; 109: 687–689.

Gunderson LL, et al. Intraoperative irradiation: a pilot study, combining external beam photons with "boost" dose intraoperative electrons. Cancer 1982; 49: 2259–2266.

Johnson DW, et al. Malignant obstructive jaundice: treatment with external beam and intracavitary radiotherapy. Int J Radiat Oncol Biol Phys 1985; 11: 411–416.

Kaiser MH, et al. Pancreatic cancer: adjuvant combined radiation and chemotherapy following curative resection. Arch Surg 1985; 120: 899–903.

Karani J, et al. Internal biliary drainage and local radiotherapy with iridium-192 wire in treatment of hilar cholangiocarcinoma. Clin Radiol 1985; 36: 603–606.

Klaassen DJ, et al. Treatment of locally unresectable cancer of the stomach and pancreas: a randomized comparison of 5-fluorouracil alone with radiation plus concurrent and maintenance 5-fluorouracil: an Eastern Cooperative Oncology Group Study. J Clin Oncol 1985; 3: 373–378.

Kopelson G, et al. The role of radiation therapy in cancer of the extrahepatic biliary system. Int J Radiol Biol Phys 1977; 2: 883–894.

Litwin MS. Primary carcinoma of the gallbladder. Arch Surg 1967; 95: 236–240.

Mittal B, et al. Primary cancers of extrahepatic biliary passages. Int J Radiat Oncol Biol Phys 1985; 11: 849–854.

Moertel CG, et al. Therapy of locally unresectable pancreatic carcinoma: a randomized comparison of high dose (6000 rad) radiation alone, moderate dose radiation (4000 rad + 5-fluorouracil), and high dose radiation (+ 5-fluorouracil). Cancer 1981; 48: 1705–1710.

Moossa AR. Pancreatic cancer: approach to diagnosis, selection for surgery and choice of operation. Cancer 1982; 50: 2689–2698.

Mornex F, et al. Radiotherapy of high bile duct carcinoma: using intracatheter iridium-192 wire. Cancer 1984; 54: 2069–2073.

Najera ME, et al. Carcinoma of the pancreas: therapeutic implications. Arch Surg 1973; 106: 293–294.

Nguyen TD, et al. Postoperative irradiation of carcinoma of the head of the pancreas area: short-time tolerance and results to precision high dose technique in 18 patients. Cancer 1982; 50: 53–56.

Passariello R, et al. Percutaneous biliary drainage in neoplastic jaundice. Acta Radiol Diagn 1985; 26: 681–689.

Qualman JS, et al. Adenocarcinoma of the hepatic duct junction: a reappraisal of the histologic criteria of malignancy. Cancer 1984; 53: 1545–1551.

Rich TA, Radiation therapy for pancreatic cancer: eleven year experience at the JCRT. Int J Radiol Oncol Biol Phys 1985; 11: 759–763.

Schuster-Uitterhoeve ALJ, et al. Radiotherapy with multiple fractions per day in pancreatic and bile duct cancer. Radiother Oncol 1986; 7: 205–213.

Shapiro TM. Adenocarcinoma of the pancreas: a statistical analysis of biliary bypass vs Whipple resection in good risk patients. Ann Surg 1975; 6: 715–721.

Tepper V, et al. Carcinoma of the pancreas: review of MGH experience from 1963 to 1973; analysis of surgical failure and implications for radiation therapy. Cancer 1976; 37: 1519–1524.

Tepper V, et al. Summary of the Workshop on Intraoperative Radiation Therapy. Cancer Treat Rep 1981; 65: 911–918.

Terblanche J. Is carcinoma of the main hepatic duct junction an indication for liver transplantation or palliative radiotherapy? A plea for the U tube palliative procedure. Surgery 1976; 79: 127–128.

Todoroky T, et al. Intraoperative radiotherapy for advanced carcinoma of the biliary system. Cancer 1980; 46: 2179–2184.

Vaittinen E. Carcinoma of the gallbladder: a study of 390 cases diagnosed in Finland, 1953–1967. Ann Chir Gynaecol 1970; 168 (suppl): 1–81.

Warren KW, et al. Primary neoplasia of the gallbladder. Surg Gynecol Obstet 1968; 126: 1036–1040.

Whelton MJ et al. Carcinoma of the junction of the main hepatic ducts. Q J Med 1969; 38: 211–229.

Whittington R, et al. Multimodality therapy of localized unresectable pancreatic adenocarcinoma. Cancer 1984; 54: 1991–1998.

Wood WC, et al. Intraoperative irradiation for unresectable pancreatic carcinoma. Cancer 1982; 49: 1272–1275.

10.5 Endoscopic Biliary Drainage (Hamburg)

H. Grimm and N. Soehendra

History

Both internal and external drainage of an obstructed bile duct is possible with endoscopy. Extracorporeal drainage is achieved by means of a nasobiliary drain, while an endoprosthesis provides internal drainage into the duodenum. The nasobiliary drain was first introduced as a method of endoscopic drainage in 1976 (Nagai et al. 1976). The first endoscopic transpapillary placement of a bilioduodenal endoprosthesis followed two years later (Soehendra and Reynders-Frederix 1979). Endoprosthesis rapidly gained significance for the drainage of malignant obstructive jaundice without stress to the patient or loss of bile. Today the nasobiliary drain, incorporating a means of lavage, is only used to treat bacterial cholangitis and litholysis (Fig. 10.5.1). A new indication for it is extracorporeal shock wave lithotripsy (ESWL), which requires repeated instillation of contrast agent to localize calculi in the bile duct.

Originally, the duodenoscope available to implant the endoprosthesis had a narrow working channel, only permitting the insertion of 5 Fr catheters. The Olympus-gastroscope GF-B2 was used to insert 7 Fr catheters. These difficulties led to modifications being introduced (Huibregtse et al. 1981, Kautz 1983). Today most prostheses are implanted with the so-called jumbo duodenoscope, which has a working channel of 3.7 to 4.2 mm, suitable for larger catheters of up to 12 Fr.

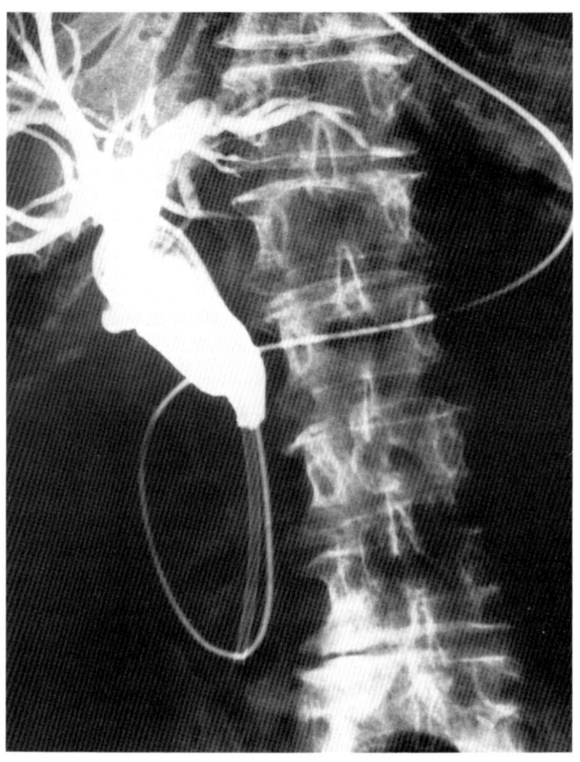

Fig. 10.5.**1 Malignant obstruction of the distal common bile duct** with coexisting purulent cholangitis. Endoscopic implantation of an endoprosthesis and a nasobiliary tube to rinse the bile duct

Table 10.5.**1 Characteristics of catheter materials**, according to Wilson-Cook Medical Inc. (with permission)

Characteristics	Teflon®	Polyethylene	Materials Polyurethane	Polyvinylchloride	Silicone
Friction Coefficient $f = \dfrac{F^*}{W}$	0.04	0.21	1.35	2.0	3.0
Hardness (Shore A Scale)	100	90	83	70	65
Moisture Absorption (% 24 h)	0	0.015	0.9	0.75	0.1
Autoclave	Yes	No	No	No	Yes
Destruction C° Temperature F°	399° 750°	93° 200°	143° 290°	93° 200°	480° 900°

*f = coefficient of friction; F = force required to move a 5 pound weight over a non-lubricated polished metal surface; W = 5 pounds, which is constant during the test

Materials and Method

To implant the prosthesis, a guide wire and a pusher catheter are necessary. Catheters are made of polyethylene, polyurethane or Teflon. Teflon is harder, and has the lowest friction coefficient (Table 10.5.**1**). It is therefore less susceptible to compression, and slides more easily. Endoprostheses come in two basic shapes: pigtail and straight.

Pigtail prostheses are tapered at the tip and curved. Tapering facilitates passage through severe stenoses. Curvature prevents displacement. The straight models have lateral flaps for the same purpose. "Double pigtail" catheters are recommended to prevent injury to the duodenal wall. The additional curve at the distal tip has proved superfluous (Fig. 10.5.**2**).

Duodenal perforations can largely be avoided if the length of the prosthesis is correct. As a rule, an endoprosthesis should not extend more than 2 cm beyond the papilla. The total length is 10 to 15 cm. A prosthesis which is too short displaces more easily in the bile duct. In order to prevent this, a reversed lateral flap is made at the duodenal end. Several side-holes, made as large as possible with a punch or scalpel according to the extent and location of the stenosis, provide optimal drainage (Fig. 10.5.**3**). Prostheses are radiopaque for fluoroscopic control. The 170 cm pusher catheter can be made of ordinary Teflon material of the same caliber. It should be of a different color from the prosthesis for easy identification during the insertion process.

The flexible guide wires (0.035 inches) familiar from angiography are suitable as mandrins. A dilator is recommended to facilitate the introduction of the guide wire (Soehendra et al. 1984). The dilator is a 7 Fr Teflon catheter, 170 cm long, which is tapered at the point (Fig. 10.5.**4**). An additional advantage is that the guide wire can turn inside it and can thus be maneuvered through complicated

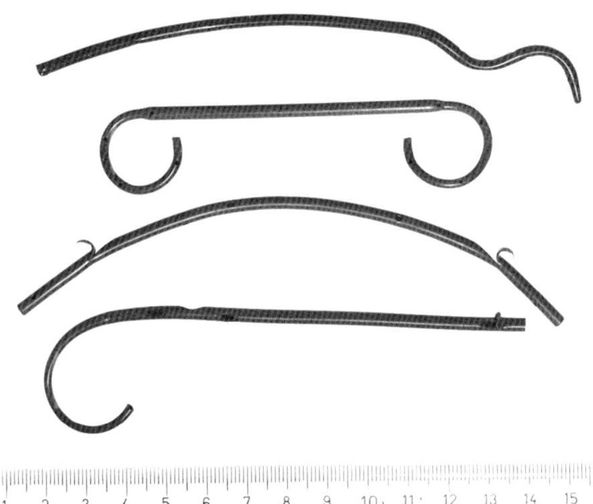

Fig. 10.5.**2 Commercially available biliary endoprostheses:** pigtail and straight forms

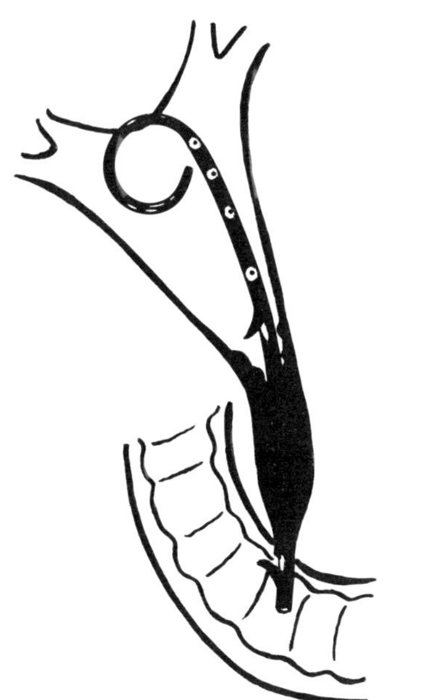

Fig. 10.5.**3 Properly-placed pigtail endoprosthesis** with several large side-holes. Two side-flaps are made on both sides of the obstruction to prevent dislocation

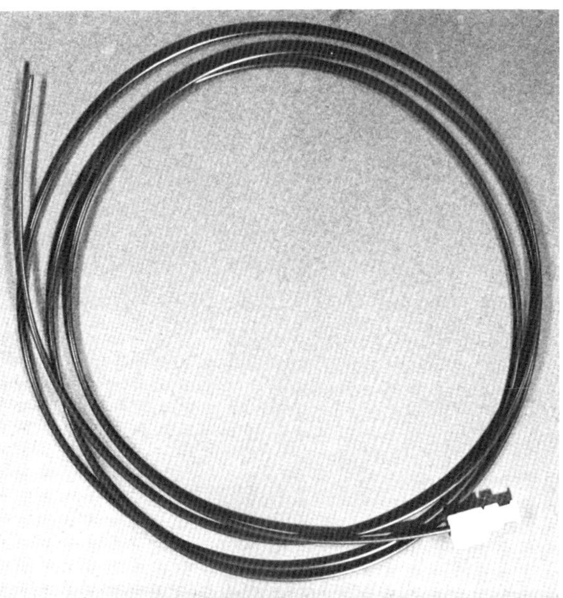

Fig. 10.5.**4 Catheter dilator** for easy insertion of the guide wire and subsequent bougienage of stenoses prior to prosthesis implantation

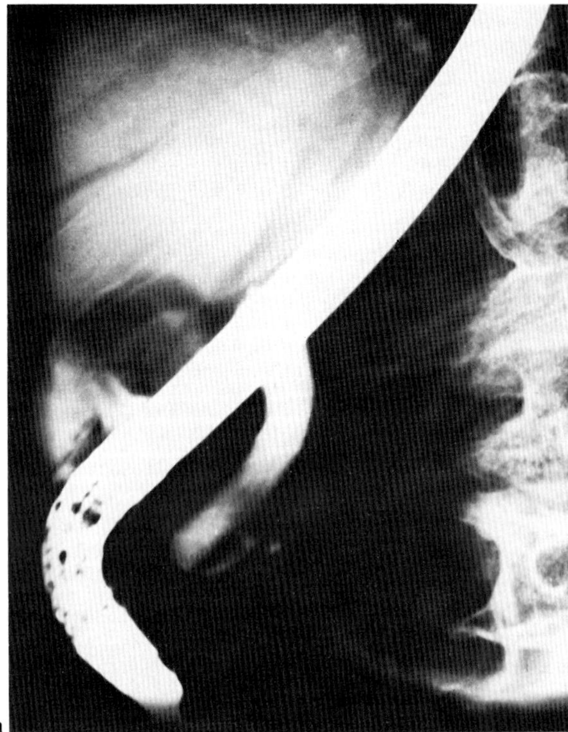

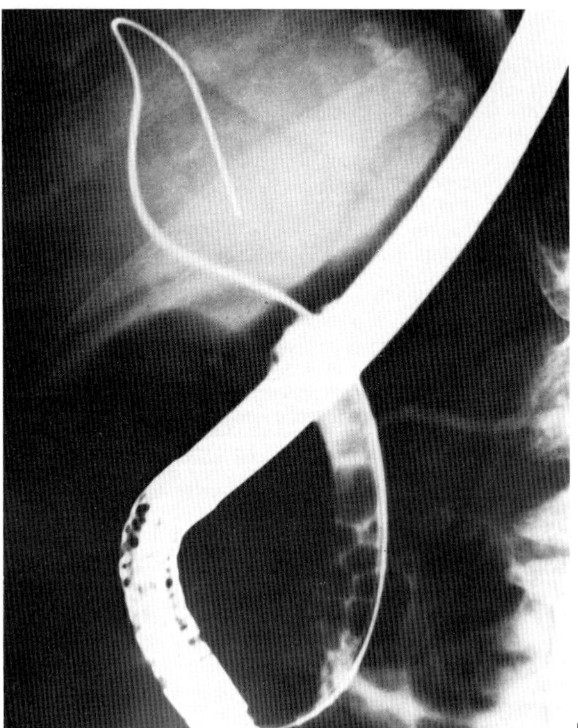

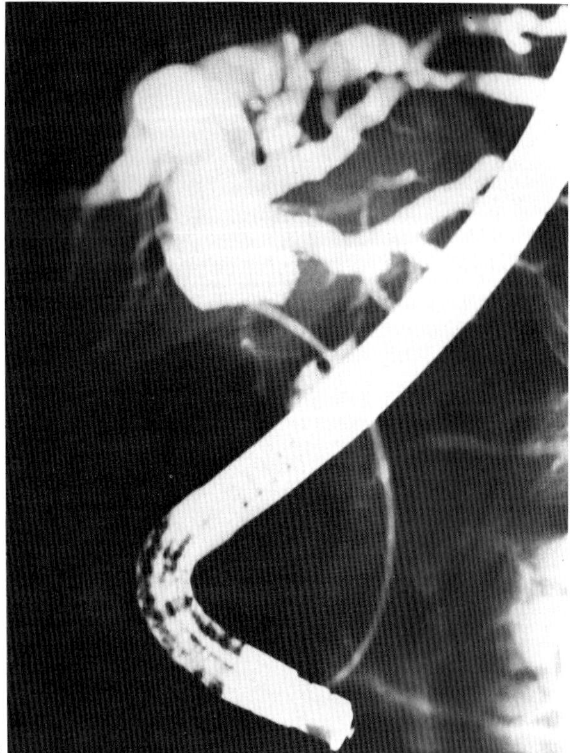

Fig. 10.5.5a   Complete obstruction of the middle part of the common bile duct due to cancer
b   After introducing the guide wire with the dilator, several bougienages are performed to allow a large stent to be placed
c   To opacify the proximal biliary tree, the dilator is used as a catheter for contrast media instillation

stenoses more easily. The insertion of a wide-channel prosthesis is also easier after dilation. After the obstruction has been passed, the dilator can serve as a catheter to opacify the intrahepatic bile ducts (Fig. 10.5.**5**) After removing the dilator, the endoprosthesis is inserted into the bile duct over the 300 cm guide wire by means of the pusher catheter (Figs. 10.5.**6**, 10.5.**7**). If the endoprosthesis is implanted over the guiding catheter (Amsterdam technique), the guide wire needs to be longer (Huibregtse et al. 1986).

The entire process of endoscopic transpapillary prosthesis implantation is based on the Seldinger principle (Fig. 10.5.**8**). In order to facilitate the procedure, it is recommended to perform a small papillotomy first.

A suitable instrument is the duodenoscope, with a 3.7 to 4.2 mm working channel, allowing the insertion of 10–12 Fr prostheses. Endoscopes with a 3.7 or 3.8 mm channel have recently been preferred, as they serve for diagnosis as well as therapy, making it unnecessary to exchange instruments. With regard to drainage effects, particularly occlusion rates, there is no significant difference between the 10 Fr and the 12 Fr prostheses. Insertion of the 10 Fr catheter is easier, however.

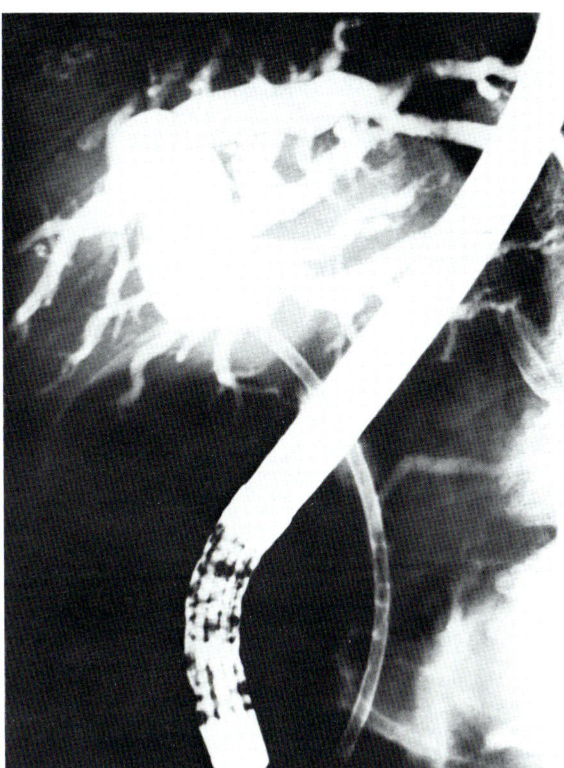

Fig. 10.5.**6** **Endoscopic transpapillary insertion of a 10 Fr stent** in a patient with common bile duct cancer

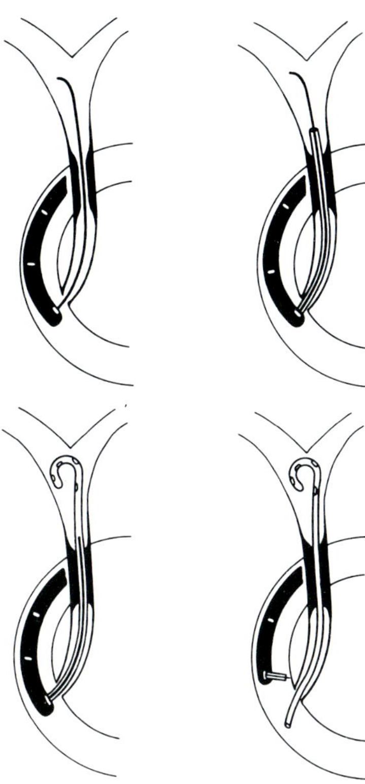

Fig. 10.5.**8** **Schematic presentation of the endoscopic transpapillary implantation of an endoprosthesis** (Seldinger principle)

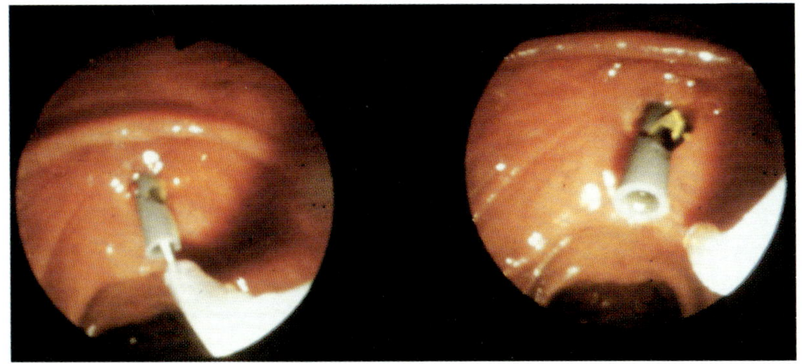

Fig. 10.5.**7** **The stenting procedure under endoscopic vision.** The endoprosthesis and the pusher are of different colors

Results

Since the introduction of the method, more than 1,500 patients have presented for endoscopic therapeutic drainage. Approximately 90 % were suffering from malignant obstructive jaundice, and the remaining 10 % from benign diseases of the biliary tract. The ratio of females to males was 6 : 4. The average age of the patients was approximately 72 years.

Prosthesis implantation in malignant obstructions was successful in 85–90 % of cases. Pancreatic carcinoma near the papilla and primary tumors of the biliary tract caused difficulties more frequently (Soehendra and Grimm 1988). Papillary invasion often makes cannulation difficult. Extreme compression and stenosis of the duodenum also make access to the papilla impossible. In carcinoma of the biliary tract, the long, kinked strictures hamper intubation (Fig. 10.5.**9**). More severe is obstruction

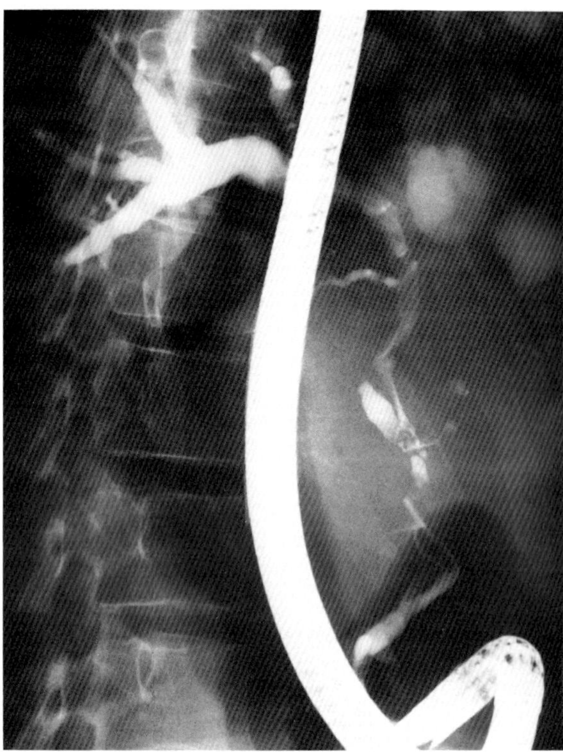

Fig. 10.5.**9** **Advanced cancer of the common bile duct** with a very severe and complicated stenosis which cannot be passed by the guide wire

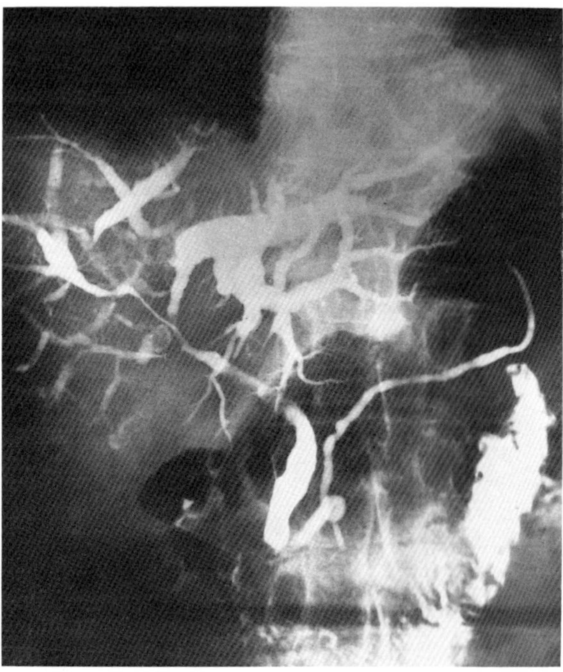

Fig. 10.5.**10** **Bile duct cancer involving both hepatic ducts** ("Klatskin tumor")

of the hepatic bifurcation, which requires separate bilateral drainage (Fig. 10.5.**10**). Endoscopic transpapillary drainage obtains good palliative results in about 90 % of patients (Cotton 1982, Grimm et al. 1988, Hagenmüller and Soehendra 1983, Kühner et al. 1984, Soehendra and Grimm 1988). The more conscientious the patient selection, the greater the success will be. Early occlusion or dislocation of the prosthesis is usually responsible for poor results.

Complications

The complication rate requiring intervention is 1.5 to 2 %, usually originating from the papillotomy. Complications are bleeding, pancreatitis, and retro-
duodenal perforation. As a rule, hemorrhage can be controlled immediately with endoscopy (Grimm and Soehendra 1983). Acute pancreatitis usually resolves after three days under conservative treatment. Retroduodenal perforation only occurs if the papillary incision is too long. Injuries to the bile duct near the tumor can be caused by the guide wire. The procedure-related mortality is 1 %.

Early complications after a successful prosthesis implantation, besides catheter occlusion and displacement, are cholangitis and cholecystitis which can manifest within a few days due to unsterile conditions and only partial drainage. Acute cholecystitis may occur in cases with distal obstruction if drainage of the common bile duct does not simultaneously relieve an existing hydrops of the gall bladder. Antibiotic prophylaxis is generally recommended. Rarely, distal displacement of the prosthesis causes duodenal perforation. These early complications occur in 1–2 % of patients (Grimm et al. 1988).

The most frequent late complication of endoscopic drainage treatment is prosthesis occlusion, usually after an average of three months. Only 20 % of these occlusions are ever registered, due to the limited life-expectancy in advanced carcinoma cases. Cholangitis develops in half of all occlusions, depending on how soon the occlusion is discovered. A timely exchange of the prosthesis can prevent further serious effects, such as cholangiosepsis and liver abscess (Fig. 10.5.**11**). A renewed rise of bilirubin in the serum indicates a reduced drainage effect (Fig. 10.5.**12**). An occluded prosthesis can usually be exchanged in the out-patient clinic.

Prostheses can displace in both directions. An endoprosthesis which has slid into the bile duct can be restored endoscopically with a forceps or a balloon catheter (Fig. 10.5.**13**). Prostheses which displace distally are usually discharged per vias naturales without complications (Fig. 10.5.**14**).

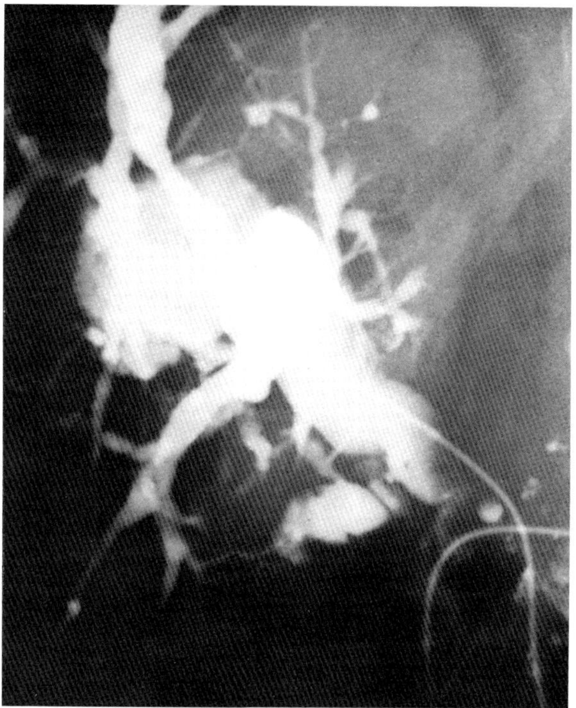

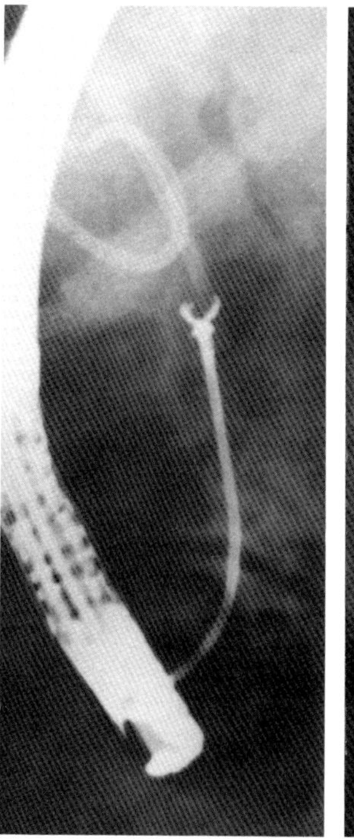

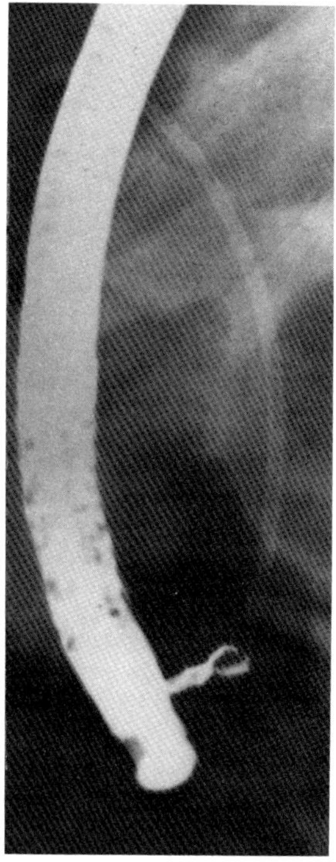

Fig. 10.5.**11   Purulent cholangitis following occlusion of the prosthesis.** Abscess in the liver. Placement of a nasobiliary tube for rinsing

Fig. 10.5.**13   Proximal dislocation of an endoprosthesis.** Endoscopic correction by means of a rat-tooth forceps (Olympus)

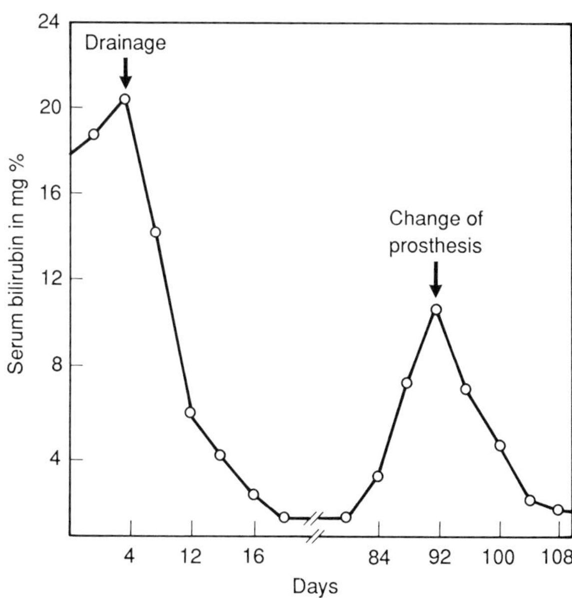

Fig. 10.5.**12   The curve of serum bilirubin levels,** demonstrating the reduced drainage effect due to clogging of the prosthesis

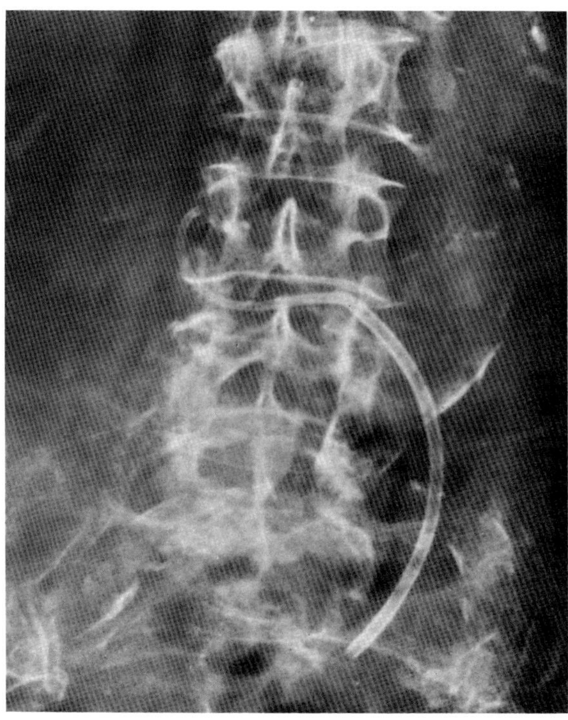

Fig. 10.5.**14   Distal dislocation of an endoprosthesis.** This usually discharges spontaneously per vias naturales

Table 10.5.**2** **Late complications of endoscopic biliary drainage** (418 followed-up patients)

Complication	n	%	Lethal
Clogging without cholangitis	37	8.9	–
Clogging with cholangitis	46	11.0	–
Cholangitis without clogging	41	9.8	4
Dislocation	6	1.4	–
Pancreatitis	12	2.9	3
Liver abscess	2	0.5	–
Cholecystitis	1	0.2	–
Total	145	34.7	7 (1.7%)

Table 10.5.**3** **Treatment protocol for malignant jaundice**, including palliative drainage

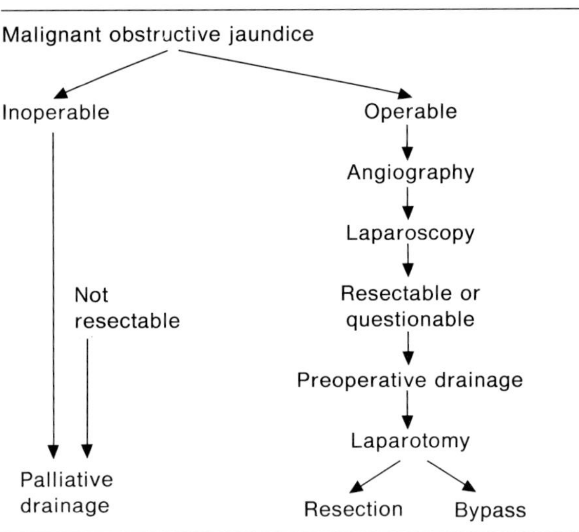

Late dislocations and other septic disturbances, and pancreatitis, occur in 5% of patients (Table 10.5.**2**).

Indications and Contra-indications

For malignant obstructive jaundice, endoscopic drainage is primarily a palliative treatment, indicated when radical surgery is impossible. Elderly patients with severe associated diseases should be admitted to endoscopic treatment if anticipated surgical or anesthetic risks outweigh expected recovery rates. If an exploratory laparotomy of younger patients rules out resection, palliative biliodigestive anastomosis is performed. Surgery is also preferred in cases with duodenal stenosis. Otherwise, palliative surgery, disregarding patient selection, has a mortality rate of over 20% (Sarr and Cameron 1982).

Preoperative drainage has yet to be proved beneficial. At present, only comparative studies based on percutaneous transhepatic drainage exist. Some conclude that preoperative treatment is beneficial (Denning et al. 1981, Nakayama et al. 1978), whereas others reject drainage due to its high morbidity (Hatfield et al. 1982, Pitt et al. 1985). More extensive statistics indicate that the endoscopic method is safer than percutaneous transhepatic drainage (Kühner et al. 1984, Riemann 1984). Prospective controlled studies must therefore be undertaken to prove whether endoscopic drainage can decrease surgical mortality rates.

Generally, insertion of a nasobiliary drain or endoprosthesis immediately following endoscopic retrograde cholangiopancreatography (ERCP) can avert infection, which endangers the seriously ill patient with extreme jaundice. Endoscopic drainage now includes differentiated procedures for treating malignant obstructive jaundice (Table 10.5.**3**).

Afterloading therapy combined with drainage is effective with malignant tumors of the central biliary duct which are often hopelessly unresectable at diagnosis (Phillip et al. 1988). This type of treatment is still in its infancy. The results, especially the survival rates, have yet to be compared to drainage treatment alone.

Icterus should be resolved prior to a scheduled oncological therapy. Often, concomitant tumor metastases compress the large biliary ducts causing cholestasis, which must be resolved. Obstructive jaundice is not necessarily always intrahepatic, in spite of diagnosed metastases in the liver, it is therefore not necessarily hopeless either. For example, our experience shows that palliative drainage treatment is still possible in about 80% of colorectal primary tumors (Grimm et al. 1988). If ultrasound examination reveals dilation of the intrahepatic bile ducts, the indication would be for ERCP followed by prosthesis implantation.

Manifest clotting dysfunction is a contra-indication to endoscopic drainage.

Treatment of multiple intrahepatic stenoses is only justified if the outcome is promising. Partial drainage only endangers patients who have cholangitis. Obstructions of the bifurcation therefore require two separate endoprostheses if both hepatic ducts are involved (Fig. 10.5.**15**).

Summary

Endoscopic drainage aims to restore bile flow, relieving such symptoms as icterus, pruritus, and impaired digestion, and preventing further complications due to the hepatorenal functional disturbance. As a symptomatic therapy, it strives primarily to improve the patient's quality of life.

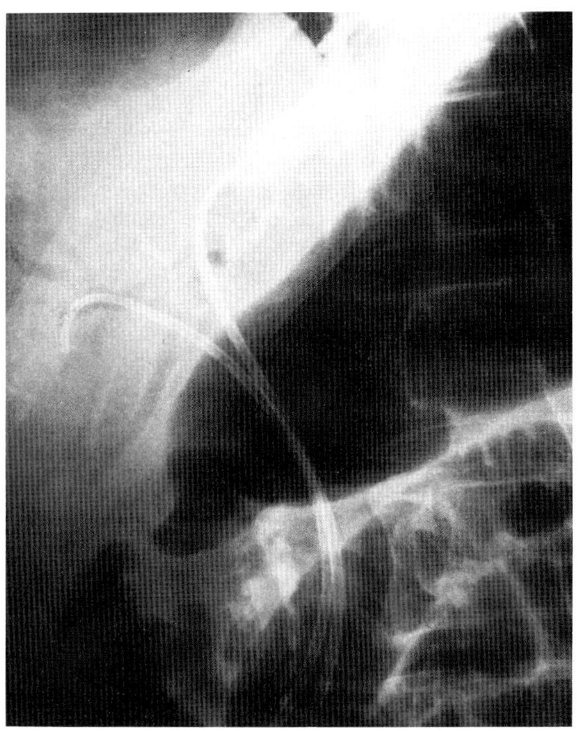

Fig. 10.5.**15** **Obstruction of both hepatic ducts** due to a carcinoma. Separate drainage by two pigtail prostheses

Successful drainage treatment can improve survival rates by preventing disease-related complications, but it cannot extend life expectancy. The average survival rate of patients presented for endoscopic drainage is 4.5 to 20.6 months, with inoperable carcinoma of the gall bladder having the shortest, and carcinoma of the papilla the longest, rates of survival. There are no significant statistical differences compared to palliative surgery (Grimm et al. 1988). Morbidity requiring intervention, and mortality, are clearly lower in endoscopic drainage treatment than in surgery. However, catheter occlusion is a problem. Thus the method requires conscientious aftercare in order to prevent the complications of cholangitis. Ethical reservations restrict this and all other palliative measures which are connected with the terminal stages of diseases. Frustrating experiments causing undue stress, and laden with complications, do not fulfill the principles of palliation. A cancer patient's short life should not be made more agonizing.

References

Cotton PB. Duodenoscopic placement of biliary prostheses to relieve malignant obstructive jaundice. Br J Surg 1982; 69: 501.

Denning DA, Ellison EC, Carey LC. Preoperative percutaneous transhepatic biliary decompression lowers operative morbidity in patients with obstructive jaundice. Am J Surg 1981; 141: 61.

Grimm H, Soehendra N. Unterspritzung zur Behandlung der Papillotomieblutung. Dtsch Med Wochenschr 1983; 108: 1512.

Grimm H, Sum PYS, Soehendra N. Erfahrungen über die endoskopische biliäre Drainage. Verdauungskrankheiten 1988; 6: 10.

Hagenmüller F, Soehendra N. Non-surgical biliary drainage. In: Classen M, Schreiber HW, eds. Clinics in gastroenterology; vol 12. London: Saunders 1983.

Hatfield ARW, Terblanche J, Fataar S, Kernoff L, Tobias R, Girdwood AH, Harries-Jones R, Marks IN. Preoperative external biliary drainage in obstructive jaundice. Lancet 1982; 11: 896.

Huibregtse K, Haverkamp HJ, Tytgat GN. Transpapillary positioning of a large 3.2 mm biliary endoprosthesis. Endoscopy 1981; 13: 217.

Huibregtse K, Katon RM, Coene PP, Tytgat GN. Endoscopic palliative treatment in pancreatic cancer. Gastrointest Endosc 1986; 32: 334.

Kautz G. Transpapillary bile duct drainage with a large-caliber endoprosthesis. Endoscopy 1983; 15: 312.

Kühner W, Frimberger E, Stölzle L, Weingart J, Ottenjann R. Transpapilläre biliare Drainage. Z Gastroenterol 1984; 19 (suppl): 57.

Nagai N, Toki F, Oi J, Suzuki H, Kozu T, Takemoto T. Continuous endoscopic pancreatocholedochal catheterization. Gastrointest Endosc 1976; 23: 78.

Nakayama T, Ikeda A, Okuda K. Percutaneous transhepatic drainage of the biliary tract. Gastroenterology 1978; 74: 554.

Phillip J, Ries G, Hagenmüller F, Classen M, Szepesi S, Manegold K. Intraluminale Strahlentherapie von malignen, hilusnahen Choledochusstenosen. Verdauungskrankheiten 1988; 6: 16.

Pitt HA, Gomes AS, Lois JF, Mann LL, Deutsch LS, Longmire WP. Does preoperative percutaneous biliary drainage reduce operative risk or increase hospital cost? Ann Surg 1985; 201: 545.

Riemann JF. Extrahepatische Cholostase – Transhepatische Drainagen. Z Gastroenterol 1984; 19 (suppl): 64.

Safrany L, Schott B, Krause S, Balint T, Portocarrero G. Endoskopische transpapilläre Gallengangsdrainage bei tumorbedingtem Verschlußikterus. Dtsch Med Wochenschr 1982; 107: 1867.

Sarr MG, Cameron JL. Surgical management of unresectable carcinoma of the pancreas. Surgery 1982; 91: 123.

Soehendra N, Grimm H. Endoscopic retrograde drainage for bile duct cancer. World J Surg 1988; 12: 85.

Soehendra N, Reynders-Frederix V. Palliative Gallengangsdrainage: Eine neue Methode zur endoskopischen Einführung eines inneren Drains. Dtsch Med Wochenschr 1979; 104: 206.

Soehendra N, de Heer K, Kempeneers I. Endoscopic implantation of bilioduodenal endoprosthesis in benign bile duct stenoses. In: Classen M, Geenen J, Kawai K, eds. Nonsurgical biliary drainage. Berlin: Springer 1984.

10.6 Endoscopic Biliary Drainage (Amsterdam)

K. Huibregtse and G. N. Tytgat

Introduction

Endoscopic retrograde cholangiopancreatography (ERCP) has become one of the major diagnostic procedures in biliary and pancreatic disease since its introduction in 1968. The further development of therapeutic endoscopy has greatly contributed to its widespread use. Endoscopic sphincterotomy and gallstone extraction, first described in 1973, opened the field for further endoscopic therapeutic procedures in the biliary and pancreatic tract. Endoscopic biliary drainage was first described by Soehendra and Reynders-Frederix (1979). This endoscopic therapeutic approach in obstructive jaundice has been adopted since by many centers around the world with great enthusiasm (Huibregtse and Tytgat 1982, 1984, Kozarek and Sanowski 1982, Classen and Hagenmuller 1984, Cotton 1984, Liquory et al. 1984, Siegel 1984). The technique has been further improved and is now well established. By and large it is now known what can be achieved technically and which types of patients and strictures are particularly difficult. Also the spectrum of possible complications, their frequency, and the way to solve them are now well appreciated. Many questions, however, are still unanswered, particularly with regard to the precise indications for operative endoscopic procedures. In general terms, endoscopic biliary drainage is the treatment of choice for very high-risk, elderly and frail patients. For younger and fitter patients, however, it is far less clear and obvious which treatment modality is best and which should be the treatment of choice. Comparative randomized controlled studies are difficult to perform, so that only very few data are available upon which to base one's medical attitude.

In this chapter, we will concentrate first on the technique, the results in different disease groups, and the complications of operative biliary endoscopic procedures. In the second part, we will concentrate on indications and reflections on the management of the patient with obstructive jaundice.

Technique

All therapeutic endoscopic procedures of the biliary tract or pancreatic duct start with a standard diagnostic ERCP. One should attempt to obtain high quality cholangiographic as well as pancreatographic documentation of any biliopancreatic malignancy. Cannulation of the papilla of Vater may be difficult or even impossible in the case of pancreatic cancer or periampullary tumors due to duodenal narrowing, papillary displacement or fixation. Atrophy of the papillary structure due to disuse of the papilla may make cannulation difficult in the case of proximally located obstructing bile duct lesions. Successful cannulation may be achieved only after precut papillotomy (incision of the roof of the papilla with a needle knife) in most of these difficult cases (Huibregtse et al. 1986a).

Following diagnostic ERCP, a standard sphincterotomy of 6 to 8 mm in length is performed. This papillotomy facilitates the introduction of the various catheters and guide wires and allows insertion of a large-bore endoprosthesis or introduction of more than one endoprosthesis. Papillotomy may also prevent occlusion of the pancreatic duct orifice by the endoprosthesis, thereby diminishing the risk of acute pancreatitis. Cytology specimens of bile duct strictures can best be taken at this stage of the procedure. Cytology brushes can be introduced easily through the papillotomy opening. A cytology brush with a metal spring tip recently became available which also allows easy passage of the brush through asymmetrical, tortuous strictures.

At present, diagnostic ERCP and papillotomy are most readily performed using a standard duodenoscope with a 2.8 mm instrumentation channel (Olympus JF1T10). This standard duodenoscope must then be replaced by a duodenoscope with a 3.7 or 4.2 mm instrumentation channel (Olympus TJF10) to insert a large caliber 10 or 12 Fr endoprosthesis. A new videoduodenoscope (Olympus TJFV10) with a 4.2 mm instrumentation channel

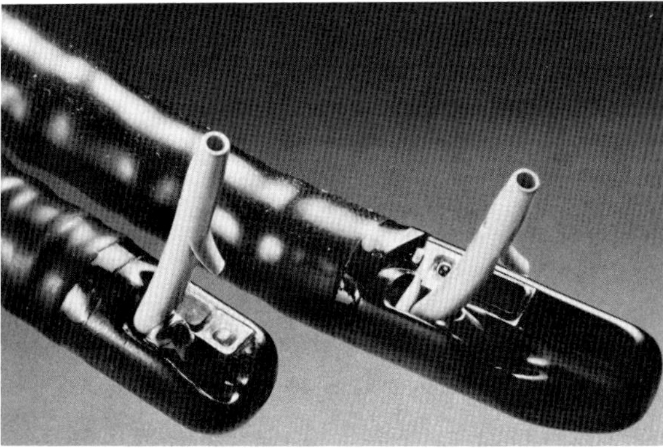

Fig. 10.6.**1**   **A TJF10 Olympus fiber duodenoscope in front of a TJFV10 Olympus videoduodenoscope.** Both endoscopes, with a 4.2 mm instrumentation channel, carry an 11.5 Fr endoprosthesis

has recently been developed which makes the change of instruments unnecessary. A special gutter in the elevator bridge stabilizes even 5 Fr diagnostic catheters, making diagnostic cannulation as easy as with the standard duodenoscope with a small caliber instrumentation channel (Fig. 10.6.**1**).

After proper positioning of the duodenoscope in the duodenum, a Teflon catheter containing a guide wire with an atraumatic flexible tip is inserted into the common bile duct up to the stricture. Usually the catheter cannot be advanced at once through and beyond the stenosis. The guide wire must then be maneuvered carefully through the stricture. This part of the procedure may be time-consuming, with repeated attempts to pass the stricture, varying the position of the endoscope and the tip of the guide wire. Sometimes it is necessary to pre-bend the tip of the guide wire, or to lengthen its flexible tip. Once the rigid part of the guide wire

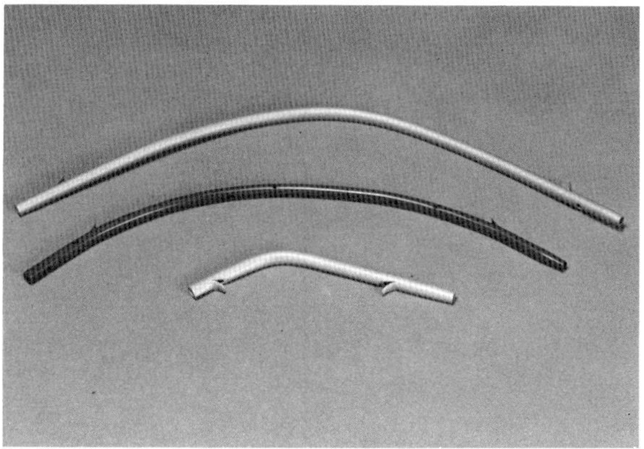

Fig. 10.6.**2 Straight endoprostheses with side flaps.** Top: 11.5 Fr, without side-holes in between the flaps. Middle: 10 Fr, with side holes. Bottom: 11.5 Fr, 9 cm

is inserted well above the stenosis, the relatively rigid catheter can be pushed through the stricture. The stiff assembly consisting of the rather rigid catheter with the stiff guide wire inside it serves as a guide for final insertion of the endoprosthesis. The endoprosthesis is pushed over the catheter with the help of a pushing catheter. Fluoroscopy is vital to ensure that the endoprosthesis moves forward in the bile duct and that the catheter is not withdrawn through the stricture during the insertion procedure. Once the endoprosthesis has been inserted so far that the distal side flap touches the papillotomy opening, it is kept in position by the pusher tube while the guiding catheter containing the guide wire is withdrawn. Finally, the distal end of the endoprosthesis is freed from the endoscope and is visible protruding from the papilla into the duodenum. The endoscope can then be removed, leaving the endoprosthesis behind. The standard endoprosthesis kit containing catheter, guide wire, pusher tube and endoprosthesis which we use is commercially available (Figs. 10.6.**2** and 10.6.**3**) (Wilson Cook Medical Inc., Winston Salem, NC USA). There are many other commercially available prostheses kits: (Surgimed (Denmark), PBN (Denmark), Biotrol (Paris), etc. In experienced hands, this endoscopic diagnostic and therapeutic procedure is successful in about 90 % of cases and takes an average of only 30–45 min.

Dilation of distal bile duct strictures prior to endoprosthesis placement is never necessary using the technique described above. Strictures at the site of the confluence may be tortuous and firm, necessitating prior dilation. For dilation we use stiff Teflon catheters with conical metal tips of increasing diameter, or dilating balloons. Special dilating catheters are now commercially available (Fig. 10.6.**4**).

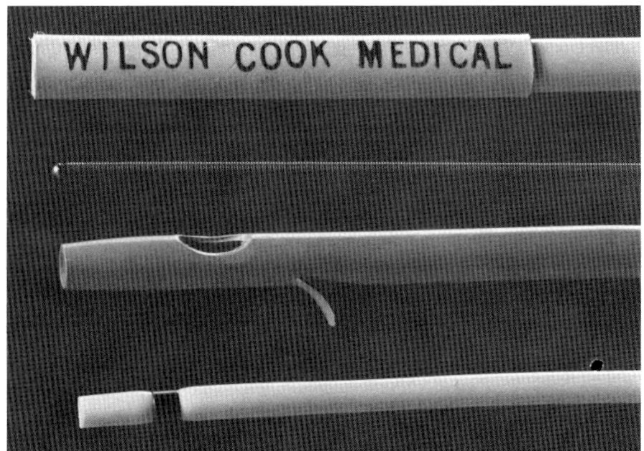

Fig. 10.6.**3 Endoprosthesis kit** consisting of pusher tube, guide wire, endoprosthesis and catheter with metal ring (Wilson Cook Medical Inc., Winston Salem, NC, USA)

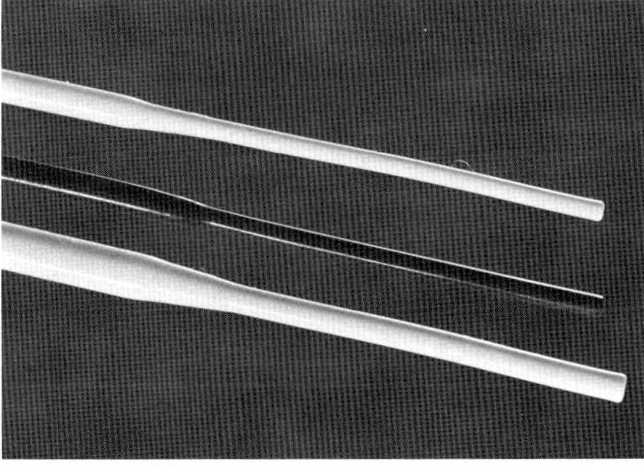

Fig. 10.6.**4 Tips of dilating catheters** of various sizes

Results

Palliation has been achieved in many patients all over the world with biliopancreatic malignancies using transpapillary endoprostheses. In our unit, about 2000 such patients have now been treated (Table 10.6.1). The overall success rate in introducing endoprostheses varies in the literature between 75 % and 90 %. In general, papillary tumors have the highest success rate (95–97 %), pancreatic and distal common duct tumors slightly less (88–92 %), while mid-common bile duct and bifurcation tumors are the most difficult (75–85 %). Failure of endoprosthesis placement might be due to duodenal compression by tumor, inability to perform a papillotomy and failure to pass a guide wire, proximal to the stricture.

Table 10.6.**1   Clinical results of endoscopic endoprosthesis** in patients with cancer (Amsterdam experience)

Type of tumor	Success rate (%)	Bilirubin (%)	Hospital mortality (%)	Median survival (months)
Ampullary	96	98	2	13.5
Pancreatic	90	97	9.5	5
Gallbladder	86	94	20	4.5
Bifurcation	89	88	23	3

With proper placement of an endoprosthesis, nearly all patients with papillary, pancreatic and distal common duct tumors have a decline in bilirubin, while bifurcation tumors are associated with a drop in bilirubin only 89 % of the time. Placement of two endoprostheses (one in each hepatic duct) may improve the clinical success rate in bifurcation tumors, but in our experience this maneuver only succeeds in about 25 % of cases. Hospital mortality in patients with papillary cancer is under 2 %, in distal strictures 7–12 %, while in mid-common bile duct and bifurcation tumors, the 30-day mortality ranges between 20 and 25 %.

For those patients in whom the endoscopic endoprosthesis was the definitive palliative treatment, median survival was 13.5 months for patients with papillary cancer, 5 months for those with distal common duct strictures, and 3–5 months for mid-common bile duct and bifurcation strictures.

Early Complications of Endoprosthesis Placement

Early complications of endoprosthesis placement may be related to the preceding small papillotomy

Table 10.6.**2   Early complications** of endoprosthesis placement (within 1 week)

Complication	Rate (%)
A: papillotomy-related bleeding	1–2
Pancreatitis	0–1
Perforation	0–1
B: Endoprosthesis-related cholecystitis	0–1
Early clogging	1–2
Acute cholangitis	7–27
Ampullary	7
Pancreatic	8
Gallbladder	12
Bifurcation	27
Mortality procedure-related	2

or to the endoprosthesis insertion itself (Table 10.6.**2**). In our experience, complications following endoscopic papillotomy have been far less frequent than the figure of 6–8 % generally quoted for endoscopic papillotomy for calculous disease, probably since the size of the papillotomy is rather small (6–8 mm). Bleeding may be seen in 1–2 % of patients, pancreatitis in 0–1 %, while perforation of the duodenum or bile duct should be exceedingly rare events.

Acute cholangitis is the most important complication of the insertion procedure itself, both in frequency and in severity. Bacterial contamination of the biliary duct system during ERCP is unavoidable. Proper disinfection of the endoscopes and any ancillary equipment is of course mandatory, but will not prevent the introduction of bacteria from the mouth and the upper gut. The introduction of bacteria into the biliary tree only leads to the development of cholangitis when biliary drainage is incomplete. As a consequence, cholangitis is more frequently seen after drainage procedures of bifurcation tumors, where adequate complete biliary drainage is difficult, than in adequately drained, more distally located bile duct strictures. Nor is it surprising that the rate of cholangitis correlates directly with the number of attempts at prosthesis insertion prior to successful insertion. In our study in 200 consecutive patients with pancreatic carcinoma, the overall incidence of cholangitis was 8 % following endoprosthesis placement (Huibregtse et al. 1986 b). However, it was only 2.7 % if successful insertion was achieved at the first attempt, while it was over 22 % if 2 or more attempts were required. It is likely that bacterial contamination was introduced into the biliary tract during the first attempt, with cholangitis ensuing 2 or more days later. With these statistics in mind, it would seem prudent to give antibiotic prophylaxis following an unsuccessful attempt at endoprosthesis insertion. In addition, the next attempt should be made at the earliest possible time, preferably the following day, to prevent major bacterial infection of the biliary tree. For bifurcation tumors, attempts at endoprosthesis placement should only be undertaken with antibiotic coverage.

Other early complications related to the endoprosthesis placement are very unusual and consist of bile duct perforation, acute cholecystitis and early clogging of the endoprosthesis by clots or tumor fragments. Mortality directly related to the papillotomy and endoprosthesis placement is an acceptable 2–4%, with cholangitis being the main cause of death. Thirty-day mortality in these patients, often with advanced cancer, ranges from 10 to 25%.

Late Complications of Endoprosthesis Placement

The main late complication is clogging of the endoprosthesis, occurring in 21–36% of cases (Table 10.6.3). In our experience, clogging may occur from 8 days to over 15 months after placement, with a mean of about 5 months. Clinically, the patients with a clogged endoprosthesis present with a flu-like syndrome, malaise, low-grade fever or recurrence of liver function abnormalities. If the significance of this syndrome is not recognized early, cholangitis and jaundice will occur. Prompt recognition of these symptoms should lead to immediate removal and replacement of the clogged endoprosthesis. Cleaning, brushing and irrigation of a clogged endoprosthesis is technically possible, but reobstruction of the endoprosthesis will quickly occur. Replacement of a clogged endoprosthesis is usually technically simple, since the preliminary papillotomy has already been accomplished (Figs. 10.6.5, 10.6.6). Replacement should require

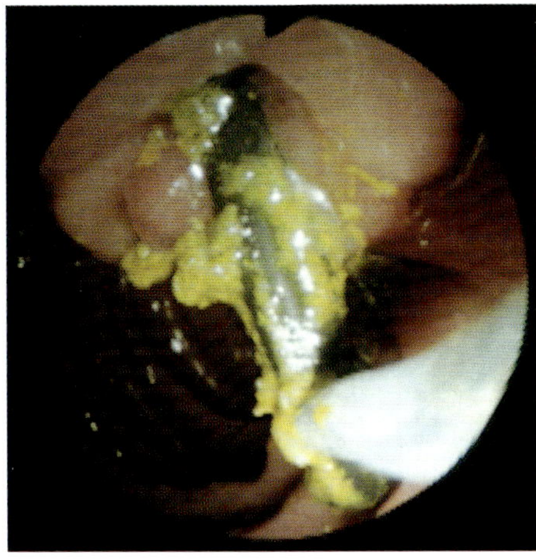

Fig. 10.6.**5** **An obstructed endoprosthesis is caught** with the dormia basket to be removed

Table 10.6.**3** **Late complications** of endoprosthesis placement

Complication	Rate (%)
Clogging	21–36
Acute cholecystitis	0–1
Migration	0–1
Perforation	1–2
Duodenal stenosis	
Ampullary cancer	23
Pancreatic cancer	7.5
Mortality	Unusual

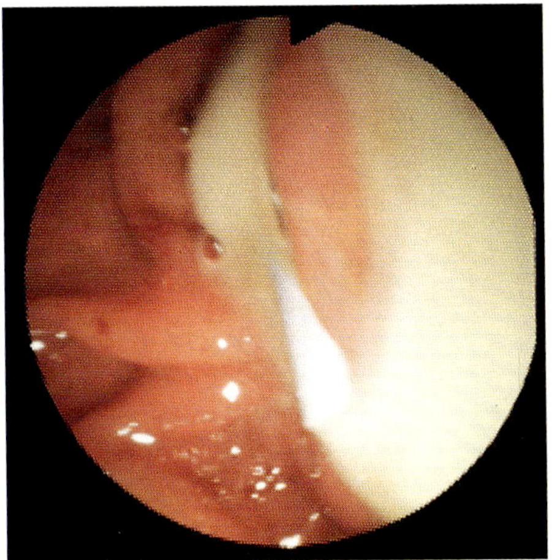

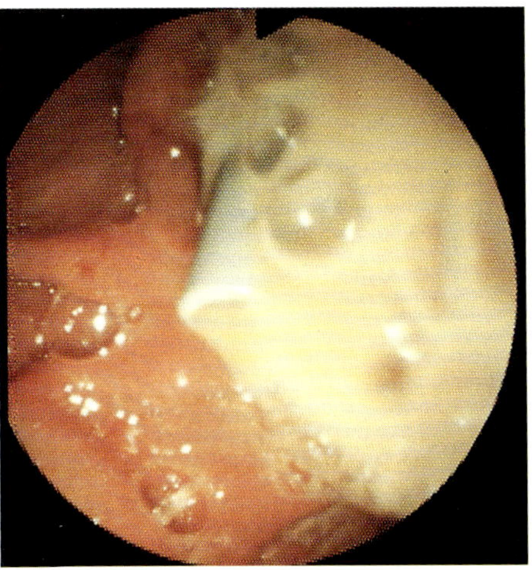

Fig. 10.6.**6** **A patient with severe cholangitis due to obstruction of the endoprosthesis**. Pure pus flows through the clean replaced endoprosthesis

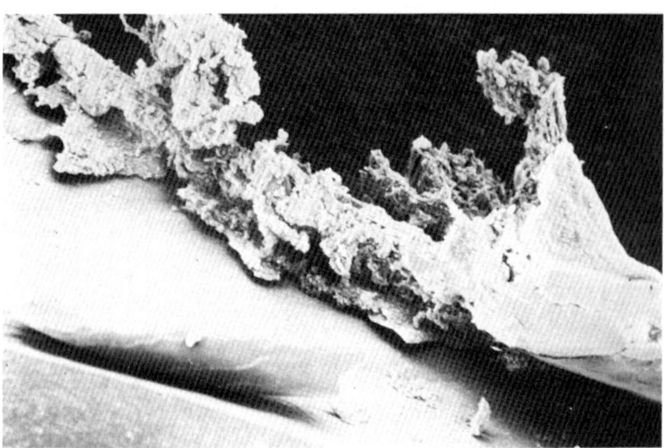

Fig. 10.6.**7 Electronmicroscopy of an endoprosthesis** which was removed 2 months after insertion. A prominent protein layer is seen at the edge of a side-hole •

no more than 15–20 min and is nearly always followed by subsidence of the symptoms of cholangitis and jaundice.

A clogged endoprosthesis contains inspissated bile, calculus-like debris and proteinaceous material (Groen et al. 1987, Wosiewitz et al. 1985). Endoprostheses removed 2 months after insertion are usually covered with a layer of protein. Especially at the site of the side-flap hole and the side-holes, this layer is very prominent (Figs. 10.6.**6**, 10.6.**7**). Bacteria are present in it, even when antibiotics have been administered continuously. It is still not clear whether this layer is produced by bacteria or whether the proteins derive from bile (Speer et al. 1986, 1988, Leung et al. 1988). It is our impression that, in all probability, this layer is the first step in the clogging process. The composition and the formation of this layer need further investigation. Clinical studies show that the patency of 10 Fr endoprostheses is longer than that of 7 or 8 Fr endoprostheses (Deviere et al. 1986). In all probability, the clogging phenomenon develops at the same speed in endoprostheses of both diameters, but the interval until complete obstruction is somewhat longer in the larger ones. Possible further solutions for the clogging problem might include the use of other materials, the use of endoprostheses without side-holes or rough surfaces, and the use of gallstone-dissolving agents, mucolytic agents or choleretic agents.

Other late complications are unusual, but include acute cholecystitis, migration of the endoprosthesis into the more proximal bile ducts or into the bowel, and duodenal or biliary duct perforation. Duodenal stenosis, although it is a direct complication of the tumor, is considered and listed in Table 10.6.**3** as a late complication. Duodenal stenosis is relatively common with ampullary carcinoma and pancreatic carcinoma, since the tumor

is contiguous with the duodenum. The incidence of late duodenal stenosis in our series of pancreatic carcinoma is 7.5%, occurring at a mean of about 300 days following insertion. This low incidence of duodenal stenosis is in all probability mainly explained by our policy of recommending surgical gastroenterostomy plus biliodigestive anastomosis in patients with duodenal compression or invasion of the duodenal wall by tumor at the time of the initial ERCP. In the literature, duodenal stenosis has been observed in 15–25% of patients with ampullary carcinoma treated by an endoprosthesis.

Mortality related to late complications is rare in our series. Prompt recognition and appropriate treatment in the case of late complications is essential to reduce late procedure-related mortality.

Indications for Endoscopic Biliary Drainage

Biliary endoprosthesis has two possible roles in patients with malignant obstructive jaundice: palliation in patients with unresectable tumor, and preoperative drainage in patients with resectable lesions.

Obstruction of the biliary tract may be associated with dysfunction of multiple organs. Energy metabolism and protein synthesis may be deranged because of hepatocyte dysfunction, anorexia, poor caloric intake and impaired digestion and assimilation of proteins, fats and carbohydrates. The mortality and morbidity associated with surgery in this condition is partly due to this dysfunction. Preoperative biliary drainage should correct these defects and lower the mortality and morbidity associated with surgery (Gouma et al. 1987). Preoperative percutaneous transhepatic drainage has been extensively studied. Nakayama et al. (1978) used preoperative drainage, and found that operative mortality was reduced compared with historical controls. Two other studies using historical controls and three studies using concurrent but non-randomized controls suggest that percutaneous preoperative drainage confers some benefit (Takada et al. 1976, Golicz et al. 1984, Denning et al. 1981, Norlander et al. 1982, Gundry et al. 1984). However, three prospective randomized trials have shown no benefit and have emphasized the complications of percutaneous drainage (Hatfield et al. 1982, McPherson et al. 1984, Pitt et al. 1985). Endoscopic stenting avoids the complications of puncturing the liver and the complications of external bile loss. Patients drained internally with an endoscopically positioned stent could spend several weeks at home allowing hepatocellular function to recover. Whether the benefits of drainage will outweigh the complications of the endoscopic procedure can only be assessed in prospective randomized trials. At present such trials are in progress. Diagnostic ERCP in patients with bile duct strictures carries a high risk of cholangitis. Most endoscopists are convinced that this risk is largely avoided by subsequent immediate drainage via a nasobiliary drain or an endoprosthesis. In all probability, this also holds true for distal strictures, where complete drainage can usually be obtained. Most endoscopists are reluctant to leave a patient with a distal stricture undrained after a diagnostic ERCP. This is the main reason why randomized results of preoperative endoscopic drainage are lacking at the present time. Endoscopic drainage procedures in bifurcation tumors carry a much higher risk of cholangitis. In addition, it is unknown, and even questionable, whether the post-ERCP cholangitis risk in these patients is decreased by endoscopic drainage procedures.

The best-evaluated role of biliary endoprosthesis is its role in definitive palliation of biliary and pancreatic malignancies. In the following section, particular technical problems, pitfalls and possible approaches for management in distal common bile duct, mid-common bile duct and bifurcation obstructions will be discussed.

Distal Common Bile Duct Obstruction

Papillary Carcinoma

A papillary carcinoma or periampullary carcinoma is an uncommon, but not rare, cause of tumor-related obstructive jaundice. In our experience, such tumors account for 8% of cases of malignant biliary obstruction. A papillary tumor may be seen endoscopically as a large, exophytic, fragile, fleshy mass lesion at the site of the papilla, or as an ulcerated firm tissue mass at the site of the papilla, or as a bulging papilla, covered with normal-looking mucosa, when the tumor growth lies mainly inside the ampulla. The differential diagnosis of such a bulging papilla includes papillary carcinoma, impacted stone, edema and a choledochocele. Correct diagnosis can only be made after papillotomy of a bulging papilla of this sort. Biopsies must be taken from the edges of the papillotomy wound for proof of malignancy. Despite extensive tissue sampling with a biopsy forceps or polypectomy snare, malignancy can only be demonstrated in 70–80% of cases. Problems with cannulation are frequent, since the orifice may be displaced to an unusual location. In addition, these tumors are extremely friable and usually start oozing as soon as they are probed with the cannula. Also, submucosal injections of contrast material commonly occur during attempts to probe the ductal stricture, since the soft, fleshy lesions allow

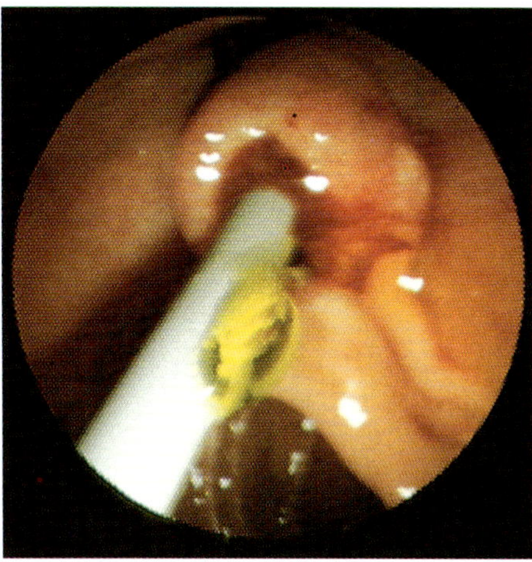

Fig. 10.6.**8** **Endoprosthesis inserted through small ampullary tumor**

cannula insertion within the tissue. It is important to inspect the surface of the tumor carefully prior to attempted cannulation. The location of the orifice can often be found by noting a spot of bile at the site of the opening into the common bile duct.

Since papillary tumors bleed easily, we prefer to place an endoprosthesis without a preliminary papillotomy if possible (Fig. 10.6.**8**). However, in at least 25–30% of cases, a precut papillotomy must be made in order to obtain access to the common bile duct or to obtain a representative tissue specimen. Once access to the biliary tract is obtained, insertion of a short endoprosthesis is usually readily accomplished, since the catheter and guide wire easily traverse the tumor (Fig. 10.6.**9**). Some endoscopists prefer a large papillotomy incision for drainage, notwithstanding the increased risk of post-papillotomy bleeding. However, restricturing of such papillotomies occurs in the majority of patients after a mean time interval of 7 months (Huibregtse and Tytgat 1984). In our series of 71 papillary carcinomas treated with endoprosthesis, the mean interval until clinical endoprosthesis obstruction was 10 months, and the mean survival was 13.5 months (Huibregtse et al. 1987a).

Duodenal stenosis is the most frequent late complication in patients treated without surgical intervention. In our series, duodenal stenosis was seen in 23% of patients.

It should be stressed that papillary carcinoma, unlike carcinoma of the pancreas, has a relatively good prognosis, with a 5-year survival after resection of 30–40%. In patients who have no evidence of metastatic disease and who are reasonable surgical candidates therefore the appropriate method of treatment is a Whipple's procedure or a local tumor resection. A biliary endoprosthesis for

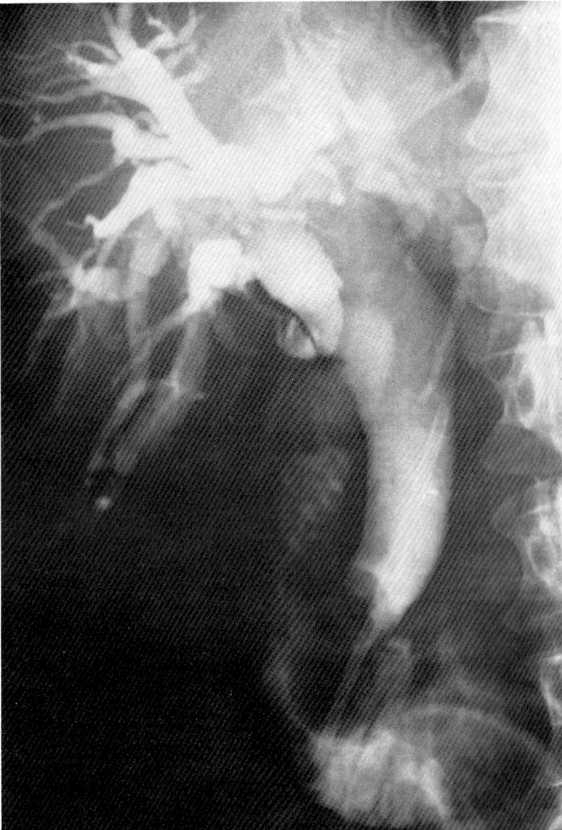

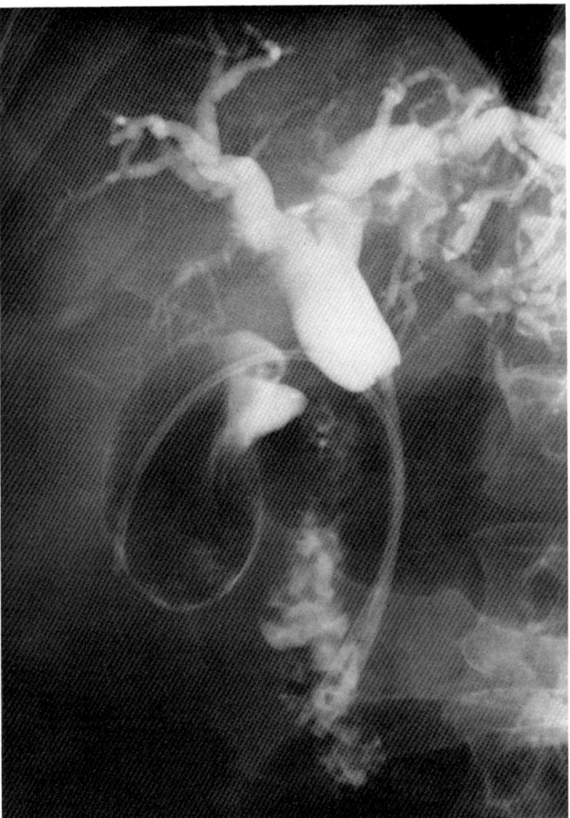

Fig. 10.6.**9 Endoprosthesis inserted through an ampullary tumor.** The tumor grows into the duodenal lumen

Fig. 10.6.**11   Pancreatic cancer occluding the common bile duct and cystic duct.** A 10 Fr endoprosthesis is introduced into the biliary tree and a 7 Fr endoprosthesis is introduced into the gallbladder

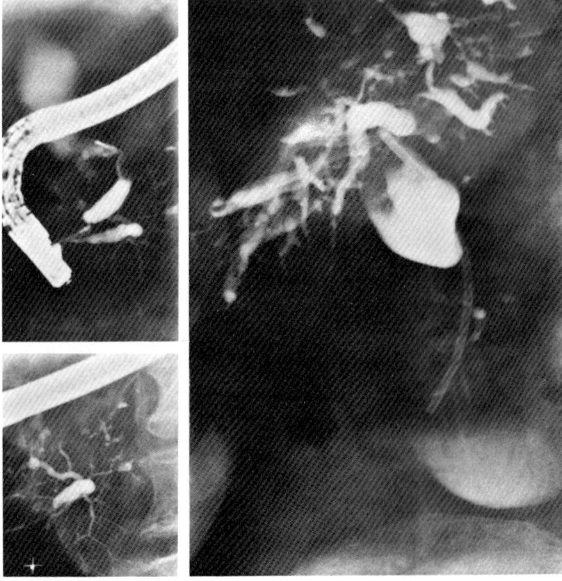

Fig. 10.6.**10   Below left:** complete obstruction of pancreatic duct by pancreatic cancer. **Above left:** stricture of the distal common bile duct with upstream dilation. **Right:** endoprosthesis has been placed, and X-ray contrast is flowing from the biliary tree into the duodenum

definitive palliation should be reserved for elderly patients with severe underlying disease and for those with advanced or metastasized cancer.

Pancreatic Cancer

Pancreatic cancer is the most common tumor leading to obstructive jaundice, and accounts for more than 50% of such cases (Figs. 10.6.**10**), 10.6.**11**, 10.6.**12**). Tumors growing near the papilla may distort the distal common bile duct and the distal pancreatic duct, so that cannulation and papillotomy may be difficult or even impossible. More sophisticated methods like needle-knife precut may be necessary to obtain access to the common bile duct. Only in a minority of cases is it difficult to pass a guide wire through the stricture, due to the stricture's sharp angulation or tortuosity. Stent placement in pancreatic cancer is successful in about 90%. Procedure-related mortality is 2%, 30-day mortality is 10%, and the hospital stay is usually limited to 2–5 days. In addition, the mean survival is aproximately six months (Huibregtse et al. 1986b, Siegel and Snady 1986).

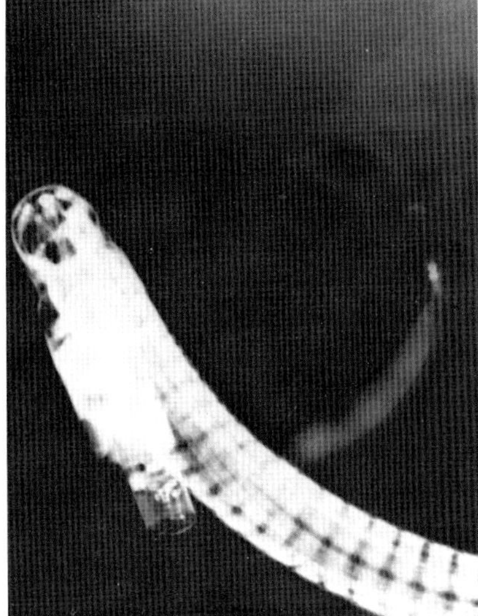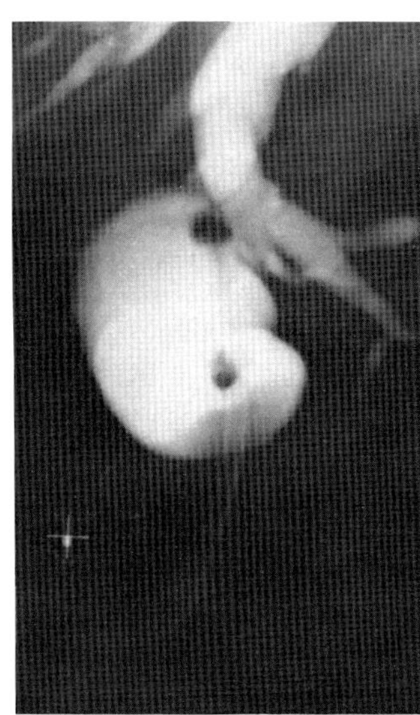

Fig. 10.6.**12** **A patient with recurrent jaundice after cholecystojejunostomy. Left:** air in the gallbladder, and failure to fill the gallbladder and common hepatic duct with contrast. **Right:** dilated common hepatic duct. No filling of the gallbladder. Proper position of the endoprosthesis

Which Patients Will Benefit from Endoscopic Endoprosthesis as a Definitive Palliation?

Carcinoma of the pancreas is a disease of the elderly. Mortality and morbidity of surgery increase with increasing age and in the presence of extensive metastatic disease. Mortality of biliodigestive bypass surgery in patients with liver metastasis and extensive metastatic disease has been reported in 43–59 % (Feduska et al. 1971, Blievernicht et al. 1980, Ubhi and Doran 1986). Age higher than 60 years was found to be a risk factor in biliary surgery (Pitt et al. 1981), and operative mortality for pancreatic resection over 65 and 70 years of age has been reported as 41 % and 58 % respectively (Lerut et al. 1984). Epidemiologic studies from England and Wales show that the median age of onset is about 70 years, with 44 % of the mean and 59 % of the women being older than 70 (Allen-Mersh and Earham 1986). In England in 1979, only 34 % of patients with carcinoma of the pancreas had surgical intervention (Fraumeni 1975). Also, in the United States of America it has been estimated that only 50 % of patients are seen by surgeons (Toouli 1986). In many surgical series, about 20 % of patients submitted to laparotomy had such extensive disease that it was not possible to perform a biliary bypass (Trede 1985). Most of these high-risk patients with resectable disease may obtain worthwhile palliation by means of biliary stents. Patients suitable for surgery with unresectable disease at present have a surgical bypass as the standard treatment. Surgical exploration has additional advantages. The tumor can be directly biopsied, the ultimate proof of irresectability can be obtained, and a prophylactic gastroenterostomy can be performed. Unfortunately, surgical bypass

has a significant mortality (18 %) in a large review of the literature (Sarr and Cameron 1984). Tumor staging and assessment of resectability has become more accurate and precise with the development of newer imaging techniques such as ultrasonography, computed tomography, angiography and endoscopic ultrasound. An exploratory laparotomy is only rarely desirable due to conflicting findings. Confirmation of malignancy can be obtained by percutaneous aspiration cytology guided by ultrasound or computed tomography (Lees et al. 1985). In addition, recently-developed cytology brushes allow endoscopic sampling from the bile duct and pancreatic duct. Endoscopic stent placement has a low early morbidity, low 30-day mortality and involves a substantially shorter hospital stay than after surgical bypass procedures. The disadvantages of stent placement are endoprosthesis clogging and late duodenal obstruction. The incidence of late duodenal obstruction is low in the endoscopic stent series, because patients with duodenal infiltration on presentation are usually referred for surgery. Whether this low incidence of duodenal obstruction will continue to be seen in younger, fitter patients as well needs to be assessed in further studies.

The results of series of endoscopic stents for carcinoma of the pancreas cannot be compared with surgical series, since most patients were referred for endoscopic treatment because they were not considered candidates for surgery. Prospective randomized trials are necessary to evaluate the usefulness of both treatment approaches. At present only one such study has been performed (Shepherd et al. 1988). In this study, 51 patients with unresectable carcinoma of the pancreas were randomized between endoscopic stents and bypass surgery. The techniques were equally successful in relieving jaundice. The 30-day mortality for endoscopic stents (8 %) was less than that for surgery (25 %). However, this was not statistically significant, presumably because of the small sample size. The length of the initial hospital admission was significantly less for stents (5 days) compared with surgery (11.5 days). Throughout the patient's lifetime the total numbers of days spent in the hospital was also significantly less for stents (8 days) compared with surgery (13 days). Additional studies are required to confirm these results. It is to be expected that further comparative studies will identify patient groups for which surgery or stenting appears to be the best treatment. It is our impression that in all probability young and fit patients will benefit more from surgery and that elderly and frail patients will benefit more from endoscopic stenting.

It should be mentioned at this point that an endoscopic biliary endoprosthesis can provide adequate preoperative drainage in the small group of patients with resectable pancreatic cancer.

Mid-Common Bile Duct Obstruction

Mid-common bile duct obstruction is usually due to a primary bile duct carcinoma or a gallbladder cancer invading the bile duct. Management is similar, regardless of the primary origin of the tumor. Obstruction of the mid-common bile duct by tumor accounts for about 15–20 % of all malignant common bile duct obstructions. Surgical bypass procedures are often very difficult in these

situations, and positioning of an endoscopic endoprosthesis seems a reansonable alternative, especially in poor risk patients or those with obvious tumor spread or recurrence after surgery (Fig. 10.6.13). In a group of 64 patients with advanced or recurrent gallbladder carcinoma proved by biopsy, good palliation was obtained in 53 patients. Thirty-day mortality was 14.5 % and overall survival about 5 months (Huibregtse et al. 1987b). Most of these tumors extend proximally into the liver. We therefore always attempt to insert two endoprostheses, one to the left liver lobe and one to the right liver lobe, before the bifurcation becomes involved.

Malignant Strictures of the Hepatic Confluence

Tumors which arise at the bifurcation grow from below into the bifurcation, or may be the result of metastatic spread from breast or colon cancer, or other sources (Okuda et al. 1977, Stellato et al. 1987). Tumors in this location account for about 20 % of cases of malignant biliary tract obstruction. Bifurcation tumors are extremely difficult to treat by any modality. Surgical access may be limited, since these neoplasms often spread proximally into the liver. On the average, only 20 % of primary biliary tumors at the hepatic confluence are resectable. Cholangitis occurs frequently in patients treated with U-tubes or hepaticojejunostomies. Palliative procedures are likewise very difficult, as the technical difficulty in stenting depends on the extent of the stricture at the hilum (Lameris et al.

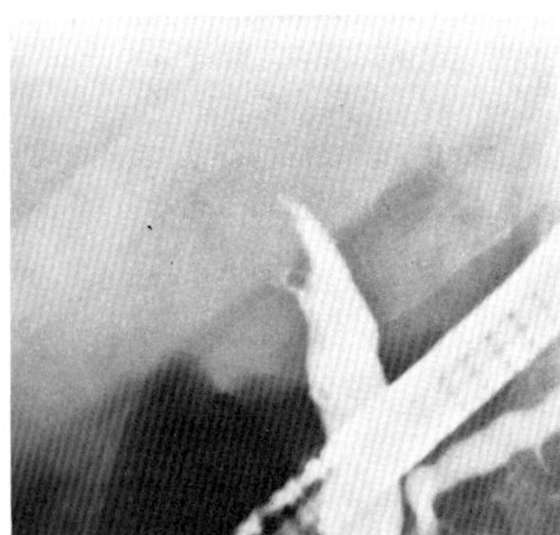
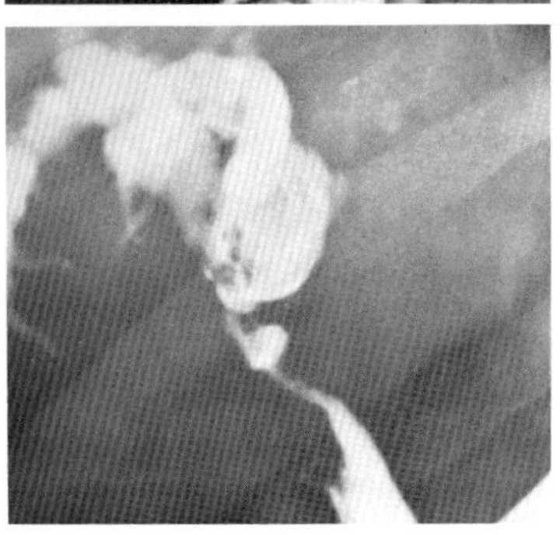
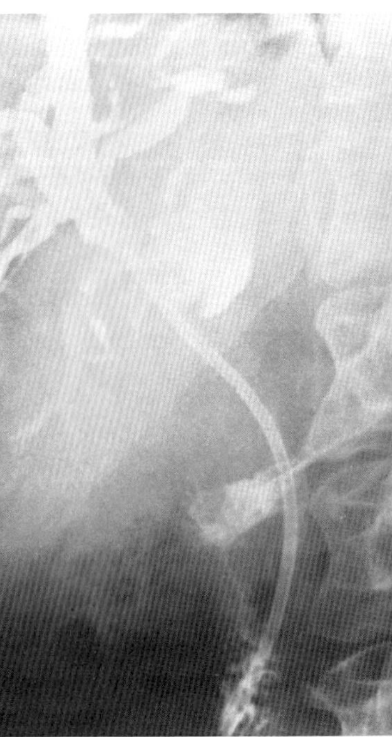

Fig. 10.6.**13** **Left:** Mid-common bile duct stricture in a patient with recurrent jaundice after surgery for gallbladder cancer. **Right:** the endoprosthesis is introduced through the stricture

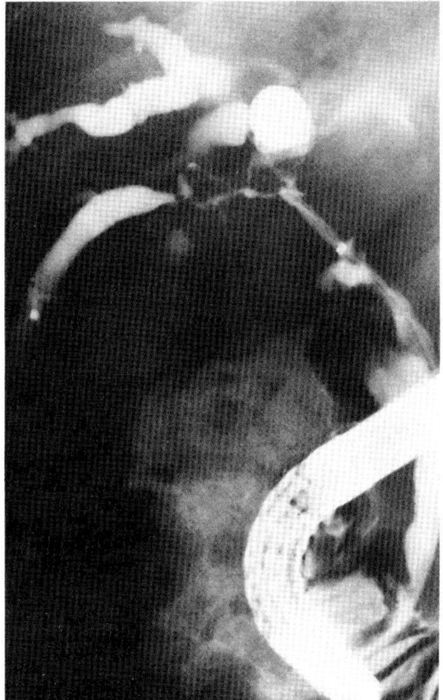 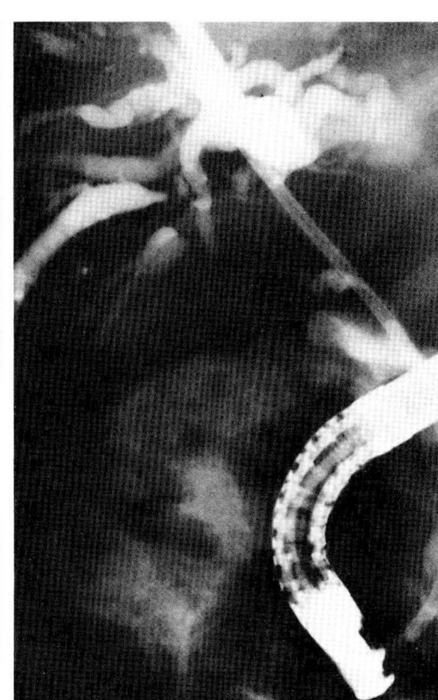

Fig. 10.6.**14   Type III stricture at the bifurcation.** The left hepatic duct is completely obstructed. Only one endoprosthesis (right) could be inserted

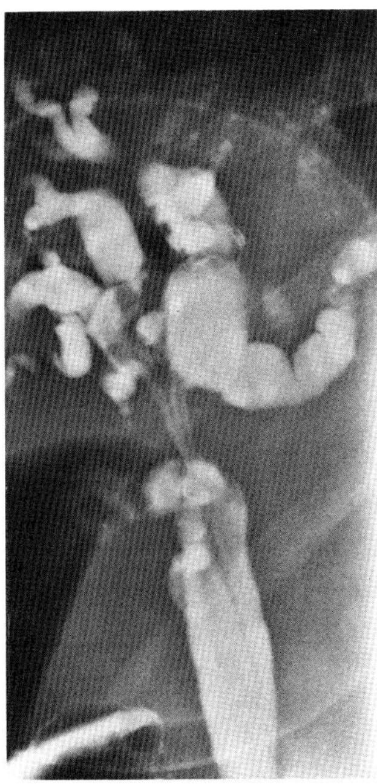 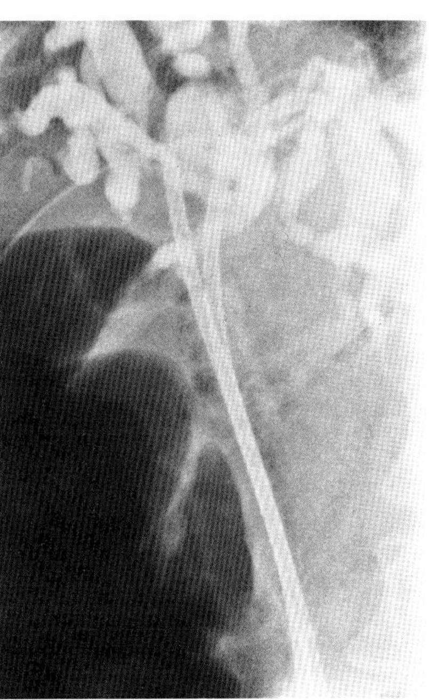

Fig. 10.6.**15   Type II stricture at the bifurcation.** Two endoprostheses (right) were placed to obtain optimal drainage

1987). Cotton (Speer et al. 1986) and Cremer (Deviere et al. 1988) have classified the strictures as follows:

Type III: strictures involving both the left and right hepatic ducts plus the intrahepatic ducts (Fig. 10.6.**14**).

Type II: strictures involving the left and right hepatic ducts (Figs. 10.6.**15**, 10.6.**16**).

Type I: strictures involving the common hepatic duct within 2 cm of the bifurcation, but not the left or right hepatic ducts (Fig. 10.6.**17**).

Type III strictures are usually associated with more extensive and often metastatic disease. As a result, stent insertion is more successful in types I and II than in type III. Consequently, jaundice is more often relieved in type I and type II. It is not surprising that survival in type I is found to be longer. In our group of 300 patients with bifurcation tumors, we were successful in inserting an endoprosthesis in 84%. A serum bilirubin decline was seen in 87% of those with an endoprosthesis inserted. Thirty-day mortality of the entire group

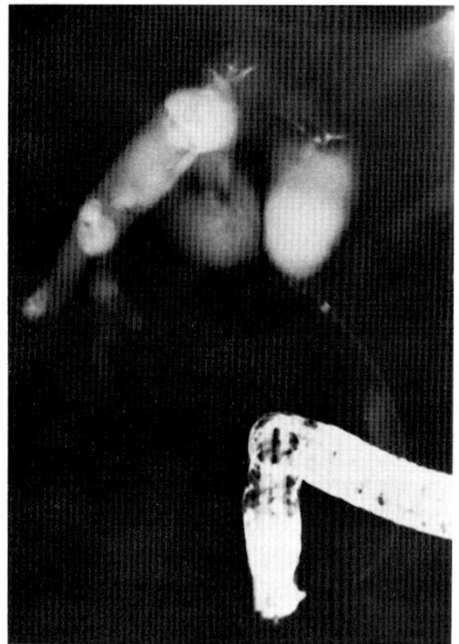

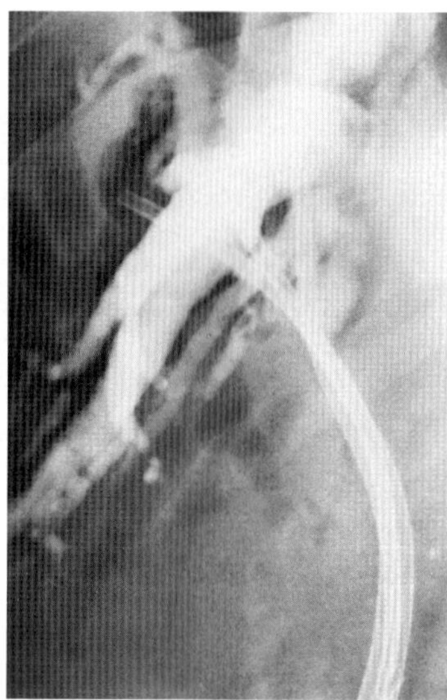

Fig. 10.6.**16 Type II stricture at the bifurcation.** Occlusion of three major ducts at the confluence. Three endoprostheses (right) were introduced for complete drainage

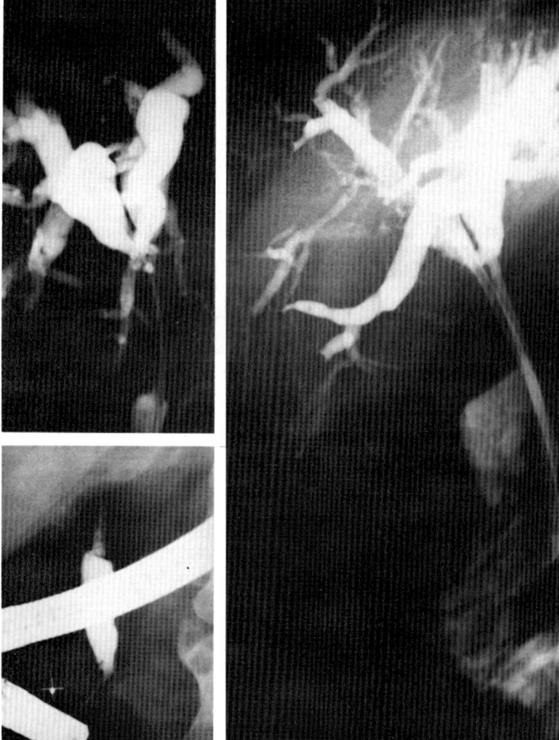

Fig. 10.6.**17 Type I stricture at the bifurcation.** Two endoprostheses (right) are inserted for proper drainage

was 25%. Mean survival was 178 days. Two endoprostheses could be inserted in only 25% of patients. We found no difference in the incidence of early cholangitis or bilirubin normalization between those with one endoprosthesis and those with two endoprostheses. The only difference was the substantially longer survival in those with two endoprostheses. In all probability this can be explained by the fact that insertion of two endoprostheses is technically much easier in smaller type I lesions. Only 20% of patients with malignancies at the site of the confluence are candidates for further surgery, in our experience. In the majority of these patients, tumor resection and hepaticojejunostomy can be performed. The choice of whether to proceed to surgical procedures should depend on factors such as age, underlying disease, the size of the tumor, extent of spread both within the biliary tract and distally, and the possibility of adequate non-surgical drainage.

Concluding Remarks

The technique of endoscopic biliary drainage is now well established, and several thousand patients have been treated using this modality. Further technical improvements are still necessary for the drainage of bifurcation tumors. The main drawback of the method is late clogging of the endoprosthesis. Further in vitro and in vivo studies need to be carried out to find out how the patency of the endoprosthesis can be secured.

The benefits of preoperative biliary drainage are not clear at present. There are many arguments in favor of preoperative biliary drainage, but clinical studies to substantiate these impressions so far are lacking. Endoprostheses are routinely inserted in most endoscopy centers after diagnostic ERCP to prevent cholangitis if stagnant bile is encountered, but the rationale and clinical benefits of this policy are still to be tested.

Further comparative clinical studies must be performed to identify patient groups which will optimally benefit from the various biliary drainage procedures. The endoscopic treatment modality will most likely be reserved for preoperative drainage and for definitive palliation in older patients with unresectable disease. Surgical palliative bypass procedures may well remain the treatment of choice in young and fit patients with unresectable disease. Percutaneous biliary interventions will be restricted to endoscopic failures (Speer et al. 1987) and to help the endoscopist by providing a transhepatically-inserted guide wire projecting from the papilla in special circumstances – the so-called "rendez-vous" procedure (Robertson et al. 1987, Sommer et al. 1987).

References

Allen-Mersh TG, Earham RJ. Pancreatic cancer in England and Wales: surgeons look at epidemiology. Ann R Coll Surg Engl 1986; 68: 154–158.

Blievernicht SE, Neifeld JP, Terz JJ, Lawrence J Jr. The role of prophylactic gastroenterostomy for the unresectable periampullary carcinoma. Surg Gynecol Obstet 1980; 151: 794–796.

Classen M, Hagenmuller F. Endoscopic biliary drainage. Scand J Gastroenterol 1984; 19 (suppl 102): 76–83.

Cotton PB. Endoscopic methods for relief of malignant obstructive jaundice. World J Surg, 1984; 8: 854–861.

Denning DA; Ellison EC, Carey LC. Pre-operative percutaneous transhepatic biliary decompression lowers operative mortality in patients with obstructive jaundice. Am J Surg 1981; 141: 61–65.

Deviere J, Baize M, Buset M, et al. Complications of internal endoscopic biliary drainage. Acta Endosc 1986; 219–231.

Deviere J, Baize M, de Toeuf J, Cremer M. Long-term follow up of patients with hilar malignant stricture treated by endoscopic internal biliary drainage. Gastrointest Endosc 1988; 34: 95–101.

Feduska NJ, Dent TL, Lindenauer SM. Results of palliative operations for carcinoma of the pancreas. Arch Surg 1971; 103: 330–333.

Fraumeni JF Jr. Cancer of the pancreas and biliary tract: epidemiological considerations. Cancer Res 1975; 35: 3437–3446.

Golicz RP, Stanley JH, Soncale CD, et al. Routine pre-operative biliary drainage: effect on management of obstructive jaundice. Radiology 1984; 152: 352–356.

Gouma DJ, Coelho JC, Schlegel JF, Li YF, Moody FG. The effect of preoperative internal and external biliary drainage on mortality of jaundiced rats. Arch Surg 1987; 122: 731–734.

Groen AK, Out T, Huibregtse K, et al. Characterization of the content of occluded biliary endoprosthesis. Endoscopy 1987; 19: 57–59.

Gundry SR, Strodel WE, Knol JA, et al. Efficacy of preoperative biliary tract decompression in patients with obstructive jaundice. Arch Surg 1984; 199: 703–706.

Hatfield ARW, Tobas R, Terblanche J, et al. Pre-operative external biliary drainage in obstructive jaundice: a prospective controlled clinical trial. Lancet 1982; ii: 896–898.

Huibregtse K, Tytgat GNJ. Palliative treatment of obstructive jaundice by transpapillary introduction of large bore bile duct endoprosthesis. Gut 1982; 23: 371–375.

Huibregtse K, Tytgat GNJ. Endoscopic placement of biliary prostheses. In: Salmon PR, ed. Gastrointestinal endoscopy: advances in diagnosis and therapy. London: Chapman and Hall, 1984: 219–231.

Huibregtse K, Tytgat GNJ. Carcinoma of the ampulla of Vater: the endoscopic approach. Endoscopy 1988; 20: 223–226.

Huibregtse K, Katon RM, Tytgat GNJ. Precut papillotomy via fine-needle knife papillotome: a safe and effective technique. Gastrointest 1986a; 32: 403–405.

Huibregtse K, Katon RM, Coene PP, Tytgat GNJ. Endoscopic palliative treatment in pancreatic cancer. Gastrointest Endosc 1986b; 32: 334–338.

Huibregtse K, Schneider B, Rauws E, Tytgat GNJ. Carcinoma of the ampulla of Vater: role of endoscopic drainage. Surg Endosc 1987a; 1: 79–82.

Huibregtse K, Schneider B, Coene PP, Tytgat GNJ. Endoscopic palliation of jaundice in gallbladder cancer. Surg Endosc 1987b; 1: 143–146.

Kozarek RA, Sanowski RA. Nonsurgical management of extrahepatic obstructive jaundice. Ann Intern Med 1982; 96: 743–745.

Lameris JS, Stoker J, Dees J, Nix GAJJ, et al. Non surgical palliative treatment of patients with malignant biliary obstruction: the place of endoscopic and percutaneous drainage. Clin Radiol 1987; 38: 603–608.

Lees WR, Hall-Craggs MA, Manhire A. Five years experience of fine-needle aspiration biopsy: 454 consecutive cases. Clin Radiol 1985; 36: 517–520.

Lerut JP, Gianello PR, Otte JB, Kestens PJ. Pancreaticoduodenal resection: surgical experience and evaluation of risk factors in 103 patients. Ann Surg 1984; 199: 432–437.

Leung JWC, Ling TKW, Kung JLS, Vallence-Owen J. The role of bacteria in the blockage of biliary stents. Gastrointest Endosc 1988; 34: 19–22.

Liquory CL, Meduri B, Canard JM, Fritsch J, Liberato M, Ingrosso M. Intubation endoscopique transpapillaire des cancers stenosants de la voie biliaire principale avec des endoprotheses de 3.2 mm. Abstracts du IVe symposium international d'endoscopie digestive 10–11 Mai, Paris, 1984.

McPherson GAD, Benjamin IS, Hodgson HJF, et al. Preoperative percutaneous transhepatic biliary drainage: the results of a controlled trial. Br J Surg 1984; 71: 371–375.

Nakayama T, Ikeda A, Okuda K. Percutaneous transhepatic drainage of the biliary tract. Gastroenterology 1978; 74: 554–559.

Norlander A, Kalin B, Sundblad R. Effect of percutaneous transhepatic drainage upon liver function and postoperative mortality. Surg Gynecol Obstet 1982; 155: 161–166.

Okuda K, Kubo Y, Okazaki N, et al. Clinical aspects of intrahepatic bile duct carcinoma including hilar carcinoma: a study of 57 autopsy proven cases. Cancer 1977; 39: 232–246.

Pitt HA, Cameron JL, Postier RG, Gadacz Tr. Factors affecting mortality in biliary tract surgery. Am J Surg 1981; 141: 66–72.

Pitt HA, Gomes AS, Lois JF, et al. Does pre-operative percutaneous biliary drainage reduce operative risk or increase hospital cost? Ann Surg 1985; 201: 545–553.

Robertson DAF, Hacking LN, Birch S, Ayres R, Shepherd H, Wright W. Experience with a combined percutaneous and endoscopic approach to stent insertion in malignant obstructive jaundice. Lancet 1987; ii: 1449–1452.

Sarr MG, Cameron JL. Surgical palliation of unresectable carcinoma of the pancreas. World J Surg 1984; 8: 906–918.

Shepherd HA, Diba A, Ross AP, Arthur M, Royle G, Collin-Jones D. Endoscopic biliary prosthesis in the palliation of malignant biliary obstruction: a randomised trial. Br J Surg 1988; 75: 1166–1168.

Siegel JH. Interventional endoscopy in diseases of the biliary tree and pancreas. Mt Sinai Med J (NY) 1984; 51: 535–542.

Siegel JH, Snady H. The significance of endoscopically placed prostheses in the management of biliary obstruction due to carcinoma of the pancreas: results of non-operative decompression in 277 patients. Am J Gastroenterol 1986; 81: 634–641.

Soehendra N, Reynders-Frederix V. Palliative bile duct drainage: a new endoscopic method of introducing a transpapillary drain. Endoscopy 1980; 12: 8–11.

Sommer A, Burlefinger R, Bayerdorffer E, Ottenjann R. Interne biliäre Drainage im "Rendezvous-Verfahren". Dtsch Med Wochenschr 1987; 112: 747–751.

Speer AG, Farrington H, Costeron JW, Cotton PB. Bacteria, biofilms and biliary sludge. Gut 1986; 27: A601.

Speer AG, Cotton PB, Dineen LP. Endoscopic stents in malignant hilar strictures, results in 70 patients. Proceedings of the 87th meeting of the American Gastroenterology Association, May 17–23, 1986, San Francisco.

Speer AG, Russell RC, Hatfield ARW, et al. Randomised trial of endoscopic versus percutaneous stent insertion in malignant obstructive jaundice. Lancet 1987; ii: 57–62.

Speer AG, Cotton PB, Rode J, Seddon AM, Neal CR, Holton J, Costerton JW. Biliary stent blockage with bacterial biofilm. Ann Intern Med 1988; 108: 546–553.

Stellato TF, Zollinger RM, Shuck JM. Metastatic malignant biliary obstruction. Am Surg 1987; 53: 385–388.

Takada T, Hanyu F, Kibayashi S, Uchida Y. Percutaneous transhepatic cholangial drainage: direct approach under fluoroscopic control. J Surg Oncol 1976; 8: 83–97.

Toouli J. Conference on pancreatic cancer. J Gastroenterol Hepatol 1986; 1: 181–189.

Trede M. The surgical treatment of pancreatic carcinoma. Surgery 1985; 97: 28–35.

Ubhi CS, Doran J. Palliation for carcinoma of head of pancreas. Ann R Coll Surg Engl 1986; 68: 159–162.

Wosiewitz V, Schrameyer B, Safrany L. Biliary sludge: its role during bile duct drainage with an endoprosthesis. Gastroenterology 1985; 88: 1706.

10.7 Therapeutic Alternatives in Liver Metastases

K. R. Aigner

Introduction

Liver metastases indicate poor life expectancy when there is no chance of curative treatment by extended resection. Survival depends on the number and size of the metastases as well as on their proliferation rate and location. As is well-known, most metastatic tumors in the liver are more or less resistant to any kind of chemotherapy. A number of treatment modalities have so far been tried, with varying success. Perfect technique and fundamental knowledge of the kind of treatment applied is mandatory to guarantee an optimal result.

When microwave-induced heat is applied to large metastases, they heat up selectively, since their neovasculature collapses at temperatures above 42 °C. However, small metastases and micrometastases are usually cooled down again by the blood stream (Skibba et al. 1988). Hyperthermic treatment by heating up the blood stream in an extracorporeal circuit is therefore virtually useless, since it is limited by the maximum tolerable blood temperature. This itself can already cause intimal damage to the perfused arteries (Aigner et al. 1985).

Among a number of local chemotherapy techniques, chemoembolization is considered a very selective and highly effective treatment for hepatic primaries and for metastases from carcinoma or melanoma. Temporary ischemia is induced by injecting microparticles (starch microspheres, Gelfoam, angiostat) and one to three drugs (mitomycin C, doxorubicin, cisplatin) into the hepatic artery (Stagg et al. 1987).

The principle of delivering high total doses of drugs to a tumorous area in order to achieve high local tissue concentrations has been put into practice in various techniques of arterial drug supply using implantable port catheters, implantable pumps (Boddie et al. 1988, Hohn et al. 1988) and isolated perfusion techniques with a heart-lung machine (Aigner et al. 1988b, 1984, Link et al. 1985). Clinical results in local chemotherapy procedures are closely related to surgical or radiological catheter techniques and knowledge of the vascularization and chemosensitivity of the tumors treated, as well as knowledge of the pharmacokinetics and pharmacodynamics of the drugs being used. Not all tumors respond to the same drug. Most drugs which are active in vitro show a steep dose–response relationship. Whether a drug is active or not can therefore not be estimated merely according to the results following intravenous application (where there is a subsequent dilution to a low concentration in the total body blood volume). As soon as the total dose increases, serum drug levels and, as a consequence, tissue levels increase too (Aigner et al. 1987). A correlation between tissue drug levels and the response, demonstrated by a decrease in tumor markers, has been observed in an ongoing study (Aigner et al. 1988a, Kemeny 1988). The easiest way to increase tissue drug levels is to administer the drug intra-arterially.

Treatment Modalities and Indications

Various local treatment modalities have been developed. Hepatic arterial infusion (HAI) is considered the easiest technique for local drug delivery. The drugs are administered via radiologically or surgically placed catheters. Fluorouracil (5-FU), mitomycin C (MMC), doxorubicin, mitoxantrone and cisplatin are well tolerated by the liver parenchyma (Aigner et al. 1988b, Aigner 1988). Total doses are usually limited by their systemic toxicity, except for 5-fluoro-2-deoxyuridine (FUDR), for which the liver has a high extraction rate. However, the high local toxicity of FUDR, which causes sclerosing cholangitis, restricts its use (Hohn et al. 1987, 1988). Although there is a high total response rate of between 60 and 80 % in HAI, the complete remission/partial remission (CR/PR) ratio is relatively low, and local recurrences also often originate from metastases showing partial response. Moreover, extrahepatic metastases develop in a large number of patients even after a good local response in the liver. A genuine advantage from HAI for survival has therefore not yet been demonstrated, although the response rate is higher, and the disease-free interval is longer than with systemic chemotherapy (Hohn et al. 1987). The quality of life is better with local chemotherapy, and patients with metastatic lesions close to the hepatic portal certainly benefit from HAI with regard to survival time, since even a slight shrinkage of the central metastases can prevent biliary obstruction. A high CR/PR ratio, with complete eradication of all tumor cells, is aimed for in HAI. The crucial point is how to increase the first-pass extraction of drugs, increasing the dosage without increasing the drug levels in the systemic circulation and thus the systemic toxicity.

Isolated liver perfusion (ILP) involves complete isolation of the liver in an extracorporeal circuit using a heart-lung machine. This technique demands surgical expertise and teamwork, and should only be applied in cases of disseminated liver disease without hepatomegaly. Hepatomegaly involves a high incidence of extrahepatic lesions which would be outside the region treated in ILP and would thus remain unaffected by the therapy.

Hepatic arterial infusion and venous drug filtration (HAI-F), a new concept, is based on hemoperfusion or ultrafiltration of drugs. A higher than normal total dose is administered intra-arterially in order to increase the area under the curve and the tissue uptake. The active load in the systemic venous outflow behind the tumor area is decreased by passing the blood through a filter (Fig. 10.7.**11**).

Hepatic Arterial Infusion

HAI can either be performed using the Seldinger technique radiologically, or surgically, using implantable devices. Arteriography via the celiac axis and the mesenteric artery is usually performed to plan the surgical approach. Since little more than 50% of patients have a normal blood supply through one hepatic artery originating from the celiac axis, accurate knowledge of the anatomy is mandatory for catheter placement.

Operative Procedure

Through a midline incision, the common hepatic artery is exposed in the hepatoduodenal ligament. Care must be taken to dissect the hepatic artery and ligate and divide collateral branches to the duodenum and stomach. Otherwise severe gastritis, duodenitis or ulcers may occur following drug delivery. The gastroduodenal artery is then ligated distally and, through a transverse incision close to the ligature, the tip of the catheter is inserted and fixed with one or two non-resorbable ligatures. The tip should be located just inside the gastroduodenal artery where it branches off from the common hepatic artery (Fig. 10.7.**1**). Valve-tip catheters (Jet Port, Implantofix) need not be flushed for prophylaxis of clotting. Homogeneous perfusion of the entire liver is then checked with fluorescein or an injection of 5–10 ml of blue dye while the common hepatic artery is clamped (Fig. 10.7.**2**). If the blue demarcation is incomplete, anatomic variations such as a substitute left or right hepatic artery from the left gastric or superior mesenteric arteries have to be excluded. Accessory left or right arteries can

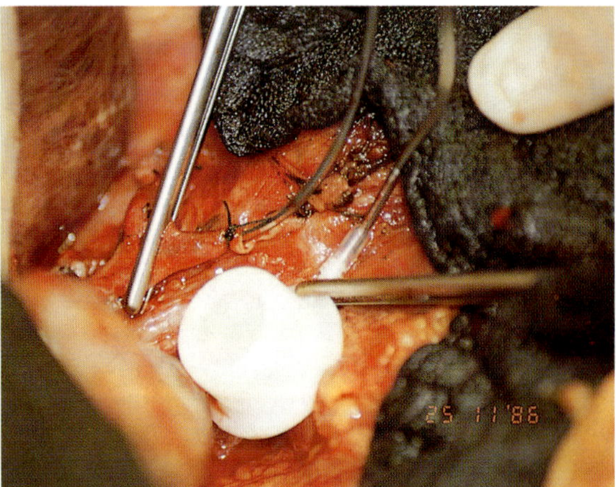

Fig. 10.7.**1   An Implantofix hepatic artery catheter** in the gastroduodenal artery which is clamped at its origin from the common hepatic artery for catheter implantation

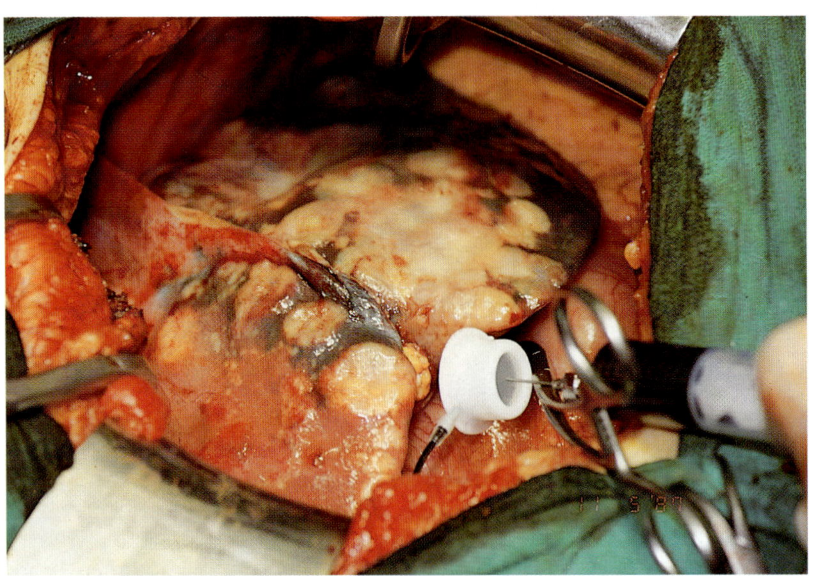

Fig. 10.7.**2   A patient with a substitute right hepatic artery.** Blue dye, injected through a catheter in the gastroduodenal artery, only appears in the left liver lobe

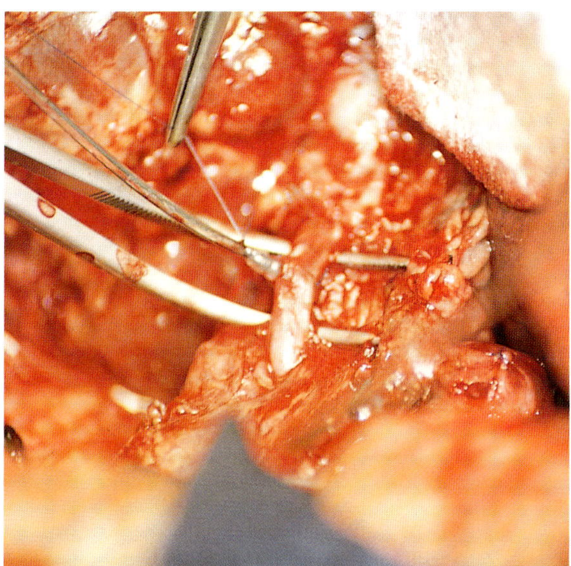

Fig. 10.7.**3** **Implantation technique for Implantofix or Jet Port valve-tip catheters** through a purse-string prolene suture in a substitute right hepatic artery without a side branch

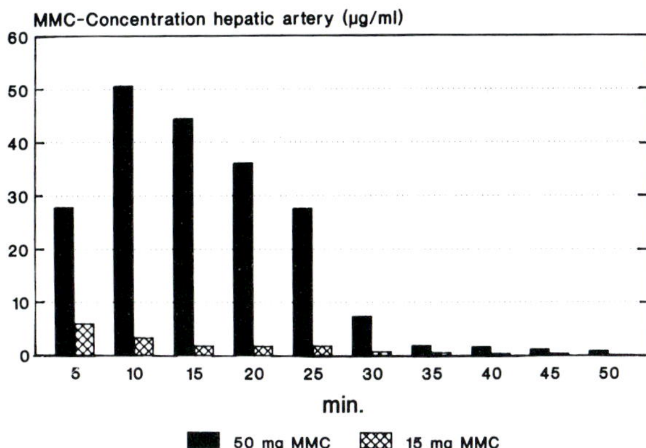

Fig. 10.7.**4** **Mitomycin C levels in the perfusate** during isolated liver perfusion with 15 or 50 mg MMC

be ligated without any danger of damage to the liver. In most cases, collaterals open immediately. Substitute left or right arteries are usually cannulated with a valve-tip catheter via a prolene purse-string suture (Fig. 10.7.**3**). If there is early branching of the left hepatic artery, the common hepatic artery is also cannulated using a purse-string suture, while the gastroduodenal artery and all visceral branches are ligated. Finally, the abdomen is closed in layers and the catheter is exited through the midline wound. The port is placed in a subcutaneous pouch in the upper third of the midline incision. Non-metal ports (e.g. Implantofix, Jet Port) do not need to be fixed to the fascia with sutures. The silicon membranes should only be punctured with so-called "Huber needles." Before implantation and after each infusion of drugs, catheters are flushed with saline/heparin (9 : 1 ml) solution. Arterial chemotherapy is given according to the protocols either as a short-term or as a continuous long-term infusion with portable external pumps. If implantable pumps (e.g. Infusaid, Medtronics) are used, the drug of choice is FUDR, and combination chemotherapy can be performed through the side ports.

Isolated Liver Perfusion

Among the various modalities available for regional cancer treatment, ILP is the most time-consuming, demanding a 4-hour operation with the heart-lung machine. The advantages, however, are that the drug can be administered via the hepatic arterial and portal route, additional hyperthermia can be used, and complete isolation makes it possible to give total doses up to amounts which are only limited by the local tissue tolerance. ILP is the method of choice for tumors with low chemosensitivity. Drug levels in the perfusate can be adjusted to any desired range, depending only on the total dose injected into the isolated circuit (Fig. 10.7.**4**).

Operative Procedure

Through an abdominal midline incision, the liver, hepatoduodenal ligament and the inferior vena cava (Fig. 10.7.**5**) below and above the liver are exposed. Access to the intrapericardial part of the inferior vena cava is achieved by a transverse incision of the diaphragm (Fig. 10.7.**6**). A tourniquet tape is placed around the vein there, and above and below the renal veins. Two tapes are placed around the portal vein for cannulation in two directions, and around the common hepatic and gastroduodenal arteries (Fig. 10.7.**7**). Cannulation of the vena cava is achieved through a longitudinal incision below the renal veins, where a special catheter (Perfufix®, B. Braun) is inserted (Fig. 10.7.**8**). This double-lumen catheter consists of two tubes, one of which collects the hepatic venous return selectively using gravity in the oxygenator of the heart-lung machine. Two lateral openings in the double-channel perfusion catheter (Fig. 10.7.**9**) collect the venous return from the kidneys. The distal portal vein cannulation catheter collecting the blood from the gastrointestinal tract is connected with a side hose of the liver perfusion catheter entering the central tube, thus bypassing the liver during isolated perfusion (Fig. 10.7.**10**). Finally, the hepatic artery is cannulated via the

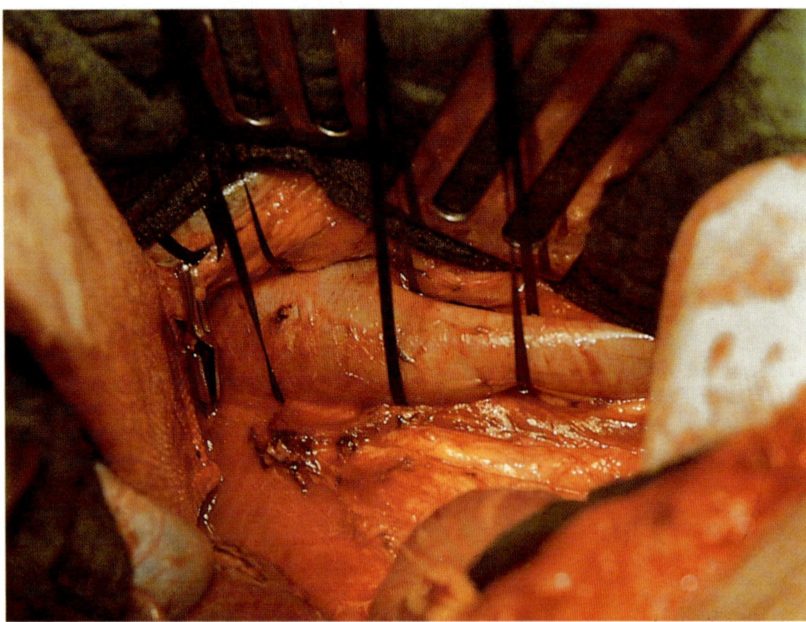

Fig. 10.7.**5 Exposure of the inferior vena cava and placement of tapes**, one above and two below the renal veins

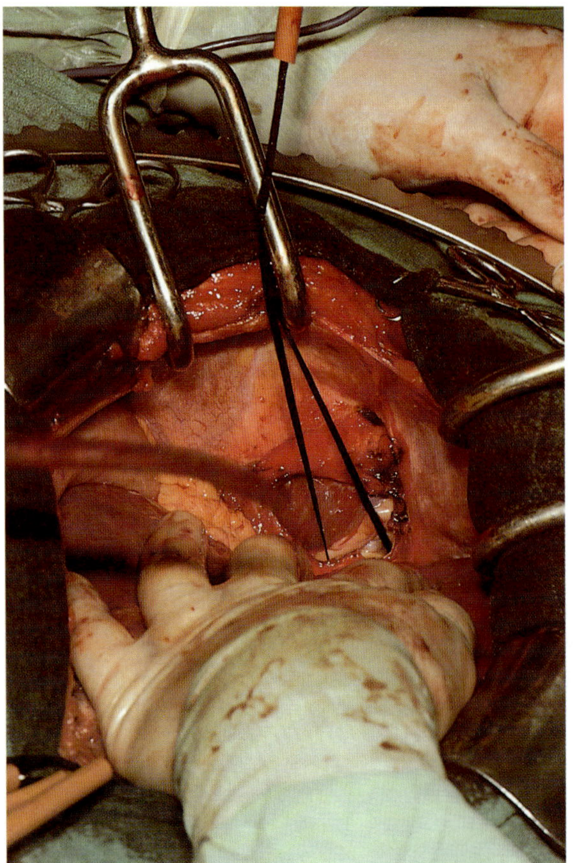

Fig. 10.7.**6 A transverse incision in the diaphragm and pericardium** and intrapericardial tourniquet tape around the vena cava at its entrance into the right atrium

gastroduodenal artery. If there are anatomic variations, double cannulations are performed.

Isolated bypass is started via the portal vein circuit. The portal venous flow with arterialized blood from the oxygenator is finally adjusted to about 300–400 ml/min while the hepatic arterial roller-pump flow rate is adjusted to about 100 ml/min. The cytotoxic drug is infused directly into the hepatic arterial line at a calculated speed in order to maintain the necessary drug concentration in the perfusate over a period of usually 30 min. Thus a very high area under the curve (AUC) is guaranteed during the first half of the isolation perfusion. During the second 30 min the drug, diluted in the perfusate, recirculates through both arterialized access lines. Thermister probes are placed in the right and left liver lobes and the tissue temperature is adjusted at 40 °C using a perfusate temperature of 41.5 °C to 42 °C. At the end of a one-hour perfusion, the liver is rinsed and remaining drugs are washed out of the vascular system. The catheters are withdrawn step-by-step, and the vessels are repaired with running sutures. Cannulation and 60 min isolated perfusion are performed under systemic heparinization of the patient with 200 IU of heparin per kg of body weight. At the end of the operation, implantation of a hepatic arterial catheter for subsequent hepatic arterial infusion is standard.

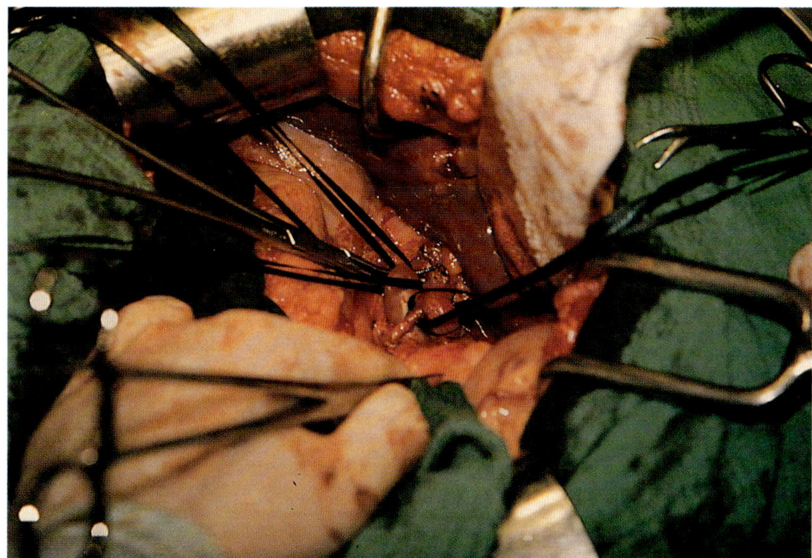

Fig. 10.7.**7** **Exposure of the porta hepatis**, with the portal vein (two tapes), the common hepatic artery (one tape) and the gastroduodenal artery

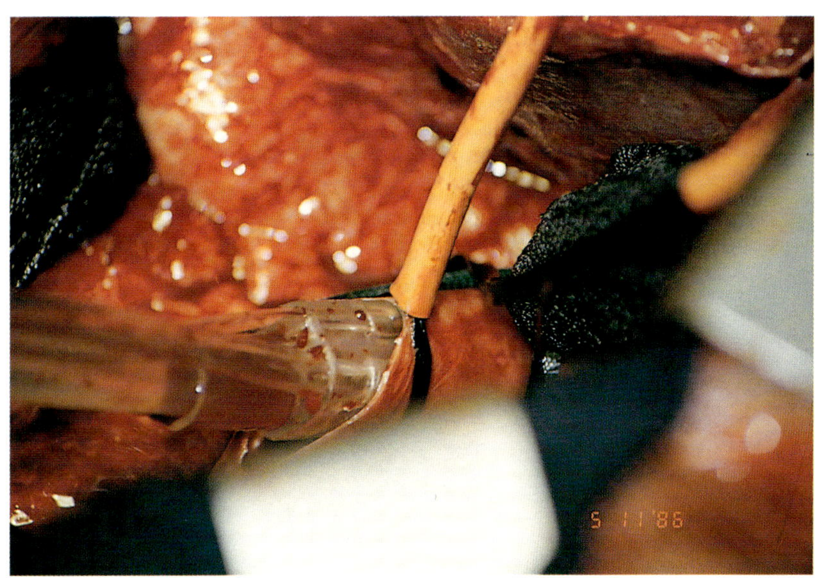

Fig. 10.7.**8** **Cannulation of the vena cava below the renal veins** with a Perfufix double-lumen catheter

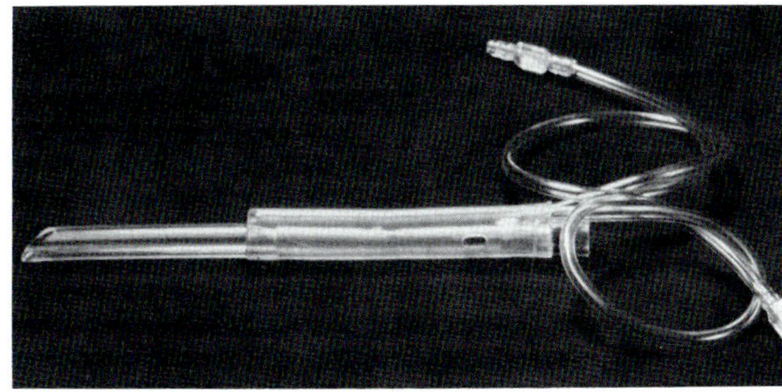

Fig. 10.7.**9** **Perfufix double-lumen liver perfusion catheter** with two lateral openings in the shunting tube

Hepatic Arterial Infusion and Filtration

Rationale of Cytostatic Filtration

By using hemofilters in regional chemotherapy it is possible to reduce the drug levels in the venous outflow behind the tumor, left over from the first pass. Thus adverse side-effects which reduce the quality of life can be avoided. In addition, by adjusting the filtration effect individually, systemic drug levels comparable to those obtained in i.v. treatment can be generated when indicated

(Fig. 10.7.**11**). In the hemofiltration circuit (Fig. 10.7.**12**), the venous blood with high cytostatic drug levels is pumped via an air trap to the hemofilter by a roller pump. Between the hemofilter and the patient, an additional air trap is fixed. By adding the substitutional volume before the hemofilter via an additional roller pump, the blood can be prediluted for higher filtration efficiency or, as demonstrated in Figure 10.7.**12**, postdiluted when the substitution inflow is behind the filter. After starting the filtration, the flow rates through the hemofilter should be slowly increased to a maximum volume of 300–600 ml/min. Cytostatic arterial infusion into the patient's tumor-affected region should be started when the filtrate flow has reached at least 70 ml/min. The total filtrate volume has to be adjusted to the desired conditions, such as the arterial drug concentration over the perfusion period and the tolerable maximum dose.

In our experience, Söring and Gambro filters have turned out to be an optimal system for cytostatic drug filtration when mitomycin C, doxorubicin, melphalan or cisplatin are used. A computerized cytostatic drug filtration hemoprocessor (Gambro, Lund) has the advantage that, once adjusted, it can run by itself. Instead of a hemoprocessor, however, a quite simple set-up consisting of three roller pumps for blood flow, filtration flow and volume substitution flow can be used as well. Volume balance is obtained by controlling the

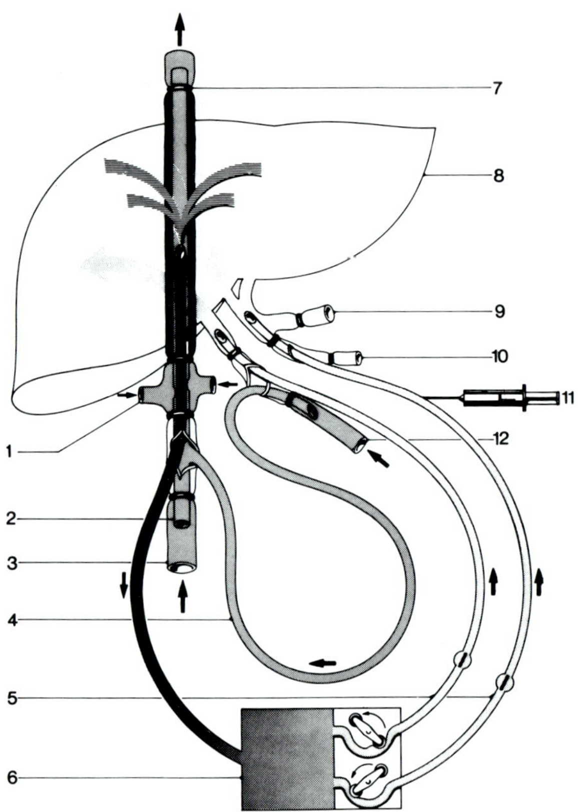

Fig. 10.7.**10   The complete isolation of the liver** in an extracorporeal circuit

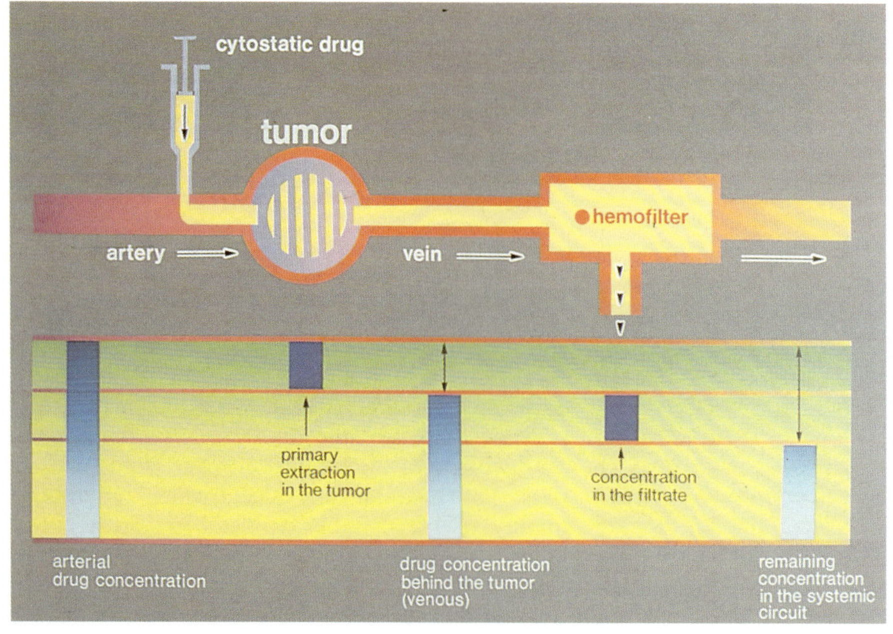

Fig. 10.7.**11   Rationale of intra-arterial cytostatic infusion with venous drug filtration** (from PfM, Cologne, Oncology II)

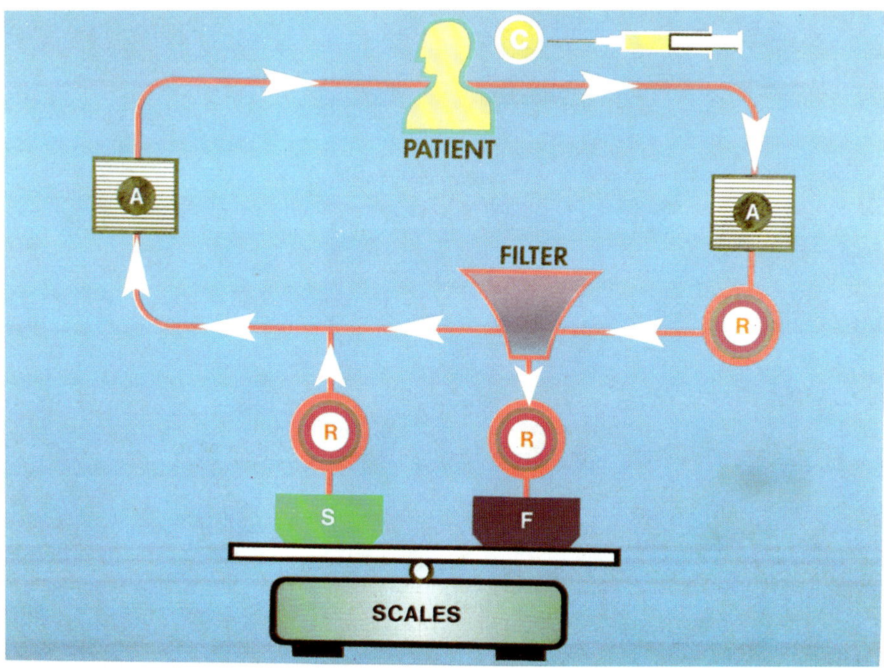

Fig. 10.7.12 System for venous drug filtration with two air traps (A), three roller pumps for blood flow through the filter (R), filtrate flow (F) and substitution flow (S). The filtrate and substitution solutions are balanced on scales

amount of filtrate and volume substitution solution on the scales. This procedure requires a greater amount of work and attention, since the patient's volume has to be balanced continuously. As a consequence, monitoring the electrocardiogram (ECG) and pulse frequency is mandatory. Leakage can be detected immediately by changes in the heart frequency.

Operative procedure

The filtration is performed with a special double-lumen catheter (PfM, Cologne), which is available in three sizes, F7, F9 and F16. The F7 and F9 catheters can be introduced into the femoral artery with the Seldinger technique, and the tip advanced to the tumor region. For intra-arterial chemotherapy of the liver with venous filtration, the tip of the catheter is positioned directly at the entrance of the inferior vena cava into the right atrium. Catheter position is controlled by X-rays at the beginning of filtration.

The large F16 catheter has to be introduced into the saphenous vein by means of a short-cut in the groin under local anesthesia (Fig. 10.7.13). Any catheter placement and filtration procedure has to be performed under systemic heparinization of the patient with 150 IU heparin/kg of body weight. After a 60 min filtration, the catheter is removed and the vessels are sutured.

Discussion

There have, up to now, been two prospective randomized trials comparing intra-arterial and intravenous chemotherapy. In both studies, colorectal liver metastases were treated with i.a. versus i.v. continuous infusion with FUDR (Hohn et al. 1987, Kemeny 1988). Although response rates and disease-free intervals were superior when FUDR was given intra-arterially, in the NCOG study (Hohn et al. 1987), the two groups were not comparable due to a cross-over of systemically treated non-responders into the arterial arm, and to local toxicity urging termination of i.a. FUDR in responders. In the Kemeny (1988) study, a significant prolongation of survival in the i.a. group was demonstrated. Furthermore, a dose–response relationship is evident when the two studies are compared, indicating that a further decrease of the FUDR dosage in order to decrease side-effects may decrease tumor toxicity as well.

It should be emphasized, however, that a study on colorectal liver metastases alone, considering only one drug whose potential efficacy is limited by local toxicity, cannot be representative of the potential advantages of the wide field of regional chemotherapy and drug targeting. In our experience in intra-arterial cancer treatment, the CR/PR

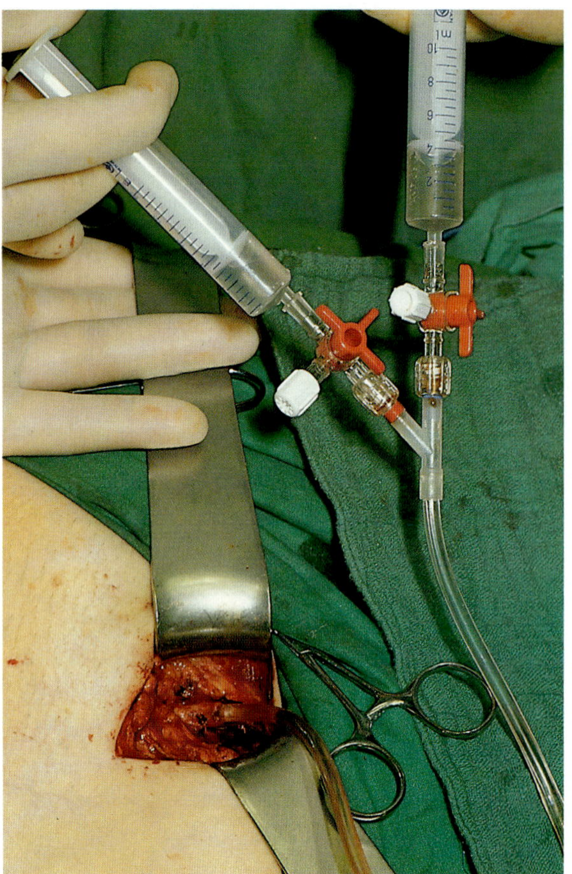

Fig. 10.7.**13 Surgical placement of an F16 filtration catheter** (PfM, Cologne) under local anesthesia through a
longitudinal incision in the groin

ratio can be further improved by using different
drugs and treatment modalities focused on the
individual situation.

The fact that tumor vascularization plays a
predominant role in any kind of chemotherapy with
regard to the maximally achievable drug levels in
tissue has not yet been taken into consideration.
There are so far no data on the required minimum
tissue levels in various histological types. The initial
experimental and clinical data indicate that there is
a marked difference in drug uptake between normal
and metastatic tissue (Aigner 1988), and between
intra-arterial and intraportal applications (Sigurdson et al. 1987).

Attention has not yet been given to chemosensitivity testing for targeted chemotherapy either. It
has been shown by Link et al. (1985) that tumor-
icidal drug concentrations and concentration X
time factors can be specifically predicted in tumor
cell colonies. In non-responding tumors, a change
of drugs in accordance with chemosensitivity tests
may result in sudden response. Currently mitomy-

cin C and doxorubicin seem to have a broad
spectrum in most tumors at concentrations achievable with high-dose local techniques as described
above. The optimal infusion or perfusion technique
recommended to achieve effective concentrations at
the tumor site can be derived from knowledge
about required minimal drug concentrations. There
have not yet been any clinical trials taking this into
account. There are impressive case reports from
many groups showing complete remissions from
hepatic arterial infusion alone. On the other hand
there are also data from isolated liver perfusion
with high doses showing minimal or no response in
a few cases, since the metastases had a poor blood
supply, as seen when blue dye was injected. These
findings indicate that regional chemotherapy has to
be considered a very specific method, which should
be only applied on the basis of tumor characteristics
such as blood supply and chemosensitivity. Long-
term survival depends on whether micrometastases
are present at the time of the initial treatment. Thus
there is a clear, early-stage dependent indication for
isolated liver perfusion. Long-term disease-free
survival of up to five years in 10.8% has been
observed in ILP for disseminated colorectal liver
metastases (Aigner et al. 1988 b). This result might
be further improved on in early-stage patients with
lesions confined only to the liver, in a study based
on predictive drug testing.

Conclusions

In non-resectable disseminated liver metastases,
regional chemotherapy may be considered a valid
therapeutic alternative. Depending on the chemosensitivity of the metastatic lesions, a local treatment modality providing medium or high drug
levels is applied. Colorectal liver metastases require
isolated liver perfusion or arterial infusion and drug
filtration in order to achieve a high CR/PR ratio.
Restitution of resectability can sometimes be obtained in primarily non-resectable hepatomas after
chemoembolization or high-dose arterial chemotherapy. Carcinomas are also very sensitive to
chemoembolization. In hepatomegaly from disseminated colorectal disease, HAI-F is preferable
to ILP. In general, intra-arterial chemotherapy
modalities offer high local efficacy with low systemic toxicity and the prospect of a good quality of
life.

References

Aigner KR. Drug filtration in high-dose regional chemotherapy.
    In: Aigner KR, Patt YZ, eds. Advances in regional cancer
    treatment: contributions to oncology. Basel: Karger, 1988:
    261–280.
Aigner KR, Tonn JC, Walther H, Link KH, Schwemmle K. The
    isolated liver perfusion technique for high-dose chemotherapy

of metastases from colorectal cancer: two years' clinical experience. In: Van de Velde CJH, Sugarbaker PH, eds. Liver metastasis: basic aspects, detection and management. The Hague: Nijhoff, 1984: 346–357.

Aigner KR, Walther H, Helling HJ, Link KH. Die isolierte Leberperfusion. In: Aigner KR, ed. Regionale Chemotherapie der Leber. Basel: Karger 1985: 43–83. (Beiträge zur Onkologie; vol. 21.)

Aigner KR, Walther H, Link KH. Pharmacokinetics and pharmacodynamics of mitomycin C (MMC) in ILP and HAI. Proceedings of the third International Conference on Advances in Regional Cancer Therapy, ICRCT 87, Ulm, 1987.

Aigner KR, Müller H, de Toma G. Mitoxantron in regional chemotherapy. In: Aigner KR, Patt YZ, eds. Advances in regional cancer treatment: contributions to oncology. Basel: Karger, 1988 a: 49–57.

Aigner KR, Walther H, Link KH. Isolated liver perfusion: surgical technique, pharmacokinetics, clinical results. In: Aigner KR, Patt YZ, eds. Advances in regional cancer treatment: contributions to oncology. Basel: Karger, 1988 b: 229–246.

Boddie AW Jr, Patt YZ, McBride CM, Wallace S, Ajani AJ, Charnsangavej C, Soski M, Levin B. MDAH surgical experience with implantable Infusaid pumps and Medtronic drug administration devices. In: Aigner KR, Patt YZ, eds. Advances in regional cancer treatment: contributions to oncology. Basel: Karger, 1988: 193–204.

Hohn DC, Stagg RJ, Rayner AA, Lewis BJ. The NCOG randomized trial of intravenous (iv) vs hepatic arterial (ia) FUDR for colorectal cancer metastatic to the liver. Proceedings of the third International Conference on Advances in Regional Cancer Therapy, ICRCT 87, Ulm, 1987.

Hohn DC, Shea WJ, Gemlo BT, Lewis BJ, Stagg RJ, Ignoffo RJ, Rayner AA. Complications and toxicities of hepatic arterial chemotherapy. In: Aigner KR, Patt YZ, eds. Regional cancer treatment: contributions to oncology. Basel: Karger, 1988: 169–180.

Kemeny N. Regional chemotherapy for cancer. Proceedings: New approaches in cancer therapy. Ulm, 1988.

Link KH, Aigner KR, Kuehn W, Roetering N, Schwemmle K. Drug testing in regional chemotherapy. Proceedings of the second International Conference on Advances in Regional Cancer Therapy, ICRCT 85, Giessen, 1985.

Sigurdson ER, Ridge JA, Kemeny N, Daly JM. Tumor and liver drug uptake following hepatic artery and portal vein infusion. J Clin Oncol 1987; 5: 1836–1840.

Skibba JL, Quebbeman EJ, Komorowski RA, Thorsen KM. Clinical results of hyperthermic liver perfusion for cancer in the liver. In: Aigner KR, Patt YZ, eds. Regional cancer treatment: contributions to oncology. Basel: Karger, 1988: 222–228.

Stagg RJ, Chase J, Lewis BJ, Ring E, Maroney T, Venook A, Hohn DC. Chemoembolization of primary and metastatic liver tumors. Proceedings of the third International Conference on Advances in Regional Cancer Therapy, ICRCT 87, Ulm, 1987.

Storm FK, ed. Hyperthermia in cancer therapy. Boston: Hall, 1983.

Index